Principles of
Surgical
Management

Principles of Surgical Management

Clive R.G. Quick

Consultant General and Vascular Surgeon,
Hinchingbrooke HealthCare NHS Trust; and
Addenbrooke's Hospital, Cambridge, UK

and

Paul Thomas

Consultant General and Colorectal Surgeon,
Whipps Cross Hospital, London, UK

with illustrations by
Philip Deakin
General Practitioner, Sheffield

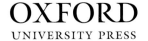

OXFORD
UNIVERSITY PRESS

OXFORD
UNIVERSITY PRESS

Great Clarendon Street, Oxford OX2 6DP

Oxford University Press is a department of the University of Oxford. It furthers the University's objective of excellence in research, scholarship, and education by publishing worldwide in

Oxford New York

Athens Auckland Bangkok Bogotá Buenos Aires Calcutta Cape Town
Chennai Dar es Salaam Delhi Florence Hong Kong Istanbul Karachi
Kuala Lumpur Madrid Melbourne Mexico City Mumbai Nairobi Paris
São Paulo Singapore Taipei Tokyo Toronto Warsaw

with associated companies in Berlin Ibadan

Oxford is a registered trade mark of Oxford University Press in the UK
and in certain other countries

Published in the United States by Oxford University Press Inc., New York

A catalogue record for this title is available from the British Library

Library of Congress Cataloguing in Publication Data

Principles of surgical management/[edited by] Clive R.G. Quick and Paul
Thomas; with illustrations by Philip Deakin.
(Oxford medical publications)
Includes bibliograhical references and index.
1. Surgery, Operative. 2. Therapeutics, Surgical. I. Quick, Clive R.G.
II. Thomas, Paul, MB BS. III. Series.
[DNLM: 1. Surgical Procedures, Operative. 2. Surgery–standards.
WO 500 P95695 2000]
RD32.P69 2000   617'.9–dc21   00-022181
ISBN 0 19 262230 7 (alk. paper)

1 3 5 7 9 10 8 6 4 2

Typeset in Minion by EXPO Holdings, Malaysia
Printed in Hong Kong

Foreword

Professor Harold Ellis CBE MCh FRCS

Most standard textbooks of surgery, (including my own), deal with surgical pathology, diagnosis, and treatment. But every surgeon, from the house officer to his Chief, knows that there is much more to the management of the surgical patient than is covered by these three headings – vitally important though they are. There is that mysterious ingredient known as 'Surgical Judgement', which experienced surgeons have acquired through long years of practical exposure and which is so difficult to pass on to the next generation of surgeons, except by example. Then there is the difficult art of counselling patients and their relatives; there is the problem of choosing between different treatment modalities; there is the care of the seriously ill patient in the operating theatre and recovery ward, with, today, the important new elements of audit and quality control. All this against a background of increasingly elderly and generally unwell patients who are being submitted to sophisticated operative procedures which had hardly been dreamed about when I was in active surgical practice. The two senior authors of this new textbook, themselves highly experienced postgraduate teachers, have done a magnificent job in covering these, and other, topics. They have taken the imaginative step of recruiting senior registrars and young consultants as their co-authors (in contrast to the usual grey haired writers of textbooks), who bring a refreshing modernity to each chapter. This is a book which will commend itself to every surgical trainee working for the higher examinations. I only wish that I had had it on my desk as I studied for my FRCS in 1951; I would have become a better rounded surgeon!

Preface

World-wide there has been a continuing trend towards sub-specialization within general surgery. This, together with shorter training programmes, has meant that the generality of surgery is often under-represented during training. This has several disadvantages for the trainee approaching appointment as a specialist or consultant surgeon: first, most surgical 'exit' exams have a high content of general surgery. Second, there are relatively few opportunities to limit practice to one sub-specialist area, and third, and perhaps most important, nearly all surgical consultants are required to cover emergency general surgery. This book has been written to cover the whole field of 'general surgery' to help overcome these disadvantages for anyone intending to specialize in general surgery and its sub-specialties. It would also be suitable for trainees in other areas of surgery who need to understand the principles of surgery. For these reasons, the book covers many topics not usually included in surgical textbooks, such as ethics and consent, maintaining standards in surgery, and handling and protecting the patient within the operating suite. In addition, areas of applied basic science important to surgeons are covered in some detail but in an easily accessible form. These include surgical microbiology, haematology and transfusion, anaesthesia and organ support, and the pathophysiology and management of pain. We make no apology for including topics on the edge of general surgery, such as the chapter on transplantation. The book as a whole has been designed to complement larger reference texts such as the *Oxford Textbook of Surgery*.

Surgeons in training at any stage need guidance in learning how to look after patients and to pass the essential examinations. We have endeavoured to explain the reasoning involved in recognizing and dealing with general surgical conditions and we have given particular attention to practical management of surgical emergencies and trauma patients. The book is also intended to serve as a practical guide to safe and effective elective surgical practice.

Our intention is to suggest logical pathways, so a patient can be conducted from an initial working diagnosis, through assessment and investigation, then if appropriate, through preparation for surgery, care in the operating theatre and afterwards. We have included details of operations trainees are likely to encounter in a standard illustrated format and, in the text, have emphasized the prevention and treatment of complications. Throughout, factors which affect surgical outcome are identified as these are fundamental to surgical audit and quality control. Chapters conclude with a few key references to classic books, papers or review articles. This is not a textbook of diagnosis nor an atlas of operative surgery but it does cover the principles of both.

The editors both work in busy hospitals and provide a general surgical emergency service as well as undertaking subspecialist elective surgery. They have each organized postgraduate surgical courses [at Cambridge and Whipps Cross]. When planning this book, we decided to involve a high proportion of authors who were senior trainees or young consultants. This was to offer a younger perspective to offset any reactionary views of the slightly older editors. To our knowledge this is the first time this mix has been used to produce a textbook of this kind. The editors have had a substantial input of the content into nearly all the chapters and have carefully scrutinized and edited the whole book in an attempt to produce a harmonious and coherent view of general surgery today.

No book can be produced without enormous effort from many people. Our thanks go to all of the authors, all of whom toiled in the face of conflicting professional pressures. Co-ordinating the many contributions has been quietly and efficiently handled by Mrs Shirley Powell, whose humour and persistence has helped move us along during the book's preparation. Finally Oxford University Press – in particular Julie Hoare and Richard Marley – have been supportive throughout.

We hope the book proves of value in the general surgical component of surgical training programmes.

Cambridge   C. Q.
London   P. T.
August 2000

Contents

Contributors

Mr John Forbes Abercrombie
Consultant Surgeon
University Hospital (Nottingham)
Queen's Medical Centre
Nottingham

Miss E. Briony Ackroyd FRCS
Consultant Breast Surgeon
Walsgrave Hospital
Coventry

Mr Niaz Ahmad FRCS
University Hospital of Wales
Cardiff
Wales

Mr Iain D. Anderson BSc, FRCS, MD, FRCS (Gen)
Honorary Consultant Surgeon/Senior Lecturer
University Department of Surgery
Hope Hospital
Salford

Dr Trevor P. Baglin MB, PhD, MRCP, MRCPath
Consultant Haematologist
Department of Haematology
Addenbrooke's NHS Trust
Cambridge

Mr I.S. Bailey FRCS
Consultant Upper GI Surgeon
Southampton General Hospital
Southampton

Mr Anjan K. Banerjee MSc, MS, DM, FRCP (Ed),
FRCS (Eng)(Gen)
Consultant Surgeon/Hon. Senior Clinical Lecturer
Royal Halifax Infirmary
Halifax, W. Yorks

Abrie Botha MD, FRCS
Consultant Surgeon
Whipps Cross Hospital
London

Dr Matthew J. Carmody MB BS FRACS
Specialist General Surgeon
Royal Brisbane Hospital
Brisbane, Australia

Dr Christine Collin
Himbleton
Droitwich
Worcestershire

Mr Mike P Corlett FRCS
Himbleton
Droitwich
Worcestershire

Mr K. Simon Cross MD, M.Med Sci, FRCS(Gen),
FRCS (Edin)
Consultant Surgeon
Vascular Unit
Aberdeen Royal Infirmary
Aberdeen

Mr Mark L. Da Costa FRCSI FRCS(Glas)
Research Fellow
Department of Surgery
Royal College of Surgeons in Ireland
Beaumont Hospital
Dublin Ireland

Mr Alun Huw Davies MA (Cantab/Oxon) DM
(Oxon) FRCS (Eng)
Consultant General and Vascular Surgeon
Charing Cross Hospital
London

Dr Patrick W. Doyle MB ChB DA(SA) FRCA
Depart. of Anaesthesia
Norfolk and Norwich Hospital
Norwich

Michael Earley FRCSI MCh FRCS (Plast. Surg),
Plastic and Reconstructive Surgeon,
Mater Miserlcordiae Hospital, Dublin

Mr W.G. Everett FRCS
Honarary Consultant Surgeon
Addenbrooke's Hospital
Cambridge

Dr Mark Farrington MA MB BChir FRCPath
Consultant Medical Microbiologist, Public Health and Clinical
Microbiology Laboratory
Addenbrooke's Hospital
Cambridge

Prof P.J. Friend MA MB Bchir FRCS MD
Professor of Transplantation
Nuffield Department of Surgery
University of Oxford

Mr Keith R. Gardiner MD MCh FRCS
Consultant Colorectal Surgeon
Royal Victoria Hospital
Belfast

Mr J. Donald Greig MB ChB MD FRCS (Ed & Glasg)
FCS (HK), FRCSEd (Gen Surg), FHKAM (Surg)
Specialist in General Surgery
Matilda and War Memorial Hospital
Hong Kong

Ms Rachel Hargest MD FRCS
Department of Surgery
University College London Medical School
London

Frances Hughes MS FRCS
Consultant Surgeon
Southend Hospital
Essex

Dr M.M. Jonas MB FRCA
Consultant in Paediatric Intensive Care & Anaesthesia
Southampton University Hospitals NHS Trust
Southampton

Mr Peter J. Lunniss BSc MCh FRCS
Senior Lecturer & Honorary Consultant Surgeon
The Royal London and Homerton Hospitals
Colorectal Development Unit
Academic Department of Surgery
London

Mr Ali Majeed FRCS
Senior Lecturer in Surgery
University of Sheffield
Royal Hallamshire Hospital
Sheffield

Miss Jane McCue MS FRCS
Consultant Surgeon
Queen Elizabeth II Hospital
Welwyn Garden City
Herts

Mr John R. McGregor MD FRCS
Consultant Surgeon
Crosshouse Hospital
North Ayrshire & Arran NHS Trust
Kilmarnock

Mr Dion Morton
Lecturer in Surgery
The Queen Elizabeth Hospital
The Queen Elizabeth Medical Centre
Edgbaston
Birmingham

Dr Rajesh Munglani
Senior Lecturer in Anaesthesia and Pain Relief
Consultant in Anaesthesia and Pain Relief
Director Pain Relief Service
Addenbrookes Hospital
Cambridge

Dr A. Oduro MRCP FRCA
Consultant Anaesthetist
Papworth Hospital
Cambs

Dr V.J. Pappachan MB Bchir FRCA
Hon. Consultant in Paediatric Intensive Care & Anaesthesia
Southampton University Hospitals NHS Trust, Southampton

Professor Henry Paul Redmond BSc MCh FRCS
Consultant Surgeon
University Hospital
Cork
Ireland

Mr Paul Rooney DM FRCS
Lecturer in Surgery
University Hospital
Queens Medical Centre
Nottingham

Mrs Sanjeev Sarin MS FRCS
Consultant Surgeon
Watford General Hospital
Watford

Miss Christobel Saunders FRCS(Gen)
Consultant Surgeon
Perth Royal Infirmary
Perth
Australia

Mr Michael Peter Saunders BSc MS FRCS
Consultant Surgeon
Eastbourne NHS Hospital Trust
Eastbourne

Dr Paul W.L. Siklos MA BSAc FRCP (Lond)
Consultant Physician
West Suffolk Hospital, Bury St Edmunds
Suffolk

Dr Howard S. Smith MBBS FRCA
Consultant in Anaesthesia and Intensive Care
Peterborough Hospitals NHS Trust
Cambridgeshire

Mr Mark Whyman
Senior Registrar in Surgery
Derriford Hospital
Plymouth

Abbreviations

Although abbreviations are defined in the text at first mention, a complete list is given here for ease of reference.

AAA	abdominal aortic aneurysm
AAGBI	Association of Anaesthetists of GB and Ireland
ADH	antidiuretic hormone
AF	atrial fibrillation
AFP	alphafetoprotein
AIDS	acquired immunodeficiency syndrome
ALG	antilymphocyte globulin
ALI	acute lung injury
ALM	acro-lentiginous melanoma
ALS	antilymphocyte serum
ALT	alanine transaminase
AMPA	2-amino-3-hydroxy-5-methyl-4-isoxazole-propionic acid
ANDI	abnormalities of normal involution and development
APC	adenomatous polyposis coli
APPT	activated partial thromboplastin time
ARDS	acute (adult) respiratory distress syndrome
ARF	acute renal failure
ASA	American Association of Anesthesiologists
AST	aspartate transaminase
ATG	antithymocyte globulin
ATLS	advanced trauma life support
ATN	acute tubular necrosis
AV	atrioventricular
AXR	abdominal X-ray
BAPEN	British Association for Parenteral and Enteral Nutrition
BCC	basal cell carcinoma
BMI	body mass index
BP	blood pressure
b.p.m.	beats per minute
BSO	bilateral salpingo-oophorectomy
BUPA	British United Provident Association
CAD	computer-aided diagnosis
CAI	community-acquired infection
CAMs	cell adhesion molecules
CAPD	continuous ambulatory peritoneal dialysis
CASS	Coronary Artery Surgery Study
CBD	common bile duct
CDC	Centers for Disease Control
CEA	carcinoembryonic antigen
CEPOD	Confidential Enquiry into Perioperative Deaths
CFA	common femoral artery
cGRP	calcitonin gene related peptide
CHRPE	congenital hypertrophic retinal pigment epithelium
CI	confidence interval or cardiac index
CIS	carcinoma in situ
CLED	cysteine lactose electrolyte-deficient agar
CME	continued medical education
CMF	cyclophosphamide, methotrexate, and 5-fluorouracil
CMV	cytomegalovirus
CNS	central nervous system
CO	cardiac output
COPD	chronic obstructive pulmonary disease
COX	cyclo-oxygenase
CPAP	continuous positive airway pressure
CPP	cerebral perfusion pressure
CRC	colorectal cancer
CRM	circumferential resection margin
CRP	C-reactive protein
CRPS	complex regional pain syndrome
CRRT	continual renal replacement therapy

CSF	cerebrospinal fluid	GIT	gastrointestinal tract
CSSD	central sterile supply department	GMC	General Medical Council
CT	computed tomography	GM-CSF	granulocyte macrophage colony-stimulating factor
CTL	cytotoxic T-lymphocyte	GOR	gastro-oesophageal reflux
CVP	central venous pressure	GORD	gastro-oesophageal reflux disease
CVVH	continuous veno-venous haemofiltration	GRP	glass-reinforced plastic
CVVHDF	continuous veno-venous haemodiafiltration	GTP	guanosine triphosphate
CXR	chest X-ray	GvHD	graft-versus-host disease
DCIS	ductal carcinoma in situ	HAC	human artificial chromosome
DHFR	dihydrofolate reductase	HAI	hospital-acquired infection
Do_2	oxygen delivery	HBV	hepatitis B virus
DPL	diagnostic peritoneal lavage	HCG	human chorionic gonadotrophin
DSA	digital subtraction angiography	HCV	hepatitis C virus
DTs	delirium tremens	HCW	healthcare worker
DTPA	diethylenetriaminepentaacetic acid	HDU	high-dependency unit
DU	duodenal ulcer	HEN	home enteral nutrition
DVI	digital vascular imaging	HIV	human immunodeficiency virus
DVT	deep venous thrombosis	HMF	Hutchison's melanotic freckle
EAA	excitatory amino acid	HNPCC	hereditary non-polyposis colorectal cancer
EBV	EpsteinBarr virus	HOC	hyperosmolar citrate
EC	Eurocollins solution	HPN	home parenteral nutrition
ECG	electrocardiogram	HR	heart rate
EEG	electroencephalograph	HRT	hormone replacement therapy
EGC	early gastric cancer	HSV	herpes simplex virus
ELISA	enzyme-linked immunosorbent assay	HSVtk	herpes simplex virus thymidine kinase
EMG	electro myograph	5-HT	5-hydroxytryptamine (serotonin)
ENT	otorhinolaryngology	HTK	histidine–tryptophan–ketoglutarate
EPMR	extraperitoneal mesh repair	HTLV	human T-lymphocyte virus
ER	oestrogen receptor	HVZ	herpes varicella-zoster
ERC	endoscopic retrograde cholangiography	ICA	internal carotid artery
ERCP	endoscopic retrograde cholangio-pancreatography	ICAMs	intercellular adhesion molecules
ERP	endoscopic retrograde pancreatography	ICC	infection-control committee
ESR	erythrocyte sedimentation rate	ICD	infection-control doctor
EUA	examination under anaesthesia	ICD 10	WHO International Classification of Diseases, version 10
FAP	familial adenomatous polyposis	ICN	infection-control nurse
FBC	full blood count	ICP	intracranial pressure
FdUMP	5-fluoro, 2-deoxyuridylate monophosphate	ICT	infection-control team
FEV	forced expired volume	ICU	Intensive Care Unit
FFP	fresh frozen plasma	IDDM	insulin-dependent diabetes mellitus
FNA	fine-needle aspiration	IFN	interferon
FNAC	fine-needle aspiration cytology	IL	interleukin
FOB	faecal occult blood	IM	intramuscular(ly)
Fr.	French gauge	INR	international normalized ratio
FSGS	focal and segmental glomerulosclerosis	IT	information technology
FSH	follicle stimulating hormone	ITU	intensive care unit
fT_4	free thyroxine	IV	intravenous(ly)
5FU	5-fluorouracil	IVC	inferior vena cava
FUTP	fluorouridine triphosphate	IVP	intravenous pyelogram
FVC	forced vital capacity	IVRA	intravenous regional anaesthesia
GCS	Glasgow Coma Score	IVU	intravenous urography
Gd–DTPA	gadolinium–diethylenetriaminepentaacetic acid	LAK	lymphokine activated killer
GFR	glomerular filtration rate	LBP	lipopolysaccharide binding protein
GGT	gamma-glutamyl-transpeptidase	LCIS	lobular carcinoma in situ
GI	gastrointestinal	LDH	lactate dehydrogenase
GIK	glucose-insulin-potassium infusion		

LFT	liver function test	PgR	progesterone receptor
LH	luteinizing hormone	PGR	pulse-generated runoff
LHRH	luteinizing hormone-releasing hormone	PLAP	placental alkaline phosphatase
LM	lentigo maligna	PNI	prognostic nutritional index
LOM	likelihood of malnutrition index	PNTML	pudendal nerve terminal motor latencies
LPS	lipopolysaccharide	PONV	postoperative nausea and vomiting
LSA	Lothian Surgical Audit	PNS	peripheral nerve stimulators
MAI	*Mycobacterium avium intracellulare*	PPF	Plasma Protein Fraction
MAP	mean arterial pressure	PPG	photoplethysmography
MAS	minimal access surgery	p.p.m.	parts per million
MBC	minimum bactericidal concentration	PR	*per rectum*
MCH	mean cell haemoglobin	PSA	prostate-specific antigen
MCV	mean corpuscular volume	PT	prothrombin time
MDR	multiple drug resistance	PTA	percutaneous transluminal angioplasty
MDU	Medical Defence Union	PTB	patellar tendon bearing
MEC	minimum effective (blood) concentration	PTC	percutaneous transhepatic cholangiography
MEN	multiple endocrine neoplasia	PTCA	percutaneous transluminal coronary angioplasty
M6G	morphine-6-glucuronide	PTFE	polytetrafluoroethylene
MHC	major histocompatibility complex	PTH	parathyroid hormone
MI	myocardial infarction	PTHrP	parathyroid hormone related protein (or peptide)
MIC	minimum inhibitory concentration	PTT	partial thromboplastin time
MMP	matrix metalloproteinase	QALYS	quality adjusted life years
MMR	mismatch repair	qds	quater die ...... (four times a day)
MODS	multiple organ dysfunction syndrome	RBC	red blood cell
MRCP	magnetic resonance cholangio-pancreatography	RBF	renal blood flow
MRI	magnetic resonance imaging	REE	resting energy expenditure
MRSA	multiresistant *Staphylococcus aureus*	RER	replication error
MSU	midstream specimen of urine	RSD	reflex sympathetic dystrophy or repetitive strain disorder
MTS	mental test score		
NCEPOD	National Confidential Enquiry into Perioperative Deaths	RtPa	recombinant tissue plasminogen activator
		SAGM	saline, adenine, glucose, mannitol
Nd:YAG	neodymium yttrium aluminium (laser)	SASM	Scottish Assessment of Surgical Mortality
NGT	nasogastric tube	SC	subcutaneous(ly)
NHS	National Health Service	SCC	squamous cell carcinoma
NK	natural killer	SEPS	subfascial endoscopic perforator surgery
NM	nodular melanoma	SFA	superficial femoral artery
NMDA	*N*-methyl-D-aspartate	SFEMG	single-fibre electromyography
NSMD	non-specific motility disorder	SFJ	sapheno-femoral junction
O	orally	SGA	subjective global assessment
OER	oxygen extraction ratio	SIMV	synchronized intermittent mandatory ventilation
OGD	oesophago-gastro-duodenoscopy	SIRS	systemic inflammatory response syndrome
OPCS	Office of Population Censuses and Surveys	SLE	systemic lupus erythematosus
PACD	perianal Crohn's disease	SMI	sustained maximal inspiration
PAF	platelet activating factor	SMP	sympathetically maintained pain
PAWP	pulmonary artery wedge pressure	SMT	spinomesencephalic tract
PBC	primary biliary cirrhosis	SMV	synchronized mandatory ventilation
PBPs	penicillin-binding proteins	SRT	spinoreticular tract
PBS	phosphate-buffered sucrose	SSM	superficial spreading melanoma
PCA	patient-controlled analgesia	STD	sexually transmitted disease
PCR	polymerase chain reaction	STIR	short tau inversion recovery
PEEP	positive end expiratory pressure	STT	spinothalamic tract
PEG	percutaneous endoscopic gastrostomy	SV	stroke volume
PGE$_1$	prostaglandin E$_1$	SVR	systemic vascular resistance
PGE$_2$	prostaglandin E$_2$	T$_3$	tri-iodothyronine
PGI$_2$	prostaglandin I$_2$	T$_4$	thyroxine

TAA	tumour-associated antigen	TPN	total parenteral nutrition
TAH	total abdominal hysterectomy	TRAM	transverse rectus abdominis muscle (flap)
TAPP	transabdominal preperitoneal repair	TRH	thyroid releasing hormone
TB	tuberculosis	TSA	tumour-specific antigen
TCD	transcranial Doppler	TSH	thyroid stimulating hormone
TCGF	T-cell growth factor	TT	thrombin time
TED	thromboembolic disease	TURP	transurethral resection of prostate
TEDBC	trial of early detection of breast cancer	Tx	thromboxane
TEM	transanal endoscopic microsurgery	UICC	Union Internationale Contre le Cancer
TENS	transcutaneous electrical nerve stimulation	US	ultrasound
TGF-	transforming growth factor-	UTI	urinary tract infection
TIA	transient ischaemic attack	VDEPT	virally directed enzyme prodrug therapy
TILs	tumour infiltrating lymphocytes	VIP	vasoactive intestinal polypeptide
TIPSS	transjugular intrahepatic portosystemic shunt	VMA	vanilyl mandelic acid
TME	total mesorectal excision	Vo_2	tissue oxygen utilization
TNF	tumour necrosis factor	VPL	ventroposterolateral thalamic nuclei
TNM	Tumour Node Metastasis system	WBC	white blood cell
tPA	tissue plasminogen activator	w/v	weight/volume

CHAPTER 1

Introduction

*Clive R. Quick, Ali Majeed, and
Paul Rooney*

1 Consent in surgical practice

1.1 Medical ethics

Surgeons aspire to practise their craft in line with the principles of the Hippocratic oath. This oath originated from the Greek school of medicine around 500 BC. The essence of these principles is as follows:

- Doctors must be instructed and registered to protect the public from amateurs and charlatans.

- Medicine is for the benefit of patients and doctors must avoid doing anything known to cause harm.

- Euthanasia and abortion are prohibited.

- Operations and procedures must be performed only by practitioners with appropriate expertise.

- Doctors must maintain proper professional relationships with their patients and treatment provided should not be governed by motives of profit or favour.

- Doctors should not take advantage of their professional relationship with their patients.

- Medical confidentiality must be respected.

The term 'medical ethics' refers to the universal principles on which medical decisions should be based and governs to a large extent the beliefs and actions that influence the day-to-day judgements of doctors. Whereas benevolence should ideally govern all medical practice, other factors such as self-interest, money, the distribution of resources, and individual skills are important motivating factors.

To a variable extent, the practice of surgery is influenced by the need for self-protection, but in trying to avoid litigation, a surgeon may overtreat or overinvestigate in ways that are not just unnecessary but even unethical. An element of self-interest is difficult to avoid but the guiding principle should be that the patient's interests are paramount.

1.2 Consent to treatment

Treatment that is against a patient's will can only rarely be justified. Clearing the airways of someone about to choke to death who is irrational because of impaired or disturbed consciousness can easily be justified on the grounds that this is what the patient would have wanted were he fully rational. Arguments for compulsory treatment when society in general is perceived to be at risk are occasionally put forward, but the damage resulting from coercion usually outweighs what it might seek to avert. However, if a patient is suffering from a highly infectious and dangerous disease, few would argue that the patient should not be allowed to refuse treatment.

Common law has long recognized the principle that every person has the right to have his or her bodily integrity protected against invasion by others. An accepted legal principle is that an adult of sound mind has the right to determine what shall be done with his own body and a surgeon who performs an operation without a patient's consent commits an assault in the eyes of the law. There has been a large volume of litigation in many countries on the consent issue and as a result the doctrine of informed consent has assumed an important role in the medical negligence debate. Fortunately, judgements in England and Canada have helped to avoid some of the problems related to consent in the United States.

1.3 When is consent necessary?

As a general rule, medical treatment, even minor treatment, should not proceed without having first obtained the patient's consent. Consent may be **expressed** or it may be **implied** as when a patient presents for examination and acquiesces in the suggested activities. A doctor may proceed without consent if the patient's balance of mind is disturbed or if the patient is incapable of giving consent because of unconsciousness. If the patient is a minor, the same principles apply, but it is always sensible to seek consent from responsible relatives or, at the very least, to check with medical and administrative colleagues that the planned action is in the patient's best interest. It is also important for opinions to be recorded in the notes, ideally before action is taken.

1.4 The unconscious patient

When treating an unconscious patient, it is best to apply the **necessity principle**. On this basis, a surgeon is justified in treating a patient without expressed consent if the value of what he seeks to protect is accepted to be of greater weight than the wrongful act he performs (i.e. treating without consent). Necessity is an adequate defence for treating an unconscious patient, provided there is no known objection to treatment. However, the treatment must not be more extensive than is essential and the surgeon must not take advantage of uncon-

sciousness to perform procedures that are not required for the patient's survival. For example, in one case, a diseased testis was removed during a hernia repair and a court held that the doctor had acted for the protection of the patient's health and possibly life, and that removal of the testis was necessary; it would have been unreasonable to put the procedure off until later. In contrast, a doctor who sterilized a patient during a Caesarean section without the patient's consent, on the grounds that it would be hazardous for her to go through another pregnancy, was deemed unreasonable and damages were awarded. Thus the principle emerges that if a doctor discovers a condition in an unconscious patient for which treatment is necessary and it would be unreasonable to postpone the operation to a later date, treatment can be justified in law.

Ambiguous wording on consent forms that require a patient to agree to any operation the surgeon considers necessary is regarded by the courts as completely worthless. For this reason a model consent form that minimizes this ambiguity was produced by the National Health Service Executive in 1990 to be used throughout the health services.

1.5 Consent in children and young people

When a minor (i.e. a child under 16 years of age) is unconscious and requiring treatment, it is wise for the doctor to obtain a close relative's consent. Such *proxy consent* will diminish the likelihood of a patient taking successful legal action, if aggrieved, provided the procedure was essential, but would not be valid if the procedure fell into the 'convenience' category. Proxy consents are only of solid value if the patient has given expressed authority to another person to give or withhold consent or when the law invests a person with these powers, for example with respect to a parent giving consent on behalf of a child. Unreasonable withholding of proxy consent, however, may justify a surgeon ignoring such a withholding.

The Family Law Reform Act of 1969 provides that a person of 16 or over may consent to medical treatment without reference to a parent or guardian and this consent may override parental objection to a particular medical treatment. On the other hand, a 16-year-old who refuses treatment is likely to have to submit to parental authority, although such a case has not been tested in the British courts.

The question of consent given by a child of less than 16 is controversial. In a recent case, the dominant opinion was that the parental right to determine whether their young child should have treatment ends if and when the child achieves sufficient understanding to enable him or her to fully understand what is proposed (Lord Scarman 1985). It follows that a doctor treating a child should attempt to obtain parental authority, but if the patient can understand what is proposed and can express his or her wishes, the surgeon may provide treatment on the child's consent alone. The decision to do so must be taken on clinical grounds and its legal acceptability depends on the severity and permanence of the therapy.

If a doctor needs to take life-saving measures for a child against the wishes of a parent, the actions may be justifiable on the grounds of necessity, bearing in mind that the required standard is that of a reasonable body of medical opinion. There may be little sympathy for parents who refuse blood transfusion on religious grounds but if doctors were able to ignore the firmly held religious convictions of adults, this would represent a major change in a free society. The legal position is that a parent's rights to control a child exist for the benefit of the child and not the parent, and these views may justifiably be overridden if the death of the child is likely. Indeed, if a child dies under these circumstances, the parents are open to prosecution for manslaughter.

1.6 Consent to testing for HIV infection

The General Medical Council (GMC) has firmly rejected HIV testing without specific consent, save in the most exceptional circumstances. They believe that specific consent is required because of the serious social and financial consequences that may follow a positive diagnosis. The GMC holds that testing without consent is permissible only when it has not been possible to obtain consent and the health of others and the patient is in danger. It also holds that the best interests of a child may permit testing even in the face of parental objection. Recent authoritative opinions on whether testing can be carried out without consent are conflicting. However, a sensible opinion is that a patient who consults a doctor gives general consent to the diagnostic tests that the surgeon considers necessary. It is true that HIV tests carry major emotional, financial, and social significance and, of course, the disease, once diagnosed, is currently incurable. The mere fact that an HIV test has been undertaken carries serious insurance implications and has to be disclosed as a condition of most policies. Although this puts HIV testing into a separate category from most tests, the law is unlikely to exclude absolutely any test for which specific consent has not been given. Anonymized HIV testing still raises ethical issues; these tests may be of epidemiological importance and involve taking blood from random groups of patients with no particular risk factors, or using blood samples obtained for other purposes. If samples are totally anonymized, the information cannot then be used for the benefit of anyone found to be positive. The Colleges of Surgeons of England and Edinburgh maintain that testing a high-risk patient before an operation requires consent but testing without consent may be performed if theatre staff suffer contamination with a patient's blood. Even in the these circumstances, it is wise to obtain the patient's consent if possible.

1.7 The consequences of proceeding without consent

A patient may be entitled to sue for damages for **battery** or claim negligence on the grounds that the doctor failed to obtain consent. There are important differences between these in law: an action for battery can arise if the plaintiff has been touched by the defendant without consent, expressed or implied. There is no need for the plaintiff to establish any loss as a result. In contrast, in an action for negligence, the patient must establish that the defendant touched him or her without consent and that this led to the injury. Thus, an action for battery is easier to prove, for example if a patient refuses to submit to a procedure but the doctor goes ahead with it. A negligence claim may arise when the plaintiff has given consent to a particular procedure but where the consent did not cover other treatments that arose during the operation or complications resulting from the operation. To succeed, a patient must prove that he would not have given consent if the appropriate information had been given beforehand and would not therefore had suffered the loss. The courts rarely use the patient's subjective view alone in determining the outcome, but try to determine the likely views of 'a reasonable patient' as well as obtaining opinions about whether the balance of risk was in favour of the treatment provided.

1.8 The concept of informed consent

This issue arose first in America in 1957, where a court concluded that a doctor had a duty to disclose any facts that are necessary for the patient to provide intelligent consent to the proposed treatment. Informed consent introduces a new element to medical treatment. It is no longer a simple matter for the patient to consent to a technical assault. Consent would now be based on a knowledge of the nature, consequences, and alternatives associated with the proposed therapy. From the ethical point of view, a person should not be exposed to a risk of damage unless he has agreed to that risk; he cannot properly agree to a treatment or make a choice between treatments without factual information. It is clear that a patient should be as fully informed as possible so that he can make up his mind in the light of the relevant circumstances. However, this view can criticized on the grounds that this leaves little scope for the doctor to exercise clinical judgement. Thus a surgeon may be permitted the therapeutic privilege of withholding information which would only distress or confuse the patient.

A **professional standard** for consent involves counselling and delivery of appropriate information. This is an integral part of normal clinical management. The extent and detail of the information supplied is a matter for the surgeon, who is always subject to a general duty of care. The quality of information provided is likely to be judged from the viewpoint of a prudent patient on the one hand, and of a prudent doctor on the other. The balance between these is perplexing. There must be a respect for the patient's legitimate interests in knowing what he is subjecting himself to, but, at the same time, there will be cases where a more paternalistic approach is appropriate. Explaining all ramifications of treatment and all possible risks would be extremely time consuming and of doubtful benefit, perhaps serving to confuse rather than inform the patient.

In the United States three-quarters of the individual states apply a professional standard to consent (see above) and one-third of these have specifically ruled out the prudent patient test which obliges the doctor to list every possible complication of the proposed procedure. A quarter of the states demand a standard for consent that would be required by the prudent patient.

In the UK, case law on consent is as follows: the doctor is not negligent if he acts in accordance with the practice accepted at the time as proper by 'a responsible body of medical opinion'. In general, the professional standard holds good, but disclosure of a particular risk may be so obviously necessary to the patient that no reasonably prudent surgeon would fail to make it. A doctor's duty clearly extends to disclosing any real risks of treatment but also to warn of any real possibility that treatment may prove ineffective.

Case law has demonstrated that a 10 per cent risk of a serious complication occurring must be disclosed but risks of 1 per cent or less need not be disclosed. In one New Zealand court judgement, factors to be considered when deciding what a patient should be told were as follows: the gravity of the condition to be treated, the importance of the benefits expected to result from the treatment or procedure, the need to encourage the patient to accept it, the relative significance of its risks, the intellectual and emotional capacity of the patient to absorb the information, and the extent to which the patient may have tacitly invited the doctor to take the responsibility for undertaking intricate or technical decisions. When questioned specifically by a rational patient about the risks of a particular treatment, a surgeon's duty must be to answer truthfully and as fully as the question demands.

It is clear that American moves towards greater patient autonomy are influencing British courts. A court decision stated that it is no longer the medical profession alone that collectively determines—by its own practices—the amount of information a patient should have in order to decide whether to undergo an operation. This implies that doctors should treat their patients as intelligent, rational people to whom important matters should be explained in reasonable detail. The term 'informed consent' is misleading and should perhaps be replaced by 'rational consent' or even 'intelligent consent'. Surgeons should be aware of a progressive change in the climate of opinion and become familiar with patients' anxieties and aspirations. It is good medicine to involve patients fully in decision making. The process of explaining likely events that will happen during and after operations gains greater patient co-operation and lowers anxiety levels. It also passes a degree of responsibility to the patient for the outcome, particularly of risky procedures. It is now standard practice to try to offer the level of information that a prudent patient would wish to know.

1.9 Practical aspects of consent to treatment

In British law, there is no such thing as informed consent. Surgeons like to feel they obtain informed consent after explaining to the patient in non-technical language the nature, purpose, and risks of the proposed investigation or treatment, together with alternatives and the likely outcome of treatment. The patient must be capable of understanding the explanation, and if this is not the case, then informed consent has not been obtained. It follows that consent cannot be obtained from patients who are unconscious or of unsound mind.

Types of consent

1. Implied: this is the most common form of consent and allows patients to be examined and investigated without obtaining written consent.

2. Expressed: the process of obtaining expressed consent involves first discussing the proposed treatment with the aim of obtaining the patient's permission to proceed. Permission can be based either on an oral or a written agreement. Most invasive investigations (such as upper gastrointestinal (GI) endoscopy or arteriography) and any operation should be preceded by written consent. If oral consent alone has been obtained, then a note to that effect should be made in the patient's record.

Obtaining consent

1. Consent should always be obtained by a medical practitioner who is sufficiently knowledgeable to be able to explain the proposed treatment, any alternatives, the likely outcome, and any significant risks.

2. The types and level of risk that need to be discussed are not well defined, but a risk of complication or potential failure to treat the condition of between 5 and 10 per cent should certainly be discussed. Operation-specific or disease-specific risks must be explained (e.g. facial nerve damage in parotid surgery, hypoparathyroidism following thyroid surgery) and an entry made in the hospital records. General risks such as deep venous thrombosis (DVT) or pneumonia are not usually discussed and this does place doubt on the efficacy of obtaining true informed consent.

3. Consent should be obtained a reasonably short time before the procedure (but see point 4, below). There is no legal limit to the period between obtaining consent and the procedure, but if circumstances change in any substantial way, then fresh consent needs to be obtained.

4. Discussion prior to consent should occur in an unhurried manner, giving the patient time to absorb the information, question the doctor obtaining consent, and to indicate treatments he does not want performed. The patient may wish to discuss aspects of what is proposed with family or friends before consenting.

5. The consent form should not be altered. If extra procedures become necessary, then a fresh consent form should be obtained.

6. In patients who are incapable of giving consent it is customary to obtain consent from a near relative. This is not essential in law but represents good practice. If life-saving treatment is required and consent cannot be obtained, then it is reasonable to carry out the minimal necessary treatment to save life or health.

Consent in children

1. Consent can be obtained from children aged 16 and over, and occasionally in those under 16. It is always sensible to liaise with parents wherever possible in children aged 17 and 18. Legal consent can be obtained from children under 16 under certain circumstances (see earlier) but efforts should generally be made to obtain parental agreement.

2. In the absence of parents, another relative or person *in loco parentis* can give consent for children.

3. Children in care: if the local authority has taken full parental rights, then the director of social services or deputy needs to sign the consent form. In circumstances where the child is in voluntary care, the parents still act as guardians and their consent should be obtained.

Jehovah's Witnesses

Adult Jehovah's witnesses will usually refuse blood transfusion, even in an extreme emergency, because of their interpretation of part of the Bible. If permission to transfuse is withheld, then blood should not be given. Failure to respond to the patient's wish may result in an accusation of battery. The moral dilemma of allowing a patient to die when treatment such as blood transfusion is likely to prevent death is uncomfortable but the law is clear on what path needs to be taken. General advice is that:

◆ A surgeon cannot refuse to treat a patient simply because the patient imposes certain conditions on that treatment. It may be possible to find a surgeon who accepts the limitations imposed and to transfer the patient to his or her care. The law has not been tested by a situation when such a surgeon cannot be found.

◆ It is wise to interview the patient in the presence of a witness and explain the risks. The outcome should be noted and the witness should sign the hospital record.

In children of Jehovah's Witnesses the position is different. If a blood transfusion is deemed necessary to save the life of such a child or to prevent harm, then the transfusion can be given and defended in law by claiming that the decision was an action taken in the best interests of the child. If parental consent is withheld and there is ample time, the child can be made a ward of court, but this is not essential simply to obtain consent.

◆ Clear explanations should be given to the parents of the risks involved. A witness should be present.

◆ If the decision to give blood is made, then a second medical opinion confirming the need for this treatment should be obtained if time allows.

◆ It is important to realize that a child subjected to transfusion against parental wishes may be rejected by the parents.

2 Medical negligence

2.1 Introduction

Claims for professional negligence against doctors in the UK have increased markedly over the past decade. This has brought omens of an American type of deterioration in doctor–patient relationships driven by fear of malpractice suits. However, it is still difficult for a patient to bring an action for medical negligence in the UK because the standards of care are still effectively defined by the profession itself and there are practical difficulties in establishing causation. Furthermore, the expense of bringing a legal action and the relative difficulty of obtaining legal aid for all but the least affluent inhibits embarking upon medical litigation. In the USA, contingency fees for lawyers and sympathetic juries tend to encourage litigation.

The reasons for increasing medical litigation are multiple. The increasing complexity of therapeutic and diagnostic procedures is placing increasing pressure on hospitals, and published 'Patients' Charters' elevate patient expectations, and perhaps there has been a change in public attitude so that doctors are no longer regarded as infallible. Extensive press coverage of medical misadventures, such as the transfusion of contaminated blood products into haemophiliacs, also makes the general public more aware of the possibility of compensation.

Actions against doctors are usually time consuming and potentially destructive and a large amount of professional time is involved in processing the claims. The period between injury and compensation can be very long. Furthermore, a single alleged incident of negligence can damage the professional reputation of a doctor out of all proportion to the seriousness of the fault. On the other hand, the patient who has been injured by an act of medical negligence has suffered in a way recognized by the law as meriting compensation. Sums required to compensate an injured victim for loss of future earnings and long-term expenses of medical or nursing care may be very large. To deny a legitimate claim or to artificially restrict the size of an award, on the other hand, could be perceived as amounting to gross injustice. In the United States, attempts have been made to limit the numbers of litigation procedures by screening out frivolous claims and by arbitration procedures which, although voluntary, are binding on the parties. There are measures along similar lines currently being implemented in the UK (the Woolf reforms).

2.2 No-fault compensation schemes

No-fault compensation provides for awards to injured patients irrespective of the need to find fault with the medical personnel. Such a scheme began in New Zealand in 1974 and worked reasonably satisfactorily in its early years. The claimant must establish that the injury resulted from medical or surgical misadventure rather than from the natural progress of a medical condition. The difficulties of distinguishing these, as well as the potential cost, have discouraged the introduction of schemes like this in the UK and they have not had the support of government. The British Medical Association, however, supports no-fault compensation but believes stricter rules should be applied. Under these, injuries would be excluded from compensation if they were not avoidable by exercising reasonable care. Thus, the concept of negligence would remain but no fault would be inferred. Many believe that the existing system of compensation may have a deterrent effect on malpractice, but since the National Health Service underwrites most settlements for malpractice in the UK, this is unlikely to be a significant factor.

2.3 The basis of medical liability

In hospital practice, an individual doctor may be suspected of being the sole perpetrator of medical negligence or it may be difficult to blame an individual because of team management. An aggrieved patient has the choice of proceeding against an individual he believes has been negligent or against a health authority, or against both in a joint action. In practice, most actions are brought against the health authority for convenience. Exactly where responsibility lies is not wholly clear from previous legal cases but there is a growing view that hospitals or health authorities are responsible for the treatment they provide. The National Health Service (NHS) is certainly the direct employer of virtually all hospital doctors, and is therefore liable for their negligence under the principle of **vicarious liability**. Indeed, the vicarious liability of hospitals has been clearly established in law for over 30 years.

Until recently, medical employees were contractually bound to be members of a defence organization and the costs of any actions were shared between the defence organization and the health authority. However, membership fees increased so dramatically with increasing litigation that Crown indemnity was given to doctors, dentists, and community physicians from January 1990. Thus the entire defence costs of negligence litigation are borne by the NHS. No special financial provision has been made for this, with the result that health authorities at times feel obliged to settle cases on the grounds of the cheapest, if not the fairest, option. This approach risks leaving medical reputations unjustly tarnished.

2.4 What constitutes negligence?

The burden of proof

In a case of alleged negligence, the court seeks to establish whether the conduct of the defendant amounted to a breach of the duty of care which was owed to the injured plaintiff (the complainant). In other words, did the standard of treatment given fall below the standard expected by the law and, therefore, was there was any fault in a legal sense? The burden of proving fault lies with the plaintiff. However, it may be that when a plaintiff attempts to pursue an action against a doctor, the law places a heavier burden in establishing a case than it requires in other personal injury litigation. An indication of this is the fact that damages are paid in 30–40 per cent of medical cases compared with 86 per cent in other personal injury cases. In

some cases, however, the courts have taken the view that the burden of proof lies with the defendant, on the basis that when an injury has been caused, which should not have occurred, some compensation ought to be paid by someone to the injured party.

What is a reasonably skilful doctor?

The essential characteristics that should be possessed by a reasonably skilful doctor have been the subject of many judicial pronouncements over the years. A surgeon does not undertake to perform a cure or to employ the highest possible degree of skill obtainable anywhere; however, he does have a duty to the patient to use due caution in undertaking treatment. A court cannot expect the highest, or even a very high, standard but it is unlikely to accept a very low standard. The standard of care required by the courts requires the doctor to exercise the ordinary skill of an ordinary doctor exercising that particular art. In other words, the ordinarily skilful doctor sets the standard by following the standard practice of the profession at the time of treatment, or at least, practices that would not be disapproved of by a responsible body of opinion within the profession. The 'custom test' refers to the legal test whereby a defendant's conduct is tested against the normal conduct of his profession. This is determined in retrospect by reference to expert witnesses and, particularly, to medical articles published around the time of the alleged malpractice. The doctor needs to have a reasonably sound grasp of modern medical techniques and to be as informed of new medical developments as the average competent doctor could be expected to be.

The circumstances in which the patient was treated are also taken into account. For example, if a doctor working on an emergency case had inadequate facilities and was under great pressure, the courts would not expect him to achieve the same results as the same doctor working in ideal conditions.

How is 'departure from normal practice' proved?

Case law has established that when a departure from normal practice is alleged, three facts need to be established:

1. There must be proof that there is a usual and normal practice.

2. It must be proved that the defendant did not adopt that practice.

3. Of crucial importance, it must be established that the course the doctor adopted was one that no professional man of ordinary skill would have taken if he had been acting with ordinary care.

However, this apparently simple set of rules is difficult to interpret consistently. For example, there are areas in surgery where more than one course of action appears correct and 'evidence-based medicine' is unable to distinguish between them. Negligence would not be inferred merely because there was a body of medical opinion against the action that was carried out. However, for a particular practice to be regarded as acceptable by a court, it must be shown to be professionally tenable and the court is the final arbiter of that. In general, the weight of expert evidence of what constitutes appropriate professional action will determine the outcome, but the court may decide otherwise.

How up-to-date must a surgeon be in law?

A surgeon is expected to have a reasonable knowledge but is not expected to know all there is to be known in a particular area. Thus failure to read a single article may be excusable, but it is not acceptable for a surgeon to disregard a series of published warnings in the medical press; it seems that attitudes are hardening in this respect. With regard to innovative techniques, the court will assess whether their use could be considered justified or was negligent, by taking into account evidence from published trials of the technique and any dangers it was known to entail. A court would be unlikely to endorse the use of an untried technique or procedure if the patient had been exposed to a risk of damage out of proportion to the likely benefits, or which had been undertaken without 'intelligent' consent. Other factors in determining the appropriateness of innovative techniques might include the previous response of the patient to conventional treatment, the seriousness of the patient's condition, and the attitude of the patient towards the use of the novel or risky treatment.

Misdiagnosis and errors of judgement

A mistake in diagnosis would not be considered negligent if the usual high standard of care had been observed. In these circumstances, a misdiagnosis would be regarded as non-culpable and an inevitable hazard of practice. As a minimum, a doctor must examine the patient and pay adequate attention to the patient's medical notes. Ordinary laboratory tests must have been employed if symptoms suggested they should be, but elaborate and expensive investigations would not necessarily be regarded as mandatory except in complicated or puzzling cases. Whether a X-ray was taken depends on the circumstances of each case.

Errors of judgement are treated similarly. Gross medical mistakes usually result in a court finding in favour of negligence. For example, an operation that removed the wrong limb or an operation on the wrong patient would always be indefensible and such cases are usually settled out of court. In cases where operating equipment or swabs have been left inside patients after operation, courts have shown that they require that some sort of standard procedure had been adopted with the intention of minimizing the likelihood of this occurring. Overall responsibility to ensure that swabs and other items are not left in the patient rests with the surgeon and may not be delegated to a nurse.

Problems of trainees

Courts require doctors to show a degree of skill that would be expected of a reasonably competent professional person. As this is, to a large degree, an objective standard, it is irrelevant how long the doctor has been qualified before the alleged incident of negligence. Most judges maintain that the public is entitled to an overall reasonable standard of competence in their medical attendants and therefore the defendant's grade would have little bearing in determining negligence. The required standard of care is likely to have been met if the trainee had sought advice or had consulted more experienced colleagues appropriately. Hospital authorities should not place too much responsibility upon junior employees because of the principle of vicarious liability; appropriate supervision of trainees is always required. A consultant could be found negligent if he delegated responsibility to a junior knowing that the junior was insufficiently experienced or was incapable of performing the duty properly for other reasons. In general, a junior doctor is required to carry out duties as instructed in order to avoid liability, but if the instructions are manifestly wrong, he or she may depart from them without incurring personal legal liability.

The concept of *res ipsa loquitur*

In a case where the plaintiff cannot identify the precise negligence that caused the injury and where the defendant can offer no explanation of the way in which the injury came to be inflicted, the court may apply the concept of *res ipsa loquitur*. This principle does not shift the onus of proof onto the defendant, as has been suggested, but it does infer negligence by the defendant. It is therefore easier for a plaintiff to succeed in a claim where *res ipsa loquitur* has been judged to apply. The doctrine might apply if the plaintiff cannot unravel the cause of an injury as a result of a procedure that he does not understand, or during which he has been unconscious. This principle may be seen to discourage the tendency of the medical profession to close ranks when one of their number has been accused of negligence.

However, the courts are markedly reluctant to apply *res ipsa loquitur* in medical negligence cases because there is a danger that negligence could be proved even though the doctors had been competent, conscientious, and careful, resulting in unfair stigma on a professional career. However, the court is likely to apply the principle if something has gone wrong which does not normally occur, the plaintiff has identified the doctor whose negligence must have been responsible for the injury, and both plaintiff and defendant are unable to explain what happened. The principle has been applied in swab cases where a patient knows nothing about swab procedures in the operating theatre and it is therefore up to the surgeon to show that he exercised due care to ensure that swabs were not left behind.

Causation

Even if negligence has been established, a patient as plaintiff must prove that the damage suffered was caused by the negligence. This may be difficult if there is a variety of possible explanations, and this is often the case. When there is doubt, damages have occasionally been awarded on the basis of probability. Thus, for the sake of argument, if 100 people underwent the procedure and 60 would be expected to develop the complication and 40 would not, the balance of probability is that the plaintiff's injury *was* the result of the action taken and the defendant would therefore be judged liable.

Injuries caused by drugs and transfusion products

In the UK, compensation for injury caused by drugs is regulated by the Consumer Protection Act of 1987. This derives from the European Directive on Product Liability, which aims to apply strict liability for most injuries caused by defective products. The drug would now be regarded as defective if it failed to reach that degree of safety which 'persons generally are entitled to expect'. In certain circumstances, the manufacturer may invoke a **development risk**. Thus, if the manufacturer can show that he could not have known of the risk at the time of injury, the company would not be liable. If a drug is beneficial to many but causes harm to a minority, a claim for compensation is unlikely to be upheld, provided the product is presented properly and warnings are appropriately given. Under the 1987 Act, blood and blood products are expected to reach the same high standards. Thus allegations regarding transmission of infection (e.g. HIV, hepatitis B and C) through contaminated blood products are likely to fall under this heading.

Criminal negligence

There has been reluctance to prosecute medical personnel for criminal negligence in the past but, with the advent of the Crown Prosecution Service, the criminal law has sometimes been applied to cases where loss of life has followed negligence. In order to establish criminal negligence, the negligence must be such that the doctor showed such disregard for the life and safety of others as to amount to a crime against the state and to represent conduct deserving punishment. The criminal law might be invoked if there was such a major deviation from the normal practice or such a reckless disregard of it that it represented a danger to the public. In general, sentences have been minimal and prosecutions have often been dropped because criminal courts are reluctant to impugn the healthcare professions.

2.5 Practical aspects of complaints about patient care

Introduction

The steady increase in the number of complaints against hospitals alleging inadequate standards of medical care has made medical staff acutely aware of the dangers of substandard practice. Fortunately only a minority of complaints reveal episodes of medical negligence, but the amount of time and concern involved in sifting the genuine problems is ever increasing. From the medicolegal viewpoint, good surgical practice should aim to minimize the prospect of medical negligence and all its harmful effects. All clinical practice should be assessed to identify potential areas of increased risk and steps taken to eliminate defects discovered in the system. The concept of 'risk management' is a new one in the health services but one that needs to be incorporated in daily surgical practice.

Concept of medical negligence leading to harm

The complexity of surgical care means that outcome in respect of cure and complications is not always satisfactory. There may be unexpected morbidity and even mortality, and the patient suffers an 'adverse outcome'. Advice to patients about treatment should be based on an assessment of the relative risk of one or more interventional treatments and of simply doing nothing. Unfortunately the information needed for this type of accurate predictive work is scanty and is usually expressed in overall mortality and morbidity rates, without adjustment for obvious inter-patient risk factors. There is a current vogue for evidence-based medicine, and, in some respects, the critical analyses of randomized controlled trials published, for example, by the Cochrane Centre has enabled many doctors to assess conflicting treatments and provide professional justification for treatments they would recommend. The Cochrane Centre necessarily has a narrow focus in some surgical areas because of its emphasis on randomized controlled trials. However, it is likely that surgical treatments will come under greater and greater scrutiny and surgeons will be expected to evaluate the evidence, learn appropriate techniques, and justify the treatments they provide.

Any 'adverse outcome' following a surgical event is likely to be detrimental to the patient but it is rarely caused by medical negligence. All episodes of 'adverse outcome' ought to be subjected to an internal 'audit' process for educational purposes and to improve the 'process' but it is vital that medical audit is conducted without medicolegal implications otherwise it is unlikely to be undertaken openly and honestly.

Medical negligence, on the other hand, does not always lead to harm but it is unlikely that a medicolegal claim will arise from an episode where no harm has been caused. The area of importance in medicolegal terms is likely to be that where both patient harm and medical negligence coincide (Fig. 1.1). In practice, many episodes of patient complaint have no bearing on clinical practice and need to be considered by the health authority responsible for other aspects of the healthcare delivery process.

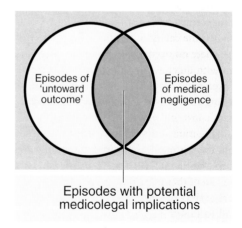

Figure 1.1 Patient harm and medical negligence. This figure identifies the area of overlap between episodes in which patients are harmed and episodes of medical negligence. The area of overlap is the problem area for potential medicolegal claims.

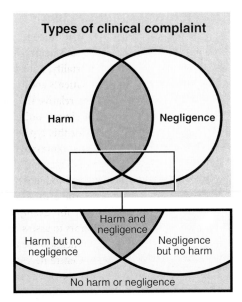

Figure 1.2 Types of clinical complaint.

Close analysis of clinically orientated complaints identify subsets that form the core of medicolegal complaints (Fig. 1.2).

The process of complaint

Many patients proceed to law only in order to find out the facts of why something went wrong. They are also likely to seek legal advice if they feel their complaint has been ignored or belittled and particularly if there appear to have been attempts to 'cover up' potentially negligent actions. In order to minimize the need for legal action, patient complaints, no matter how trivial, should be dealt with swiftly, sensitively, and openly. It often helps for the surgeon to talk through the events with the patient or relatives, often with a 'friend' of the patient present, perhaps provided by a local patient group, and with a witness present to record the conversation.

If a clinical complaint reaches the point where legal opinions are sought, then the category of complaint needs to be decided. Complaints where no negligence or patient harm have occurred can be dealt with quickly. For example, accusations of rudeness or offhand treatment may simply require an explanation and an apology. If harm has occurred as a result of obvious negligence, then an out of court settlement may be the most prudent course. Most legal contention is likely to involve cases where harm has occurred but there is dissension about whether it occurred accidentally or as a result of negligence.

It is self-evident that measures that prevent adverse outcomes and discourage risky practices are likely to reduce the damage to patients and to raise the quality of surgical practice. These, in turn, should reduce the number of indefensible claims surgeons are called upon to face. However, the number of complaints is unlikely to fall because of a rise in patient expectations and an upsurge in litigation in society in general.

Handling patient complaints

As complaints become more ubiquitous, surgeons need to understand the methods of handling these sensitive issues. The natural response of involved clinicians is often concern, anxiety, and perhaps a degree of anger. These emotions can complicate the issue, particularly if the complaint has arisen unexpectedly. The theoretical analysis outlined earlier can be useful to assess the seriousness of the complaint and to predict whether a legal claim is likely to follow. Each complaint needs to be appraised objectively and medicolegal opinions obtained early in the course of events if legal action seems likely.

Phase 1

The first official contact is usually through a letter of complaint to the health authority and then directed to the senior clinician for comment. Managerial experts can determine how specific the complaint is and whether it involves a clinical event. There are often several complaints in the initial letter, mentioning nursing care, food, medical care, and discharge procedures, for example. If there is a clinical element to the complaint, it is often wise to meet the complainant early on rather than enter into a long correspondence. This should be undertaken with a witness present who can also take notes. Explanation of what actually happened and why will often settle the complaint. A summary of what was said and agreed should be approved and then sent to the patient.

Phase 2

If the complaint cannot be resolved satisfactorily by discussion, then the case may need to be handed over formally to legal representatives. Clinicians need to be aware of the legal procedures to defend their own interests. Most legal work involving clinical complaints in the UK is now handled by the hospital trusts, but it is worth remembering that the trust's interests may not coincide with those of the individual clinician and it may be wise to consult one's own medical defence society early in potential legal claims.

Practical strategies for avoiding clinical complaints

1. Surgeons should maintain a quality of patient care that will stand up to peer review. This requires knowledge of what is currently 'best practice', an understanding of the alternatives, and a reasonable grasp of cure and relapse rates, as well as the potential complications of treatment.

2. Information about which surgeons are on emergency call at any one time must be clear and unambiguous to all hospital staff, and each person named must be available or have provided proper alternative cover.

3. All emergency patients seen in hospital should have the benefit of the appropriate level of expertise. The level of responsibility to be carried by each level of junior staff must be clearly defined and, when appropriate, more senior staff consulted whenever greater experience is needed. Each patient admitted to hospital needs to be under a named and available consultant.

4. Surgeons should explain the risks of procedures using the principles of consent discussed earlier. They should also anticipate potential problems to do with incipient deterioration: developing complications, the need for a further operation, and anticipated failure to cure, for example, and warn patient and relatives as early as possible.

5. The patient and relatives should be provided with regular progress reports, ensuring that the information is accurate and can be understood. It is wise to involve senior staff in this process, particularly in sensitive situations such as children or staff under treatment.

6. The consultant in charge should be informed as soon as there is any suggestion of complaint or litigation.

The last word

Patient complaints have become a regular feature of surgical life and should no longer be necessarily interpreted as a slur on professional conduct. Indeed, cases settled out of court are often of greater gravity than those reaching court because the treatment involved is regarded as so obviously indefensible. When patients complain, polite, speedy, and honest handling of the complaint will often circumvent the need for litigation.

3 Classification of surgical procedures

3.1 Introduction

Every surgical trainee has a mental classification of operative procedures which he is eager to build on. The range of procedures that a trainee has carried out has always been used as an indicator of 'surgical experience'. Indeed, a log of surgical procedures that have been observed or personally performed is now a prerequisite for entry to most postgraduate surgical examinations. There used to be little need for more senior surgeons to maintain a log of their operative work except on a personal basis, but the introduction of strict economic control of surgical work and the need to audit the outcome of surgical procedures has changed this. In the United States, the number of index procedures performed, both as a total and as a rate, is used to categorize a surgeon's clinical practice. Surgeons performing more than certain threshold numbers of operations are classified as specialists and those who do not are called generalists or as 'having an interest', depending on numbers. This classification of a surgeon may mitigate the legal expectation of quality of outcome after a particular operation, with higher standards expected of specialists.

The need to quantify procedures, measure their magnitude and effectiveness, and, in addition, identify operations with specific risks, has produced several classifications. These can be used for both audit and resource allocation.

3.2 Classification of interventional therapeutic manoeuvres

Introduction

Not all surgical practice involves open surgery. Technological advances have resulted in the evolution of less-invasive methods of treatment. As each new method is introduced, it should first be the subject of tightly controlled pilot studies. If these appear satisfactory, its place in the existing range of therapeutic procedures should be established prospectively, by comparing it directly with the best existing method. However, in practice this has not been the way the efficacy of new methods has been established. Most new operations, for example coronary artery bypass grafting, were tried out as a last resort on patients where other methods were inappropriate. Others, such as laparoscopic cholecystectomy, were modifications of techniques used in other specialties, in this case gynaecology. In the latter case, early enthusiasts were carried along by their own eagerness and a public encouraged by press coverage to believe that 'new was best'. Only much later were randomized studies carried out, with results often at odds with those claimed by non-randomized trials.

Types of interventional therapeutic manoeuvre

These are summarized in Table 1.1.

Table 1.1 Types of interventional therapeutic manoeuvre

Open incisional surgery
Minimal access surgery
Interventional endoscopy
Interventional radiology
Lithotripsy

Open incisional surgery

This is the largest group of operative procedures. The types and classifications are dealt with below.

Minimal access surgery

This is the term currently employed to embrace 'keyhole surgery' or minimally invasive surgery, usually performed using rigid laparoscopes or thoracoscopes. As indications, both experimental and in daily practice, have expanded, a wide variety of additional types of access for diagnostic and therapeutic manipulation have developed. These include multiple 'ports' in abdominal laparoscopic surgery for access by retractors, staplers, diathermy probes, etc., and small incisions through which a specially gloved hand can be inserted. The basic principle is that minimal access surgery is potentially useful where the usual open access causes damage to the patient that is out of proportion to the size of the operation actually perormed. Another justification would be that improved visibility enables the operation to be performed better than the open variant. In some cases, heated discussion develops between minimal access enthusiasts and open surgery enthusiasts but it should always be

possible to perform appropriately monitored trials to sub-
stantiate or refute claims. It should also be remembered that
minimal access surgery requires special training and prolonged
supervision before trainees can operate independently. This type
of surgery is often more costly in terms of equipment and
operating time than open surgery and this must be taken in
to account when assessing the advantages of one or other
technique.

Interventional endoscopy

Interventional endoscopy, such as injecting bleeding
oesophageal varices or bleeding peptic ulcers, were perhaps the
first modern examples of minimal access surgery. Details of the
principles and scope of the methods is covered in Chapter 20.

Interventional radiology

The ability to target needles, guide wires, and therapeutic
devices using contrast radiology, ultrasonography, or computerized tomography has enabled radiologists to play a major
part in the treatment of gastrointestinal, peripheral vascular, and
biliary tract diseases (Table 1.2).

Lithotripsy

Focused beams of high-energy ultrasound can be directed to
stones localized by ultrasonography in the renal tract. Thus,
stones obscured by bony landmarks (e.g. lumbar pedicles or the
sacrum) cannot be dealt with easily by this method. Therapeutic
ultrasound breaks the stones into smaller particles which are

Table 1.2 Examples of procedures in interventional radiology

General	Percutaneous core biopsy or fine-needle aspiration for cytological examination of abdominal swellings
	Percutaneous biopsy of enlarged lymph nodes, thyroid swellings, and other head and neck masses
	Percutaneous therapeutic aspiration of fluid collections and abscesses; now the first-line treatment for many abdominal and pelvic abscesses
Arterial	Percutaneous transluminal balloon angioplasty of arterial stenoses and occlusions; may include stenting of certain arterial lesions. Stenting is beginning to be used for treating aortic and other aneurysms
	Intra-arterial or intravenous thrombolytic infusion
	Embolization of bleeding tumours, arteriovenous malformations, and preoperative devascularization of vascular lesions
Biliary	Balloon dilatation of biliary strictures
	Transhepatic insertion of biliary stents
	Drainage of pancreatic pseudocysts
Urological	Percutaneous placement of nephrostomies for obstructed systems
	Transrectal ultrasound-guided biopsy of suspected prostatic carcinomatous nodules
	Percutaneous balloon dilatation of pelvi-ureteric junction obstruction

then allowed to pass out in the urine. Some urologists routinely
insert ureteric stents prior to treatment. Occasionally, the debris
needs to be removed endoscopically. Techniques of lithotripsy
have evolved rapidly. The first-generation machines required the
patient to be partially immersed in a water bath and anaesthetized as pain was a prominent feature of treatment. Recent
machines have dispensed with both of these, allowing treatment
on an outpatient basis.

Lithotripsy has been used for the treatment of biliary stones
but with a lesser degree of success. In most centres, this method
of treatment has been discarded because of the high incidence of
recurrence. The main reasons appear to be the difficulty of
achieving complete clearance of stones and the propensity for an
already diseased gallbladder, or a predisposing biochemical
abnormality, to form new stones.

Other percutaneous treatment methods

With improved imaging and endoscopic equipment, the range
of percutaneous treatment methods is ever expanding. It is now
routine to remove percutaneously renal stones that are
unsuitable for lithotripsy. The technique involves creating a
direct percutaneous track from the loin to the renal pelvis,
dilating it to a suitable size, shattering the stones with various
electromechanical probes under endoscopic vision, and
removing the fragments with grasping instruments.

Experimental studies are being conducted which employ percutaneous application of thermal or light probes to treat
malignant lesions (e.g. liver metastases). Thermal methods
involve placing a heating or freezing probe accurately in the
centre of the lesion and heating it under careful thermal control
to destroy the lesion by coagulation. In light treatment, sensitizing drugs taken up only by the target tumour are given as
pretreatment, then a light guide is passed into the tumour to
activate the drug to damage the malignant cells.

There are a range of treatments for benign enlargement of the
prostate for patients too unfit for surgery. Many types, such as
freezing and microwave treatment, have been rejected as
ineffective but thermal needle probes show promise for
alleviating prostatic obstruction and allowing indwelling
catheters to be removed. Expanding metal stents have also been
used to relieve prostatic obstruction but these tend to drift or
obstruct and have not proved generally effective.

3.3 Clinical methods of classifying operative and interventional procedures

Introduction

Classifications are used as a form of shorthand when describing
individual cases or groups of cases. They can be useful for
epidemiological or clinical research projects to provide non-
parametric variables for descriptive statistics. However, in order
for a classification to be robust, it must have the authority of
respected academic or professional bodies or be widely
employed in practice (such as the BUPA classification of
operation severity).

Urgency of operation

The National Confidential Enquiry into Perioperative Deaths (NCEPOD) has recommended that operations on non-elective patients admitted to hospital should be classified into groups according to the level of urgency of the operation. These groups are:

Emergency

Those patients who need life-saving procedures, such as surgery for abdominal trauma with an unstable patient or for ruptured abdominal aneurysm. This level of urgency requires transfer of the patient to the operating theatre after minimal investigation, often directly from the resuscitation room.

Urgent

Identified as those patients needing an operative procedure but who need to be resuscitated fully before surgery and where the condition allows time for resuscitation. This group has been a major cause for concern in several NCEPOD studies, which have reported that many patients who died in the perioperative period had been operated upon without adequate prior attention to resuscitation and correction of fluid balance. A common subject for this was obstructed groin hernia. Death was often a result of the adverse effect of this on the patient's cardiovascular and renal function. This group of patients is best dealt with by preparing the patient by correcting fluid balance and other supportive measures, then operating during the day in a designated emergency operating theatre.

Scheduled

These are patients admitted as emergencies with a condition that can be managed initially without an operation but who require surgery in the near future. Examples of this include irreducible hernia which reduces after admission or biliary colic requiring cholecystectomy. The principle is that these patients should be scheduled to be operated upon on the next available operating list, ideally during the same admission.

Elective

Patients who have specific surgical requirements identified during an emergency admission but who do not need operation with any great degree of urgency. The level of urgency is the same as would be given to similar conditions diagnosed in the outpatient department.

Magnitude of operation

Healthcare insurers and the British Medical Association have scaled operative procedures according to the extent of surgery for the purpose of calculating remuneration. The scales are based on OPCS (Office of Population Censuses and Surveys) classification of operations which is used nationally for statistical purposes. The British United Providence Association (BUPA) coding is the best known and most widely used. This is not an official classification nor is it particularly scientific, but it serves a useful rule of thumb function when looking at workload.

There are five main categories:

(1) minor (e.g. removal of a simple skin lesion or lateral submucous sphincterotomy);

(2) intermediate (e.g. inguinal hernia repair);

(3) major (e.g. cholecystectomy);

(4) major plus (e.g. right hemicolectomy);

(5) complex major (e.g. grafting of abdominal aortic aneurysm (AAA)).

Another way of looking at workload is to use 'hernia equivalents'. Thus, if an inguinal hernia takes 30 minutes (or any other time period locally acceptable), a minor operation might be half a unit, a cholecystectomy two units, a colectomy three or four units, and an AAA graft six to eight units. Clearly, problems would arise if tight time schedules became mandatory, but use of some form of workload calculation can be helpful when negotiating for more operating sessions or reallocation of old ones. Similarly, emergency operative workload can be assessed and used as a negotiating tool.

3.4 Classification of the effectiveness of surgical treatment

Introduction

When planning surgical treatment, it is helpful to try to assess the aims of therapy. In general, these are the relief of symptoms or cure of the condition. Realistic appraisal of the likelihood of cure, particularly of malignant disease, is helpful when discussing likely outcomes with patients and relatives, as well as communicating the anticipated result of surgery to general practitioners.

A classification of effectiveness

Curative

Most elective surgical procedures for benign conditions might be expected to cure the underlying condition (e.g. hernia repair, excision of benign lesions, TURP, joint replacements, or varicose veins). However, it should be remembered that many such operations are by nature palliative. All operations suffer from complications and will often have a failure rate and a recurrence rate, which can both be anticipated statistically. Recurrence rates have been shown to vary between different surgeons and in different countries. Part of evidence-based medicine is to tease out the factors involved and to promote the acknowledged most effective techniques. It should be remembered, however, that some 'recurrences' are in fact new primary cancers. For example, metachronous cancers are common in colonic cancer because of a field change in the colonic mucosa.

Many malignant conditions are cured by surgery. Predictions can be given on the basis of tumour type, staging, and the potential effectiveness of adjuvant therapy.

Potentially curative

This applies to operations performed for malignant disease where it seems likely that the local extent of disease has allowed complete excision. The biological nature of most malignant disease does not allow a 'cure' to be confidently claimed immediately after treatment because of the possible existence of undiagnosable micrometastases. However, the biological behaviour of different malignancies can be predicted statistically so that the chances of 'cure' of a Dukes A carcinoma of colon is far better than for a Dukes C, for example. Results of therapy are often presented in terms of 5-year or 10-year survival or a particular disease-free interval. Adjuvant treatments such as radiotherapy, chemotherapy, or hormonal therapy are often added to surgical procedures, with the intention of improving cure rates, or at least extending the disease-free life span.

The potential period for recurrences or metastases after surgery varies between different malignancies. Colonic cancer can usually be regarded as cured 5 years after surgery, whereas carcinoma of the breast can reappear 40 years or more after treatment and can never confidently be regarded as cured. However, the longer the period after treatment, the smaller the chance of recurrence.

Palliative

In malignant disease, this applies to operations where it has not been possible to excise the tumour because of extensive local infiltration or because of the presence of distant metastases. The best palliation varies, but should be designed to cause minimal interference with the patient's quality of life while giving maximum relief from distressing symptoms. In antral gastric carcinoma, the best palliative treatment is often resection. This removes a large bulk of necrotic tissue, relieving gastric outlet obstruction and removing a source of steady haemorrhage which causes anaemia. Where the common bile duct is obstructed by carcinoma of the head of the pancreas, endoscopic stent placement can be extremely effective at relieving obstructive jaundice. Palliative treatment may include pain-relieving measures;for example, percutaneous coeliac ganglion block using absolute alcohol is very effective for the pain of pancreatic cancer.

No procedure

There are two main reasons for this: rarely, a condition is diagnosed at operation which is best treated by non-surgical means (e.g. tuberculosis, lymphoma). More commonly, malignant disease is found to be so far advanced that no useful procedure is possible. With improved imaging methods and the increased use of staging laparoscopy, such 'open and close' operations are largely a thing of the past.

3.5 Microbiological classification of wounds

Introduction

Classifying wounds at operation enables prediction of the statistical probability of wound infection. There are four categories:

Clean, wound infection rate 1.5 per cent

Operations where there is no incision through a microbially colonized viscus, no infection is encountered, and there has been no breach in aseptic technique. Examples include inguinal herniorrhaphy, excision of a lipoma, and total hip replacement. In medical audit terms, an infective local complication following an operation in this category would be regarded as unexpected and probably avoidable.

Clean-contaminated, wound infection rate 8 per cent

Clean-contaminated operations occur when a microbially colonized viscus is entered in a controlled manner. Examples include elective sigmoid colectomy, cholecystectomy, and vaginal hysterectomy. The incidence of postoperative infection can be reduced by the judicious use of prophylactic antibiotics. In medical audit terms an infective complication would be regarded as expected but probably avoidable.

Contaminated, wound infection rate 15 per cent

This occurs when a microbially colonized viscus is entered surgically with incomplete preparation, there is spillage of infected material or a break in aseptic technique. Examples include cholecystectomy for acute cholecystitis and sigmoid colectomy with defunctioning colostomy. Traumatic wounds less than 4 hours old also fall into this group.

Infected or dirty, wound infection rate 40 per cent

Operations are infected or dirty when pus or a perforated viscus is encountered at operation. Traumatic wounds over 4 hours old also fall into this group. Infected or dirty operations are generally performed to remove the cause of infection and sometimes to provide external drainage for an abscess. Examples include drainage of a perianal abscess and laparotomy for generalized bacterial peritonitis resulting from a gastrointestinal (particularly colonic) perforation.

4 Coding of diseases and operative procedures

4.1 Why code?

There is a need to measure the incidence of diseases and their treatments in both hospitals and community for the purposes of financial management, resource allocation, and epidemiology. This has stimulated the development of various coding systems—international, national, and local. When diagnoses and operations are reduced to codes, they can be manipulated statistically and meaning derived from the figures.

If all surgical cases could be coded effectively as regards diagnosis, operation, and complications, it would then be possible to accumulate information about the number of diseases or procedures occurring in a locality, which could, in turn, be used to assess the health of the local population and the need for healthcare resources. This occurs in hospitals and health authorities, but clinicians should remember that such coding can be imprecise. It is useful in the grand scheme of things but may prove useless for individual cases.

For medical audit, accurate coding could be used to categorize the numbers and the severity of illness for each patient and give an idea of outcome. In practice, the restrictions already mentioned apply to a variable degree and, in many units, simpler local codes have proved more useful for this focused application.

4.2 Design and limitations of coding systems

The principles of coding are complex (as discussed below) and most systems fall down because of their attempts to be comprehensive, with insufficient attention to their use in individual specialty units. This results in unnecessary complexity, a varying degree of obscurity and a general lack of user-friendliness. In addition, it is often difficult to find a suitable code for an individual case. It often happens that two cases given the same codes are not truly comparable because the coding system lacks the necessary sophistication.

All hospitals are required to code the diagnoses, operations, and procedures of all their patients. The standard system in UK is ICD 10 (WHO International Classification of Diseases, version 10) and OPCS 5 (Office of Population Censuses and Surveys Classification of Operations and Procedures, version 5). Both of these coding systems have been in use for many years and have been updated progressively with successive releases. However, they both betray their early origins by their inflexible numerical codes. Hospitals all have coding departments with the coding performed by clerical personnel, usually based on perusal of the hospital notes or discharge summaries. Several published studies have shown error rates in coding as high as 15 per cent. This can be attributed to poor clinical input but, more importantly perhaps, to unnecessarily complex or obscure codes. Clinicians will never use these coding systems for clinical purposes unless they can be made much more intelligible.

The Read coding system (discussed below), a 'superset' of ICD 10 and OPCS 5, is used increasingly in general practice and is making inroads into hospitals. However, despite its intention to simplify the process, it has added a further layer of complexity to the existing systems. In particular, the attempt to refine diagnoses by breaking down existing codes into subcodes (Read level 5) is destined to fail in some cases because the problem lies with unsatisfactory existing codes. In many cases, several of these codes could be put together as a single code (e.g. surgery on the abdominal aorta) and the detail put into level 5. There are, however, limitations on the ability to change ICD 10 and OPCS 5 codes because of their different origin and usage elsewhere.

4.3 Design of coding systems

When designing a coding system, the following factors need to be considered:

- Is it purely for administrative purposes or is it intended to be clinically useful (e.g. for medical audit, research, trainee log books)? Can the two functions coexist in a single coding system?

- Comprehensibility versus simplicity—is the system to be used locally in a single specialty or is it for universal use? If it is intended to be comprehensive throughout medicine, it must be possible for individuals to use a 'cut-down' or restricted subset of codes appropriate to their own clinical practice, and to be able to access wider fields when necessary.

- In a comprehensive system, codes need to be available for all recognizable disease processes and therapies, tending to make them unwieldy. Read codes have attempted to simplify this by introducing a hierarchical structure, described below. However, a better solution would be for each specialty to look at its own practice and produce codes based on real-life practice, unshackled by existing coding systems, and to incorporate the various specialties into a comprehensive system. This process is in progress for the Read codes, but it is likely that ghosts of the old system will remain and impair its usefulness.

- Is the coding system easily understood and intuitive to use? Clinicians should be able to employ the codes without having to attend special courses or spend long hours learning systems.

- Can it easily be used on a computer? Easy navigation and rapid and reliable searching are essential features.

- Will it cross-refer ('map') to existing systems (e.g. ICD 10 diagnostic codes, OPCS 5 operation codes)? Codes are a method of communication between groups and if different codes are used and there is no interface between the different systems, then communication is not possible. Employing the power of modern computers to match old and new systems can be relatively straightforward, given the will and the necessary expenditure of programming time. This is an essential step and would allow comparability of clinical practice and the incidence of diseases and frequency of treatments between different units and between different time periods.

- Any new coding system needs to be able to expand so that new codes can be added without disturbing the position of current terms and their codes. The problem with ICD and OPCS is that they are numerical codes, presumably designed for an earlier era when computers could only handle numbers.

4.4 The Read codes

This structure allows diagnoses or operations to be redefined, or for new conditions to be added to the existing hierarchy; if no suitable code group exists, a new one can be started. However, in practice, the coding system is hamstrung by the need to 'map' to previous coding systems for retrospective and comparative

Table 1.3 Illustration of the hierarchical structure of Read and ICD diagnostic codes

Read code	Description	ICD code
B	Neoplasms	140–239
B1	Malignant neoplasms of GIT	150–159
B11	Malignant neoplasm of stomach	151
B111	Carcinoma of pylorus of stomach	151.1
B1111	Carcinoma of pyloric canal	(151.1)

analysis, and by the continuing need to retain the original numerical codes.

An attempt to produce a comprehensive coding system, the Read codes, was made by a Loughborough-based GP, James Read, and subsequently taken up by the NHS executive. The system is used by many GPs but is used less widely by hospitals. The Read coding system incorporates and attempts to improving on the ICD 10 diagnostic coding system and the OPCS 5 operation and procedure coding system, and incorporates other classifications such as the British National Formulary. Read has reclassified these systems into a five-level hierarchical structure, which allows the coding to begin with a few broad groups and then branch down through the levels to a very specific coding for an individual (Table 1.3). Read level 4 corresponds exactly to existing ICD and OPCS codes but has added an additional fifth layer to classifications to allow further refinement of these codes. As mentioned earlier, problems arise when the existing codes are unsuitable. Several level 5 codes are the daughters of each level 4 code; adding subcodes to unsatisfactory codes does not overcome the embedded problems of the original system. A further disadvantage of the Read system is that it has added many thousands of new codes, increasing complexity.

Most users of ICD, OPCS, and Read find that the codes rarely match what they do in practice, so they end up giving less-than-satisfactory classifications to their cases, which considerably reduces their usefulness. National coding continues as a necessity but it is too complex, too clunky, and too imprecise in its present incarnations to carry full professional endorsement.

5 Screening for surgical disease

5.1 Introduction

Screening is defined as the application of a test in an asymptomatic population to identify individuals at increased risk of a disease, with the aim of preventing or reducing morbidity or mortality.

Medical screening today is distinct from traditional medical practice in that it aims to detect disease before symptoms present and, perhaps more importantly, before an individual decides to seek medical advice. Screening has ethical constraints and responsibilities attached to it because a person in whom a screened abnormality is detected moves in a short space of time from a position of apparent well-being to becoming a patient requiring investigation and perhaps an operation for what may be a potentially disabling disorder.

When screening, we must be sure that we are neither identifying conditions that are either effectively untreatable (e.g. lung cancer) or else insignificant. In the latter case this may induce anxiety in individuals and perhaps in the population at large. Screening must therefore be concerned with the worthwhile prevention of disease. Intrinsic to this is that we should screen only for disorders that have an effective intervention for detected abnormalities.

Benefits of screening come about if there is an improved prognosis for screen-positive individuals, improved cure rates, less radical treatment, and perhaps saving of resources. Further benefits accrue if there is worthwhile reassurance for those with negative tests. However, there are also a number of potential disadvantages. For example, a longer period of morbidity for patients whose prognosis is unaltered by the intervention, overtreatment of dubious and insignificant abnormalities, increased resource costs, false reassurance for individuals with false-negative results, anxiety during the process of screening and particularly for those with detected abnormalities, morbidity for individuals with false-positive results and, of course, any hazard associated with particular screening tests (e.g. mammography or colonoscopy).

Justifying a new screening programme

Before embarking upon any screening programme, funding bodies and particularly health authorities have to be convinced that the programme is viable and can be justified. In this respect, the guidelines set out by Wilson and Jungner in 1968 are a useful starting point. These authors stated 10 principles:

1. The disease screened for must be important numerically and in its capacity to cause morbidity and mortality.

2. The natural history of the disease should be well understood and the disease recognizable at an early stage.

3. Treatment of the early stage disease using currently available methods should be known to produce a survival advantage.

4. A test which is both specific and sensitive for early stage disease should be available.

5. This test should be acceptable to the population and allow for a high level of participation.

6. Facilities should be available to make the diagnosis and to treat the early stages of the disease.

7. There should be strong evidence that the screening test can result in reduced mortality and morbidity within the targeted population.

8. The benefits of screening must outweigh the disadvantages.

9. The benefits for the individuals should be achieved at a reasonable cost to society.

10. If implemented, the programme must be audited to ensure that the expected benefit is observed in practice.

Other potential intrinsic biases in screening studies

Length bias

The biological characteristics of a disease often dictate the eventual outcome despite the extent of spread or size of lesion at the time of diagnosis or surgery. In malignant disease, it has been clearly documented that poorly differentiated tumours fair far worse than those that are well or moderately differentiated. Screening is liable to detect the slower growing and less aggressive lesions (e.g. small aneurysms, moderately or well-differentiated cancers) because they are present within the screening population for longer. When assessing the results of any such study, it is possible that any observed survival advantage was due to screening, but the effect may merely reflect the relatively non-aggressive nature of these more benign lesions. This phenomenon is referred to as **length bias**.

Lead time bias

Any apparent increase in survival accruing from the early diagnosis of lesions by screening may be misleading because screening will tend to detect lesions at an earlier stage some months or years before the normal presentation. However, the final outcome of both screened and symptomatic cases may be unchanged, leading to the perception of an increase in survival. This phenomenon is known as **lead time bias** (Fig. 1.3).

Volunteer bias

Medical research of any kind, including screening programmes during the research phase, usually involves the participation of volunteers. Volunteer bias is a potential source of error, however, and the 'healthy volunteer effect' is the main reason why screening studies have to be analysed on an 'intention to treat basis'. Health-conscious individuals are more likely to participate in screening programmes and the natural history of the disease in the volunteer population is almost certain to be different from that of a population with a less positive attitude towards health. Indeed, it has been well documented that people who refuse invitations for screening have a higher all–cause mortality than people who attend for screening. Under these circumstances, mortality data would be biased in favour of a screened group compared with an unscreened group. Similarly, if regular attenders for health checks are randomized to receive screening tests or not, any real advantage of screening may not be apparent as the control group may already have a favourable prognosis. A number of studies already fall foul of such volunteer bias.

Sensitivity and specificity

For a screening programme to be successful it must be directed at a suitable disease and based upon a reliable and acceptable test. A suitable test must have a high sensitivity and a high specificity. The **sensitivity** of a test relates to the proportion of subjects with the disease who have a positive test (how well does the test detect abnormalities?) and the **specificity** is expressed as the proportion of individuals without the disease who have a negative test. Thus a highly specific test has a low false-positive rate.

The most important value to be derived from a pilot study of a screening test is the **predictive value**. The predictive value is the probability that a person with a positive test has the disease, or the probability that a person with a negative test does not have the disease. The predictive value of a test is determined by the sensitivity and specificity of the test and by the prevalence of the disease, as shown in Table 1.4.

In Table 1.4, sensitivity = $a/(a + c)$; specificity = $d/(b + d)$, and predictive value = $a/(a + b)$. An example makes this clear: consider a test with a sensitivity and specificity of 90 per cent. In scenario 1, we are planning to screen 1000 persons for a fairly common disease which has a prevalence of 10 per cent. Table 1.5 shows typical values.

Table 1.4 Derivation of sensitivity, specificity, and predictive value of a test for a disease

		Disease status	
		Positive	Negative
Test result	Positive	a	b
	Negative	c	d

Table 1.5 Scenario 1: screening for a fairly common disease

		Disease status		
		Positive	Negative	Total
Test result	Positive	90	90	180
	Negative	10	810	820
	Total	100	900	1000

Table 1.6 Scenario 2: worked example of calculation of sensitivity, specificity, and predictive value of a test for a disease with a 1 per cent incidence

		Disease status		
		Positive	Negative	Total
Test result	Positive	9	99	108
	Negative	1	891	892
	Total	10	900	1000

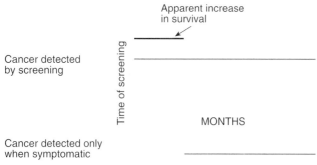

Figure 1.3 Lead time bias in screening. The apparent prolongation of survival for screened patients where the outcome is inevitable is shown.

This means that only 50 per cent of those with a positive test actually have the disease (therefore 50 per cent might have unnecessary breast biopsies or colonoscopies). Tests for faecal occult blood generally have much lower sensitivity and specificity even than this.

In a different screening programme we might be planning to screen 1000 people for an uncommon disease with a prevalence of about 1 per cent (scenario 2, Table 1.6). The results mean that only 8 per cent of those with a positive test actually have the disease and 92 per cent are at risk of having unnecessary breast biopsies, colonoscopies, etc.

In control trials for screening of cancer, the trial population is usually divided into a test and a control group. The test group is further divided into those who undergo the test (the acceptors) and those who refuse the test (the non-responders). Screen-detected tumours are those diagnosed following a positive test. **Interval tumours** are those found in a test-negative subject who presents with symptomatic neoplasia during the period after the test or prior to a retest. It is often assumed that interval lesions were missed by the test but, in many cases, the tumour may have been present but too small to detect or may have arisen *de novo* and undergone accelerated biological behaviour.

Current areas of screening

In western Europe there are three main areas for screening relevant to the surgeon, although many others are in place for screening neonates for congenital disorders, such as congenital dislocation of the hip. 'Surgical disorders' include breast cancer, colorectal cancer, and abdominal aortic aneurysms. At present there are national screening programmes only for breast cancer and cervical cancer, and these apply to age-limited populations only.

5.2 Breast cancer screening

In the UK there are approximately 26 000 new cases of breast cancer each year. Breast cancer is responsible for 16 000 deaths per year, which represents almost 20 per cent of all female cancer deaths. The UK has one of the highest mortality rates from breast cancer worldwide. These statistics led to the setting up of mammographic screening in the UK.

Screening for breast cancer by mammography every 1–3 years has been shown in some studies to reduce breast cancer mortality substantially in women aged between 50 and 70. Belief in this statement is founded upon the UK trial of early detection of breast cancer (TEDBC, described below) and the Swedish Two-County trial of screening for breast cancer.

The outcome for breast cancer patients is determined by several factors, including histological grade, tumour size, hormone receptor status, and nodal status. The last carries the greatest prognostic importance.

For screening in breast cancer to be effective, diagnosis has to occur at an early stage. A prerequisite for decreasing mortality is that this also proves to be at a biologically early stage to permit an effective treatment. Ideally, lesions that would later metastasize would be detected at a preinvasive stage. Many believe that ductal carcinoma in situ (DCIS) may be such a condition. To begin to achieve this, screening compliance must be high and a high-quality diagnostic service with exemplary mammographic images must operate. Major advances in diagnostic technique are likely to be required before substantial gains can be made. Tumours that would lead to death if not treated at a truly early stage are the ones of greatest importance. Whether this can be achieved by current methods remains unproven.

The UK trial of early detection of breast cancer (TEDBC)

The TEDBC study was based on examining women between the ages of 45 and 64, initially in two districts, Edinburgh and Guildford, and later in two further districts, Huddersfield and Nottingham. The Edinburgh and Guildford arm invited every women in this age range to be screened every year for 7 years. The Huddersfield and Nottingham arm invited every women in the age range to learn breast self-examination and provided them with a self-referral breast clinic. Three other districts, Dundee, Oxford, and South Basingstoke, served as control groups. The entire study population being followed up was 240 000 women, in which breast cancer incidence and cancer mortality comparisons can be made. The interim results of the study (known as UK TEDBC 1988) were published by Forrest in 1991. After 7 years, this showed an apparent 20 per cent reduction in mortality in the screened populations compared with controls, but this was not statistically significant. There was no difference in mortality between the breast self-examination groups and the controls.

On closer examination of the data, it can be seen that the sensitivity for mammography in this study was in the order of 95 per cent but the sensitivity of self-examination was only 71 per cent. Mammographic sensitivity was found to be poor below the age of 55 and it was only after this age that sensitivity improved. This was in contrast to the Swedish trial, where the increase in sensitivity occurred at the earlier age of 50. However, it is clear from these data that screening by physical examination is less sensitive than screening by mammography.

The likelihood of an unaffected women being referred for further investigation because of a screen-detected abnormality is one of the unwanted side-effects of screening. The TEDBC showed that between 3 and 8 per cent of women fell into this category. It is possible, therefore, that a large proportion of women referred for breast screening may have anxiety induced by the false-positive result. This has been addressed in one study in Guildford which found that the level of psychological morbidity amongst women referred for investigation was less than that found in symptomatic women referred for investigation and that this anxiety was transient.

The Swedish Two-County trial

This Swedish trial employed purely mammography for screening. The study was based on 133 000 women aged between 40 and 74 years. Of the total number, 77 000 were randomized to the study group and 56 000 were randomized to the control group. Compliance rates of screening were high, with 93 per cent participating between the ages of 40 and 49 at the first screen, dropping to 66 per cent for the second round of screening for the older population. The study found that the rate of detection of tumours less than 2 cm diameter was significantly greater in the mammographic group than the control group, and there were also significantly fewer cases with nodal metastases in the mammographic group. After 10 years of follow-up, this translated into a survival advantage for individuals who had been screened between the ages of 50 and 69. There was no decrease in the relative risk of dying from breast cancer in the 40–49 age group and only a small reduction in the 70–74 age group. After 10 years' follow-up, 2454 women had developed breast cancer. The study provided evidence for a 30 per cent reduction in mortality from breast cancer among women invited for screening compared with the control group.

The Swedish Two-County studies have clearly shown a reduction in the clinical stage of breast cancer at diagnosis.

Mammography below the age of 50

These two European studies have provided evidence that mammographic screening may reduce morbidity and mortality from breast cancer in patients over the age of 50. However, a substantial proportion of women are at risk of breast cancer between the ages of 40 and 49. So far, only one screening study has addressed this issue. The Canadian National Breast Screening Study enrolled 50 000 women aged between 40 and 49 years up to 1988. After at least 7 years follow-up, there was no indication that mammography plus physical examination of the breasts resulted in any reduction in mortality from breast cancer. On this basis, it would appear that with current methodology, screening by mammography is not indicated for women below the age of 50.

Familial breast cancer

It has been estimated that 5 per cent of breast cancer is due to highly penetrant dominant genes. Affected patients are more likely to develop cancer at an early age, bilateral disease is more common, and there is a strong family history of disease, with several relatives likely to be affected. Genetic research has found three important genes for breast cancer, all on chromosome 17, known as *BRCA1*, *BRCA2*, and *BRCA3*, and there may be more yet to be discovered. DNA testing may be appropriate for a small number of families, but there are ethical constraints, and counselling should be undertaken before offering testing. In addition, one live relative with breast cancer is needed to locate the abnormal gene.

Breast cancer is common and therefore identifying individuals at risk can be complex. A woman's risk increases with increasing age and risk of a strong genetic influence is assessed both by age and by number and closeness of affected relatives and the age at which they developed the disease. Thus a woman with two affected first-degree relatives may have a lifetime risk of developing breast cancer of 1 in 4. By the age of 70 years of age the same woman's risk becomes much less and is

no greater than for unaffected 70-year-olds. Some guidelines for referral to a family history clinic for breast cancer have been put forward (Evans *et al.* 1994). The main guidelines are as follows:

- One first-degree relative with breast cancer below age 40.
- One first-degree relative with breast cancer before age 50 plus another relative on the same side of the family with cancer of colon, ovary, endometrium, or sarcoma.
- One first-degree relative with breast cancer aged 50–65 and one further close relative with cancer of breast, colon, endometrium, or sarcoma before age 50.
- One first-degree relative with cancer of breast and a second primary malignancy, with at least one cancer developing before age 50.
- A dominant history of familial breast cancer.

Audit and quality control in breast cancer screening

Screening programmes for breast cancer have been introduced following randomized trials. Based on those trials, figures for performance and quality of service have been set. These are set out in Table 1.7.

In the UK, there are 90 individual screening programmes. On a regional level, each is overseen by a regional coordinator who submits an annual statistical return to a central evaluation unit. For the year 1991–92, all the above targets were being met or exceeded.

Interval breast cancers

Breast cancers diagnosed between screening visits are known as interval cancers. These have generally proved to be more aggressive in their biological behaviour than screening-detected cancers. Woodman *et al.* (1995) described an interval breast cancer rate in the north-west region of the UK, 2 years after initial screening, of 15.8 per 10 000 screened. The interval cancer rate for the Swedish Two-County study was 9.4 per 10 000. Other studies have also shown high interval cancer rates. The Dutch study from Nijmegen and the Stockholm study from Sweden had interval cancer rates of 15.7 and 19.2 per 10 000

Table 1.7 Target figures for performance and quality of service for breast cancer screening

Aspect of breast screening	Target
Compliance with screening	Greater than 70%
Number of recalls	Less than 10%
Number of technical recalls	Less than 3%
Number of cancers detected	More than 50 per 10 000 screened
Number of cancers less than 15 mm in diameter	More than 25 per 10 000 screened
Proportion of ductal carcinomas *in situ*	More than 10% of all cancers
Biopsy rate	Less than 1.5% of women screened
Malignant : benign biopsy ratio	Between 1 : 1 and 1.5 : 1

patients, respectively. This must be set against rates of cancer detection by screening of 2.9/1000 and 3.9/1000. These data question the sensitivity of the mammography employed, and several factors may account for this:

◆ For cost reasons, the UK National Health Breast Screening Programme relies on a single oblique mammographic view of each breast every 3 years, with each film being read by one radiologist. It has been shown that two-view mammography can obtain 20 per cent higher rates of breast cancer detection than single-view mammography and to this end the UK Co-ordinating Committee on Cancer Research set up a one-view versus two-view trial. The results are awaited. Further, using high-resolution mammography films may improve detection and this has already been implemented without additional cost.

◆ Further improvement in quality can be achieved by 'double reporting', where two radiologists review the radiographic images independently. In this way, 15 per cent more cancers may be detected, although this method may lead to reduced specificity (Elmore *et al.* 1994).

◆ Between 50 and 60 per cent of interval cancers occur in the third year after initial screening. The Swedish Two-County Trial argues that intervals of 2 years rather than 3 should be adopted as the standard screening interval, an approach already used in other countries but not in the UK. Clearly, decreasing the screening interval has cost implications on a system already stretched.

In general, it is reassuring to note that the National Breast Screening Programme has demonstrated clear internal monitoring and a satisfactory quality assurance programme. This internal monitoring has detected a higher than expected incidence of interval cancers and steps have to be made to deal with this unexpected finding.

Cost effectiveness evaluation of breast cancer screening

Cost effectiveness comparisons can be made through 'cost per life-year saved' calculations or via an estimate of 'number needed to treat to save one life'. Cost per life-year saved calculations have the disadvantage that they are sensitive to local healthcare costs. 'Number needed to treat' analyses do not suffer from this drawback. Comparisons in 'number needed to treat' between different health intervention programmes tend to be more robust and can also be used for comparisons between different countries.

It has been calculated that the benefit of breast cancer screening is one life saved per 10 000 women screened (Querci della Rovere 1995). This compares to one life saved per 2000 men screened in the Huntingdon aneurysm screening project (see below).

The last word

Breast screening was started in UK to try to reduce the rising incidence and death rate from breast cancer. The national screening programme has radically improved diagnostic techniques and has encouraged specialist programmes for the management of breast disease with harmonization of treatment methods based on evidence. Nevertheless, the hoped-for dramatic fall in breast cancer incidence has not come about and many question whether the beneficial impact of mammographic screening has been illusory and whether the money could have been better spent on improving treatment for symptomatic breast cancer.

5.3 Screening for infrarenal abdominal aortic aneurysms

Incidence and prevalence of abdominal aortic aneurysms

An abdominal aortic aneurysm is a dilatation of the main abdominal artery which will inevitably progress and rupture unless the patient dies of another disease. Most aneurysms do not cause symptoms until they rupture. Those that are discovered are usually found by chance on abdominal examination, or radiography or ultrasonography for an unrelated condition. Virtually all small aneurysms and most potentially lethal aneurysms therefore remain undetected, and published figures for incidence and prevalence probably grossly underestimate the size of the problem. In particular, many patients die in the community after sudden collapse, with the death recorded as due to myocardial infarction. An unknown proportion of these actually died of aortic rupture.

Aortic aneurysm disease killed at least 5500 people in 1994 in England and Wales. Eighty per cent of these patients were male and 75 per cent of these patients were both male and over 60 years of age. Six per cent of males over the age of 65 have been shown to have aortic aneurysms; 2 per cent of males over the age of 65 have aortic aneurysms larger than 4 cm.

There has been a threefold increase in the incidence of aortic aneurysms between 1951 and 1980 but the factors involved are unknown. Possible culprits include a rise in the elderly population, the increased prevalence of smoking, and perhaps dietary factors.

Rupture of an aneurysm is a common and often unrecognized cause of death. It is responsible for at least 1.2 per cent of all deaths in men over 65 and 0.6 per cent of deaths in women over 65. Office of Population Censuses and Surveys figures indicate that 1 in 70 men who die between 60 and 84 do so from a ruptured aneurysm. The condition is rare in people under 50 and increases markedly with age. A number of studies have looked at the growth rate of aortic aneurysms, which seems to vary between 0.2 and 0.6 cm/year. Only 2 per cent of aneurysms that rupture are less than 4 cm in size; 10 per cent are between 4 and 5 cm and the rest are greater than 5 cm. Apart from age, other risk factors for aortic aneurysms are family history of aortic aneurysms, hypertension, ischaemic heart disease, peripheral vascular disease, connective tissue disorders such as Marfan's syndrome, and predisposing factors associated with these conditions.

Risks associated with the untreated disease

Before surgery for aneurysm was introduced, only 18 per cent of known aneurysm patients survived 5 years, whereas 85 per cent of unaffected people of similar age survived. Males who rupture an aneurysm have only a 20 per cent chance of undergoing a successful operation. Only 1 in 10 women survive rupture. In Swansea, 260 ruptured aneurysms were identified over 9 years in the hospital and in the community. Only 101 reached hospital and only 52 (20 per cent) survived after an operation. In contrast, the mortality for elective operation for aneurysm should be less than 5 per cent.

The risk of rupture increases with aneurysm size but even small ones (under 4 cm) rupture. Large aneurysms (over 6 cm) have a 50 per cent chance of rupture in 1 year, but in one series of small aneurysms, rupture caused 31 per cent of the deaths, 40 per cent of them within 2 years. Collin *et al.* (1988) showed that the annual death rate in men between 60 and 64 is increased by 230 per cent if a small aneurysm is present.

Potential benefit of surgical intervention

Over the past 30 years, mortality from ruptured aneurysm has hardly improved, but there has been a steady decline in mortality after elective operations, with about 5 per cent mortality quoted from the better centres. It has to be remembered, however, that not all units can emulate this standard. Poor survival figures are rarely published, but mortality rates of up to 20 per cent have been published by candid units. Mortality levels of this magnitude would militate against a screening programme, which, in recommending treatment for asymptomatic people, can only be justified if there is a low perioperative mortality. After successful aneurysm surgery, long-term survival is only about 20 per cent less than for unaffected people (mainly from cardiovascular disease), and the quality of life, even in patients over 80, is as good as before operation in at least 85 per cent.

Operating on ruptured aneurysms is difficult and costs twice as much as elective operations, whether the patient lives or dies. This is because patients invariably present as emergencies and demand immediate surgery. Any delay dramatically increases the mortality and such patients do not travel well to other hospitals. Operation should be performed by a trained vascular surgeon and a consultant anaesthetist. Large quantities of blood for transfusion are required (an average of 27 units in one series, compared with four for elective cases) and patients spend long periods in intensive care. Operation is often complicated by sepsis syndrome and renal failure, requiring time-consuming and costly treatment. Staff are placed under stress by these emergency procedures, especially when operation has to be performed during the night, and this is likely to affect adversely the unit's ability to deal with concurrent emergencies.

For elective operations, in contrast, the patient can be properly assessed and optimized, for example undergoing cardiac investigation. The best qualified and most experienced staff can perform the operation during the daytime and the results, in terms of mortality and complications, bed stay, and patient satisfaction are correspondingly better. The development of endovascular stenting may decrease the morbidity of treatment to even lower levels.

Results of screening studies

Introduction

The dire results of treatment of ruptured AAA have led to calls for screening for aortic aneurysms on a national level. Abdominal examination and plain X-rays are known to miss at least 50 per cent of aneurysms, but ultrasonography is highly reliable. Pilot studies have been set up in Oxford (briefly), Birmingham, Cheltenham, Chichester, and Huntingdon in the UK, using abdominal ultrasonography as the mode of screening. Other studies have been conducted elsewhere in the UK and particularly in Denmark and Canada.

The benefits of ultrasound scanning are that it is cheap, simple, safe, acceptable, portable, virtually 100 per cent sensitive with no false negatives, and virtually 100 per cent specific with no false positives, and therefore has virtually a 100 per cent positive predictive value. These results are marred only by the occasional patient who cannot be scanned for technical reasons and by the occasional confusion of an iliac aneurysm for an aortic aneurysm. It should be said that ultrasound is a useful screening test but characterizing the aneurysm requires other modalities, usually computed tomography (CT) scanning.

The size of the aortic aneurysm is easy to measure accurately ultrasonographically. It has been postulated that a single scan of the aorta would be sufficient to identify patients who are at risk of aortic aneurysm disease. This evidence has been put forward in a recent paper by Emmerton, which reports a study of 223 men who were first examined by ultrasound in 1988 and, at that time, were found to have no aortic aneurysm. Five years later, 166 of the 189 repeat scan measurements were within 3 mm of the original value and two patients were found to have an aortic diameter of 3 cm or greater, thus suggesting that a single scan at aged 65 would exclude over 90 per cent of patients at risk of future significant aneurysmal dilatation. This has beneficial economic and practical implications for a national programme.

The Chichester study

One of the longest running series of screenings for aortic aneurysms has been located in Chichester, where a pilot study has been running for more than 8 years. During this time nearly 9000 people aged between 65 and 80 years have been screened. Males and females were randomized into screened and non-screened groups. Aortic aneurysms greater than 3 cm in diameter were found in 356 individuals, and surgery was offered to patients with symptomatic aneurysms or those that grew at a rate of 1 cm or more per year, or those greater than 6 cm in diameter. Based on these criteria, 43 patients underwent surgery during the study period (equivalent to 4.8 patients per 1000 screened). Scanning accuracy approached 100 per cent, with diameter measurements precise to within half a centimetre. Where screening was repeated, measurements were found to be reproducible. Patients could be screened without preparation and the procedure was shown to be well tolerated, safe, and painless.

The Gloucester study

In another pilot screening study, O'Kelly and Heather invited all males aged between 65 and 74, in four general practices in Stroud, to screening (O'Kelly and Heather 1988). The study was conducted by a nurse coordinator and a senior radiographer. The attendance rate was 76 per cent (905 out of 1195 invited). Small aneurysms were found in 71 (7.8 per cent), who are being followed up with repeat scans. Aneurysms over 4 cm were found in 14 (1.5 per cent), who were successfully operated upon. They estimated their screening costs at £3 per scan. Calculating the cost : benefit analysis by extrapolating to their whole health district of 300 000, screening all of the target population (i.e. males reaching their sixty-fifth birthday) would cost £19 200 for the first year. This is estimated to cost £300 per potential lethal condition detected and £5500 per life saved.

The Huntingdon study

The Huntingdon screening project was begun in 1991 and still continues. The aim was to screen the entire male population of the health district over the age of 50. So far 90 per cent of this population has been screened, with an overall 76 per cent participation (81 per cent aged 54–84). Only those over 84 years were reluctant to be screened. Of the 13 000 people invited for screening, 10 000 attended. Of these, 454 were found to have small aneurysms (≥3 cm) and 56 had large aneurysms (≥5 cm). The prevalence of small aneurysms was 2.5 per cent at 60 years and 10 per cent at 70 years, with little rise after that age. Large aneurysms were present in 1 per cent of men aged 65 (none below 55), 2.5 per cent at 75, and 7 per cent at 85 years. In a parallel study of deaths from ruptured AAA in Huntingdon over a 10-year period, involving both community and hospital mortality, death rates of 7 per 10 000 person years in men were found, compared with 1 per 10 000 person years in women.

The results of a quasi-randomized study of the effects of screening on the incidence and mortality of ruptured AAA have been favourable. In those invited for screening (i.e. on an intention to screen basis) the mortality was 2.8 per 10 000 person years (95 per cent confidence interval (CI), 1.3–5.2) compared with 7.0 per 10 000 person years (95 per cent CI, 5.1–9.4) in controls. This represents a 60 per cent reduction in incidence. The mortality of ruptured AAA was reduced by 55 per cent in those invited for screening.

Overall, 93 patients have been referred with large aneurysms for consideration of surgery, 73 found at first screen and 19 with aneurysms that expanded during follow-up.

Cost-utility analysis can be calculated using the demonstrated reduction in ruptured aneurysms set against the costs of screening plus the cost of additional elective aneurysm operations, less the reduced costs occasioned by fewer emergency AAA operations. Accurate calculations in Huntingdon have shown that the cost of an elective AAA operation averages £4000, the cost of an emergency AAA operation is £5200, and the cost per live patient after emergency operation is £7700. The average age of rupture was 75 years and life expectancy at that age is 8.3 years. This is reduced by 20 per cent in patients operated on for AAA. Calculating all this results in a cost per life year gained as a result of screening of £1059. This compares favourably with estimated costs per life year gained for breast cancer screening of £2500–£3000 and for cervical cancer screening of £10 000.

Follow-up strategies for screen-detected aneurysms

Follow-up strategies for people screened have not yet become standardized and different screening programmes operate different routines. However, a reasonable strategy might be that after screening the whole population once, more than 90 per cent would not have an enlarged aorta and would not require screening for another 5 years, if ever; 5–10 per cent would have a small aneurysm, which could be screened 6 monthly or annually; while 2–3 per cent would have aneurysms requiring consideration of operation.

In the UK MRC small aneurysm trial, 1000 patients aged 60–76 with aneurysms between 4–5.5 cm were randomized to surgery or ultrasound surveillance for an average of 4.6 years. This study showed no mortality difference between the groups at 2, 4, or 6 years and thus may influence the indications for surgery. If aneurysms below 5.5 cm do not need operation, those detected can continue surveillance. However, as more data emerges about which small aneuryms will expand and when they might rupture, it may prove beneficial to operate earlier in younger patients or those predicted to expand.

Recommendations regarding screening for AAA

A population screening programme for abdominal aortic aneurysm could save much of the money currently spent on emergency operations for ruptured aneurysms. In the early stages, more elective aneurysm operations would be performed. This would probably stabilize at 1.5 to 2 times the current rate. Whether or not a national programme should be advocated remains the subject of debate and will be determined by the results of continuing studies, as well as further contemplation of the socio-economic benefits or disadvantages that may accrue from such a study. Meanwhile, pilot projects will continue.

5.4 Screening for colorectal cancer

Colorectal cancer and the target population for screening

Colorectal cancer was responsible for approximately 25 000 deaths in England and Wales in 1992 and the incidence is increasing throughout the developed world. Surgical treatment for colorectal cancer has improved only a small amount over the past 3 decades and prognosis remains relatively poor in the UK, with between 30 and 40 per cent of patients surviving 5 years. However, in the United States the equivalent survival is closer to 50 per cent.

This high rate of surgical 'failure' has led to calls for a primary prevention programme with screening for the disease. Screening for colorectal cancer has to be aimed at a population with a relatively high risk. The incidence of colorectal cancer is known to increase dramatically with age; calculations have shown that a 50-year-old person has a 5 per cent risk of developing colorectal cancer by the age of 80 and a 2.5 per cent risk of dying from the disease. A cost-effective screening programme could reasonably be restricted to a population over the age of 50. Within the general population, there are other high-risk groups of individuals with detectable predisposing factors: people at risk of familial colorectal cancer.

Familial colorectal cancer

First-degree relatives of colorectal cancer patients have a lifetime risk of dying from the disease 4–5 times greater than that of the general population. This was first shown in the UK by Lovett and, more recently, by Stephenson. Between 10 and 20 per cent of patients with colorectal cancer have a positive family history of the disease, but identifying this is insufficient to identify the entire group at risk. However, a strategy for screening family members of index cancer patients has been devised and found to be feasible within the practice of a colorectal surgeon, although the value of it remains unproven. Despite this, several family history registries exist and screening programmes are taking place within the UK. These are based on assigning risk to prospective candidates for screening and offering screening according to this risk. Holston (1991) looked back at pedigrees and identified patterns based on the age and the number of relatives with colorectal cancer (Table 1.8). These ranged in risk from the high-risk autosomal dominant inherited forms of colorectal cancer to the lower-risk familial cases detailed below.

Using these risk factors in a clinical setting seems to work well in identifying patients and helps to provide cut-off levels for patients who require colonoscopy or investigation. There are no national guidelines, but a consensus seems to be that individuals with a risk of 1 : 10 ought to be investigated fully by colonoscopy. So far, there have been few reports of such screening programmes. Numbers have been small and there have been poor yields, as demonstrated by data reported from Guildford and from Nottingham. Thus, the effect of such screening remains unproven.

Hereditary non-polyposis colorectal cancer (HNPCC)

In addition to the more diffuse familial tendencies, there are well-recognized specific dominant inherited forms of colorectal cancer. The most consequential of these is **hereditary non-polyposis colorectal cancer** (HNPCC) previously known as Lynch syndrome. This is an autosomally dominantly inherited

Table 1.8 Risk assessment in familial colorectal cancer (after Holston et al. 1991)

Three first-degree relatives (any age)	Risk = 1 : 2
Two first-degree relatives (any age)	Risk = 1 : 6
One first-degree relative (under 45 years)	Risk = 1 : 10
One first-degree and one second-degree relative (over 45 years)	Risk = 1 : 12
One first-degree relative (over 45 years)	Risk = 1 : 17

condition in which large bowel cancer is prevalent. Colonic cancers present at a young age and are often right-sided. Patients with the disorder often develop other cancers affecting mainly the endometrium, stomach, and urinary tract. Patients with this disorder do characteristically have colonic polyps but fewer than 100 polyps per patient. Identifying those affected by this syndrome has been made easier as a result of an international collaborative meeting which produced the **Amsterdam criteria**. These propose that patients with three first-degree relatives in two succeeding generations with colorectal cancer, at least one below the age of 50, should be regarded as having hereditary non-polyposis colorectal cancer.

Three genes are now known to be responsible for HNPCC (*hMSH1*, *hMSH2*, and *hMLH1*). Diagnosis could be made by genetic screening but watertight criteria are not yet available. There are reports of linkage to chromosome 2, but there are at least two genes for HNPCC in this area and genetic studies were only informative for two-thirds of the large pedigrees studied. Plans to make testing for these genes available on a commercial basis are under way in the USA.

Familial adenomatous polyposis coli

Familial adenomatous polyposis coli is a rare condition and accounts for only a small proportion of colorectal cancers. However, screening for this condition is based upon a family history and endoscopic surveillance, together with the discovery of more than 100 colonic polyps. Other phenotypic markers are present, for example mandibular osteomas and congenital hypertrophic retinal pigment epithelium (CHRPE). These markers have been used to predict reliably the presence of disease before the polyps appear. However, the gene defect that causes familial polyposis, the *APC* gene, has now been localized on the short arm of chromosome 5 and has recently been characterized and sequenced. There are a large number of mutations of this gene, giving rise to several different phenotypic syndromes, all now encompassed under the term familial adenomatous polyposis coli. Characterization of the *APC* gene now means that familial members can be tested for the mutation. This spares those at low risk from repeated colonoscopic follow-up.

Screening techniques:faecal occult blood tests

Large bowel cancers and large adenomas usually bleed from the surface into the colon. Thus, the finding of blood within faeces may herald one or other of these disorders. This has led to the introduction of a range of faecal occult blood tests. The most widely used has been Haemoccult® (Rohm Pharma). This test consists of a filter paper impregnated with guaiac, which undergoes phenolic oxidation changing it to blue in the presence of both haemoglobin from the stool and hydrogen peroxide in the test reagent. The positive reaction depends on the pseudoperoxidase activity of haemoglobin.

False reaction to Haemoccult® tests

Unfortunately other materials possess peroxidase activity, for example fresh fruit and cooked vegetables, and these can produce false-positive reactions. A positive test can also occur in the presence of non-haemoglobin peroxidases found in meat or from inconsequential blood losses from the bowel wall. False-negative reactions can be caused by agents such as vitamin C, which can interfere with the oxidation reaction in the presence of haemoglobin.

Newer tests for faecal occult blood

Nasal and gastrointestinal blood loss is normally between 0.5 and 1.0 ml/day. Haemoccult® is able to detect losses of 10 ml/day in 67 per cent of cases and 20 ml/day in 80–90 per cent of cases. Newer occult blood tests include more sensitive peroxidase-based tests, an immunochemical test specific for haemoglobin (Haemselect®), and a haematoporphyrin assay (Haemoquant®). These last two tests are not affected by pseudoperoxidase activity but do require the subject to adhere to a strict dietary protocol. The sensitivity of Haemselect® was examined in a recent study, where 1489 subjects were tested with both Haemoccult® and Haemselect®. The positivity rate was 1.1 per cent for Haemoccult® and 9.7 per cent for Haemselect®. Nine cancers were discovered as a result of testing by Haemselect® but only one of these was positive to Haemoccult®. Similarly, 49 patients with adenomas were identified, 48 of whom were Haemselect® positive compared with only 8 Haemoccult® positive.

Although greater sensitivity of Haemselect® was evident from this study, the test had a much lower specificity, which resulted in substantially increased endoscopic work. For this reason, this assay has not yet been tested in a population screening study. Most large population screening studies have used Haemoccult®. Despite its limited sensitivity for carcinoma, Haemoccult® has a high specificity for blood, with very few false positives caused by dietary intake. It is likely to remain the preferred test for mass screening trials for colorectal carcinoma. It is capable of identifying 1–2 per cent of the population at high risk of concealing an asymptomatic carcinoma or adenoma.

Results of screening studies

Six prospective randomized trials have been initiated, but only one has been fully reported. Three European studies have reported only interim results.

The New York study of detecting faecal occult blood

This trial was conducted by the Memorial Sloan Kettering Cancer Centre and the Preventative Medicine Institute Strang Clinic between 1975 and 1984 in a setting of a comprehensive preventative medical examination. Unfortunately, the sample size was too small to detect even a moderately significant reduction in mortality, particularly when 43 per cent of all those patients who were enrolled were excluded from the analysis as having been screened previously. The study was not randomized although the subjects were well matched. Compliance was high, at 80 per cent for first-time screening candidates, but fell to 20 per cent after 1 year. The low overall compliance led to the detection of only 5 out of 31 cancers by screening. Although

there was a significant improvement in survival for the study group, the overall reduction in mortality was not significant.

The Minnesota study

The Minnesota study began in 1975 and was designed to compare annual and biannual Haemoccult® screening with an unscreened control group. The study provided the first evidence that screened subjects had earlier-stage disease at diagnosis. As in the New York study, participants were volunteers between 50 and 80 years old but, unlike that study, participants were randomly allocated to one of three groups, with 1500 people in each group. Screening finished in 1982 but had to be restarted in 1986 to increase the power of the study. After 13 years' follow-up, a significant reduction in morality was found for the annually screened group compared with controls (ratio = 0.67; 95 per cent CI, 0.5–0.87). No additional benefit was found in those screened biannually.

This is the only study so far to show a reduction in mortality; however, the data so far presented are insufficient to guide recommendations for mass screening. First, it is surprising that more cancers were detected in the control group than in either screened group. The differences in mortality between screened and unscreened groups can accounted for by the low number of patients presenting with distant metastases in the annually screened group. This study used rehydrated Haemoccult® tests, which produced a very high positivity rate, with the consequence that almost 38 per cent of patients screened annually had at least one colonoscopy during the study. Thus reduction in mortality was more likely to have been a function of the colonoscopic examinations rather than the Haemoccult® screening.

The Swedish Göteborg study

Two cohorts of 51 000 patients between 60 and 64 years were enrolled in this study between 1982 and 1987. Screening for faecal occult blood was with Haemoccult® and, in contrast with other studies, investigation of test-positive subjects was by flexible sigmoidoscopy and double contrast barium enema. The sensitivity for detecting carcinoma with this combination of investigations was 93 per cent.

Compliance was 66 per cent at the initial screening. Seven years on, 101 carcinomas had been diagnosed in the screened group and 128 in the control group. The number of adenomas in each group during the 7-year follow-up was identical. The study further indicated that screening and rescreening of this population had little influence on the stage of carcinomas found in the test group compared with the control group over the 7 years of follow-up.

The Danish Funen study

This began in 1985 and was similar in design to the Nottingham study described below. Compliance was 67 per cent at initial screening and this increased to 91 per cent and 95 per cent respectively for the subsequent screening rounds. There was a low positivity rate of only about 1 per cent because of the use of unhydrated tests and imposition of dietary restrictions. Fifty per cent of the cancers detected by screening were Dukes stage A. Up to 1992, 58 patients had died from colorectal cancer in the test group and 71 in the control group, a reduction of 18 per cent; this is not statistically significant. The main problems in this study were poor test sensitivity and unexplained variances in the mortality data; while 70 per cent of patients with screen-detected cancer had died of the disease, only 43 per cent with interval cancers and non-responders with cancer had died of colorectal cancer.

The Nottingham study

This study is the largest and the only study with sufficient sample size and power to detect a difference in mortality. The trial is nearing an end and a report on mortality differences are keenly awaited. However, a number of preliminary findings have been reported.

The Nottingham study consisted of 155 034 people aged 50–74, randomly allocated into test and control groups. Screening was with Haemoccult® every 2 years. The results are given in Table 1.9. Compliance was low at the start of the study but has averaged around 60 per cent overall. Two interim indicators of success for the study were as follows: first, the proportion of stage A cancers was significantly lower in the control group, at 14 per cent versus 47 per cent in the screen-detected group (28 per cent in the whole study group). Secondly, there was a greater proportion of stage D cancers (with distant metastases as distinct from nodal metastases) in the control group compared with the screen-detected group—21 per cent versus 6 per cent. However, there was no significant difference when compared to the whole study group. No difference in mortality was demonstrated when the study was reported in 1991. This may be because the test was inadequate and compliance was too low, as well as the fact that large numbers with advanced and untreatable disease were found in both groups. The results regarding cancers detected in the screened group are given in Table 1.9.

The most recent results of the Nottingham and Funen studies have been published (Kronborg et al. 1996; Hardcastle et al. 1996). Both studies show a 15–18 per cent reduction in colorectal cancer mortality. Cost per life year saved was comparable in both series at US$10 000–20 000. However, the compliance was very low in both studies: 38 per cent in Nottingham and 46 per cent in Funen. Set against this background, screening for colorectal cancer comes out favourably.

Recommendations as regards faecal occult blood screening

It is likely that a growing number of at-risk individuals will place an increasing demand upon surgical and genetic services because of a discerned genetic susceptibility to colorectal cancer. There is no real evidence for any benefits for this type of screening but the widescale introduction of family history clinics on a regional level may mean that screening of this population is inevitable. It is important that such screening should be carried out in conjunction with a genetic counsellor and a clinical geneticist.

Population screening for colorectal cancer cannot yet meet the criteria set out at the beginning of this section. Improved and more specific tests, and perhaps methodology to improve compliance, may change this in the future. As with other screening programmes, tight standards would have to be set in the areas of compliance, positivity rates, colonoscopy rates, and interval cancer rates.

Bibliography

Consent and medical negligence

Mason and McCall Smith (1994). *Law and Medical Ethics*, Butterworths, Oxford.

Screening

General

Cole, P. and Morrison, A.S. (1980). Basic issues in population screening for cancer. *JNCI*, **64**, (5), 1263–72.

Wilson, J.M.G. and Jungner, G. (1968). *Principles and practice of screening for disease*, WHO Public Health Paper, 34. WHO Geneva.

Table 1.9 Cancers detected in the 1991 Nottingham screening study (with permission of J.D. Hardcastle)

	Initial screen	First re-screen	Second re-screen	Third re-screen	Fourth re-screen
Number of subjects offered screening	77 226	46 371	43 727	36 570	10 113
Acceptors	41 114	32 191	26 425	18 589	5169
	(54.5%)	(69%)	(60%)	(51%)	(51%)
Test positive	843	415	271	256	80
(%)	(2.0)	(1.3)	(1.0)	(1.4)	(1.5)
Neoplastic disease detected:					
Carcinomas	89	55	32	38	9
(per 1000)	(2.2)	(1.7)	(1.2)	(2.0)	(1.7)
Adenomas	461	199	125	93	61
Neoplasia missed by investigation	6 cancers	1 cancer	None known	None known	None known

Breast cancer and screening

British Medical Journal Editorial (1995). What should be done about interval breast cancers? Two view mammography and possibly a shorter screening interval. *BMJ*, **310**, 203–4.

Elmore, J.G., Wells, M.P.H., Lee, C.H., Howard, D.H., and Feinstein, A.R. (1994). Variability in radiologists' interpretation of mammograms. *N. Engl. J. Med.*, **331**, 1493–9.

Evans, D.G.R., Fentiman, I.S., McPherson, K., Ashbury, D., Ponder, B.A., and Howell, A. (1994). Familial breast cancer. *BMJ*, **308**, 183–7.

Frisell, J., Eklund, G., Hellstrom, L., and Somers, A. (1987). Analysis of interval breast carcinomas in a randomised screening trial in Stockholm. *Breast Cancer Res. Treat.*, **9**, 219–25.

Moss, S.M., Eilman, R., Coleman, D., and Chamberlain, J. (1994). Survival of patients with breast cancer diagnosed in the United Kingdom Trial of Early Detection of Breast Cancer. *J. Med. Screen.*, **1**, 193–8.

Nystrom, L., Rutqvist, L.E., Wall, S., Lindgren, A., Lindqvist, M., Ryden, S., *et al.* (1993). Breast cancer screening with mammography:overview of Swedish randomised trials. *Lancet*, **341**, 973–8.

Querci della Rovere, G., Bird, P.A. (1998). Sentinel-lymph-node biopsy in breast cancer. *Lancet*, **352**, 421–2.

Querci della Rovere, G., Benson, J.R., Warren, R. (1995). Screening for breast cancer, time to think–and stop? *Lancet*, **346**, 437–9.

Tabar, L., Fagerberg, C.J.G., Gad, A., Baldetorp, L., Holmberg, L.H., Grontoff, O., *et al.* (1985). Reduction in mortality from breast cancer after mass screening with mammography. *Lancet*, **i**, 829–32.

Tabar, L., Fagerberg, G., Duffy, S.W., *et al.* (1992). Update of the Swedish Two County Programme of Mammographic Screening for Breast Cancer. *Radiol. Clin. North Am.*, **30**, 187–270.

Woodman, C.B.J., Threlfall, A.G., Boggis, C.R.M., and Prior, P. (1995). Is the three year breast screening interval too long? Occurrence of interval cancers in NHS breast screening programme's north western region. *BMJ*, **310**, 224–6.

Aortic aneurysm screening

Allen, P.I.M., Gourevitch, D., and McKinley, J. (1987). Population screening for aortic aneurysms. *Lancet*, **2**, 736.

Anonymous (1997). Screening brief: ruptured abdominal aortic aneurysm. *J. Med. Screen.*, **4**, 112.

Choksy, S.A., Wilmink, A.B., Quick, C.R. (1999). Ruptured abdominal aortic aneurysm in the Huntingdon district: a 10-year experience. *Anna. RCS. Eng.*, **81**, 27–31.

Collin, J., Araujo, L., and Lindsell, D.A. (1988). A community screening programme for abdominal aortic aneurysms. *Eur. J. Vasc. Surg.*, **2**, 83–6.

Law, M.R., Morris, J., and Wald, N.J. (1994). Screening for abdominal aortic aneurysms. *J. Med. Screen.*, **1**, 110–15.

Morris, G., Hubbard, C., Quick, C.R.G. (1994). An abdominal aortic aneurysm screening programme for all males over the age of 50 years. *Eur. J. Vasc. Surg.*, **8**, 156–60.

O'Kelly, T.J. and Heather, B.P. (1988). The feasibility of screening for abdominal aortic aneurysms in a district general hospital. *Ann. R. Coll. Surg. Engl.*, **70**, 197–9.

Scott, R.A.P., Gudgeon, A.M., Ashton, H.A., Allen, D.R., and Wilson, N.M. (1994). Surgical workload as a consequence of screening for abdominal aortic aneurysm. *Br. J. Surg.*, **81**, 1440–2.

Vardulaki, K.A., Prevost, T.C., Walker, N.M., Day, N.E., Wilmink, A.B., Quick, C.R. *et al.* (1999). Incidence among men of asymptomatic abdominal aortic aneurysms: estimates from 500 screen detected cases. *J. Med. Screen.*, **6**, 50–4.

Vardulaki, K.A., Prevost, T.C., Walker, N.M., Day, N.E., Wilmink, A.B., Quick, C.R., Ashton, H.A. *et al.* (1998). Growth rates and risk of rupture of abdominal aortic aneurysms. *Br. J. Surg.*, **85**, 1674–80.

Wilmink, A.B., Quick, C.R. (1998). Epidemiology and potential for prevention of abdominal aortic aneurysm. [Editorial review; 130 refs]. *Br. J. Surg.*, **85**, 155–62.

Wilmink, A.B., Quick, C.R., Hubbard, C.S., Day, N.E. (1999). The influence of screening on the incidence of ruptured abdominal aortic aneurysms. *J. Vasc. Surg.*, **30**, 203–8.

Colorectal cancer screening

Hardcastle, J.D., Chamberlain, J., and Sheffield, J. (1989). Randomised controlled trial of faecal occult blood screening for colorectal cancer. Results for first 107 349 subjects. *Lancet*, **i**, 1160–4.

Hardcastle, J., Chamberlain, J., Robinson, M., *et al.* (1996). Randomised controlled trial of faecal-occult-blood screening for colorectal cancer. *Lancet*, **348**, 1472–7.

Hart, A.R., Wicks, A.C.B., and Mayberry, J.F. (1995). Colorectal cancer screening in asymptomatic populations. *Gut*, **36**, 590–8.

Kronborg, O., Fenger, C., Olsen, J., Jørgensen, O., and Søndergaard, O. (1996). Randomised study of screening for colorectal cancer with faecal-occult-blood test. *Lancet*, **348**, 1467–71.

Mandel, J.S., Bond, J.H., Church, T.R., Snover, D.C., Bradley, G.M., Schuman, L.S., *et al.* (1993). Reducing mortality from colorectal cancer by screening for faecal occult blood. *N. Engl. J. Med.*, **328**, 1365–71.

Winnawer, S.J., Schottenfeld, D., and Flehinger, B.J. (1991). Colorectal cancer screening. *JNCI*, **83**, 243–53.

CHAPTER 2

Setting the standards of surgical practice

J.D. Greig and Clive R. Quick

If politics is the art of the possible, research is surely the art of the soluble.

Sir Peter Medawar

1 Why do we need standards?

Standards in surgery are both consciously and unconsciously part of everyday surgical practice. Standards of access to care, waiting times to consultation and to elective operation are regularly debated in the media and are subject to much angst within government. Indeed, an excessive amount of attention is given to these subjects, with far less attention to the vital matters of the management of emergency admissions, the quality and outcome of operations, and the calibre of perioperative care.

Up until 15 or so years ago, relatively little attention was paid to the quality of care. The population was uncomplaining and there was something of a culture of the pioneer about much surgical practice—struggling against the odds with little training and minimal critical comment while attempting to do a good job.

There has been a gradual change away from this, with recognition that improving the quality of everyday care (perhaps aided by medical audit) is every bit as important as devising new and momentous treatments by research.

Standards are important for a variety of reasons. It is intrinsic to the surgeon as a vocational craftsman to want to do a good job and to gain the best and most trouble-free outcomes. In order to do the best job, a surgeon has to be familiar with what is the best and may need to be taught how to achieve it. The old apprenticeship scheme worked well provided the trainer took his responsibilities seriously and provided the apprenticeship lasted long enough. It was perceived to work best at a time when junior surgeons were able to operate on patients without fear of criticism if things went wrong, but, understandably, this is no longer acceptable. With the public becoming ever more aware of differing standards, and with public and professional tolerance for substandard results much lower than before, the old system no longer stands scrutiny. Furthermore, the old system could not be reconciled with the centrally stated intention of shortening surgical training.

To replace the old system requires a much greater investment in practical teaching, such as basic surgical skills workshops, anastomosis workshops, and the like. In addition, with limited exposure to operative surgery and shortened training, surgeons will have to focus earlier on subspecialty interests and not expect to practise across the entire field of general surgery.

Other reasons for setting standards within surgery include the need to demonstrate that we as a profession are examining our own practices and accomplishing what we set out to achieve. This will help to retain the respect and confidence of our public and, where necessary, to demonstrate to lawyers that we are practising both optimally and ethically.

1.1 What is optimal practice?

The basis on which we practise surgery is defined by the prevalent opinions within the surgical community of what is optimal practice. Surgeons often have strong individual opinions, which are likely to be based predominantly on their experience and training, tempered by reading, continued medical education, and professional meetings. Trying to alter patterns of patient care is frustratingly difficult. It is relatively easy to obtain information on current methods and their results and to discuss these with colleagues and even to agree on what is best. However, implementing change can be slow and difficult. Although this may seem reactionary to outside observers (such as newspaper columnists), it would be reckless to change methods that not only work but can be demonstrated to be working by medical audit methods. It is absolutely correct that change should be considered carefully and introduced gradually unless there is overwhelming evidence that current practice is unsatisfactory. However, subjective opinions about the efficacy of certain treatments may be incorrect, and surgeons must be prepared to have their clinical freedom challenged by informed opinion and to modify their behaviour if it is found wanting. In some instances, this will require a certain amount of retraining or hands-on experience. Public awareness of raw differences in results and consequent perceptions of substandard care and 'out-of-datedness', as well as other negative views of medicine, are now part of popular enlightenment. Surgical practice needs to be aware of changing standards and changing perceptions and endeavour to remain ahead of the game.

Despite the current high standards in surgical practice in the United Kingdom, practices do vary widely. Examination of morbidity and mortality data has enabled suboptimal practices to be identified because of poorer surgical outcomes, but when interpreting comparisons between individual surgeons or institutions, cities or regions, other comparabilities must be taken into account. Like must be compared with like, and factors such as the nature of the population and the disease epidemiology must be taken into account. Objective assessment of procedures and the quality of patient care can take these and other factors into account, using appropriate research and medical audit method-

ologies. This evidence and peer consensus should be the starting point of generating acceptable standards of practice.

1.2 How are improved methods evaluated?

In order to show that a particular aspect of patient management has improved, and thus to set new standards, it must be evaluated carefully and compared with existing practices. While this may seem Utopian, the example of 'the greatest uncontrolled medical experiment of all', namely the introduction of laparoscopic cholecystectomy, was undoubtedly at the expense of a doubling of the incidence in common bile duct injuries. The proper view should be that the safety of the many outweighs the current enthusiasm of the few.

There have been few prospective randomized trials that have properly evaluated laparoscopic cholecystectomy, one of the common major surgical procedures. A recent study from Sheffield, however, showed no benefit for laparoscopic surgery in terms of duration of hospital admission and time to return to work, but did show lower perioperative analgesic requirements.

It is encouraging to see that laparoscopic hernia repair is not likely to be allowed to escape peer review in the same way, with the establishment of a Medical Research Council multicentre trial comparing the existing standard of open hernia repair with the prospective standard of laparoscopic repair. Indeed, many of the randomized trials comparing laparoscopic versus open hernia repair have now identified advantages for laparoscopic repair, but with the caveat that these may only be realized in the hands of hernia subspecialists.

1.3 An ethical surgical practice

The essence of an ethical surgical practice is one conducted in accordance with principles of conduct that are generally considered correct (by peer groups, judgements at law, and published data). It embodies doing the best for the patient in the circumstances, not taking advantage of the patient, and not allowing financial and other mundane considerations to be dominant. Setting the highest standards of surgical practice can best be achieved by critical analysis of each stage of management. This includes the referral process, investigation, diagnosis, operative and non-operative treatment, and post-hospital discharge care. The instrument of analysis may be research (when comparing one treatment with another) or medical audit (when analysing aspects of practice against existing or idealized standards). This can provide the observer (in this case, the surgeon), with objective evidence of the effects that changes may have on patient management.

2 Research in surgery

2.1 Research and experimentation on humans

There have been important changes in attitudes to human research over recent decades. At one time experimentation using human subjects proceeded almost without comment. However, for a variety of reasons there has been a gradual increase in legislation and ethical constraint on human experimentation. These reasons include: reactions against paternalistic medicine; development of many new drugs and therapies; the ability to effect genetic manipulation and the potential to use fetal tissue for transplantation. At the same time, as the scope for interference with the rights of the individual has broadened, there has been increasing public concern and debate about erosion of the rights of the individual.

The first international set of accepted ethical guidelines was known as the *Nuremberg Code* and this was a direct result of the war crimes trials after the Second World War. Later, the medical profession publicly endorsed these principles in the *Declaration of Helsinki* drawn up by the World Medical Association in 1964 and revised in 1975. The Royal College of Physicians of London too has published a comprehensive set of guidelines, entitled *Research involving patients* (1990), which explains and expands the principles established at Nuremberg. All of these codes have in common that they appreciate the need for human experimentation while accepting that this can only be accomplished at the expense of some of the subject's rights to self-determination. Progress in medicine usually depends upon some form of clinical trial but a sensible balance must be found between progress and basic human rights.

2.2 Experimental treatment

This is a contentious subject. Medicine is not always entirely scientific and many advances are made fortuitously or by intuition. The difficulty then arises of distinguishing courageous innovation from unethical experimentation. The resolution often depends on the quality of outcome.

2.3 Research versus experimentation

Research implies the use of a predetermined protocol and a clearly defined end point. Experimentation, by contrast, involves a more speculative approach, usually towards an individual subject. An experiment may be modified to take account of the individual's response, whereas a research programme is likely to lock the researcher into a particular course of action until the results and general effectiveness of the treatment is revealed at the end of the study. Research includes **clinical research**, aimed at improving treatment of a patient or a group of patients, and **non-therapeutic research**, in which the aim is to extend scientific knowledge, although this may eventually have wider application. When research is applied to sick patients, it is essential that vigorous controls be applied to non-standard treatment of a vulnerable group. Any degree of risk permitted in research must be in proportion to the expected beneficial outcome. Research subjects may fall into one of four categories: individual patients, groups of patients suffering from a particular condition, patients with other conditions, and healthy volunteers.

2.4 Risks of research

The *Declaration of Helsinki* and the Royal College of Physicians guidelines on human research state that a risk : benefit analysis must be undertaken in each case and patients should be involved only when the benefit clearly outweighs the inconvenience, discomfort, or possible harm the protocol may impose. The Royal College of Physicians distinguishes different risk levels for research as follows:

1. Research involving 'less than minimal risk' is of the level involved in giving a sample of urine or obtaining a single venous blood sample from an adult.

2. Research involving 'minimal risk' is when there is a moderate chance of a mild reaction or side-effect and a remote chance of serious injury or death.

3. If the level of risk rises above this, then the College takes the view that patients should be involved only if the following conditions are satisfied:
   ◆ the risk remains small in comparison with the consequences of the disease itself;
   ◆ the disease is serious;
   ◆ the knowledge gained from the research is likely to be of great practical benefit;
   ◆ there is no other means of obtaining the knowledge;
   ◆ the patient gives fully informed consent.

2.5 Design of research and experiments

All research requires careful planning because badly planned research sacrifices ethical justification and the findings are scientifically useless. It is obligatory for each British health authority to establish an ethics committee with the function of examining and sanctioning each experimental or research project before it is launched. These committees generally include medical members, other professionals such as lawyers, church leaders, or statisticians, and lay members. Ethics committees have even greater power in the United States.

2.6 Random sample testing

Using tissue or blood samples removed for one purpose for a different purpose could contain an element of invasion of a patient's privacy; for example, finding things out about the subject without consent. This might include the geographical distribution of abnormal genes or cultural alterations in body chemistry. Justification for such projects rests on the consequences of a positive finding; at one extreme is HIV, with dire consequences for the positive individual, and at the other extreme, the search for a particular gene which is unlikely to make any difference to the individual. However, great care would be needed before embarking upon a survey of abnormal genetic markers which, if known, would influence the advisability of having children. Other research studies which might have adverse effects if published include estimation of blood alcohol in a community. If specimens are used without expressed consent, preservation of anonymity must be a determining condition.

The disposal of surplus human material is seldom addressed in law. The patient may object to a part of his body being exposed in a museum jar but at most, could insist on it being returned to him. Without that request it may be assumed to be abandoned. There are no property rights in a dead human body and it is assumed that there are none in dead human tissue. However, if body tissue assumes commercial importance—as in the development of cell lines in cell culture—then other views may prevail in future court actions.

3 Clinical trials

3.1 Controlled trials

Many biomedical experiments involve controlled trials in order to decide whether a new drug or treatment is better than an existing one or no treatment at all. The treatment is given to a group of patients or healthy volunteers and not given to a similar group. The subtleties of experimental design are crucial to the success of the project but even the best-designed trials have built-in moral uncertainties. On the one hand, a relatively untried treatment which may do harm is given to one group while, on the other hand, a treatment which may be of considerable benefit is withheld from a similar group. The vital question is, 'would a patient improve faster if treatment was not restrained by the treatment protocol?'

In therapeutic controlled trials, the health of the patient must be paramount. A prerequisite for any controlled trial is therefore that all arms are entirely ethical and each treatment tested should have an equal chance of benefiting the patient. The trial must provide its answer as rapidly as possible and be capable of termination as soon as adverse effects become apparent. Any patients affected should be transferred to an alternative treatment regimen. There is a good case to be made out for independent observers or the local ethics committee itself maintaining responsibility for monitoring the trial from this standpoint.

3.2 The use of placebos

The mere taking of tablets may lead to subjective improvement—the placebo effect—which needs to be considered whenever a new drug or procedure is on trial. It would clearly be improper to use placebo controls if pain was a feature of the condition under treatment. Placebo trials are unethical if there is a suitable alternative to the experimental treatment available from existing treatment methods. In most instances, the purpose of using placebos is to analyse the effect of a treatment on symptoms rather than on the progress of the organic disease, or to disguise from the researchers the fact that one group of patients is being treated and the other is not.

3.3 Informed consent regarding research

The basis of ethical research is that the participation of the subject is freely entered into and autonomous; thus the standard of information should be higher, if anything, than for regular treatment. Patient consent must be based on four lines of explanation:

- the purpose of the experiment;
- the potential benefits to the patient and society;
- the risks involved;
- the alternatives open to the subject.

Two further common problems with trial consent are:

1. Who should impart the information—the patient's doctor or the researcher?

2. Should the patient have the benefit of a friend to help interpret information?

Patients may have difficulty understanding the alternative treatments, particularly if the doctors involved also find this perplexing. In practice, giving full explanations to the patient to obtain fully informed consent may render some controlled trials next to impossible to undertake.

3.4 Avoiding claims for personal injury

Researchers must take precautions to avoid claims against them for battery or medical negligence. These include obtaining advance approval of an ethics committee and informing the patient or subject fully of his or her rights (or lack of them), before enrolment.

3.5 Clinical trials—details

Introduction

Before a new therapeutic or surgical treatment can be accepted into medical practice, it needs to be shown to be better than existing methods in one or more respect. These improvements might be, for example, that it is more powerful, cheaper, safer, or it causes less pain. Information about novel surgical techniques spreads rapidly, but some of those eager to try the new and exciting procedure may rush to apply it without the attention to detail and level of skill traditionally associated with the surgical pioneer. This was manifest in the early experiences of laparoscopic surgery. The risks of this precipitate attitude have been recognized and formal training is now mandatory for surgeons wishing to perform new and technically demanding techniques.

Drug trials

The pharmaceutical industry is obliged to determine drug efficacy and tolerability before releasing new agents onto the market. This process involves a number of phased studies. The initial animal bioavailability and toxicology studies are known as Phase I trials. Following these, human dosages are determined and Phase II trials initiated. These are carried out in a small number of informed human volunteers. Only then is it feasible to determine the likely efficacy of the product within the human species.

Once human safety and efficacy has been established, Phase III trials are initiated. These prospectively study the effect of introducing the drug or treatment into an established therapeutic regimen. The efficacy, predictability, and side-effects of the new agent or therapy then need to be compared with the standard therapy. These trials involve a large amount of data collection on a moderate number of patients. To recruit patients in sufficient numbers, it is often necessary to combine the results from a number of centres so the results can be statistically meaningful. These trials are often 'blinded' to minimize bias, so that the patient, the observer, and the investigator do not know to which arm of the trial an individual has been allocated.

Once a new therapy or treatment has been shown to offer distinct advantages and has been approved and debated by peer review, the drug joins the medical armamentarium. At this stage it may enter a Phase IV trial with continuing prospective data collection and analysis from patients commenced on the new treatment. This is necessary to identify rare side-effects or complications.

This structured approach to the introduction of new pharmacological agents into clinical practice could be used as a model for new surgical treatments or practices. Central legislation in this area is likely to become codified but it remains the surgeon's responsibility to ensure that risky innovative treatments are introduced in an acceptable, logical, and coordinated way.

3.6 Surgical trial design and conduct

Trial design

In designing a clinical trial, a researcher must carry out a great deal of groundwork and forward planning. The area to be investigated is first established, then background work performed to establish the depth of current knowledge, after which the potential contribution of the proposed study should be defined. Only then is it possible to identify the hypothesis being tested that leads to the design of the study. The design process determines the need for a pilot study and defines the practical details of the study.

Retrospective studies

Retrospective studies, which analyse previously recorded data, can produce useful data in appropriate circumstances and may also be used as pilot studies in advance of a prospective study. A retrospective study may give some idea of the results to be expected, and in so doing, provide justification for a more refined prospective study. It may also allow the trial design to be streamlined. Retrospective studies can be criticized on several counts:

- a suitable control group is hard to find;
- some vital data may be missing from the case notes;
- there are many potential flaws in retrospective analysis;
- conclusions are usually strictly limited.

Prospective studies

Prospective studies, which involve sequential data collection from a recruited cohort, generally achieve the most worthwhile data. A prospective study design ensures that relevant data are all accrued chronologically and that patients are entered into the trial as they become available. The disadvantage is that it may take many months (or even years) to recruit enough patients to give sufficient power to the study.

Longitudinal and cross-sectional studies

Longitudinal studies are most often used to study the effects of therapy on a predetermined population or to examine epidemiological changes in populations. This is in contrast to **cross-sectional studies**, which take a 'snap shot' at a particular time and place. Cross-sectional studies lend themselves most readily to epidemiological research and are most commonly used to monitor the incidence and location of diseases and treatment.

Maintaining the objectivity of a trial

The objectivity of any trial needs to be protected and for this, the gold-standard remains the **double-blind randomized trial**. Randomization removes the natural tendency for bias to enter the project, particularly when new treatments are compared with tried and tested techniques. Without formal randomization planned in advance, **investigator bias** could lead to the wilful inclusion or omission of patients from one or other arm of the study. Proper randomization requires the use of randomization tables or an appropriate computer program.

The second important factor in retaining objectivity is to conceal which arm of the study each individual belongs to (treatment A versus treatment B, or treatment versus no treatment) from both the patient and the investigator. This is practicable with pharmaco-therapeutic studies but is rarely possible with surgery, unless there are no obvious differences between invasive treatments. The double-blind technique attempts to eliminate any personal preferences the doctor may have for a particular treatment by keeping those assigned to the therapeutic group secret. This dictates that the patient's normal treating doctor cannot be the researcher and makes it implicit that the ethical justification for the trial has been agreed in advance by the patient's own doctor. This sometimes makes it difficult to implement randomization in particular trials.

Single-blind studies in which the patient does not know which arm he has been allocated to can be useful if double blinding is impossible; if patients are unaware of their treatment, the therapeutic effect of any placebo is maximized.

Many doctors dislike randomized trials for their own patients because they fear the doctor–patient relationship may be jeopardized, and in particular, that proper informed consent cannot be obtained. However, if the doctors involved believe their patients will not be disadvantaged whichever arm they are allocated to, and that it is important to know whether one or other treatment is better, they are likely to support the trial. Where there is doubt, however, attempts to initiate randomized trials suffer from difficulties with recruiting patients, for example mastectomy versus local resection for breast cancer.

Case-control studies

Sometimes it is desirable to study the effects of a given treatment in a particular environment. In such trials, like must be compared with like and a **case-control study** should be employed. Matching of individuals for (for example) height, weight, sex, age, diet, parity, and disease severity allow meaningful comparisons to be made when looking for small or subtle differences between groups.

Practical elements in carrying out a controlled trial

Once the study design has been established, the practicalities and necessary extent of data collection must be determined. A practicable cohort size which has sufficient power to show differences between treatments must be determined and the data to be collected must be determined.

To ensure success, responsibility for the practicalities of data collection, storage, and analysis must be allocated to dependable individuals. The reliability, sensitivity, and specificity of the data collected need to be established from previously published work or by means of pilot studies. The researcher needs to have an idea of the expected results and to be able to demonstrate that these are likely to differ significantly from those in a control population. After that, it is necessary to establish inclusion and exclusion criteria, the population size and characteristics to be studied, and then to determine how the data will be analysed and presented statistically. The planning, execution, and analysis of any proposed trial should be carried out in consultation with a medical statistician versed in trial methodology and analysis, and a realistic timetable must be set.

Other considerations include the identification of suitable individuals to carry out the research. These key people must be suitably remunerated and have the time, facilities, information, practical and emotional support, and financial means to achieve their goal. Specialized equipment and training may be needed, as well as the means to fund unanticipated overheads such as travel, publishing costs, and conference expenses. It is clear that worthwhile research often proves expensive in resources and manpower and should not be undertaken simply for the sake of the curriculum vitae.

4 Other methods of improving quality

4.1 Referral patterns

Patient expectations and successive healthcare reforms have necessitated closer cooperation between hospital and community heathcare providers. The greater involvement of general practices in determining care for their patients, as well as the itemized remuneration of some aspects of primary community care, has encouraged much straightforward surgery to be performed by general practitioners. The newer concept of polyclinics aims to decentralize specialized care and provide it within the community (although for many people these aims are unrealistic). The expansion of day-case surgery for hernias, varicose veins, and the like shifts part of the cost of treatment onto community services. In providing a well-integrated and effective surgical service, it is important that guidelines such as collaborative care plans are developed jointly by surgeons and primary-care providers. Even if recent healthcare reforms disappear, these principles remain good.

'Prevention is better than cure' is only partially true. Very little that is worthwhile comes out of many 'health checks' or 'medicals' and activity of this sort and screening in general bears close scrutiny for its potential benefits and disadvantages (see Chapter 1, Section 5). Surgical screening relies on identifying, monitoring high-risk groups of patients, and treating abnormalities discovered. Screening attempts to identify treatable disease at an early pathological stage, and some success has been achieved in detecting early breast cancer and pre-rupture abdominal aortic aneurysm. The rapid pace of developments in molecular and genetic biology will ultimately enable populations at risk from many different diseases to be identified. Some will require lifelong screening and others even prophylactic surgical intervention. Genetic studies will also be able to identify individuals who do not carry disease genes and are therefore not at risk. Both of these are potentially beneficial but much ethical debate needs to be conducted before any such diagnostic method can be embraced.

4.2 Patient education

There is little reason for patients in the United Kingdom to be unaware of disease or to neglect it. The National Health Service provides healthcare free at the point of delivery to all comers. This idealistic philosophy has been blamed for spiralling costs and inefficiencies in the service. Unlike countries with non-government-financed healthcare, the onus for well-being and disease awareness in the UK has not traditionally been the responsibility of the consumer. However, greater openness about health matters such as cancer, patient charters, and the public discussion of health matters are gradually changing this. Problems arise when patient expectations rise above what the resources of government-funded healthcare can provide. Hospital and community clinicians have a duty to educate the public and this can have the beneficial effect of passing some responsibility for individual health back to the individual. When not scare-mongering or 'doctor bashing', the popular media can have major beneficial influences on consumer living patterns. They could be employed more effectively to advance preventative programmes.

4.3 Protocols and guidelines

Peer-group opinions and initiatives such as the National Confidential Enquiry into Perioperative Deaths (NCEPOD) have compelled surgeons to look closely at the appropriateness of their practice. In another approach, **evidence-based medicine** requires analysing clinical results via large prospective studies or meta-analyses of the published data. This has become increasingly popular to generate diagnostic and therapeutic guidelines or algorithms. Although perhaps useful in the educational and clinical setting, established protocols of this type are in danger of being used as examples of 'standard practice' by the judiciary and must be viewed with caution. The term **protocol** is dangerously restrictive of clinical judgement and should be replaced with the term **guideline**. If used sensibly, such guidelines can improve practice, for example by reducing unnecessary investigations.

4.4 New modes of investigation

New techniques of investigating disease are continually being developed and gradually become part of everyday practice. Improved cross-sectional imaging, miniaturization, and computerization are having increasing influences on healthcare practice. Computerized radiology now enables clinicians to work in a filmless department and to modify images in real time. For example, digital subtraction techniques reduce the volume of contrast needed for angiography and demonstrate better detail. In addition, three-dimensional images of internal organs can be generated to help pre-plan operations stereoscopically. This has particular uses in neurosurgery, vascular surgery, and hepatic and pancreatic surgery. Colour flow Doppler ultrasound allows flow disturbances in blood vessels to be detected deep within the body without resorting to direct invasion and sometimes avoids the need for angiography. These investigative techniques also enable detailed assessment of blood flow to specific organs and have proved useful in vascular, transplant, neurological, and obstetric surgical practice.

4.5 Computer-aided diagnosis

The clinical diagnosis of surgical pathology can prove elusive. Abdominal pain, for example, can be a symptom of many different pathologies. Techniques such as computer-aided diagnosis (CAD) may have a role to play in clinical management of patients as well as in teaching surgical trainees. CAD is limited by the skill and expertise of the programmers, but in West Lothian, a CAD system has been developed by Mr A. Gunn over many years and contains the largest database of the features of abdominal pain in Europe.

The skills trainees employ in determining the aetiology of abdominal pain in the Accident and Emergency department can be assessed by the feedback obtained from CAD analysis. Trainees can learn to improve their diagnostic and investigative skills interactively by referring to the diagnostic standards extracted from the database. This has proved to have a high predictive value for the origin of the symptoms and signs of abdominal pain. However, it should be remembered that the computer depends on the input from clinicians used in constructing the program and does not itself set the standards.

4.6 Direct access and day-case surgery as means of quality improvement

Direct access

With the current system of healthcare, emphasis is placed on service efficiency and value for money, and lessons learned in the United States over the past decade are gaining credence in the UK. 'One-stop' or open-access diagnostic services such as endoscopy may avoid the need for outpatient consultation, reduce the waiting time for patients and generally provide necessary treatment rapidly and efficiently on the first visit to hospital. On the down side, patients are not necessarily the best judge of where they should be referred and excessive numbers of 'worried well' may attend such clinics inappropriately.

Day-case surgery

Improvements in anaesthesia have brought many operative procedures into the province of day surgery. Day surgery is often perceived to be cheaper than inpatient care but any real cost benefit must be minimal. However, patients generally prefer to convalesce in their own surroundings and unblocking acute beds by day surgery can reduce waiting lists. The political value of this apparent 'streamlining' of care is high but there are disadvantages to day surgery. For example: specified day-case lists must be kept full; there is a high administrative cost; part of the care burden is shifted to GPs and the nursing burden on general wards increases because the 'light' cases have been removed. Furthermore, many patients undergoing, for example, day-case hernia repair, would prefer an overnight stay in hospital to allow the early pain and immobility to be managed in optimum conditions.

The efficient use of beds may be enhanced by the introduction of 'care hotel' beds for convalescent patients. These have the advantage of keeping patients 'on site' for review while reducing the service costs as patients are deemed to require low levels of nursing care. Care hotels have been implemented successfully in USA and Scandinavia, but examples in the UK have yet to make much impact.

5 Conclusions

Current clinical surgical practice varies widely in the UK. This may arise from the lack of properly directed and nationally approved clinical training. The traditional idea of 'see one, do one, teach one' no longer finds favour with the consumer and is unacceptable to the purchasing authorities. Surgeons are therefore charged with the task of setting the standards of surgical practice. Failure to do so will result ultimately in standards being imposed by government bodies perhaps not best qualified to do so. The 'surgical personality' may mislead surgeons into believing that they are providing the 'best' care possible for their patients, even if this is based largely on subjective opinions. This brings a diversity of current clinical practice with all the richness that entails, but with the drawback that the highest standards may not be propagated sufficiently widely. Too standardized a training risks stifling innovation and creativity, but there is no doubt that in certain areas, there is a 'best' way to perform a procedure. The danger is that a firmly established national training method is difficult to change when better methods arrive. Nevertheless, it is the surgical profession's responsibility to establish acceptable clinical standards.

The acquisition of basic and specialist surgical skills comes first, but the need for properly directed and controlled research remains the life-blood of future surgery. In the past, research has been used in many cases as a determinant of suitability to pursue a surgical career. However, large-scale research studies should ideally be performed only by those interested in academia and who are prepared to undertake the onerous task of developing, monitoring, gaining funding, and progressing a research programme.

The acquisition of a higher degree by the surgical trainee was once essential to progress through higher surgical training. In the restructured and shortened Calmanized training programmes, the necessity for a higher degree has been reduced except for trainees wishing to pursue an academic career or a particular avenue of research. Similarly, the view of 'publish or perish' may need to be modified. It must be in the interests of all surgeons to be able to spot problem areas in clinical practice and to solve some of them. The ability to read the medical literature critically is mandatory and the discipline involved in testing whether you have discovered something new, and in writing it up to convince ones peers, can be a worthwhile exercise. However, it should not replace time spent on clinical activities.

Trainees should all be encouraged to participate in a period of clinical or laboratory-based research, ideally within a 'taught course' leading to an M.Sc., for example. This provides exposure to research method and brings an appreciation of the intricacies of establishing aims, methods, statistical analysis, data presentation and interpretation, discussion of the results which is concise and focused, and altogether a wider general appreciation of the surgical literature. This equips the surgeon to analyse his or her own performance critically against current standards and any proposed new standards. Furthermore, a surgeon trained in these methods who is considering changing current practice can thoroughly assess the results of new trials and published studies and decide whether the data interpretation is reliable and robust, and the conclusions relevant.

Standards cannot be set unless current practice is monitored and assessed. Auditing of clinical results serves as a quality control for clinicians but data thus collected must be handled with care and not be allowed to fall into the hands of 'non-experts'. If the trend towards standard setting and performance indicators set by politicians and managers is to be resisted, surgeons must take this responsibility themselves. Greater understanding and cooperation between clinicians and NHS managers needs to develop to establish workable policies that are not threatening clinically; this can only be based on understanding of their respective roles and a degree of trust.

Surgeons should be prepared to monitor their results and to review the data critically. They may need to accept the logic of tertiary referral centres and other such changes in responsibility, but this will not come easily to general surgeons used to a broad, non-superspecialist practice. If properly set up, regional or supraregional centres, where resources and training are concentrated for the management of complex cases, must be beneficial to patients and surgeons. Indeed, there is a growing medicolegal imperative that states that tertiary referrals should be made when apparently insoluble problems arise. These centres have to be adequately funded and prepared to always accept appropriate referrals.

The future of the surgical profession lies in its own hands. Failure to accept the need for critical appraisal will result in this responsibility being applied from outside the profession. This can be resisted by a willingness to set high professional standards and strive to maintain them.

Bibliography

Andersen, B. (1990). *Methodological errors in medical research.* Blackwell Scientific Publications, Oxford.

Beauchamp, T.L. and Childress, J.F. (1983). *Principles of biomedical ethics.* Oxford University Press, Oxford.

Cuschieri, A. and Baker, P.R. (1977). *Introduction to research in medical sciences.* Churchill Livingstone, Edinburgh.

Hartley, R.J., Keen, E.M., Large, J.A., and Tedd, L.A. (1990). *On-line searching:principles and practice.* Butterworth, London.

Levine, R.J. (1986). *Ethics and regulation of clinical research.* Urban and Schwarzenberg, Baltimore-Munich.

McLean, S.A.M. (1995). Research ethics committees:principles and proposals. *Hlth Bull.,* 53, 243–8.

Mathie, R.T., Taylor, K.M., and Calman, J.S. (1989). *Principles of surgical research.* Butterworth, London.

Murrell, G., Huang, C., Langdon, C., and Ellis, H. (1990). *Research in medicine. A guide to writing a thesis in the medical sciences.* Cambridge University Press, Cambridge.

Wager, E., Tooley, P.J.H., Emanuel, M.B., and Wood, S.F. (1995). Get patients' consent to enter clinical trials. *BMJ,* 311, 734–7.

CHAPTER 3

Maintaining and improving the standards of surgical practice

J.D. Greig and C.R.G. Quick

1 Introduction

The principal aim of healthcare should be to prevent illness or at least to provide healthcare that is timely, appropriate, effective, efficient, and acceptable to the patient. It should also result in a favourable outcome in both the short term and the long term. At the same time, recovery after treatment should be uncomplicated and complete, while treatment should not predispose to secondary disorders (for example, susceptibility to infection or new malignancies following chemotherapy).

Measuring outcomes of healthcare is a growth industry, prompted largely by the upward spiralling of costs in healthcare world-wide. In order to create an efficient healthcare system, the health needs of a population need to be known so that the system can be appropriately resourced. In addition, the effectiveness of the care provided needs to be evaluated continually, so that resources can be directed to areas that bring about the greatest 'health gain' or the most appropriate relief from disease. The term 'health gain' is used more and more to decide whether particular treatments or screening programmes should be funded.

1.1 Terminology of the effectiveness of healthcare and outcomes

Efficacy

A treatment is efficacious if it succeeds on a given set of patients under standard conditions (e.g. a controlled clinical trial).

Effectiveness

This describes a treatment that works beneficially in regular clinical practice on a broad range of patients under a wide range of conditions. The **clinical effectiveness** of an intervention is a measure of the benefits to a population, whereas the **outcome** of a treatment relates to its effects on an individual.

Efficiency

The efficiency of a treatment relates to cost minimization, producing the maximum output for a given input. This is sometimes measured in 'cost per case'. Efficiency says little about the quality of what is being produced. Throughput may be high, such as in short hospital stays after surgery, but the impact of that care may be shifted to another sector. For example, in day-case surgery, there is a shift in activity from hospital to community. In broad terms the efficiency determines whether the investment in healthcare is worthwhile. **Cost effectiveness** includes efficiency along with some measure of quality.

Acceptability of treatment

This is a term of increasing relevance as the notion of the doctor as an authority figure recedes. Treatment must be acceptable to patients, their healthcare advisors, and to members of the healthcare team providing it.

Appropriateness of care

A term that has a different perspective when seen from different points of view; for example, the patient, the national treasury, the insurer, the doctor involved in research, and the GP.

Outcome of healthcare

This is simply the end result of a disease or intervention, although the term is increasingly being used in attempts to evaluate the performance of surgeons and other clinicians. However, it may not involve treatment, in which case the natural history may be the determining factor. The outcome has no implicit value, but the term is used to identify the benefits to the patient of healthcare (i.e. a favourable or an adverse change in health status). It is important to explore whether the perceived change in health really does result from the intervention and would not have happened in the natural evolution of the disorder.

Measurement of outcome on a broad front is difficult and fraught with drawbacks. In order to measure change, a measurement has to be made before the intervention takes place, ideally before the patient was ill. The measurement needs to be accurate, reproducible, and simple, and can often be achieved by employing a well-designed patient questionnaire. The point at which the effects of treatment should be measured and for what period the observation should continue remain subjects for discussion, and these vary according to the nature of the underlying pathology and its natural history.

In the context of measuring outcome and sustaining favourable outcomes, clinicians collectively should first determine the acceptable standards for patient care. For example, what is an acceptable rate of infection after uncomplicated inguinal hernia repair? At the same time, methods need to be implemented by which standards can be monitored and maintained, and a framework for improvement should be put in place. Ideally, these mechanisms should apply to the entire work

of a department, with special emphasis from time to time on areas of concern. Methods that address these aims are threefold:

◆ effective auditing of clinicians' working practices and implementation of recommended changes;

◆ continuing medical education through practical and educational elements; the former includes workshops and specified training sessions and the latter, scientific meetings and courses;

◆ anticipatory risk and care management planning using guidelines, patient education, and, where appropriate, employing a multidisciplinary approach to disease in hospitals and community (e.g. breast cancer, management of obstructive jaundice).

2 Surgical audit

Research is concerned with discovering the right thing to do; audit with ensuring that it is done right.

Richard Smith

It has been argued that every doctor can audit his or her own work and there is no need for other doctors to become involved. However, in practice, time constraints are usually too great for introspection and there is also a tendency to be overoptimistic about one's own practice. Medical or clinical audit is a means by which doctors can be accountable collectively for the quality of medical care. To achieve this, and to provide the educational objectives, requires a forum to be created in which doctors can scrutinize each other's work in a non-threatening and constructive manner. In a formal clinical audit of a particular topic, a group of doctors can meet and collectively agree what their objectives are in providing the aspect of care under discussion (i.e. agree the standards for **indicator based audit**). Data are then collected prospectively in a standard form and then peer review is employed to examine non-conforming cases and to decide why they do not conform. This approach is more likely to succeed than individual doctors giving subjective judgements of what is appropriate or acceptable. In essence, clinical audit examines the quality of care provided and seeks to measure it against standards of care which have already been established, or more often, against standards generated by those involved in the treatment.

Medical audit can be a powerful tool for improving the quality of medical care and for enhancing education of doctors. However, to be successful, it needs to be carried out in a formal and systematic manner. Early attempts to formalize the process with morbidity and mortality meetings to review collected figures (e.g. death rates or duration of hospital stay and individual problem cases) provided glimpses of what could be achieved, but provided little in the way of structured conclusions because patients are not uniform items to which general criteria can easily be applied and the results of intervention can become confused by concomitant medical illness, such as chronic respiratory insufficiency, diabetes, or heart disease.

Informal subjective mechanisms, such as morbidity and mortality meetings, are intrinsically flawed because they depend on total honesty in presenting and discussing one's own adverse outcomes. They do not allow for human nature and its extraordinary ability to forget or fail to learn from and disseminate knowledge about adverse events and errors. The meetings are based on complications affecting individuals, but usually fail to address recurring problems, such as rates of wound infection, or aspects of care seen from the patient's point of view. These include delays in treatment, offhand consultations, poor pain control, and failure to explain.

Systematic medical audit is not the same as financial audit nor is it about saving money. It is about improving the quality of delivery of healthcare by scientific analysis of often quite small and clearly defined aspects of the delivery of healthcare. The process embodies motivation for the right reasons (improving patient care rather than self-aggrandizement or denigrating other departments or specialists), being specific about objectives and measures of quality to be used, accepting the principles of peer review, and being committed to change current practices should weaknesses be revealed. All of this has to be carried out while maintaining the confidentiality of doctors and patients. Medical audit works by encouraging the natural tendency of all doctors to heal the sick and soothe the dying to the best of their ability. This includes knowing the results of their work and how it concurs with current literature.

There are many potential pitfalls in the audit process which need to be considered before an audit study is begun. The audit may breach medical ethics or produce inaccurate data and, as a result, produce inappropriate changes in patient management. Items that need to be addressed include:

- the type of audit needed;

- data collection—completeness, accuracy of recorded data, methods of recording data, avoiding duplication;

- maintaining confidentiality of patients and the anonymity of the clinicians;

- outcome measures to be used in assessing quality;

- implementing change—if a better way is found to manage patient care, how can clinicians be convinced of the need for change? They first need to believe that the audit process has been accurate and reliable. After that, what steps need to be undertaken to ensure that change occurs?

2.1 Medical research versus medical audit

The purposes of medical audit are several:

- to compare present practitioners and performance systems with defined measures;

- to show how well research-based 'good care' is put into practice;

- to demonstrate the quality of medical care provided.

Surgical research usually looks at a single problem, with an encapsulated project to determine the relationships between structure or process and outcome by analysing complex data. Clinical audit uses outcomes as indirect evidence that structure and process were appropriate by analysing data through an ongoing process of collection. The average doctor is likely to make only tiny strides in improving the care of patients through medical research, but every doctor has the opportunity to improve the way his or her patients are cared for by critically examining his or her own practices against current expectations or standards.

Medical audit shares certain characteristics with medical research, as with any scientific approach to measurement. These include the need to define explicit objectives of the evaluation, to apply valid measurements, to establish precise definitions of the concepts to be measured, to analyse data by scrutinizing it in accordance with agreed and acknowledged methods, and to interpret data fairly and without bias. Carried out systematically and scientifically, medical audit can show how actual practice matches up to predefined standards. Patient care under scrutiny in this way can improve knowledge, develop guidelines for management, and pinpoint areas where education needs to be concentrated.

After collecting the data, the latter part of the audit process is what distinguishes audit from research. Given a commitment to change practises if shown to be necessary, analysing the data to identify problems and their causes, implementing action to achieve improvements, and following up, usually by repeat audit after a defined interval, is what can make medical audit into a quality assurance mechanism. There is a natural tendency to stop audit when the data collection is complete (after quality has been assessed). Unless these data are segregated into instances of acceptable care and unacceptable care, it is unlikely that quality will be improved as a result of the assessment.

Clinicians need to be trained in audit method and they need to be helped to design audits that are scientifically sound. Otherwise the population samples that are used may be inappropriate and the data collected by unsatisfactory sampling methods, resulting in analyses that are unsound.

2.2 Subjects for audit

Subjects for detailed audit scrutiny should be selected for their ability to reveal something about the quality of patient care currently provided and with the potential to discover means of improving that patient care. A group considering topics for audit should consider the frequency with which the proposed condition or treatment occurs, the level of risk to patients without treatment or as a result of treatment, any areas where there is concern about whether treatment is up to date, areas where patient care crosses specialties, and, finally, to take account of topics of particular interest to the doctors and other health professionals involved in care.

Single-subject audits do not require large groups of patients. Systematic observation of 20–50 patients will usually reveal sufficient information to analyse and plan improvements. A homogeneous group needs to be defined by diagnosis, by surgical or drug treatment, by investigation, or even by day of the week.

For the subject selected, specific objectives should be identified. These focus on important aspects of the process of care (including resources employed), appropriateness of tests or treatments, outcomes of treatment. They may include aspects of care as seen from the patient's point of view, such as delays in treatment, offhand consultations, poor pain control, and failure to explain. The first objective of the study should be to define what represents good-quality care in the subject selected. It should not be to prove a firmly held point of view. This objective is achieved by discussion and agreement about what quality their own treatment should achieve by a group of health professionals involved.

By setting objective and measurable standards of care which have all been agreed by the group, fruitless future discussion can be avoided about what represents 'a good standard of care' in terms of appropriate clinical behaviour or judgement. A standard of care specifies what and how patient care should be provided as determined by professional knowledge and judgement. This is developed into an audit indicator which specifies how that standard should be audited and incorporates a measurable criterion and specifies a percentage of cases that would be expected to reach that standard. For example, perhaps 100 per cent of patients referred for palliative radiotherapy for lung cancer should receive their first treatment in no more than 10 days after referral, or wound infection rates after appendicectomy should be no more than 3 per cent. These indicators (also known as criteria) may be based on published results or on previous local results, or by setting standards that the group would hope to achieve by running pilot studies.

2.3 Criterion-based or indicator-based audit

Key elements

- ◆ Looks in detail at a relatively small aspect of medical care in a carefully structured way.

- ◆ Accepts that there is often more than one equally valid way of achieving the solution to a problem.

- ◆ Requires clinicians and audit officers to take time to plan the audit, discuss the results, and implement change.

- ◆ It is important that information about whether criteria have been met is capable of being retrieved reliably by non-medical audit officers.

Construction of audit criteria or indicators

There are several ways of constructing indicators, but each method has four common components to be agreed:

- ◆ the standard that represents quality in the aspect of care under audit;

- ◆ the percentage of cases expected to conform to that standard—cases that fail to conform to this are subjected to detailed analysis to find out where care is substandard; in most cases, the percentage is 100 per cent or 0 per cent (i.e. all cases conform or none conforms);

- ◆ permitted exceptions to the defined aspect of care, which are clinically acceptable and are known in advance to account for failing to conform;

- ◆ definitions and instructions about where to look for data, such as the values that determine concordance with the indicators.

Samples of audit criteria (indicators) include one or more of the following list, which is not exhaustive.

Outcome-orientated criteria

- ◆ Mortality;

- ◆ individual complications;

- ◆ degree of relief of symptoms;

- ◆ short-term results of specific treatments;

- ◆ adverse events;

- ◆ health status at discharge;

- ◆ patient level of knowledge about his or her condition;

- ◆ extent of ability to live independently after discharge;

- ◆ longer-term health status or functioning;

- ◆ degree of patient satisfaction.

Process-orientated criteria

- ◆ Appropriateness of assessment;

- ◆ diagnosis, treatment, recognition, and response to indications for treatment;

- ◆ technical performance of a procedure;

- ◆ patients' rights.

Resource-orientated criteria

- ◆ Examination of the use of equipment, beds, support services, money;

- ◆ day-case surgery versus overnight stay versus formal inpatient stay;

- ◆ community based evaluation of health screening programmes.

Avoiding the 'surgeon H' phenomenon

Analysis of non-conforming cases by peers involves judgement of whether variation between cases represents acceptable or unacceptable care. Certain circumstances may account for variations without flagging the substandard card. These include a faulty indicator which omitted an important exception or inappropriate definition, a complex case which did not conform but still represents appropriate care, and a mistake in data collection.

The infamous Glasgow-based paper which examined clinical outcome by individual (but unnamed) surgeons in terms of mortality and morbidity following colorectal surgery, was audit based and generated furious debate within the profession. On the one hand, it showed that there was considerable inter-surgeon variation in outcome for a particular disease group of patients, which was especially poor in the hands of 'surgeon H'. On the other hand, it generated substantial criticism directed at the authors because of the methods utilized to collect, sample, and analyse the data. Furthermore, the media and politicians misinterpreted the highly publicized outcome data from this study, and this generated a background of suspicion and fear by the public that they might be treated by a 'surgeon H'. The public clearly has a right to know that clinicians have reached an acceptable standard and practice within it, but this right should not become a witch hunt by media and politicians. Informed interpretation of outcome data is required before releasing information as sensitive as this to the general public. Often however, the motivation to adopt this altruistic advice is dictated by other issues and concerns. The original intention of the Glasgow study was well meaning, but the distorted or selective interpretation of its results are a salient example of the need for the profession to ask the right questions and draw the correct conclusions when it audits itself in order to influence healthcare favourably in the future.

Peer-group review of medical audit data

When unacceptable variations in care are revealed, the peer group may look for patterns that explain the variation. This is often a single factor, such as patient education, one type of patient, or one area of the hospital. Problems with data will also become apparent, such as missing information, lack of discharge summaries, lack of dates, inaccurate coding, or lost or missing records. Variations may be due to a particular practitioner, but if not, those attributable to institutional or community factors need to be acted upon.

Using audit indicators may be seen as time consuming, technical, and narrow as regards overall patient care, but it has several advantages over raw data analysis or informal meetings. For example, valid conclusions can be reached about important aspects of patient care, sufficient to support implementation of remedial action. Simple yes–no decisions about concordance with audit indicators can be made by trained clerical or audit assistant staff, saving doctors' time. If necessary, large numbers of cases can be screened by this method to sort out those that vary from the standards for further discussion. Cases that need review can be agreed in advance by medical peers, for example, those that fail to meet the agreed indicators. Thus there should be no disagreement about which cases are to be discussed. Furthermore, the process of developing audit indicators is an educational experience in itself for those who participate, which

simplifies future audits and encourages an atmosphere of self-criticism by individual, department, unit, or region.

Analysis and discussion should reveal how to rectify demonstrated weaknesses in cases that deviate from the expected results. They may be due to poor coordination (for example between the outpatient department and admissions department), poor performance, deficiencies in resources (hardware, personnel, time for clinicians, surveillance, medical records), or specialized treatments being attempted inappropriately when they should have been referred to specialists. Improvements may result from simple changes in organization; for example, change in appointment timing, further training, or concentration of particular cases in specialist hands (local or elsewhere).

2.4 Confidentiality and anonymity

Patients whose care is being evaluated and the professionals whose judgement, behaviour, and performance are being examined through medical audit are entitled to privacy. This is the only way to persuade clinicians to be entirely honest. Thus any documentation pertaining to medical audit must protect the identities of patients and those professionally involved. Non-identifiable codes rather than names should be used on forms and computers, with only one holder of the translation. Confidential integrity can be maintained by avoiding recording names, initials, dates of birth, and dates of treatment in minutes of audit meetings, and reports should be general rather than specific in their findings. A written confidentiality policy should be agreed that applies to every care setting where medical audit is conducted.

2.5 The audit cycle

Despite its value for improving quality and its popularity in the United States and other countries such as Saudi Arabia, medical audit was initially unpopular with grant-giving bodies and medical journals in UK, so there was little stimulus to initiate it or to develop the mechanisms. However, the White Paper and Act of Parliament, *Working for patients*, gave the stimulus by providing central funds to establish departments of medical audit. It also mandated that all doctors should be involved in the medical audit process.

This initiative led to vigorous activity by many people to develop and implement systematic and refined methods of peer review acceptable to those involved, with the clear aim of improving all aspects of current patient care. The Royal Colleges now insist that their approval of training posts in hospitals depends on junior doctor involvement in medical audit.

The scope of medical audit has expanded to involve professions allied to medicine, community care, and general practice, and the broader brief has been renamed clinical audit. This is generally described as a cycle composed of several stages. It is a raft of methods of improving current performance by determining what is ideal (setting standards, as discussed in Chapter 2), analysing the real situation (measuring current performance), and finding ways of shifting practice from the real to the ideal. Finally, the cycle is closed by re-auditing the perceived improvement in practice after an interval, to assess the effectiveness of the change that has been implemented and to ensure that changes have occurred with beneficial results.

2.6 Examples of how audit may improve the quality of medical care

◆ Reduction of risk of morbidity or mortality;

◆ improved effectiveness of care, such as streamlined processes of treatment;

◆ improvement in diagnosis—availability, appropriateness, or quality;

◆ improved timing of care—reduced delay, better planning, efficient use of facilities;

◆ better use of resources—equipment, beds, support services, money;

◆ consumer satisfaction—patients and referring doctors;

◆ access to care—availability of diagnostic services and treatment;

◆ documentation and records—improved recording of the process of care;

◆ identifying educational needs by audit activity (e.g. pain management).

2.7 Introducing audit into surgical practice

Most surgical units now practise some form of surgical audit to improve the quality of practice. The most common method is regular peer-group morbidity and mortality meetings, where deaths and complications over a recent period are discussed. Even the most conscientious doctor tends to forget the failures and to remember the successes, and data for these meetings are time consuming to collect and unreliable in retrospect, therefore each case needs to be written down as the patient is treated. It is best to record all adverse events, even if doubt exists as to whether they represent complications; the meeting can decide whether they qualify. Many units now have computer systems to help in data collection, but it is easy to imagine that computer data collection is surgical audit. For this purpose, the computer is only a sophisticated data store, allowing rapid retrieval of cases that match selection criteria.

Effective audit can be conducted without computers, and computers cannot compensate for inadequate methods. Even with complete data, there are pitfalls which impair the educational value of morbidity and mortality meetings. Meetings can become threatening if conducted in a way that appears to victimize doctors presenting their problem cases. It is important that meetings are conducted in a non-judgmental way in order to encourage participants to bring all possible cases for discussion and not be tempted to conceal or 'forget' embarrassing

ones. Meetings need to be chaired by a senior clinician, either rotating members of the surgical department or even bringing in, for example, a general physician, who could give unbiased comment. The chairman should be responsible for ensuring clear presentations, guiding and summarizing discussion, leading the meeting to reach conclusions about whether adverse events were unavoidable (e.g. a patient admitted to die of terminal cancer) or potentially avoidable, and if avoidable, whether any general change of policy could be brought about to minimize risk in the future. General conclusions should be published and circulated to participants for later reference. It may also be appropriate for the chairman to produce a brief report of what was discussed and be responsible for implementing any changes recommended. All clinical staff should give these meetings priority, officially adjusting clinical commitments if necessary. There should be a sign-in register. The format of audit meetings should be varied to include notes reviews, topic reviews presented by juniors or seniors, discussions about criterion-based projects, and clinico-pathological conferences.

Key elements of mortality and morbidity meetings

◆ Avoid witch hunting (constructive versus destructive criticism);

◆ continual observation of activities in the surgical unit;

◆ recent activity should be reviewed so that cases known to junior doctors;

◆ establish guidelines for future management when problems are pinpointed;

◆ meetings must be consultant led, otherwise there will be no incentive for juniors to attend and no worthwhile conclusions will be reached;

◆ ideally, the chairman should be from a different specialty;

◆ thorough preparation of cases should occur in advance, remembering confidentiality;

◆ a report (respecting confidentiality), which needs to be implemented, should be produced after each meeting; an audit officer could check on implementation by re-audit at intervals;

◆ include conclusions in standing orders for department;

Specific areas in surgical practice which may be audited

◆ Common conditions (e.g. management of varicose veins);

◆ expensive (e.g. palliative chemotherapy for cancer);

◆ dangerous (e.g. oesophagectomy);

◆ topics giving cause for local concern (e.g. waiting times for outpatient appointments for breast lumps).

General rules for successful medical audit

◆ Keep it simple and avoid overambitious studies;

◆ arrange the next meeting with clinicians each time;

◆ keep track of progress along the audit cycle and re-audit;

◆ produce regular reports.

Problems in setting up an audit programme

◆ Where to start;

◆ lack of interest or cooperation from clinicians—they need to see the point;

◆ large hospitals and entrenched ideas—start small, with keen clinicians, then seek out others gradually;

◆ computers and compatibility—decide which word processor, database, or spreadsheet to use and find ways of exchanging data;

◆ training for audit assistants—may need outside help;

◆ medical records—inability to find records or reluctance to find records;

◆ money—staff, hardware, and budgets—the unit will usually have funded the initial cost out of monies distributed nationally; important topics may attract regional or central funding.

Initiating an audit programme

◆ Set up a central office for 'quality' that is accessible, reliable, and informative, which clinicians will eventually not be able to do without;

◆ train staff of appropriate levels and keep a list of part-timers able to help;

◆ computers are valuable tools but need to be used appropriately;

◆ medical records officers and medical secretaries should be encouraged to participate;

◆ the audit chairman needs to be enthusiastic and objective without being didactic, and to encourage keen clinicians in all specialties to attend; meetings should be minuted and reports produced;

◆ junior staff should take part and help to produce audits they find satisfying;

◆ cross-specialty audits should be encouraged (e.g. Accident and Emergency/orthopaedics, pathology/surgery/anaesthetics;

◆ audits between hospital and community or general practitioners can be useful;

◆ feedback is vital—publish results of audits locally (and nationally).

Structuring a medical audit report for the district audit committee

Before submitting a report, the local audit committee needs to know which doctors are involved in audit, that regular meetings are held and attendances recorded, what issues have been considered and what action taken, and whether there are any unresolved issues. Additional information is required about the nature of studies being undertaken, the protocols produced to effect a change in practice, the outcome after the audit cycle has been closed in terms of improvement to practice and/or patient satisfaction, and, finally, whether any statistics have been generated for wider debate.

The reports should be produced at specified intervals, arbitrarily 6 monthly, and include a summary of each meeting held. There should not be any reference to individual patients nor specific peer criticism on record. Discretion must be used in describing inadequacies in patient management. Reports are better if they are structured by specialty, listing the chairman, meetings, and attendances. Where there is more than one speciality involved in the audit, then a cross-specialty report would be more appropriate. A report needs to specify whether a comment refers to one case, a specially prepared review of a subject, or a formal project or study, and whether the effect of the report has been assessed.

Reports may need to be given to several bodies—district health authority, hospital management board, community health council. Structured reporting, relating achieved improvements in care, as in the list following, can be efficient and effective for these purposes. Bruce Campbell recommended that reports should contain information relating to:

◆ reduction of risk (morbidity and mortality);

◆ effectiveness of care (indicate how intended benefits to patients have been achieved);

◆ improvement in diagnosis (availability or appropriateness or quality of diagnosis);

◆ timing of care (reduction of delays, good planning, use of facilities);

◆ better use of resources (use of equipment, beds, support services, money);

◆ consumer satisfaction (patients and referring doctors);

◆ access to care (availability of diagnostic services and treatment);

◆ documentation and records (improvement in recording the process of care);

◆ educational needs identified by audit activity (e.g. pain control);

◆ participants in meetings should be asked to highlight important issues by specialty and an audit officer can coordinate cross-specialty matters.

Lothian Surgical Audit (LSA)

Edinburgh and the Scottish Lothians have led the way in pioneering medical audit in the United Kingdom. The origin of LSA can be traced to 1946 when Sir James Learmonth inaugurated weekly mortality meetings in the Royal Infirmary of Edinburgh, which expanded in scope to include the whole of Edinburgh and eventually the Lothian Region. These continue today in the form of morbidity and mortality meetings with presentation of audit and research projects by individual units on Saturday mornings at the Royal College of Surgeons of Edinburgh during university term-time. Their success is gauged by a regular attendance of 50–60 surgeons plus their trainees.

In addition, true surgical audit was pioneered in Lothian in the late 1970s by Tony Gunn, Vaughan Ruckley, and Rosamund Gruer. Between 1978 and 1982 they looked at 16 areas of surgical practice and devised a unified system whereby all operations were coded by central coders for later analysis. The system was used initially as a research tool. However, because of its success and applicability, in 1983 the emphasis changed to enable surgeons to code their own operations based on a 40-organ system. From its inception, data was stored on computer. Up to 1995, a massive database of over 300 000 operations has been stored in this way.

In the government White Paper *Working for patients*, the fundamental work of Lothian Surgical Audit was recognized for its peer-review structure, and to a degree formed the model recommended for other areas. LSA resulted directly in the establishment and organization of specialized units in vascular surgery, urology, and others. In addition, LSA established early on that audit at unit level could inspire changes in individual practice. LSA now has to examine its objectives while continuing the audit. An example can be seen in the Lothian and Borders Colorectal Cancer Audit and similar ventures, such as the examination of the management of oesophageal and gastric cancers.

3   Day-case surgery as an example of regional audit

3.1   The cost-effectiveness of day-case surgery

Introduction

In the past decade there has been a major drive to increase throughput of surgical patients in all specialities by means of day surgery. The intention is to reduce waiting lists, improve consumer satisfaction, and reduce inpatient hospital costs. Judging whether these objectives have been achieved requires established standards of care for individual procedures and the ability to compare day-case and inpatient care for the same condition against the same standards. Several subsidiary aspects related to utilization of resources and the process and outcome of care also need to be studied in the audit process.

Appropriateness

- ◆ Is day surgery the best way of performing all those procedures regularly performed that way?
- ◆ Are inappropriate patients or patients with inappropriate conditions being brought forward for day-case surgery?

Quality of care

- ◆ Patient satisfaction—preference for type of surgery, opinion as to the way they were prepared and treated, opinion about outcome.
- ◆ Can day cases be done with shorter time on waiting lists?
- ◆ Are the results from day surgery and inpatient surgery comparable (e.g. quality of repair for hernia, complication rates and severity, recognition and treatment of complications)?
- ◆ Are day patients exposed too early to housework, looking after children, or a demand for mental activity when they should be resting away from the home environment?

Information

- ◆ What is the quality of transfer information provided to patients, general practitioners, and practice nurses? Are doctors working on day surgery satisfied with the quality of case notes? These should be compared with regular notes and with discharge notes and summaries.
- ◆ Are protocols for case selection, preoperative assessment, patient information, and follow-up adequate?
- ◆ Are there proper protocols for readmitting patients with inadequate analgesia or wound/procedure complications?

Cost

It is recognized that there is a need for senior staff to anaesthetize and to perform surgery and that certain procedures, such as hernia repair, may be carried out under local anaesthesia. Given this extra cost:

- ◆ Is day-case surgery cheaper than inpatient care for equivalent cases?
- ◆ Where is the money spent in day surgery compared with overnight low-dependency admission? (Is the average bed day cost of any use for comparison?)
- ◆ Is there a hidden cost per day case, such as extra transport, administration, clerical staff, nurse and general practitioner visiting costs, both in terms of finance and health professionals' time? Other costs for the patient may include spouse required to be off work or extra paid care needed at home and for the hospital services, as well as additional need for outpatient follow-up.

The true costs of running a day-case unit are perhaps best discovered by examining established units or by consulting private hospitals and insurance companies about their relative costs. Specific groups may gain special advantage or disadvantage from day surgery. For example, different age groups, or repeat procedures such as cystoscopy or laser treatment.

Views to be canvassed

These include:

- patients;
- consultants, both surgical and anaesthetic;
- hospital nurses;
- hospital management and financial services;
- general practitioners;
- practice and community nurses and managers.

3.2 Aspects of day-case surgery

Case selection

- What proportion of cases with a given condition or range of conditions is excluded from day surgery and why (age, infirmity, home circumstances)?
- Does this have a bearing on the viability of day-case surgery for certain conditions?
- What proportion of patients presenting for day surgery prove to be inappropriate and have to be rejected?
- What cost to efficiency does this involve?

Preparation of the patient

- Are schemes of preoperative physical assessment adequate and safe? Is documentation foolproof?
- Is psychological preparation of the patient adequate? Do patients know what to expect?

Operation and anaesthesia

- Informed consent is required.
- Are differences in surgical technique required?
- Are special anaesthetic techniques required, and if so, how do they differ from inpatient techniques? Are they equally satisfactory (e.g. can regional techniques be used on day cases)?
- Are there cost differences between methods of anaesthesia?
- A shorter period is often spent in the recovery room as patients are given general anaesthesia designed to ensure they awake rapidly. Procedures performed under local anaesthesia require less time in recovery. Both of these have the potential for increasing throughput of patients.

In-hospital postoperative care

- How much nursing care is required for day cases as compared with inpatients?

- Analgesia—is it satisfactory over the whole recovery period in both groups?
- Is more analgesia required for early transport home?

Transport

- Are special arrangements needed?
- Are costs different?
- Is transport satisfactory from the patient's point of view (analgesia, pain on movement)?

Home care

- Adequacy for day cases and inpatients.

Follow-up and rehabilitation

- What factors affect rate of recovery to normal living, such as pain, mobility, psychological factors?
- Do any problems occur that would not have happened in hospital, such as pain and damage during transport, falls, DVT due to inadequate mobilization?
- Were any problems not recognized or managed correctly at home (e.g. bleeding)?
- Were there any unplanned visits to general practitioners, casualty, outpatients in either group?
- Do histology and other follow-up reports reach general practitioners in a timely manner?

Each of the stages of setting up a day-case unit in terms of efficiency and cost effectiveness can be subjected to a detailed audit analysis in turn, as outlined above. However, closure of the audit loop with reference to day-case surgery can only be achieved after a unit has been running for a period of time. After that, comparisons can be made between day care and inpatient care for comparable conditions and decisions made on the grounds of economy, efficacy, and effectiveness, as well as patient satisfaction about whether the unit should remain open and about the type of cases to be treated and how.

4 National surgical morbidity and mortality surveys

4.1 Introduction and CEPOD

There are several continuing national surveys assessing mortality within particular areas of patient care. These include confidential enquiries into neonatal, maternal, and anaesthetic deaths; the Scottish Assessment of Surgical Mortality study; and the National Confidential Enquiry into Perioperative deaths (NCEPOD). None of these is a true audit since denominators are not used. Nevertheless, they can provide invaluable information to help in improving the quality of care.

These surveys report annually and each has produced valuable information on healthcare and has highlighted deficiencies. As a result, changes to overcome these deficiencies have been implemented with the backing of national bodies. Assessing the efficacy of these changes is itself a continuing process, but all involved in the fields targeted have noticed beneficial changes. The conception, inception, and prosecution of the original 1987 CEPOD report will be considered in more detail.

The Confidential Enquiry into Perioperative Deaths (CEPOD)

The study was designed to describe aspects of the delivery of surgical and anaesthetic care in Britain by reference to perioperative deaths. It was conceived in 1983 jointly by the Association of Surgeons of Great Britain and Ireland and the Association of Anaesthetists, and a pilot study was first performed involving three health districts—Darlington, Exeter, and Middlesex.

This was followed by CEPOD which reviewed all deaths within 30 days of a surgical operation (all specialties) in three regions (Northern, South West and NE Thames) throughout 1986. 500 000 operations were reviewed, in which there were 4000 deaths (0.8 per cent); 79 per cent of deaths occurred in patients over 65 years of age. A local reporter notified deaths, and the consultant surgeon and anaesthetist involved with that patient's care each completed a very detailed questionnaire. These responses were reviewed by a panel of assessors who gave their joint opinion as to:

◆ cause of death;

◆ avoidable elements;

◆ departures from ideal practice;

◆ whether the patient should have been operated upon;

◆ whether death could be attributed to surgery or anaesthesia;

◆ the choice of operation and quality of management;

◆ appropriateness of grade of staff;

◆ any failure of organization or equipment;

◆ any failure to apply knowledge.

Reviewers also reached conclusions as to the cause of mortality in each case from the following list:

◆ surgery, and/or anaesthesia, and/or presenting 'surgical' disease, and/or intercurrent disease (co-morbidity);

◆ inappropriate operation;

◆ inappropriate preoperative management;

◆ inappropriate grade of surgeon/anaesthetist;

◆ failure of organization or equipment;

◆ drug effect;

◆ technical failure: lack of knowledge, care or experience; fatigue/physical or mental impairment.

The initial report was published in December 1987 and the principle findings were as follows:

◆ there was 95 per cent cooperation in this voluntary study;

◆ gross discrepancies were found in facilities available to different consultants and their expectations;

◆ the quality of hospital notes was often inadequate to enable questionnaires to be completed;

◆ patient's weight was often not recorded, urine was often not tested, and prophylaxis against thromboembolism and hepatorenal failure were neglected;

◆ few deaths had been reviewed collectively;

◆ results of the peer review were rarely requested from the CEPOD committee.

The most common diagnoses in patients who died were fractured neck of femur (12 per cent); intestinal obstruction (7 per cent); aortic aneurysm (5 per cent); peptic ulcer (5 per cent); and colonic cancer (5 per cent). The most common cause of death was bronchopneumonia (13.5 per cent); congestive heart failure (11 per cent); myocardial infarction (8.5 per cent); pulmonary embolism (8 per cent); and respiratory failure (6.5 per cent). Most deaths occurred in the elderly, who were often subjected to long operations when in poor condition. Surgical assessors considered surgery culpable in 30 per cent of deaths, with failure of preoperative management found in one in three patients; the grade of surgeon was inappropriate in one in five patients; and there were avoidable elements in one in five patients. The assessors also determined that 6.5 per cent of cases should not have had an operation; anaesthetic deaths only accounted for 1.8 per cent; progression of surgical disease contributed to death in 67.5 per cent; and progress of co-morbid disease was relevant in 44 per cent of patients.

Anaesthesia and CEPOD

Everyone knows there is a great deal of operative intervention out of hours, when the need of the patient is not as urgent as the timing implies.

British Journal of Anaesthesia

When juniors were responsible for anaesthetizing patients who died, consultants were asked for advice in only 21 per cent of cases. Anaesthetists were not satisfied with preoperative preparation in 14 per cent of cases, yet they still allowed the operation to proceed. The role of anaesthesia in surgical deaths was commendably small—perhaps a result of the three previous anaesthetic mortality studies. The simple message that arose was that adequate preoperative resuscitation of patients prior to surgery would have been of benefit in many cases when the precipitating admission pathology was not life-threatening. Furthermore, surgery should not be undertaken in the middle of the night unless the patient has a bleeding diathesis, a perforated viscus, or abdominal trauma.

Principal findings related to poor surgical practice

The elementary pharmacology of local anaesthetics was misunderstood and resulted in 172 deaths. Unfortunately, further detail was absent from the report about this astounding finding. Only 36 per cent of leaking aneurysms were operated on by consultants and nearly half of deaths after oesophagectomy were surgeon-related. Of the operations performed for colorectal cancer, 13 per cent were carried out at night, for which no clear justification could be found, and five patients with pseudo-obstruction died after unnecessary operations. Just over half of the 60 deaths after hernia operations were attributable to surgery and one-third had inadequate resuscitation. Nineteen patients died after surgery for acute biliary disease: five after operations for pancreatitis. There was frequently a lack of appropriate antibiotics, and an inappropriate grade of surgeon carrying out difficult surgery in many.

Educational lessons from CEPOD

Many of the substandard practices identified could be put down to a lack of education in particular fields. These included:

◆ when and how to investigate;

◆ when to give prophylaxis, against both infection and thromboembolism;

◆ when to delay operation in order to resuscitate;

◆ when not to operate;

◆ when to call the consultant;

◆ management of head injuries;

◆ managing co-morbid disease;

◆ managing the elderly;

◆ keeping accurate records;

◆ safe use of local anaesthetics;

◆ local protocols for referral, handover, and transfer;

◆ organizing effective audit or morbidity and mortality meetings (i.e. structured meetings of all clinicians involved, reviewing poor outcomes together, non-judgementally, and then adjusting their practice accordingly).

4.2 National Confidential Enquiry into Perioperative Deaths (NCEPOD)

Following the initial CEPOD report, the study was consolidated into the continuing national CEPOD study (NCEPOD). The NCEPOD report for 1990 was published in 1992. This study focused on comparisons between patients who lived after surgery and patients who died within 30 days of surgery. These were randomly chosen for sampling and analysis. The study was authoritative and comprehensive; only 10 of the 7000 clinicians whose work could have been sampled refused to participate. This was the largest sample of surgical and anaesthetic cases ever to be randomly and jointly audited by both disciplines.

During 1990, 18 817 deaths were reported within 30 days of surgery, of which one-fifth were selected randomly to be assessed. Marked improvements in standards were observed in comparison with the 1987 CEPOD report. For example, 89 per cent of the preoperative decision-making was consultant based, compared with only 63 per cent in 1987; and 67 per cent of operating was done or supervised by consultants, compared with 47 per cent in the 1987 report. The report continued to highlight deficiencies in data collection, the standard of clinical notes, dabbling surgeons, and the absence of prophylaxis against thromboembolism. Above all, it signalled to the general public and central government that the medical profession could and would audit itself and there was no need for the imposition of external audit.

4.3 Scottish Assessment of Surgical Mortality (SASM)

It is difficult to understand why Scotland was not included in NCEPOD, but the origins appear to lie within the realms of the Scottish Office. The intention to assess deaths in Scotland was initiated by a Conference of the Royal Colleges and a standing committee under the chairmanship of Professor Spence. Mortality data were collected in Glasgow and Edinburgh from 1988 until the early 1990s. At that point, Greater Glasgow Health Board (the largest in the UK) decided to initiate its own in-depth study, termed the Greater Glasgow Mortality Study. Simultaneously, an East Scotland group based in Edinburgh set up a comparable study involving Dundee, Aberdeen, and Inverness. SASM became a reality in 1993 when East and West Scotland pooled resources to form a unified body, with mechanisms to assess all surgical deaths in Scotland rather than just a random sample of deaths and this is its fundamental difference from NCEPOD.

There are an average of 5000 deaths annually in surgical wards in Scottish hospitals. All deaths are examined without selection and include patients who have undergone operations and also, of particular interest, those who have not. Furthermore, the assessors have access to the case records and therefore the report is not anonymized prior to assessment as in NCEPOD. However, the final report, which is distributed to all surgeons and anaesthetists, is anonymized to make it extremely difficult to ascertain the place of a particular death. The success of this mortality study in honestly reporting deaths and the quality of assessment is manifest by high compliance (99 per cent in the East of Scotland and 80 per cent in the West of Scotland). The importance of this work has been recognized by government and it is now centrally funded.

5 Quality control and risk management

With ever-reducing junior hospital doctors hours, it is even more imperative that the written clinical record for all patients is kept up to date, informative, and can demonstrate the current management strategy. This applies to both the original clerking and the continuation notes. Furthermore, there must be adequate handover of patients at house officer, middle grade, and senior levels during periods of absence and at the end of full or partial shifts. This means that briefing includes details of particularly ill patients and those with intricate management problems. Communication needs to be thorough and effective, both verbally and in writing.

5.1 Communication points in the clinical record

◆ Is each entry signed legibly and the name given in block capitals?

◆ Are blood results written in notes?

◆ Has a hand written note been made in the continuation notes regarding the operation and principal findings, with clear postoperative instructions?

◆ Are the instructions for antibiotic and deep venous thrombosis prophylaxis clearly indicated?

◆ Are the operation and anaesthetic notes completed and readily available?

◆ Have discussions with relatives (and patient) been documented in notes, with particular reference to poor prognosis, withdrawal of active treatment, knowledge of whether patients or relatives have been told about malignancy?

◆ In high operative risk patients, has the consultant documented prior to surgery that this is so and discussed it with relatives?

◆ Have all laboratory and radiographic results been filed before the formal discharge summary is completed?

◆ Was a hand-written discharge summary completed and sent within 48 hours?

◆ Was a final discharge summary sent within 10 days?

◆ Was the diagnosis clearly recorded in the summary?

◆ If the patient died, was the cause of death given on the certificate recorded in the notes?

5.2 Information technology and the medical record

The general expansion in information technology (IT) has the potential for major beneficial changes at ward level regarding the admission, management, and discharge documentation for any patient. However, medical IT lags far behind its application in industry. This is for a variety of reasons, including: lack of investment in programming, lack of standardization, poor communication between incompatible computer systems, and, until recently, the lack of a unique patient identifier to allow cross-disciplinary studies. A major factor against widespread computerization is the need for speed and convenience. Doctors are generally hard-pressed and any system that demands extra processes or that proves unreliable will simply not be used.

The technical ability has long been available to allow information systems to perform sophisticated tasks, but implementation has been slow and patchy compared with other countries, such as Denmark. Systems can allow direct screen access to haematological, biochemical, radiological, and pathological results on ward patients, rather than the house officer having to telephone for results or wait for delivery of printed reports. Graphic tablet technology could allow hand-written entries to be recognized and translated into printed text, avoiding possible illegible continuation or clerking notes. Computerized pharmacy packages have already been piloted in an effort to reduce errors on ward prescribing, encourage the use of generic drugs or drugs listed on a hospital formulary, and to warn of potential drug interactions. Pilot schemes are under way to manage patients throughout with a paperless admission but there is a long way to go. Caution is needed, however, as fail-safe back-up of information is required in the event of a computer crash. Eventually, graphic tablets may give way to voice recognition technology, which will further encourage rapid and accurate documentation of salient information.

Instant printed discharge summaries can be produced from a common source admission documentation held on a central file server for hospital admissions, with, for example, a one-line summary entered by the resident about diagnosis and treatment for the general practitioner. These could replace the poorly produced, illegibly hand-written house officer discharge summaries that are a source of annoyance to general practitioners. Computerized drug menus in the instant discharge package could display drugs dispensed from pharmacy with correct drug doses, and this could highlight simultaneously potential drug interactions and unwelcome polypharmacy.

Within 5 years most health centres will be connected by email (electronic mailing). Instant and formal discharges could be instantly emailed to the patient's general practitioner, whereas the printed letter ('snail-mail') would arrive days later. Patient confidentiality and security against computer viruses and 'hackers' is crucial in planning by hospital information technologists. As with any new system, the effectiveness of change in documentation and dissemination of information will have to properly audited at each stage to demonstrate that standards are maintained or improved.

5.3 Risk management

The process of risk management is widespread in aviation and in industry and is beginning to make an impact in medicine. The principles include anticipation of risk, pre-emptive activities to reduce risk, monitoring of adverse events, and development of appropriate preventative strategies. Many hospitals have risk management groups, often incorporated within clinical audit and quality control departments. Risk management is an integral part of daily surgical practice, but formal structures, including education, which are supported by management have the potential to reduce risk to staff, patients, and the hospital budget from unnecessary medicolegal claims. Particular areas of risk include:

- The elderly: surgeons are having to deal with an ever increasing elderly population, no matter what improvements are made in anaesthetic and surgical techniques and technology. However minor the surgery, the operation needs to be carefully explained to the patient, highlighting any appreciable operative risk. The likelihood of co-morbid disease is high in patients of advanced age, although chronological age by itself is less important than biological age.

- Emergency surgery: this carries a higher risk of complications and death than elective surgery, and this needs to be borne in mind when preparing patients for operation and seeking consent. Special attention should be given to appropriate resuscitation, seniority of staffing, and specialism to reduce risk.

- Day surgery: proper patient selection is vital to the success of day-surgery procedures. Local protocols to determine suitability of patients are usually worked out together with anaesthetists, and the most appropriate choice of anaesthesia is determined before surgery. Appropriate preoperative assessment, intraoperative and postoperative monitoring are essential to detect early anaesthesia- or surgery-related complications. Even under local or regional anaesthesia, monitoring standards need to remain high.

Intensive care unit training for surgical staff

It is widely recognized that surgical trainees should undertake a period of ICU training. Many training schemes include an optional period in an ICU. The trainees learn the principles of intensive care management and the management of extremely ill patient, together with the necessary techniques, such as central line insertion and tracheostomy. They learn to recognize signs that signify improvement or deterioration in a patient's condition. This experience helps when returning to ward management, enabling the trainee to identify patients early with signs of postoperative deterioration, for example sepsis, respiratory failure, cardiovascular instability, or problems with fluid balance management. Early consultation with an intensive care specialist may prevent irreversible deterioration in the patient's condition by timely intervention on the ward or by treatment in an ICU or high dependency unit (HDU).

Joint anaesthetic and surgical management of critically ill patients

The ICU and HDU should not be the exclusive domain of either surgeon or anaesthetist and patients benefit from clinical input from both specialties. This joint approach may begin before operation in high-risk patients identified by the surgeon and discussed with a senior anaesthetist regarding optimal preparation before surgery. This may produce a change of surgical approach, a more realistic expectation of outcome, further preoperative investigations or, in the case of emergencies, resuscitation, perhaps in the ICU or HDU. In the postoperative period, discussion may involve stepping the patient down from ICU to HDU or the ward, with an appropriate level of anaesthetic input. At its least complicated, this may mean epidural analgesia or patient-controlled analgesia, and monitoring oxygen therapy and fluid management.

Operative risk assessment

There are many scoring systems to assess risk and provide prognostic information that can be applied to surgical practice; each has its own particular advantages and disadvantages. Examples include POSSUM and APACHE, which both require many variables to be collected and analysed. In general, these complex methodologies are most useful for looking retrospectively at outcomes in groups of patients. A simpler rule of thumb assessment is the American Association of Anesthesiologists (ASA) scheme, which gives an idea of a patients' prospective ability to withstand surgical intervention, providing the anaesthetist and surgeon with a level of risk that the patient will be exposed to. ASA assessment offers a semi-objective number, which aids the subjective risk assessment. The principal disadvantage of ASA grading is that it is, in reality, subjective. However, a patient given a high ASA grade is likely to succumb on the table and this will colour the intentions regarding surgery.

ASA grades

- ASA 1: the patient has no organic, physiological, biochemical, or psychiatric disturbance. The pathological process for which operation is to be performed is localized and does not entail a systemic disturbance.

- ASA 2: mild to moderate systemic disturbance caused by either the condition to be treated surgically or by other pathophysiological processes.

- ASA 3: severe systemic disturbance or disease from whatever cause, even though it may not be possible to define the degree of disability with precision.

- ASA 4: severe systemic disorders that are already life-threatening and not always correctable by operation.

- ASA 5: a moribund patient who has little chance of survival and who would be submitted to operation only as a last resort. Some anaesthetists use ASA 5E in patients expected to die within hours

Combined management of patients with anaesthetists and other specialists gives the responsible clinician an opportunity to discuss difficult management problems with colleagues. This may supply ideas about management not previously considered or support for treatments which may end in an adverse outcome.

6 Continuing medical education

When a simple spirit animates a College, there is no appropriate interval between the teacher and the taught—both are in the same class, the one a little more advanced than the other.

Sir William Osler

After appointment to a senior post, maintaining or improving the quality of patient care depends on acquiring and disseminating new knowledge by reading journals, attending conferences, carrying out research and audit, writing papers, and teaching undergraduate and postgraduate students and trainees. With rapid developments in medicine, greater expectations by the general public, and the growing tendency to apportion blame, clinicians are expected to remain aware of current developments and to demonstrate that they do so. The need to ensure that clinicians have time to pursue these activities by continued medical education (CME) was clearly recognized by the profession and politicians. The Royal Colleges of Medicine initiated and agreed the general supporting principles of CME in 1993, followed closely by the Royal Surgical Colleges. The conclusions and recommendations produced by the first College report on CME are outlined below.

6.1 Conclusions and recommendations for CME by the Royal Surgical Colleges

◆ Participation of clinicians in a structured programme of CME is a professional responsibility which the public is entitled to expect and which will be reflected in high-quality patient care.

◆ All career grade trainees with clinical responsibility for patients engaged in NHS or university practice should participate in a programme of CME.

◆ CME activities should be approved in both the setting of their clinical units and hospitals (internal CME) and also outside their hospitals in meetings which would normally entail the taking of study leave (external CME).

◆ In order to fulfil requirements for participation in CME, clinicians should take their study leave entitlement.

◆ Time required to fulfil CME activities should be protected, and should amount to 100 hours/year.

◆ The colleges should establish a system of CME approval for courses and meetings which operate to agreed criteria; at present a simple scoring system with no weighting for various activities.

◆ An individual's CME programme should be balanced and orientated to the professional commitments of that individual.

◆ Where they do not already exist, the colleges will appoint college tutors who will take responsibility for ensuring an appropriate educational climate in their hospitals and the clinical units within these hospitals.

◆ Regional advisors should take overall responsibility for CME activities within their regions and this will include support for college tutors, regular hospital visits, and the receipt of individual CME returns.

◆ Each college will establish a CME office, appoint a CME director, appoint and train regional advisors and college tutors, and maintain CME records.

◆ The colleges will issue certificates of participation in CME on a 5-yearly basis to individuals, and maintain a register of clinicians who have been issued with a certificate. This register will be available for inspection.

◆ The colleges will undertake provision of their own programmes of CME in general surgery and medicine and will be involved closely with the specialist societies in the provision of specialist CME.

◆ CME activities organized by the colleges, centrally and regionally, and by the specialist societies in liaison with colleges, will meet agreed criteria.

◆ The colleges believe that the proposals will provide a satisfactory system of CME for clinicians and are opposed to a system of formal re-examination.

◆ CME cannot operate without adequate resourcing, the contractual provision of fully funded study leave, and protected internal CME time, which requires the unequivocal support by central government.

CME for most clinicians will mean documentation of what they are already doing and provide a stamp of approval. CME of this type is preferable to the alternative of recertification, perhaps 5-yearly. CME will help ensure that standards are maintained and indeed improved.

6.2 Source material

Maintaining and improving surgical standards can be achieved by education and training in a threefold manner:

(1) education by the written word;

(2) education by verbal communication;

(3) education by practical workshops and training.

Written word

Peer-reviewed journals

These provide a week-to-week, or month-to-month update on current surgical research, review articles, surgical workshops, and interesting case reports about aspects of patient management. The information in journals is as relevant to the most junior and the most senior surgeons, although what is extracted and applied varies according to the experience and speciality of the reader. The prime general journals include the *British Medical Journal*, *The Lancet*, and the *New England Journal of Medicine*. The popular surgical journals in the UK and Europe include the *British Journal of Surgery*, *Journal of the Royal College of Surgeons of Edinburgh*, *Annals of the Royal College of England*, and *European Journal of Surgery*. In the United States the main journals are the *Annals of Surgery*, *American Journal of Surgery*, *Archives of Surgery*, and the *Journal of the American College of Surgeons* (formerly known as *Surgery, Obstetrics and Gynecology*). Within the generality of surgery, there are speciality and subspecialty journals of greater importance to groups of surgeons than the mainstream journals indicated above.

Submitting articles to journals which are subject to peer review encourages constructive self-criticism (retrospective and prospective studies of patient management), stimulates laboratory-based research (basic medical science papers), broadens one's reading (review articles), and helps set, maintain, and improve standards (new techniques, patient care, investigation and assessment, their introduction or evaluation). Critical review of published literature is important, as studies with fundamental flaws may pass peer review but have faulty implications if taken at face value. This may be carried further by acting as a referee for a journal for articles prior to acceptance, or in local journal clubs where articles are chosen to be discussed in depth. Although most current surgeons have higher degrees, many will argue that their research has little influence on their current practice. Changes in surgical training may make this type of research towards a thesis unnecessary except for the highly motivated.

Searching for articles on specific topics used to be tiresome and involved drifting through endless volumes of *Index Medicus*. The process has been greatly facilitated by computer technology that allows on-line searches of medical libraries, *Index Medicus* and the Internet via a vast number of resource-based libraries from the comfort of one's own home.

Books

Books provide in-depth discussion and illustrations on every aspect of surgery and its specialties. They may be used as reference guides or to update on an aspect of care. However, books take an appreciable time to reach the shop after the writing and are often out of date. Recommended textbooks may not have undergone recent or thorough updating and many are written by people who are not in the forefront of medical knowledge. Certain core textbooks are used by surgeons for reference and each will have his or her favourites. Alternatively, some publishing houses produce series of relatively cheap books which provide up-to-date information about surgical practice.

Computer-based learning

Textbook updates, illustrative and reference textbooks are being produced in a CD-ROM format to allow rapid access to information. From an educational point of view, a well-produced CD-ROM can allow interaction with the source material, which may consist of text, audio or video sequences. The *Oxford Textbook of Surgery* is a major reference work recently added to the ever-growing list of CD-ROMs. Laparoscopic and open surgery lend themselves very well to interspersing text and illustrations with short video sequences to emphasize points of technique. However, CD-ROMs are not the last word in educational material. They are not as convenient as textbooks, and production costs are so high that poor-quality material is the norm. The Internet is a rapidly growing resource and it seems likely that in time, the most current material will be published there, with a simple and cheap 'pay by access' system. Already, there is a wealth of free resource material, which when located, can readily be re-accessed by storing the appropriate 'bookmark' on computer.

Guidelines

Clinical guidelines, practice policies, protocols, and codes of practice are mechanisms by which standards can be set. Many are generated locally but the Cochrane Collaboration is a national body that critically reviews randomized controlled trials in specified fields and produces scrupulous meta-analyses that weigh the strength of evidence for different treatments for the condition under study. These results are widely available and can provide the basis for local guidelines.

If monitored properly, guidelines can be maintained and improved with use. However, they could be misused as inflexible policy rules designed to change and control the behaviour of clinicians and institutions, and even to ration healthcare. There is a real danger that on a superficial level, or to the non-medical observer, guidelines are seen as absolute rules that remove the need for clinical judgement. There are many instances of guidelines lacking an evidence basis or proven clinical effectiveness. For example, in the case of cancer surgery, protocol-driven treatment is used as an argument to force all cancer services into cancer centres or cancer units. The evidence in colonic cancer, however, is that if a surgeon can demonstrate comparable morbidity and mortality with his peers, without necessarily being a specialist coloproctologist, the biology of the disease rather than the surgeon is the major determinant of long-term survival. This also applies to the biology of other cancers, for example in the breast. There is a need to recognize that superspecialist services give better results in certain areas, such as oesophageal cancer, but that the generalist can achieve excellent results in most areas.

However, many clinicians do not adhere to recommended management guidelines, and when complications result in litigation, deviation from basic standards is likely to be viewed as negligent. In British law courts currently, written guidelines cannot be cross-examined and are therefore classed as hearsay evidence. This means that courts cannot determine what is reasonable and proper care by referring to them, and British judges have confirmed this in two recent cases in which they did not automatically equate established guidelines with reasonable and proper medical practice. Expert witness testimony, for all its weaknesses, is still the backbone of determining current practice.

Verbal communication

Forum discussion

These may take place at a basic level on the ward when discussing a patient's management with one's colleagues. Or it may imply discussion at unit/hospital/local/regional/national meetings, which include journal clubs, case presentations, reviews of specific topics, and presentation of research or audit projects. Meetings are organized to cater for specialities or subspecialities, often employing the format of topic-based symposia.

Surgical meetings and working parties

Broad national update meetings include the Association of Surgeons of Great Britain and Ireland, and more purely research-orientated national meetings include the Surgical Research Society. In addition, speciality meetings such as the Vascular Surgical Society and the British Orthopaedic Association take place regularly and provide a forum for trainees to present their work. Working parties under the auspices of the Senate of Surgery, the individual Royal Colleges, or the specialist associations play their part in setting surgical standards and reporting changes to their sponsoring body which affect the day-to-day practice of surgery.

Courses

Attending accredited meetings will accrue CME points and facilitate learning new techniques, updating the clinician's knowledge, or provide information on community and hospital support services or institutions. One aspect that is becoming an educational necessity is attending management courses for clinicians at various levels. These provide information on healthcare systems, markers of quality assurance that are in place, and explain the mechanisms by which informed decisions are made within the Health Service about managing healthcare resources, budgetary planning, and ensuring continuity of care.

The intercollegiate FRCS examination

The introduction of an exit examination created what was seen as another hurdle for surgical trainees at the end of training. The purpose of the examination was to ensure that certain standards had been met before completing higher surgical training and gaining a certificate of accreditation. The examination is still undergoing changes as it comes to terms with the differences between old-style senior registrars and the new Calman registrars. The latter are likely to reach the examination earlier. The problem lies in ensuring that the exam is seen as fair and yet sufficiently testing for both groups of candidates.

The intercollegiate FRCS examination consists of a 1-hour clinical exam and three half-hour vivas. One viva is on emergency surgery, trauma, and critical illness; another is on general surgery or a special interest within surgery, such as vascular surgery, transplantation, or endocrine surgery. The third viva is academic and the candidate is required to take his or her three best published papers to the viva for discussion. In addition, log books will be reviewed and discussed.

Satellite and video-conference communications

At undergraduate level initially, the **Superjanet project** uses land-lines and a satellite link to provide data, audio, and video communication links between several British universities, including London, Edinburgh, Manchester, Newcastle, and Cambridge. This has enabled inter-university video conferencing to avoid the need for participants to travel, access to research data between centres and to resource materials.

Rapid improvements have been made in telephone and fibre-optic technology, with very fast digital ISDN lines readily available at reasonable prices. This will enable video links and video conferencing to replace at least some scientific meetings. In surgery, remote sites can be linked, for example, to demonstrations of new techniques in an operating theatre. A lecture given in one place can easily be transmitted simultaneously to several places, with any member of any of the audiences able to question the speaker remotely.

6.3 Practical workshops and training

Surgical skills laboratories

Candidates wishing to take the MRCS examination of the Royal College of Surgeons of England already have to provide proof that they have attended a College-approved basic surgical skills course. The Royal Surgical Colleges have jointly agreed that all basic surgical trainees, irrespective of specialty interest, will have to attend a basic surgical skills course and reach a required standard before progressing. It is planned that skills courses will be organized at higher and speciality levels. Workshops will be directed at teaching anastomotic techniques using animal material and anatomical approaches for particular operations such as femoro-distal bypass surgery.

Endoscopic and laparoscopic training.

Computer-based endoscopic simulators are already available to assist training in colonoscopy but need refinement and development. Laparoscopic training in the initial stages is usually undertaken on abdominal models, first carrying out simple hand–eye coordination exercises and progressing to more complicated tasks. Computer simulations have also appeared recently. These employ regular laparoscopic instruments which are manipulated to perform task simulations on a monitor screen. Sensors attached to the instruments allow the instruments to be represented on the screen. This is not true virtual reality nor is there any instrumental feedback. However, it is a useful first stage and has proved helpful in marking different candidates' performance of standard tasks and also testing for improvement after training courses. It is also able to detect particular types of error, for example poor left-sided coordination. 'Body form' models using synthetic organs require laparoscopic dissection to locate and remove the target tissue. These are more expensive but provide a more realistic operative environment than, for example, peeling grapes with laparoscopic instruments. In many countries, laparoscopic training is permitted on anaesthetized animals and some trainees prefer to travel to one of these courses before proceeding to advanced training.

Virtual reality training

This is at a very early stage in surgery but it holds the promise that new trainees will learn basic surgical skills and more experienced surgeons will learn specific procedures before operating on a patient. Current virtual reality, however, lacks the tactile feedback that surgeons need to perform a technique.

Advanced trauma life support (ATLS)

Since its inception in the United States in the late 1970s and in Europe in the 1980s, ATLS courses have been an important element in improving the standards of trauma care. Their importance has been recognized by many consultants who have attended these arduous but realistic courses. The courses provide a core manual, and place the candidate in several 'real-life' situations where action is required. The participants are assessed throughout the courses and marked on their performance. The Royal Colleges already make attending an ATLS course mandatory before completing basic surgical training

7 Conclusions

There is a commitment within the National Health Service to quality development. Quality in healthcare is about finding the best ways of meeting the legitimate needs of patients. These needs are best identified using input from health economists and epidemiologists, from providers of the service (the clinicians), and the recipients of the service (patients). It will then be up to the NHS executive through its purchasers (health authorities) to make sure that resources are used appropriately to meet those requirements.

There seems little point in developing new standards if existing standards are not being met. In developed countries, we have the luxury of progressively improving standards, since basic health needs have long been met. Several mechanisms for improving standards have been discussed, but in essence, clinical audit can be used to ensure that standards set by research are being met and that optimal clinical procedures defined by research are properly implemented.

Figure 3.2 summarizes the relationship between research, audit, and education. For the profession (and the public) to recognize an advance in clinical care depends on well-structured research; implementing the research requires education, and ensuring that education has been effective requires clinical audit. Clinicians need to understand the factors involved in quality management and to lead the debate to define quality standards for their patients and the health service as a whole.

Bibliography

Davis, E.B. and Schmidt, D. (1995). *Using the biological literature. A practical guide.* Marcel Dekker, New York.

Department of Health (1989). *Working for patients.* HMSO, London.

Dixon, N. (1990). Practical principles of medical audit. *Postgrad. Med. J.*, **66**, (Suppl), S17S20.

Frostick, S.P., Radford, P.J., and Wallace, W.A. (1993). *Medical audit. Rationale and practicalities.* Cambridge University Press, Cambridge.

Hobsley, M., Johnson, A., and Treasure, T. (1993). *Current surgical practice series.* Edward Arnold, London.

Hopkins, A. (1990). *Measuring the quality of medical care.* Royal College of Physicians Publications, London.

Hopkins, A. (1995). *Professional and managerial aspects of clinical audit.* Royal College of Physicians Publications, London.

Jacyna, M.R. (1992). Audit assesses quality: but what is quality? A clinician's view. *Hospital Update*, 822–4.

Kinn, S., Lee, N., and Millman, X. (1995). Using computers in clinical audit. *BMJ*, **311**, 739–42.

Pollock, A. and Evans, M. (1993). *Surgical audit.* Butterworth-Heinemann, Oxford.

Royal Colleges of Physicians of the United Kingdom (1994). *Continuing medical education for the trained physician. Recommendations for the introduction and implementation of a CME system.* Royal Colleges of Physicians of the United Kingdom, London.

Royal College of Surgeons of England (1989). *Guidelines to clinical audit in surgical practice.* Royal College of Surgeons of England, London.

Taylor, I. *Progress in surgery series.* Churchill Livingstone, Edinburgh.

CHAPTER 4

Principles of anaesthesia and intraoperative monitoring

Howard Smith

1 Introduction: types of anaesthesia and choice of anaesthetic technique

Some form of anaesthesia is required for almost every surgical procedure. Whatever method is chosen, it should cause minimal stress to the patient and allow normal physiology to be maintained. The choice of technique lies between anaesthetizing part of the body (regional anaesthesia) and the whole body (general anaesthesia). Methods other than general anaesthesia may be supplemented with intravenous sedation.

A combination of a regional anaesthetic and a balanced general anaesthetic can minimize postoperative respiratory and cardiovascular depression, thus reducing postoperative morbidity. For example, caudal anaesthesia provides excellent analgesia after perineal operations and intercostal nerve blocks allow more comfortable breathing and coughing after an abdominal operation. Close liaison between surgical and anaesthetic staff before, during, and after operation, and careful selection of appropriate drug combinations for each case greatly facilitate postoperative recovery.

2 General anaesthesia

2.1 Aims of general anaesthesia

The primary aim of general anaesthesia is to produce temporary lack of response to noxious stimuli (unconsciousness) with lack of awareness and an absence of recall of the perioperative events later. Other aims include effective analgesia and facilitating surgical access. The latter can achieved, for example, with muscle relaxation for certain types of surgery or by minimizing surgical bleeding using deliberate hypotension for middle-ear surgery.

Three main classes of drugs are used in anaesthesia:

◆ drugs rendering the patient unconscious (i.e. anaesthetic agents-intravenous and inhalational);

◆ analgesics (plant alkaloids and synthetic derivatives);

◆ neuromuscular blockers (depolarizing and non-depolarizing).

The ideal anaesthetic causes minimal side-effects and allows rapid and safe recovery and may use a combination of drugs from the three categories.

> *Case example: A 76-year old man with a history of heavy smoking, chronic obstructive airways disease, and a productive cough, presents for TURP. The lumbar spines are easily felt and a spinal anaesthetic is deemed safest, given his chest condition. This is performed successfully and the patient is positioned on the operating table with full anaesthesia below T12 dermatome. The surgeon passes the resectoscope and starts the operation. The patient, however, persistently coughs, making prostatic venous bleeding impossible to control. The surgeon decides to insert a suprapubic catheter, but the patient experiences discomfort and a general anaesthetic has to be added.*

Comment: a better technique would have been to paralyse and ventilate the patient and to perform a caudal epidural for postoperative analgesia. Bronchial suction could have been performed throughout the anaesthetic, coughing would have been avoided, and surgery made easier.

In its early days, general anaesthesia had to be performed with a single agent (e.g. chloroform or ether). To produce passable operating conditions, the patient often suffered from side-effects because of the high concentrations of the one agent. Modern balanced anaesthesia employs combinations of drugs, gaining optimal effects from each class of drug and avoiding toxicity or side-effects. This type of anaesthesia is inevitably more complex but has facilitated enormous surgical advances.

2.2 Problems of anaesthesia in particular areas

Emergency anaesthesia

The main problems are due to inadequate preparation of the patient. Sick patients may have, for example, fluid and electrolyte imbalances, hypovolaemia from plasma or blood loss, a full stomach, hypoxaemia from untreated respiratory or cardiac disease, septic shock due to ruptured or gangrenous viscera, or cerebral damage from trauma. In general, surgery is best delayed until resuscitation is well under way. This means trying to achieve near normal blood pressure, urine output (at least 0.5 ml/kg/h), central venous pressure, blood oxygen saturation, and plasma electrolytes. There is little point in performing heroic surgery if the patient succumbs from untreated co-morbidity. Close cooperation between surgeon and anaesthetist is essential and should be at consultant level for patients in ASA grades 3–5 (Table 4.1) (NCEPOD recommendations). For patients with a potentially full stomach, nasogastric aspiration is desirable and, at induction of anaesthesia, precautions should be taken to

Table 4.1 American Society of Anesthesiologists (ASA) physical status

1	Healthy patient
2	Mild systemic disease[a]: no functional limitations
3	Severe systemic disease[a]: functional limitation
4	Severe systemic disease[a]: constant threat to life
5	Moribund patient not expected to survive 24 hours with or without operation

[a] Whether or not the systemic disease is the disease for which the patient is undergoing surgery.

prevent regurgitation of stomach contents (cricoid pressure). If endotracheal intubation proves difficult or impossible, anaesthetists should have a well-rehearsed 'failed intubation drill'.

Paediatric anaesthesia

Here the main problems are due to the small size of the patient and limited physiological reserve in the respiratory and cardiovascular systems. They become cyanosed very quickly if there is any respiratory inadequacy during anaesthesia. It is helpful to have two pairs of expert hands available should problems arise.

Small children lose heat rapidly because of their large body surface area to weight ratio. Precautions should be taken against cooling, including raising the ambient temperature in theatre, wrapping exposed parts of the body in wadding, using warming or thermoreflective blankets, and avoiding leaving the child uncovered. Sophisticated monitoring devices often fail on very small children and more reliance is placed on clinical observation by the anaesthetist. Anaesthetizing a small child takes skill, care, and time for it to be done safely. Judgement of correct fluid replacement may depend on clinical signs such as capillary perfusion rather than central venous pressure measurement. During the first few months of life opiates should be avoided as metabolism of these drugs is impaired and respiratory depression occurs easily. Children are usually apprehensive when going to theatre. This can be mitigated by kindness and reassurance from theatre staff and the presence of a calm parent. Unfortunately some parents are so afraid themselves they transfer their anxiety onto the child.

Applying eutectic mixtures of local anaesthetic cream to the hands preoperatively aids painless venepuncture. As an alternative, rapid induction of anaesthesia is possible with modern inhalational anaesthetics, and can be achieved within 1 minute using sevoflurane. Postoperative analgesia in small children is best supplemented by peroperative infiltration of the wound with local anaesthetic where practicable.

Cardiothoracic anaesthesia

Cardiac surgery is most commonly performed for coronary artery disease or for valvular lesions in adults and for congenital defects in children. Anaesthetic technique is modified to avoid or minimize the adverse cardiovascular effects of the drugs and to support the heart if necessary with inotropic or chronotropic agents. Invasive monitoring is mandatory to detect adverse effects as they occur. Techniques of general anaesthesia can help minimize myocardial oxygen demand and prevent myocardial ischaemia.

Core temperature is often deliberately reduced to about 28 °C for cardiopulmonary bypass and this changes the pharmacokinetic properties of some drugs, as does dilution of drugs in the priming fluid of the bypass circuit. During reversal of anaesthesia following cardiac bypass procedures a hypertensive response is common and this may require vasodilator therapy. The marked physiological instability of postoperative patients initially requires postoperative high dependency or intensive care.

Thoracotomies pose particular difficulties, such as pulmonary ventilation/perfusion mismatch (which causes hypoxaemia) due to patient posture as well as surgical manipulation of the lungs. Some procedures require induced collapse of one lung and this requires placement of a double lumen endotracheal tube. These tubes can also protect one lung from transfer of infected secretions to the other (e.g. in bronchiectasis). Cardiac output can be impaired by surgical manipulation and the anaesthetist needs to be continually aware of the heart rate and stroke volume. Other special considerations include the need for appropriate analgesia after thoracotomy (which is a particularly painful surgical approach) and the fact that some patients have advanced pulmonary disease likely to complicate recovery.

Anaesthesia for neurosurgery

Positioning of the patient in neurosurgery poses special problems of access (surgical access to the patient can be difficult in the prone or sitting position) and a high risk of venous air embolism because the surgically open cranium is higher than the heart in these positions. Embolism can be recognized early by monitoring end-tidal carbon dioxide levels and carrying out trans-oesophageal cardiac Doppler ultrasound. The anaesthetist can manipulate the physiology of the patient to minimize the risk of air embolism by maintaining central venous pressure, by administering slight positive airways pressure (PEEP), and by avoiding nitrous oxide gas which would tend to make the gas embolus larger. If embolism should occur, a right heart catheter allows aspiration of the gas.

Raised intracranial pressure (ICP) can be treated effectively on a temporary basis by mildly hyperventilating the patient. This reduces arterial P_{CO_2}, inducing cerebral vasoconstriction and reducing cerebral blood volume. The anaesthetist can also help reduce raised ICP by manipulating central venous pressure and mean inflation pressures, and by administering drugs such as intravenous anaesthetics, sedatives, or diuretics.

Lowering the blood pressure can be invaluable during cerebral aneurysm surgery, where haemorrhage would otherwise make surgical access difficult. Specialized techniques of stereotactic brain surgery sometimes involve light sedative infusion so that the patient can easily be woken up to communicate with the surgeon and anaesthetist.

Anaesthesia for abdominal surgery

Relaxation of the abdominal wall muscle and artificial ventilation are usually necessary for intra-abdominal surgery. Modern anaesthetic techniques can facilitate this without compromising spontaneous respiration or impairing protective cough reflexes after operation. Postoperative analgesia can be most effectively achieved using patient-controlled analgesia, epidural analgesia, or intercostal regional analgesia. Regular intramuscular opiate injections give less dependable results and are not ideal. For major surgery, a short stay on a high dependency unit may be an advantage as this can ensure complete pain relief with safety.

The anaesthetist can assist with the management of fluid and electrolyte disturbances, including preoperative resuscitation. Central venous pressure measurement may be required. This allows close monitoring of fluids and provides the best route for administration of certain drugs, such as inotropes. Septic patients, such as those with faecal peritonitis, are likely to need intensive care with full supportive therapy for several days or weeks and often present with the systemic inflammatory response syndrome or multiple organ dysfunction syndrome.

Laparoscopic surgery usually involves inflating the abdominal cavity with carbon dioxide and often placing the patient in a steep head-down tilt. Absorption of the CO_2 into the bloodstream leads to a temporary rise in Pa_{CO_2} and end-tidal CO_2. The latter can readily be observed on the gas monitor during surgery. There may also be a rise in blood pressure due to the positive inotropic effect of CO_2. Inflating the abdominal cavity causes lung volumes to be decreased, with atelectasis of the bases, and there is increased risk of regurgitation of gastric contents into the respiratory tract. For all of these reasons, laparoscopic surgery patients are most safely managed with intubation and ventilation. Peritoneal irritation causes postoperative discomfort, so that adequate systemic analgesia and antiemetic therapy should be given, ideally peroperatively. The surgeon can help by performing bilateral rectus sheath blocks in diagnostic laparoscopy or by applying local anaesthetic directly to the fallopian tubes in tubal surgery. Non-steroidal anti-inflammatory drugs given perioperatively reduce the requirement for additional analgesics.

Anaesthesia for head and neck surgery

The anaesthetist has to provide adequate anaesthesia for head and neck surgery without interfering with surgical access. This may involve oral or nasal endotracheal intubation, which provides a high level of safety for the airway. Laryngeal masks are increasingly being used where less stringent airway protection is required. Wiring of the jaws for some maxillofacial surgery is a particular risk during emergence from anaesthesia because of the danger of vomiting and laryngospasm. These patients should be nursed in a high dependency area until fully awake, with wire cutters at hand.

For operations where it is vital to minimize bleeding, such as in middle-ear or dacrocystorhinostomy surgery, a head-up posture with mechanical ventilation gives optimum conditions. Hypotensive anaesthesia provides additional benefits where haemorrhage is likely to interfere with access. Thyroid surgery carries a small risk of postoperative bleeding with a risk of causing tracheal compression and laryngeal oedema. Thus, hypotensive techniques are best avoided for thyroid surgery to give the surgeon the best chance of securing lasting haemostasis.

For parotid surgery, muscle relaxation can be avoided during the period the surgeon needs to stimulate branches of the facial nerve to locate them.

2.3 Anaesthesia for co-morbidity

Anaesthesia and obesity

There is a high association of obesity with diabetes, hypertension, and an increased risk of dying from heart disease or stroke. Gross obesity also increases perioperative anaesthetic and surgical morbidity and mortality. Particular difficulties include patient manipulation, obtaining venous access, and maintaining good airway control. Spontaneous respiration is compromised by the weight of fat on the chest and upper airways during anaesthesia. Obesity can be so severe as to lead to CO_2 retention (Pickwickian syndrome) and this type of patient carries a great risk of right ventricular failure. Mechanical assistance with ventilation is usually necessary, postoperative physiotherapy more difficult, and postoperative pneumonia more likely. There is an increased volume and acidity of gastric contents and a higher risk of hiatus hernia and intraoperative regurgitation. Even measuring the blood pressure can be technically difficult. In general, elective surgery is best postponed until weight loss can be achieved. Patients with a body mass index (BMI) greater than 35 should not be accepted for day-case surgery.

Anaesthesia in patients with cardiovascular disease

Whatever type of surgery is undertaken for patients with cardiovascular disease, it is important to remember that the disease is often widespread. Thus, a patient admitted for a femoropopliteal bypass is likely to be at increased risk of myocardial infarction or stroke from coexisting atherosclerosis of coronary or carotid arteries. The aim should be to keep physiological parameters as near normal as possible in the perioperative period. A history of recent myocardial infarction (within 6 months) greatly increases the chances of perioperative reinfarction and this carries a high mortality, so surgery should be delayed if possible until the highest risk period is past. Patients who have had recent coronary artery bypass surgery and are symptom-free, however, can be treated as normal. Patients with angina or hypertension (diastolic >110 mmHg) should be stabilized on effective medical treatment before anaesthesia. Fast atrial fibrillation should be treated preoperatively as anaesthetic agents reduce the cardiac output more than when the heart is in sinus rhythm. Valvular lesions should be covered with suitable antibiotics according to local recommendations.

Patients with cardiac failure cause most concern. They have limited cardiac reserve and the negative inotropic effects of anaesthetic agents adversely affect cardiac output. These patients should be admitted to hospital prior to surgery for echocardiography, several days' bed rest, chest physiotherapy, and medical treatment for cardiac failure. Diuretic therapy may be all that is needed. With careful preoperative preparation, there is a better chance that the anaesthetist will be able to support vital organ function during the stress of surgery. Heart failure can also develop during operation.

Case example: A 75-year-old former heavy smoker presented for elective aortic aneurysm surgery. He had a history of two previous myocardial infarcts, the second a large inferior infarction 1 year before. There were no preoperative signs of heart failure but towards the end of surgery and following 5 units of transfused blood, his blood pressure began to decline despite a high central venous pressure. An infusion of dobutamine reversed this trend. In addition to the cardiac ischaemia, other possible contributing factors to the deterioration were hypothermia, metabolic acidosis, and citrate chelation of ionized calcium from the blood transfusion.

Anaesthesia for a ruptured aortic aneurysm poses special problems. At induction of anaesthesia, muscle relaxation can remove the tamponading effect of the abdominal wall and cause further massive and rapid bleeding. Patients should be prepared awake on the operating table, using local anaesthesia for arterial, central venous lines, and urinary catheter. Two large-bore peripheral cannulae should be in place and connected to pressurized units of blood via warming devices. When everything is ready, the patient is anaesthetized and the surgeon proceeds to clamp the aorta as soon as possible. The blood bank should be warned they may need to supply fresh, frozen plasma (FFP), cryoprecipitate, or platelet concentrates later in the operation because of the loss of clotting factors by haemorrhage and the dilution of remaining clotting factors by massive transfusion. Renal protection with mannitol, frusemide, or inotropes is usually needed, and patients require a period of stabilization in intensive care. The three major life-threatening complications are persistent bleeding, acute renal failure, and bowel ischaemia.

Patients with cardiac pacemakers should not have unipolar diathermy used close to the site of the pacemaker. However, modern pacemakers are not affected by unipolar diathermy at distant sites. Bipolar diathermy is safe in all circumstances.

Anaesthesia in respiratory system disease

Smoking-related diseases account for most of the problems. Smokers have an increased risk of postoperative pneumonia. They are also more difficult to anaesthetize due to ventilation/perfusion mismatch in the lungs and coughing and bronchospasm during anaesthesia. Ideally, smoking should be stopped 6 weeks before surgery to allow the bronchial mucosal ciliary function to recover. During this period, smokers must expect to experience a more productive cough!

Patients with reversible obstructive airways disease are best given bronchodilator therapy just before coming to theatre, and the anaesthetist will choose drugs to minimize histamine release. When severe bronchospasm occurs during anaesthesia, it can be treated with intravenous bronchodilators and by deepening anaesthesia with the volatile inhalational agent. Severely emphysematous patients who are dyspnoeic at rest pose a particular anaesthetic challenge. If elective surgery is essential, regional analgesic techniques may not be appropriate because of intraoperative coughing, the inability to lie flat, and potential respiratory muscle paralysis resulting from high bilateral epidural or intrathecal blockade. With the advent of more rapidly metabolized muscle relaxants and inhalational anaesthetics which are less fat-soluble, a general anaesthetic technique with mechanical ventilation may be preferable. It allows excellent surgical conditions as well as tracheobronchial toilet with little postoperative respiratory depression. Regional analgesic supplementation gives good postoperative pain control without respiratory depression.

Anaesthesia and metabolic disorders

Electrolyte and acid–base status abnormalities should be corrected before surgery. If not, low plasma sodium (<120 mmol/l) can cause fits; potassium or magnesium imbalance causes cardiac dysrhythmias or prolonged recovery from muscle relaxants; and a base deficit of greater than 10 mmol/l induces poor cardiac output. Complete preoperative correction of these abnormalities may not be possible, for example in the presence of ischaemic bowel injury. In such cases, the patient should be prepared as well as possible and the surgery should proceed with the hope that the surgery will remove the precipitating cause and allow full resuscitation.

Diabetes mellitus is the most common endocrine disorder during surgery and its management should be understood.

Perioperative care of the diabetic patient

This is often thought to be complex but in reality it is relatively straightforward. Most diabetics should be managed on continuous intravenous glucose together with a sliding-scale insulin infusion. The only exceptions are diabetics on oral hypoglycaemic agents or diet-controlled patients undergoing minor operations. In general, all should be placed first on operating lists and all should be kept in hospital for the night after surgery.

Non-insulin-dependent diabetics

◆ Minor surgery. If blood sugar is adequately controlled (< 11 mmol/l) and the patient is not ketotic, chlorpropamide should be omitted for 24 hours before operation and other hypoglycaemic agents omitted on the day of surgery. The patient is starved as for non-diabetics and blood glucose is monitored during the operation. Provided the patient is not vomiting after operation, hypoglycaemic therapy is restarted with the first meal.

◆ Major surgery or patients with poorly controlled diabetes. Poorly controlled diabetics are defined for this purpose as those with a blood sugar of 11–17 mmol/l or who are ketotic. In these patients and in anyone undergoing major surgery, management requires glucose and insulin infusion.

Insulin-dependent diabetics

These patients should ideally be admitted on the day before surgery and started on glucose infusion and sliding-scale insulin on the morning of surgery after the usual period of starvation. If control is poor, glucose and insulin infusions can be started on the day before surgery. Postoperatively, blood glucose is monitored hourly at first, and 2-hourly when stable, until the patient is eating normally without nausea or vomiting. Normal subcutaneous doses of insulin are then restarted.

Some insulin-dependent diabetics undergoing minor surgery in the afternoon can be admitted on the morning of surgery following a light breakfast and a half dose of short-acting insulin. Glucose and insulin infusions are then usually started about 11 a.m.

Sliding-scale insulin administration

Glucose is administered in a 5 per cent solution with 20 mmol KCl/litre at 125 ml/h (adult). A separate insulin infusion is made up with 50 units of soluble insulin (e.g. Actrapid®) in 50 ml of normal saline. The insulin infusion is changed every 24 hours. Glucose and insulin are given via the same intravenous cannula, but with a non-return valve placed in the glucose line to prevent backwash of insulin into the line. Control of blood glucose should aim at a level of 7–17 mmol/l. The usual insulin dose per hour according to blood glucose levels (mmol/l) is as follows: 0 for less than 4 mmol/l, 0.5 units for >4–7 mmol/l, 1 unit for >7–11 mmol/l, 2 units for >11–17 mmol/l, 4 units for >17–28 mmol/l, and 6 units for greater than 28 mmol/l. It should be remembered that these patients are insulin dependent and require insulin for normal metabolic processes. Thus, they should not be left without insulin for long periods and the concentration of glucose infusion may need to be increased to allow insulin to be given.

3 Monitoring in anaesthesia

A monitor is one who informs, warns, or gives advice. Monitoring involves acquiring information, overseeing, or supervising. It is important to monitor patients throughout induction and maintenance of anaesthesia and recovery because most anaesthetic incidents and deaths are due to human error. Most of these are due to simple faults where lack of simple precautions or a lapse in clinical alertness has taken place. Major anaesthetic accidents can lead to extremely expensive malpractice settlements and this provides a great incentive to improve anaesthetic safety. The death rate where anaesthesia plays a part is approximately 1:10 000 anaesthetics in the UK, but deaths solely attributable to anaesthesia are probably in the order of 1:200 000 procedures. The death rate solely attributable to anaesthesia has fallen over the past 40 years even without the current trend for aggressive monitoring. However, high-quality monitoring undoubtedly contributes to safer and more complex anaesthesia and surgery.

The Closed Claim study of the Professional Liability Committee of the American Society of Anesthesiologists suggested that 31 per cent of all insurance settlements for anaesthetic complications involved respiratory problems and that 55 per cent of these had been inadequately monitored. It was concluded that in 40 per cent of claims, pulse oximetry and capnography could have prevented the initial mishap.

In this ASA study the following caused most of the deaths:

- complications of tracheal intubation;
- respiratory inadequacy following myoneural blockade;
- inadequate postoperative care and observation;
- hypovolaemia.

Anaesthetic mishaps can occur in all ASA grades of patients, elective or emergency, but the most unfit patients are least able to compensate for complications.

3.1 Recommendations for minimum safe monitoring

The Harvard Medical School recommendations were published in 1986 and adoption of them by the American Society of Anesthesiologists caused insurance companies to reduce premiums for those working in suitably equipped hospitals. In ASA grade 1 and 2 patients, most of the anaesthetic incidents were ventilatory problems. The study showed that once basic monitoring was adopted, the incidence of anaesthetic-related accidents fell.

The Association of Anaesthetists of GB and Ireland (AAGBI) published a document on monitoring in 1988 and revised it in 1994. Its main recommendations are given below. *They should be applied wherever an anaesthetic is given, in recovery areas, and where anaesthetized patients are being transferred.* The Association guidelines emphasize that using monitoring devices should not absolve the anaesthetist from making standard clinical observations. Although there is no conclusive evidence that more extensive use of monitoring equipment reduces morbidity and mortality, it is believed it will encourage higher-quality patient care. The most effective monitor is still the constant presence of a skilled and vigilant anaesthetist. Other factors contributing to increased patient safety include improved training and better anaesthetic drugs.

Summary of AAGBI recommendations
Presence of the anaesthetist

The anaesthetist should always be present throughout any general anaesthetic, and for local anaesthetics where there are appreciable risks of unconsciousness or cardiovascular or respiratory complications. Responsibility should only be handed over to another anaesthetist or, in a dire emergency, another medical practitioner. The anaesthetist should continually check equipment, depth of anaesthesia, and the patient's physiological state until the patient has been transferred to recovery staff. *Non-anaesthetists practising local anaesthetic or sedative techniques must be aware of the potential complications and how to treat them.*

Clinical observations should include:

- colour and eye signs;
- response to surgical stimulus;
- movement of chest;
- movement of reservoir bag;
- palpation of pulse;
- auscultation of heart and breath sounds.

Monitoring devices
Continuous monitoring using:

- pulse plethysmography;
- O_2 saturation;
- ECG;
- capnography (end-tidal CO_2) and expiratory volume;
- airways pressure;
- body temperature probes;
- anaesthetic agent analysers;
- neuromuscular function monitor if muscle relaxants are used.

Special monitoring of oxygen supply
The following should always be present to detect supply failure:

- a low-pressure warning device in the supply line with an audible alarm;
- an O_2 analyser with an audible alarm when hypoxic mixtures can potentially be administered.

Monitoring for special circumstances (e.g. major arterial surgery or neurosurgery)

- Intra-arterial pressure;
- central venous pressure;
- pulmonary artery wedge pressure;
- urine output;
- measurement of blood loss;
- oesophageal stethoscope;
- intracranial pressure monitoring;
- biochemical and haematological analyses.

With minimum safe monitoring in mind, can there be too much monitoring? There is good evidence that no more than 3–5 sensory variables can be assimilated effectively. If sensory input is overloaded, this can work against patient safety. Anaesthetists should always check or calibrate the equipment before they use it and should remain sceptical about what a monitor is displaying, particularly if it does not agree with clinical findings. Alarm systems can be turned off deliberately or inadvertently, or they can be set off by other electrical or electronic devices. Ergonomics are important, as with aircraft controls. Displays can be confusing—in some instances, an analogue display is more intuitive and in others a digital display is preferred. Ideally, information displays should be concentrated near the patient's head but this is rarely practicable.

3.2 Comments on monitoring

Pulse oximetry

Users of pulse oximetry need to be aware of a range of potential drawbacks:

- The reading may not reflect true cellular O_2 levels in raised intracranial pressure or methaemoglobinaemia. In carbon monoxide poisoning, the display is likely to show a falsely high O_2 saturation.

- At hypoxic levels oximetry is less reliable; there is a wide variation in accuracy.

- Readings can be incorrect if there is hypotension, vasoconstriction, or during large swings in pulse volume with mechanical ventilation or patient movement.

- The changes in oxygen saturation at the finger may lag a minute or more behind central changes.

- Smokers very often have low O_2 saturations.

- Burns caused by the probe have been reported—regular changing of the probe site is recommended, especially in hypoperfusion and with small children.

Capnography

Measurement of inspired and expired carbon dioxide is the most reliable method of detecting misplaced endotracheal tubes, pulmonary embolism, decreased cardiac output, or malignant hyperpyrexia. Hypotension causes a fall in end-tidal CO_2 due to poor lung perfusion.

Apnoea or disconnect alarms

Circuit disconnection is still one of the most common anaesthetic incidents. These monitors are used to measure pressure changes in the breathing circuit and are mandatory during artificial ventilation.

Blood pressure monitors

Non-invasive methods such as mercury columns, oscillotonometers, aneroid sphygmomanometers and automatic non-invasive blood pressure machines of various types are all in use, but the last type frees the anaesthetist to perform other tasks. Invasive methods are mostly used during major surgery (e.g. arterial, cardiothoracic, neurosurgery) and for those surgical patients likely to need intensive care postoperatively.

ECG

Pulse oximetry has now replaced the ECG as the principal method of monitoring. The ECG is useful for monitoring the heart rate and for detecting arrhythmias. Lead 2 is the most useful vector as it shows P waves most clearly, recording parallel to atrial depolarization. Lead V5 can indicate developing ventricular ischaemia but is not wholly reliable.

Body-core thermometry

This is indicated when large-volume blood transfusions are needed, during long operations with open body cavities, during deliberate or accidental hypothermia, for neonatal surgery, and for patients potentially susceptible to malignant hyperpyrexia.

Neuromuscular blockade monitors

Peripheral nerve stimulators (PNS) are helpful where neuromuscular blockers are in use. They contain either constant current or constant voltage generators, delivering a monophasic rectangular pulse of 0.1–0.2 milliseconds. When surface electrodes are used, the output is about 60 mA to ensure supramaximal stimulus. The initial stimulation threshold should be tested during induction and before the patient is paralysed. Peripheral nerve stimulators can be used to indicate when further doses of neuromuscular blockers are necessary and to assess reversibility of blockade. Intraoperative sequences of four stimuli are applied and the responses and any post-tetanic facilitation observed. When all four produce a response, reversal will be swift and complete. With only one, reversal will be incomplete despite neostigmine, and if none is seen, the block is pharmacologically irreversible at that moment.

EEG and evoked potentials

The processed EEG by Fast Fourier transformation, or the change in the ECG in response to external auditory stimuli, can be measured and gives some indication as to depth of anaesthesia. This is an area of current research and may lead in the future to a widening use of such monitoring during anaesthesia. The subject is complex because many outside factors affect the electrical activity of the brain apart from depth of anaesthesia. These include surgical stimulation, the age and gender of the patient, the drugs used, the body temperature, and the acid–base status.

Microprocessors have played an integral part in the monitoring boom; they can be programmed to perform repetitive tasks with great precision; they can store and retrieve historical monitoring trends and control sophisticated alarm functions.

3.3 The pre-anaesthetic 'cockpit drill'

Although not strictly monitoring, the importance of this is difficult to overstate. No airline pilot would take off without a 'pre-flight check', nor should the anaesthetist. In practice, this takes 10–15 minutes. A careful check of all the equipment must be performed by a trained assistant before every list, followed by another check by the anaesthetist. This should include inspecting the bulk gas supply, the reserve cylinders, flow meters and vaporizers, gas delivery systems (e.g. circle absorbers or rebreathing systems for integrity and leaks), emergency oxygen supply, scavenging system, suction, airway equipment, drugs, syringes, and monitoring equipment. Each department should have its own protocol.

4   Recovery from anaesthesia

The anaesthetist is responsible for the patient until full protective reflexes have returned. Inadequate recovery facilities are still responsible for the occasional anaesthetic death. There should be a dedicated area which is large enough and properly equipped with oxygen, suction, ECG, blood pressure devices, and pulse oximetry. There needs to be sufficient suitably qualified recovery staff to deal with the daily projected throughput of the operating theatres, and close liaison should be maintained between anaesthetist and recovery staff. Recovering patients on the ward, in the corridor, or elsewhere is indefensible. The period of recovery from anaesthesia can be used to assess the severity of the patient's pain and to provide appropriate analgesia. The anaesthetist can often administer intravenous opiates or regional analgesic injections in the recovery unit.

Rarely, patients need to be ventilated in the recovery area until full recovery has occurred. Delayed recovery used to be due to the effects of neuromuscular blockade but is nowadays caused more often by poor cardiac, respiratory, hepatic, or renal function. The following is an example.

> *Case example: A frail 75-year-old woman with treated left ventricular failure entered the recovery area after an anterior resection of the rectum. She had been extubated following surgery. A peripheral nerve stimulator demonstrated full pharmacological reversal of neuromuscular blockade. However, she breathed weakly with bilateral poor air entry. In recovery, she was sat up and given oxygen via a facemask but soon drifted into unconsciousness with very little air entry and weak gasping respirations. Pulse oximetry demonstrated a falling oxygen saturation of 85 per cent (normal 96–99 per cent). She was therefore reintubated in recovery, ventilated, and given intravenous frusemide for acute left ventricular failure. She made a slow recovery over the next 18 hours on intensive care. Further surgery (her request for colostomy closure) was strongly resisted by surgeon and anaesthetist. Two years later she died during such an operation.*

5   Local anaesthesia

5.1   General properties of local anaesthetics

A secondary or tertiary amine hydrophilic group is joined to an aromatic lipophilic group by means of an alkyl chain with an ester or amide linkage. Local anaesthetics are weak bases with a pH of 7.7–9.5 and have limited solubility in water. They are used as salts (e.g. hydrochlorides) which are acidic and more water soluble. When injected, ionized and non-ionized fractions appear in the tissues. The non-ionized form is probably responsible for penetration through the tissues and transmission across the nerve membrane. Addition of sodium bicarbonate to local anaesthetics speeds up the onset of conduction blockade,

probably by increasing the amount of drug in the non-ionized form.

Both forms are probably responsible for blocking the neuronal membrane sodium channels by interacting with a channel receptor. Alteration in sodium permeability causes several changes that block nerve transmission: the excitation threshold is raised, the rate of rise of the action potential is retarded, and propagation of the action potential is slowed. Local anaesthetics may also block acetylcholine–activated channels in a similar way at neuronal synapses.

In summary, local anaesthetics reduce the transient increase in sodium permeability in nerve fibre membranes necessary for the initiation and conduction of action potentials.

The ability of local anaesthetics to block sodium channels makes them potentially toxic, particularly to the central nervous system and the myocardium. Their record of safety is mainly due to dilution and rapid metabolism of the drug. Central nervous system toxicity causes restlessness, tremor, convulsions, and respiratory paralysis. Cardiovascular toxicity is manifest by negative inotropism and vasodilatation. Protocols to deal with side-effects and the necessary drugs must be to hand wherever local anaesthetics are given.

5.2   Duration of action

The duration of action of local anaesthetics is determined mainly by the rate of removal from the site of action by blood flow. For certain applications requiring prolonged local anaesthesia, adrenaline (epinephrine) is added to cause vasoconstriction. The mode and rate of metabolism of local anaesthetics also affects the duration of action. For esters (cocaine, procaine, and amethocaine (tetracaine)), metabolism is mainly via plasma cholinesterase, and for amides (lignocaine (lidocaine), mepivacaine, bupivacaine, prilocaine and cinchocaine) it is by oxidative dealkylation and hydrolysis in the liver.

Note regarding the addition of adrenaline to local anaesthetic agents

The two main purposes of adding adrenaline (epinephrine) are:

◆ reducing surgically induced bleeding;

◆ prolonging the effect of local anaesthetics other than long-acting agents given epidurally (e.g. bupivacaine).

Adrenaline should **never** be added to agents used for intravenous regional anaesthesia nor for infiltration in digits, penis, or nose where arterial spasm may cause necrosis.

The usual concentrations of adrenaline are 1:200 000 for general infiltration and 1 : 80 000 for dental use.

5.3   Local anaesthetics in common use

Cocaine

First used for local anaesthesia over 100 years ago, cocaine is an alkaloid derived from the leaves of the South American shrub

Erythroxylum coca. Cocaine also has the property of blocking reuptake of noradrenaline (norepinephrine) at adrenergic nerve terminals, giving it vasoconstrictor (alpha-adrenergic) effects. This makes it beneficial for topical use on the nasal mucosa or in the eye, where it is still regularly employed. However, the toxic and addictive properties of the drug have led to its being replaced by newer, synthetic, local anaesthetics without the intrinsic vasoconstrictor effects. Cocaine is now employed only for topical analgesia in the eye or nose in a 1–20 per cent solution.

Lignocaine (lidocaine)

Lignocaine was first synthesized in 1943 and is very stable. It is metabolized in the liver and adding adrenaline (1 : 200 000) prolongs its effect from 30 minutes up to 1–2 hours. It has no intrinsic vasoconstrictor effects. Toxic side-effects are primarily on the cardiovascular and central nervous systems but these are rare. The maximum safe dose is 3 mg/kg, or 7 mg/kg with adrenaline.

Concentrations used are:

◆ Infiltration: 0.5–2 per cent with or without adrenaline.

◆ Topical anaesthesia (e.g. spraying vocal cords): 4 per cent solution.

◆ For nerve blocks and extradural analgesia: 1–2 per cent with or without adrenaline.

◆ For urethral analgesia: 1–2 per cent in jelly.

◆ For hyperbaric spinal anaesthesia ('heavy lignocaine') it may be made up in glucose solutions.

Bupivacaine

This was first used in 1963. It is very stable (it can be autoclaved) and is metabolized in the liver. The maximum safe dose is 2 mg/kg. A 0.5 per cent solution is equivalent in potency to 2 per cent lignocaine (lidocaine). However, it is cardiotoxic and should not now be used in intravenous regional anaesthesia. The duration of action is approximately 3–6 hours, largely due to its powerful binding to nerve tissue. It comes in strengths of 0.25, 0.5, and 0.75 per cent, with or without adrenaline (epinephrine) 1 : 200 000. Adrenaline reduces its potential toxicity and cuts down bleeding. This drug is used extensively in anaesthetic practice, and can be mixed with lignocaine if a more rapid onset is required. It also has a wide sensory : motor blockade differential. Thus, a 0.25 per cent solution, which is an effective blocker of sensory transmission, causes little paralysis. For most peripheral nerve blocks a 0.25 per cent solution is adequate.

Prilocaine

This is similar to lignocaine (lidocaine) but less toxic. It has been used since 1959 and is very stable. It is metabolized rapidly in liver, kidneys, and lungs, and it is the preferred drug for intravenous regional anaesthesia as a 0.5 per cent plain solution (5 mg/ml) at a dose of 2–3 mg/kg body weight. Prilocaine is supplied in concentrations of 0.5, 1, 2, and 3 per cent with octapressin, and 4 per cent. The last two are used primarily in dental anaesthesia. The maximum safe adult dose when infiltrated is 4–6 mg/kg (with adrenaline (epinephrine) 8–9 mg/kg). Methaemoglobinaemia can occur at higher doses and intravenous methylene blue should be available as the antidote.

5.4 Regional anaesthesia

Introduction

This section highlights some of the more common techniques in UK anaesthetic practice but is not an exhaustive list. Regional anaesthesia may be by:

◆ topical application;

◆ infiltration;

◆ single or combined nerve blocks;

◆ plexus blocks;

◆ central epidural or intrathecal blockade;

◆ a combination of the above.

Benefits of regional anaesthesia are:

◆ Avoiding or supplementing general anaesthesia or systemic analgesia, allowing preservation of the cough reflex and minimal cardiovascular and respiratory disturbance.

◆ Excellent pain relief, both peri- and postoperatively.

◆ Reduced CNS stimulation and adverse physiological effects of pain during operation.

◆ Blockade of sympathetic fibres, thus causing vasodilatation (usually a side-effect but may be useful in microvascular or arterial/venous surgery).

◆ Reduction in the incidence of postoperative deep venous thrombosis and pulmonary embolism with central techniques.

Whenever regional anaesthesia is employed, the operator must know the anatomy of the nerves to be blocked and be aware of the upper dose limits and toxic reactions. Preparations should be made to treat toxic effects immediately and effectively. The operator/anaesthetist is discouraged when there is a risk of toxic or adverse reactions (e.g. intravenous regional anaesthesia or epidural or spinal techniques).

Techniques of regional anaesthesia

Topical

Local anaesthetics can be applied to mucous membranes (e.g. in eye or nasal surgery). Eutectic mixtures of lignocaine (lidocaine) and prilocaine have been found very effective in anaesthetizing skin prior to venepuncture, and this is especially useful in paediatric practice. After circumcision, local analgesia can be effected by applying local anaesthetic gel to the glans.

Infiltration

This is effective for procedures like carpal tunnel release, excision of a ganglion, or hernia repair. Infiltration of an arthroscopic tract with 0.25 per cent bupivacaine is highly effective.

Almost any local anaesthetic can be used and adrenaline (epinephrine) can be used to prolong the duration of action. However, infiltration is best performed with a long-acting agent such as bupivacaine, noting the dose limit of 2 mg/kg. In practice, 0.25 per cent without adrenaline is used and the dose limit means that sufficient volume can be given for most procedures. Infiltration around surgical wounds ensures postoperative analgesia for at least 4 hours, and by avoiding opiates in general anaesthesia, the anaesthetist can ensure that patients wake up clear-headed.

Single or combined nerve blocks

Femoral nerve block

Approximately 20 ml of local anaesthetic solution is injected into the neurovascular compartment lateral to the artery and just distal to the inguinal ligament. This is particularly useful for relieving the pain of femoral fracture and total knee replacement.

Combined nerve blocks

An ankle block of the deep peroneal, superficial peroneal, sural, saphenous, and tibial nerves is useful for foot surgery if the patient is unfit for general anaesthesia or spinal or epidural techniques.

Femoral, obturator, lateral cutaneous, and sciatic nerve blocks for lower-limb surgery are specialized anaesthetic techniques, which require practice to be effective; a peripheral nerve locator is helpful.

Regional anaesthesia for inguinal herniorrhaphy involves local infiltration of the skin incision site, a block of the ilioinguinal and iliohypogastric nerves as they descend medial to the anterior superior iliac spine and deep to the external oblique muscle, and infiltration of the neck of the hernia sac when exposed. About 60–90 ml of 0.5 per cent prilocaine with adrenaline 1 : 200 000 are required, up to doses of 6–8 mg/kg. It is important to check whether the patient is experiencing pain during the procedure as peroperative supplementation may be necessary. Epidural or spinal techniques are simpler and perhaps more effective for inpatient use but the block has to extend up to at least the T10 dermatome to be effective, or higher if the discomfort of peritoneal handling is to be avoided. This is likely to delay the discharge of short-stay patients.

Intercostal nerve blocks are highly effective for the pain of fractured ribs, open cholecystectomy, or midline incisions if bilateral. They are simple to perform but pneumothorax is a potential complication and they may have to be repeated.

Techniques for relieving the pain of thoracotomy include cryoanalgesia of intercostal nerves under direct vision at thoracotomy, thoracic epidural analgesia, intrapleural infusion, and paravertebral blocks. A catheter can be passed into the potential paravertebral space for longer-term unilateral thoracic analgesia; a unilateral block causes less thoracic sympathetic blockade and hypotension and less respiratory muscular embarrassment than the bilateral block of an epidural technique.

Intravenous

A German surgeon, August Bier first described intravenous regional anaesthesia (IVRA) in 1908. It is useful for upper-limb surgery where exsanguination and a tourniquet are desirable. Neither adrenaline (epinephrine) nor bupivacaine should be used. Bupivacaine has been associated with death due to premature release of the tourniquet. The more potent agents such as bupivacaine depress cardiac contractility at the lowest concentrations and recovery is slowest. They have a greater myocardial uptake and cardiac resuscitation is difficult.

The recommended local anaesthetic for IVRA is prilocaine in a 0.5 per cent solution up to 3 mg/kg. This allows volume of about 30–40 ml to be used for a 70 kg adult. To prevent unwanted leakage of local anaesthetic past the tourniquet, it is recommended to inject into a distal vein over at least 90 seconds, with a tourniquet pressure of at least 300 mmHg after exsanguination with an Esmarch bandage. A double cuff can be used so that after initial inflation with the proximal cuff for 10–15 minutes, the distal cuff can be inflated over a relatively anaesthetic area and the proximal cuff deflated. However, these narrow cuffs require relatively higher pressures, which may defeat the purpose. For safety, there should always be an intravenous cannula placed in the contralateral arm and drugs and equipment available to deal with central nervous system and cardiovascular toxicity.

The main advantages of the block are ease of administration, rapidity of onset, reliability of block, and very low failure rate.

Plexus blockade

There are several approaches to the brachial plexus: the interscalene, the supraclavicular, and the axillary. Although the interscalene approach allows cervical plexus block and surgery to the shoulder, the latter two are more commonly used. The supraclavicular approach is useful for all surgery on the arm from the shoulder joint distally.

Localization of the brachial plexus with a peripheral nerve locator is useful for the supraclavicular approach as the plexus crosses the first rib, close behind the subclavian artery. Failed blocks are common because of injection outside the neural sheath. Complications include pneumothorax and subclavian artery puncture. Approximately 30 ml of local anaesthetic are used and the block takes 15–30 minutes to be effective. Onset is slower with bupivacaine than with lignocaine (lidocaine) but the block can be very long lasting (>12 hours).

The axillary approach is useful in operations on the hands and lower arm where a tourniquet is not necessary. The approach avoids the risk of pneumothorax. The musculocutaneous, radial, and axillary nerves are difficult to block with this technique unless distal spread of the local anaesthetic is prevented by pressure on the neurovascular sheath distal to the injection. Approximately 30 ml of local anaesthetic are injected into the neurovascular sheath, or an epidural catheter can be introduced into the sheath to provide longer-term block. Autonomic blockade is a side-effect causing vasodilatation, which is, however, beneficial for microvascular or arteriovenous surgery. The main complication is puncture of the axillary artery.

Central

Spinal (subarachnoid) and epidural techniques

These techniques have a high success rate. Employing isobaric or hyperbaric solutions, different analgesic agents, and different positions of the patient can vary duration and extent of blockade. Injection of any drugs into the spinal canal requires meticulous care in drawing up, labelling, and administration.

Epidural techniques

Epidural anaesthesia is slower in onset than spinal anaesthesia and therefore physiologically less challenging. It is of great benefit postoperatively as prolonged analgesia can be sustained by periodic 'topping-up' or continuous infusion of local anaesthetic. Epidurals are most useful for:

◆ relief of labour pains and operative obstetrics;

◆ regional anaesthesia for thoracic, abdominal, pelvic, and lower-limb surgery.

The particular benefits are that the patient can be awake and there is little cardiovascular or respiratory disturbance. The chief disadvantage is that the nerve block is bilateral and may reach a high level. This causes widespread vasodilatation and the blood pressure may have to be maintained with intravenous fluids and sympathomimetics. Thus, an epidural may not be ideal for the patient in heart failure. Artificial respiratory support may be required.

A further complication occurs if the epidural catheter migrates through the theca into the subarachnoid space and a bolus dose of local anaesthetic causes a 'total spinal block'. The patient is likely to stop breathing and become profoundly hypotensive with fixed, dilated pupils. This demands immediate induction of artificial ventilation and measures to raise blood pressure until the effect has worn off.

The height of the block is determined by the volume injected, while the intensity of block is governed by the concentration of local anaesthetic. It is not necessary to paralyse a patient by using a high concentration to achieve satisfactory anaesthesia. Epidural opiates are now commonly added to a weak local anaesthetic solution (e.g. 0.125 per cent bupivacaine) and employed as a continuous infusion for postoperative pain relief. Agents that are more fat-soluble (such as fentanyl and diamorphine) are safer than less-soluble drugs (such as morphine), having less upward spread and a lower risk of respiratory centre paralysis. However, even this small risk means that the techniques should not be practised unless the patient can be monitored in a high dependency unit or given special nursing on a ward.

Caudal epidural anaesthesia is an invaluable technique for surgical areas supplied by the sacral plexus (e.g. in prostate, circumcision, anal, and other perineal operations). The volume of solution injected through the sacral foramen determines the level of the block.

Intrathecal (spinal) anaesthesia

These techniques were first used in the early part of the 20th century. Drugs and equipment at the time made them easier than epidural techniques. They are popular for operations below the waistline (e.g. transurethral resection of prostate, leg amputations), where lengthy surgery is not anticipated.

It is often mistakenly thought that patients with cardiac or pulmonary disease should have spinal anaesthesia in preference to general anaesthesia. Spinal anaesthesia offers relative simplicity and rapid onset of profound block with good muscle relaxation, but has the disadvantage for these compromised patients of hypotension and potential respiratory depression. The onset of hypotension is extremely rapid and has to be treated with fluid administration and intravenous sympathomimetics (e.g. ephedrine).

Spinal analgesia is usually performed through the lumbar intervertebral interspace at L3/4 or L4/5. Approximately one-tenth of the volume needed for epidural analgesia is required. The spread, depth, and duration of block are affected by the volume of drug, the positioning of the patient, the density (baricity) of the drug, and the type of local anaesthetic used. Osteoporosis of the lumbar spine, vertebral collapse, or calcification can make spinal anaesthesia technically difficult.

Postprocedure spinal headache is common following inadvertent dural puncture at epidural, or following spinal analgesia in obstetric surgery. It is less common in the elderly general surgical patient. It may be due to leakage of cerebrospinal fluid through the dural perforation, and typically presents as a severe bilateral headache, worse on sitting, and perhaps with photophobia. Patients find it distressing and obstetric patients often find they cannot feed their babies because of it. A 'blood patch' of 20 ml of the patient's own venous blood can be injected into the epidural space and, probably by sealing the leak, causes dramatic and permanent improvement. It has little morbidity of its own.

5.5 Supplementation

With any regional anaesthetic technique, it is possible to provide anxiolytic, amnesic, or analgesic supplementation. Benzodiazepine sedation may induce unconsciousness and respiratory depression in the frail, elderly patient and care must be exercised with dosages. There is a wide range of individual responses to these drugs, as with opiates. A patient who is partially demented and uncooperative may be made worse by intravenous sedation. Opiates can be given intravenously alone or in combination with benzodiazepines to supplement regional analgesia, bearing in mind that the effect will be synergistic and smaller doses of each drug will be required. Minimum monitoring requirements must be observed.

6 Complications of anaesthesia

Complications of anaesthesia are essentially the responsibility of the anaesthetist. The exception is local anaesthesia administered by the surgeon. Much of the preoperative assessment for an anaesthetic, whether spinal, epidural, or general, is a joint venture between members of the surgical and anaesthetic teams, who by anticipating complications can prevent many of them.

6.1 Common complications of anaesthesia

Complications of local and regional anaesthetic techniques

- Injection site: pain, haematoma, delayed recovery of sensation (direct nerve trauma), infection;

- ischaemic necrosis: if vasoconstrictors used in digits or penis;

- systemic complications: CNS depression or fits, dizziness, tinnitus, nausea, and vomiting;

- bradycardia and asystole, severe hypotension or postural hypotension; similar effects are produced by premature release of a Bier's block cuff;

- failure of anaesthetic: anatomical difficulties or technical failure;

- headache: loss of cerebrospinal fluid (CSF) in epidural or spinal techniques;

- epidural bleeding (especially if the patient is on anti-coagulants);

- unintentionally wide field of anaesthesia:

  (1) in epidural anaesthesia, injection of local anaesthetic into the wrong tissue plane may give a spinal anaesthetic;
  (2) in spinal anaesthesia, if the anaesthetic agent flows too far rostrally, respiratory paralysis and unconsciousness may occur;

- permanent nerve or spinal cord damage: injection of incorrect drug;

- paraspinal infection: introduced by the needle;

- idiosyncratic or allergic reactions (very rare).

Complications of general anaesthesia

Respiratory

Laryngeal spasm

Laryngeal spasm is usually due to stimulation in the upper airway when the patient is too lightly anaesthetized. It has become less prevalent with the use of the laryngeal airway.

Bronchospasm

Usually seen at induction of anaesthesia in the susceptible patient (i.e. bronchitic or asthmatic). Deepening anaesthesia (the volatile anaesthetic agents have relaxant properties on smooth muscle), or the use of bronchodilators is required.

Aspiration of gastric contents

Pulmonary aspiration of as little of 20 ml of gastric contents with a pH of 2 can lead to severe adult respiratory distress syndrome. This can be fatal. A period of starvation pre-operatively of 3–4 hours for liquids and 6 hours for solids is standard practice.

Technical problems

Blocked or misplaced endotracheal tubes, and disconnected breathing circuits are still frequently reported in anaesthetic accidents.

Cardiovascular

Hypo- or hypertension

Most of the inhalational or intravenous anaesthetic drugs have hypotensive properties. Intubation causes a marked vasopressor effect.

Cardiac ischaemia

As the patient cannot complain of angina when anaesthetized, it is important to minimize the work of the heart during surgery in those at risk by not allowing systolic hypertension or tachycardia. Myocardial oxygen supply and demand should be matched.

Posture, positioning, instrumentation

Pressure effects—neuropraxia due to direct pressure or traction on superficial nerves or plexuses can occur. Basal atelectasis of the lungs and ventilation/perfusion defects occur in abdominal surgery. Direct trauma to the mouth or pharynx (e.g. damaged teeth, lacerations to soft palate, uvula or pharynx, vocal cords, etc.) can be caused by instrumentation.

Postoperative nausea and vomiting (PONV)

Postoperative nausea and vomiting is of multifactorial aetiology. Patients who are undergoing certain types of surgery, such as middle-ear operations or gynaecological surgery, are more prone to it. Women, children, and anxious patients are more susceptible. Opioids administered peroperatively can stimulate the vomiting centre, and on the other hand they have an anti-emetogenic effect by producing adequate analgesia. Many drugs have been used to try to prevent PONV, including dopamine antagonists such as phenothiazines, metoclopramide, and domperidone, antihistamines, and 5-HT3 antagonists. Extrapyramidal effects can occur with the dopamine antagonists, and can be quite frightening for the patient and relatives, although they are easily treated. The newer 5-HT3 antagonists are promising and can be more effective than traditional drugs for either surgery known to stimulate vomiting, or for preventing PONV due to patient-controlled analgesia with intravenous opioids.

Organ failure

Liver

The risk of 'halothane hepatitis', where repeated exposure of a patient to halothane leads to an antibody/antigen reaction on the surface of liver cells with resultant fatal massive necrosis, is now reduced by using alternative inhalational agents that are minimally metabolized (e.g. desflurane, isoflurane).

Renal

Renal failure can occur peroperatively due to profound hypotension or inadequate fluid management. A renal protection regimen employing maintenance of adequate central venous filling pressure, intravenous fluids, and other measures such as mannitol, frusemide, or inotrope infusions may be employed.

Neurological

Epilepsy

Some anaesthetic agents may increase epileptiform activity, others have a protective effect.

Delayed recovery

Peroperative stroke, or raised intracranial pressure from undiagnosed cerebral tumour may (rarely) be the cause. More commonly delayed recovery is due to poor cardiac output.

Awareness during surgery

This was mainly a worry in obstetric anaesthesia a few years ago where patients were kept deliberately light to avoid adverse effects on the baby. Older inhalational volatile anaesthetics such as trichloroethylene were poor anaesthetics but good analgesics. During the past 15 years or so it has been shown that maintaining a small percentage of halothane, or one of the newer inhalational anaesthetics, throughout a surgical obstetric procedure incurs no harm to mother or baby, and almost completely excludes the possibility of awareness under anaesthesia. A general surgical patient should not experience awareness or pain under anaesthesia; however, if it occurs, it is almost always due to faulty technique (e.g. the use of neuromuscular blockers without adequate anaesthetic and analgesic agents) or equipment malfunction. Volatile anaesthetic agent concentrations must now be monitored and this further minimizes the risk of awareness. With the current vogue for developing total intravenous anaesthesia, careful consideration has to be given to the infusion rates of these drugs to avoid potential awareness.

Inherited disorders

Malignant hyperpyrexia

Malignant hyperpyrexia is a disorder of muscle which renders it peculiarly sensitive to certain anaesthetic agents. These include certain volatile anaesthetic agents and suxamethonium. The effect is a fatal rise in body temperature unless immediate remedial action is taken, such as whole-body cooling and intravenous dantrolene.

Pseudocholinesterase deficiency

This results in sensitivity to drugs that use pseudocholinesterase for their metabolism, such as succinylcholine and mivacurium (muscle relaxants). Such patients may have to be ventilated for several hours postoperatively following a single dose of such drugs.

Hypothermia

Long operations with extensive fluid loss, large-volume transfusions of cold blood, and inhalation of cold, dry anaesthetic gases all cause hypothermia. Warming blankets, blood warmers, heat, and moisture exchangers are employed.

Bibliography

Monitoring in anaesthesia

Association of Anaesthetists (1988). *Recommendations for standards of monitoring during anaesthesia and recovery.* Association of Anaesthetists, London [revised 1994].

Buck, Devlin and Lunn (1987). *The report of a confidential enquiry into perioperative deaths.* The Nuffield Provincial Hospitals Trust, London.

Eichhorn *et al.* (1986). Standards for patient monitoring during anaesthesia at Harvard Medical school. *JAMA*, **256**, 1017–20.

Harrison, G.G. (1978). Death attributable to anaesthesia. A 10-year survey (1967–76). *Br. J. Anaesth.*, **50**, 1041–6.

Lunn and Mushin (1982). *Mortality associated with anaesthesia.* The Nuffield Provincial Hospitals Trust, London.

Regional anaesthesia

Pinnock, C.A., Fischer, H.B.J., and Jones, R.P. (1996). Peripheral nerve blockade. Churchill-Livingstone, Edinburgh.

CHAPTER 5

Minimizing perioperative risk

Ian Bailey and Clive R. Quick

1 Introduction

The aim of surgical diagnosis and treatment is to cure disease and to palliate symptoms caused by disease. This usually involves a variety of healthcare workers and carries a range of potential hazards for them and for their patients. All surgical treatments should be considered in terms of their potential harm as well as their potential benefit.

Some hazards are intrinsic to the surgical procedure or disease and are unavoidable. Other hazards are partially or entirely avoidable, and damage resulting from exposing a patient to such a hazard reflects bad practice. Those caring for patients have a duty to try to minimize unavoidable injury and to prevent, at all costs, the avoidable. For surgical patients, the surgeon has primary responsibility for this. A fundamental requirement is good communication between the surgeon and patient as well as between all members of the healthcare team. Breakdown in effective teamwork is responsible for many of the avoidable adverse events affecting patients;for example, failing to recognize that a patient is allergic to aspirin.

It is increasingly evident that providing optimal care depends on the allocation of resources locally. Surgeons strive to secure the best resources for their patients but need to recognize the circumstances where the patient is at less risk of harm if transferred to another unit with better resources for dealing with that particular condition.

The resources required to treat a surgical patient safely vary with the patient and the condition. For example, the requirements for local anaesthetic day-case hernia repair are entirely different from those required for open cardiac bypass surgery. This chapter does not discuss detailed individual requirements. This information is largely available in consensus documents developed by individual specialties about minimal standards of provision. Although not yet carrying the force of law, surgeons need to be aware of these documents and to try to ensure that the environment in which they care for patients is appropriate. In some cases, it is better to refuse to undertake certain procedures when resources are unsafe than to risk legal challenge if adverse events should occur.

As in other areas of medicine, surgeons are being increasingly pressurized to increase efficiency. While this may be financially desirable, it is essential that patients are not exposed to unnecessary risk in order just to meet financial targets. Surgeons need to take a stand and make managers aware, verbally and in writing, when drives for efficiency compromise safety.

2   General hazards

As doctors, we know that 'to err is human' and we need to be constantly vigilant of our own actions and those of our colleagues. The two major sources of error in medical practice are communication failures and drug-prescribing errors.

Badermann reported that 26 per cent of 100 consecutive cases referred to the Medical Protection Society stemmed from communication failure. Doctors must communicate; this means setting up systems to ensure that all who need to know, do know, and mechanisms to ensure that they have understood what is being communicated. This applies to all members of the healthcare team—nurses, anaesthetists, and locums (especially). The same principles apply to patients and colleagues. Problems often arise because a doctor assumes someone else knows what is going on, but ultimately it is the consultant's responsibility to ensure that communication systems do not fail.

Drug prescribing is fraught with dangers. Errors occur for the following reasons: wrong drug, wrong dose, unexpected drug interactions, or failure to elicit a history of allergy or idiosyncrasy. Drug errors can be eliminated only by great vigilance on the part of the prescribing doctor, the dispensing pharmacist, and the administering nurse. Doctors need to interact with the patient (Table 5.1) and to at least consider a checklist for each drug-prescribing episode (Table 5.2). The illustrative checklists are exhaustive and need to be modified in the light of the circumstances and the patient's level of understanding.

Table 5.1 What to tell patient about their drugs (modified from *Drugs and Therapeutics Bulletin*, 1981, **19**, 734)

1. Name of the drug
2. Purpose of drug: how it will treat the disease or symptoms?
3. How can the patient tell if it is working and what to do if it appears not to be working
4. When and how to take it, e.g. before or after meals
5. What to do if a dose is missed
6. For how long to take the drug
7. Important side-effects and appropriate actions to be taken
8. Possible effects on driving or work, and precautions
9. Interactions with alcohol, foodstuffs, other drugs

Table 5.2 Questions to ask yourself about a drug to be prescribed (after Herxheimer 1976)

Name	What is the approved/generic name?
Class	To what class does the drug belong?
Aim	What is the aim of each drug prescribed?
Efficacy	What observations can be made to assess whether the aim has been achieved?
Dosage	What route, dosage, and interval are to be prescribed and why?
Options	Are there alternatives as regards efficacy, safety, cost?
Duration	For how long should treatment continue? Why, how, and when to stop the drug
Excretion	How is the drug eliminated; consider confounding factors?
Side-effects	What, when, and how often do these occur and are they acceptable?
Interactions	What are they and how can they be avoided?
Patients' ideas	What does the patient know about the drug?

3   Preoperative preparation

3.1   Clerking the patient

Traditionally within the National Health Service, surgical patients are clerked by a pre-registration house officer. This clerking is performed in a well-established and relatively structured manner. Clerking is designed to identify the symptoms related to the patient's presenting complaint, the history of these symptoms, and their place within the patient's previous medical history. The clerking is also designed to assess any co-morbidity and to establish the social context of the patient's disease and the hospital admission, and to record a detailed drug history. During this exercise, many factors must be considered and placed in the context of the proposed treatment.

Such a complex exercise should not be the sole responsibility of the most junior and inexperienced member of the surgical team. With appropriate training, instruction, and lines of communication, the clerking exercise can act as a filter for identifying areas of concern that require more detailed and specialist attention. Performed assiduously, it will avoid giving patients drugs to which they are allergic, avoid having to deal with unexpected (but previously recognized) co-morbidity during anaesthesia and surgery, and minimize the risk of exposing hospital staff to potentially dangerous infections (e.g. hepatitis B, HIV).

3.2   The surgeon's role

Surgeons should be much more than simply operating technicians. They are involved in diagnosis, treatment planning, treatment delivery, and continuing aftercare. Patients attending hospital for a surgical procedure should all have been seen by the operating surgeon before arriving in the operating department.

If this is not possible, the surgeon must see the patient before induction of anaesthesia and confirm that the correct patient is going to have the correct procedure. Before operation, the surgeon should run through a checklist. For example:

1. Has the patient been correctly identified?

2. Has the correct diagnosis been made and confirmed by appropriate investigations?

3. Has the appropriate treatment been scheduled, bearing in mind the diagnosis and any co-morbidity?

4. Has the patient been appropriately informed and given properly informed consent?

5. Are the notes unambiguous with regard to the above four points?

6. Has the operation site been marked?

7. Is the patient's identification correct on the published operating list and is the planned operation correctly described on the list?

8. Are the appropriate resources (e.g. intensive care unit (ITU)) and personnel available for the safe performance and conclusion of the patient's operative management?

9. Can any factors be modified to reduce the risk to the patient?

Using a checklist helps the surgeon minimize the risk to the patient. However, other safety mechanisms must be in place locally to prevent the unforgivable accident of a patient undergoing the wrong operation. It is hard to believe that within the modern hospital environment such an accident could occur, but despite all the precautions of nurses completing theatre checklists and the formal handing over of patients from one member of the surgical team to another, these accidents still occur with astonishing regularity. Surgeons should be quite clear that responsibility for such errors lies with the person performing the wrong procedure—the surgeon (Table 5.3).

3.3 The anaesthetist's role

Preoperative assessment by the anaesthetist is a vital part of any surgical patient's care. The structure of patient care often gives

Table 5.3 Recommended checks to prevent wrong operation errors

1. Record the diagnosis, side, and operation in the notes

2. Mark the operation site before operation and premedication

3. Publish a carefully checked operating list and ensure the list is re-written and changes are fully notified

4. Ensure correct patient identification

5. Use written handover on leaving the ward, arrival in the theatre complex, and arrival on the operating table

6. Identify potential dangers (e.g. highlighting patients with the same name on a list or ward)

7. Identify key personnel responsible at the various levels in a published hospital policy

insufficient time for pre-anaesthetic assessment and surgeons are often tempted to pressurize their anaesthetic colleagues into foreshortening this phase. Surgeons should be mindful of the complex and specialist nature of anaesthetic care and should give their anaesthetist sufficient time to assess the patients preoperatively and, where appropriate, be prepared to defer surgery until other investigations, resuscitation, or treatments are undertaken.

3.4 Patient optimization

A patient's condition should be optimized preoperatively as far as possible to minimize the risks of the peri- and postoperative period. This process is complex and may be multidisciplinary. Its takes place within three categories:

(1) factors related to the disease and the procedure (e.g. bowel preparation for left colonic surgery);

(2) general risks associated with surgery (e.g. thromboembolism prophylaxis);and

(3) management of co-morbidity.

It is important to recognize that the outcome for the patient is often determined in this period of preoperative assessment and management. There is a danger that the process could be rushed to the detriment of outcome. Indeed, for high-risk patients, a randomized controlled trial has shown that aggressive preoperative preparation in intensive care has a substantial beneficial effect on postoperative morbidity and mortality (Boyd *et al.* 1993). As a result of this and other studies, as well as criticisms voiced in successive NCEPOD reports, public and professional momentum is gathering to offer considerably more intensive preoperative preparation to high-risk patients, particularly those presenting as emergencies with, for example, strangulated hernia. Although this appears to increase resource utilization, the reduced postoperative morbidity and mortality would be likely to offset this to a large extent.

3.5 Day surgery

In the current world-wide climate of financial pressure on hospitals, patients are increasingly admitted to hospital on the day of operation. This may compromise proper preoperative assessment unless planned facilities such as pre-admission clinics are universally utilized and adequately supervised. For day surgery (i.e. patients admitted and discharged on the same day) preparation time is limited and only patients that fulfil predetermined criteria should be offered this service. Criteria vary from unit to unit but the following normally apply (Royal College of Surgeons 1985):

◆ the patient should be ASA grade 1 or 2 (Table 5.4);

◆ the planned procedure should take less than 1 hour;

◆ adequate analgesia should be offered;

◆ suitable home support should be available.

Table 5.4 American Society of Anesthesiology grading (ASA)

Class	Operative mortality (%)
1 Normally healthy individuals	0.1
2 Mild systemic disease	0.2
3 Severe systemic disease not incapacitating	1–2
4 Patient with incapacitating systemic disease threatening life	7–10
5 Moribund patient who is expected to die in 24 hours with or without surgery	>10

3.6 Emergency surgery

Patients requiring emergency surgery are particularly at risk of complications, many of which are avoidable. Once it has been decided that emergency surgery is necessary, the anaesthetist should be contacted and informed about:

- the likely surgical diagnosis;
- the magnitude of the proposed surgery;
- the urgency of the surgery;
- any known risk factors (e.g. hypertension, anticoagulants).

There is sometimes a conflict between preoperative resuscitation and the need to correct the underlying pathology surgically. These cases often present first to junior surgeons and anaesthetists who need to be aware of particular difficulties and, where appropriate, seek senior advice and assistance early in the management process.

4 Avoiding hazards in the operating theatre

4.1 Introduction

The period between a patient entering the operating department and leaving the recovery unit is a potentially hazardous one for the patient as well as for the staff attending the patient. The normal defence mechanisms and avoiding reflexes that a fully conscious patient is able to employ to avoid injury and other harmful activities are obtunded and the patient relies on the care and trained actions of a large number of staff to replace these (Table 5.5).

Table 5.5 Avoidable hazards within the operating theatre

Wrong procedure
Anaesthetic mishaps
Surgical mishaps
Handling injury (patient and staff)
Equipment failure
Cross infection (patient and staff)

4.2 Wrong procedure

All hospitals should ideally have written policies to avoid this error. Several levels of checking should occur and great care must be taken when the order of published operating lists is changed. Essentially, if the surgeon has seen the patient before operation and goes through the previously described checklist, this error should never occur (*Theatre safeguards* 1985).

4.3 Anaesthetic mishaps

Local, regional, and general anaesthesia are all associated with well-recognized complications. It is beyond the scope of a surgical textbook to discuss these in detail; however, surgeons should be aware of the main dangers of anaesthesia and methods of avoiding such dangers. Most anaesthetic mishaps fall into the categories of critical incidents or injuries to teeth. Tooth injuries comprise about half of the non-hypoxic/death incidents reported to the medical defence organizations. However, various other injuries still occur (Table 5.6).

More serious injuries are classified as **critical incidents**. These are of major concern to anaesthetists, and substantial changes in anaesthetic practice and monitoring have been introduced in recent years to reduce this risk (Table 5.7) (Buck *et al.* 1987). These changes include improved training and supervision in an attempt to reduce human errors (Table 5.8) and improved

Table 5.6 Non-death/hypoxic anaesthetic mishaps (information from the MDU 1970–82)

Injury	Percentage occurrence
Teeth	52
Nerve damage	9
Extradural foreign body	7
Thrombophlebitis/minor injury	7
Awareness under anaesthesia	7
Spinal cord damage	4
Pneumothorax	3
Extravasation	2
Lacerations/fracture (falls)	2
Blood cross-match errors	1
Burns	1
Others	5

Table 5.7 CEPOD-identified causes of anaesthetic-related death

Failure to apply knowledge
Lack of care
Failure of organization
Lack of experience
Lack of knowledge
Drug effect
Equipment failure
Fatigue

Table 5.8 Human error as a cause of anaesthetic critical incident

Type of error	Percentage of total
Drug error	24
Misuse of anaesthetic machine	22
Airway problem	16
Ventilation system failure	11
Fluid therapy error	5
Intravenous disconnection	6
Monitoring failure	4
Other	12

monitoring equipment used to check patient well-being during anaesthesia and recovery from anaesthesia.

As a result of these precautions, anaesthesia has become highly technological. In response to these expensive developments in instrumentation, various bodies have issued guidelines for minimum standards of anaesthetic monitoring. In the United Kingdom, the Association of Anaesthetists of GB and Ireland (AAGBI) published an advisory document in 1988 (see Chapter 4). The recommendations apply wherever an anaesthetic is given, as well as to recovery areas and where anaesthetized patients are being transferred. They emphasize that use of monitoring devices should not distract the anaesthetist from making basic clinical observations. Although there is no conclusive evidence that more widespread use of monitoring equipment reduces morbidity or mortality, it is believed that it will encourage a high standard of patient care. The most effective monitor is still the constant presence of a skilled and vigilant anaesthetist. Better drugs also contribute to increased patient safety.

The increased emphasis on continuous monitoring of the anaesthetized patient has also changed the physical conduct of anaesthesia in many hospitals. In the United Kingdom it has been traditional to construct theatre complexes with an anaesthetic room adjacent to the theatre. The patient is anaesthetized in the anaesthetic room and then moved to the theatre. This transfer is potentially hazardous and, in practice, the monitoring equipment must be completely portable or else be duplicated in the anaesthetic room and the theatre, which is expensive. For this reason many anaesthetists are now inducing anaesthesia on the operating table (Association of Anaesthetists 1988).

4.4 Surgical mishaps

Surgical mishaps within the operating theatre range from the acutely dramatic disaster of uncontrolled haemorrhage to the harder to define 'inadequate' surgery leading to delayed but theoretically avoidable recurrence of the pathology. The prevention of surgical harm is dependent on adequate surgical training, continuing education, audit, and definition of standards in surgery (Chapter 2). Individual surgeons, institutions, and the surgical profession as a whole must strive to improve their performance in this area. Surgeons have had clear evidence

of wide variation in results of surgical treatment for many years but they have generally been slow to change their working practices. However, gradual changes are occurring with improvements in audit, specialization, training, and continuation of medical education after specialist accreditation.

4.5 Handling and positional injuries

Moving patients within the hospital and theatre is potentially hazardous, particularly when the patient is anaesthetized or partly recovered from anaesthesia.

Transfer of patients to the theatre

Ideally, patients should be brought to theatre on their own beds. However, to do so safely, these must be height adjustable, easily manoeuvred, and with the ability to tilt the head down (in the event of vomiting). They should have brakes and side guard rails. Transfer to the table may be performed by several methods:

♦ The fully conscious patient may move over while assisted and observed by assistants.

♦ The patient may be lifted by theatre attendants on a canvas stretcher.

♦ The patient may be slid sideways on a stretcher using a proprietary sliding board or lateral rolling device. These are preferred as they protect theatre staff from lifting hazards. In some theatres, trolley-top transfer systems are used. Here, the patient is transferred to a special trolley which incorporates the operating table top. After induction of anaesthesia, the trolley is wheeled over the table base and the top lifted off by hydraulic elevation of the table base.

♦ Patients with pelvic or lower-limb fractures are best induced on their beds and transferred to the table only once.

Moving and positioning the anaesthetized patient

Handling and positioning a patient in theatre is a team effort. The anaesthetist is in overall charge, aided by operating-room assistants and by the surgeon for final adjustments. Theatre and recovery nurses also play an important part. Whenever a patient is moved, it is important to ensure in advance that access is possible all around the patient, that the necessary number of assistants are available to move and position the patient safely (this varies with the complexity of the positioning and on the patient's weight). All involved need to understand and perhaps rehearse what is to be achieved and any necessary equipment should be assembled in advance. Everyone involved needs to be alert to prevent accidents, particularly at critical moments such as transfer from trolley to operating table. Lifting aids should be used whenever possible (e.g. patient slides or rollers and hoists).

Theatre staff are also at risk during these activities. Back injuries and strains are common in portering and nursing staff, and have long-term consequences. Training is therefore important and EC directives require a nominated person to coordinate and monitor lifting and handling in each hospital.

Injuries and hazards of moving and positioning patients

Damage to the cervical spine

This may occur if the unsupported head is allowed to fall backwards or sideways. This is a particular risk in unconscious patients or those with rheumatoid arthritis of the cervical spine. Examples include the head extending unwittingly beyond the canvas stretcher or during changing the position of the patient without supporting the head.

Falls to the floor

These usually occur only if several things go wrong simultaneously. For example, the brakes may not be locked on the receiving trolley or operating table, allowing one or other to roll sideways during transfer. Brakes should be applied before transfer and an assistant should stand on the opposite side to steady the table and receive the patient. If the assistants are not strong enough, a heavy patient ends up being dragged rather than lifted and pushing the table away, resulting in falling through the gap. The canvas may tear, or the table top may tilt if inadequately secured. If guard rails are not in position on a trolley, a semiconscious patient may shift and fall from a narrow trolley or bed.

Damage to upper limbs

Damage to upper limbs can occur during transfer and positioning. Elbows may be bruised or even olecranon fractures caused when poles for the canvas are inserted forcefully. Fingers may become trapped between operating table joints during positioning, and care of the shoulder is required during positioning of the arms, particularly when they are placed out on arm boards. Lower-limb damage can also occur and particular care is needed in placing diseased hips into flexed abduction.

Infusion-line injuries

Traction on infusion lines, tubes, and catheters can cause tissue injury or interfere with monitoring or intravenous therapy, or both. Steel needles of butterfly type are prone to cut out during transfer and have largely been superseded by plastic cannulae (up to 40 per cent of steel needle infusions are no longer functional by the time the patient reaches the recovery room). Protection of cannulae requires careful checking of all lines prior to moving the patient. Complex cases may have several cannulae to protect, with peripheral and central venous lines, arterial cannulae, and epidural catheters all at risk.

Drains and catheters

Drains and catheters are at similar risk. Drainage tubes may separate from their containers, compromising sterility, and glass bottles may be broken. Also, drains are placed for specific therapeutic reasons and loss of a drain may require re-induction of anaesthesia and re-operation.

Chest drains require special attention as detachment allows air to enter the pleural cavity causing pneumothorax, or, if the container is raised above the patient, fluid from the underwater drain may siphon into the chest. Formerly, it was advised that chest drains be clamped before transfer but this is potentially dangerous, especially in the presence of a broncho-pleural fistula, as a tension pneumothorax can develop with alarming speed. Clamping is now generally condemned but avoiding it demands greater care be devoted to transfer without clamping.

Urinary catheters usually have a balloon retention device, and traction can pull them out while still inflated, traumatizing the urethra or bladder.

Injuries during surgery

During surgery in any position the patient is at risk form various physical injuries (Fig. 5.1).

Peripheral nerve injuries

Peripheral nerve injuries after anaesthesia are probably caused by nerve ischaemia and can occur after as little as 30 minutes in an adverse position. Examples include:

♦ ulnar nerve compression at the medial epicondyle by pressure on the edge of a mattress;

♦ facial nerve damage by pressure from a face mask;

♦ the radial nerve is poorly protected where it spirals posteriorly around the humerus, and may be injured by a metal post clamped to the operating table;

♦ the brachial plexus is vulnerable to traction on the arm. If the arm needs to be placed at right angles to the patient, the hand should be **pronated** and the patient's head turned towards the arm. If an arm inadvertently falls off the table, both brachial plexus and shoulder capsule may be stretched.

Eye injuries

Pressure on the eyes from a badly fitting face mask during operation diminishes intraocular pressure which may later rebound. Intraocular lens implants may be displaced and direct corneal damage may occur. Irritant fluids such as antiseptics, sprays, or gastric acid may be spilled on the cornea, causing chemical injury. The eyelids are usually taped gently shut during operation to prevent direct corneal trauma and drying. Corneal drying causes damage after about 10 minutes. Epithelial breakdown predisposes to infection and perhaps corneal scarring.

Direct pressure effects

Under anaesthesia, the patient's normal protective responses are lost and without proper padding, the weight of parts of the body may cause pressure necrosis of particular areas of skin. This chiefly affects the occiput, the sacrum, and the heels. The heels of patients with lower-limb ischaemia are particularly at risk and need special attention until recovery is complete.

Pressure on calves on the operating table may cause deep venous thrombosis by compression of veins, trauma to the vein wall, and stagnation of blood. Elevation by pads under the ankle, graduated compression stockings, and pneumatic compression devices all reduce this risk.

Supine position

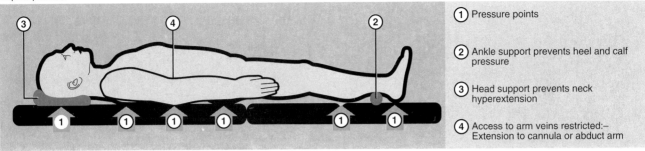

① Pressure points

② Ankle support prevents heel and calf pressure

③ Head support prevents neck hyperextension

④ Access to arm veins restricted:– Extension to cannula or abduct arm

Lithotomy position

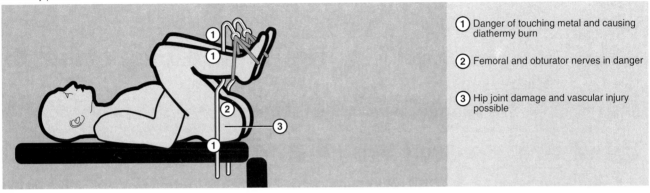

① Danger of touching metal and causing diathermy burn

② Femoral and obturator nerves in danger

③ Hip joint damage and vascular injury possible

Lloyd-Davies position

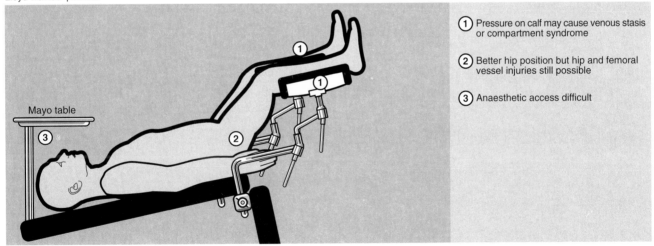

① Pressure on calf may cause venous stasis or compartment syndrome

② Better hip position but hip and femoral vessel injuries still possible

③ Anaesthetic access difficult

Figure 5.1 During surgery in any position the patient is at risk from various physical injuries.

Surgeons need to be aware that leaning on anaesthetized patients may cause injury.

Joint injury

In rheumatoid patients, the odontoid ligament may already be eroded, and with careless passive neck movements, this allows the odontoid peg to penetrate the cervical cord, with disastrous results. Preoperative X-rays in flexion and extension should be performed in rheumatoid patients.

In any patient, if the normal lumbosacral lordosis is not supported, postoperative backache may result. Inflatable wedges or pads may be used to prevent this.

If the ankles are lifted too high on a support, hyperextension injury to the knee may occur, especially if assistants lean on the legs during operation.

Burns

Occasionally patients receive burns while on the operating table. These are often due to faulty positioning of the patient. Diathermy burns occur if the patient comes into contact with

Lateral +/– Break

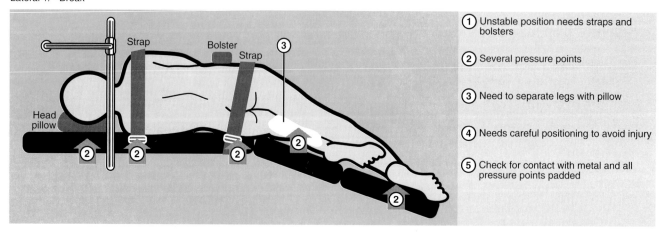

① Unstable position needs straps and bolsters

② Several pressure points

③ Need to separate legs with pillow

④ Needs careful positioning to avoid injury

⑤ Check for contact with metal and all pressure points padded

Prone position

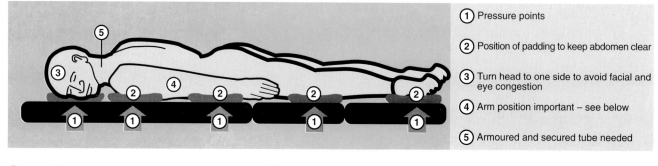

① Pressure points

② Position of padding to keep abdomen clear

③ Turn head to one side to avoid facial and eye congestion

④ Arm position important – see below

⑤ Armoured and secured tube needed

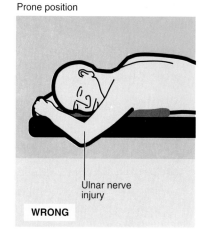

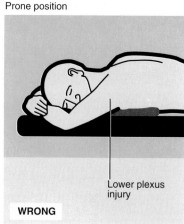

Figure 5.1 Continued

bare metal of the operating table or its attachments, and constant vigilance is required to prevent this injury. Other diathermy burns can occur if the earth plate is placed in a faulty position or in inadequate contact. In general, hairy skin-contact areas should be shaved and single-use disposable electrodes employed and correctly applied. If the patient is moved extensively after placement of the pad, it is important to check that the pad has not shifted.

Supine position

Most patients will spend some time in the supine position during anaesthesia and surgery. Anaesthesia is usually induced in a supine patient and most operations are carried out in this position. In this position, handling and manipulation of the patient is minimized, physiological upsets related to position are minimal, and most physical hazards to the patient are easily avoided. However, supine patients are at risk of aspirating gastric contents (particularly in emergency operations for intestinal obstruction and Caesarean sections) and induction of anaesthesia must not be performed in this position unless the table or trolley is capable of being rapidly tilted head downwards and pharyngeal suction is to hand.

Patients generally lie supine on a flat operating table with arms by the side of the body, across the chest, or supported in an abducted position on arm boards. A soft pad is placed under the ankles to lift the calves just off the table. Some surgeons prefer the alternative 'lawn chair position' with gentle flexion of the hips and knees, usually by placing a pillow beneath the knees. This is anatomically neutral and distributes support along the entire dorsal surface of the body. It may prevent postoperative backache by straightening the lumbar spine.

A moderate head-down tilt of up to 20° in the supine position is often used for lower-limb surgery and for abdominal pelvic surgery. For varicose vein operations, this reduces the lower-limb venous pressure and for operations such as anterior resection of the rectum, it helps keep bowel out of the field by gravity. The Trendelenberg position (1890) is an obsolete variant, using extreme head-down tilt of about 35–40°, formerly used for abdominal gynaecological or pelvic surgery. Modern muscle relaxants have rendered this position unnecessary.

Reverse Trendelenburg, or head-up tilt, is often used for major head and neck surgery. Steep angles are sometimes used and the patient is prevented from slipping off the table by foot supports. Reverse Trendelenburg facilitates operating in intracranial, middle-ear, and plastic surgical procedures by reducing venous pressure in the head. It also potentiates the effects of hypotensive anaesthetic techniques. Air embolism is a risk if veins are inadvertently opened.

Lithotomy positions

The lithotomy position is a modification of the supine position in which the knees and hips are flexed and the hips adducted to provide surgical access to the perineum. The name is derived from its early application in the perineal approach to cutting for bladder stone. The modern lithotomy position is often combined with a minor degree of head-down tilt, which aids access and visibility to the perineal area, particularly the anal canal.

The lithotomy position is widely used in gynaecology, urology, and anorectal surgery, including abdomino-perineal resection of the rectum. In its simplest form and for short procedures, the ankles are supported in canvas stirrups on vertical poles attached to the side rails of the operating table and the caudal section of the operating table is removed. For longer operations and where precise leg positioning is needed, a more elaborate variety of limb support such as the Lloyd-Davies type is preferred (Fig. 5.1).

For simultaneous access to abdominal pelvic organs and perineum (e.g. abdomino-perineal resection or pelvic pouch procedure) the Lloyd-Davies position, described in 1939, is usually employed. Multijointed leg supports allow precise positioning of the limbs, require a lesser degree of hip and knee flexion, and provide greater support for the calves in semi-cylindrical padded rests. Access to the perineum is achieved largely by abduction rather than flexion of the hips. This allows the abdominal surgical team to work on the abdomen at the same time as the perineal operator works on the perineum. The latter can assist the abdominal surgeon from between the legs at first and later operate independently on the perineum.

Access is improved by placing a firm support such as a sandbag under the sacrum and by adjusting the patient so the sacrococcygeal junction projects just beyond the end of the table. The operating table is tilted about 20° head-down.

The scrub nurse may use a Mayo table across the patient's chest but this restricts surgical access to the abdomen and anaesthetic access to the head. Many surgeons prefer the nurse to use an instrument trolley at the left side of the patient's head, with the anaesthetist working from the right.

Induction of anaesthesia in the lithotomy position

Anaesthesia is induced with the patient lying flat. A double-length breathing circuit is used to allow the patient to be moved down the table. The patient's arms are usually placed across the chest. The posts and stirrups are next attached symmetrically to the table under the supervision of the surgeon. Two assistants should do this while the anaesthetist is responsible for controlling the head and neck. Ideally, the patient should have been placed with hips level with the stirrups. If not, the patient is gently lifted down the table on the canvas into the correct position. The calves must not be allowed to rest on the end of the table. The legs are then lifted together, one by each assistant and secured in the supports or stirrups. The patient may need shifting laterally so the perineum is midway between the poles. The caudal end of the table is then folded down or removed. A sandbag may be placed under the sacrum and the perineal position may need adjusting. Force should never be used as any perceived immobility may be due to joint deformities, stiffness, or light anaesthesia.

Musculoskeletal injury is more likely in lithotomy than supine positions. The hips, knees, and back are at risk when moved passively under general anaesthesia because a greater range of movement may be attempted than a conscious patient would use. Thus, when preparing a patient likely to placed in the lithotomy position, an appropriate history and perhaps test movements should be performed beforehand. Sacroiliac or hip joint strain may occur if poor technique is used, and a prolapsed intervertebral disc may be exacerbated by forward flexion of the lumbar spine. The average incidence of postoperative backache (1/3) is about the same as for the simple supine position, but increases in proportion to the duration of operation. If the patient has restricted hip or knee flexion, this can usually be accommodated by angling the pillars forwards, but if there is bilateral fixed adduction deformities of the hips, difficulties arise and an alternative means of access to the perineum, such as a left lateral or face-down position, may have to be employed.

The **sciatic nerve** is immobile at the sciatic notch and at the point where the common peroneal branch passes around the fibular neck. Forced hip flexion, particularly if prolonged, is likely to damage the nerve at either of these points. Straight-leg variants of the lithotomy position should be avoided as they are more likely to cause sciatic nerve damage. Intramuscular buttock injections must not be given in the lithotomy position as the sciatic nerve is displaced laterally. The common peroneal nerve is also at risk if an assistant leans on a leg placed outside a pole, crushing it against the fibula. The saphenous nerve above the knee may similarly be compressed against the poles, which should be enclosed in foam padding along their entire length to prevent this, and the legs positioned so that pressure is minimal.

Vascular injury is unfortunately relatively common and may be disastrous. Compression and damage to the calf veins is probably the most common and most dangerous hazard of the lithotomy position. Poles should be foam padded and leg position adjusted to avoid pressure. Assistants must be discouraged from leaning on the legs. In the Lloyd-Davies position, the calf supports should be padded and their orientation carefully adjusted (and checked by the surgeon) to ensure there is no undue or uneven pressure on the calf or popliteal fossa. In long operations, intermittent calf compression boots may be helpful.

Reports of trauma from muscle crush injury have been published and compartment syndrome should be considered in patients complaining of leg pains after prolonged 'legs-up' procedures. Many patients undergoing surgery in the Lloyd-Davies position are elderly and have concurrent iliofemoral arterial disease. Acute occlusive thrombosis of these disease segments may occur and particular attention should be paid to the peripheral pulses before and after surgery.

Lateral position

This position is used in pulmonary and oesophageal thoracic surgery, renal surgery, hip replacements, and some neurosurgical procedures. Percutaneous skeletal fixation is used for some neurosurgical procedures, using special head-supporting devices. It should be remembered that the lateral position is intrinsically unstable and places pressure on unusual anatomical sites.

The head should be supported on a soft pillow to avoid necrosis of the underlying ear and to prevent brachial plexus traction injury. The upper arm should be supported in a padded arm rest. A sheepskin or evacuatable mattress should be placed under the patient to spread the load evenly and prevent necrosis of the skin over the lower iliac crest. Bony prominences in the lower limbs should be supported by pillows, particularly near the common peroneal nerve around the neck of the fibula. An evacuatable mattress consists of a plastic cover filled loosely with polystyrene beads. Once the patient has been positioned, air is evacuated from the mattress, solidifying the beads and maintaining the patient safely in the set position. Careful handling is needed to place a patient safely into the lateral position. Before moving the patient, it is important to check that all necessary equipment is available, including pillows, and the table brakes are applied.

The table break point should be positioned just caudal to the lower rib margin. Positioning requires two strong assistants and a third to position the legs. They should all stand on the same side so the patient can be rotated away from them. One looks after the chest, the second the pelvis, and the third the legs. All lift and rotate together to place the patient on the edge of table nearest them. The pillows are placed and the breathing hoses temporarily secured. The upper arm is lifted into its support and bandaged in place and the underlying arm is flexed at the elbow

and taped in place. The hips are then flexed and a seat support placed against the ischial tuberosities and a strap applied across the upper pelvic crest or an abdominal strut placed to prevent the patient rolling forwards.

A diathermy plate is applied to the uppermost thigh or to the chest wall and pillows are placed between knees and ankles to support the semiflexed limbs. Finally an anaesthetic screen is placed across the head end.

Thoracic surgical lateral positions

It is important that the upper arm support and screen are placed to allow the anaesthetist good access to the double lumen tube. An inflatable air cushion below the chest may be used to expand an intercostal incision. Sometimes the surgeon prefers the patient to lean 10–15° towards him.

Renal and extraperitoneal lateral positions

The nephrectomy position is full lateral with the table broken 20° each way above and below the flank with the dependent leg flexed at hip and knee. The older kidney bridge is no longer necessary and the lateral jackknife position is deprecated as it interferes with blood flow. For the extraperitoneal approach to the hilum of the liver and head of pancreas, a **semilateral position** is often preferred. Sandbags are placed under the pelvis and chest on the right side and the table broken as for nephrectomy. The right arm is positioned away from the surgical field across the chest and the other arm is alongside the body or out on a board.

Prone positions

Prone positions are used for surgery on the posterior aspect of the patient. They carry greater risk than other postures and good positioning is vital to prevent pressure necrosis, joint injuries, and to minimize venous pooling and bleeding.

Patient support should exert pressure only on bony areas, avoiding compressing large blood vessels in the groins and abdomen, the liver and inferior vena cava (the epigastrium must be free of pressure from the costal margin downwards), and the jugular veins in the neck. The back and neck should remain in a single plane and the head should be in a neutral position as overextension of the cervical spine may cause cervical cord damage in patients with spinal degeneration or rheumatoid arthritis. The face must rest on the forehead only and be properly padded. Eye pressure must be avoided to prevent central retinal artery thrombosis as well as glaucoma in susceptible patients. The eyes must also be protected against contact with skin preparation solutions, aerosols, the patient's own saliva, and vomitus, using pads and adhesive tape.

The arms should be in the normal prone sleeping position above the head and not on lateral arm boards. Radial and ulnar nerve damage can occur if the arms are allowed to hang over the side of the table in this position. In head and neck surgery, the arms may need to be placed beside the body. Areas of skin in contact with supports must be protected by foam pads or soft pillows. These include bony prominences such as the anterior superior iliac spine, knees, and feet. In women, a pillow should be used to support the chest and the breasts should be displaced laterally. The knees are supported on a soft pad and the lower legs raised higher than the knees with one or two pillows to protect the toes, as well as the lateral cutaneous nerve of thigh and external popliteal nerve at the neck of the fibula.

Anaesthetic access is an important consideration in the prone position. The patient is usually induced supine and venous access and central venous cannulation placed in this position, often with extension sets added. Spontaneous respiration is not appropriate because ventilatory function is impaired in the prone position. An armoured endotracheal tube is used and securely fixed; adhesive strapping may come off because of salivary dribbling. If mouth packs are used, their presence should be written on the patient's forehead. ECG leads and blood-pressure cuffs are best disconnected and reattached after positioning is completed.

Positioning should be coordinated by the anaesthetist. Two strong men and, ideally, two more assistants are needed. One strong person supports and turns the chest, the other turns the pelvis and legs, the third assistant stands opposite them to place the chest and pelvic supports during the turn. The fourth assistant looks after the legs. To turn the patient, the table brakes are secured and the table head support is lowered, with the anaesthetist supporting the head. The patient is lifted and rolled from supine on the trolley to prone on the prepared table in one smooth movement. Alternatively, the patient can first be rotated towards the third assistant and placed in a lateral position on the side of table nearest the lifters. In this case, the patient's lower arm is straight underneath and the assistants' arms remain under the patient. Pillows are placed under the chest and pelvis. The patient is lifted again, turned, and the pillows adjusted and the lower arm taken through. Final adjustments consist of placing the patient's head on a soft pad or pillow under the forehead, the arms are supported above the head, and a pillow placed under the knees and the ankles. The anterior abdominal wall, particularly the epigastrium, should not touch the mattress even during maximum respiratory excursion. The diathermy plate is applied and monitoring and venous access checked.

At completion of the operation, the patient is returned to the supine or lateral position before extubation. This may be done after transfer to the recovery trolley. The patient should not be transferred directly to a bed as handling is difficult and may cause back strain in the assistants.

4.6 Equipment failure

Care in theatre is becoming increasingly technical. This raises the possibility of injury through equipment malfunction. Theatre-equipment-related injury is usually a consequence of human error and inappropriate use of technology. Common errors include failure to use equipment as instructed and deliberate disconnection of alarms. Diathermy equipment, electrical heating devices, and lasers have all been reported to cause severe injury to patients, and surgeons and theatre staff should be fully trained in their use and abuse. Temperature-control devices are becoming used increasingly in major

Table 5.9 Temperature-control methods

Control of ambient theatre temperature
Warming of infusions and washout solutions
Heated mattresses
Recovery-room patient heating devices and 'space blankets'

prolonged surgery, and prevention of hypothermia should be a major concern to surgeon and anaesthetist. Various methods have been employed and are listed in Table 5.9.

Hypothermia

Inadvertent hypothermia is a considerable danger to children and to adults undergoing prolonged surgical procedures. Hypothermia is a largely avoidable injury to surgical patients. Reduction in core temperature causes alteration in drug metabolism, impairment of coagulation, and, during the post-operative period, an increase in tissue oxygen requirements and consequent acidosis and increased myocardial work. In the elderly and in patients with cardiorespiratory disease, acidosis and increased myocardial work and oxygen requirements may cause major complications after surgery.

4.7 Infection risks

Minimizing the risks of infection within the surgical environment should be a major concern of all theatre staff. In the pre-antibiotic era, bacterial infection was a serious hazard to both patients and staff, with operations reported with mortalities of 300 per cent caused by bacterial contamination of surgeons and assistants through sharps injuries. Bacterial infection remains a major problem for patients but should not now cause problems for staff. However, operating theatre environments should continue to be kept stringently clean, with proper filtering and ventilation.

Global excessive use of antibiotics has led to the emergence of resistant bacterial strains (e.g. multiresistant *Staphylococcus aureus*, MRSA) and surgeons should continually review antibiotic usage in individual patients and generally. Viral infection has become an important concern for all patients and staff involved with invasive procedures. Human immuno-deficiency virus (HIV), hepatitis B, and hepatitis C viruses are serious hazards for patients and staff, and extreme care is required to prevent accidental cross-infection.

HIV and AIDS

AIDS is not yet curable. Many infected individuals remain well for years but most will develop AIDS and die as a result of infection. Therefore prevention of infection is paramount.

The viruses infect and destroy T4-helper lymphocytes, persist indefinitely, and paralyse the immune system. After HIV exposure, a self-limiting infectious mononucleosis-like illness usually results, and the patient's serum later becomes positive for anti-HIV antibody (thus the patient is infectious before sero-conversion). There is then a variable period of up to 10 years of subclinical infection, during which the T4 lymphocyte count falls and the patient remains infectious. Later, persistent generalized lymphadenopathy occurs. Progression to AIDS is marked by the development of opportunistic infections. These include oral and oesophageal candidiasis, chronic diarrhoea caused by *Cryptosporidium* and other unusual organisms, *Pneumocystis* and bacterial pneumonias, tuberculosis, cytomegalovirus (CMV) retinitis, and *Cryptococcus* meningitis.

Patients carrying HIV may present to surgeons with incidental conditions during the subclinical period (for example, male homosexuals with perianal disease) or with opportunistic infections after developing AIDS. Any patient may carry the virus, and a negative HIV antibody test does not mean that the patient is not infectious if exposed recently to risk of infection. HIV infection is now endemic throughout the world, with particularly high prevalence in certain geographical areas and populations.

Theatre staff should assume that all patients treated are HIV positive and apply **universal precautions** to minimize the risk of infection of staff. However, this is often impracticable and most institutions operate a policy of damage limitation by applying some sort of screening. In high-risk geographical areas, all patients admitted for emergency surgery should be assumed to be infected. Screening of elective cases is based firstly on the history. This includes questions about sexual behaviour, drug abuse, travel to HIV endemic areas, contact with hepatitis B, and the possibility of previous transfusion of infected blood. Examination for needle puncture sites is essential as history about intravenous drug use is often unreliable. High-risk patients should be counselled and offered an HIV test. Surgeons should bear in mind that a negative test does not exclude active infectious disease.

HIV antibody tests are required in transplant donors and before blood, sperm, or milk donation. However, despite this, infection in organ recipients has been reported because testing took place before seroconversion.

Hepatitis B

Hepatitis B is a DNA virus that has a long incubation period of 2–5 months (during which cases are infectious); 5–10 per cent of cases become carriers with persistent HBV infection, and occasionally fulminant hepatitis occurs. Laboratory diagnosis relies on detection of the HBV surface antigen (HB_sAg), usually by ELISA. Patients with this antigen in their serum are infectious. Acute and active infection can be distinguished from chronic carriage in HB_sAg-positive people by detecting IgM antibodies against the core antigen (anti-HB_cAg); presence of the 'e' antigen (HB_eAg) in serum indicates that the individual is particularly infectious. Previous immunization or infection results in antibodies to the surface antigen (anti-HB_sAg). Patients with these antibodies are *not* infectious.

Hepatitis B infection is endemic in many populations, with high incidences seen in South-East Asia, Africa, eastern Europe, and the Americas. Homosexuals and intravenous drug abusers are also at high risk. The agent is highly infectious and staff in

theatres are at high risk of infection from needlestick injuries and other sources of contamination. Vaccination with genetically engineered HB_sAg against HBV is safe and highly effective, and must be given to all clinical and other staff at risk of inoculation with HBV-containing blood, including all surgeons. Seroconversion should be checked after the three-dose vaccination course and, if an adequate antibody titre is demonstrated, vaccination is repeated at 5-yearly intervals. Antibody levels greater than 100 IU give long-lasting immunity but these people should still have booster doses at 3–5 years. People with antibody levels of 50–100 IU should be revaccinated after a year and those with 10–50 IU and non-converters remain at risk of infection and should be vaccinated again. The latter group may require hepatitis B immunoglobulin prophylaxis in the event of a sharps or needlestick injury. If they still fail to convert, they should be tested for hepatitis B e antigen and, if positive, avoid invasive procedures until they become no longer e antigen positive. Transmission of HBV in both directions between surgeons and patients has been documented on numerous occasions, and successful vaccination will abolish this risk.

Hepatitis C

Hepatitis C virus causes a relatively mild hepatitis. Before blood screening, it was identified after about 1 per cent of blood transfusions. The incubation period is about 6–8 weeks. Tests for HCV have only recently become available but, because seroconversion takes up to 6 months after jaundice, they are useful for screening blood for transfusion but not for acute diagnosis. The risk of hepatitis C infection has become of increasing concern in recent years. Intravenous drug abusers are often infected, with up to 85 per cent prevalence. However 45–50 per cent of infected cases appear to be sporadic. Many infections are subclinical (75 per cent), and when considered with the late development of seropositivity, screening is seen to be unreliable. The major clinical problem with hepatitis C infection is chronic hepatitis. Fifty per cent of new, non-alcohol-related cases of chronic active hepatitis and cirrhosis are now attributed to previous hepatitis C infection.

Hepatitis D or the **delta agent** is an incomplete virus that can only multiply in the presence of HBV, which acts as a 'helper' virus. Thus the delta agent may cause exacerbations of HBV infection in patients who are already HB_sAg-positive.

Screening for infection
Screening staff

Potential trainees may consider screening for hepatitis B e antigen and, if positive, avoid a career involving surgical or invasive procedures. These personnel may eventually lose their positive status spontaneously or be treated with interferon. Surgeons and staff at personal risk of HIV should undergo confidential testing. Insurance companies will not penalize healthcare workers who have serological tests for HIV and hepatitis B, although the consequences of positive testing may be far-reaching. The General Medical Council, the Department of Health, and the Medical Defence Union recommend that staff who think that they have been at risk of infection should be confidentially tested for HIV and hepatitis B and counselled appropriately. If HIV or e antigen positive, performing invasive procedures must be stopped. These include operative surgery, repair of traumatic injuries, angiography, obstetric deliveries, and any form of dental treatment.

The status of hepatitis C infection is not yet clear, but it is likely that similar restrictions will be placed on those who are seropositive.

Screening patients

Screening of patients is a contentious issue. In fact, screening to identify all infected patients is not possible. Emergency surgery and treatment must often be performed before the results of serological tests could possibly be available, and tests during seroconversion may be inappropriately reassuring. Furthermore, the logistics of mass screening and consequent mass counselling are formidable.

Preventative precautions

Every patient and member of staff is at risk during every invasive procedure. However, the risks for the whole population are tiny (Table 5.10). To minimize risk, basic general precautions are necessary in all situations, with specific measures employed in high-risk situations.

General precautions

1. Staff should be vaccinated successfully against hepatitis B.

2. Apply basic hygienic practices, including hand washing between patients, appropriate disposal of dressings, and covering wounds and skin breaks with waterproof dressings.

3. Take precautions to avoid contamination of skin or clothing with blood.

4. Protect mucous membranes of eyes, mouth, and nose from blood splashes.

5. Take care to prevent wounds, cuts, and abrasions in the presence of blood.

6. Avoid using sharps whenever possible.

Table 5.10 Comparative risks for adverse outcomes for healthcare workers (HCW) and patients (USA) (adapted from Wenzel 1993)

	Risk/10^6 exposures:
HCW risk of HBV infection after HB$_e$Ag needlestick	1:230 000
HCW risk of HIV infection after HIV needlestick	1:2800
HCW risk of HIV infection after mucous membrane exposure	<1:2800
Risk of death by car accident	1:250
Risk of death by anaesthetic complication	1:100
Risk of HIV after 1 unit of blood	1:1025

Table 5.11 Universal precautions to prevent contamination and infection of theatre scrub staff

- Cover cuts and abrasions with waterproof dressings
- Do not pass or receive sharps from hand to hand—the giver should lay them on a table and the receiver should pick them up
- Avoid using hand needles and avoid picking up needles by hand that have passed through tissues (no-touch technique). Avoid using sharps near fingers, particularly in blind areas
- Dispose of all sharps safely. Suture needles and scalpel blades should be collected on sticky pads and others placed in purpose-designed sharps containers
- Disposables and clinical waste should be placed in yellow clinical waste bags for incineration

General precautions (cont.)

7. Ensure safe handling of sharps (e.g. no hand-to-hand transfer), and safe disposal of used sharps.

8. Clear spilled blood promptly and disinfect surfaces.

9. Ensure safe disposal of contaminated waste.

10. In the theatre, practice universal precautions (Table 5.11).

Precautions in known high-risk situations

In patients with known infection, it is sensible to take extra precautions. The same precautions should be followed in emergency surgery and in situations of potentially high risk when the patient's infectivity is unknown.

1. Avoid operation if possible.

2. Consider endoscopic surgery.

3. The minimum number of people should be in theatre and only experienced surgeons and other staff should be present.

4. Observe a high level of theatre discipline, if possible with rehearsal and teaching in advance.

5. Remove unnecessary equipment from theatre to reduce the burden of later decontamination.

6. Scrub staff should use double gloves (and change outer gloves if damaged). Special coloured indicator undergloves can be used; a third layer of linen gloves or special gloves with woven metal threads may be used to prevent scalpel injury (but not needle penetration). High-efficiency masks, eye protection (goggles or transparent face shields), boots, impervious gowns (or waterproof sleeves and plastic aprons beneath) extending below the level of the top of the boots may also be used.

7. Drapes should be waterproof and disposable.

8. The patient's skin should be cleaned of blood at the end of the operation and dressings employed with an impervious outer layer to contain exudate. Only closed wound drainage should be employed and open wound drainage avoided.

9. Everyone handling used instruments, dressings, and linen, as well as those involved in disinfecting equipment and surfaces, should wear plastic aprons and disposable gloves.

10. All linen and theatre clothing should be sealed in water-soluble plastic bags, double bagged, and labelled 'infected linen'.

11. Despite the lack of evidence for spread in anaesthetic tubing, it is sensible to use disposable anaesthetic circuitry and high-efficiency heat and moisture exchange filters, all of which should be changed between cases. Filters are interposed between the expiratory limb of the circuit and the ventilator to prevent ventilator contamination. Ventilator components should be decontaminated by autoclaving.

12. There is probably no need for high-risk patients to be operated on at the end of a list, but the theatre floor should be disinfected after operation with a chlorine disinfectant (e.g. hypochlorite solution with 1000 p.p.m. available chlorine; surfaces splashed with blood should be disinfected with a similar, weaker solution.

Despite all precautions, contamination and inoculation incidents will occur. These create immense anxiety and the surgeon must be clear how to manage the incident.

Managing an inoculation incident

An inoculation incident occurs when a break in the skin sufficient to cause bleeding is contaminated with blood or tissue fluid, or there is a splash of blood or tissue fluid into the mouth or conjunctivae. Deep injuries with a contaminated hollow needles carry the greatest risk, particularly for hepatitis. Other injuries with solid sharps, mucosal splashes, and minor sharps injuries without bleeding do not warrant detailed investigation or prophylactic measures, but should be reported.

After a needlestick injury, a surgeon, scrub nurse, or assistant should stop operating, remove gloves and wash the area with detergent surgical scrub. The wound should be encouraged to bleed and then covered with a waterproof dressing before regloving or handing the operation on to someone else.

At-risk incidents in high-risk patients should be reported in writing and handled by someone qualified to offer professional advice (e.g. occupational health doctor, AIDS physician, medical microbiologist). Counselling of the staff member is required and, where possible, the serological status of the source patient should be checked, after counselling and with consent if possible, but without consent if necessary (see Chapter 1). Blood from the staff member should be stored and possibly tested later.

If the source patient is hepatitis B positive, non-immunized surgeons should start a course of active immunization and be treated with passive hepatitis B immune globulin. If vaccinated, antibody levels should be checked and if below 100 IU, a booster dose of vaccine should be given. If the source patient is HIV positive or refuses to be tested, the staff member should be tested for HIV at 3 and 6 months and should use safe sex techniques until proved negative at 3 months. The staff member should not donate blood for 12 months, until the final test is negative. Because of the small risk of seroconversion, operating may continue unless a flu-like illness develops, when further testing should be done.

Zidovudine may modify the risk of infection after an inoculation incident, although the evidence is weak. No major reactions have developed to prophylactic use of the drug, but minor reactions such as nausea and anaemia may occur. The drug has most chance of averting infection if given within 2 hours, and starter packs should be available in the theatre in high-risk areas. Counselling should then be undergone to decide whether to continue the drug. If the source patient is positive, 250 mg 4-hourly (five times a day) should be given for 28 days and blood count checked every fortnight and discontinued if the source patient is negative.

4.8 Recovery hazards

During recovery from anaesthesia, the patient remains vulnerable and needs special care. Note that 20 per cent of all cases of death and serious neurological damage due to anaesthesia occur in the recovery room. Full patient monitoring should be continued in the recovery area. The British Association of Anaesthetists recommends that patients should have the same standards of monitoring in recovery as in the operating theatre. In practice, this means the minimum of a pulse oximeter.

Extubation

Many anaesthetists prefer to extubate the patient in the supine position. In this position, the patient does not require special support, coughing and straining on the tube is less likely to occur (movement may induce this), laryngoscopes and suckers are easier to use, and a face mask is easily applied. Furthermore, if reintubation becomes necessary, it is easier than in any other position. However, in the patient with a high risk of vomiting, the lateral position with moderate head-down tilt is safer for extubation. The endotracheal tube (or laryngeal mask) is often left in position during transfer to recovery, and recovery nurses remove it when the patient is judged to be sufficiently awake. This applies particularly if intubation has been difficult, if recovery is delayed, or if the airway is at special risk of soiling by gastric contents, blood, or other body fluids. The anaesthetist remains in charge of the patient until recovery is complete. If laryngeal masks are used, removal is usually effected in recovery and often by the patient themselves, having regained full reflexes. As the laryngeal mask does not enter the larynx, the patient is not as stimulated as they would be by an endotracheal tube and will tolerate its presence until widely awake. The airway is protected with it in place. An unconscious patient cannot cooperate nor protect themselves, thus, after extubation, the patient should be turned to the full lateral position before transfer from the operating room.

The recovery period is undoubtedly a hazardous one for the patient. When there is risk of gastric reflux (e.g. intestinal obstruction or during pregnancy), patients are safest in the lateral position, but may otherwise be recovered in the supine position. Good access to the head end of the patient is essential and the head should not be pushed against a wall. Bed headboards should be detached and not replaced until the patient is ready to leave the recovery room. Patients with respiratory difficulties or a degree of left ventricular failure are best sat up in bed in the recovery unit as this improves oxygenation.

4.9 Avoiding toxic hazards

Anaesthetic gases

Theatres should all be equipped with anaesthetic gas scavenging apparatus to avoid potential teratogenic effects to pregnant theatre staff during the first trimester, and to avoid fatigue in theatre staff caused by inhaling exhaled anaesthetic agents. Scavenging is either passive, where the patient's exhaled gases pass through a tube in the wall to the atmosphere, or active where they pass out under gentle negative pressure from a vacuum system or fan extractor. Active systems require inbuilt safety systems to prevent negative pressure acting on the patient's airway.

Sterilizing solutions

Glutaraldehyde is the best agent for cold sterilization of endoscopes. It has effective activity against bacteria, viruses, and mycobacteria, while causing little damage to the instruments. In the past, it has been handled in the open but studies have demonstrated unwanted effects in exposed workers, even with concentrations well below 0.2 p.p.m., the recommended limit. Moreover, symptoms increase with duration of exposure. In one series, there was an excess of nose and throat symptoms and rashes on the hands. In another, airway obstruction, rhinitis, eye irritation, and allergic asthma were reported. Patch testing is usually negative, suggesting that the agent is more often a direct irritant than an allergen, although a few show positive patch tests without cross-reactivity with formaldehyde. Unfortunately, alternative disinfectants such as formaldehyde or chlorhexidine may cause similar unwanted effects. Therefore, exposure to glutaraldehyde should be reduced by taking precautions in the way it is used. Rubber gauntlets and long aprons should be worn. Containers of activated glutaraldehyde should be kept tightly covered and the agent only handled in areas designed to take airflow away from the user.

Radiation hazards

In the UK it is now necessary for all healthcare workers who use or prescribe the use of X-ray irradiation to undergo a formal radiation protection training course. These courses inform healthcare workers of the risks and safeguards needed to use X-rays safely in clinical practice and are mandatory.

Bibliography

Aitkenhead, A.R. and Smith, G. (ed.) (1990). *Textbook of anaesthesia*. Churchill Livingstone, Edinburgh.

Anderton, J., Keen, R., and Neave, R. (1988). *Positioning the surgical patient*, (1st edn). Butterworths, Sevenoaks.

Anonymous (1992). Risks to surgeons and patients from HIV and hepatitis: guidelines on precautions and management of exposure to blood or body fluids. *BMJ*, **305**, 1337–43.

Association of Anaesthetists (1988). *Recommendations for standards of monitoring during anaesthesia and recovery*. The Association of Anaesthetists, Bedford Square, London.

Badermann, H. (1976). *Communication in medicine*. MPS annual report 1976, pp. 23–7.

Boyd, O., Grounds, M., and Bennet, D. (1993). A randomized clinical trial of the effect of deliberate perioperative increase of oxygen delivery on mortality in high-risk surgical patients. *JAMA*, **270**, 2699–707.

Buck, Devlin, and Lunn (1987). *The report of a confidential enquiry into perioperative deaths*. The Nuffield Provincial Hospitals Trust, London.

Nuffield Trust (1984). *Doctor to doctor writing and talking about patients*. Nuffield Trust, London.

Royal College of Surgeons of England: Commission on the Provision of Surgical Services (1985). *Guidelines for Day Case Surgery*.

Theatre safeguards (1985). A joint document from RCS, nurses' and defence organisations.

Wenzel, R. (ed.) (1993). *Prevention and control of nosocomial infection*. Williams and Wilkins, Baltimore.

CHAPTER 6

Managing co-morbid medical conditions in surgical patients

Paul Siklos and Mike Corlett

1 Introduction

Surgical intervention is carried out with the intention of either a cure or an improvement in the patient's quality of life. Any decision to operate must depend on the nature of the presenting condition as well as an assessment of the relative risks and benefits of the operation. This chapter addresses the risks to the 'surgical' patient that may accrue from additional or co-morbid 'medical' problems.

'Medical' conditions affect the surgical patient in the following ways:

♦ A consequence of the medical condition may require surgical intervention (e.g. a foot problem in a patient with diabetes).

♦ A patient with a chronic co-morbid medical condition may require an operation unrelated to the medical condition, and the operation may thus be complicated by the underlying condition or its medical treatment (e.g. rheumatoid arthritis).

♦ A pre-existing condition may be exacerbated by anaesthesia or operation (e.g. chronic bronchitis, ischaemic heart disease).

♦ A previously undiagnosed condition may become evident under the stress of operation (e.g. postoperative myocardial infarction, Addison's disease).

Attempts have been made to quantitate operative risk to aid the decision as to whether an operation at a given time is likely to be in the patient's best interests. The best documented is the American Society of Anesthesiologists' (ASA) Physical Status Classification. The overall individual operative risk cannot be derived directly from the ASA score because it is altered by the magnitude of the operation itself. The five categories of the ASA score are:

♦ Class 1: a normal healthy patient.

♦ Class 2: a patient with mild systemic disease.

♦ Class 3: a patient with severe systemic disease which is not incapacitating.

♦ Class 4: a patient with incapacitating systemic disease which is a constant threat to life.

♦ Class 5: moribund patient not expected to survive 24 hours with or without an operation.

Unfortunately this simple scoring system is not as useful as was hoped, despite several revisions. This is mainly because of disparity in scores given by different assessors when grading the same patient. When anaesthetists were presented with the same case histories, 59 per cent was the best rating consistency that was achieved. Other reasons for inaccuracy include the fact that the following factors are not brought into the assessment:

1. Difficulty in measuring outcomes: successfully allocating numerical values to particular risk factors depends on being able to measure the outcomes of operations. If this proved to be possible in a large number of patients with known risk factors, a databank could be generated and used to predict outcomes. Unfortunately, although mortality is easy to measure, degrees of morbidity are not.

2. Patient-related factors: age, nutritional status, functional state of specific organs.

3. Surgical management factors: the experience and expertise of the surgeon and the quality of the 'back-up' team undoubtedly affect outcome but are difficult to define and quantify. More than 30 years ago, teaching hospitals were shown to have lower case-fatality ratios than non-teaching hospitals for several common conditions and even now there appears to be a survival advantage when certain complex operations are performed in particular (often larger) units. The reasons are probably many and diverse, but one at least has been shown to be important: for each complex operation, there appears to be a threshold number of cases that needs to be performed in a unit each year in order to maintain clinical excellence. This has been demonstrated using medical audit techniques for several operations (e.g. ruptured abdominal aortic aneurysm, carotid artery surgery, colorectal anastomoses). The number of cases per surgeon or per unit required remains a matter of discussion and will probably vary for different operations and for different complexities of the same operation. However, the range probably falls between 10 and 50 cases/year.

Despite the difficulty of quantifying individual risk before operation, what is meant by a 'high-risk' patient is generally understood. This chapter deals with several well-recognized risk factors and also describes some related postoperative complications. Specialist problems in neurosurgery and cardiothoracic surgery are outside the scope of this book.

2 Obesity

2.1 Introduction

Clinically significant obesity is defined as a body weight greater than 20 per cent of **ideal body weight**, or body mass index (Quetelet index) greater than 30 (the body mass index is calculated by dividing weight in kilograms by height in metres squared, with the normal range extending between 20 and 25). Using these criteria, approximately 15 per cent of people in UK are obese; this proportion doubled between 1980 and 1991. In the United States, obesity has been estimated to be responsible for 8 per cent of all health costs. In UK, the *Health of the Nation* initiative recognized obesity as a key target. A combination of ready access to highly palatable and refined foods and (perhaps more important) a modern inactive lifestyle has probably caused the increased prevalence of overweight individuals.

Clinically significant obesity is associated with 2–3 times the risk of perioperative death or morbidity (Table 6.1), although those with only moderate obesity probably have a more modest increase in risk. Ischaemic heart disease is prevalent in obesity (particularly **central obesity** as defined by a waist–hip ratio significantly greater than unity in men or 0.8 in women).

Table 6.1 Special risks faced by obese patients undergoing anaesthesia and surgery

Increased incidence of associated medical and surgical disorders	More likely to require operative treatment	Gallstones
		Osteoarthritis of hips and knees
		Varicose veins and haemorrhoids
	Likely to increase risk of postoperative management problems and complications	Hypertension Ischaemic heart disease (particularly central obesity)
		Oesophageal reflux with risk of aspiration
		Diabetes
		Nocturnal hypoventilation/ostructive sleep apnoea
Diagnosis is more difficult	Clinical signs	Difficult to elicit and interpret
	Blood tests	Difficult venepuncture may not yield satisfactory blood sample for analysis
	Imaging	Special tests such as ultrasound and scintigrams are difficult to interpret
	Recognizing complications	Complications such as hypovolaemia and pulmonary embolism may not be detected
General anaesthesia is more difficult	Venous access	Intravenous cannulae are more difficult to site
	Intubation	Endotracheal intubation is more likely to be necessary protect the airway from aspiration and because high pressures are often required for ventilation. A short, thick neck makes intubation difficult
	Drugs	Altered distribution of drugs means that the doses of many drugs may have to be modified
	Duration	The operation and hence the anaesthetic is likely to last longer
Surgery presents a technical challenge to the surgeon	Access and visibility are more difficult	Organs often lie further from the surface Tissue planes and structures are obscured by surrounding fat
Postoperative complications are more common	Pulmonary complications	Reduced vital capacity due to diaphragmatic splinting causes underventilation of the lung bases, sputum retention, and consequent hypoxia from underventilation and shunting. There is an increased incidence of postoperative atelectasis and chest infection
	Cardiovascular complications	Demands on the cardiovascular system are increased, with higher incidence of cardiac failure
	Thromboembolism	There is an increased incidence of venous thrombosis and pulmonary infarction
	Wound problems	Abdominal incisions often need to be longer and wound closure is less secure because of fatty infiltration and stretching of abdominal wall
		Large 'dead space' in adipose tissue predisposes to haematoma, wound infection, and dehiscence

2.2 Management of obesity in patients needing operation

Obesity is potentially preventable but it is unlikely that substantial weight will be lost preoperatively on the advice of the surgeon as a result of a change in lifestyle, even with the help of a dietician. However, some patients may be motivated to lose weight by the thought that they will not have their operation (particularly on the gallbladder or hip) unless they do. All obese patients should have their blood glucose measured and have an electrocardiogram before operation.

A recent study found the incidence of wound infection increased by 18 per cent in obese patients (43 per cent incidence)

compared with non-obese patients (25 per cent incidence) undergoing emergency abdominal operations.

3 Elderly

Approximately one in four patients admitted to a surgical ward is over 65 years of age and about 10 per cent are aged over 75 years. In ophthalmology and orthopaedic wards up to half of the patients are over the age of 65 years and surgical operations on patients in their 70s and 80s are becoming everyday events.

The risk of postoperative complications increases with age for two reasons:

1. The elderly frequently have several concurrent medical problems.

2. Ageing is associated with decreased functional reserve in many organ systems. This leads to a declining ability to respond to the physiological consequences of a surgical procedure.

The following organ systems are affected:

◆ **Cardiovascular system.** Changes lead to a decrease in cardiac output and a reduced ability to compensate for hypovolaemia or fluid overload. These changes include: hypertrophy and increased stiffness of the left ventricle, which impair ventricular filling in diastole; calcification of aortic and mitral valve rings, often with valvular incompetence; increased peripheral vascular resistance and stiffness (reduced compliance) of large arteries.

◆ **Kidney.** Reduction in nephron numbers, renal blood flow and glomerular filtration rate cause deterioration in renal function so that creatinine clearance may fall. This is not reflected in the plasma creatinine because the muscle mass also tends to be reduced in the elderly. The capacity for handling fluid overload is impaired and reduced renal tubular concentrating adequacy reduces the ability to compensate for fluid loss.

◆ **Respiratory system.** There is a reduction in pulmonary reserve because the thoracic cage is more rigid and of smaller volume; respiratory muscle strength and stamina are reduced; the lung parenchyma is stiffer and there is a reduction in alveolar numbers. Measures of pulmonary function are decreased and arterial oxygen tension is reduced. In addition the numbers and activity of respiratory cilia are reduced, making it more difficult to clear the airway of secretions. The elderly thus have an increased risk of postoperative respiratory complications such as pneumonia.

◆ **Nervous system.** There is a reduction in cerebral blood flow with ageing as well as deterioration in coordination, visual and hearing ability, and short-term memory. Although elderly patients may function well in familiar environments, the alien environment of a hospital may precipitate an acute confusional state which may hamper recovery.

◆ **Drug handling.** Lean body mass declines with age and the percentage of fat increases. Plasma volume and total body water decrease and plasma albumin decreases. These variations in body composition derange drug distribution. Excretion and clearance may be altered as hepatic and renal function decline and there may be decreased receptor sensitivity to some drugs but increased sensitivity to others. As a general rule, medication for the elderly needs to be prescribed in smaller doses.

3.1 Preoperative assessment of elderly patients

Physiological status

Assessment of organ systems that have functions expected to deteriorate with age involves a series of standard investigations (depending on local preference) such as plasma urea and electrolytes, blood count, chest radiograph, and electrocardiogram. The extent of investigation will depend on previously identified co-morbid conditions and the type and extent of the operation planned.

Disease status

Pathological processes affecting several systems often coexist. In addition, there may be iatrogenic problems caused by multiple medication.

Functional status

The success of postoperative rehabilitation depends upon the elderly surgical patient's ability to perform common everyday tasks. **Activities of daily living** should be assessed (self-care, mobility, continence, housework, and activities outside the home such as shopping and gardening).

Nutritional status

Inadequate nutrition affects surgical outcome by increasing the likelihood of complications and delaying wound healing. Preoperative nutritional assessment includes a brief history of eating habits, identification of recent weight loss of more than 10 per cent, assessment of body habitus (body mass index), and measurement of plasma proteins and folate. Measuring grip strength has been shown to be an indication of protein nutritional state and this influences postoperative recovery. If malnutrition is confirmed and the operation can be postponed, a period of nutritional augmentation should be considered. There is little evidence that 7–10 days of nutritional support improves operative outcome in simple protein/calorie malnutrition, but other vitamin and mineral deficiencies and dehydration should undoubtedly be corrected before surgery.

Cognitive status

Preoperative cognitive function should be documented to help evaluate any postoperative confusional state. Simple clinical assessment includes orientation to person, place, and time; the ability to list five items in a class (for example cities or fruit), and the ability to remember three objects or an address after a short period. The 10-item abbreviated mental test score (MTS) is a standard.

4 Respiratory disorders

4.1 Introduction

Postoperative respiratory problems occur in up to 15 per cent of surgical patients, and in elderly general surgical patients this may increase to between 20 and 40 per cent. Up to one-third of all postoperative deaths in patients over the age of 65 years are due to respiratory causes.

The major postoperative complication in patients with normal lungs is atelectasis (Table 6.2) leading to pneumonia. In the majority of cases, small airways closure is the primary event and if there is subsequent infection then pneumonia develops. In the minority of cases (and often when there is chronic bronchitis) the primary event is retention or aspiration of respiratory secretions with subsequent airway closure, atelectasis, and pneumonia.

The basal airways of the lungs are on the point of closure and are kept open by sustained maximal inspirations (SMIs) which occur 5–10 times an hour. If these SMIs are abolished, then airways closure and atelectasis will occur. In addition, the stiffer the lung and the smaller the functional residual capacity, the more likely are the small airways to close on expiration.

4.2 Preoperative risk factors for respiratory complications

- Age (particularly over 75 years);
- male sex;
- smoking;
- obesity;
- reduced exercise tolerance due to breathlessness;
- incision near diaphragm (upper abdominal/lower thoracic);

- history of respiratory disease;
- peak flow less than 250 l/min.

4.3 Prevention and treatment of atelectasis

Classic physiotherapy techniques concentrate on expiratory manoeuvres and encouragement of coughing in order to clear the chest of secretions. These methods are probably inappropriate where retention of secretions is not the major problem and where an increase in expiratory effort may contribute to airway closure. It is probably better to concentrate on inspiratory encouragement (deep breathing) where standard techniques fail to produce sputum. Patients should be encouraged to take deep inspirations 10 times during every hour. Those at high risk have been shown to benefit from incentive spirometry devices.

4.4 Preoperative clinical problems

Chronic obstructive pulmonary disease (COPD)

Chronic bronchitis and emphysema are common and predispose to postoperative complications because the lungs are stiff, there is poor respiratory reserve, and there is increased sputum production. Treatment of any reversible component of airflow limitation and infection is important.

Cigarette smoking

Smokers have up to seven times more postoperative respiratory problems than non-smokers. This is due partly to the increased incidence of chronic obstructive pulmonary disease and also to the reduction in bronchial ciliary activity. The latter can be reversed by abstaining from smoking, preferably for at least 4 weeks before surgery.

Acute respiratory infection

Infection itself may reduce resistance to surgical trauma and predispose to further infection. There will be an increase in respiratory secretions and possibly also infection-induced bronchospasm, all of which will increase the likelihood of postoperative complications.

Asthma

Bronchoconstriction, bronchial wall oedema, and increased bronchial secretions (the elements of asthma) predispose to postoperative atelectasis and infection. In addition, inhaled anaesthetic agents, endotracheal intubation, and operative 'stress' may trigger further bronchoconstriction in a patient with airways hyperreactivity.

It is important that asthma be treated aggressively preoperatively. Many patients will know their optimum peak flow rate and, if possible, operation should be postponed until this value is consistently recorded. There is often diurnal variability of airways resistance and one hallmark of uncontrolled asthma is a dip in the peak flow rate in the early morning; this may predict those patients that will react adversely to surgery.

Table 6.2 Factors predisposing to atelectasis

Increased lung stiffness	Increasing age
	Chronic lung disease
	Smoking
Reduced functional residual capacity	Obesity
	Supine position during and after operation
	Pain from incision
Abolition of SMI	Oversedation
	Pain from incision

It may be wise to change to a long-acting inhaled broncho-dilator (e.g. salmeterol) preoperatively. Inhaled nebulized bronchodilating drugs may be given during the operation if necessary. Intravenous steroids may be required, particularly if the patient has been taking high-dose inhaled steroids preoperatively.

4.5 Preoperative assessment of a patient with lung disease

- History of past and present lung disease;
- smoking history;
- medication;
- clinical assessment of exercise tolerance by asking the patient about daily activity and, if necessary, seeing how far he can walk (around the hospital corridors) in a given time;
- chest radiograph;
- peak flow rate measurements before and after inhaled brochodilator;
- vitalography;
- arterial blood gas measurements are often useful as a baseline, particularly if there is evidence of carbon dioxide retention.

4.6 Perioperative management of the patient with lung disease

- Stop smoking from time of booking for elective surgery;
- preoperative and early postoperative deep breathing and possibly physiotherapy;
- appropriate drug therapy;
- nebulized beta-agonist;
- intravenous steroids;
- antibiotics for evidence of infection (not prophylactic).

Avoid: overtransfusion with blood and crystalloid; excessive narcotic analgesia; oxygen therapy at concentrations greater than 24 per cent if there is evidence of carbon dioxide retention; epidural anaesthesia/analgesia; intravenous theophylline because of potential interactions with anaesthetic agents.

Transfer to intensive care if risks of postoperative ventilatory failure are high.

5 Non-cardiac surgery in patients with heart disease

5.1 Introduction

In patients undergoing a surgical operation, the cardiovascular system is subject to multiple stresses from the operation and the anaesthetic. Myocardial contractility and respiration may be depressed and there may be fluctuations in arterial blood pressure, ventricular filling pressure, blood volume, body temperature, and the activity of the autonomic nervous system. Complications such as haemorrhage, fever, and infection add to the burden. Patients with heart disease, even if well-compensated beforehand, may be unable to meet these demands, with the result that myocardial ischaemia and heart failure may develop. Cardiovascular complications make up a substantial proportion of the morbidity and mortality associated with surgical operations, and the dangers of the disease for which the operation is proposed must be balanced against the risks of operation.

There is a higher risk of cardiac complications in patients with heart disease who have other co-morbid conditions, such as renal insufficiency, abnormalities of liver function, electrolyte disturbances, or hypoxaemia. Morbidity is also greater in obese subjects.

The type of anaesthesia and the nature of the operation will influence the level of risk:

- Spinal and epidural anaesthesia include sympathetic blockade. Systemic vascular resistance may fall by up to 15 per cent, venodilatation causes reduction in right ventricular preload, and the stress to the cardiovascular system may be as great as that caused by general anaesthesia.

- Different operations cause differing levels of physiological disturbance. For example, ophthalmic operations are usually safe even with severely compromised cardiac function, whereas abdominal aortic aneurysm surgery (myocardial stress due to aortic cross-clamping and blood loss) and other abdominal or thoracic operations are potentially much more stressful to the system.

Some apparently minor procedures are associated with increased risk. For example, transurethral prostatectomy, previously thought to be relatively harmless, has been shown to result in a higher than expected rate of cardiovascular complications, largely due to volume overload from absorbed irrigant fluid and lowered plasma sodium concentration.

Although the duration of anaesthesia can be correlated with the risk of cardiovascular mortality, this may be because long operations often result from intraoperative difficulties and complications such as excess blood loss. In addition, the longest operations usually involve the abdomen or chest. There is evidence to suggest that careful preoperative assessment and, in appropriate cases, invasive haemodynamic monitoring during operation significantly reduce the risks.

An emergency operation increases the risk of cardiovascular complications by up to four times compared with a similar operation carried out electively. However, the National Confidential Enquiry into Perioperative Deaths reports (NCEPOD) have clearly demonstrated that patients undergoing emergency surgery, particularly at night, have frequently been under-resuscitated and operated on and anaesthetized by doctors in training without direct supervision.

5.2 Assessment of cardiovascular risk

The leading cause of death after surgery is myocardial infarction. Some patients require an urgent life-saving operation and estimating the theoretical operative risk would be an academic exercise since failure to operate will result in the patient's death. Often, however, the timing and perhaps type of an operation depend on assessment of risk. Analysis of preoperative factors contributing to increased cardiac complications after major non-cardiac surgery has identified those that can predict peri-operative risk. When these factors are weighted, based on their relative significance as predictors of cardiac outcome, a multi-factorial index can be developed, as shown in Table 6.3.

On the basis of the above data the authors recommend that only truly life-saving procedures should be performed on patients with risk scores greater than 26. Patients with index scores between 13 and 25 have sufficient cardiac risk to justify medical assessment and delay of operation (if possible) because over half of the 'points' that contribute to the overall score (e.g. raised jugular venous pressure) may be reversed preoperatively with appropriate medical management.

Pooled data from four studies that have used the above cardiac risk index give the following major complication rates (myocardial infarction, pulmonary oedema, ventricular tachycardia, or cardiac death):

- Class I (0–5 points), 1.6 per cent.
- Class II (6–12 points), 5.0 per cent.
- Class III (13–25 points), 16.0 per cent.
- Class IV (> 26 points), 56.0 per cent.

The decision of whether or not to operate on a given patient must take into account a number of factors, including the operative versus the non-operative risk as well as the patient's own wishes. The operative risk includes the non-cardiac risk of a given operation and also the cardiac risk, and the above is intended to help in calculating the latter risk. It is important that the cardiac risk score is not rigidly applied and used as a guide to assess overall operative risk.

5.3 Ischaemic heart disease

Chronic stable exertional angina

These patients tolerate most surgical procedures well. Assessment should take account of current exercise tolerance but note that the frequency of anginal attacks may not reflect the severity of the ischaemic heart disease. This is because patients reduce their activity to avoid angina, and may have other conditions that limit ambulation, such as joint disorders or peripheral vascular disease. If a patient is able to climb stairs, carry shopping, perform household chores such as bed-making and vacuum cleaning, and dig the garden, there is likely to be little cardiovascular risk.

Unstable angina

This a serious risk. Angina is unpredictable, occurring with progressively decreasing amounts of exercise or even at rest. Attacks usually last longer than 15 minutes. These patients often progress to myocardial infarction even without the stress of a non-cardiac operation. The angina should be treated aggressively in hospital and even minor elective surgery should be postponed.

A history of myocardial infarction

A history of myocardial infarction (MI) is important. Studies in the 1970s showed a 30 per cent risk of reinfarction or cardiac death when patients had an operation within 3 months of myocardial infarction. The risk fell to about 15 per cent between 3 and 6 months postinfarction and to around 5 per cent after 6 months. The 5 per cent risk seemed to remain constant thereafter.

More recent data suggest that improved intraoperative monitoring and modified anaesthetic techniques have substantially reduced the risk, but it is still common practice (and probably sensible) to delay elective surgery for 6 months after MI.

In the Coronary Artery Surgery Study (CASS) in the USA, patients with angiographically documented coronary disease were randomized to medical management or CABG surgery. After urological, orthopaedic, breast or skin operations, 30-day mortality was under 1% in both groups. After abdominal, thoracic, vascular or head and neck surgery, 30 day MI plus mortality was 1.7% in the CABG group (mortality 0.8%), and 3.3% in the medical group (mortality 2.7%).

If a life-saving emergency procedure is necessary in a patient after recent myocardial infarction, the decision to operate can be reached almost regardless of the cardiac risk. The decision is more perplexing in operations of intermediate urgency. If a patient has evidence of good left ventricular function (as demonstrated by exercise tolerance, submaximal exercise ECG, MUGA scan), surgery can be undertaken with only a small increase in risk.

Table 6.3 A multifactorial index to predict cardiac risk in non-cardiac surgery (adapted from Goldman *et al.* 1977)

Factor	Points
Age >70 years	5
MI in previous 6 months	10
Third heart sound or raised jugular venous pressure	11
Significant aortic stenosis	3
Cardiac rhythm other than sinus	7
>5 premature ventricular contractions per min documented preoperatively	7
General status: $Po_2 < 8$ or $Pco_2 < 6.5$ (kPa)/Plasma potassium <3 mmol/l. Plasma urea >18 mmol/l or creatinine >265 mol/l	3
Features of chronic liver disease/Patient bedridden from non-cardiac cause/Intraperitoneal, intrathoracic, or aortic operation	3
Emergency operation	4
Total	53

Patients who have had successful coronary artery revascularization

Except perhaps in the first month after bypass surgery, these patients usually tolerate major non-cardiac surgery very well.

Preoperative assessment of patients with cardiac disease

In all patients

- Check for a history of myocardial infarction and angina.

- Assess exercise tolerance clinically.

- Resting ECG. In a study of 200 patients, a perioperative cardiac event occurred in 23 per cent of patients with an abnormal preoperative ECG but only in 2 per cent with a normal ECG. Pathological Q-waves indicate a previous MI but are not by themselves of prognostic importance. A pre-operative trace is also useful for comparing with a post-operative one in the event of a subsequent suspected MI.

In patients with either a severe cardiac condition or if very major surgery is intended:

- An exercise ECG, usually on a treadmill, adds little more information than a resting ECG and clinical assessment, and should not be part of the standard work-up. Poor exercise tolerance (less than 2 minutes' exercise) seems to correlate better with peri- and postoperative cardiac complications than ECG changes.

- Gated ventricular scintigram (using the radioisotope MUGA) measures left ventricular ejection fraction and correlates well with perioperative cardiac morbidity and mortality. Several groups have found it particularly useful in assessing patients for abdominal aortic surgery.

- In patients at risk, continuous 24-hour ECG monitoring before operation has been used to detect ischaemic changes in the ST segment. Some patients demonstrate frequent 'silent' (i.e. painless) episodes of ischaemia. In these patients, there is a ninefold increase in the risk of a postoperative ischaemic event. This form of monitoring is not yet advocated for regular use.

Perioperative therapy

The guiding principle during the perioperative period is to keep myocardial oxygen consumption as low as possible and to maintain the best possible coronary artery perfusion.

Patients with ischaemic heart disease may be taking 'triple therapy' in the form of a beta-blocker, a calcium-channel blocker, and a nitrate. This therapy should be continued unless there is evidence of heart failure, in which case the calcium-channel blocker or beta-blocker, or both, should be stopped. Most patients will be taking a daily dose of aspirin (75–300 mg). Aspirin predisposes to perioperative haemorrhage and for certain operations (e.g. AAA surgery), should be stopped 2 weeks before operation.

If a patient is taking no treatment, it is advisable to cover the operative period with a nitrate. This is best prescribed as a transdermal preparation given intermittently to prevent tolerance (i.e. with a 'nitrate-free interval' of about 6 hours in 24, usually overnight). Aspirin can also be started if there are no contraindications.

Perioperative angina

If a surgical patient develops angina either before or after operation, the immediate care is to advise the patient to sit up (lying down increases the venous return and may worsen angina, while standing up may exacerbate the tendency of the nitrate to lower the systemic blood pressure) and use sublingual trinitrin, either by spray or tablet (no matter what other treatments they are receiving). If the pain does not settle within a few minutes, a further dose of sublingual nitrate may be given and if this is not effective, advice of a physician should be sought with the possible diagnosis of myocardial infarction in mind.

Postoperative myocardial infarction

MI may be difficult to recognize because patients may have pain from the operation and are likely to be receiving analgesia that suppresses cardiac pain. Tachycardia, fever, and hypo-tension may be wrongly attributed to blood loss, pulmonary embolism, or infection rather than to myocardial infarction. A high index of suspicion should be maintained in every high-risk patient.

Seventy per cent of postoperative MIs occur within 6 days of operation, the majority by the third day. The infarction is often painless and may present as hypotension, cardiac failure, or cardiac arrest. Diagnosis can often be made on ECG (parti-cularly if there is a preoperative trace for comparison) and with the results of plasma CKMB measurement. This cardiac iso-enzyme of creatine kinase is elevated at about 8–16 hours after myocardial infarction and has the advantage that it is not significantly elevated by surgical procedures.

Initial treatment should be with aspirin (300 mg chewed and then swallowed) which helps to limit infarct size. Recent surgery is a contraindication to fibrinolytic therapy but intravenous beta-blockade or even primary percutaneous transluminal coronary angioplasty (PTCA) may be appropriate. Urgent medical advice should be sought and the patient is likely to require monitoring in a unit with facilities for inotropic support and antiarrhythmic treatment if needed.

5.4 Hypertension

Patients with hypertension have an increased risk of cardiac complications during or shortly after surgery compared with those whose blood pressure has always been normal. Much of this increased risk is due to the presence of associated ischaemic heart disease and left ventricular dysfunction, the rest being due to swings of blood pressure during the operation.

Blood pressure may be acutely raised in association with the anxiety of hospital admission and impending operation, and will settle with relaxation or sedation. The recording may be inaccurate in a fat arm unless a wide cuff (usually 'alternative adult') is used. Patients with blood pressures less than about 170/110 mmHg and with no evidence of end-organ damage usually tolerate surgery without significant risk.

More severe and poorly controlled hypertension conveys a significantly increased risk of perioperative MI and stroke, particularly if there are swings in blood pressure. Operation should be postponed if possible and the blood pressure treated more effectively. If there is severe hypertension and an operation is required urgently then control of the blood pressure is best achieved with an intravenous infusion of sodium nitroprusside with careful haemodynamic monitoring.

Treated hypertension

Medication should be continued as withdrawal may lead to rebound hypertension and some drugs (particularly beta-blockers) are 'cardioprotective'. Hypotension may occur postoperatively, particularly if there is reduction in plasma volume.

Thiazide diuretics are commonly prescribed for hypertension and may cause volume depletion and abnormalities of plasma electrolytes, particularly in the elderly. Plasma urea, creatinine, and electrolytes (particularly K^+) should be measured in these patients before operation, in addition to assessing the patient for the presence of ischaemic heart disease.

Preoperative assessment of the hypertensive patient

- A series of blood pressure recordings should be taken (using a wide cuff if the patient has a fat or muscular arm). A cuff that is too narrow will give an artificially raised pressure reading but a too wide cuff will not give a falsely low reading. Therefore use a wide cuff if there is any doubt.

- Bed rest and sedation.

Clinical evidence of end-organ damage
- Examination of retinal vessels for hypertensive change.
- Chest radiograph for cardiomegaly and pulmonary oedema.
- Electrocardiogram for left ventricular hypertrophy and 'strain'.
- Plasma creatinine, urea, and electrolytes; proteinuria.

Treatment of postoperative hypertension

- Check the blood pressure readings yourself.

- Look for and correct causes such as cessation of preoperative antihypertensive medication, urinary retention, fluid overload, pain, anxiety, and hypoxaemia. Greatly elevated blood pressure may be controlled with intravenous nitroprusside or hydralazine or with a nifedipine capsule (5 mg) broken sublingually.

- Remember that undetected phaeochromocytoma is a very rare but well-documented cause of greatly raised blood pressure and if suspected treat with combined alpha- and beta-blockade (labetolol).

5.5 Cardiac failure

Congestive cardiac failure is a major determinant of perioperative risk, irrespective of the underlying disorder. The mortality associated with surgery increases as myocardial function (as measured by left ventricular ejection fraction for example) declines. The risk appears to correlate with the patient's cardiac function at the time of the operation (rather than the most severe state that the patient has ever experienced) so it is well worth treating cardiac failure aggressively prior to a planned operation. However, overtreatment, particularly with diuretics, will cause problems such as hypovolaemia and electrolyte imbalance, adding further to the risks of anaesthesia.

Preoperative assessment of a patient with cardiac failure

- History of breathlessness and fatigue, the two major symptoms of cardiac failure.

- Examination to include raised jugular venous pressure, peripheral oedema, tender hepatomegaly, tachycardia, third heart sound, lung crackles that do not clear with coughing, and hypotension.

- ECG.

- Chest radiograph, which may show cardiomegaly, pulmonary oedema, or pleural effusion.

- Plasma urea, creatinine, and electrolytes.

- Echocardiogram to exclude valvular heart disease and to assess left ventricular function.

- More detailed assessment of left ventricular function (MUGA; see above).

Preoperative treatment of cardiac failure

- Identify and correct any precipitating causes, such as arrhythmia, hyperthyroidism, valvular heart disease, anaemia, negatively inotropic drugs (beta-blockers, calcium-channel blockers) and non-steroidal anti-inflammatory drugs (NSAIDs), which cause fluid retention.

- Oral frusemide (furosemide) with a maximum daily dose of 80 mg to avoid dehydration.

- Oral captopril, starting with a test dose (6.25 mg) with careful observation for hypotension.

- Digoxin, particularly if atrial fibrillation with an uncontrolled ventricular response (i.e. resting heart rate, measured at the cardiac apex, not the radial artery, exceeding 100 b.p.m.).

Treatment of postoperative heart failure

Identify causes such as myocardial infarction and fluid overload. Then as above, except that frusemide (furosemide) and the vasodilator (nitrate rather than captopril) are given intravenously, preferably with haemodynamic monitoring on the cardiac care unit.

5.6 Cardiac arrhythmias

Arrhythmias often reflect underlying heart disease and are markers for the likelihood of perioperative cardiac complications. For example, the frequency of ventricular premature contractions (ectopics) correlates with left ventricular dysfunction in patients with coronary artery disease, and specific antiarrhythmic treatment does not alter the prognosis. However, uncontrolled tachycardia or bradycardia may cause heart failure and therefore do require treatment.

Tachycardias

Atrial fibrillation (AF)

Chronic

A common finding, particularly in the elderly (up to 20 per cent of patients over the age of 70 years will have AF as their usual cardiac rhythm). AF usually reflects ischaemic heart disease but may be a feature of valvular heart disease, cardiomyopathy, or hyperthyroidism. Patients are at risk of systemic embolization from the left atrium and there is increasing evidence that anticoagulation with warfarin can reduce this risk even when AF is not due to mitral stenosis. Such anticoagulation could be reduced perioperatively if necessary (e.g. to an international normalized ratio (INR) of about 1.5).

AF with a controlled ventricular response (i.e. ventricular rate around 90/min at rest with no apical–radial deficit) causes few haemodynamic problems. The ventricular rate is often controlled by drugs that affect conduction through the atrioventricular node, such as digoxin, verapamil, beta-adrenergic blockers, amiodarone, or a combination of these. It is wise to omit atropine from the premedication as this may cause an increase in the ventricular response by increasing conduction through the atrioventricular node.

Intermittent

AF may complicate an acute event such as pulmonary embolus or MI, and may also be associated with acute pneumonia or hyperthyroidism.

Precipitating causes must be sought and treated. Specific treatment is aimed at reducing the ventricular response. Cardioversion under these circumstances is seldom successful. Digoxin may be given intravenously, as may verapamil (in the absence of cardiac failure and prior treatment with beta-blockers) or amiodarone, the latter being useful as there is no negative inotropic effect and there may be conversion to sinus rhythm. Anticoagulation with heparin should be considered.

Sinus tachycardia

This is usually a physiological response to hypotension, sepsis, fluid overload, heart failure, anxiety, or thyrotoxicosis. Treatment of the underlying cause is appropriate.

Atrial tachycardia

Usually has the same significance as AF (see above). May be a feature of digoxin toxicity, particularly if there is atrioventricular (AV) block. The plasma digoxin concentration should be measured and the digoxin withheld until the result is known.

Ventricular tachycardia or fibrillation

This may be the end result of any severe metabolic (usually hypoxic) insult to the myocardium or myocardial infarction. This will usually present as 'cardiac arrest' and electrical cardioversion or cardiopulmonary resuscitation is required.

Bradycardias

Sinus bradycardia

Sinus bradycardia may be caused by vagal overactivity precipitated by procedures such as anal dilatation. Excessive beta-adrenergic blockade may contribute. Treatment is with atropine (glucagon or isoprenaline if beta-adrenergic blockade is the cause).

Heart block

Complete (third-degree) atrioventricular heart block may be present preoperatively or develop acutely intraoperatively. The heart is unable to meet the increased demands placed upon the cardiovascular system by anaesthesia and operation because the heart rate is slow and fixed. A temporary transvenous pacemaker should be inserted.

The development of complete heart block may be anticipated in some patients who have preoperative **bifascicular block** (usually right bundle branch block and left axis deviation on the electrocardiogram) and a temporary pacing wire should be inserted prophylactically. Cardiological advice should be sought.

Permanent pacemakers

The presence of a permanent cardiac pacemaker usually poses no problem for patient, surgeon, or anaesthetist. All modern pacemakers have a sensing and pacing function ('demand') so that pacing will be inhibited if the system senses electrical activity from the heart. Diathermy may be interpreted thus and the pacemaker inhibited, but this should not cause a problem provided the 'bursts' of diathermy are kept short. The pacemaker box itself is very robust and although permanent damage is most unlikely, it is wise to keep the diathermy current as far away from the box as possible.

5.7 Valvular heart disease

Patients with valvular heart disease are subject to the following hazards:

1. **Heart failure.** The risks depend on the functional state of the myocardium, and patients with only mild limitation of activity will tolerate surgery well. Any degree of heart failure should be treated preoperatively. Patients with symptomatic aortic and mitral stenosis are prone to sudden death or pulmonary oedema and the valve lesion should ideally be corrected before non-cardiac surgery. Balloon valvuloplasty is a possibility for patients whose condition precludes corrective valve surgery. The echocardiogram is an excellent non-invasive method of assessing heart valves and should be

performed preoperatively when there is any doubt about the significance of a heart murmur.

2. **Infective endocarditis.** Appropriate antibiotic prophylaxis must be given for operations that are likely to cause bacteraemia in patients who are susceptible (see Table 6.4).

3. **Arrhythmias.** Particularly atrial fibrillation.

4. **Thromboembolism.** The risks are well documented in mitral stenosis and patients are usually anticoagulated with warfarin.

Prosthetic heart valves

The two major problems are:

1. A greatly increased risk of infective endocarditis (a highly dangerous condition). There should be a lower threshold for employing antibiotic prophylaxis (Table 6.4).

2. Anticoagulation. Tissue prosthetic valves (porcine heterografts such as Hancock and Carpentier–Edwards) have a very low risk of thromboembolism and do not require anticoagulation therapy (except during the first three postoperative months while the sewing ring becomes endothelialized). The mechanical prostheses (Starr–Edwards (caged ball) and Bjork–Shiley (tilting disc), for example) do require permanent anticoagulation to prevent embolism and thrombosis of the valve. Ideally the anticoagulation should be carried through the operative period, but often the risk of haematoma and haemorrhage dictates that anticoagulation be reduced. It is important to liaise with the haematology department, but, in general, warfarin may be discontinued for 3 days prior to surgery and restarted 3 days afterwards without a significant risk of prosthetic valve thrombosis. Prostheses in the mitral position are more liable to thrombosis and it is often wise to cover the perioperative period with intravenous heparin, which can be easily controlled.

Antibiotic prophylaxis of infective endocarditis

Infective endocarditis is a life-threatening condition and treatment of confirmed endocarditis is lengthy and may be

Table 6.4 Antibiotic prophylaxis (adult doses)

Dental extractions, scaling, or periodontal surgery

(1) Patients without special risk

  Local or no anaesthesia

  (a) Not allergic to penicillin: amoxicillin 3 g single oral dose 1 hour before procedure

  (b) Allergic to penicillin: erythromycin 1.5 g orally 12 hours prior to procedure plus 0.5 g 6 hours later

  OR

  Clindamycin 600 mg orally as one dose 1 hour prior to the dental procedure

  General anaesthesia

  (c) Not allergic to penicillin: amoxicillin 1 g IM just before induction and 0.5 g orally 6 hours later

  OR

  Amoxicillin 3 g orally 4 hours before anaesthesia and a further 3 g by mouth as soon as possible after operation

(2) Patients with special risk

  (d) Patients not allergic to penicillin and who have not received penicillin more than once in the previous month: amoxicillin 1 g IM PLUS gentamicin 120 mg IM just before induction AND amoxicillin 0.5 g orally 6 hours later

  (e) Patients allergic to penicillin or who have had penicillin more than once in the previous month: vancomycin 1 g by slow IV infusion over 60 minutes PLUS gentamicin 120 mg IV just before induction or 15 min before the surgical procedure

Application of an antiseptic such as chlorhexidine to the gingival margins reduces the severity of bacteraemia and may be used to supplement antibiotic prophylaxis

Maintaining good dental heath and hygiene is very important in those at risk of infective endocarditis

Surgery or instrumentation of the upper respiratory tract

As above (a)(e) but any postoperative antibiotic may be given parenterally if swallowing is difficult

Genitourinary surgery or instrumentation

For patients with sterile urine, cover should be directed against faecal streptococci as (d) and (e) above. If the urine is infected, then the regimen should also cover the organisms involved

Obstetric and gynaecological procedures

Cover is suggested only for those patients with prosthetic valves and is as (d) and (e) above

Gastrointestinal procedures

Cover for patients with prosthetic valves as (d) and (e) above

---

Based on the recommendations from the Endocarditis Working Party of the British Society for Antimicrobial Chemotherapy. More detailed antibiotic regimens (including doses for children) may be found in: 'Antibiotic prophylaxis of infective endocarditis.' *Lancet*, 1990, **i**, 889.

complicated by drug toxicity. Cardiac surgery may be needed for acute complications or to correct the destructive results of infection after recovery. Prevention is therefore a very worthy objective and strategies are directed at those at risk. These strategies include short-course chemoprophylaxis to protect against bacteraemia in relation to certain medical, surgical, and dental procedures. The use of chemoprophylaxis is based on certain assumptions with regard to infective endocarditis:

♦ There should be a cardiovascular abnormality which is readily identifiable clinically with a known risk of infection.

♦ Bacteraemia should be a frequent event following a given procedure.

♦ Target organisms should be predictably susceptible to the proposed antibiotic regimen, which should be safe and effective in controlling the bacteraemia.

The debate continues concerning the effectiveness of established programmes for endocarditis prophylaxis. Most patients presenting with infective endocarditis have no history of a bacteraemia-producing event and the level of protection of those at risk may be only about 10 per cent. Despite this, well-defined and internationally accepted chemotherapeutic prophylaxis regimens for infective endocarditis are available (Table 6.4) and should be used.

Patients at risk

1. Those individuals whose endocardium is damaged or rendered defective by acquired or congenital disease and who have not received penicillin more than once in the previous month. Endocardial lesions particularly at risk are those where there is a **jet effect** produced by blood flowing from a zone of high pressure to one of relatively low pressure. These include:

   ♦ coarctation of the aorta;

   ♦ patent ductus arteriosus;

   ♦ arteriovenous fistula;

   ♦ ventricular septal defect;

   ♦ aortic and mitral valve regurgitation;

   ♦ mitral valve prolapse where there is also regurgitation.

2. Those patients with special risk who should be referred to hospital:

   ♦ patients with prosthetic heart valves;

   ♦ patients who have had a previous episode of infective endocarditis;

   ♦ patients who are to have a general anaesthetic and who are allergic to penicillin or who have had penicillin more than once in the preceding month.

3. Patients with prosthetic joints may be at increased risk from late infection related to dental treatment. There are, however only a few anecdotal reports of infection of prosthetic joints by oral bacteria despite the hundreds of thousands of these operations performed over the past 30 years or so. The American Academy of Oral Medicine has stated that 'there is insufficient scientific evidence to support routine antibiotic prophylaxis for patients with prosthetic joints who are receiving dental care'.

Guidelines

The Endocarditis Working Party of the British Society for Antimicrobial Chemotherapy has subsequently revised the guidelines shown in Table 6.4 (*Lancet*, 1992, **i**, 1292–3), the differences being as follows:

♦ Oral clindamycin should replace erythromycin as the treatment of choice for patients allergic to penicillin who are not to have a general anaesthetic.

♦ Teicoplanin 400 mg intravenously should replace vancomycin.

♦ Amoxicillin should be given intravenously rather than by the intramuscular route.

For further up-to-date details, consult current versions of the *British National Formulary*.

6 Cerebrovascular disease

Atherosclerosis of the cerebral vessels will make the brain susceptible to hypoperfusion and subsequent infarction. There may be occlusive vascular disease and, in addition, the atherosclerotic cerebral circulation may lose its capacity for autoregulation of blood flow with respect to changes in systemic blood pressure. Patients are thus at risk of cerebral infarction during the perioperative period from hypoxia, hypotension, hypovolaemia, or increased blood viscosity.

The presence of cerebrovascular disease should be suspected in the following categories of patient:

♦ with previous stroke;

♦ with episodes of transient cerebral ischaemia (transient ischaemic attacks, TIA);

♦ who have ischaemic heart disease or peripheral vascular disease;

♦ who have carotid artery bruit.

Management of cerebrovascular disease

♦ Elective operation should be postponed for at least 2 months after a stroke.

♦ Low-dose aspirin (75 mg a day) should be given to patients with a history of TIA (if not already taking it).

♦ Carotid artery duplex Doppler ultrasound should be performed on patients with clinical evidence of cerebrovascular disease in the carotid territory (TIA or non-disabling completed stroke) with a view to angiography and carotid endarterectomy if the stenosis is 70 per cent or greater (results of the European and American Multicentre studies).

◆ The management of asymptomatic carotid artery bruit is as yet unknown, but hypotension should be avoided as far as possible in patients with cerebrovascular disease.

7 Renal disorders

Normal urine excretion is approximately 1–1.5 litres/day. Renal blood flow is 25 per cent of the cardiac output, the highest flow rate per unit weight of any organ. The kidneys are particularly susceptible to the effects of hypoperfusion since the renal extraction of oxygen (ratio of oxygen delivery to oxygen consumption) is only about 8 per cent.

The normal metabolic responses to injury (and surgery) include catecholamine production. This causes vasoconstriction and secretion of antidiuretic hormone (ADH) and aldosterone, starting within minutes of the injury or operation. A degree of postoperative oliguria can therefore be regarded as normal. Increased secretion of ADH and aldosterone lasts for 24–36 hours after injury. Even under conditions of maximal ADH secretion, an obligatory volume of urine is still produced provided normal glomerular filtration rate (GFR) is maintained. If the GFR falls, then urine volume is likely to fall below 0.3 ml/min. For an average patient, a state of **oliguria** is generally defined as a urine output below 20 ml/hour.

In a fit person, the loss of up to 30 per cent of the estimated blood volume (750–1500 ml for a 70 kg person) can be compensated for by the combined actions of catecholamines, ADH, and aldosterone, and therefore the blood loss does not necessarily require replacement. Greater than 30 per cent loss leads to hypotension, hypothermia, oliguria, and anxiety, and volume replacement is required. In an unfit patient, the loss of circulating volume is less readily compensated for and volume replacement is likely at an earlier stage.

Surgical patients are particularly at risk of hypovolaemia and hence perioperative renal impairment or failure. Patients may present to the surgical firm already dehydrated, bleeding, or septic. Intraoperative fluid and blood loss may be large and postoperative fluid depletion may occur because of inadequate replacement. Preventing hypovolaemic renal damage, whether due to blood loss or to fluid depletion, involves careful fluid management in the preoperative, intraoperative, and postoperative phases of surgical care.

7.1 Preoperative fluid management

In a patient with potential fluid problems, preoperative management requires sufficient intravenous fluid administration to reverse the signs of volume depletion. In effect, the pulse rate should be stabilized below 100/min and blood pressure above a systolic pressure of 100 mmHg. The urine output should be between 30 and 50 ml/hour without administration of diuretics (which cause an inappropriate diuresis).

Note that patients with established chronic renal failure may have an inappropriately high urine output.

Fluid can be administered if necessary at up to 2 litres/hour but ideally should be given at a rate of no more than 1 litre/hour to minimize the risk of overexpanding the plasma volume and causing left ventricular failure.

Severe levels of anaemia should be corrected to allow adequate transport of oxygen to the tissues. Traditionally, a haemoglobin concentration of 10 g/dl was regarded as optimal but recent work has suggested that 8 g/dl is satisfactory if fluid balance and anaesthetic monitoring is correct. Hyponatraemia in the presence of dehydration requires infusion of physiological saline. Without dehydration, hyponatraemia implies dilution and saline infusion should be avoided. Hypernatraemia requires 5 per cent dextrose infusion.

Intravenous potassium chloride (KCl) should not be given at a rate greater than 40 mmol/hour without continuous ECG monitoring; higher rates may be necessary if gastrointestinal losses have been great as a result of obstruction or prolonged ileus. Higher concentrations of KCl should be given via a central vein to allow dilution by greater blood flow.

Obstructive jaundice

Patients with obstructive jaundice are often chronically dehydrated as a result of vomiting and anorexia. Furthermore, bacterial overgrowth tends to occur in the biliary tree because of obstruction, and in the intestinal lumen due to a lack of bile salts. This can cause bacteraemia or endotoxaemia during surgical manipulation of the biliary tract. Endotoxaemia is detectable in over 50 per cent of patients with obstructive jaundice. In renal terms, this causes redistribution of blood away from the cortex, risking tubular and cortical necrosis. In addition, patients with obstructive jaundice may excrete conjugated bilirubin in the urine, which diminishes glomerular perfusion and is directly toxic to tubular cells. Disordered coagulation may also increase the risk of operative haemorrhage and hypovolaemia. All of these factors together increase the likelihood of renal failure in jaundiced patients—the so-called **hepatorenal syndrome**.

Preventing renal failure in jaundiced patients requires appropriate antibiotic cover prior to surgery and maintenance of good hydration, with an continuous diuresis of at least 40 ml/hour. Some authorities argue that 100 ml of 20 per cent mannitol should be used to maintain a diuresis and improve renal protection.

Preoperative biliary decompression has not proved beneficial as regards risk of renal failure in patients offered surgery, but should be performed where possible to optimize the patient's condition in other respects.

7.2 Intraoperative fluid management

Intraoperative fluid management generally requires replacement of blood loss in excess of 500 ml. Otherwise extracellular fluid loss (third space shift) should be replaced with electrolyte solutions such as physiological saline or Hartmann's solution (favoured by anaesthetists but controversial nevertheless) to help prevent renal ischaemia. Volumes of fluid replacement should be judged by the extent of the surgery performed and the results of intraoperative monitoring of pulse rate and blood pressure, aided by central venous pressure monitoring and monitoring of pulmonary arterial wedge pressure (Swan–Ganz catheter) where appropriate. Central venous pressure (CVP) monitoring gives a measure of right ventricular filling pressure (i.e. preload) and is normally 0–4 mmHg. Pulmonary arterial wedge pressure is an indication of pulmonary arterial diastolic pressure or left ventricular filling pressure; 5–10 mmHg is normal. In patients with actual or potential heart failure, the normal balance between left and right atrial pressures may be lost, hence the need to monitor both sides of the heart.

7.3 Postoperative fluid management

Postoperative fluid management requires blood, colloid, or crystalloid solutions as appropriate to replace operative losses and the continued depletion of extracellular fluid after surgery (e.g. loss at the operation site, intestinal sequestration). Fluid replacement is administered so as to maintain pulse, blood pressure, and urine output at acceptable levels. CVP monitoring may be indicated if simple measures such as a volume challenge do not remedy developing abnormal vital signs. Some intensivists believe that renal blood flow may be protected by administering dopamine in a 'renal' dose of 2.5–5 μg/kg body weight, but this remains controversial.

Insensible fluid losses can be replaced with 5 per cent dextrose. The normal volume is 500–1000 ml/day, but it is important to note that this is substantially increased by increasing levels of pyrexia. In addition, measured urine output and the estimated gastrointestinal losses should be replaced. Even though the metabolic response to surgery causes renal conservation of sodium, physiological saline should be included in the postoperative fluid regimen, usually in a ratio of 1 : 2 with 5 per cent dextrose. This is particularly important after GI surgery. Potassium is usually given at a rate of 40 mmol/day plus the estimated gastrointestinal loss (in uncomplicated cases this is about 20 mmol/day).

Prevention of septic shock by early recognition and intervention is crucial. Any infective source should be identified and treated (e.g. abscess drainage, débridement of dead or ischaemic tissue, aggressive management of anastomotic leakage). Antibiotics should be given empirically initially, the choice depending on the likely pathogens; and more specifically when the results of cultured specimens are available. Fluid resuscitation requires large volumes to replace fluid loss and to replace temporarily the circulating volume lost as a result of vasodilatation and increased capillary permeability. Ideally, monitoring should be performed in an intensive care or critical care unit and requires CVP and perhaps Swan–Ganz catheters. Early recognition of sepsis and aggressive intervention are likely to prevent or reverse early renal failure.

7.4 Renal failure

One of the main aims of perioperative fluid management is to minimize the risk of acute postoperative renal failure; if this requires dialysis, it carries a mortality rate in the order of 50 per cent.

Acute renal failure (ARF) is defined as an abrupt reduction of renal excretion of waste products causing **azotaemia** (i.e. a rise in plasma urea and creatinine). Acute renal failure can be classified into anuric (< 50 ml/day), oliguric (< 400 ml/day), non-oliguric (400–1000 ml/day), or high output (> 1000 ml/day).

Acute renal failure may be pre-renal (hypoperfusion secondary to shock, depleted circulating volume or vascular occlusion), intrarenal (intrinsic renal parenchymal disease, e.g. acute tubular necrosis, ATN), or post-renal (obstructive).

Acute tubular necrosis

Acute tubular necrosis (ATN) is defined as an acute reduction in renal function secondary to ischaemic insult or nephrotoxins. ATN leads to either oliguric or non-oliguric renal failure. Complete anuria suggests there is total renal vascular occlusion or obstructive uropathy.

Differentiation between pre-renal and renal failure relies on a number of clinical- and laboratory-based factors. Renal hypoperfusion (pre-renal) must be suspected when there is dehydration, hypotension, or cardiac failure. Appropriate invasive monitoring may be required. In cases of pre-renal failure, re-establishment of the circulating volume usually results in a return of normal renal function within 3 days. If this does not occur, this suggests ATN has occurred either because of pre-renal failure or as a result of nephrotoxic agents (assuming there is no pre-existing renal parenchymal disease).

Laboratory tests may help differentiate between pre-renal problems and ATN. A greater rise in plasma urea compared with creatinine suggests pre-renal failure, as proximal tubular reabsorption of sodium and water enhances passive urea reabsorption. The actions of ADH and aldosterone cause retention of sodium and water, resulting in a urine with a high osmolality (>500 mosmol/kg), whereas in ATN osmolality will be similar to that of plasma (<350 mosmol/kg), since the ability to concentrate the urine is lost. The failure to concentrate the urine in ATN also leads to a high urinary sodium concentration (> 40 mmol/l) whereas pre-renal failure leads to a low urinary sodium (< 20 mmol/l).

Oliguric ATN is described as passing through four phases. The first is the **initiation phase**, where it may still be possible by intervention to convert the problem into non-oliguric ATN, for example by administration of mannitol (25 g) or sometimes frusemide (furosemide) 80–160 mg to help 'flush out' the tubules. It must be stressed that in an oliguric patient, a fluid challenge should be tried before administering diuretics.

The second phase is the **oliguric phase**, during which plasma creatinine, urea, potassium, and phosphate all rise and metabolic acidosis occurs. Hypercatabolism is often a feature of septic, post-traumatic, and postoperative patients and is likely to aggravate these changes. Nutritional support with carbohydrates and essential fatty acids is important where appropriate. The oliguric phase lasts between 2 days and 3 weeks and may require temporary haemofiltration or dialysis.

The third phase is the **diuretic phase**, during which a progressive increase in urine volume occurs. At this stage, it is important to replace water and electrolyte losses.

The final phase is the **recovery phase**, during which most patients make a full recovery and, although there is occasional residual damage, chronic renal failure as a result of ATN is rare. It should be noted that these phases are somewhat theoretical but provide a basis for clinical expectations.

Treatment of renal failure caused by hypovolaemia should include the above attempts to return vital signs to normal; in this case, CVP monitoring is mandatory to prevent fluid overload. Frusemide (furosemide) may also improve renal cortical blood flow and may help to relieve tubular obstruction.

Treatment of established renal failure requires fluid restriction to replace the measured volume of fluid lost plus 500 ml/day. Regular reappraisal of vital signs and CVP readings enable fluid administration to be adjusted and to prevent dehydration or overload developing. Sodium (as physiological saline) is administered as indicated by plasma levels, and potassium will usually require restriction. Acidosis, as monitored by blood gas analysis, may need to be controlled by administering bicarbonate solutions. Antibiotics are given if appropriate (avoiding nephrotoxic drugs) and any infective source is treated.

Haemodialysis or haemofiltration is indicated when one or more of the following metabolic changes is detected: blood urea greater than 35 mmol/litre, plasma creatinine greater than 900 μmol/litre, plasma potassium greater than 6.5 mmol/litre (and not responding to other methods such as calcium Resonium® or dextrose and insulin), and acidosis with a pH of less than 7.1. Furthermore, volume overload on its own will require dialysis when stimulation of renal excretion is not possible.

7.5 Obstructive uropathy

Anuria in a surgical patient may result from obstruction of urine outflow rather than renal failure, and will eventually lead to renal failure if untreated. If a urinary catheter is already *in situ*, blockage will cause anuria and requires catheter washout or replacement. Suspected obstructive uropathy should be investigated by ultrasonography of the urinary tract, which will identify obstruction in both upper and the lower urinary tracts. Intravenous urography may be indicated if renal function is nearly normal and isotope excretion studies may be required to determine renal blood flow and glomerular filtration rates.

Treatment of obstructive uropathy depends on the level of obstruction and may require bladder catheterization, ureteric stenting, or percutaneous nephrostomy drainage of the renal pelvis or pelvices.

8 Substance abuse

8.1 Alcohol abuse

It is important to detect patients who abuse alcohol for the following reasons:

- they are prone to cirrhosis with its attendant problems of hepatocellular dysfunction and portal hypertension;
- they may be suffering from malnutrition;
- alcohol potentiates the effects of general anaesthetics and opiate analgesics and the inebriated patient needs smaller doses;
- chronic alcohol abuse induces liver enzymes and higher doses of anaesthetic and sedating agents may be required;
- they may suffer the effects of alcohol withdrawal;
- complications such as hypoglycaemia, subdural haematoma, and cardiomyopathy may occur.

Patients should always be asked how much alcohol they drink and this is best recorded as units of alcohol a week. One unit of alcohol is equivalent to:

- half a pint of beer;
- one measure (pub) of spirits;
- one glass of wine;
- one glass of sherry.

The alcohol content of beer and wine varies so this is only an approximation.

Doctors recommend 'safe' levels of alcohol consumption as follows (although recent government recommendations increased these limits, with little support from the medical profession)

- 21 units a week for a man (recently increased to 28);
- 14 units a week for a woman (recently increased to 21).

Clinically significant problems are unlikely unless a patient is drinking more than 50 units a week. Remember that patients almost always underestimate their consumption of alcohol!

An alternative method of detecting the problem drinker is by using the **CAGE** questionnaire as follows. A state of alcohol dependence is likely if the patient gives positive answers to two or more of the following questions:

1. Have you ever felt that you should **C**ut down on your drinking?

2. Have people **A**nnoyed you by criticizing your drinking?

3. Have you ever felt **G**uilty about your drinking?

4. Have you ever had a drink first thing in the morning to steady your nerves or get rid of a hangover (**E**ye-opener)?

In addition, pointers to alcohol abuse may include an unstable work or marital history, or work in an occupation, such as publican, which carries a high risk. Evasive answers to questions about alcohol or symptoms such as morning headache, nausea, and vomiting also point towards alcohol excess.

Examination may reveal tremor, bruising, rib fractures, features of hepatic cirrhosis, or clinical depression. Laboratory tests often show a raised mean corpuscular volume (MCV) and elevated γ-glutamyl-transpeptidase (GGT), but specificity is low.

Alcohol withdrawal syndrome

Early symptoms (3–12 hours after last drink) are due to sympathetic overactivity and include tremor, sweating, anxiety, nausea, and insomnia. Seizures may occur between 10 and 60 hours; they are generalized and precede or accompany **delirium tremens (DTs)**. It is important to exclude hypoglycaemia as a predisposing factor.

After about 72 hours, around 5 per cent of patients with withdrawal symptoms will develop DTs. Symptoms include severe tremor, confusion and disorientation, agitation, visual hallucinations (typically seeing coloured insects), and paranoid ideas. These symptoms are more severe in the elderly and often occur in the early hours of the morning. Mortality may be as high as 10 per cent, often from a cardiac arrhythmia.

Management of withdrawal

Giving alcohol is the most effective method of treating life-threatening features of alcohol withdrawal in critically ill postoperative patients. This is rarely needed, but may be administered orally or intravenously.

Vitamin B preparations, particularly thiamine (e.g. Pabrinex®) should be given daily for 7 days via the intramuscular route or slowly intravenously over 10 minutes as serious adverse reactions are more common when given rapidly intravenously.

Chlordiazepoxide (up to 40 mg orally three times daily) is useful for a moderately severe withdrawal syndrome as it is thought to be less likely to cause dependence than chlormethiazole. For severe withdrawal, chlormethiazole is useful in the short term for DTs, particularly if there are seizures. It may be given orally (four capsules four times daily initially) or infused intravenously. For control of seizures, diazepam (as Diazemuls®) is given intravenously.

Haloperidol may be used to control troublesome hallucinations; alpha-adrenergic blockers (clonidine) may help tachycardia and hypertension, and a beta-adrenergic blocker (propranolol) may decrease the risk of arrhythmia.

It is often helpful to involve the local liaison psychiatry service and it is important to inform the general practitioner when the patient is discharged from hospital.

9 Neurological disorders

9.1 Myasthenia gravis

In this disease, there is a defect of myoneural transmission caused by antibodies to the acetylcholine receptors on the motor end plate. The result is weakness and fatiguability of skeletal muscle. These patients are particularly sensitive to neuromuscular blocking agents but have a normal response to opiate analgesics and other drugs.

Patients are usually taking anticholinesterase drugs (e.g. pyridostigmine) and often steroids and should continue these

until about 2 hours before operation. The anaesthetist must be made aware of the condition and the patient is usually ventilated postoperatively until adequate spontaneous tidal volume returns. Anticholinesterase treatment should be continued, via nasogastric tube if necessary. A standard perioperative regimen for steroids is also required.

9.2 Myalgic encephalomyelitis

This condition is known by a number of names, including postviral fatigue syndrome and chronic fatigue syndrome. There is considerable discussion as to the cause of the condition (and even whether it exists as a clinical entity). It is likely that there is a spectrum of disorders persisting for at least 6 months with the hallmark of postexertional fatigue and myalgia. There is a risk that any trauma (including general anaesthesia and surgery) will precipitate a relapse or deterioration in symptoms, and operative intervention should be kept to a minimum.

9.3 Parkinson's disease

Parkinson's disease is a progressive disorder of the central nervous system, characterized by:

◆ tremor

◆ rigidity

◆ akinesia

◆ postural instability.

The abnormality that causes the clinical disease is degeneration of the dopaminergic neurons in the substantia nigra of the midbrain. By the time of presentation there is a loss of about 80 per cent of the neurons and a corresponding reduction in striatal dopamine. The mainstay of treatment is replacement of the dopamine deficiency with **levodopa**, usually combined with a dopa-decarboxylase inhibitor (which does not cross the blood–brain barrier) to minimize peripheral side-effects.

The following are clinical features in response to medication, which may be used for assessment of severity and which impact on the effectiveness of treatment:

1. A single dose may be missed without obvious deterioration in symptoms.

2. Symptoms recur between doses and medication has to be given more frequently (five or six times a day).

3. Symptoms (particularly akinesia) become a problem in the morning after a night's sleep and no medication.

4. Duration of response shortens with episodes of 'freezing'.

5. Response to each dose becomes short-lived and unpredictable. 'On–off' reactions occur, dyskinesia may be a problem, and there may be autonomic symptoms.

It is clearly important to know which stage the disease has reached in the patient requiring surgery. Medication has to be given orally and, if possible, the usual regimen should be continued. Patients with stage 1 or stage 2 disease are unlikely to develop significant symptoms if medication is stopped temporarily, while those with stage 5 disease will pose considerable problems.

Treatment

Anticholinergic agents

These agents are infrequently used now because of their side-effects and relatively poor efficacy (although tremor may be helped). If this is the patient's sole anti-Parkinsonian treatment, it can be discontinued safely.

Preparations of levodopa (usually either Sinemet® or Madopar®)

Levodopa is the standard therapy and the clinical severity of the disease can be assessed by knowing the dose of levodopa that controls symptoms. There are now slow-release preparations which are useful when given at night, and these may be useful if given before surgery.

Dopamine receptor agonists

These compounds (lisuride, pergolide, and bromocriptine) stimulate the dopamine receptors directly. They tend to be used in conjunction with levodopa to prolong its effect in patients with more severe disease.

Adverse effects of levodopa and dopamine receptor agonists include:

◆ nausea and vomiting;

◆ postural hypotension;

◆ hallucinations, vivid dreams, psychosis, acute confusional state;

◆ dizziness, drowsiness;

◆ involuntary movements.

The dose should be reduced (or the drugs discontinued) if any of the above are postoperative problems.

Selegiline

This is an inhibitor of monoamine oxidase B, the enzyme mainly responsible for the metabolism of dopamine in the brain. It is used in conjunction with levodopa to potentiate and prolong its effects. In addition there was some evidence that selegiline used as monotherapy may delay the progression of the disease, but this now seems unlikely. Selegiline can probably be stopped if necessary without significant adverse effects.

Apomorphine

This is a potent dopamine agonist which is given parenterally and is therefore a great advantage in patients with severe Parkinson's disease who are unable to take medication orally. It may be given subcutaneously or by continuous intravenous infusion, usually requiring co-administration of domperidone to prevent vomiting.

For the 'drug-dependent' patient with Parkinson's disease who has had an operation and is taking fluids enterally (either orally or via a nasogastric tube), freshly prepared solutions of the dispersible preparations are of use. If a patient is unable to take fluids enterally after operation, the parenteral route of administration of L-dopa is not available as L-dopa is poorly soluble and needs to be maintained in a very acidic solution. In addition L-dopa is not absorbed through the rectal mucosa. Subcutaneously injected apomorphine covered by domperidone suppositories to prevent nausea may be needed.

9.4 Multiple sclerosis

Patients with multiple sclerosis (MS) may need operations that are incidental to their disease, or which are necessary to treat complications such as pressure ulcers, which require plastic surgery in patients with paraplegia, or tendon division for contractures. There is no clear evidence that regional or general anaesthesia contributes to an exacerbation of the disease, although there is a relationship between deterioration of clinical condition (usually reversible) and postoperative pyrexia, as demyelinated nerves exhibit an increased sensitivity to an increase in core temperature.

10 Haematological disorders

10.1 Anaemias

Introduction

In most anaemic patients, blood transfusion can be withheld until the anaemia has been characterized. Exceptions to this are active bleeding or the need for emergency surgery with a very low haemoglobin concentration. This is because the hazards of blood transfusion may outweigh the benefits (see Chapter 9). In addition, the nature of stored and transfused blood impairs its oxygen-carrying capacity.

Several factors other than simple haemoglobin concentration are involved in oxygen transport to the tissues; these include cardiac output, tissue perfusion, oxygen saturation, and viscosity of blood. Blood viscosity falls with falling haemoglobin concentration and volume flow is therefore increased. When considering transfusion, a balance between flow and oxygen-carrying capacity occurs when the haemoglobin concentration is about 10 g/dl. In general, transfusion is unnecessary if the haemoglobin is stable above 8 g/dl.

Macrocytic anaemia

1. Megaloblastic anaemias are due to lack of either vitamin B_{12} or folate. The anaemia is by nature chronic and the patient is rarely haemodynamically compromised despite haemoglobin concentrations as low as 3 g/dl. Transfusion (and operation) should be avoided if possible because cardiac failure may easily be precipitated. If transfusion is considered essential, then small aliquots (even of only 50 ml) of packed cells should be used with diuretic 'cover'.

2. Normoblastic macrocytosis is commonly due to alcohol abuse and should alert one to the possibility of alcohol-associated problems.

Normocytic anaemia

1. May occur in acute haemorrhage and transfusion may be appropriate.

2. Is often secondary to systemic (and usually chronic) inflammatory disorders and renal failure. The cause of the anaemia should be sought because the underlying condition may be important in the consideration of operative intervention. Transfusion should be avoided.

Microcytic anaemia

1. Usually due to chronic blood loss (if there is malabsorption, folate will also be low). The site of bleeding should be identified. Transfusion may be appropriate if haemoglobin concentration is very low and further blood loss is anticipated. Otherwise treat with oral iron.

2. Uncommonly due to **thalassaemia** when the serum ferritin concentration is high (rather than low as in blood loss).

Polycythaemia

1 **Polycythaemia rubra vera** is a myeloproliferative disorder characterized by an increase in red cell mass and an increase in platelet numbers and white blood cells (except in its early stages). Complications include an increased tendency both to thrombosis (particularly if the platelet numbers are increased) and, paradoxically, to haemorrhage. Operation should be postponed if possible until haematological control has been achieved with myelosuppression (busulfan or hydroxyurea). If emergency operation is required and the haematocrit is substantially above 50 per cent, then pre-operative venesection with fluid volume replacement may be appropriate. Remember that the platelet count rises following this blood loss as any other.

2. Secondary polycythaemia ('stress polycythaemia') occurs when there is an abnormal stimulus to red blood cell formation. This usually occurs with hypoxia associated with chronic lung disease and, occasionally, is due to primary overproduction of erythropoietin. In secondary polycythaemia, there is no rise in platelet or white cell counts and the main problem is the increased risk of thrombosis. Venesection may be required if the haematocrit is substantially above 50 per cent; if possible, the operation should be postponed until the cardiovascular system has stabilized after venesection.

10.2 Bleeding disorders

These are covered in Chapter 9.

11 Endocrine disorders

11.1 Diabetes mellitus

Introduction

Diabetes is common, affecting about 2 per cent of the British population. About half of all diabetics will need surgery during their lifetime and three-quarters of them will be over 50 years of age at the time.

Diabetic patients are potentially at high risk during anaesthesia and surgery. In addition to metabolic instability, they are more likely to have atherosclerosis of coronary and peripheral arteries, including carotid arteries, they may have a depressed response to infection, and may have renal impairment.

The effects of insulin and types of diabetes

The main action of insulin is anabolic, directing fuels into body stores. It inhibits hepatic mobilization of glucose, gluconeogenesis, and ketogenesis, as well as peripheral lipolysis and protein degradation. The actions of insulin are diametrically opposed to many of the hormonal responses to stress and trauma. Thus, catecholamines and glucagon increase hepatic generation of glucose and increase lipolysis and, at the same time, catecholamines inhibit insulin secretion. Cortisol enhances protein degradation, while growth hormone promotes lipolysis and increases resistance to insulin. The extent of these hormonal responses is in proportion to the severity of the insult.

The net result of the hormonal response to injury is to increase metabolic rate, to increase catabolism of body tissues, and to inhibit insulin secretion and increase insulin resistance, thus raising blood glucose. In the diabetic patient, these changes are relatively unopposed due to the relative deficiency of endogenous insulin and proceed unchecked, causing harm to the patient. The insulin-dependent patient *must* have insulin and the non-insulin-dependent patient should be treated as insulin dependent in the event of major surgery or trauma.

Diabetes results from an absolute or relative lack of insulin. Insulin-dependent diabetes mellitus (IDDM), also known as type I or 'juvenile onset' diabetes, usually manifests below the age of 30 and is characterized by an absolute insulin deficiency. These patients are truly dependent on administered insulin, which must be maintained *even if the patient is not eating* in order to prevent catabolism. Type I diabetics are at particular risk of becoming ketoacidotic.

Non-insulin-dependent, or type II diabetes, also known as 'maturity onset diabetes' usually develops in older, often obese patients. This is not in any way a 'mild' form of diabetes, as these patients are still prone to develop any of the same complications as type I patients. Indeed, peripheral neuropathy may be more common in this group. These patients have both a reduced β-cell secretory capacity for insulin and an increased resistance to insulin. Circulating plasma insulin concentrations are often normal for age and sex, but low for body weight. Perioperatively, these patients need only glycaemic control as they do not become ketoacidotic.

The aims of managing the diabetic patient undergoing surgery

In a diabetic patient needing an operation, the principle is first to optimize glycaemic control over the perioperative period, avoiding swings in blood glucose, particularly hypoglycaemia; and second to optimize metabolic control to avoid ketoacidosis. Patients should be reviewed critically as to their fitness and the timing of surgery. For an elective operation in an insulin-dependent patient, the local diabetic team should be involved at an early stage so that diabetic control can be optimized before surgery. Ideally, meticulous control should be attempted for 4–6 weeks before operation, particularly in a patient not previously under specialist diabetic care.

The potential mortality and morbidity for patients with diabetes undergoing surgery is high. However, despite this, several developments have meant that operative outcome is little worse than for patients without diabetes; these include better perioperative diabetic control, new antibiotics, and improved anaesthetic techniques.

Problems in patients with diabetes

1. Increased incidence of atherosclerosis causing ischaemic heart disease (with a tendency for myocardial infarction to be painless or 'silent'), peripheral and cerebral vascular disease with greater risk of stroke and lower-limb ischaemia.

2. Microvascular disease, particularly causing nephropathy.

3. Autonomic neuropathy leading to cardiovascular instability and increased risk of cardiac arrest.

4. Increased incidence of postoperative infection. Immune responses may be impaired and increased blood glucose concentration is known to reduce granulocyte function.

5. Predisposition to pressure sores, particularly when there is peripheral neuropathy.

6. Stress and infection raise insulin demand by causing insulin resistance. Patients presenting as emergencies are likely to have poor glycaemic control.

7. Enteral restriction and postoperative vomiting upset the balance between calorie intake and diabetic therapy.

8. Wound healing is impaired because of hyperglycaemia and loss of the anabolic effects of insulin.

9. Diabetic ketoacidosis (particularly in children) may present with abdominal pain, raised serum amylase activity, and polymorphonuclear leucocytosis, making diagnosis of intra-abdominal disorders difficult. Conversely, peritonitis may be present despite minimal pain. As a rule, vomiting precedes abdominal pain in diabetic ketoacidosis, whereas the reverse is true in the surgical 'acute abdomen'. Emergency laparotomy in a patient with ketoacidosis is highly dangerous and should be avoided until the patient is stabilized. It should be remembered that an 'acute abdomen' may be due solely to ketoacidosis.

Preoperative assessment of patients with diabetes

Glycosylated haemoglobin should be measured to demonstrate the quality of diabetic control over the previous month or two and should ideally be below 8 per cent. For major surgery, plasma creatinine should be measured, as renal impairment may be revealed. Proteinuria in the absence of urinary infection implies nephropathy and, if suspected, potentially nephrotoxic drugs should be avoided or closely monitored. An ECG should be performed to look for signs of myocardial ischaemia, which is often painless ('silent') in patients with diabetes. ECG alone is an insensitive test for myocardial ischaemia and more sophisticated investigations are likely to be needed prior to major surgery (see Section 5, above). Blood pressure may be elevated and treatment for this may be required.

The optic fundi should be carefully examined with pupils dilated. Untreated proliferative retinopathy is a contraindication to elective surgery because of the risk of vitreous haemorrhage. Sensory and autonomic neuropathy should be sought. Autonomic neuropathy may lead to cardiorespiratory arrest under anaesthesia, to postoperative urinary retention, and to prolonged gastric 'ileus' after operation. Patients with sensory neuropathy of the feet are particularly at risk of pressure sores.

Principles of management

◆ Blood glucose measurements should be used to assess control. Urine glucose measurements are inevitably retrospective and do not reflect the current blood glucose level. In addition, a urine test negative for glucose means nothing in respect of hypoglycaemia or any other blood sugar value below the renal threshold for glucose (usually about 10 mmol/l).

◆ Good preoperative glycaemic control should be achieved so the patient can arrive at the operating theatre with a blood glucose between 5 and 15 mmol/l. This usually requires the patient to be admitted to hospital 24–48 hours before the planned operation.

◆ Hypoglycaemia must be avoided (blood glucose < 3 mmol/l); this is far more harmful than moderate hyperglycaemia.

◆ Frequent monitoring of blood glucose (fingerprick capillary or venous blood sample) and electrolytes should be performed in the perioperative period.

◆ The operation should be planned for as early as possible in the day.

Protocols for the management of diabetic patients for surgery

Patients controlled on diet alone

No special treatment is necessary but blood glucose concentrations should be monitored frequently and insulin/glucose infusion given if blood glucose is greater than about 15 mmol/l.

Patients controlled on oral hypoglycaemic drugs

Metformin should be discontinued as it may cause lactic acidosis when there is metabolic stress. If possible, chlorpropamide (which has a very long half-life) should be stopped at least 48 hours before operation and substituted by a short-acting sulphonylurea such as tolbutamide or glipizide. For minor operations, this sulphonylurea should be omitted in the morning and reintroduced when usual diet is resumed. For major operations the sulphonylurea is omitted and the patient managed perioperatively as if insulin dependent (see below). When usual diet is resumed, the oral agent is reinstated. If recovery is likely to be prolonged, subcutaneous intermediate-acting insulin twice daily will be required (e.g. Mixtard®).

Patients requiring insulin

Most hospitals and anaesthetic departments have their own guidelines for managing patients who require insulin and therefore only the general principles are covered here.

If the patient is truly insulin-dependent, adequate doses of insulin must be given to prevent excess catabolism and ketoacidosis. Under the stress of operation and anaesthesia (and any complications), the daily requirement for insulin will be up to 20 per cent more than the usual dose. The dose of insulin should ALWAYS be increased during stress, with additional carbohydrate given to prevent hypoglycaemia.

Most patients are able to continue their usual twice-daily regimen (a combination of rapid- and intermediate-acting insulin) until the day of operation.

Minor and intermediate surgery

For this purpose, minor and intermediate surgery is defined as surgery that will allow the patient to take the next scheduled meal after the operation. The principles of management are similar to those described below for major surgery.

For morning operation, breakfast and the morning dose of insulin are both omitted. Blood glucose is monitored at 8 a.m. and if less than 5 mmol/l, an infusion of 5 per cent glucose should be commenced. Blood glucose is measured on return from operation and a small subcutaneous dose of insulin given if necessary. The usual dose of insulin is given in the evening

For afternoon surgery, a light breakfast is given with half the normal dose of insulin in the form of intermediate-acting insulin. The normal evening dose of insulin is administered.

If surgery is unexpectedly delayed or prolonged, or if the patient is unable or unwilling to eat, blood glucose should be monitored frequently and an insulin infusion begun at the first hint of loss of control.

Major surgery

Many regimens have been employed for managing diabetics who need insulin infusions who are having operations, but only two have proved consistently satisfactory. These are:

(1) independent infusions of glucose and insulin solution;

(2) combined glucose–insulin–potassium infusion.

Table 6.5 Sample sliding scale for controlling insulin dosage when using independent infusions of glucose and insulin

Blood glucose (mmol/l)	Infusion rate (ml/hour, equivalent to units/hour)
<2	Nil
2–3	0.5
4–8	1
9–12	2
13–16	4
17–20	6
>20	8

A 50 ml syringe containing 50 units of soluble insulin is used.

A doctor should be called if the patient has a blood glucose below 2 mmol/l, above 20 mmol/l, or fails to fall below 15 mmol/l with therapy, or is rising progressively.

Both have their adherents but the former has the advantage of flexibility, with the ability to vary either the insulin dose or the fluid input, and the latter has the disadvantage that the composition of the mixture may need to be modified by trial and error to achieve satisfactory control. In either case, no subcutaneous insulin is given on the day of the operation.

Independent infusions of glucose and insulin solution

Insulin dosage is determined by reference to a sliding scale, with doses varied according to blood glucose measurements. Sliding scales are not immutable and may be varied according to local preference, or for individual patients not controlled satisfactory by the chosen regimen (see the sample in Table 6.5).

Infusion is controlled by a syringe pump. A 50 ml syringe contains 50 units of soluble insulin made up with normal (physiological, 0.9 per cent) saline. Ten per cent glucose solution is infused in parallel through a Y-cannula. If the patient becomes hypoglycaemic, insulin infusion is discontinued but is recommenced as soon as hypoglycaemia has been corrected.

Combined glucose–insulin–potassium infusion

Intraoperative and immediate postoperative control is achieved by infusing glucose solution containing insulin and potassium chloride (GIK). A starting regimen (**Alberti**) might be as below, but the precise composition of the infusion and the infusion rate is determined for an individual patient by preoperative blood glucose level and by frequent blood glucose and electrolyte measurements during the perioperative period.

Typical Alberti regimen Infusate of glucose–insulin–potassium solution containing 15 units of soluble insulin and 10 mmol potassium chloride in 500 ml of 10 per cent dextrose solution. This is infused at a rate of 100 ml/hour, commencing early on the morning of surgery. Blood glucose is monitored and the insulin content of the infusion bag adjusted in 5 unit increments to maintain the blood glucose between 7 and 11 mmol/l. This requires the bag to be replaced each time the dose is varied. The infusion is continued until the patient is able to eat and subcutaneous insulin can be given; the infusion should continue for at least an hour after the first subcutaneous dose is given. The required dose may be similar to the patient's preoperative dose, but if in doubt, the total intravenous dose for 24 hours should be summed and that dose given as two divided doses of intermediate-acting insulin, 60 per cent in the morning and 40 per cent in the evening.

If fluid restriction is necessary, 20 per cent or 50 per cent glucose can be infused via a central venous line, with appropriate additions of insulin and potassium.

When the patient is mobile, eating normally, and free of infection, the usual dose of long- and short-acting insulin is given twice daily. If there are continuing complications (restricted oral intake, infection, or vomiting), then intravenous insulin should be given continuously using a sliding scale of blood glucose.

The insulin-dependent diabetic presenting as a surgical emergency

The diabetes may be markedly out of control at the time of presentation because of vomiting, infection, stress, and the inability to maintain usual treatment. The operation should be delayed as long as possible while the metabolic upset is rectified. This involves rehydration with intravenous normal saline, intravenous infusion of insulin, and potassium replacement where appropriate. In correcting the metabolic abnormality, it is wrong to withhold insulin should the blood glucose become low in the presence of ketoacidosis (as determined either by arterial blood pH measurement or in the presence of significant ketonuria). The patient requires intravenous glucose to correct the hypoglycaemia and insulin to correct the ketoacidosis.

Patients not previously known to be diabetic

If metabolically deranged, the patient should be treated as insulin dependent. A patient with impaired glucose tolerance may present with frank diabetes precipitated by the stress of operation or illness. These patients are probably best treated with small doses of insulin perioperatively to improve the metabolic response to surgery. After operation, the glucose tolerance should be assessed to determine the need for further treatment.

Follow-up of patients with diabetes

Diabetic patients should be reviewed after major surgery by a specialist in diabetes to ensure that control is maintained. Patient compliance varies, and the less careful patient easily becomes hypoglycaemic when returning to the less controlled conditions outside hospital.

11.2 Thyroid disease

Hypothyroidism

Patients maintained on replacement therapy

The usual replacement dose of L-thyroxine (T_4) is 150–200 μg/day. The half-life of thyroxine is around 5 days, and the replacement for the whole week may be given as a single dose if the patient will be unable to tolerate enteral medication. Intravenous tri-iodothyronine (T_3) should not be used for replacement.

Patients thought to be hypothyroid when presenting for surgery

The best clinical sign of hypothroidism is slow relaxation of tendon reflexes (particularly supinator and biceps). This is confirmed by finding an elevated plasma thyroid stimulation hormone (TSH) level (primary hypothyroidism). Operation should be postponed if possible because hypothyroid patients are susceptible to myocardial dysfunction, have a decreased ability to handle a fluid load, and are more sensitive to depressant drugs. If surgery must be performed urgently, it is best to proceed and to start treatment after operation. Tri-iodothyronine has a rapid onset of action but is best avoided because the rapid change in metabolic rate may cause problems (particularly cardiac).

Hyperthyroidism

Introduction

Thyrotoxicosis is common, affecting up to 3 per cent of the female population and 0.25 per cent of males. In patients with uncontrolled or undiagnosed hyperthyroidism, the stress of operation may precipitate a 'thyroid storm'. It is therefore important to exclude thyroid overactivity preoperatively and to postpone the operation if possible until the patient is euthyroid. There is debate as to whether beta-blockade in isolation can prevent thyroid storm and it is best to use additional treatment with antithyroid drugs (carbimazole or propylthiouracil) and iodine. Patients scheduled for partial thyroidectomy should be rendered euthyroid before operation.

Signs and symptoms

The signs and symptoms of thyroid overactivity are listed in standard texts and will not be repeated. It is important to remember that lethargy (rather than hyperactivity) is fairly common and elderly patients may present solely with features of cardiac dysfunction (particularly atrial fibrillation with an uncontrolled ventricular response). Weight loss is often an important diagnostic feature.

Biochemical diagnosis

A useful screening test for thyroid dysfunction is the highly sensitive thyroid stimulating hormone (TSH) assay. TSH is completely suppressed (< 0.03 mU/l) in hyperthyroidism (except when the very rare pituitary thyrotropinoma is the cause) and often remains suppressed for some time after the patient has become euthyroid.

An assay of free thyroxine (fT_4) is a useful confirmatory test and fT_4 will be raised in thyroid overactivity. Measurement of the free hormone avoids incorrect diagnosis of hyperthyroidism caused by increased concentrations of thyroid-binding proteins (euthyroid hyperthyroxinaemia) caused by the oral contraceptive pill or pregnancy, for example.

Measurement of fT_4 and TSH give an accurate assessment of thyroid function in most cases and the thyroid releasing hormone (TRH) test is almost never necessary. If further assessment of thyroid function is required, then an isotope uptake scan of the gland is helpful.

Cause of thyrotoxicosis

Once the diagnosis of thyrotoxicosis has been established, it is important to determine the aetiology. Correct long-term management depends on identifying the cause of thyroid over-activity as antithyroid drugs will have no effect on the course of conditions other than Graves' disease, although they can be used to render the patient euthyroid in the short term.

Common causes

◆ Autoimmune thyroid disease (Graves' disease);

◆ toxic single thyroid nodule;

◆ toxic multinodular goitre.

Rare causes

◆ Factitious (abuse of liothyronine (T_3), particularly for weight loss);

◆ thyroiditis—usually 'viral';

◆ metastatic thyroid carcinoma;

◆ trophoblastic tumours (choriocarcinoma, some testicular tumours, struma ovarii);

◆ Jod–Basedow effect (hyperthyroidism precipitated by iodine in, for example, radiographic contrast media or iodine-containing drugs such as amiodarone).

Features of Graves' disease

The features of Graves' disease are:

◆ small, diffuse goitre;

◆ tendency to severe thyrotoxicosis;

◆ dysthyroid eye signs;

◆ pretibial myxoedema;

◆ clubbing (rare);

◆ family history of organ-specific autoimmune disorders;

◆ circulating thyroid autoantibodies.

11.3 Adrenal insufficiency

Secondary adrenal insufficiency

The most common cause of adrenal insufficiency is hypothalamo-pituitary–adrenal suppression secondary to corticosteroid treatment for 'steroid-sensitive' conditions. The daily therapeutic dose is usually greater than the endogenous production of corticosteroids (20–30 mg hydrocortisone a day) and is usually in the form of prednisolone or dexamethasone. The dose of these drugs which is equivalent to the daily physiological output is 7.5 mg of prednisolone and 1 mg of dexamethasone. Larger doses cause a range of problems, including greater susceptibility to infection, poor wound healing, and a susceptibility to gastrointestinal haemorrhage and electrolyte imbalance. In addition, some normal responses to infection, such as pain and pyrexia in peritonitis, may be suppressed, making the clinical diagnosis difficult. After corticosteroid treatment has ceased, adrenal responsiveness may be suppressed for months. These patients should be treated as described below unless stimulation tests show that normal responsiveness has returned.

Management of suspected secondary adrenal insufficiency

Minor surgical procedures: hydrocortisone hemisuccinate 100 mg intramuscularly with the premedication, and restart usual oral dose after operation. More major procedures: hydrocortisone hemisuccinate, 100 mg intramuscularly with the premedication and 6-hourly intravenously thereafter until the normal oral dose can be resumed. There has been a recent suggestion that patients who have been taking 10 mg or less prednisolone daily do not require an increase in perioperative dosage, but further evidence is required before abandoning this prophylactic treatment for this group.

Any unexplained postoperative cardiovascular collapse should be treated with a further dose of intravenous hydrocortisone. However, since most of these episodes are due to unrecognized blood loss, myocardial infarction, or septicaemia, these causes should be excluded.

Primary adrenal insufficiency

A patient with primary adrenal failure is likely to be taking a replacement dose of hydrocortisone. The adrenal glands will not be able to respond to stress by increasing production of corticosteroids, so the above regimens should be used in the perioperative period.

11.4 Disorders of calcium metabolism

Introduction

Ionized calcium concentration in the extracellular fluid is maintained within a very narrow range by calcium-regulating hormones. These include calcitonin, parathyroid hormone, and 1,25-dihydroxyvitamin D. The calcium ion (approximately 50 per cent of total plasma calcium) is involved in many vital physiological processes, including muscle contraction, nerve conduction, blood coagulation, and cell secretion. It also acts as an important intracellular 'second messenger'.

The ionized calcium concentration may be influenced by surgery in several ways:

1. Following transfusion of citrated whole blood or fresh, frozen plasma, there may be a substantial fall in ionized calcium concentration as a result of calcium ion chelation by citrate.

Plasma total calcium concentration is unaffected and the adverse effect of citrate is usually short-lived because it is rapidly cleared by hepatic oxidation. A citrate-induced tendency to haemorrhage caused by massive blood transfusion is reduced by intravenous administration of 10 ml of 10 per cent calcium gluconate.

2. Acidosis as a result of major surgery causes an increase.

3. Changes in plasma albumin cause a reciprocal change in ionized calcium concentration.

4. The corticosteroid stress response inhibits the intestinal absorption of calcium, as well as new bone formation and renal retention of calcium.

5. Transient hypocalcaemia is a well-recognized complication of parathyroid and thyroid surgery. Mechanisms include damage to the blood supply or the substance of the parathyroid glands, or a phase of bone repair in parathyroid bone disease ('hungry bones').

6. Surgery on the gastrointestinal tract may reduce the absorption of calcium.

7. Acute pancreatitis causes hypocalcaemia, the extent of which is a prognostic guide.

8. Acute renal failure causes hypocalcaemia but the metabolic abnormality requires dialysis rather than calcium replacement.

The effects of hypocalcaemia

Hypocalcaemia may cause hypotension and increased muscular excitability, including cardiac irritability. Hypotension may be due to impaired vascular smooth muscle tone. Calcium infusion has been shown to increase mean arterial pressure and cardiac index in acutely ill hypocalcaemic patients and should be borne in mind in these patients following major surgery or trauma.

Hypocalcaemia is suspected clinically by eliciting symptoms such as perioral tingling and acroparaesthesiae (tingling in hands and feet) and by demonstrating latent tetany with:

1. **Chvostek's sign.** The facial nerve is irritable in the presence of hypocalcaemia and will respond with contraction of the facial muscles if the facial nerve is tapped anterior to the ear with a patella hammer. A modification of this test (when the zygomatic prominence is tapped with the patella hammer and the angle of the mouth contracts) may be more specific.

2. **Trousseau's sign.** A sphygmomanometer cuff is inflated over the forearm to above the systolic blood pressure and the hand observed for about 2 minutes. A positive response (latent tetany) is involuntary flexion of the fingers and thumb to form the '*main d'accoucheur*' (obstetrician's hand). The pathophysiology of this response is not understood as occlusion of the blood supply to the forearm will cause acidosis which ought to protect muscle from hypocalcaemic spasm. It is possible that the increased plasma albumin concentration caused by the increased intravascular pressure binds more calcium and leads to a reduction in ionized calcium.

Hypercalcaemia

Recognized causes of hypercalcaemia include:

♦ primary hyperparathyroidism;

♦ malignant disease;

♦ vitamin D intoxication;

♦ sarcoidosis;

♦ hyperthyroidism, hypothyroidism, Addison's disease;

♦ Paget's disease of bone, particularly with immobilization;

♦ chronic renal failure associated with taking calcium and vitamin D supplements or treatments with drug mixtures containing calcium carbonate (used to replace aluminium hydroxide as a phosphate binder because aluminium toxicity was thought to contribute to renal bone disease and possibly dementia);

♦ tertiary hyperparathyroidism requiring parathyroidectomy.

From a practical point of view, the main differential diagnosis of clinically significant hypercalcaemia is between primary hyperparathyroidism and malignancy; the other causes account for less than 10 per cent of cases.

Malignant hypercalcaemia

Malignancies commonly associated with hypercalcaemia include:

♦ carcinoma of the breast;

♦ squamous cell carcinoma of the lung (much less common in adenocarcinoma and rare with anaplastic or oat-cell carcinoma);

♦ haematological malignancies, particularly myeloma;

♦ squamous cell cancers of the head and neck, including proximal oesophagus;

♦ rare tumours, such as cholangiocarcinoma and VIPomas (pancreatic tumours secreting vasoactive intestinal polypeptide);

♦ renal cell and ovarian cancers;

♦ some common tumours, such as carcinoma of the colon and carcinomas of the female genital tract occasionally cause hypercalcaemia.

Pathophysiology of malignant hypercalcaemia

Malignant hypercalcaemia is due to a combination of bone resorption and renal tubular calcium retention. This is usually accompanied by reduced intestinal absorption of calcium (in contrast to the hypercalcaemia of hyperparathyroidism).

Three syndromes may coexist in an individual patient:

1. **Humoral hypercalcaemia.** Circulating factors are responsible for the abnormalities of calcium and phosphate metabolism. There is an increase in both osteoclastic bone resorption and

renal tubular reabsorption of calcium, mediated by factors that include:

(a) Parathyroid hormone related protein (or peptide) (PTHrP). Hypercalcaemia resulting from malignancies that had not metastasized was thought to be due to parathyroid hormone (PTH) itself, produced ectopically by the tumour. It is unlikely that this ever occurs; more likely, it is due to PTHrP which, in malignancy, mimics the action of PTH.

(b) Other bone-resorbing polypeptides, such as transforming growth factor-α (TGF-α), tumour necrosis factor (TNF) and interleukin-1.

2. **Osteolytic metastases.** Hypercalcaemia often occurs in patients with widespread osteolytic metastases, particularly from breast cancer. The malignant cells themselves may absorb bone directly but it is more likely that osteoclasts are stimulated by factors produced by tumour cells.

3. **Myeloma and other haematological malignancies.** Hypercalcaemia commonly occurs in myeloma, usually in the presence of extensive osteolytic bone disease. The mechanism for bone destruction is osteoclastic, with myeloma cells producing local factors that activate adjacent osteoclasts. **Lymphotoxin** has been identified and may be the major mediator of bone destruction in myeloma. Hypercalcaemia associated with various types of lymphoma is likely to be multifactorial; one possible factor is that lymphoma cells may somehow activate vitamin D.

Indications for treatment of malignant hypercalcaemia

Hypercalcaemia is potentially life-threatening by virtue of its action in causing dehydration and cardiac arrhythmias. It frequently causes unpleasant symptoms such as nausea, abdominal pain, and extreme malaise. Hypercalcaemia can occur relatively early in the course of the cancer (of the breast, for example). At this stage, lowering the plasma calcium allows time to start specific anticancer treatment. Hypercalcaemia, however, may be a preterminal event; at this stage, treatment of hypercalcaemia is often required for symptom relief or to buy time for a patient to settle his or her affairs. In terminal illness, any treatment of hypercalcaemia may be inappropriate.

The level of hypercalcaemia is important in assessing the need for treatment:

- Severe: patients who are symptomatic or where the corrected plasma calcium concentration is greater than 3.5 mmol/l require urgent treatment.

- Moderate: asymptomatic patients in whom the corrected calcium concentration lies between 3.0 and 3.5 mmol/l require less urgent treatment.

- Mild: asymptomatic patients with plasma calcium concentrations below 3.0 mmol/l may not require treatment, but note that the natural history of malignant hypercalcaemia is of progression and the change from mild to severe may be rapid.

Practical treatment of malignant hypercalcaemia

In theory, it is possible to determine the relative contribution of bone and kidney to the hypercalcaemia and modify treatment accordingly. In practice this is rarely useful and the following treatment tends to be used in all cases:

1. **Rehydration.** Dehydration accompanies and worsens the hypercalcaemia. Between 3 and 4 litres of normal saline given intravenously over 24 hours will lower the plasma calcium and improve symptoms. Rehydration does not modulate the underlying mechanisms and the fall in plasma calcium is transient.

2. **Calcitonin.** This inhibits bone resorption and also has an effect on the distal renal tubule, promoting calcium loss via the kidney. Salmon calcitonin (400 international units) is given intramuscularly 6- to 8-hourly for 48 hours. A fall of plasma calcium concentration of around 0.5 mmol/l is expected within hours but this lasts for only about 48 hours, probably because of downregulation of calcitonin receptors in bone cells.

3. **Bisphosphonates.** These bind to bone and inhibit osteoclast resorption of bone. The onset of action is slow (24–48 hours) but the calcium-lowering effect may persist for several weeks. The most commonly used bisphosphonate is disodium pamidronate. This is given after rehydration as a slow intravenous infusion of between 15 and 90 mg, depending on the plasma calcium concentration. Sodium clodronate has a similar action and has the potential advantage that it can subsequently be given orally.

4. **Antitumour therapy.** This is the main hope for long-term therapy as reduction of tumour mass helps to control the hypercalcaemia.

5. **Other treatments.**

- Frusemide (furosemide) is no longer recommended. Although it increases renal tubular excretion of calcium, it also increases dehydration. In addition, the required dose is more than 100 mg/hour.

- Corticosteroids are usually ineffective in lowering the plasma calcium, but may have an antitumour effect in certain lymphomas.

- Intravenous phosphate may cause the side-effect of extraskeletal calcification, and mithramycin (a cytotoxic antibiotic that inhibits bone resorption), has a range of side-effects that make it unsafe to use in the face of safer and more effective alternatives.

The most efficacious therapeutic approach to treatment of severe or symptomatic hypercalcaemia is initial rehydration followed by a combination of calcitonin and bisphosphonate.

Primary hyperparathyroidism

Until the 1970s the usual presentation of primary hyperparathyroidism was with renal stones or nephrocalcinosis; up to half of these patients had bone disease. Non-renal, non-osseous presentations accounted for only 5 per cent of cases. Since the advent of biochemical screening, numbers of patients identified with primary hyperparathyroidism have increased and the presentation has changed.

Nowadays, fewer than 10 per cent of hyperparathyroid patients have renal or bone disease and 80 per cent are asymptomatic or have vague ill health. Eighty per cent are female and more than 50 per cent are over 70 years old. The pathology of the parathyroid glands has not changed, however, with a single adenoma as the cause in 90 per cent and generalized hyperplasia in most of the remainder. Parathyroid carcinoma as a cause is very rare. Because of this transition to an older and less symptomatic population, there is increasing opinion that the approach to these patients should be non-surgical. A controlled trial to compare surgical and conservative management would be interesting but difficult to undertake, and the indications for surgery in primary hyperparathyroidism continue to be the subject of debate.

Summary of the treatment of primary hyperparathyroidism

◆ Surgery is the only therapy demonstrated to influence hyperparathyroidism.

◆ Renal stones and bone disease respond well to successful parathyroid surgery but the more non-specific effects, such as hypertension and an elevated cardiovascular death rate, malaise, fatigue, lethargy, and psychiatric symptoms, are often unchanged.

◆ Conservative management with careful observation of symptoms and plasma calcium concentrations appears to be safe and will detect patients who are developing significant problems before serious complications develop.

The best surgical centres cure 90–95 per cent of patients, but rates as low as 75 per cent have been reported.

Indications for parathyroidectomy

◆ Patients under 40 years of age, independent of symptoms or complications. Family screening is important.

◆ Patients over 40 years with specific complications, such as bone or stone disease.

◆ Patients with corrected plasma calcium concentrations greater than 3.0 mmol/l.

◆ Patients over 40 years with severe non-specific symptoms should be considered for surgery.

Diagnosis of primary hyperparathyroidism

The following are common features of primary hyperparathyroidism:

◆ Hypercalcaemia: the corrected plasma calcium concentration is persistently above the reference range but not usually much greater than 3.0 mmol/l.

◆ The hypercalcaemia is of long duration. This may be determined prospectively by observation or retrospectively by review of the case notes, with evidence of raised plasma calcium concentrations in the past.

◆ There is no evidence of malignancy. The hypercalcaemia of malignancy usually presents with obvious clinical evidence of primary or secondary malignancy.

◆ There is evidence of elevated plasma parathyroid hormone (PTH). This can now be measured reliably and should normally be suppressed in the presence of hypercalcaemia. If levels are measurable or elevated, this is good evidence of hyperparathyroidism, as PTH assays do not usually measure PTHrP, the humoral agent involved in malignant hypercalcaemia. In hypercalcaemia of malignancy, PTH is above the limit of assay detection in fewer than 25 per cent of cases and the PTH in these cases is rarely as high as seen in primary hyperparathyroidism. PTHrP can be assayed, but this is not yet widely available.

◆ There is low plasma phosphate, due to PTH-mediated phosphaturia.

◆ There is hyperchloraemic acidosis.

Rarely, there is radiological evidence, such as periosteal bone resorption of phalanges and the lamina dura of tooth sockets.

Parathyroid localization

Identification of an overactive parathyroid gland may help in diagnosis, but localization is particularly useful preoperatively. In general, parathyroid localization is disappointing and neck exploration by a competent surgeon is the best option. However, the following techniques are being used, depending upon local practice and availability:

◆ High-resolution ultrasound.

◆ Thallium–technetium subtraction scanning. Thallium accumulates in tissue with high blood flow, including thyroid and parathyroid. Technetium accumulates only in the thyroid. The technetium scan is subtracted from the thallium scan, leaving an image of the parathyroid concentration.

◆ Computed tomography: high resolution with contrast injection.

◆ Magnetic resonance imaging.

◆ Selective venous catheterization and sampling for PTH.

◆ Arteriography.

11.5 Phaeochromocytoma

Diagnosis

Phaeochromocytoma is a rare cause of hypertension, occurring in about 0.1 per cent of an unselected population with 'essential' hypertension. It is one of the treatable causes of hypertension as 90 per cent of tumours are benign (surgically curable) and the remainder are amenable to radiopharmaceutical or chemotherapeutic treatment. Paroxysmal hypertension with associated headache and sweating should arouse clinical suspicion, but the exclusion of the diagnosis rests on screening tests.

The most widely used test is detection of increased urinary vanilyl mandelic acid (VMA). Most major series have suggested that the sensitivity of this test is about 70 per cent and dietary restrictions are required to minimize the number of false positives.

Direct measurement of plasma and urinary catecholamines has become more generally available and it is likely that measurement of urinary catecholamine excretion will become the screening method of choice. Plasma and urine catecholamine excretion is also useful in confirming the cause of elevated urinary VMA excretion and in cases where clinical suspicion is high but VMA excretion is within the reference range.

Having confirmed an increase in catecholamine production, the next step is to localize the site of production. The radionuclide MIBG is selectively taken up by neuroendocrine tissue and is the best initial investigation. Computed tomography can then be used to give a clearer localization of the tumour.

Bibliography

Ritchie, J.L. (on behalf of the ACC/AHA Task Force on Practice) (1996). American College of Cardiology/American Heart Association Guidelines for Perioperative Evaluation of Noncardiac Surgery. *Circulation*, **93**, 1278–317.

Goldman, L. *et al.* (1977). Multifactorial index of cardiac risk in non-cardiac surgical procedures. *NEJM*, **297**, 845–50.

Turner, M. and Haywood, G. (1998). Pre-operative assessment of cardiac risk for non-cardiac surgery. *JRCP London*, **32**, 545–7.

CHAPTER 7

Surgical infection

Mark Farrington

1 Introduction

Before considering the prevention, investigation, and treatment of surgical infection, it is important to know the range of microbes that are of surgical relevance and to understand the principles of the pathogenesis of infection. The terms 'microbe', 'micro-organism', and 'organism' are generally used interchangeably for plants or animals that cannot be seen without microscopes and do not form organized multicellular tissues. Microbes of significance to the surgeon belong to one of four groups: bacteria, fungi, protozoa, and viruses.

2 Microbes of surgical importance

A limited and highly selective classification of organisms is given in the section that follows, concentrating on those relevant to surgical practice and serving only as an *aide-mémoire* and reference while reading this book. Standard textbooks of microbiology should be consulted for more detailed information.

2.1 Bacteria

Classification

Aerobes and anaerobes

It is convenient to divide bacteria by their abilities to grow in the presence or absence of oxygen because of their fundamentally different antibiotic sensitivities and cultural requirements in the laboratory: **facultative anaerobes** (usually called 'aerobes') multiply regardless of the partial pressure of oxygen, whereas **obligate anaerobes** (usually called 'anaerobes') require very low oxygen concentrations or its complete absence. A few clinically significant organisms require oxygen, the **obligate aerobes**.

Gram staining

Gram-stain reactions provide the next key division. Gram-negative cell walls allow the crystal violet/iodine primary stain (which is blue) to be washed out of the organisms, which then take up the red counterstain.

Gram-negative bacteria are more sensitive than Gram-positives to drying, alkali, oxidizing agents, and lysis by complement and antibody, but less sensitive to acids, detergents, and many antiseptics and solvents.

Gram-negative and Gram-positive organisms

Gram-negative organisms have an outer cell membrane, never form spores, and contain and release **endotoxin** (a complex lipopolysaccharide structural component of the outer membrane that is responsible for most of the signs and symptoms of septic shock and the sepsis syndrome). Gram-positive organisms (and Gram-negatives) may release **exotoxins**, which are non-structural products, often enzymes, that are sometimes responsible for specific features of an organism's pathogenicity (such as *Clostridium difficile* cytotoxin, and *Streptococcus pyogenes* hyaluronidase which may aid spread through the tissues).

Morphological types

Bacteria are also divided morphologically in to **cocci** (round cells), **rod-shaped** cells (or **bacilli**), and others, including spiral and 'cocco-bacillary' forms.

The classification of surgically important bacteria is summarized in Table 7.1.

2.2 Fungi

Most fungi stain Gram-positive and many will grow on conventional bacteriological media. Types of surgical importance include:

1. Yeasts. These include *Candida albicans* (intestinal and vaginal commensal, an opportunist pathogen that causes mucosal and, increasingly commonly, systemic infection), and *Cryptococcus neoformans* (an environmental organism which is an opportunist pathogen, causing meningitis in immunosuppressed patients, especially those with AIDS).

2. Filamentous fungi (*Aspergillus* spp., moulds).

2.3 Parasites and protozoa

Infections of surgical importance caused by parasites and protozoa include:

1. Tissue infections, including *Toxoplasma gondii*, *Strongyloides stercoralis*, *Entamoeba histolytica*.

2. Intestinal infections, including *Cryptosporidium* sp., *Schistosoma* spp., *Entamoeba histolytica*.

3. Urinary tract infections, including *Schistosoma haematobium*.

4. Lung infections, including *Pneumocystis carinii* (recently reclassified as a fungus), *Echinococcus granulosus*.

2.4 Viruses

Introduction

Viruses are a very large group of infectious agents that are obligate parasites of other organisms; they contain DNA or RNA but not both. Relatively few cause conditions presenting to routine surgical practice, but those that are blood-borne are potentially transmissible among patients and surgeons, and a number of viruses are important causes of infection in organ transplant recipients.

Classification

1. Blood- and tissue-borne (hepatitis B virus (HBV), the other hepatitis viruses, the human immunodeficiency virus (HIV), and Creutzfeldt–Jakob disease).

2. Viruses and organ transplantation (including cytomegalovirus (CMV), Epstein–Barr virus (EBV), herpes simplex virus (HSV), herpes varicella-zoster (HVZ)).

3 Introduction to surgical infection and its definitions

3.1 Terminology

There is much confusion and disagreement about the meaning of many clinical terms used in infectious diseases. The following section gives explanations favoured by this author.

All body surfaces are **colonized** with many species of bacteria and fungi that comprise the **normal commensal flora** (Table 7.2). These organisms do not cause disease while body defences are intact, indeed they may help to resist colonization from external **pathogens** by production of inhibitory substances (called bacteriocines) and by occupying epithelial binding sites. Many usually commensal bacteria are capable of causing **infection** (that is, causing clinical illness) when general or local defences are compromised; these organisms are called **opportunist** pathogens (examples include *Staph. epidermidis* and *Pseud. aeruginosa*). A knowledge of the organisms commonly found at particular body sites is valuable when tracing the primary source of infection. For example, *Bacteroides fragilis* isolated from a blood culture implies a colonic source, whereas *Prevotella bivius* would suggest gynaecological sepsis.

A **virulent** organism is readily capable of causing infection, even in some immunologically normal individuals, by possession of virulence factors such as those allowing adhesion to host epithelia (e.g. surface pili of *Esch. coli* that adhere to uroepithelium) and by production of toxins (e.g. *Clost. difficile* enterocyte toxins). Certain microbial isolates from any site inevitably cause

Table 7.1 Classification of surgically important bacteria

---

facultative anaerobes (AEROBES)

1. Gram-positive

(a) Staphylococci (cocci)	(i) Coagulase positive. The major pathogen, *Staph. aureus,* is identified by the production of *coagulase*, which coagulates plasma
	(ii) Coagulase negative. Important members of this group include *Staph. epidermidis* and relatives (skin commensals and opportunist pathogens, especially of foreign bodies; frequently multiply antibiotic-resistant), and *Staph. saprophyticus* (causes urinary tract infection in young females)
(b) Streptococci (cocci)	(i) Pyogenic. These include the β-haemolytic streptococci of Lancefield groups A, C, and G, which cause wound and throat infection. Lancefield grouping is based on cell-wall antigens. The 'Lancefield group A β-haemolytic streptococcus' is synonymous with *Strep. pyogenes*. The group B β-haemolytic streptococcus causes neonatal infections and maternal sepsis, and also pyogenic infections, especially in diabetics. *Strep. milleri*, a normal gastrointestinal and urogenital commensal, may carry Lancefield antigens of groups A, C, F, G, or none. It is an important cause of abscesses, which often also contain other normal flora from these sites (such as non-sporing anaerobes)
	(ii) Faecal. These include *Enterococcus faecalis* and *Ent. faecium*, gut commensals causing urinary tract and a variety of opportunist infections. These organisms are innately resistant to many antibiotics, and hospital strains are rapidly acquiring even broader resistance, including to vancomycin.
	(iii) Pneumococcus. Otherwise known as *Strep. pneumoniae*, a normal upper respiratory commensal causing respiratory tract infection and meningitis
	(iv) Viridans and non-haemolytic groups. Oral and gut commensals, uncommonly pathogenic except as causes of infective endocarditis
(c) *Bacillus* spp. (rod-shaped)	Most commonly isolated as contaminants, with a propensity to multiply in wound and biliary drainage bags
(d) Diphtheroids (including *Corynebacterium* spp.); rod-shaped organisms	Skin and upper respiratory commensals, rarely opportunist pathogens (e.g. IV line and CSF shunt infection)

2. Gram-negative

(a) Coliforms (rod-shaped). Otherwise known as the Enterobacteriaceae; commensals of the large bowel	(i) Usually community-acquired. This group includes *Escherichia coli*, *Proteus,* and *Klebsiella* spp., which tend to be antibiotic sensitive
	(ii) Usually hospital-acquired. These include *Enterobacter*, *Citrobacter*, *Serratia*, and *Providencia* spp. and are usually more antibiotic resistant. Not commonly found as normal flora in fit individuals
	(iii) Enteric. *Salmonella* and *Shigella* spp. are the most important members of this group, causing gastrointestinal and systemic infections
(b) Pseudomonads (mostly rod-shaped). Sometimes called 'non-fermenters', are mostly obligate aerobes that are common in moist environments, eg sink traps and wash mops, but are mostly rare commensals in normal individuals	Examples include *Pseudomonas* and *Stenotrophomonas* spp., which are opportunist pathogens. *Acinetobacter* spp. are skin commensals that may cause nosocomial urinary tract (UTI) and other infections
(c) Curved rod group	Including *Vibrio* spp. (e.g. *V. cholerae*, causing cholera, and *V. vulnificus* causing necrotizing wound infections after contact with sea water), and *Campylobacter* spp. causing diarrhoea
(d) Fastidious group	This group includes *Haemophilus* spp. (small, rod-shaped commensals of the upper respiratory tract, causing acute-on-chronic bronchitis and invasive infections in children), *Pasteurella multocida* (an oral commensal of dogs and cats causing bite wound infection and septicaemia), *Moraxella catarrhalis* (coccus, causing acute-on-chronic bronchitis), and *Neisseria* spp. (cocci, including the meningococcus and gonococcus)
(e) *Legionella*	*Legionella pneumophila* and its relatives; environmental organisms that cause pneumonia in susceptible hosts

---

obligate anaerobes

Virtually all are sensitive to metronidazole

1. Non-sporing, Gram-negative rods and cocci

(a) *Bacteroides* spp. and their relatives	(i) Colonic. *Bact. fragilis* and relatives such as *Bact. vulgatus* and *Bact. thetaiotaomicron*. Resistant to penicillin
	(ii) Oral/skin/urogenital. Including *Bact. asaccharolyticus*, *Prevotella melaninogenicus,* etc. These used to be frequently sensitive to penicillin, but resistance is now much more common

(continued overleaf)

Table 7.1 *continued*

(b) Others	Including *Fusobacterium* spp.
2. Non-sporing, Gram-positive	
(a) Cocci	*Peptococcus* ('anaerobic staphylococci') and *Peptostreptococcus* spp. ('anaerobic streptococci'). Common commensals of mucosal surfaces, and components of mixed infections associated with these mucosae
(b) Branching rods	Including *Actinomyces israelii*, the cause of actinomycosis, which is resistant to metronidazole
3. Sporing, Gram-positive rods	
(a) *Clostridium* spp.	Faecal commensals, mostly non-pathogenic, but including *Clost. perfringens* (gas gangrene, food poisoning), *Clost. difficile* (antibiotic-associated diarrhoea), *Clost. botulinum*, and others
MYCOBACTERIA. Usually slow-growing organisms with waxy cell walls that mostly require special culture techniques and are stained only by the ZiehlNeelsen or auramine stains	(i) Tuberculous mycobacteria (*Myco. tuberculosis*, *Myco. bovis*) (ii) Non-tuberculous mycobacteria. Many species, including *Myco. avium-intracellulare* (systemic infection in AIDS) and *Myco. marinum* (fish-fancier's ulcer, etc.)
OTHER BACTERIA	Including mycoplasmas, chlamydias, and rickettsias

Table 7.2 Normal bacterial flora of the human body

External sites	Internal sites
Hands: the same as normal skin elsewhere plus transient flora, especially *Staph. aureus*	**Nose:** *Staph. aureus, Staph. epidermidis*, corynebacteria, *Neisseria* spp., viridans streptococci
Normal skin colonists: *Staph. epidermidis*, corynebacteria	**Stomach:** sterile unless achlorhydric
Moist skin areas: as skin elsewhere (but concentrations are higher) plus *Acinetobacter* spp., coliforms, faecal streptococci, *Clostridium* spp., anaerobic cocci, and *Candida* spp.	**Biliary tract:** sterile, but occasional intestinal flora via ampulla or portal circulation
	Urethra, vagina: *Staph. epidermidis*, 'oral/skin' anaerobes, *Lactobacillus* spp., viridans and other streptococci, *Candida* spp.
	Naso- and oropharynx, mouth, and oesophagus: as nose plus 'oral/skin' non-sporing anaerobes, but without *Staph. aureus*
	Small intestine: 'faecal' anaerobes, coliforms, faecal streptococci, *Candida* spp.
	Large intestine: as small intestine, but much higher concentrations (10^{12} organisms per gram)

disease, and therefore will always justify intervention. Examples include *Myco. tuberculosis, Strep. pyogenes*, and HIV. More commonly, a decision has to be made whether an isolate is significant and, if so, how best to treat it.

3.2 Sources of infection

Introduction

A **source** of infection may be animate or inanimate. **Fomites** are mobile sources, non-human, and usually inanimate (e.g. a hypodermic needle). A **reservoir** of infection is a continuing source where multiplication can occur (such as a contaminated bottle of hand emollient cream, or a septic lesion on the hand of a staff member). Organisms pass to patients and staff via **routes** of infection (such as through the air, or on hands) and gain entry to

the body by way of a **portal** of infection (such as *Neisseria meningitidis* through the upper respiratory tract, or *Staph. aureus* via a surgical wound). Pathogenic microbes may colonize an individual (who then becomes a **carrier**) without causing overt illness, and may thence be passed on to others (by **cross-infection** or **cross-colonization**). **Autoinfection** (or **self-infection**) occurs when an infection is caused by organisms normally colonizing the host.

Hospital-acquired infection

In epidemiological surveys, the term **hospital-acquired** infection (HAI, or **nosocomial** infection) is often restricted to infections that become apparent after a patient has been in hospital for over 48 hours. Before that time they are likely to have been **community-acquired** (CAI). Of course, infections presenting after hospital discharge (especially after short-stay, or day surgery) should usually be considered HAI. An **outbreak** of infection implies clustering in space and time, and usually requires the same species (and type) of organism to have been isolated from two or more patients. **Typing** of organisms refers to any method of classifying microbes below species level.

3.3 Sepsis

Sepsis implies an infective process which may be local (usually implying pus formation) or generalized, although in common usage the term sepsis tends to be used to describe systemic sepsis, while local sepsis is termed infection. **Bacteraemia (fungaemia)** is best defined simply as the isolation of bacteria (fungi) from a blood culture, whereas **septicaemia** (or systemic sepsis) should be reserved as a clinical description implying a febrile, shocked patient who may (but not necessarily) be bacteraemic. The **sepsis syndrome** is now well defined as a constellation of clinical signs including fever, tachycardia, tachypnoea, sustained hypotension, and multiple organ dysfunction (including the adult respiratory distress syndrome, renal and hepatic failure, and confusion).

4 Surgical patients and the microbiological risks they run

4.1 Introduction and infection rates

How large is the problem? Surveys of infection in hospital are either 'snapshots' of the position at one time (**prevalence surveys**) or are longitudinal surveys of infection rates as a percentage of admissions or deaths-and-discharges over a defined period (**incidence surveys**).

Recent prevalence studies of infection in hospitals reveal that about 20 per cent of patients are infected, with about half this proportion having community-acquired infection. A multi-centre study in the UK in 1980 found that UTI was the most common hospital-acquired infection (prevalence about 2.8 per cent), and wound infection (1.7 per cent), lower respiratory infection (1.5 per cent), and skin infection (1.2 per cent) were less frequent. The most common organisms causing HAI were *Esch. coli* (26.1 per cent), *Staph. aureus* (17.6 per cent), *Proteus* spp. (11.2 per cent), *Klebsiella* spp. (7.2 per cent), and *Pseud. aeruginosa* (7.0 per cent). This study was repeated in 1993–94, with surprisingly similar results.

Incidence rates are usually lower than prevalence rates, because infected patients tend to stay in hospital for longer and therefore are more likely to be counted in a prevalence survey. Overall incidence rates of infection of about 5 per cent of hospitalized patients have generally been found.

4.2 How and why are infections established?

Multiple factors determine whether clinically significant infection will develop once bacteria gain access to a site. These include both microbial and host variables. All serious infections evolve through the stages of acquisition, colonization, multiplication, pathogenesis, and dissemination within the host or to other hosts. Organisms are acquired via the airborne route or by direct contact, and immediately come into contact with host defences, which include mechanical, phagocytic, humoral, and

Table 7.3 How surgical procedures compromise local and general defence mechanisms

Adverse effect of procedure	Defences compromised	Notes
Skin incision	Skin barrier	Epithelial keratin; antibacterial fatty acid secretions
Haematoma formation and devascularized areas in wound	Access by opsonins and phagocytes	Complement and immunoglobulins are both important in the formation of abscesses
Splenectomy	General impairment of phagocytosis	Susceptibility to infection with capsulate organisms (pneumococci, meningococci), especially in childhood. Specific immunization and penicillin prophylaxis indicated
Foreign body insertion: arterial grafts, orthopaedic prostheses, meshes	Local impairment of phagocytosis	Organisms attached to prostheses have low metabolic rates within the sheltering biofilm. Here they have shelter from humoral and cellular defences (and to antibiotics)
Tracheal intubation	Mucociliary elevator, cough reflex	Colonizing flora blown into bronchial tree
Urinary catheterization	Urine flow	Ascending infection between catheter and urethral mucosa. Risks of external contamination of catheter bag
Intravenous catheterization, CAPD	Skin	Foreign body plus breach of integument. Prime route of infection is via junctions in infusion system
H_2-blocker use	Gastric acidity	Bacterial overgrowth in stomach, which can be aspirated into the lungs of artificially ventilated patients. *Salmonella* spp. cause particularly severe enteric disease in achlorhydria
Antibiotic use	Normal colonizing flora	Mucosal binding sites exposed, allowing attachment of potentially pathogenic flora. Reduced 'bacterial interference'

cytotoxic systems. Many surgical procedures compromise these local and general defences (Table 7.3).

4.3 Local factors that promote wound infections

Experiments on animals have demonstrated the role of local factors in promoting wound infections. Thus, the inoculum of *Staph. aureus* necessary to initiate infection in skin is reduced by a factor of about 10^3 simply by inserting a subcutaneous non-absorbable suture, which acts as a foreign body. Microbial factors are also important. For example, in the same model, there is a need to inoculate about 10^3 more *Staph. epidermidis* than *Staph. aureus* cells to produce infection.

Pathogenic bacteria release many toxins and other substances to their surroundings, but relatively few can be incriminated in specific pathological processes. Of those that can, obvious examples include cholera toxin's effects on enterocytes, and Gram-negative endotoxin initiating the cascade of mediators leading to septic shock. In contrast with these examples, both *Staph. aureus* and *Staph. epidermidis* strains produce a range of enzymes but none, or no particular combination, correlates clearly with the capability of causing invasive infection.

More is becoming clear, however, about the key bacterial factors involved in initiating the processes of colonization and infection, namely those that promote adhesion to host cells. For example, certain strains of *Staph. aureus* are particularly successful at colonizing the nasal mucosae of volunteers and these prove to be avid binders of mucosal fibronectin.

5   Prevention of surgical infection

It is helpful to discuss minimizing infection in surgical patients under two headings: preventing infection in hospital patients in general, and reducing rates of surgical wound infection.

5.1 General prevention of hospital infection: the control of infection service

All NHS hospitals are now required to designate a consultant as the infection control doctor (ICD), who is directly responsible to the hospital trust board, via the chief executive, for all aspects of infection control within the unit. This direct responsibility allows the ICD, when necessary, to recommend and enforce actions that may be unpopular with clinical colleagues—such as closing a surgical ward during an outbreak. Most ICDs are microbiologists. One or more infection control nurses (ICNs) work with the ICD, and together they form the infection-control team (ICT). Most hospitals have an infection control committee (ICC) with wide representation, usually including a consultant surgeon, which is responsible for strategic issues in infection control, such as setting policies and receiving reports from the ICT.

Controlling infection in hospitals is an important but sometimes thankless task! Recent studies in the USA, however, suggest that a properly constituted and active ICT reduces the risk of HAI by about 30 per cent, and is highly cost-effective. Infection control services always face a problem of image: good infection control does not interfere with the smooth running of clinical departments, and therefore the ICT is not noticed when things are going well. Unfortunately, detection of episodes of HAI often then results in the ICT coming to prominence by their recommendations, which often temporarily restrict freedom of clinical action.

Functions of the ICT and ICC

- Monitoring infection in hospital and community;

- investigating and reacting to proven and potential outbreaks; by advising hospital staff on appropriate practices, isolating patients, and screening staff and patients;

- educating all hospital staff about the control of infection;

- establishing local policies (for example, to cover isolation, antibiotic treatment and prophylaxis, and antiseptics and disinfectants) and auditing their implementation;

- advising on the design, use, and monitoring of various hospital units; these include theatres, wards, and central sterile supply departments (CSSDs).

Typing of organisms

Various typing methods are useful epidemiologically, and are frequently used by the ICT to investigate whether a suspected outbreak involves the same bacterial or viral strain. Some of these methods are based on:

- antibiotic resistance patterns;

- possession of immunologically distinct structures (such as surface polysaccharide 'O' antigens in salmonellae);

- biochemical variations (called **biotyping**; such as patterns of enzyme activity in gonococci);

- patterns of sensitivity to lysis by different bacteriophages (such as staphylococcal phage typing);

- plasmid contents, and gel electrophoresis patterns seen after enzymatic digestion of bacterial DNA;

- amplification of type-specific microbial DNA sequences by the polymerase chain reaction (PCR).

Many of these methods are performed only in research and reference centres, but most laboratories are able to perform basic typing procedures for common pathogens.

Cross-infection

Organisms

Important organisms that regularly cause cross-infection between surgical patients in hospital are *Strep. pyogenes*, *Staph. aureus* (including multiresistant *Staph. aureus*; MRSA), *Clost. difficile*, and multiply resistant coliforms and other Gram-negative organisms. All of these may be spread on staff hands, regardless of any other routes that are sometimes important.

Handwashing between each patient contact is therefore the single most effective infection control measure. Hands may be transiently contaminated from carriage sites on the staff member (such as *Staph. aureus* from the nose), or organisms acquired while performing clinical procedures on patients or with contaminated equipment.

Other microbes that are worthy of special note include *Myco. tuberculosis*, hepatitis B virus, and HIV. The first is spread via the airborne route, and the viruses by direct inoculation of blood or other body fluids.

Strep. pyogenes may colonize the upper respiratory tract or minor skin lesions of patients and staff who may have no obvious signs of infection, or only intermittent signs. *Strep. pyogenes* is readily transmissible by direct contact or via the air. Cases or carriers require 10 days of effective therapy for reliable clearance (with a penicillin or macrolide), and 'standard' isolation for the first 2–5 days is normally required for patients in hospital.

Results of surveys vary, but probably about half of all sporadic *Staph. aureus* surgical wound infections are acquired during the operation by aerial spread from normal carriage by theatre staff members. The remainder are from carriage by the patients themselves. In addition, outbreaks of surgical wound infection can occasionally be traced to chronic carriage of particularly virulent strains of *Staph. aureus* by a member of theatre staff.

MRSA strains are no more likely to cause clinical infections than methicillin-sensitive strains of *Staph. aureus*, but some MRSA appear to be well adapted to spread among patients and staff, and all are awkard to treat and eradicate. Control becomes expensive and virtually impossible once many patients and staff have become colonized and infected, and many hospitals abroad and some in the UK have given up the struggle. Once MRSA is endemic in a unit, overall infection rates rise, and vancomycin and teicoplanin usage becomes an expensive necessity. MRSA strains that are clinically partially resistant to vancomycin ('VISA' strains) have been reported mainly in Japan, and it is to be hoped that a number of currently investigational antibiotics will prove useful for treating such infections. Mupirocin rapidly clears staphylococcal carriage from the nose, and treated colonized staff can return to work after 24–48 hours' therapy if they do not have colonized skin lesions. Repeated screening is required before anyone who has carried MRSA in a wound or other abnormal area can be considered clear, and some patients are impossible to clear.

New broad-spectrum antibiotics have partially solved the problems of cross-infection with multiply resistant Gram-negative organisms, such as gentamicin-resistant *Klebsiella* spp. that were common in urological and intensive care wards in the 1970s and early 1980s. It is now rare to have no rational choice of antibiotic therapy for Gram-negative bacteria. Control of hand-borne bacterial spread remains of prime importance, but antibiotic restriction, attention to disinfection of 'wet' medical apparatus such as ventilator humidifiers, and institution of closed urinary drainage are also required. Recently, more frequent resistance to new agents has begun to appear (to 'second-' and 'third-generation' cephalosporins in *Enterobacter*

spp. *Acinetobacter* spp., and *Klebsiella* spp. and to quinolones in *Klebsiella* and *Pseudomonas* spp.) so vigilance is still required.

Antibiotic-associated diarrhoea

Clost. difficile produces at least two toxins that damage colonic epithelium to cause 'antibiotic-associated diarrhoea' and 'pseudomembranous colitis'. Carriage in normal individuals is rare, but it survives (probably as spores) in the hospital environment around patients with *Clost. difficile* associated diarrhoea, and it can be transmitted between patients on hands and via unsterile equipment, such as sigmoidoscopes. Once established as a bowel colonist, overgrowth can occur in patients given almost any antibiotic that achieves antimicrobial concentrations sufficient to 'unbalance' the colonic flora. The relative risk of diarrhoea appears greatest with cephalosporins of the second and third generations. Management includes stopping all existing antibiotic treatment, 5–7 days of oral metronidazole or vancomycin therapy, and isolation of the patient. Relapse occurs in up to 25 per cent.

Isolation

Physical separation of patients to prevent transmission of infectious agents has been practised since the time of Florence Nightingale. Details of methods vary, but most centres distinguish between **source** isolation (that is, isolation of a patient known or suspected to be carrying or infected with a transmissible pathogen) and **protective** isolation (separation of an uninfected but particularly susceptible patient from contact with opportunist pathogens in food, air, or carried by staff or other patients). Full protective isolation is only justified for a very few patient categories, such as the profoundly neutropenic. Isolating patients may also isolate them from clinical care, and ward routines will be disrupted, so isolation must only be used when it is clearly justified. In most hospitals the infection control doctor has authority over isolation facilities.

Several categories of source isolation can be identified, and Table 7.4 describes those that are commonly used.

5.2 Prevention of surgical wound infection

Introduction

Microbiologists and surgeons are not always in agreement about what constitutes a wound infection, and there are almost as many definitions as there are surgeons operating. Because of this variation, comparisons between published series need care, and practicable and unambiguous definitions should be agreed before research studies or audits are started. The most appropriate definition will depend upon the type of operation performed and may be linked to the method of surveillance used, but the following are useful guidelines:

Definitions of wound infection

A **wound infection** is a clinical event, of significance in the management of the patient and requiring local or systemic treatment. Purulent discharge is a cardinal sign, and it is not

Table 7.4 Modes of isolation for infection

Type of isolation	Relevant organisms	Characteristics
'Standard'	Air- and hand-borne pathogens (e.g. MRSA, *Strep. pyogenes*, *Herpes zoster*, tuberculosis)	Single room with lower air pressure than ward and dedicated lavatory and washing facilities. Door closed. Gloves and plastic apron worn inside room (consider mask), discarded before exit and hands washed. Linen and waste separately bagged for disposal/washing. Wash horizontal surfaces in room after patient discharged
'Enteric'	Hand-borne pathogens (e.g. *Salmonella* spp., undiagnosed diarrhoea, multiply resistant Gram-negative bacteria)	Single room with dedicated lavatory and washing facilities. Gloves and plastic apron worn when touching patient, discarded before exit and hands washed. Linen and waste separately bagged for disposal/washing. Wash horizontal surfaces in room with detergent/disinfectant after patient discharged
'Strict'	Especially virulent pathogens (e.g. Lassa fever, rabies)	Transfer patient to specialist isolation unit

The 'enteric' category is sometimes extended to include blood-borne organisms spread by direct inoculation (such as HIV and hepatitis B virus) and is then called 'excretion/secretion/blood' isolation. Patients carrying these viruses should be nursed out of isolation unless they are especially likely to bleed, or have other infections, such as tuberculosis.

necessary (but may be helpful) for a positive culture to be obtained.

Thus, an unequivocally 'infected' wound discharges macroscopic pus; a non-purulent wound with serous discharge or 1.5 cm surrounding inflammation is best classified as 'probably infected', to become 'infected' if culture of a swab reveals a significant pathogen that responds to an appropriate antibiotic. Other, more sophisticated schemes have been devised, such as the 'ASEPSIS' score (calculated by summing a variety of individually minor characteristics, such as presence of serous discharge and low-grade fever). This approach needs intensive surveillance, and presupposes that the underlying causes of minor and major wound problems are the same. However, such scores have been shown to be consistent between different observers.

An **operative wound** includes the parietal incision itself, and any internal site of operative manipulation. Thus, empyemas occurring after pulmonary lobectomies should be classified in the same group as any parietal wound infections, but any pneumonias after colonic resection should not. This distinction is particularly important when comparing the relative efficacy of prophylactic antibiotic regimens.

Classification of wounds

Once satisfactory definitions are established, the next important factor is wound classification, shown in Table 7.5. Infection rates in the clean-contaminated, contaminated, and infected groups vary considerably between different departments and operators, but a clean wound infection rate of less than 2 per cent should be the goal of every surgeon. Several studies have shown that the most reproducible results are obtained when independent trained observers assess wounds prospectively by regular inspection. This is usually too time-consuming for regular audit purposes, but is the gold standard for published research studies.

Preoperative, peroperative, or postoperative wound infection (and how to tell)

Although it was fashionable in the past to blame ward dressing procedures and other late events for many postoperative wound

Table 7.5 Classification of wounds (infection rates used are those reported by Cruse and Foord, 1980)

Category	Description (examples)	Rate
Clean	No incision through microbially colonized viscus, no infection encountered, and no break in aseptic technique (herniorrhaphy, resection of lipoma, total hip replacement)	1.5%
Clean-contaminated	Microbially colonized viscus entered in controlled manner (elective sigmoid colectomy or cholecystectomy, vaginal hysterectomy)	7.7%
Contaminated	Microbially colonized viscus entered with incomplete preparation, spillage, break in aseptic technique, or in the presence of inflammation (emergency cholecystectomy or sigmoid colectomy with defunctioning colostomy). Also, traumatic wounds less than 4 hours old	15.2%
Infected or dirty	Pus or perforated viscus encountered at operation, or traumatic wound over 4 hours old	40.0%

infections, the great majority are now recognized to have become established in the theatre. Delayed presentation is not an infallible guide to a postoperative origin; for example, in a multicentre study of hip and knee replacement infections, cases of *Staph. aureus* sepsis presenting up to 16 months after operation were shown probably to have been implanted in theatre.

Of course, organisms acquired by the patient via cross-infection on the ward preoperatively ('cross-colonization') may be implanted in the wound in theatre, and these give the appearance of a postoperative origin. Preoperative colonization may partly explain the common observation that the longer a patient spends in hospital before operation, the higher is the risk of wound and other infection. Recent studies have documented the rapid acquisition of resistant 'commensal' organisms by patients; for example, multiply resistant strains of coagulase-negative staphylococci appear on the skin of patients preoperatively in cardiothoracic units. These are further selected by antibiotic prophylaxis, and some go on to cause prosthetic valve endocarditis.

Most undrained, non-oozing surgical wounds seal and become quite resistant to exogenous infection within hours. Suction drains inserted via separate stab incisions seem not to predispose to postoperative infection (and certainly reduce its incidence when fluid collections are present). However, particular care is needed when certain types of wound are dressed. For example, suction generated by breathing and the heart beat may draw contaminated material in to a median sternotomy incision, and several outbreaks of sternal wound infection with Gram-negative rods have been traced to unsterile cleansing of the days-old incision.

5.3 Reducing the risks of wound infection

Wound infection may be avoided by reducing the inoculum of organisms introduced into the wound and by reducing the chances that organisms implanted will survive and multiply.

Reducing the inoculum

Sterilization, asepsis, and disposable equipment

Bacteria reach surgical wounds by direct contact with skin (of staff or the patient) or contaminated equipment, and via the air from these sites and from environmental dirt. Numerous procedures have been designed to clear these sources and interrupt these routes. **Sterilization** implies the total removal or killing of all microbes contaminating an article (such as by autoclaving a tray of instruments), but **disinfection** is best defined as rendering an article sufficiently microbially safe for its intended purpose. In practice, this usually means that living, vegetative forms of bacteria are killed, but that bacterial spores are not. For example, exposure of a cystoscope to low-temperature steam is satisfactory because spore-forming bacteria do not cause urinary infection, but an arthroscope must be sterile because spores are significant in tissue infection.

Asepsis (or **aseptic technique**) involves all the practical measures taken to avoid ingress of microbes to a susceptible site (such as instrument sterilization, theatre ventilation, and no-touch technique), or to kill or remove them from that site (such as skin antisepsis and wound cleansing). A **sterilant** is a liquid or gas that can sterilize under appropriate conditions, and a **disinfectant** is a fluid that can disinfect. An **antiseptic** is a disinfectant that can be used on living tissue.

Table 7.6 Some methods of sterilization

Process	Examples	Notes
Autoclaving	Metal theatre instruments	Steam under pressure in porous load. Machines must comply with Department of Health HTM10 regulations. 121° C for 15 minutes at 15 psi and 134° C for 3 minutes at 30 psi are common combinations. Extra time is needed for heating, 'safety time', and cooling. Vacuum cycle autoclaves ensure evacuation of air and exposure to pure steam
Hot-air oven	Ophthalmic instruments	e.g. 180° C for 30 minutes. Preferred for some instruments with delicate edges
Ethylene oxide	Plastic catheters, sutures during manufacture	Toxic gas used in chamber with controlled humidity. Penetrates many plastics. 'Airing' time needed after each cycle
Ionizing radiation		Commercial process, usually irradiation
Glutaraldehyde (some new alternatives are coming onto the market that may prove as effective and safer, e.g. Dexit and Nu-Cidex)	Urological instruments	Liquid used is buffered at 2–2.5% concentration. Use within expiry date. Sterilization needs 3 hours (UK regulations) followed by rinsing. Useful for certain delicate equipment, but glutaraldehyde usage should be avoided whenever possible because of toxicity and expense
Low-temperature steam plus formaldehyde	Sigmoidoscopes	70–80° C at reduced pressure with steam inside chamber. Sometimes problems of polymerization of formaldehyde inside instruments

A number of novel physical processes (e.g. gas plasma sterilization) are employed by some equipment new to the market; experience is limited with these methods, and local CSSD and microbiology staff should be consulted before they are considered for purchase.

Reusable surgical equipment for use in sterile body sites should be sterilized between uses, and this is best performed in a hospital **central sterile supply department** (CSSD). Here, proper control of decontamination, packing, sterilization, and storage can be assured, although the delays inherent in transport to and from the CSSD may require the purchase of extra sets of equipment. Recent requirements of the UK Medical Devices Agency may mandate that the majority of surgical instruments are either disposable or are cleaned and sterilized in CSSDs where a full audit trail may be maintained. Table 7.6 summarizes the features of important methods of sterilization, Table 7.7 lists the properties of some methods of disinfection, and Table 7.8 describes some important antiseptics. For disinfecting or sterilizing equipment, processes involving wet heat in an autoclave are generally preferred because these are usually cheapest, safest, and the most thorough and easily controlled. Details of construction of the articles to be sterilized and disinfected may dictate that other methods be used. Before specifying or purchasing new types of surgical equipment it is important to seek the advice of the ICD and CSSD manager about suitable decontamination procedures.

Disinfection and antisepsis in general

The reliability and speed of most disinfecting processes are improved by prior cleaning, and many chemical disinfectants are inactivated by organic materials.

Using mixtures of agents

Antiseptic and disinfectant cocktail mixtures should generally be avoided because many combinations mutually inactivate. Useful alliances include:

◆ adding alcohol to chlorhexidine or povidone-iodine to reduce the risks of contamination and possibly improve bactericidal and virucidal activity;

◆ adding cetrimide to aqueous chlorhexidine (Savlon®) to improve cleansing properties—useful in management of traumatic wounds.

Multiple-use containers are liable to contamination each time they are topped up, therefore antiseptics should be supplied at working concentrations in small, single-use containers with attached dispensers if needed.

Table 7.7 Some methods of disinfection

Process	Examples	Notes
Low-temperature steam	Rigid cystoscopes	About 73 °C at reduced pressure for 10 minutes
Hypochlorite	Blood spills	Cheap, but corrosive for metals. Otherwise best used at 10^4 p.p.m. available chlorine for blood spills, and 10^3 p.p.m. for surfaces
Phenolics (e.g. Clearsol)	Faecal spills	Cheap. Little inactivation by organic substances. Can be mixed with neutral detergents
Glutaraldehyde, or peracetic acid	Bronchoscopes	Four minutes before and after each use, providing the instrument is clean. Increased to 60 minutes if HBV or mycobacteria likely, or the patient is immunosuppressed
Alcohols	Some small, delicate articles	Wiping injection ports (see Table 7.8). Other antiseptics best reserved for use on skin

Table 7.8 Properties of some commonly used antiseptics

Antiseptic	Notes
Alcohols (ethyl, methyl, isopropyl)	Broad spectrum, flammable, moderately expensive. Most active against bacteria at 70% concentration
Chlorhexidine	Good activity against Gram-positive bacteria, but only moderate against Gram-negatives. Persistent action, moderately expensive, non-toxic
Povidone-iodine	Broad spectrum, moderately expensive, some hypersensitivity and local tissue toxicity. Rapidly inactivated by blood and tissue fluid
Chlorinated lime and boric acid (EUSOL)	Broad spectrum, moderately expensive, considerable tissue toxicity
Sodium hypochlorite solution	Broad spectrum, cheap, locally toxic
Hexachlorophene	Cumulative action against Gram-positive bacteria. Systemically toxic for neonates. Moderately expensive
Triclosan	Similar to hexachlorophane, but less toxic
Quaternary ammonium compounds (cetrimide in Savlon)	Weak Gram-negative activity, readily contaminated by pseudomonads. Detergent action, cheap, non-toxic
Hydrogen peroxide	Slow and weak bactericidal activity, cheap and spectacular

Avoiding infection in theatre

Skin antisepsis

Human skin carries a **long-term commensal flora** on its surface and within sweat glands and follicles. In all areas this consists of coagulase-negative staphylococci and diphtheroids. In moist sites the flora is more diverse and includes Gram-negative organisms, yeasts, and occasionally *Staph. aureus*. Skin that comes in to contact with the outside world (principally the hands) acquires a varied **transient surface flora**. Transients may progress to deeper, prolonged colonization if the skin is damaged, especially with eczema. Some bacterial strains survive longer on skin than others.

Skin commensals only become major pathogens in prosthetic implant infection. Staff may acquire significant numbers of transients on their hands by touching colonized patients, contaminated areas of the environment, or heavily colonized areas of their own body (such as *Staph. aureus* from the anterior nares). Large numbers of transients can be exchanged even during quite minor procedures, such as taking temperatures or blood pressures. Surgical incisions that pass through or near heavily contaminated areas of the body (axillae, umbilicus, groins, perineum) are especially prone to contamination, and preoperative skin antisepsis of these areas should be especially thorough.

Different requirements apply to skin disinfection for the operative team and for the patient.

Operating team

Hand antisepsis for the surgeon should be rapid, and able to be repeated many times per day without skin damage. Ideally the agent chosen should have a prolonged action, to suppress regrowth of commensals and multiplication of organisms that have penetrated holed gloves.

All transient organisms, and a large proportion of the resident flora, are removed by a 2-minute wash with a suitable antiseptic. Chlorhexidine gluconate 4 per cent with surfactant (Hibiscrub®, ICI), or povidone-iodine 7.5 per cent with surfactant (Betadine® surgical scrub, Napp) probably offer the best balance of properties, with chlorhexidine giving more prolonged anti-bacterial action and less skin sensitization. The word 'scrub' is a misnomer; scrubbing brushes damage the epidermis and should only be used (if at all) to clean under the nails.

Patient

In most routine surgery a single, thorough antiseptic application is adequate. Alcoholic chlorhexidine or alcoholic povidone-iodine are most often used—povidone-iodine is easily seen on the skin, but causes more hypersensitivity reactions, has less persistent activity, and is rapidly inactivated by blood. Rubbing 70 per cent alcohol to dryness with the gloved hand is equally effective and cheaper. Care is needed to avoid pooling of alcoholic agents if electrocoagulation is used, but aqueous antiseptics are slower to act, prone to contamination and, paradoxically, often more expensive. Aqueous agents are necessary for use on mucous membranes, and the same antiseptic in alcoholic solution should be used on the adjacent skin.

Before critically clean (especially prosthetic vascular) operations, additional preoperative antiseptics can be applied on the ward to the area of the planned incision and sites of heavy bacterial colonization. This procedure (sometimes called 'whole body disinfection') has been shown to reduce contamination of the wound during the operation, but it has given variable results

Table 7.9 Equipment for reducing wound contamination in theatre

Value	Equipment	Comment
Proven effective	Ultraclean, laminar-flow air supply	Only use is orthopaedic prosthetic surgery. Gives a small additive effect to antibiotic prophylaxis. Very expensive
Unproven but rational	Normal plenum-filtered air supply	Dilution effect on airborne organisms
	Gloves	Frequently holed, but they reduce transmission of organisms to patient. Double-gloving reduces blood access to surgeon's skin in 'high-risk' cases
	Masks	Deflect forceful expirations that carry bacteria. Recently proven to reduce airborne contamination, but no evidence of improved wound infection rates. Skin squames may be rubbed off the face by a mask
	Caps, hoods	Restrain long hair, but little evidence airborne spread reduced. May rub off squames
	Gowns	Limit contact spread when dry, but only Ventile (and similar) gowns reduce skin squame dissemination
Dubious or proven ineffective	Adhesive plastic wound drapes	Hold towels in place, but bacteria multiply beneath
	Sticky floor mats	Exchange dirt between passing feet and wheels
	Plastic overshoes	No evidence wound infection reduced. Hands contaminated as they are put on
	Separate, designated theatre trolleys	Organism counts in theatres not reduced

when clean and prosthetic surgical infections have been assessed prospectively. To avoid inactivation, the same antiseptic should be applied in aqueous solution on the ward and in alcohol in the theatre.

Depilation may produce an aesthetically satisfying operative field, but razor shaving has been repeatedly shown to increase postoperative sepsis rates in many types of surgery. Use of electric clippers gives an intermediate risk, but the only entirely microbiologically safe method of hair removal appears to be by use of depilatory creams. Delays of more than 12 hours between depilation and incision further increase the risk; rapid bacterial colonization of the razor-damaged epidermis presumably increases the number of organisms inoculated to the wound during the operation.

Theatre procedures for reducing wound infection rates

Many ingenious pieces of equipment have been introduced in an effort to reduce microbial exposure of the surgical wound (Table 7.9). Most of these are designed to prevent exogenous contamination, many are expensive, and very few have been proved to be effective. Patients with large numbers of organisms present on the skin surface at the time of incision have been shown to have a significantly higher count in the wound before closure, and the use of plastic adhesive wound drapes only reduces these by a maximum of one-third. Bacterial multiplication occurs in the moist conditions under adhesive drapes, therefore they may be useful to hold other drapes and equipment in position, but are not justifiable microbiologically. Surprisingly, although glove punctures are common (between 11 and 47 per cent of gloves per operation) and under experimental conditions thousands of skin commensals pass through a punctured glove, very few organisms from the operating team's skin can be detected in the wound. In support of this, Cruse and Foord (1980) found that punctured gloves were not associated with an increased rate of postoperative infections.

Sources of organisms in theatre

Most organisms in theatre air come from the skin of staff and patients, therefore staff numbers present during operations should be kept to the minimum, they should move around as little as possible, and anyone with a septic lesion or sore throat should be firmly excluded. Outdoor clothing carries and disseminates more organisms than clean theatre wear, hence theatre clothing should not be worn outside the theatre area, except in an emergency. Trouser cuffs should be elasticated or tucked into boots.

Reducing bacterial survival

General measures

A number of operative procedures may reduce wound infection rates by encouraging normal tissue defences to destroy implanted bacteria. Closing 'dead spaces', controlling haemorrhage, using drains when indicated, and avoiding leaving devascularized or damaged tissues are obvious, but excessive use of suture material or diathermy to control bleeding points have also been clearly linked to an increased risk of infection.

Principles of antibiotic prophylaxis

Antibiotics are commonly used prophylactically in surgery, with the aim of preventing multiplication of pathogenic microbes introduced to a susceptible area.

In surgical practice, prophylaxis should involve high-dose antibiotic administration just before the period of exposure (i.e. with the anaesthetic), with maintenance of effective concen-

Table 7.10 Some indications for prophylaxis in surgery

Procedures	Common pathogens	Suggested prophylaxis (alternative agents, commonly used)
Uncomplicated appendicectomy, vaginal hysterectomy	Local anaerobic normal flora	Metronidazole, IV or PR
Elective colorectal, gastric or oesophageal malignancy, emergency gastric	Non-sporing anaerobes, coliforms, streptococci	Benzylpenicillin (BP) + gentamicin + metronidazole (cefotaxime + metronidazole) (see Song and Glenny, 1998)
Perforated abdominal viscus	Non-sporing anaerobes, coliforms, streptococci (as above)	BP + gentamicin + metronidazole (cefotaxime + metronidazole) These combinations may be continued for treatment
Biliary tract, elective gastric	Coliforms, streptococci (staphylococci)	BP + gentamicin (cefotaxime)
Open-heart, prosthetic vascular, neurosurgery, renal transplantation	Staphylococci	Flucloxacillin + gentamicin (cefotaxime or vancomycin)
Prosthetic joint (and most other prosthetic implants)	Staphylococci	Flucloxacillin (vancomycin)
Amputation of ischaemic leg	Clost. welchii	Penicillin (metronidazole)
TURP, lithotripsy, ERCP, and other instrumentation (prophylaxis against septic shock, and infective endocarditis in those with damaged heart valves)	Coliforms, faecal streptococci	BP + gentamicin (but note prior urine culture and sensitivity results if available)

trations throughout the procedure and for a short period after. Single-dose prophylaxis has usually been shown to be just as effective as longer courses. Prophylaxis is readily justified in procedures that commonly lead to infection (such as in colonic surgery), and is rational in those where infection is rare but catastrophic (such as in aortofemoral bypass surgery using a prosthesis) (Table 7.10). Before making a choice of regimen, it is important to define the common causative pathogens by prospective observation, and (ideally) prophylactic efficacy should be assessed by blinded, placebo-controlled or comparative trial. Proof of effectiveness is much more difficult to obtain when postoperative infection is rare, but high-quality meta-analyses of multiple small trials have recently shown the effectiveness of perioperative prophylaxis for colorectal surgery and implantation of orthopaedic prostheses (see Song and Glenny, 1998; Gillespie and Walenkomp, 1998).

Intravenous administration of prophylactic antibiotics is usually indicated in hospital, but oral agents are more convenient for minor procedures in the community. For most surgical indications it is relatively easy to define the risk period, which is usually a matter of minutes or hours, hence the duration of prophylaxis need only be brief. Short courses reduce drug costs, avoid side-effects, and limit the exposure of the patient's normal microbial flora to antibiotics. Increasingly, single-dose prophylaxis is becoming the accepted standard. Additional doses of agents with a short half-life may need to be given during long operations.

Improvement in prophylactic antibiotic usage is necessary because audit in the UK shows that 30–40 per cent of all prescriptions are for prophylaxis rather than treatment, and 50 per cent of these courses are given for longer than 48 hours. Prophylaxis carries (inevitable) disadvantages and risks: hypersensitivity and adverse drug reactions; drug and administration costs; and promotion of resistance. These need to be outweighed by the (only potential) advantages. Prophylaxis can never be a substitute for good surgical, aseptic, and antiseptic technique.

6 Treatment of infection

Effective treatment of established infection requires:

◆ re-establishment and reinforcement of host defences (such as the drainage of abscesses, removal of foreign bodies, maintenance of nutritional status, and the recovery of the neutrophil count by reducing immunosuppressive drugs);

◆ the use of antibiotics and antiseptics;

◆ in the future, use of agents such as anti-TNF antibodies to modify the systemic sepsis response may become established.

6.1 Antibiotics

Introduction

Strictly defined, an **antibiotic** is 'a substance produced by one micro-organism that kills or inhibits the growth of another micro-organism in high dilution'. This excludes metal ions, phenols, alcohols, acids, peroxides, and similar non-specific toxins. In practice, most antibiotics used today are partially or completely man-made, and are probably better called 'antimicrobial agents'.

Selective toxicity against microbial but not human cells is the object of antibiotic usage, and most agents are therefore targeted at structures or metabolic pathways unique to bacteria, such as the cell wall and membrane, or protein synthesis and DNA replication. Sensitivity tests and antibiotic 'activity' can be measured in many ways *in vitro* in the laboratory (Table 7.11), but the results are sometimes not closely related to how an antibiotic will perform in human patients. Important patient-related variables include changing antibiotic concentrations with time, serum protein binding, access to privileged sites (such as across the blood–brain barrier), penetration to abscesses, interaction with the immune and phagocytic systems, and the presence of foreign bodies. It is therefore not surprising that

Table 7.11 Laboratory measures of antibiotic sensitivity and activity

Test (time needed after specimen arrival to produce result)	Notes
Disc diffusion sensitivity (24–48 hours)	Zone of inhibition around antibiotic-impregnated paper disc after overnight incubation, compared with that of a standard organism
Breakpoint sensitivity (24–48 hours)	Growth, or not, of a spot inoculum on agar containing known concentrations of antibiotic
Minimum inhibitory concentration, MIC (48–72 hours)	Least concentration of antibiotic that prevents bacterial growth. Performed in broth or on solid agar media. Controlled by comparison with known organisms
Minimum bactericidal concentration, MBC (72–96 hours or more)	Least concentration of antibiotic that kills 99.9% of bacterial inoculum. Usually done by subculturing the broth media that were used in MIC determination onto solid agar
Serum bactericidal titre 'serum-versus-organism' (48 hours)	Highest dilution of patient's serum (containing the treatment antibiotic) that prevents growth, or kills, a known inoculum of the organism causing the infection. Wide variations in technique and interpretation in different laboratories

Table 7.12 Simple penicillins

Agent	Characteristics
Benzylpenicillin	Cheap, parenteral only. Short half-life, therefore give 2–4 hourly for serious infections. Large doses can be given (e.g. in meningitis or *Strep. pyogenes* cellulitis up to 24 megaunits/day)
Penicillin V	Cheap, oral only. Sometimes poor absorption in adults
Procaine penicillin (and others). Depot preparations	IM administration for prolonged therapeutic levels
Ampicillin, amoxicillin, other esters	Amoxicillin is better absorbed by mouth than penicillin V or ampicillin

All achieve good urinary and biliary levels.

Table 7.13 Targeted and broad-spectrum penicillins

Agent	Characteristics
(Flu)cloxacillin	Resistant to staphylococcal beta-lactamases. Usually satisfactory alone for mixed staphlococcal/streptococcal sepsis
Augmentin® (co-amoxyclar	Amoxicillin combined with clavulanic acid (an inhibitor of many beta-lactamases). Adds many staphylococci, coliforms, *Bacteroides* spp. and haemophili to amoxicillin's spectrum. More likely to cause diarrhoea than amoxicillin
Piperacillin-kazobactam	Piperacillin combined with an inhibitor of many beta-lactamases. Adds pseudomonads and other Gram-negative bacteria to co-amoxyclav's spectrum.
Imipenem-cilastatin, meropenem	Active against all organisms except some faecal streptococci and pseudomonads.

patients' responses occasionally confound the predictions of the microbiology department.

Antibiotics that kill bacteria *in vitro* are termed 'bactericidal' agents and those that just inhibit their growth 'bacteriostatic', but this distinction is not always maintained *in vivo* and is not very important when choosing optimal therapy.

A practical guide to some available antibiotics

Within each group of antibiotics, many variants are available that differ usually only slightly in spectrum or pharmacological properties. In any one hospital only one or two of each group need be generally available. There still remain many indications for well-established agents such as benzylpenicillin and gentamicin, which have predictable side-effects and are cheap (see Table 7.12). New antibiotics are enthusiastically promoted by commercial interests, but are expensive and rarely shown to be superior for common indications. They should be reserved whenever possible for specific and uncommon problems.

Beta-lactams include penicillins, cephalosporins, monobactams and their relatives, all of which contain the **beta-lactam ring nucleus** with varied side-chains and rings. All interfere with cell-wall production by inhibiting enzymes called **penicillin-binding proteins** (PBPs). Bacterial resistance may result from:

◆ production of beta-lactamase **enzymes** that hydrolyse the beta-lactam ring (e.g. *Staphylococcus* spp.) or bind the antibiotic molecule (e.g. *Enterobacter* spp.);

◆ alteration of penicillin-binding protein to reduce antibiotic binding (e.g. methicillin-resistant *Staph. aureus*);

◆ exclusion of the beta-lactam from the organism by alterations to permeability of the outer membrane (e.g. *Pseud. aeruginosa*).

Hypersensitivity is the only common beta-lactam side-effect. Maculopapular rash and fever are more often seen with ampicillin/amoxicillin. Anaphylaxis to the beta-lactam ring is rare, and cross-allergy between penicillins and cephalosporins occurs in less than 10 per cent of patients (probably in about 1 per cent). Many patients' claims of being allergic to penicillins

are not correct, and careful trial of therapy may be worthwhile for infections when a beta-lactam is clearly indicated.

Simple penicillins

A summary of the simple penicillins is given in Table 7.12. **Sensitive bacteria** include most streptococci (*Strep. pyogenes*, *Strep. pneumoniae*, viridans group), *Clostridia*, *Neisseria*, treponemes. Lancefield group B streptococci and faecal streptococci are less sensitive, and combination with gentamicin is indicated for severe infections with these organisms. Resistance is increasing in many *Bacteroides* spp. and other anaerobes, and enterococci. Ampicillin/amoxicillin is still active against 75–85 per cent of haemophili, but in UK hospital practice about 90 per cent of coliforms and *Staph. aureus* are now resistant.

Table 7.14 Varieties of cephalosporins

Agent	Characteristics
'Oral' cephalosporins (e.g. cefalexin, cefradine, cefadroxil)	Broader anti-Gram-negative and antistaphylococcal spectrum than ampicillin because they are more beta-lactamase stable. Useful for UTI, but generally achieve low tissue levels and not usually adequate substitutes for parenteral cephalosporins once a patient has recovered enough for oral treatment
'Gram-negative' cephalosporins (e.g. cefuroxime, cefotaxime, ceftriaxone)	Parenteral, expensive. Usefully very broad Gram-negative spectrum, retaining adequate antistaphylococcal activity. Penetrate CSF. High incidence of *Clost. difficile* diarrhoea
'Extended spectrum' cephalosporins (e.g. ceftazidime, cefpirome)	As above, but ceftazidime adds good antipseudomonal activity, and cefpirome is active against many enterococci and enterobacters

Targeted and broad-spectrum penicillins

These agents and combinations are usually more expensive than standard penicillins, but are useful for particular indications (Table 7.13).

Cephalosporins

Classification of these antibiotics into 'generations' is popular, but not a reliable guide to their spectra of activity or uses. New agents appear regularly; for example, the latest to appear have 'extended' spectra and are available orally (Table 7.14). All currently available examples are inactive against enterococci and *Listeria monocytogenes*, and almost all have poor activity against *Pseudomonas* and *Bacteroides* spp. *Enterobacter* spp. and their relatives tend to become resistant during therapy.

Monobactams

These are new class of agent, with monocyclic beta-lactam rings. Aztreonam has been available for the longest; this is an expensive parenteral agent with a broad anti-Gram-negative spectrum, but no activity against Gram-positive or anaerobic organisms. Care is therefore needed in its use because most surgical infections may involve one or both of these sorts of bacteria. In addition, aztreonam may be safe to use in most patients who are hypersensitive to penicillins and cephalosporins.

Aminoglycosides

Aminoglycosides are parenteral, oral, or topical agents, with a narrow therapeutic index (a small range between therapeutic and toxic serum concentrations). Important predictable adverse reactions include renal failure (usually reversible) and ototoxicity (primarily to the vestibular component of VIII). Major dosage modification is necessary in the young and elderly, in small and large patients, and in those with impaired renal function. In these groups, regular serum assay (at least twice weekly) is required. Courses should be kept as short as possible consistent with good efficacy. Despite these warnings, aminoglycosides are extremely valuable agents for prophylaxis and for treatment of serious infections (Table 7.15), and they have not been supplanted by recent developments in other groups. Aminoglycosides are particularly useful for single-dose or short-course prophylaxis because serum assay is not needed.

Aminoglycosides have no useful activity against anaerobes or haemophili, and should not be used alone against staphylococci or streptococci. These drugs interfere with bacterial protein synthesis at the ribosomal level. Resistance may be mediated by production of inactivating enzymes, alteration of the ribosome binding site, or by exclusion of the antibiotic by the cell membrane.

Monitoring aminoglycoside treatment

The therapeutic index of aminoglycosides is very low and the pharmacokinetics of the drugs vary widely between patients (i.e. tissue distribution and renal handling). Half-life for the same drug in different patients—even with normal renal function—may vary from 30 minutes to 8 hours. This makes accurate prediction of the required doses difficult and reinforces the need for careful monitoring in order to maintain therapeutic levels and at the same time avoid toxic effects.

The drugs are excreted almost completely unchanged by the kidney. This has two implications: first, septic patients are likely to have impaired renal function and are therefore likely to reach toxic levels rapidly, but may have greatest need of the drugs; secondly, the drugs are nephrotoxic (usually reversible) with the result that they may impair their own clearance from the body. This may result in irreversible ototoxicity.

The doses of these drugs have very little relationship with their therapeutic effect, but there is a predictable relationship between the serum concentration and the therapeutic effect. In practice, effective serum concentrations have been calculated by observing their therapeutic clinical effects. For gentamicin used on a twice- or thrice-daily regimen, a peak serum concentration of 5 μg/ml or more is recommended 15 minutes after intravenous infusion or 1 hour after an intramuscular dose. To prevent ototoxicity the peak level should not exceed 10 g/ml and the trough level (just before the next dose) should not exceed 2 g/ml. Once-daily dosing regimens are becoming popular, but effective and practicable dosing and assay guidelines are yet to be fully established. Frusemide (furosemide) is also ototoxic and should be avoided in combination with aminoglycosides. Bumetanide is a suitable substitute if a loop diuretic is needed.

After a week of treatment, aminoglycoside tissue levels often begin to rise without corresponding rises in serum levels. Thus, if long-term treatment is required, special care is needed (for example, in the treatment of osteomyelitis, infective endocarditis, or an infected arterial graft).

Patients with normal renal function usually start with a loading dose of 120 mg gentamicin then continue an initial maintenance dose of 80 mg three times daily. After 24 hours two blood samples should be taken, one just before the next dose and one 15 minutes (IV) or 1 hour (IM) after the next dose. The levels from these are used to calculate both future doses and frequency. For details of once-daily treatment and monitoring, readers are referred to the latest edition of the *British National Formulary*.

Table 7.15 Aminoglycoside antibiotics

Agent	Characteristics
Gentamicin, netilmicin, tobramycin (note spelling!)	Minor differences in spectrum of activity and likelihood of side-effects. Useful for serious Gram-negative infection. Used in combination with beta-lactams for staphylococcal sepsis and streptococcal endocarditis
Amikacin	Expensive, but stable to some aminoglycoside resistance mechanisms; therefore useful as a reserve agent
Neomycin, framycetin	Topical (ear drops, Naseptin® nasal cream) and oral use ('bowel decontamination', hepatic failure)
Streptomycin	Intramuscular use for tuberculosis

Sulphonamides and trimethoprim

These are broad-spectrum agents, available individually or in a fixed-dose combination, co-trimoxazole. Both block the enzymatic synthesis of tetrahydrofolate, essential in bacterial DNA synthesis. Human cells can absorb preformed tetrahydrofolate directly without need for synthesis. Marrow suppression is seen occasionally but the most common side-effect is a Stevens–Johnson reaction to the sulphonamide component.

By inhibiting consecutive enzymes in the pathway, sulphonamides and trimethoprim have a theoretical synergistic antimicrobial effect, but this is now thought to be clinically insignificant. For most indications, trimethoprim is best used alone and, in this form, is less likely to produce side-effects. Co-trimoxazole is now recommended only for a few specialized indications (e.g. *Pneumocystis* pneumonia). Resistance of organisms to sulphonamides is mediated by alteration of target enzymes and by exclusion of the molecule from the organism. Resistance rates in coliforms from community-acquired UTIs range between 15 and 50 per cent, in hospital-acquired UTIs between 25 and 75 per cent, and in respiratory *Haemophilus* infection, up to 15 per cent.

Trimethoprim is available for oral or parenteral use, and is commonly recommended as first-line therapy for minor lower urinary tract infection (coliforms) and acute exacerbations of chronic bronchitis (*Haem. influenzae*, pneumococci). Trimethoprim or co-trimoxazole are not recommended for therapy of significant streptococcal or staphylococcal infections (including *Enterococcus faecalis* UTI, and pneumococcal pneumonia). Sulphonamides are rarely used alone nowadays; previously important indications, such as meningococcal prophylaxis and neurosurgical therapy and prophylaxis, have been overtaken by rising resistance rates.

Quinolones

These agents represent important advances in antimicrobial pharmacology. Ciprofloxacin, norfloxacin and the other new 4-quinolones inhibit bacterial DNA replication. All are expensive, especially as parenteral preparations. Most coliforms, even those resistant to multiple other agents, are exquisitely sensitive, and *Pseudomonas aeruginosa* is sufficiently sensitive to allow oral therapy of those (relatively few) infections with this organism that require treatment (such as hospital acquired urinary tract infection and osteomyelitis). Gaps in the quinolone spectrum include anaerobes and most streptococci. Attempted therapy of staphylococcal infections often encourages resistance. Resistance to the new quinolones is rising in hospital and appearing in a few community-acquired infections, especially in *Klebsiella* spp. Quinolones rapidly remove sensitive Gram-negative organisms from the commensal flora, and this may be useful in 'selective decontamination' of the gut flora in immunosuppressed patients and certain patients in intensive care units. Initial parenteral therapy can usually be converted rapidly to oral therapy, with considerable cost savings. Topical preparations are available for ophthalmic use, but there is concern that their widespread use may encourage the emergence of resistance.

Macrolides and lincosamines

Macrolides inhibit protein synthesis, and resistance may be due to molecular exclusion or to alteration of the ribosomal target. For many years erythromycin has been the surgeon's drug of first choice for treating Gram-positive infections in patients allergic to penicillin. It should be remembered, however, that macrolides do not reach therapeutic concentrations in the urine or CSF. Resistance rates vary throughout the UK, but average 10 per cent in *Staph. aureus* and 8–12 per cent in pneumococci. Erythromycin also has important applications in Legionnaires' disease and other 'atypical' pneumonias and *Campylobacter* diarrhoea, and it has moderate anti-anaerobic activity. New macrolides, such as clarithromycin and azithromycin, are expensive but usefully improve on erythromycin's activity against *Haem. influenzae*, and are much less likely to cause gastrointestinal upset.

Clindamycin is the only commonly used member of the lincosamines, a group closely related to the macrolides. This agent has an unfortunate propensity to cause *Clost. difficile*-associated diarrhoea when given in high dose, but occasionally its broad-spectrum Gram-positive and anaerobic spectrum is valuable, for example in oral therapy of lower-limb cellulitis in arteriopaths. It is still widely used for abdominal surgical prophylaxis in the United States.

Vancomycin and teicoplanin

These are expensive parenteral agents that remain active against almost all Gram-positive bacteria by interfering with cell-wall formation. Vancomycin must be given by slow intravenous injection to avoid histamine release ('red person syndrome'), and dose modification in renal failure and serum assay are required. Oral vancomycin is as effective (but much more expensive than metronidazole) in *Clost. difficile*-associated diarrhoea. Teicoplanin has minor differences in spectrum and can be given intramuscularly. There is debate about the need to perform serum assays of teicoplanin. Both drugs are valuable in the treatment of MRSA infections.

Metronidazole and other imidazoles

Virtually all anaerobic bacteria are sensitive to metronidazole, but facultative anaerobes and strict aerobes are resistant. Oral, rectal, and intravenous preparations are available. Important indications include the treatment and prophylaxis of anaerobic sepsis, and a variety of parasitic infections including giardiasis, trichomoniasis, and *Entamoeba histolytica* infection. An Antabuse® effect is seen with alcohol, and prolonged use (over 4–6 weeks) may cause peripheral neuropathy. Other imidazoles are more expensive and have broadly similar antibacterial spectra, but may differ in antiparasitic efficacy.

Mupirocin

This is a natural product, available for topical use only, with excellent anti-Gram-positive activity. Common indications include treatment of skin sepsis such as impetigo, and clearance of nasal carriage of pathogens such as MRSA.

Fusidic acid (Fucidin®)

Fucidin® may be used orally in severe staphylococcal infection, preferably in combination with another agent such as flucloxacillin, erythromycin, or vancomycin to reduce the risk of the emergence of resistance. It is highly active against intracellular and extracellular staphylococci, and has a long half-life. Intravenous use is commonly associated with hepatic toxicity, so the oral route should be used whenever possible, and liver function should always be monitored. Topical use is popular for minor skin sepsis in domiciliary practice, but this may induce resistance. An ophthalmic preparation containing high concentrations is available, designed to achieve a broad anti-bacterial spectrum; this is a good second-line choice to chloramphenicol.

Tetracyclines

These are inexpensive, broad-spectrum antibiotics, but they find few applications in current surgical practice. They act by inhibiting bacterial protein synthesis at the ribosomal level, but resistance is frequent among common bacterial pathogens. Chlamydial infection is the most common indication, but occasionally tetracyclines are helpful when other agents are contraindicated because of hypersensitivity and resistance. Some cases of chronic lower-limb cellulitis respond well to oral tetracyclines.

Other agents

Rifampicin, traditionally reserved for mycobacterial therapy, has excellent antistaphylococcal activity and is sometimes used in combination with other agents (flucloxacillin, vancomycin) for severe infections.

A number of agents active against multiply-resistant Gram-positive bacteria (such as MRSA) have recently been released, or are about to be. These include Synercid® and Linezolid®, and it is to be hoped that they prove effective and safe.

Systemic use of chloramphenicol, a cheap, broad-spectrum antibiotic, is decreasing because of its rare association with idiosyncratic aplastic anaemia. It penetrates to give useful concentrations in the CSF, whether there is meningeal inflammation or not, therefore it is sometimes recommended for treatment of meningitis and for neurosurgical prophylaxis. However, other antibiotics, such as cefotaxime, have largely supplanted chloramphenicol as first-line choice. Chloramphenicol remains useful as cheap, reliable, topical ophthalmic therapy.

Several antimicrobial agents are available exclusively for urinary tract infections, but their usage is declining. Nitrofurantoin is occasionally helpful for treatment and long-term prophylaxis, but *Proteus* spp. are inherently resistant. Nalidixic acid is a long-established quinolone antibiotic with a limited spectrum, and Mandelamine® releases formaldehyde in the urine as a weak broad-spectrum agent (*Proteus* spp. are resistant).

Candida infections in hospitalized surgical patients are increasing in incidence, especially in those who have received prolonged antibiotic therapy after major abdominal procedures; early use of adequate doses of fluconazole improves outcomes. Because of expense or toxicity, most other antifungal agents (such as amphotericin B and liposomal amphotericin) are best reserved for specialist indications, and their use discussed with local microbiologists.

Principles of antibiotic treatment

Table 7.16 summarizes the ideal management of a potentially infected patient.

A few clinical syndromes are reliably caused by organisms of predictable sensitivity, enabling definitive therapy from the beginning. These include erysipelas and scarlet fever (*Strep. pyogenes*), and gas gangrene (*Clost. perfringens*). Microbiological diagnoses in some others may be reliably confirmed by rapid tests at presentation, such as a Gram stain of CSF in meningococcal meningitis, but often initial therapy is empirical or 'blind'.

Once a microbiological diagnosis is made, there is very rarely a single antibiotic indicated in preference to all others, and

Table 7.16 Principles of antibiotic treatment

Timing	Actions	Think...	Resulting therapy
At presentation	Provisional diagnosis (is infection likely?)		
	Take all specimens for microbiological diagnosis	Are non-antibiotic measures indicated or sufficient? (e.g. surgical drainage of an abscess or resection of devitalized tissue in 'synergistic gangrene')	
	Perform any rapid tests: • Gram stain (pus, CSF) • Urine microscopy • Latex agglutination, etc.	Has the patient received any prior antibiotic treatment (may indicate likely resistances of superinfecting organisms)	Empirical (blind') therapy if indicated
Day 1	24-hour culture results, further rapid tests, direct sensitivities	Alter empirical therapy?	
Day 2 and later	Definitive culture and sensitivity results		Definitive therapy (may be provisional therapy plus or minus some antibiotics, or be completely different)
		Is the patient clinically better?	Stop therapy as soon as possible consistent with response

alternatives should always be made available to cope with hypersensitive patients and unusually resistant pathogens. Voluntary local 'antibiotic policies' seek to restrict clinical freedom of choice between the many possible rational alternatives; they bring advantages of economy and simplicity, and can provide guidance on the local prevalence of resistance in common pathogens. Such policies require regular updating and are valuable outcomes of joint medical audit meetings between surgeons and microbiologists.

Specimens taken after antibiotic treatment has begun, even a few hours after, may be grossly misleading because of the overgrowth of resistant microbes that develops rapidly on mucosae and skin once the sensitive normal flora has been killed.

Combinations of antibiotics that may be useful

1. For 'broad-spectrum cover', especially for empirical treatment of severe infection. These combinations should be modified, and the spectra usually narrowed, as soon as more information has become available. An example for severe community-acquired sepsis of unknown aetiology is flucloxacillin plus gentamicin plus metronidazole.

2. For 'synergy', when the activity of two or more agents used together exceeds the sum of the activities of the two used separately. This is rarely of clinical use, but can be valuable in certain specific problems, such as the treatment of streptococcal endocarditis with penicillin and gentamicin.

3. To overcome resistance, such as the combination of amoxicillin with clavulanic acid (an inhibitor of many bacterial beta-lactamases) in co-amoxiclav (Augmentin®).

4. To prevent the emergence of resistance during therapy, such as in the treatment of tuberculosis.

5. To treat known or suspected mixed infections, when use of a single drug is inappropriate. For example, benzylpenicillin plus metronidazole plus gentamicin for abdominal sepsis when a mixed faecal flora is likely.

Many antibiotics have limited penetration to certain privileged body areas (Table 7.17), and certain agents have poor entry to other sites or are relatively inactive once they have penetrated.

Routes of administration

Intravenous

Generally recommended for the initial therapy of serious infection. Some agents can only be given by this route. Increasing evidence favours switching to oral therapy for most conditions once the patient has made a favourable response. Intravenous administration is an expensive route, because of high drug costs and the time and skills needed to administer treatment. It also carries the risks associated with continuous intravenous access.

Intramuscular

Satisfactory for single dose prophylaxis, but painful if repeated doses needed, and contraindicated with bleeding diatheses. Poor absorption in shock, and risk of infection at the injection site. Depot preparations are sometimes useful (e.g. procaine penicillin).

Oral

Cheap and effective for minor sepsis, for gastrointestinal infections, and for continuation therapy. The patient must usually be conscious and not be vomiting or have diarrhoea, and the drug should be acid stable and be absorbable. Unabsorbed antibiotic has a maximal effect on the normal gut flora via this route.

Topical

Satisfactory for minor local infections, but the risks of inducing resistance in bacteria and hypersensitivity in patients are highest. Antiseptics, or antibiotics not related to those used for systemic therapy (e.g. mupirocin), are preferable.

Rectal

Safe, cheap, and effective for certain agents (e.g. metronidazole) in the absence of diarrhoea.

Intrathecal

Now reserved for agents that do not cross the blood–brain barrier (e.g. aminoglycosides, vancomycin) for certain neurosurgical infections, and streptomycin in tuberculous meningitis.

Table 7.17 Penetration of antibiotics

Privileged sites (effective agents)	Particular gaps in penetration or activity (ineffective agents)
Brain, CSF (high-dose benzypenicillin (BP), cefotaxime, ceftazidime, chloramphenicol, trimethoprim, sulphonamides, rifampicin, quinolones)	Pneumonic lung (aminoglycosides)
Eye (high-dose BP, flucloxacillin, cefotaxime, ceftazidime, rifampicin, quinolones)	Gut lumen (aminoglycosides and vancomycin after parenteral administration)
Abscess, empyema (surgical drainage is virtually essential)	Urine (erythromycin)
Inside phagocytes (quinolones, rifampicin, fucidin, some new macrolides)	Most tissues (many oral cephalosporins, nalidixic acid)
Foreign bodies (vancomycin, ? plus the 'inside phagocytes' list)	

Instillation, lavage

May be useful for some difficult-to-treat infections (e.g. of vascular prostheses) when conventional therapy has failed. Problems of systemic absorption (of aminoglycosides) and potential for local hypersensitivity (to beta-lactams). Antibiotic lavage of the peritoneal cavity or abscess cavities has not been shown to be more effective than saline lavage plus appropriate systemic antibiotics.

Duration of therapy

Treatment duration has received little attention in many areas of antimicrobial therapy, and course lengths recommended by even the most eminent authorities are often based on educated guess-work. Two useful principles for immunocompetent patients are:

1. Treat *long-standing* infections, or those where *abscess formation* is known or likely, until the patient is clinically better *and* measurable variables (white cell count, erythrocyte sedimentation rate (ESR), C-reactive protein (CRP), etc.) have returned to the normal range.

2. Treat *acute infections* until the patient is clinically better, then add a few extra days. Keep the patient under observation for signs of metastatic sepsis if bacteraemia was likely.

Course lengths have been studied for some infections of surgical relevance, including:

◆ minor *Staph. aureus* infection or transient bacteraemia: 1–2 weeks;

◆ *Staph. aureus* IV line sepsis and transient bacteraemia: at least 2 weeks;

◆ serious *Staph. aureus* infection: 4 weeks;

◆ *Staph. epidermidis* infection of long IV lines: 5 days' vancomycin if the line needs to remain *in situ*;

◆ uncomplicated UTI: 24 hours to 3 days of most agents;

◆ pyelonephritis or other complicated UTI: 2 weeks for most agents, but perhaps less for quinolones;

◆ *Clost. difficile* diarrhoea: 5 days' oral metronidazole.

6.2 Unwanted effects of antimicrobial agents

For any drug, unwanted effects may be predictable and dose-related, or else idiosyncratic. Reactions are more common in certain groups of patients, such as those with renal or liver failure or the very young or old. Five types of reaction can be distinguished:

1. Direct toxic effects: these include renal tubular damage and VIIIth nerve damage with aminoglycosides, and liver damage with rifampicin.

2. Allergic reactions: such as rash or anaphylaxis with ampicillin.

3. Superinfection: for example, *Clost. difficile*-associated diarrhoea with cefotaxime.

4. Complications of administration: such as thrombophlebitis with intravenous agents.

5. Interaction with other drugs: for example, ciprofloxacin plus aminophylline may cause neurological reactions.

Cost

Antibiotic costs are a substantial component of a hospital's pharmacy budget, because at any one time about 25 per cent of inpatients will be receiving antibiotics and up to 50 per cent will receive one or more courses during their hospital stay. About 60–70 per cent of inpatient prescriptions are for therapy and the remainder for prophylaxis. Prospective surveillance in hospitals suggests that at least 15 per cent of antibiotic prescriptions in the UK are inappropriate. Drug costs for single doses of different antibiotics range from 4 pence to about £40, and some antifungal agents cost £400 per day. Considerable financial savings can therefore be made by adhering to a structured hospital antibiotic policy. Antibiotic usage can be an important subject for medical audit.

Antibiotic use and resistance

Widespread use of an antibiotic in any community inevitably increases the prevalence of resistance to the agent used, as well as to other agents that are subject to the same resistance mechanisms. Thus, heavy use of a 'second-generation' cephalosporin such as cefuroxime on a urology ward selects for coliforms that are also resistant to 'third-generation' agents such as ceftazidime. Furthermore, resistance will also be encouraged to unrelated antibiotics whose mechanisms are coded on the same genetic elements. For example, excessive use of trimethoprim on a urology ward may increase the prevalence of coliforms resistant to gentamicin because both genetic determinants are found on the same plasmid. Many microbiology laboratories monitor the prevalence of resistance to first-line antibiotics among common pathogens, and are therefore well placed to recommend how the most reliable empirical agents should be used.

Treatment failure or relapse

These have many possible causes, but useful general questions to consider include:

◆ **Compliance:** is the patient taking the drug?

◆ **Absorption:** is the drug entering the body (e.g. vomiting, diarrhoea)?

◆ **Dose:** is this adequate?

◆ **Culture:** was the sample representative of the microbes present at the true site of infection?

◆ **Drainage:** is drainage of a collection, relief of obstruction, or removal of a foreign body or necrotic tissue required?

◆ **Incidental causes:** is the continuing fever caused by factors unrelated to the original infection (e.g. 'antibiotic fever', deep venous thrombosis)?

◆ **Superinfection**: is a different organism involved, at the same or a different site (e.g. IV line, urinary tract or chest infection, *Clost. difficile* diarrhoea)?

◆ **Inadequate course**: was treatment stopped too soon?

◆ **Resistance**: has resistance developed in the original pathogen? (This is usually less common than the other causes.)

6.3 Principles of management of other common perioperative infections

Urinary tract infections

In the normal urinary tract, only the distal urethra has a commensal flora, which comprises a mixture of perineal skin and faecal organisms. **Bacteriuria** is the term given to the presence of bacteria in bladder urine, and this may be accompanied by symptoms of infection. Overall, bacteriuria is most common in the young sexually-active female. It most often comprises facultative organisms from the colonic flora. Normal production of urine and complete bladder emptying continually flush away organisms that penetrate upstream to the bladder or upper tracts. Bacteria commonly infecting normal patients carry specialized adhesins (such as **pili**) that bind to the uroepithelium. Many surgical patients, however, have physically abnormal urinary tracts or are catheterized. Hospital-associated bacteria infecting this group tend to have other specializations that include multiple antibiotic resistance, enhanced binding to plastic materials, and prolonged survival on staff hands.

There is disagreement over the terminology of urinary tract infection (UTI). **Lower urinary tract infection** (or **cystitis**) implies the presence of bacteria in the bladder urine associated with symptoms of dysuria, frequency, and lower abdominal pain. **Upper urinary tract infection** and **acute pyelonephritis** are best defined clinically to include loin pain, dysuria, frequency, and sometimes fever. Blood cultures may be positive in these cases, but the value of bacteriological methods to localize acute upper-tract infection are controversial. Such methods include searching for antibody-coated bacteria.

Microscopy is usually performed on uncentrifuged urine, sometimes stained with methylene blue to highlight cellular morphology. Most laboratories report semiquantitative counts of pus cells (indicating host response), red cells, organisms, casts, and epithelial cells (indicating likely perineal contamination, which is much more common in the female).

Midstream specimens of urine (MSU) are taken via the bacterially colonized urethra so it is essential to culture on a selective medium (usually **cysteine lactose electrolyte-deficient agar** (CLED), which inhibits swarming of *Proteus* spp.), and to quantitate the results. A growth of one or two species at concentrations of 10^5 organisms/ml or higher correlates with bladder infection in normal females. This level is convenient to use in the laboratory and is usually assumed to be valid for all other types of patient and specimens.

Escherichia coli, *Staph. saprophyticus*, and *Proteus mirabilis* cause over 90 per cent of urinary infections in domiciliary practice. Although resistance to older antibiotics (such as trimethoprim and ampicillin/amoxicillin) is now 25–60 per cent, these organisms are uncommonly resistant to more recent agents such as oral cephalosporins or co-amoxiclav (8–20 per cent), and rarely to norfloxacin or ciprofloxacin (1–5 per cent). Up to 30 per cent of bacteriologically proven cases of cystitis will resolve spontaneously within 10 days if untreated, therefore trials of the effectiveness of antibiotic therapy for this condition need careful design.

Table 7.18 shows that the picture is more complex for hospital-associated UTIs. Here urinary tract structural abnormalities, instrumentation, multiple antibiotic usage, and cross-infection are common. However, *E. coli* remains the most common isolate.

Table 7.18 Prevalence of organisms in hospital-associated urinary tract infections

Organism	Prevalence	Notes
E. coli	40%	Up to 95% ampicillin/amoxicillin resistance and 80% trimethoprim resistance
Proteus spp.	15%	*P. vulgaris* and relatives are often resistant to cephalosporin and sometimes to gentamicin
Klebsiella spp.	15%	All are ampicillin/amoxicillin resistant. Occasional outbreaks of gentamicin resistance. Recent problems with multiple cephalosporin resistance
Enterobacter spp., *Serratia* spp., *Citrobacter* spp.	10%	Cephalosporins are unreliable for this group
Pseud. aeruginosa	5%	Occasional multiple resistance
Enterococcus faecalis	5%	Increasing ampicillin/amoxicillin and high-level gentamicin resistance. Outbreaks of vancomycin resistance increasing
Staph. aureus and *Staph. epidermidis*	5%	*Staph. epidermidis* is often multiply resistant. Infection is often associated with catheters, stents, nephrostomies, etc.
Candida spp.	5%	Associated with catheters, multiple antibiotics, diabetes. May resolve with catheter removal

Instrumentation in the presence of infected urine commonly produces bacteraemia, therefore antibiotic prophylaxis is indicated (single-dose penicillin plus gentamicin is a rational choice, unless urine culture suggests otherwise).

Urethral catheterization rapidly results in colonization of the bladder urine, reaching nearly 100 per cent in about a week, although the rate is reduced by closed drainage and careful aseptic technique. Treatment of bacteriuria in catheterized patients should be avoided unless they are systemically affected by the infection, because colonization inevitably returns and involves progressively more resistant organisms. Symptoms and signs of infection are unusual without provocation, such as that provided by catheter blockage or reinsertion. Attempts at long-term prophylaxis of catheter-associated UTI with antibiotics (or antiseptics added to the drainage bag) have not proved successful.

Treatment of catheter-associated, complicated, or septicaemia-associated UTI is best guided by results of urine culture, but penicillin plus gentamicin (or, possibly, a parenteral cephalosporin alone) is a good empirical choice. Prolonged remission from recurrent symptomatic infections with coliforms or pseudomonads in patients with structural abnormalities can sometimes be obtained by 7–10 days oral treatment with a new quinolone. However, this should be used prudently because increasing resistance will follow indiscriminate use. Apparent primary treatment failure is often caused by unrecognized obstruction (e.g. stone, renal abscess, or cyst) and less commonly by resistant pathogens (Table 7.19). Response in diabetics is generally slow.

Perinephric abscess most commonly follows urinary obstruction, and coliforms such as *E. coli* and *Proteus* spp. are the usual isolates. Because of their copious production of the urease enzyme, which alkalinizes urine and precipitates salts, *Proteus* spp. most frequently infect renal stones and resulting obstructive lesions. Occasional cases of perinephric abscess are blood-borne (especially *Staph. aureus*), or contain a mixed faecal flora (anaerobes, *Strep. milleri*, and coliforms). The latter often implies there has been a colonic perforation with direct spread to the underlying kidney. Most cases require drainage plus appropriate antibiotics.

Respiratory tract infections

Chest infection is an important cause of postoperative fever, and the likely infecting organisms can often be predicted from knowledge of the patient's past and recent history.

1. Apparent chest infection presenting during the first 24 post-operative hours in previously fit subjects is commonly caused by mucous plugging of the lower airways. Vigorous physiotherapy will often avoid the need for antibiotic therapy.

2. Patients with chronic bronchitis usually suffer postoperative chest infections with the flora that chronically colonizes their airways; usually pneumococci, *Haem. influenzae*, and *Moraxella catarrhalis*. Mild cases will usually respond to oral therapy with amoxicillin or clarithromycin, but more seriously ill patients are better given a short course of a parenteral cephalosporin.

3. Previously ill patients who have been in hospital for more than a few days (especially if they are being ventilated, have acute respiratory distress syndrome (ARDS), and have already received antibiotics) are prone to colonization and chest infection with a wide range of organisms, including coliforms and pseudomonads. True Gram-negative pneumonia is rare, and is overdiagnosed by criteria that rely only on new chest X-ray shadowing, fever, and the isolation of organisms from respiratory secretions. Nevertheless, it is wise to include such isolates within the spectrum of empirical therapy, and therapeutic advice should be sought from the local microbiologist. The best way to prove ventilator-associated pneumonia is by quantitative culture of fibre-optic broncho-alveolar (or non-guided broncho-alveolar) lavage aspirate.

4. If aspiration of upper respiratory or stomach contents is suspected, a combination such as cefotaxime plus metronidazole is recommended to cover anaerobic involvement.

5. Legionella infection occurs especially in the immuno-suppressed, and hospital-acquired legionellosis should be borne in mind, particularly if an 'outbreak' of pneumonia occurs. Erythromycin is currently the drug of choice.

Intravenous line infections

Infections of intravenous access devices are rising in incidence, being responsible for over 10 per cent of all bacteraemias in the UK and for about half of all cases of hospital-acquired endocarditis. Over 80 per cent are caused by *Staph. aureus* and *Staph. epidermidis*, and the remainder involve a variety of Gram-negative organisms, *Enterococcus faecalis,* and *Candida* spp. Most infections are acquired by infection of the skin entry site or contamination of junctions in the infusion system when these are opened, but a small proportion are introduced during line insertion, seed the line from bacteraemias from other sources, or spread directly from contamination of infusion fluids.

Staph. epidermidis has special abilities to cause persistent infection of IV lines, although the bacteraemia it then causes is

Table 7.19 Return of bacteriuria after treatment can be caused by reinfection or relapse with the following characteristics

Reinfection	Relapse
Different species, strain, or type of organism (e.g. by antibiotic sensitivity, serotype)	Same species, strain, and type
More common	Less common
Urinary tract usually structurally normal	Suggests persisting urinary tract abnormality (stone, stricture, diverticulum, chronic prostatitis). Investigation may need upper tract localization (selective ureteric catheterization after bladder washout)
Long-term antibiotic prophylaxis as a last resort	Avoid long-term prophylaxis

rarely associated with severe symptoms. Initial electrostatic attraction between the organism and the plastic catheter is followed by production of a tough, inert extracellular biofilm matrix (or 'slime'), which binds the two together and protects the slowly multiplying staphylococci from host defences and antibiotics. Most peripheral line infections will be adequately treated by removal of the catheter. For long-line infections with *Staph. epidermidis*, vancomycin appears to retain the greatest activity. However, infections that do not respond to 5 days' treatment (and most infections with other species) usually require the line to be changed.

Other important surgical infections

Actinomycosis

Caused by the Gram-positive, branching anaerobe *Actinomyces israelii*. This is almost always a chronic mixed infection involving other anaerobes and facultative aerobes, including *Strep. milleri*, *Bacteroides* spp, and other fastidious organisms. Actinomycosis occurs most commonly at sites where the organism is a commensal, namely large-bowel-associated abscesses and in gynaecological sepsis. Dental abscess and sinuses are now much less common than previously described. In most cases of actinomycosis it is likely that an initial mixed infection, perhaps resulting from a perforated viscus, is contained locally by host defences, then *Act. israelii* later multiplies at the expense of the other flora. Characteristically the infections are surrounded by dense fibrous tissue, and may discharge granular pus ('sulphur granules', which consist of microcolonies of *Act. israelii*). Histological and Gram-stain appearances are characteristic. Therapy should include adequate surgical drainage, and antibiotics should be aimed at the likely mixed infecting flora: amoxicillin plus metronidazole is one possible combination. Four to six weeks' treatment is normally needed (prolonged metronidazole therapy should be avoided because of the risks of peripheral neuropathy). *Act. israelii* is resistant to metronidazole.

Bite-wound infections

Human and animal mouths are heavily colonized with a wide range of bacteria that may be pathogenic when inoculated into a bite, and severe systemic infection is not rare. The mainstays of antibacterial therapy are débridement, vigorous cleansing with antiseptic, and antibiotic treatment if clinically indicated. Staphylococci, streptococci, and anaerobes are common mouth flora, and animals harbour several small, Gram-negative, fastidious organisms with sinister reputations for causing septicaemia after quite minor bites. These include *Pasteurella multocida* and *Capnocytophaga canimorsus* (also called 'DF-2'). Suitable antibiotics to cover the necessary spectrum include co-amoxiclav, or parenteral cefotaxime plus metronidazole.

Blood-borne viruses and surgery

Introduction

The major blood-borne viruses of surgical significance are the hepatitis viruses (especially hepatitis B, C, and the delta agent) and HIV. All may be spread by inoculation of unscreened blood or blood products, by sharing undisinfected needles between intravenous drug misusers, and by sexual transmission. Intravenous drug misusers, male homosexuals, and nationals of certain countries (for example, Central African states) are considered to be at 'high risk' for carriage of HBV and HIV. During clinical procedures carrier patients may infect their medical attendants, and transmission in the reverse direction may also occur.

Creutzfeldt–Jakob disease

The agent of Creutzfeldt–Jakob disease, a rare progressive dementia, is classified as a 'prion' which is resistant to routine sterilization procedures. It has been transmitted to patients by neurosurgical equipment and organ transplantation, and to experimental animals via blood. In hospital, suspected cases should be notified immediately to the ICT and CSSD. The agent can be inactivated only by autoclaving at 132 °C for 18 minutes, and under some circumstances instruments should be destroyed rather than reused.

Hepatitis

Hepatitis B is a DNA virus that has a long incubation period of 2–5 months (during which time cases are infectious); 5–10 per cent of cases become carriers with persistent HBV infection, and occasionally fulminant hepatitis occurs. Laboratory diagnosis relies on detection of the HBV surface antigen (HB$_s$Ag), usually by enzyme-linked immunosorbent assay (ELISA); patients with this antigen in their serum are infectious. Acute and active infection can be distinguished from chronic carriage in HB$_s$Ag-positive people by detection of IgM antibodies against the core antigen (anti-HB$_c$Ag). Possession of the 'e' antigen (HB$_e$Ag) in serum indicates that the individual is particularly infectious. Previous immunization or infection results in antibodies to the surface antigen (anti-HB$_s$Ag). Patients with HB$_s$ antibodies are *not* infectious.

Vaccination (the vaccine contains genetically engineered HB$_s$Ag) against HBV is safe and highly effective, and must be given to all clinical and other staff at risk of inoculation with HBV-containing blood. This includes all surgeons, and is now a legal requirement for all staff performing 'exposure-prone procedures'. Seroconversion should be checked after the three-dose vaccine course and, if an adequate antibody titre has resulted, vaccination should be repeated at 5-yearly intervals. Transmission of HBV in both directions between surgeons and patients has been documented on numerous occasions, and vaccination will abolish this risk.

In the past, **hepatitis C virus** (HCV) used to cause a relatively mild hepatitis after about 1 per cent of blood transfusions, with an incubation period of about 6–8 weeks. Tests for HCV have only recently become available and, because seroconversion takes up to 6 months after jaundice, they are useful for screening blood for transfusion but not for acute diagnosis. **Hepatitis D** or the **delta agent** is an incomplete virus that can only multiply in the presence of HBV, which acts as a 'helper virus'. Thus the delta agent may cause exacerbations of HBV infection in patients who are already HB$_s$Ag-positive.

HIV and AIDS

The **human immunodeficiency viruses** (HIV-1 and -2) infect and destroy T4-helper lymphocytes, persist indefinitely, and paralyse the immune system. After HIV exposure, a self-limited infectious mononucleosis-like illness usually results, and the patient's serum later becomes positive for anti-HIV antibody (thus the patient is infectious before seroconversion). There is then a variable (up to 10 years) period of subclinical infection, during which time the T4 lymphocyte count falls and the patient remains infectious, then persistent generalized lymphadenopathy occurs. Subsequent progression to AIDS is marked by the development of opportunistic infections. These include oral and oesophageal candidiasis, chronic diarrhoea caused by cryptosporidium and other organisms, pneumocystis and bacterial pneumonia, tuberculosis, CMV retinitis, and cryptococcus meningitis.

Patients carrying HIV may therefore present to surgeons with incidental conditions during the subclinical period (for example, male homosexuals with perianal disease), and with opportunistic infections after development of AIDS. Any patient seen by any surgeon may therefore carry the virus, and a negative HIV antibody test does not mean the patient is non-infectious if they have been exposed to the risk of HIV recently. Depending upon the local prevalence of carriage, it may be worthwhile at the moment to distinguish 'high-risk' groups for special precautions, but it is likely that 'universal precautions' will be adopted by most units in the near future. For surgical operations (where some sharps injuries are inevitable) these include double-gloving and wearing woven Kevlar or other gloves, wearing face shields to prevent splashing mucosal surfaces, and avoiding sharp instruments wherever possible. Nowadays all staff need to cover skin lesions and scratches with impermeable dressings, to discard sharps into proper disposal bins, and to disinfect surfaces and equipment that may be contaminated with blood. Fortunately, HIV appears to be less infectious than HBV by inoculation (the relative risks after a percutaneous inoculation are about 0.3 and 30 per cent, respectively) and it is more susceptible to disinfection by glutaraldehyde, hypochlorite, alcohols, and heat. Advice for HIV-infected clinical staff will doubtless change as more information about risks becomes available, but transmission to patients during routine dental work has been documented. At the moment, HIV-1 antibody-positive workers should not have close, ungloved contact with patients' mucosae or perform invasive procedures.

Bibliography

Clinical microbiology

Gruneberg, R.N. (1981). *Microbiology for clinicians.* MTP Press, Lancaster. [Entertaining and highly practical guide to preventing, investigating, and treating infection, but becoming dated.]

Surgical infection

Taylor, E.W. (1992). *Infection in surgical practice.* Oxford University Press, Oxford. [Good mixture of practical experience and scientific background, with excellent lists of references for further reading. Tends to be dogmatic in areas of uncertainty.]

Infectious diseases and microbiology, including antibiotic usage

Wilks, D., Farrington, M., and Rubenstein, D. (1995). *The infectious diseases manual.* Blackwell, Oxford. 1995. [Practical, up-to-date 'Michelin Guide' to diagnosis and management of infections.]

Hospital-acquired infection

Ayliffe, G.A.J., Collins, B.J., and Taylor, L.J. (1990). *Hospital-acquired infection:principles and prevention.* Wright, Sevenoaks. [Up-to-date brief summary of all aspects of the control of HAI.]

Wound infection

Cruse, P.J.E. and Foord, R. (1980). The epidemiology of wound infection. A 10-year prospective study of 62,939 wounds. *Surg. Clin. North Am.,* **60**, 27–40. [One observer continuously surveyed an entire hospital's surgical wounds over a 10-year period. Standard criteria were used, and many conclusions were reached about the remediable causes of infection that are still valid today.]

Gillespie, W.J. and Walenkamp, G. (1998). Antibiotic prophylaxis in patients undergoing surgery for proximal femoral and other closed long bone fractures.

The Cochrane Library, issue 4. [Systematic review of use of prophylactic antibiotics for prosthetic orthopaedic surgery. Contains many evidence-based recommendations of direct clinical relevance.]

National Academy of Sciences-National Research Council (1964). Division of Medical Sciences, Ad Hoc Committee of the Committee on Trauma: Post-operative wound infections: the influence of ultraviolet radiation of the operating room and various other factors. *Ann. Surg.,* **160** (Suppl. 2), 1–192. [Seminal paper on the classification of surgical wounds and the avoidance of infection at the operative site.]

Centers for Disease Control and Prevention (1999). Guideline for Prevention of Surgical Site Infections. *Amer. J. Infect. Control,* **27**, 97–134 (and online at *www.cdc.gov/ncidod/hip*). [Evidence-based guidelines for preventing all types of surgical wound infection].

Song, F., Glenny, A.M. (1998). Antimicrobial prophylaxis in colorectal surgery: a systematic review of randomized controlled trials. *Health Technol. Assess.,* **2**, 1–87.

CHAPTER 8

Nutrition and nutritional support in surgical practice

K. Gardiner

1 Introduction

The importance of artificial nutritional support for patients with critical illness has been demonstrated convincingly in many studies over the past 20 years. More recently there have been significant shifts in nutritional management with regard to nutrient composition, route of administration, and organization of delivery:

1. There is increasing evidence that the enteral route of administration is often possible in critically ill patients and is associated with reduced complications and lower costs than parenteral nutrition. Enteral nutrition has been facilitated by technological improvements in access devices and equipment for nutrient delivery.

2. There has been increasing interest in the formulation of new enteral and parenteral diets designed for individual diseases or to support specific organ systems. Glutamine, arginine, branched-chain amino acids, n-3 fatty acids, ornithine, and nucleotides have all attracted interest as specific nutrient substrates designed to prevent muscle protein breakdown, maintain gastrointestinal integrity, or to modify inflammatory and immune responsiveness.

3. It has been recognized that a multidisciplinary team approach to nutritional support, involving clinician, nurse, dietician, and pharmacist, can reduce the incidence of feeding complications and improve the overall quality of care.

This chapter reviews the definition, incidence, aetiology, and clinical significance of malnutrition for the surgical patient, before discussing the benefits and hazards of nutritional support.

2 Malnutrition

In 1976, Butterworth described malnutrition in the hospital patient as a 'skeleton in the hospital closet' which could be greatly improved by modest revisions of attitude, administrative effort, and financial support. Before we can evaluate Butterworth's hypothesis a clear idea of what is meant by the term 'malnutrition' is necessary.

2.1 What is malnutrition?

Malnutrition occurs where there is an imbalance between the intake of, and the need for, nutrients as a result of decreased dietary intake, altered use of nutrients, or increased requirements.

Protein–energy malnutrition (and its associated vitamin and mineral deficiencies) is the most common disturbance in nutrition found in hospital patients, although a variety of selective nutrient deficiencies can occur as a result of different diseases and treatments.

2.2 Recognizing malnutrition

Protein–energy malnutrition is usually recognized by assessing dietary intake, general cellular or muscular dysfunction, or body composition. However, it is important to note that reported changes in dietary intake are notoriously inaccurate. General cellular dysfunction may be reflected by certain changes in cellular immune function (e.g. total lymphocyte count), whereas muscular dysfunction may lead to a reduced ability to perform basic activities (Table 8.1). Changes in body composition are determined by comparison with norms derived from well-nourished populations (weight loss, plasma albumin or prealbumin concentrations, skinfold thickness, or muscle circumference; see Table 8.2).

Weight loss, accurately measured, is an essential global marker of poor nutritional status. Errors in determining weight loss based on a single measurement of body weight are greater if the predicted rather than the patient's own recall of his or her

Table 8.1 Tests of muscle function

Test	Method
Handgrip strength	Hand dynomometry
Respiratory function	Forced inspiratory and expiratory pressure; forced inspiratory and expiratory volumes[a]

[a] Assumes previously normal pulmonary compliance and airway resistance—which is often not the case.

Table 8.2 Anthropometric measures

Measure	Method	Meaning
Body weight loss	Accurate scales	Loss of fat, muscle, and fluid
Skinfold thickness	Calipers on skin over triceps, biceps, and iliac crest	Estimate of subcutaneous fat
Mid-arm muscle circumference	Arm circumference and triceps skinfold thickness allows arm muscle circumference to be calculated	Estimate of lean body mass

well weight is used. However, recalled weight loss has also been shown to have poor sensitivity and predictive power: on this basis, one-third of patients with more than 10 kg weight loss would be unrecognized and a quarter having lost less than 10 kg would be wrongly considered to have lost at least 10 kg.

The problem with any of these measurements is that the fraction of surgical patients considered malnourished can vary from 15 per cent to over 30 per cent, depending on which indicator is used. Single indicators can be evaluated rapidly but have been criticized as they are affected by numerous non-nutritional factors. For example, albumin concentration will be affected by albumin infusion, hepatic failure, or a protein-losing enteropathy.

2.3 Clinically significant malnutrition

As there is not one absolute criterion for malnutrition, the usefulness of these tests is often measured by their ability to predict nutrition-related complications. Thus **clinically significant malnutrition** could be defined as a deficit in nutrition that is associated with an adverse clinical outcome, and the correction of which reduces the risk of those nutritionally associated complications. This has led to evaluation of these measurements (either alone or in combination) as predictors of in-hospital or postoperative complications such as infections, wound dehiscence, respiratory failure, or death.

In surgical patients, a plasma albumin concentration of less than 35 g/l was found to be associated with a 4.6-fold increase in complications. In critically ill patients, a low plasma albumin predicted a 9.7-fold increase in death. When both plasma albumin and total lymphocyte count were low, there was a 19-fold increase in deaths. Absolute weight loss of 4.5 kg in the 6 months before surgery was associated with a 19-fold increase in mortality. One problem in using protein or other laboratory measurements is establishing the relationship between their measurement and the likelihood of protein–energy malnutrition in an individual as opposed to the reference population. However, individual anthropometric measurements have performed poorly as predictors of adverse clinical outcomes.

In an attempt to improve the diagnosis of malnutrition, multifactorial indices of malnutrition, such as the likelihood of malnutrition index (LOM), the prognostic nutritional index (PNI), and the subjective global assessment (SGA), have been developed (Table 8.3). Patients with a high LOM index have longer hospital stays and increased mortality rates. In patients undergoing non-emergency gastrointestinal surgery, an increase in PNI was associated with an increased incidence of sepsis and death. Other investigators have found that the PNI is no better than measurement of albumin concentration or weight loss in predicting nutrition-related complications. The SGA has been found to be reproducible between independent observers and can be used to categorize patients into low-, moderate-, and high-risk categories. However the SGA has not been shown to be consistently better than the PNI in the prediction of postoperative complications.

Table 8.3 Multiple indicators as an index of malnutrition

Likelihood of malnutrition index (LOM)	Prognostic nutritional index (PNI)	Subjective global assessment (SGA)
Plasma albumin concentration	Plasma albumin concentration, serum transferrin concentration	Weight change
Anthropometrics (weight and height, triceps skinfold thickness, mid-arm muscle circumference)	Triceps skinfold thickness	Dietary intake change
Lymphocyte count	Delayed type hypersensitivity	Gastrointestinal symptoms for >2 weeks
Haematocrit		Functional capacity
Plasma vitamin concentration (folate, vitamin C)		Underlying disease
		Effect on metabolic stress
		Physical findings (loss of subcutaneous fat, muscle wasting, ankle and sacral oedema, ascites)

It therefore appears that many types of data (historical, clinical, biochemical, and anthropometric) are useful in making the diagnosis of malnutrition, and a synthesis of these sources of information will aid prediction of nutrition-related complications.

2.4 Is malnutrition found among surgical patients?

Using indices of malnutrition, the prevalence of mild malnutrition has been estimated to be 48 per cent among hospital patients, and 31 per cent are severely malnourished. Many patients are already malnourished when admitted to hospital. In addition, serial estimations have shown that patients may become increasingly malnourished during their stay in either medical or surgical wards.

Food intake after major surgery is invariably low—whether by elderly patients undergoing orthopaedic surgery or any patients after thoracic, gynaecological, or gastrointestinal surgery. Typically, patients are not allowed to drink or eat during the first postoperative days. Thereafter liquid diet, bland diet, and finally normal food are consumed. At the day of discharge from the hospital, most patients still have an inadequate nutritional intake. After gastrointestinal surgery, average in-hospital weight loss is 3–5 kg, with half the weight loss being lean body mass.

Little is known about how much patients eat after being discharged from the hospital, but long-term studies have shown that after elective colonic surgery, patients do not regain their preoperative weight until 3–4 months after the operation.

2.5 Why is malnutrition found in surgical patients?

Malnutrition is found among two groups of patients—those with uncomplicated starvation and those who are septic, injured, or with active inflammation with a hypercatabolic state in addition to some degree of starvation.

Malnourishment found on admission may be due to decreased intake of food, malabsorption, or the hypermetabolism

Table 8.4 Groups of surgical patients at risk of malnutrition

Gastrointestinal surgery	Serious illness	Elderly
'Ileus'	Burns	Self-neglect
Intestinal failure	Trauma	
Short bowel syndrome	Sepsis	
Inflammatory bowel disease	Unconscious patient	
High intestinal fistula		
Congenital intestinal disorders		

associated with illness. As mentioned above, food intake in hospital is often insufficient because meals are missed because of multiple procedures requiring temporary starvation and because of lack of provision of nutrition in the postoperative period. Decreased nutrient intake may also result from poor appetite, difficulty in swallowing (e.g. nasogastric tube, oesophageal cancer), or handicaps such as arthritis, motor neurone disease, or multiple sclerosis. Careful nursing supervision is necessary at meal times or patients with poor appetite may pass unnoticed and corrective action is not undertaken. Patients with intestinal disease or having undergone intestinal resection are most obviously at risk of malabsorption (Table 8.4). Hypermetabolism may be caused by burns, major trauma, surgery, or septic illness.

In any individual patient the clinical features may be those of simple starvation, of hypermetabolism, or a mixture of the two:

Metabolic response to starvation

In starvation, a decrease in plasma insulin and an increase in plasma cortisol and growth hormone allow the body to mobilize and oxidize fat, skeletal muscle protein, and glycogen stores to provide glucose and ketone bodies for brain metabolism and fatty acids for skeletal, cardiac, and respiratory muscle metabolism. Decreased energy intake is followed by a lowered metabolic rate, modulated through changes in thyroid hormone metabolism and the activity of the sympathetic nervous system.

Metabolic response to trauma, inflammation, and sepsis

The initial stimulus for metabolic change is provided by the release of hormones from the hypothalamic–pituitary axis as well as release of catecholamine, glucagon, and corticosteroids. Basal metabolic rate increases, sodium and water are retained, blood glucose concentration rises, and negative nitrogen balance develops. In an extreme case, products of local tissue ischaemia and inflammation circulate and this, combined with translocation of enteric bacterial endotoxin, leads to activation of the cytokine cascade, initiating the **systemic inflammatory response syndrome** (SIRS). Release of cytokines (interleukins and TNF) and free radicals causes an increase in tissue oxygen consumption, metabolic rate, and catabolism. In addition, cardiac output, resting energy expenditure, and carbon dioxide production increase. If these changes persist, the hypermetabolic/**multiple organ dysfunction syndrome** (MODS) develops. Prominent features of MODS are glycogenolysis, gluconeogenesis, insulin resistance, nitrogen depletion, and malnutrition.

In **hypermetabolism**, energy expenditure and catabolism are greatly increased—as opposed to starvation where they are decreased or unaffected. In starvation, the predominant fuel utilized is carbohydrate, whereas in hypermetabolism a mixed fuel source is required. Production of hepatic glucose is increased, with loss of normal biofeedback mechanisms. Consequently, the proportion of calories obtained from glucose compared to an equivalent state of starvation is reduced. This leads to hyperglycaemia with recycling of the glucose as lactate. Another contributing factor to hyperglycaemia is increased **gluconeogenesis**. In part, alanine effluxing from skeletal muscle drives this, as does a carbon flux arising from increased lactate production. Initially, overall fat use is increased with increased lipolysis, increased oxidation of triglycerides and fatty acids, and enhanced lipid clearance from the bloodstream. Eventually fat utilization diminishes and triglyceride clearance gradually decreases.

The principal changes in protein economy include:

- increased hepatic synthesis;

- increased total protein catabolism (increased production of ammonia, urea, creatinine, and uric acid);

- reduced total body synthesis.

Amino-acid efflux is increased, with flow from mobile amino-acid pools (skeletal muscle, gut) to the liver. Glutamine is used by the gut as an energy source, and branched-chain amino acids become important fuels for skeletal and heart muscle. The liver initially increases its clearance of this heavier amino-acid load. As organ failure intervenes, catabolism increases, amino-acid clearance decreases, and protein synthesis shifts to the production of inflammatory mediators at the expense of visceral and transport proteins. Protein depletion and impaired immune function develop in association with rampant malnutrition.

When the stress of an operation or serious illness is added to starvation, the processes of gluconeogenesis still occur. In these circumstances, gluconeogenesis is important in providing glucose for wound as well as cerebral metabolism. Lipolysis provides ketone bodies to support cerebral metabolism as well as that of skeletal, cardiac, and respiratory muscles. Although insulin levels are increased, there is relative insulin resistance due

to the outpouring of cortisol and growth hormone. During the initial **stress** and **ebb** phases over the first 24 hours after operation, the metabolism is little increased but there is mobilization of fuel substrates. During the next 3–4 days in the **flow** phase there is increased metabolism, increased catabolism with protein loss, and wound healing at the expense of other tissues. Following this, the anabolic **recovery** phase occurs, during which there is protein gain if a protein source is supplied to the body.

2.6 Does malnutrition have any effect on the outcome of surgical illness?

Although an affirmative answer to this question is implied by the definition of clinically significant malnutrition used above, it is worth examining the evidence that malnutrition adversely affects the function of different organs and the overall outcome of illness episodes. Mild and moderate degrees of malnutrition seem to be tolerated by surgical patients, but those who have experienced a weight loss of 10–15 per cent show impaired wound healing, immunity, and muscle function, which may increase the risk of developing postoperative complications.

Wound healing

Low plasma albumin or transferrin concentrations were predictive of delayed wound healing in elderly patients requiring repetitive vascular surgical procedures and in patients requiring lower extremity amputations for vascular disease.

Immune function

The malnourished patient develops impaired immune resistance to infection with anergy developing after 7 days of nutritional deprivation. Luminal deprivation of nutrients has been shown to alter the immune and barrier functions of the gut, but these will be discussed later.

Muscle function

Weakness of the respiratory muscles impairs coughing, increases the risk of pneumonia, and may make it more difficult to wean malnourished patients from a ventilator. Cardiac muscle function is also impaired, with reduced cardiac output and a liability to cardiac failure. Mobility is reduced, delaying recovery and predisposing to thromboembolism and bedsores.

Psychological effects

Semistarvation results in apathy, depression, loss of morale, and loss of will for recovery. Inability to concentrate means that the patient cannot benefit from instruction about the techniques needed for self-care. A general sense of weakness and illness can also impair appetite and the ability to eat, so perpetuating malnutrition.

Morbidity, mortality, and length of hospital stay

Severe protein–energy malnutrition in surgical patients is associated with:

◆ delayed resumption of an adequate oral food intake;

◆ an increased incidence of postoperative complications (a twofold increase in minor and a threefold increase in major complications);

◆ a greater risk of dying (up to fourfold);

◆ an extended length of hospital stay;

◆ an increased financial cost (up to 50 per cent).

However, data on length of hospital stay are difficult to interpret as they may be affected by many other factors, such as age, liver disease, malignancy, social circumstances, and variations in discharge policy by different medical staff.

2.7 What should be done about malnutrition in surgical patients?

Action regarding malnutrition needs to be three-pronged. First, measures to prevent or minimize the development of hospital-acquired malnutrition. Secondly, measures to improve the identification of patients on admission who are malnourished or who are at risk of developing malnutrition. Thirdly, measures to provide nutritional support to these patients promptly, safely, and effectively.

Hospital-acquired malnutrition may be reduced by encouraging oral intake, avoiding unnecessary fasting (after emergency admission or postoperatively, for example), minimizing the surgical stress response (e.g. minimal access surgery, optimal pain relief), and by modifying techniques of postoperative pain relief (e.g. epidural local anaesthesia has less effect on intestinal motility than morphine or pethidine).

The simplest method of preventing malnutrition is to persuade the patient to eat more by providing frequent small meals, appetizing dishes of favourite foods, or more nutritious items than the usual diet. However, at present this is often not given a high-enough priority by hospital managers (in many hospitals the catering budget/patient/day is only £1.50–£2.50), nor by the ward staff, where the serving of meals is increasingly delegated to untrained personnel. Techniques of artificial nutritional support, such as providing fortified liquid drinks or administration of liquid nutrients through an enteral tube or parenteral feeding, only become necessary if simple measures fail or are inappropriate.

Two controlled trials have compared food intake via a traditional postoperative regimen (including a nasogastric tube until flatus is passed) with a new tube-free regimen that includes early introduction of food. In this regimen, the nasogastric tube was removed at the end of the operation and the patient allowed to drink aqueous liquids, including protein drinks, on the first postoperative day. The next day patients received a full liquid diet and solid food if they asked for it. After both colonic surgery and radical hysterectomy, most patients consumed 1000 ml the first day and asked for and tolerated solid food on the third day. The average daily intake was higher with the new regimen and these patients consumed an average of 25–30 g protein/day and

energy corresponding to 50 per cent of their basal metabolic rates during the first four postoperative days.

One of the main problems in improving the recognition of malnutrition is that clinicians and nurses are not trained to look for it. This situation has developed because nutrition has been regarded as a Cinderella subject in medical schools, and therefore undergraduate and postgraduate education in nutrition has lagged behind nutritional research. Surveys in England and Scotland have shown poor knowledge of nutrition topics among senior medical students and junior doctors. The key to improving care is the education of nurses, medical students, and medical staff about nutritional assessment and support. The cause of nutrition is likely to be further advanced by the recognition of nutrition as a discipline by medical schools, Royal Colleges, and professional associations.

One method of improving recognition of malnutrition is the use of nutritional risk assessment scores on admission; this has received much recent attention (Table 8.5). Of course, screening for malnutrition will carry a cost—the time taken to assess patients by the nurse and dietician/nutrition team and the cost of the nutritional support for the malnourished patients identified. However, delay in identifying protein–energy malnutrition is associated with an extended length of hospital stay and therefore cost.

Slow progress in tackling the problem of malnutrition within hospitals is due in part to diffusion of responsibility and lack of coordination between disciplines in the recognition and treatment of malnutrition. The King's Fund Centre Report of 1992 drew attention to the extent of the problem and led to formation of the **British Association for Parenteral and Enteral Nutrition** (BAPEN) and positively encouraged the development of a multidisciplinary team approach to the provision of nutritional support. These teams involve clinicians, nurses, dieticians, and pharmacists, with the aim of organizing the delivery of nutritional treatment in a cost-effective manner.

3 Nutritional support

3.1 What is nutritional support?

Nutritional support depends on giving a balanced formulation of energy, protein, minerals, and vitamins by either the enteral or parenteral route as treatment for malnutrition or to prevent the development of malnutrition.

3.2 Does the provision of nutritional support have any effect on outcome of surgical illness?

Although malnutrition has been shown to have an adverse effect on the outcome of illness in surgical patients, it is important to evaluate whether nutritional support can restore nutritional deficits successfully or improve outcomes, before the effort and expense can be justified.

Table 8.5 Nutritional risk scores to assess state of nutrition (based on one devised by the nutrition team at The Royal Victoria Hospital, Belfast)

A Nutritional Risk Assessment Score Sheet

Name........................ Hospital number........................ Date of assessment........................

Feature					Nutritional assessment score
Weight	Usual weight	Weight loss of up to 10% or 3 kg over past 3 months	Weight loss of more than 10% or 3 kg over past month	Extremely thin, emaciated, or cachectic	
	1	2	3	4	
Body mass index	>20	18–19	15–17	10–14	
	1	2	3	4	
Appetite	Normal	Reduced: leaves up to half food and drinks offered	Poor: leaves most of food and drinks offered	Little or no appetite: refuses meals or unable to eat	
	1	2	3	4	
Ability to eat	Normal and independent	Cannot eat without assistance	Chewing and swallowing difficulties	Unable to eat or drink	
	1	2	3	4	
Intestinal function	Normal	Feels nauseated	Diarrhoea and/or vomiting	Profuse diarrhoea and/or vomiting	
	1	2	3	4	
Medical condition/ treatment	No interruption to food intake	Pre/post minor surgery or mild GI disease	Pre/post major surgery or severe GI disease	Burns, cancer, multiple injuries, severe infection	
	1	2	3	4	
				Total score	

Interpretation of nutritional assessment score:

    0–8   minimal risk
    9–16   moderate risk
    17–24   high risk

Action for patients at minimal risk: weigh and review score weekly.
Action for patients at moderate or severe risk: refer to dietician or nutrition team.

Preservation of nutritional status

Oral nutritional supplements have been shown to reduce post-operative weight loss after various elective gastrointestinal operations.

Wound healing

The literature concerning the effect of nutritional support on wound healing is inconclusive. A decrease in wound infections but not in anastomotic leakage has been reported in patients receiving intravenous nutrition prior to surgery. However, a decrease in wound infections with preoperative parenteral nutrition has not been confirmed by a subsequent study. Improved wound healing in surgical patients receiving intravenous nutrition has also been reported, but the Veterans Affairs TPN Cooperative Study failed to find evidence of a beneficial effect of preoperative parenteral nutrition on wound dehiscence, decubitus ulcer formation, or wound infection. Albina (1995) concluded that most surgical and accidental wounds will heal adequately despite moderate preoperative malnutrition and postoperative fasting.

Immune function

There is evidence that provision of specific nutrients (arginine, nucleotides, and n-3 polyunsaturated fatty acids) improves immune function in postoperative, traumatized, and septic patients. There is also evidence to support the use of glutamine-supplemented parenteral nutrition as compared with standard parenteral nutrition for its beneficial effects on gut barrier function and microbial colonization.

Muscle function

Improved muscle function can be seen in patients receiving nutritional support before any measurable increase in muscle mass is detectable. Oral dietary supplementation significantly increased hand grip strength after a range of elective gastrointestinal operations. Restoration of function in the form of the ability to walk after surgery for hip fracture was improved by nutritional support in malnourished elderly subjects. Feeding liquid nutritional supplements to underweight orthopaedic patients with femoral neck fractures improved their average energy intake and shortened their mobilization time.

Postoperative complications

Oral nutritional supplements reduced postoperative weight loss and significantly reduced morbidity after different types of elective gastrointestinal operations. Immediate enteral feeding via a jejunostomy reduced septic complications after acute abdominal surgery and after major burns.

Length of hospital stay

The effect of nutritional support is more difficult to assess as regards duration of hospital stay, as providing this support for a useful period (7 days) may lengthen hospital stay. In addition, access for nutrition itself may cause complications which delay hospital discharge. However, a review of the literature indicates that providing nutritional support can result in a reduction of hospital stay of between 5 and 16 days in appropriate cases (BAPEN 1994).

In summary, patients who are moderately or severely malnourished will benefit from nutritional support through improved muscle function (early mobilization, reduced postoperative fatigue) and reduced postoperative complications.

3.3 How much support is required?

Few uncomplicated surgical patients require more than 2000 kcal/day to achieve positive energy balance and a supply of 35–40 kcal/kg/day is sufficient to match the energy requirements of most septic patients. Resting energy expenditure (REE) can be approximated using the Harris and Benedict equations:

Box 8.1 Harris and Benedict equations for calculating resting energy expenditure

Males:

REE = 66 + (13.7 × body weight in kg) + (5 × height in cm) − (6.8 × age in years).

Females:

REE = 665 + (9.6 × body weight in kg) + (1.7 × height in cm) − (4.7 × age in years).

Nomograms have been constructed to predict the effect of different diseases on REE, but these apply better to groups of patients than to individuals.

Metabolically stressed patients appear to have a proportionately greater need for nitrogen compared with energy. Nitrogen requirements can be estimated from measurements of 24-hour urinary nitrogen or urinary urea nitrogen excretion. This is not routinely calculated and most patients will receive an energy and nitrogen supply based on the severity of their illness (Table 8.6) (Silk 1995).

Table 8.6 Nitrogen and energy requirements

Illness severity	Nitrogen requirement (g N/kg/day)	Calorie requirement (kcal/kg/day)
Reduced intake	0.17	28.6
Moderate injury or sepsis	0.26	34.3
Severe injury or sepsis	0.34	34.2–42.9

3.4 Preoperative or postoperative nutritional support?

Nutritional support might be expected to restore deficiencies more effectively when given preoperatively rather than postoperatively, owing to the increase in metabolism associated with surgical trauma. If this were the case, it would be reasonable to delay surgery for a stable patient who is not suffering from sepsis, necrosis, or bowel obstruction.

Many studies have tried to address this question but, unfortunately, most have been severely criticized either because they were retrospective, were lacking a control group without nutritional support, or involved too few patients. In other studies, the nutritional support was found to be of inadequate duration or inappropriate composition. Only 4 of the 11 studies that supplied preoperative nutritional support for an adequate period (more than 7 days) showed significant benefits—a reduced incidence of postoperative complications, septic episodes, and intra-abdominal abscesses. This beneficial effect was more pronounced in the most severely depleted patients.

Nutritional support can therefore be advocated preoperatively in patients who are severely malnourished (weight loss greater than 10 per cent). It is probable that malnourished patients for whom chemotherapy or radiotherapy is planned will also benefit from preliminary nutritional support, but further studies are necessary.

3.5 How should nutritional support be given?

The adage 'if the gut works, use it' is supported by a series of studies that have examined nutritional parameters, intestinal structure and function, complications, outcome, and cost.

Parenteral and enteral nutrition regimens have been shown to be equally effective in promoting nitrogen balance, preserving body weight, and promoting protein synthesis in unselected patients. However, critically ill patients tolerate enteral feeding less well and may take 4–5 days to attain caloric targets.

Administration of nutrition by the parenteral route alone for a period of 2–3 weeks is associated with significant decreases in intestinal mucosal thickness and villous and microvillous heights. In addition to this evidence of intestinal mucosal atrophy, parenteral nutrition is also associated with disturbances in intestinal function: decreased intestinal mucosal brush-border enzyme activity, decreased amino-acid transport by jejunal brush-border membrane vesicles, and increased intestinal permeability to lactulose. Thus enteral nutrition is seen to promote growth of the intestinal mucosa and maintain intestinal absorptive, metabolic, and barrier functions. The mechanisms underlying the beneficial effects of enteral nutrition on the gut are unknown, but may relate to a direct effect of enteral nutrients on enterocytes, and/or indirect effects due to increased release of gut hormones, improved mesenteric blood flow, or maintenance of a favourable intestinal microflora.

Compared with parenteral nutrition, aggressive enteral feeding with a high-protein diet reduced septic morbidity and improved nutritional status and survival in burned children. In a randomized trial in injured patients, early enteral nutrition with an elemental diet reduced septic complications, such as pneumonia and intra-abdominal abscesses, and improved outcome. A lower sepsis rate in intensive care unit patients who received most of their nutrition via the gastrointestinal tract has also been reported. The incidence of bacterial infections and the number of days in the intensive care unit were significantly lowered in patients with head injuries by early enteral feeding. Enteral feeding was found to blunt the acute-phase response and attenuate the hepatic reprioritization of protein synthesis found after major trauma. There were significantly fewer infective complications in patients randomized to receive enteral feeding after major trauma than in those receiving parenteral feeding. The favourable effects on enteral nutrition on general health may be related to a reprioritization of hepatic protein synthesis and/or preservation of intestinal mucosal integrity, so preventing bacterial translocation from the gut.

The mean daily costs for enteral nutrition have been shown to be substantially lower by 2–10 times than for parenteral nutrition. In addition, studies have shown that the cost of treating complications is virtually always lower for enterally fed than for parenterally fed patients.

Therefore, unless there is a specific contraindication to the use of the gastrointestinal tract, the enteral route should be first choice for nutritional support (Table 8.7). Concurrent enteral and parenteral nutrition is advised in patients who are unable to attain their caloric targets via the enteral route, as provision of even 10 kcal/day of enteral nutrients maintains the beneficial effects of the enteral route. A trial of enteral nutritional support is therefore indicated if the gastrointestinal tract is accessible and enteral feeding is not contraindicated (Table 8.8).

Table 8.8 Contraindications to enteral feeding

Intestinal obstruction
High-output fistula
Intractable vomiting
Intractable severe diarrhoea
Severe malabsorption
Ischaemic intestine

4 Enteral nutrition

The method of administration will depend on the patient's ability to eat or drink (Fig. 8.1) and the composition varies with the presence and extent of hepatic, renal, pulmonary and intestinal dysfunction.

4.1 Method of administration

Enteral feeds may be administered as oral supplements, drink feeds, or tube feeds. **Oral supplements** are usually prescribed for patients with near-normal gastrointestinal function to provide additional nitrogen (containing 3 g N/250 ml and 1 kcal/ml) or energy (containing 1.8 g N/250 ml and 1.5 kcal/ml). They are often marketed as 200–250 ml liquid portions but may also be semisolid or solid. **Drink feeds** are usually prescribed for patients who cannot eat solid food but can ingest liquids and have a near-normal intestine. These feeds are nutritionally complete, providing 15–20 g N, 1900–2500 kcal and all of the daily requirements of trace elements and vitamins in a volume of 1.5–2 litres. Both oral supplements and drink feeds need to be palatable and are usually based on a polymeric diet. If the patient is unable to swallow sufficient calories because of disease (oral, pharyngeal, or oesophageal cancer; multiple sclerosis; or cerebrovascular accident), upper gastrointestinal surgery, altered level of consciousness, or lack of palatability of elemental diet (Crohn's disease) then **tube feeds** may be indicated.

Tube feeds

The access route for the **tube feed** is mainly determined by its probable duration. The majority of hospitalized patients require nutritional support for less than 4 weeks and this can usually be

Table 8.7 Advantages of enteral nutrition

Intestine	Body
Maintains	Reduces
intestinal mucosal mass	hypermetabolic response to injury
barrier function	infectious complications
activity of amino-acid transporters	Improves
activity of brush-border enzymes	systemic immunity
Prevents disruption of normal gut flora	survival
Promotes intestinal healing after injury	

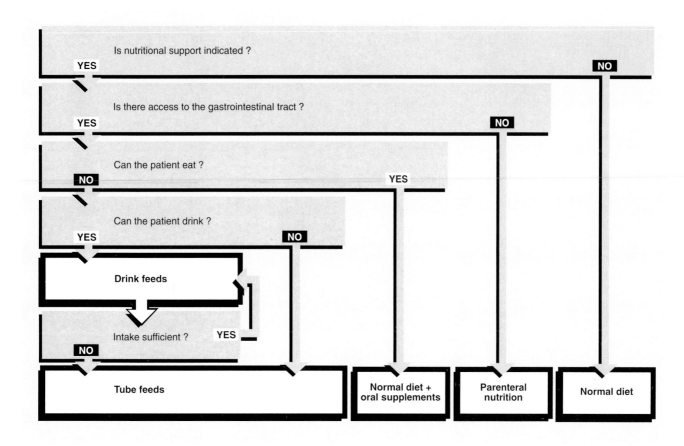

Figure 8.1 Choice of method for administering nutrition.

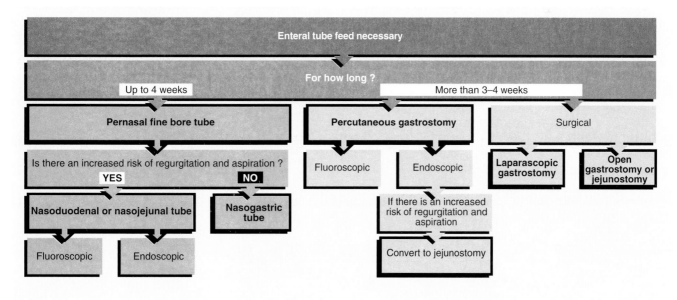

Figure 8.2 Choice of method for administering enteral tube feeding.

given by a **fine-bore nasogastric tube** (Fig. 8.2). Fine-bore tubes are made of polyurethane or silicone elastomer and are much better tolerated and less likely to cause gastro-oesophageal reflux or ulceration than standard nasogastric tubes. Common problems with enteral feeding using this route are shown in Table 8.9. In patients at increased risk of aspiration as a result of

Table 8.9 Enteral feeding via fine-bore nasogastric tubes

Problem	Complication	Prevention
Malposition	Intrapulmonary aspiration, pneumothorax, pharyngo-oesophageal perforation	Test aspirate pH (<3) Inject air and auscultate X-ray (necessary if impaired consciousness, cough, or gag reflex)
Gastro-oesophageal regurgitation	Intrapulmonary aspiration	Postpylorus placement (fluoroscopic or endoscopic) Nurse at angle of 45°
Tube blockage	Frequent replacement of tube	Twice-daily tube flushing with water
Unplanned extubation	Frequent replacement of tube	Secure tube fixation and regular examination

recumbent position, old age, abdominal surgery, diabetes, or hypothyroidism, the incidence of pulmonary aspiration of feed can be reduced by achieving postpyloric placement. This usually requires a 110-cm-long fine-bore tube and the aid of either fluoroscopy or endoscopy. The endoscope can be used to visualize the positioning, to insert a guidewire for later advancement of the fine-bore tube, or to pull or push a tube into the small bowel. Double-lumen tubes have also been developed. In these, the aspiration ports of one lumen are positioned in the stomach for gastric decompression while the distal lumen is positioned in the upper jejunum for feeding.

Surgical jejunostomy

Longer term or indefinite feeding is better achieved by either surgical (open or laparoscopic) or percutaneous tube placement (Fig. 8.2). A **surgical jejunostomy** may be performed either as a separate procedure or during the course of an abdominal operation. Jejunostomy should be considered during a laparotomy for patients who are malnourished, traumatized, or undergoing major upper gastrointestinal surgery (oesophagec-

tomy, gastrectomy, or pancreatectomy) where anastomotic leakage may lead to a requirement for prolonged nutritional support. Jejunostomy is contraindicated if there is distal intestinal obstruction, radiation enteritis, or small intestinal Crohn's disease.

Jejunostomy access may be obtained by Witzel, button, or needle jejunostomy techniques. Common to these techniques is the identification, at laparotomy, of a point 20–25 cm distal to the ligament of Treitz where a purse string suture is inserted. The Witzel jejunostomy technique involves an enterotomy at this site, insertion of a feeding tube into the jejunum, tying of the suture, and then approximating the edges of a proximal seromyotomy over the tube to create a tunnel (Fig. 8.3). The feeding

Table 8.10 Complications of surgical jejunostomy

Intraperitoneal leakage of feed and peritonitis

Wound infection

Small bowel obstruction

Unplanned removal

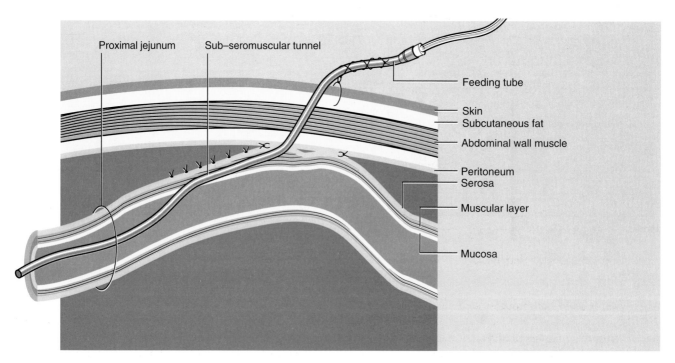

Figure 8.3 Witzel jejunostomy technique.

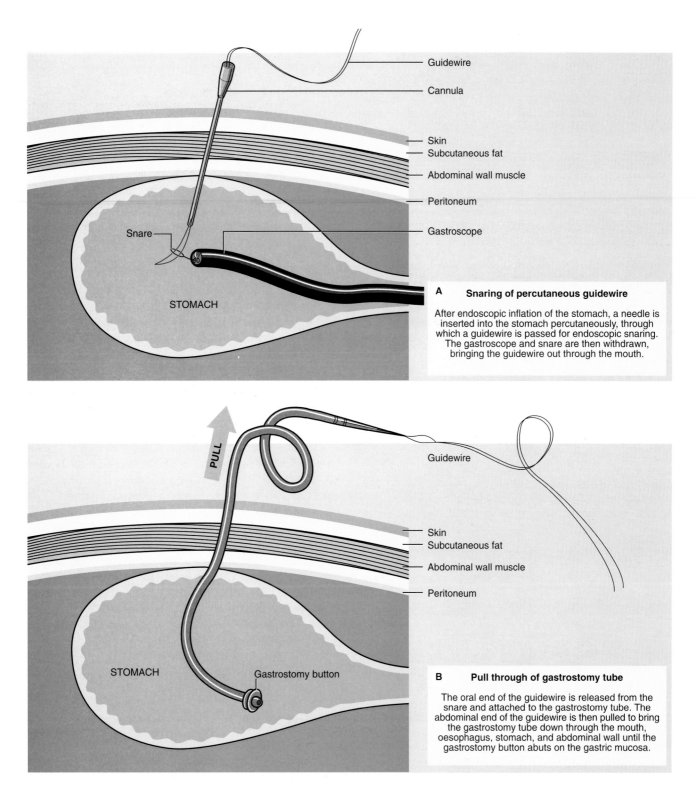

A   **Snaring of percutaneous guidewire**

After endoscopic inflation of the stomach, a needle is inserted into the stomach percutaneously, through which a guidewire is passed for endoscopic snaring. The gastroscope and snare are then withdrawn, bringing the guidewire out through the mouth.

B   **Pull through of gastrostomy tube**

The oral end of the guidewire is released from the snare and attached to the gastrostomy tube. The abdominal end of the guidewire is then pulled to bring the gastrostomy tube down through the mouth, oesophagus, stomach, and abdominal wall until the gastrostomy button abuts on the gastric mucosa.

Figure 8.4 Technique of percutaneous endoscopic gastrostomy (PEG).

tube is then brought out through a separate stab incision with the proximal edges of the tunnel carefully sutured to the peritoneal aspect of the anterior abdominal wall. This technique substantially reduces feeding-related aspiration pneumonia. The button jejunostomy avoids the need for an externally protruding catheter, is as effective, and is associated with a lower incidence of inadvertent tube dislodgement, leakage around the tube, and tube blockage. In the needle catheter jejunostomy technique, a 14-gauge, 5-cm needle is inserted through the pursestring suture to create a submucosal tunnel. A 5-Fr. catheter is then introduced through the needle into the jejunum, before the needle is withdrawn and the catheter is brought out through the abdominal wall. As in other techniques, the jejunum is sutured onto the peritoneal aspect of the anterior abdominal wall. This technique is quick and easy to use but has a higher rate of tube occlusion due to the smaller diameter of the catheter; this makes the technique unsuitable for long-term use. Complications of surgical jejunostomies are given in Table 8.10.

Percutaneous gastrostomy can be performed endoscopically (percutaneous endoscopic gastrostomy; PEG) or fluoroscopically. With both methods the stomach is insufflated with air (endoscopically or via a nasogastric tube) before percutaneous puncture. PEG tubes may be inserted using a direct stab technique or a per-oral pull-through technique (Fig. 8.4). With the direct stab technique, the endoscope is passed into the stomach which is then inflated with air. The cannula is then inserted into the stomach directly through the anterior abdominal wall, a guidewire is passed through the cannula, and the PEG tube inserted through a peel-away sheath. Major psychotic illness, dementia, coagulopathy, peritonitis, and ascites are considered contraindications to PEG tube insertion. The technique carries a morbidity of less than 10 per cent (Table 8.11), a mortality of 2 per cent, and a failure rate of 5 per cent. Failures result from an inability to transilluminate the stomach as a result of previous extensive upper gastrointestinal surgery or extreme obesity. PEG tubes that can be removed by external traction have advantages in terms of ease of use and cost.

For patients who require indefinite enteral access, skin-level gastrostomy **buttons** can be placed in mature ostomies and confer a cosmetic benefit for the patients, as well as being less likely to be pulled out, clogged, or dislodged. A subcutaneous

Table 8.11 Complications of percutaneous gastrostomy

Complications	Comment
Infection	
Local infection	Reduce incidence with prophylactic
Intra-abdominal wall abscesses	antibiotics
Necrotizing fasciitis	
Streptococcal bacteraemia	
Extravasation of air or feed	
Pneumoperitoneum	Resolve spontaneously
Subcutaneous emphysema	
Leakage of feed	Laparotomy
Peritonitis	
Misplacement	
Intracolonic	If prolonged vomiting or diarrhoea,
Gastrocolic fistula	confirm tube position by X-ray
Displacement	Avoid excess local pressure on gastric wall
Gastro-oesophageal regurgitation and aspiration	Convert to percutaneous gastrojejunostomy. Nurse at an angle of 45°
Blockage	Prevent by twice-daily water flush. Clear using papain or chymotrypsin injection

jejunostomy technique has been described where a port is placed in the subcutaneous fat and connected to the jejunal catheter so that the patient has no external tube (Payne-James *et al.* 1995).

4.2 Enteral feed composition

The feed formulation for individual patients will depend on their requirements for energy and nitrogen as well as on the presence and severity of cardiopulmonary, hepatic, renal, or gastrointestinal dysfunction.

Enteral diets may be categorized as polymeric, predigested, disease-specific, or organ-specific. **Polymeric diets** are usually given to patients with normal or near-normal gastrointestinal function and contain whole protein as the nitrogen source, together with a partial hydrolysate of corn starch and triglycerides as the energy source, electrolytes, minerals, trace elements, vitamins, and some also contain fibre. **Predigested diets** (elemental or semi-elemental) are prescribed for patients with nutrient malabsorption and contain partially or completely hydrolysed protein, partially hydrolysed corn starch, a small amount of long-chain triglycerides, electrolytes, minerals, trace elements, and vitamins. Elemental diets contain free L-amino acids, have no potential for antigenicity, and have been shown to have primary therapeutic efficacy in acute Crohn's disease. The recognition that the intestinal mucosal brush border possesses dipeptide and tripeptide transporters has led to increasing use of semi-elemental diets that contain partial hydrolysates of protein. It should be assumed that patients requiring predigested enteral diets will have malabsorption of micronutrients as well as macronutrients, and therefore 100 per cent of the recommended daily allowance of trace elements and vitamins are included in the diet.

There is experimental evidence that polymeric diets are superior to elemental feeds in preventing atrophy of the intestinal mucosa, maintaining mucosal protein and DNA content, secretory IgA production, a normal balance of intestinal microflora, and mucosal barrier function. Adding a fibre source to the polymeric diet is also thought to be beneficial by regulating bowel function, and maintaining small and large intestinal epithelial morphology and barrier function.

Disease-specific diets

Disease-specific diets have been described for patients with cardiopulmonary disease, renal failure, or hepatic failure. For patients with respiratory failure, a diet where the proportion of carbohydrate relative to fat is reduced should be considered. This will reduce the production of carbon dioxide as, for a given amount of oxygen consumed, more carbon dioxide is produced from the metabolism of carbohydrate than from fat or protein. Patients with liver disease and encephalopathy tend to retain sodium, have a reduced ability to assimilate triglycerides, and have increased plasma concentration of aromatic amino acids, which may act as false neurotransmitters. A diet low in sodium, with a mainly carbohydrate energy source and containing a modified mixture of L-amino acids (low in aromatic amino acids and rich in branched-chain amino acids) has therefore been recommended. These diets also contain 100 per cent of vitamin and trace element requirements and are usually energy-dense (1.2–1.5 kcal/ml), as some degree of fluid restriction is often required.

A relatively recent development in nutritional support has been the use of specific nutrient substrates as supplements to standard enteral diets with the aim of supporting the function of individual organs. These **organ-specific diets** are claimed to be beneficial in the support of systemic immune responsiveness and gut mucosal barrier function, and in modulation of neuro-endocrine and cytokine responses as well as Kupffer cell function. In particular, there has been considerable interest in the utilization of specific substrates to maintain intestinal muco-sal integrity as a barrier to bacteria and endotoxin (selective gut nutrition). Substrates suggested as capable of maintaining intestinal integrity include amino acids (glutamine, arginine, and ornithine), fatty acids (short chain and n-3 polyun-saturated), and nucleotides. Arginine, nucleotides, n-3 polyun-saturated fatty acids, and glutamine have all been evaluated as potential immunomodulators. Some of these diets contain more than one new substrate (Impact®: arginine, nucleotide, and n-3 polyunsaturated fatty acid) which makes it more difficult to decide which of the nutrients is actually beneficial. The position that these diets will occupy in the nutritional armamentarium remains to be determined.

4.3 Enteral feeds and their problems

Patients receiving enteral feeds require careful monitoring of fluid and calorie intake, weight, plasma biochemistry (potassium, phosphate, and glucose), and vitamin and trace-element concentrations (if on long-term feeding). In addition to compli-cations associated with feeding tubes (Tables 8.9–8.11), patients may also encounter gastrointestinal (Table 8.12) or metabolic complications related to the feeds. The type and frequency of these complications depends on the underlying disease state, method of access and delivery (gravity versus pump feeding), type of feed, and metabolic state. Aspiration into the respiratory passages may be due to incorrect tube placement, severe gastro-oesophageal reflux, or delayed gastric emptying.

Metabolic complications of enteral nutrition are similar to those associated with parenteral nutrition but are usually less severe because of the homeostatic properties of the intestinal tract. Metabolic complications can be classified as disturbances of electrolyte and sugar balance, deficiencies of vitamins or trace elements, and **tube-feeding syndrome**. Commonest of the electrolyte abnormalities are hyperkalaemia (renal insufficiency, postoperative), hyponatraemia, and hypophosphataemia (hypermetabolic patients, e.g. trauma, surgery, sepsis). The tube-feeding syndrome is caused by hypertonic dehydration with elevated plasma concentrations of sodium, chloride, and ammonia, and is due to inadequate fluid replacement.

5 Parenteral nutrition

Parenteral nutrition is reserved for those patients in whom the gastrointestinal tract is not functional or is inaccessible and who are malnourished or who are likely to become malnourished (Table 8.13). Parenteral nutrition should be established as soon as these conditions are recognized and should be continued for as long as necessary. Parenteral nutrition is contraindicated for patients with terminal disease where there is no specific treatment goal, and carries greater risks in patients with cardiac failure, acidosis, or diabetes.

5.1 Methods of administration

Peripheral veins have, until relatively recently, been considered unsuitable for administration of parenteral nutrition because the hypertonic nutrient solutions frequently caused peripheral

Table 8.12 Enteral feeds and gastrointestinal complications

Symptom	Cause	Solution
Diarrhoea	Reduced intestinal absorptive capacity	◆ Slow transit (loperamide) ◆ Replace fluids via intravenous line
	Hyperosmolar feed (elemental diet)	◆ Change to predigested formula
	Too rapid or irregular administration	◆ Reduce feeding rate ◆ Give as pump-controlled continuous infusion
	Bacterial contamination (prolonged infusion, ascending contamination)	◆ Handle feeding system with sterile gloves ◆ Minimize handling using large-volume reservoirs, closed administration system and sterile gloves ◆ Daily change of infusion set
	Low feed temperature	◆ Warm to room temperature
	Drugs (e.g. antacids, digoxin, propranolol, antibiotics) Intolerance of lactose (alactasia) ◆ Intolerance of lipids (pancreatic or hepatobiliary disease or postgastrectomy)	◆ Stop or administer parenterally ◆ Low-lactose formulae ◆ Replace long-chain triglycerides with medium-chain triglycerides
Constipation	Inadequate fluid replacement	◆ Increase fluid replacement
Reflux, vomiting, and bronchial aspiration	◆ Proximal position of tip of tube ◆ Too rapid infusion rate	◆ Three-hourly gastric aspiration during first 24 hours of enteral feeding to assess tolerance ◆ 45° elevation of head and chest

Table 8.13 Indications for parenteral nutrition

Postoperatively

(enteral feeding contraindicated for more than 5 days)

Short bowel syndrome

Gastrointestinal fistulae

Prolonged paralytic ileus

Acute pancreatitis

Multiple injuries involving viscera

Major sepsis

Severe burns

Inflammatory bowel disease

Table 8.14 Complications of attempted cannulation of central veins

Structure	Injury
Arteries	Haematoma
	Laceration (haemothorax, haemomediastinum)
	Arteriovenous fistula
Lymphatics	Laceration of thoracic duct
Lung	Pneumothorax
Nerves	Brachial plexus injury
	Recurrent laryngeal nerve injury
Heart	Arrhythmia

vein thrombophlebitis. Improvements in catheter design and alterations in nutrient composition have made peripheral parenteral nutrition a feasible alternative to the central venous route for patients who require supplemental or near-total parenteral support for short periods.

Peripheral parenteral nutrition can be used in patients where the requirement for nutritional support is short term (1–4 weeks) and there are adequate peripheral veins. In addition, peripheral veins may be used when central veins are inaccessible due to local surgery, local injury, or thrombosis, or when central venous catheterization is contraindicated because of a high risk of fungal or bacterial sepsis (e.g. purulent tracheostomy secretions, immune deficiency states, history of repeated septic episodes). The most common indication for peripheral parenteral nutrition is to build up reserves of marginally depleted patients pre- and postoperatively. The particular concerns regarding peripheral parenteral feeding are: progressive thrombophlebitis and obliteration of peripheral veins; its low caloric density necessitating the administration of large fluid volumes; and its lack of nutritional balance.

Central parenteral nutrition will be required for patients who have high requirements for fluids (short bowel syndrome) or calories and nitrogen (hypercatabolic), or who require parenteral nutrition in the longer term. Central parenteral nutrition is achieved by cannulation of a tributary of one of the large veins draining into the superior vena cava (cephalic, external jugular,

internal jugular, or subclavian) or inferior vena cava (long saphenous vein). Access may be achieved by either percutaneous puncture or a cut-down technique. Percutaneous puncture of central veins has a low complication rate in experienced hands but some complications can be fatal. Complications can be classified as due to incorrect placement (Table 8.14) or incorrect handling (embolism with air, guidewire, or catheter). The cephalic, jugular, and saphenous veins can be readily exposed under local anaesthetic in adults.

It is usually assumed that tributaries that access the superior vena cava should be the first choice, as these achieve a higher flow rate and carry a lower risk of infection. A tunnelled line inserted into the right subclavian vein via the infraclavicular approach (Fig. 8.5) is often preferred for central parenteral nutrition. Tunnelled lines are said to have a lower incidence of infection and restrict movement less, use of the right side avoids risk of injury to the thoracic duct and avoid some of the problems of jugular venous lines which are difficult to dress adequately and tend to restrict neck movements.

Central venous catheters need to be firm during insertion yet soft, of low thrombogenicity, and resistant to kinking during use. Most are made from polyvinyl chloride, polyurethane, polytetrafluoroethylene, or silicone elastomer. Catheters now often have integral clamps (to reduce catheter damage) and subcutaneous Dacron cuffs (to prevent inadvertent removal and reduce ascending-track infection). Single-lumen catheters are preferred for parenteral nutrition as multiple-lumen catheters are more likely to become infected because of increased handling.

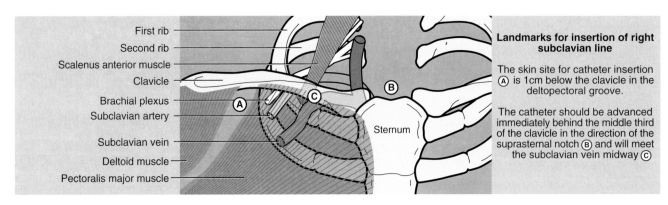

Figure 8.5 Landmarks for insertion of right subclavian line.

However, scheduled changing of multiple lumen catheters every 72 hours has been shown to reduce sepsis rates to an incidence comparable with single-lumen catheters. Catheters that are heparin- or antibiotic-bonded are currently under evaluation.

Implantable central venous catheter systems are of little benefit for short-term parenteral nutrition as they require surgical insertion and removal, but may be useful in patients requiring home parenteral nutrition who wish to undertake regular swimming. The catheter is inserted in the same way as for a conventional catheter and is then tunnelled to a reservoir that sits in a subcutaneous pocket over a bony point.

5.2 Composition of parenteral nutrition

Parenteral nutrient solutions need to provide adequate calories, protein, essential fatty acids, electrolytes, vitamins, and trace elements (zinc, copper, manganese, and chromium). Approximate caloric needs can be calculated using the Harris–Benedict equations, as described in Box 8.1, and are usually supplied as dextrose or a combination of dextrose and fat. Crystalline L-amino acids are the source of nitrogen in parenteral nutrition. Fluid and electrolyte requirements depend on pre-existing abnormalities, ongoing losses, and on the presence of cardiac, renal, or pulmonary dysfunction. Vitamin and trace element supplements are available commercially and designed to be added directly to parenteral nutrition solutions.

Dextrose monohydrate is inexpensive but has a low caloric density (3.4 kcal/g). Therefore, if caloric targets are to be met by dextrose alone without fluid overload, it is necessary to administer highly concentrated dextrose solutions (15–35 per cent dextrose). As adult peripheral veins can only tolerate dextrose in a concentration of 8–10 per cent, these highly concentrated dextrose solutions must be administered by central venous cannulae.

Intravenous **fat** may be administered as a source of essential polyunsaturated fatty acids (linoleic, arachidonic, and linolenic acids) or of isotonic non-protein calories. The essential fatty acids are required for the maintenance of cell membrane stability and for prostaglandin synthesis. Exogenous supplementation is necessary only for linoleic acid as both arachidonic acid and linolenic acids can be synthesized from this. Commercially available fat emulsions are composed of soybean oil or a combination of soybean and safflower oils, and include egg-yolk phospholipids as emulsifying agents and glycerin to maintain tonicity. These oils contain triglycerides composed of long-chain fatty acids, principally linoleic acid. Parenteral fat emulsions are supplied as 10 per cent (1.1 kcal/ml) and 20 per cent (2 kcal/ml) emulsions in 50–500 ml containers. The high caloric density of fat emulsions (9 kcal/g) is beneficial in patients who are fluid-restricted, glucose-intolerant, or have only peripheral venous access. The parenteral administration of fat is contraindicated in patients who have severe egg allergies or abnormalities of fat metabolism due to hereditary disorders or pancreatitis.

There has been a hesitancy about the inclusion of lipid emulsions in parenteral nutrient solutions. Some authorities have considered essential fatty-acid deficiency to be too rare to justify the routine use of fat emulsions. In addition, fat emulsions are more expensive and less protein-sparing than dextrose, have suppressive effects on the reticuloendothelial system, and may give rise to fatty infiltration of the liver.

These criticisms have led to a search for a lipid source that is less toxic and used more efficiently. Two of the alternatives considered are a medium-chain and long-chain triglyceride mixture and the use of structured lipids. Medium-chain triglycerides are hydrolysed rapidly and absorbed in the intestinal tract. Administration of a solution containing a mixture of medium-chain and long-chain triglycerides produces fewer circulating triglycerides and non-esterified fatty acids than solutions containing only long-chain triglycerides, which suggests more favourable fat utilization. Structured lipids are man-made and have been synthesized from a combination of long-chain triglycerides and coconut oils. There is some experimental evidence that structured lipids improve nitrogen retention, reduce infection rates, and improve survival. These effects are assumed to be the result of lowered production of inflammatory and immunosuppressive eicosanoids.

The use of a combination of dextrose and fat as the calorie source has been reported to confer several advantages (Table 8.15). If such a combination is used, a minimum of 100–150 g/day of glucose should be administered (to inhibit gluconeogenesis from protein sources) and fat should provide no more than 30 per cent non-protein calories (to avoid overwhelming the body's fat-clearance capacity).

Parenteral solutions should contain all the essential **amino acids** and provision of a well-balanced mixture of the amino acids used in protein synthesis promotes positive nitrogen balance. The essential amino acids should provide about 40 per cent of the total amino nitrogen. A daily intake of 12–16 g of nitrogen with the appropriate non-protein calories is necessary to limit protein breakdown and support synthesis of structural and functional proteins. Nitrogen requirements will be higher in young men with a large body frame or in those subjected to traumatic or septic insults.

Requirements of 2000 kcal and 14 g nitrogen/day for an uncomplicated surgical patient may be met with a dextrose–amino-acid solution with or without added fat. The calorie to nitrogen ratio should be in the range of 100–150 : 1 (Table 8.16).

Table 8.15 Advantages of a dual-energy source of non-protein calories

More physiological
Prevents essential fatty-acid deficiency
Improves protein synthesis
Reduces hepatic dysfunction
Decreases generation of CO_2
Reduces the risk of hypophosphataemia
Reduces energy expenditure
Less stimulation of the sympathetic system

Table 8.16 Standard regimens to provide 2000 kcal and 14 g nitrogen

	Regimen
Dextrose	
with fat	250 g
without fat	500 g
Nitrogen	14 g
Fat (soybean oil)	100 g
Sodium	70–115 mmol
Potassium	60–100 mmol
Calcium	7.5–11 mmol
Magnesium	9.5–19 mmol
Phosphate	20–40 mmol
Chloride	103–160 mmol
Zinc	40 μmol

Electrolyte content is varied according to daily biochemical results. Additives required include trace elements (e.g. 1 × 10 ml ampoule of Additrace®) and vitamins (e.g. 1 vial MV1–12).

Such a standard parenteral solution has been shown to be suitable for 70–80 per cent of surgical patients. Standard solutions are cost-effective as they permit bulk purchase, reduce pharmacy workload, and minimize waste. An initial rate of infusion of 40 ml/h is advised when standard 15–25 per cent dextrose-based formulations are used. Once parenteral nutrition tolerance has been established, the rate can be increased to achieve the calorie target. Fat is usually included in solutions for peripheral parenteral nutrition to achieve calorie requirements (up to, but not more than, 60 per cent of total calories) and to decrease fluid volume requirements.

All-in-one ('big bag') systems for parenteral nutrition are widely used in the UK. The solutions are prepared in a single container in a sterile environment in the hospital pharmacy or by a commercial company. This system allows modification of the solution depending on an individual's electrolyte requirements, reduces the risk of infection, makes administration easier and more evenly balanced. Simultaneous infusion of dextrose and amino acids promotes optimal nitrogen balance. The main concerns of all-in-one systems relate to the stability of lipid emulsions and chemical incompatibilities.

Disease-specific parenteral solutions have been designed for patients who have been injured, are catabolically stressed, or have renal or hepatic dysfunction. Branched-chain amino-acid-enriched solutions have been advocated for patients with trauma, catabolic stress, and hepatic dysfunction, where low plasma concentrations of branched-chain amino acids have been described (leucine, isoleucine, and valine). However, clinical trials with these solutions in patients with hypercatabolism or hepatic failure have not demonstrated any improvement in nitrogen balance or mortality compared to standard amino-acid formulations. Parenteral solutions containing only essential amino acids have been suggested for patients with acute renal failure, to prevent the development of hyperuraemia, but again have not been shown to be effective.

As with enteral nutrients, there has been considerable interest in the parenteral administration of **organ-specific** solutions, with the aim of maintaining intestinal mucosal integrity or altering inflammatory and immune responses. Glutamine has attracted most attention as a substrate for maintaining intestinal function. None of the commercially available amino-acid solutions contain glutamine, due to its instability in aqueous solutions. This has led to the synthesis of short-chain peptides

Table 8.17 Biochemical monitoring of patients on parenteral nutrition

	During first week or until metabolically stable	After one week or when metabolically stable	Long-term (home)
Sodium	Daily	Alternate days	6 weeks
Potassium	Daily	Alternate days	6 weeks
Chloride	Daily	Alternate days	6 weeks
Total CO$_2$	Daily	Alternate days	6 weeks
Urea	Daily	Alternate days	6 weeks
Creatinine	Daily	Alternate days	6 weeks
Glucose	Daily	Alternate days	6 weeks
Phosphate	Daily	Twice per week	3 months
Calcium	Alternate days	Weekly	3 months
Magnesium	Alternate days	Weekly	3 months
Total protein	Alternate days	Weekly	3 months
Albumin	Alternate days	Weekly	3 months
Lipid profile	Twice weekly	Weekly	3 months
Liver function	Twice weekly	Weekly	3 months
Selenium, iron, copper	Only if deficiency suspected	Monthly	3 months
Vitamins A, C, E, B$_{12}$	Only if deficiency suspected	Monthly	3 months
Zinc	Weekly	2 weeks	3 months

Table 8.18 Biochemical problems in patients on parenteral nutrition

Problem	Most common cause	Investigations	Action
Hypophosphataemia ($PO_4 < 0.5$ mmol/l)	Refeeding after a period of malnutrition		Consult clinical chemist
Hypernatraemia ($Na^+ > 150$ mmol/l)	Negative water balance	Plasma osmolality; urinary electrolytes and osmolality	Review fluid balance Correct dehydration
Hyponatraemia ($Na^+ < 130$ mmol/l)	Fluid overload; diuretic use	Plasma osmolality; urinary electrolytes and osmolality	Treat cause
Hyperglycaemia	Metabolic stress		Review calorie administration; consider starting insulin

containing glutamine (alanyl-glutamine, glycyl-glutamine) for use in parenteral nutrient solutions. Parenteral solutions containing alanyl-glutamine improved nitrogen balance in patients with severe accidental trauma, and maintained intramuscular glutamine concentrations close to preoperative values in patients undergoing elective colorectal resection for carcinoma.

5.3 Problems associated with parenteral nutrition

Patients receiving parenteral nutrition require careful monitoring of their fluid balance (daily), weight (daily), temperature (6 hourly), line entry site (daily), full blood picture (daily), and appropriate biochemistry (Table 8.17). In addition to complications that may occur at the time of central catheter placement (described above), administration of parenteral nutrition may also be complicated by catheter infection, blockage or leakage, central vein thrombosis, and metabolic abnormalities (Table 8.18).

Central line infection may be caused by invasion of microorganisms along the path of the catheter from its entry site or by invasion through the catheter lumen from the infusion system. Central line infection may be as common as 12.5 per cent in patients given parenteral nutrition on general wards. Such an infection is a major and life-threatening complication which is often difficult and expensive to treat. The risks of line infection may be reduced if the lines are inserted by only one designated and experienced clinician under full aseptic conditions, are tunnelled subcutaneously, and dressed by a small number of trained nurses following an agreed aseptic protocol. The line infection rate can be further reduced if solutions are put together inside a laminar flow cabinet by experienced pharmacy staff, if no additions are made outside the pharmacy, if solutions and giving sets are changed only by experienced nurses using a strict technique, and if the central line is used exclusively for intravenous nutrition.

A wide range of biochemical problems may occur in patients receiving parenteral feeding. The most common abnormalities relate to disturbances in plasma sodium, phosphate, and glucose concentrations. Disturbances in acid–base balance, plasma lipid concentrations, liver function, and deficiencies of essential fatty acids or trace elements should be discussed with a clinical chemist.

As enteral nutrition, either orally or by feeding tube, becomes tolerated, parenteral nutrition can be weaned off. Weaning is usually done by reducing the delivery of the parenteral feeding at a rate of 20–40 ml/h/day until a rate of 40 ml/hour is reached, when the parenteral nutrition can be discontinued.

6 Hazards of nutritional support

A recent meta-analysis has shown that patients treated enterally experience fewer complications than those treated parenterally (41 versus 52 per cent). This difference is due mainly to the frequency of infective complications (16 versus 35 per cent). In addition, complications associated with enteral feeding are usually not life-threatening and are easier and less costly to treat.

It can be concluded:

(1) that wherever possible the enteral route should be used;

(2) if parenteral nutrition is necessary, the central lines should be inserted by an experienced operator;

(3) the central lines should only be looked after by trained staff according to strict protocols and should not be used for any other purpose.

It has been shown that the incidence of central line sepsis can be reduced tenfold (27 to 2.5 per cent) by the introduction of nutritional support teams (King's Fund Centre 1992). This was estimated to produce a cost saving of between £1650 and £5000 per episode of line infection at 1992 prices, depending on whether the patient was occupying a general ward or high-dependency unit bed.

7 Multidisciplinary nutritional support teams

Although the indications for and techniques of artificial nutritional support are well established, national surveys have shown great diversity in nutritional support practices in UK hospitals. One of the main deficiencies identified was a lack of organization of nutritional support in at least two-thirds of hospitals. A coordinated multidisciplinary team approach to nutritional support reduces the incidence of complications due

Table 8.19 Members of a nutritional support team

Member	Main responsibility	Shared role
Clinician	Liaise with the patient's clinical team Place central lines and feeding tubes Prescribe parenteral nutrition	Supervision of nutritional support Training of staff, patients, and carers
Nurse	Prepare, teach, and supervise protocols for the care of central lines and enteral feeding tubes Assist with, or perform, placement of central lines and feeding tubes Liaise with relatives and the community team for patients requiring home nutritional support	Audit outcome
Dietician	Assess dietary intake Assess nutritional status Calculate nutritional requirements Design enteral feeding regimen	
Pharmacist	Provide enteral feeds and sterile parenteral nutrition solutions Advise on compatibility of nutrient mixtures and on drug reactions	

to central vein catheterization, catheter sepsis, and metabolic disturbance, as well as reducing cost. Cost reduction is achieved by more appropriate prescribing of parenteral nutrition, reducing complications, reducing waste, using less expensive preparations, and reducing length of hospital stay.

A typical nutritional support teams consists of four members with overlapping responsibility—clinician, dietician, nurse, and pharmacist (Table 8.19). Teams also need to have close liaison with a bacteriologist, infection-control nurse, and chemical pathologist. Some nutritional support teams provide an advice and staff-training service only. In other hospitals all patients requiring artificial nutritional support will be concentrated on a single ward, with nutritional care being restricted to team members. There is evidence that a team that controls and supervises enteral tube and parenteral feeds leads to better quality of care than a team that only advises. However, it has been found that clinical colleagues cooperate best when an advice service is offered with a willingness to undertake a patient's nutritional care on request.

Nutritional support teams have taken on a range of responsibilities, including those of improving recognition of malnourished inpatients, providing advice on the appropriate method of nutritional support for individuals, providing a coordinated central line and feeding tube insertion service, day-to-day monitoring of patients on artificial nutritional support, training and supervising patients requiring home artificial nutritional support, and auditing the outcome of artificial

nutritional support. The potential advantages of a nutritional support team are shown in Table 8.20.

8 Home nutritional support

Refinements in the techniques of enteral and parenteral nutrition have allowed patients dependent on artificial nutrition to escape from an institution to independence, a home environment, increased activity, and more normal relationships. Domiciliary treatment frees a hospital bed and reduces costs. However, it is limited by a patient's or carer's manual dexterity and ability to understand the technique, its potential complications and how to deal with these complications. Home nutritional support is not indicated for patients whose underlying illness is likely to progress rapidly with deteriorating quality of life.

Home parenteral nutrition (HPN) was first described in 1970. It is relatively expensive, demanding on both patients and carers, and associated with potentially serious complications, such as catheter-related sepsis, central vein thrombosis, and hepatobiliary disease. However, HPN has been used successfully to maintain the nutritional status of patients for many years, replacing or supplementing oral nutrition. Home enteral nutrition (HEN) is considerably safer and cheaper (the cost of nutrient solutions and materials necessary for catheter care result in HPN costing up to 10 times as much as HEN).

8.1 Home parenteral nutrition

The indication for HPN is intestinal failure, as a result of either a short or diseased gut where nutritional, water, and electrolyte deficits cannot be corrected by the enteral route (Table 8.21). Patients with a short bowel length, generally less than 150 cm as an end jejunostomy, or of less than 60 cm with residual colon, will require supplemental HPN—as well as intravenous fluid and electrolyte supplementation—for a variable period. More controversial indications are AIDS and intestinal obstruction due to cancer.

Table 8.20 Advantages of nutrition team

Action	Outcome
Guidelines for use of nutritional support	Avoid unnecessary treatment Reduce complications Reduce cost

Simplify treatment regimens
  Standardize nutrients
  Standardize equipment
	Enable bulk purchase
	Reduce cost

Monitor use of nutritional support	Reduce waste Improve outcome

Table 8.21 Indications for home parenteral nutrition

Short bowel syndrome	Intestinal disease
Primary	Stenoses and fistulae
trauma	radiation enteritis
volvulus	Crohn's disease
ischaemia	
Secondary	Obstruction
radiation enteritis	idiopathic pseudo-obstruction
Crohn's disease	

Life has been significantly improved for patients receiving HPN as a result of simplified administration systems (all-in-one bags), improved mobility (cyclical nocturnal feeding), and reduced complications (training programmes and oral nutrient intake). Oral feeding reduces the incidence of biliary sludging, gallstones, fatty liver, and vitamin or trace-element deficiency, while also promoting intestinal adaptation. Patients with cardiac or renal failure or who require more than 3.5 litres fluid daily are not suitable for cyclical HPN.

Vascular access for HPN is most commonly by a silicone elastomer, central venous, tunnelled catheter placed via the subclavian vein into the superior vena cava. Both externalized catheters and implanted reservoirs are suitable. There is some evidence that infection rates and patient acceptance are better with implanted reservoirs. Patients on HPN require storage space for disposables, hygienic work surfaces and washing facilities, appropriate equipment (trolley, pump, refrigerator), an established routine for nutrient delivery, a phone link with the treating team, and regular review for monitoring of nutritional status.

The main complications of HPN are tunnel or catheter infection (one every 2.5 years), catheter blockage (one every 5.5 years), catheter migration (one every 10 years), and central venous thrombosis (one every 20 years), as well as metabolic complications (biliary tract disease, liver function disturbance, osteopenia). Complications of HPN, in particular catheter-related infection, are inversely related to the treating team's experience with HPN. It has therefore been proposed that these patients should only be looked after by multidisciplinary teams in specialist centres with considerable experience of both parenteral and enteral nutrition, with established protocols for patient selection, management, and funding. Complete autonomy in HPN techniques usually requires 3 weeks of training of the patient by an experienced team. The ideals of a HPN programme are a negligible rate of catheter-related sepsis, fewer than 4 per cent deaths due to HPN administration, and a duration of hospital readmission for HPN complications that is less than 4 per cent of the time spent at home.

Quality of life for patients on HPN is poorer in those who are single, over 65, or with systemic disease. Weaning from HPN within a year is possible in about 40 per cent of patients as a result of improvement in underlying disease, intestinal adaptation, or surgical intervention. The 5-year survival for patients on HPN for intestinal failure due to benign disease is 62 per cent, but depends on disease category, being best for those with Crohn's disease and worst in radiation enteritis.

8.2 Home enteral nutrition

Improvements in feeding tubes and pumps and the commercial development of sterile complete enteral feeds have facilitated safe and cost-effective management of many patients in their own homes. HEN is indicated for patients who have anorexia or swallowing difficulties and for those with impaired intestinal absorption where overnight administration maximally utilizes absorptive capacity and encourages adaptation (Table 8.22). Cyclical feeding, where possible, has significant advantages over continuous feeding in promoting psychological well-being and in improving nitrogen retention with less fat deposition.

For HEN, fine-bore nasogastric tubes are preferred for those who require short periods of nutritional support (Crohn's disease, cystic fibrosis) whereas PEG tubes are more convenient for patients with swallowing disorders. Small, portable pumps powered by rechargeable batteries enable patients who require continuous nutrient infusion to be mobile, whereas large, non-portable pumps are satisfactory for those who require overnight feeding alone. Most patients are adequately nourished with polymeric whole-protein feeds, which are considerably cheaper than the elemental diets necessary for some patients with Crohn's disease or the branched-chain amino-acid-enriched solutions advised for those with chronic liver disease and encephalopathy.

Patients and their carers require careful explanation of the reasons for treatment as well as training in the insertion of nasogastric tubes, care and use of infusion pumps, handling of enteral feeds, and instruction about recognition and treatment of complications. Patients on HEN require monitoring of their nutritional status, psychological adaptation, and underlying disease, and are therefore best managed in major centres where

Table 8.22 Indications for home enteral nutrition

Inability to eat	Anorexia	Inadequate intestinal function
Neurological disorders	Malignancy	Crohn's disease
cerebral palsy	Chronic renal failure	Short bowel syndrome
cerebrovascular accidents	Chronic infection	intestinal infarction
motor neurone disease	Crohn's disease	trauma
Malignancy of mouth or oesophagus		

a multidisciplinary nutritional support team can provide telephone advice 24 hours a day.

9 Conclusions

Malnutrition is prevalent among surgical patients in hospital, particularly in those with cancer, critical illness, or gastro-intestinal disease. Malnourished patients often have more adverse clinical outcomes when compared with normally nourished individuals with the same diagnoses. Available enteral and parenteral feeding techniques can deliver nutritional support both safely and efficaciously to these malnourished patients.

Unfortunately, in UK clinical practice, there remain deficiencies in identifying malnourished patients and in the appropriate application of established principles of nutritional support. It is expected that this will be improved by the setting up of nutritional support teams in more UK hospitals as a result of the driving force of the British Association for Parenteral and Enteral Nutrition (BAPEN). Nutrition assessment should become a mandatory part of the admission assessment of patients to surgical wards, and nutritional support is an essential component of the therapeutic options of surgeons. It is likely that there will be continuing extensive research into novel nutritional substrates that may modify the outcome of disease.

Bibliography

Albina, J.E. (1995). Nutrition and wound healing. In *Nutrition for the Hospitalized Patient*. M.H. Torosian (ed.), pp 57–83. Marcel Dekker, New York.

Albina, J.E. (1998). Problems of total parenteral nutrition. *Arch. Surg.*, **133**, 679–80.

American Gastroenterological Association (1995). Medical Position Statement: guidelines for the use of enteral nutrition. *Gastroenterology*, **108**, 1280–301.

American Society for Parenteral and Enteral Nutrition Board of Directors (1986). Guidelines for the use of total parenteral nutrition in the hospitalized adult patient. *J. Parent. Ent. Nutr.*, **10**, 441–5.

American Society for Parenteral and Enteral Nutrition Board of Directors (1993). Guidelines for provision of nutritional support. *J. Parent. Ent. Nutr.*, **17** (Suppl. 1).

Babineau, T.J. and Blackburn, G.L. (1994). Time to consider early gut feeding. *Crit. Care Med.*, **22**, 191–3.

Baumgartner, T.G. and Cerda, J.J. (1993). Enteral nutrition. *Curr. Opin. Gastroenterol.*, **9**, 284–91.

Bhandarkar, D.S., Evans, D.A., and Taylor, T.V. (1994). Minimally invasive techniques for gaining access to the gut. *Min. Inv. Ther.*, **3**, 13–17.

Bower, R.H. (1990). Nutritional and metabolic support of critically ill patients. *J. Parent. Ent. Nutr.*, **14**, 257S–259S.

Bowling, T.E. (1995). Enteral-feeding-related diarrhoea: proposed causes and possible solutions. *Proc. Nutr. Soc.*, **54**, 579–90.

British Association for Parenteral and Enteral Nutrition (1994a). *Enteral and parenteral nutrition in the community.* BAPEN, Maidenhead.

British Association for Parenteral and Enteral Nutrition (1994b). *Organization of nutritional support in hospitals.* Working Party of the British Association for Parenteral and Enteral Nutrition, Maidenhead.

Buzby, G.P., Williford, W.O., Peterson, O.L., Crosby, L.O., Page, C.P., Reinhardt, G.F., Mullen, J.L. (1988). A randomized clinical trial of total parenteral nutrition in malnourished surgical patients. *Am. J. Clin. Nutr.*, **47**, (Suppl): 357–65 [*The VA study*]

Cerra, F.B. (1990). How nutrition intervention changes what getting sick means. *J. Parent. Ent. Nutr.* **14**, 164S–169S.

Clevenger, F.W. (1993). Nutritional support in the patient with the systemic inflammatory response syndrome. *Am. J. Surg.* **165**, 68S–74S.

Detsky, A.S. (1995). Evaluating a mature technology: long-term home parenteral nutrition. *Gastroenterology*, **108**, 1302–4.

Doyle, F.M. and Kennedy, N.P. (1994). Nutritional support via percutaneous gastrostomy. *Proc. Nutr. Soc.*, **53**, 473–82.

Elia, M. (1995). Changing concepts of nutrient requirements in disease: implications for artificial nutritional support. *Lancet*, **345**, 1279–84.

Elia, M. and Jebb, S.A. (1994). Nutrition. *Medicine International*, **22**, 381–420. The Medicine Group, Abingdon.

Gardiner, K.R., Kirk, S.J., and Rowlands, B.J. (1995). Novel substrates to maintain gut integrity. *Nutr. Res. Rev.*, **8**, 43–66.

Grant, A. and Todd, E. (1987). *Enteral and parenteral nutrition*, (2nd edn). Blackwell Scientific Publications, Oxford.

Grant, J.P. (1991). Total parenteral nutrition. *Curr. Pract. Surg.*, **3**, 38–43.

Grant, J.P. (1994). Nutritional support in critically ill patients. *Ann. Surg.* **5**, 610–16.

Grant, J.P. (1995). On enteral nutrition during multimodality therapy in upper gastrointestinal cancer patients. *Ann. Surg.*, **221**, 325–6.

Grimble, G.K., Payne-James, J.J., Rees, R.G.P., and Silk, D.B.A. (1990). *Nutritional support—theory and practice.* Medical Tribune UK Limited.

Hansell, D.T. (1989). Intravenous nutrition: the central or peripheral route? *Inten. Ther. Clin. Monit.*, 185–90.

Heyland, D.K., Cook, D.J., and Guyatt, G.H. (1993). Enteral nutrition in the critically ill patient: a critical review of the evidence. *Inten. Care Med.*, **19**, 435–42.

Heyland, D.K., Cook, D.J., and Guyatt, G.H. (1994). Does the formulation of enteral feeding products influence the infectious morbidity and mortality rates in the critically ill patient? A critical review of the evidence. *Crit. Care Med.*, **22**, 1192–202.

Hill, G.L. (1992). *Disorders of nutrition and metabolism in clinical surgery—understanding and management.* Churchill Livingstone, Edinburgh.

Howard, L., Ament, M., Fleming, C.R., Shike, M., and Steiger, E. (1995). Current use and clinical outcome of home parenteral and enteral nutrition therapies in the United States. *Gastroenterology*, **109**, 355–65.

Jenkins, A.P. and Thompson, R.P.H. (1994). Enteral nutrition and the small intestine. *Gut*, **35**, 1765–9.

King's Fund Centre (1992). *Working party on the role of enteral and parenteral feeding in hospital and at home. A positive approach to nutrition as treatment.* King's Fund Centre.

Lipman, T.O. (1995). Bacterial translocation and enteral nutrition in humans: an outsider looks in. *J. Parent. Ent. Nutr.*, **19**, 156–65.

Lo, C.W. and Walker, W.A. (1989). Changes in the gastrointestinal tract during enteral or parenteral feeding. *Nutr. Rev.*, **47**, 193–8.

Lowry, S.F. (1990). The route of feeding influences injury responses. *J. Trauma*, **30**, S10–S15.

Lundholm, K., Hyltander, A., and Sandström, R. (1992). Nutrition and multiple organ failure. *Nutr. Res. Rev.*, **5**, 97–113.

McCarthy, M.C. (1991). Nutritional support in the critically ill surgical patient. *Surg. Clin. North Am.*, **71**, 831–41.

McMahon, M.M., Farnell, M.B., and Murray, M.J. (1993). Nutritional support of critically ill patients. *Mayo Clin. Proc.*, **68**, 911–20.

Mainous, M.R. and Deitch, E.A. (1994). Nutrition and infection. *Surg. Clin. North Am.*, **74**, 659–76.

Manning, E.M.C. and Shenkin, A. (1993). Parenteral nutrition in the hospitalized patient. *Curr. Opin. Gastroenterol.* **9**, 292–7.

Maynard, N.D. and Bihari, D.J. (1991). Postoperative feeding. Time to rehabilitate the gut. *BMJ*, **303**, 1007–8.

Meguid, M.M., Blackburn, G.L., Jeejeebhoy, K.N., and Ogoshi, S. (1995). The skeleton in the hospital closet—20 years later: malnutrition in patients with GI disease, cancer and AIDS. *Nutrition, Supplement*, **11**, 192–254.

Moran, B.J. (1994). Access methods in nutritional support. *Proc. Nutr. Soc.*, **53**, 465–71.

Payne-James, J., Grimble, G., and Silk, D. (1995). *Artificial nutritional support in clinical practice.* Arnold, London.

Plester, C.E. and Fearon, K.C.H. (1995). Nutrition in the surgical patient. *Surgery*, 160–3. The Medicine Group, Abingdon.

Powell-Tuck, J. (1994). Management of gut failure: a physician's view. *Lancet*, **344**, 1061–4.

Raper, S. and Maynard, N. (1992). Feeding the critically ill patient. *Br. J. Nursing*, **1**, 273–80.

Reed, C.R., Sessler, C.N., Glauser, F.L., and Phelan, B.A. (1995). Central venous catheter infections: concepts and controversies. *Inten. Care Med.*, **21**, 177–83.

Reynolds, N., McWhirter, J.P., and Pennington, C.R. (1995). Nutritional Support Teams: an integral part of developing a gastroenterology service. *Gut*, **37**, 740–2.

Saunders, C., Nishikawa, R., and Wolfe, B. (1993). Surgical nutrition: a review. *J.R. Coll. Surg. Edinburgh*, **38**, 195–204.

Silk, D. (1995). Nutrition for gastroenterologists: when, how and for how long? *Europ. J. Gastroenterol. Hepatol.*, 7, 491–532.

Silk, D.B.A. and Grimble, G.K. (1994). Gut mucosal nutritional support—enteral nutrition as primary therapy? Proceedings of the Abbott Ross Research Conference, Vevey, Switzerland 28–30 June 1992. *Gut*, **35**, (Suppl. 1), S1–S80.

Solomon, S.M. and Kirby, D.F. (1990). The refeeding syndrome: a review. *J. Parent. Ent. Nutr.*, **14**, 90–7.

Torosian, M.H. (1995). *Nutrition for the Hospitalized Patient—Basic Science and Principles of Practice.* Marcel Dekker, New York.

Truswell, A.S. (1992). *ABC of Nutrition.* BMJ Publishing Group, London.

Twomey, P.L. and Patching, S.C. (1995). Cost-effectiveness of nutritional support. *J. Parent. Ent. Nutr.*, **9**, 3–10.

van den Broeck, J. (1995). Malnutrition and mortality. *J. Roy. Soc. Med.*, **88**, 487–90.

Veterans Affairs TPN Cooperative Study Group (Buzby, G.P., Blouin, G., Colling, C.L. *et al.* 1991). Perioperative total parenteral nutrition in surgical patients. *N. Engl. J. Med.*, **325**, 525–32.

Ward, B.A. (1992). Parenteral nutrition. *Curr. Opin. Gastroenterol.*, **8**, 296–301.

CHAPTER 9

Surgical aspects of haematology

T.P. Baglin

1 Laboratory investigation

1.1 Sample identification

It is essential that all samples sent to the laboratory are identified correctly. In the case of samples sent for red cell compatibility testing, with a view to transfusion therapy, the need for correct labelling cannot be emphasized strongly enough. The majority of fatal transfusion reactions are the result of clerical errors (see below). All samples should be labelled with four points of identification: **first name, surname, hospital number, date of birth**. The destination for the result should be clearly indicated to prevent delays, and relevant clinical details indicated to assist interpretation of results and the need for further laboratory evaluation.

In the accident and emergency department, a number of casualties may all be candidates for transfusion therapy. In such an emergency, incompatible transfusions due to wrong identification can easily occur. If hospital numbers are not immediately available, it is essential that the casualty department can label patients with unique accident patient identification numbers so that samples taken will be identified correctly. Transfusions must be commenced only after a bedside check to ensure that the correct blood product is given to the correct patient.

1.2 The cellular components of the blood

The blood is the transport medium of the body. The average human body weighing 70 kg contains 6 litres of blood (10.5 pints). At rest, 60 per cent of the blood volume is contained in the systemic venous system, 20 per cent in the systemic arterial system, and 20 per cent in the pulmonary system. In the normal state, the cellular components of the blood constitute slightly less than one-half of the blood volume, the red cells making up more than 99 per cent of the cellular volume.

The cellular constitution of the blood can be determined rapidly and accurately by electronic cell counters present in most haematology laboratories in the United Kingdom. In addition to measuring the total haemoglobin concentration, the red cell count and individual cell sizes are measured and a mean cell volume (MCV) and mean cell haemoglobin (MCH) are calculated. These 'red cell indices' (MCV and MCH) are useful in ascertaining the possible cause of any anaemia that may be present. For example, a low MCV and MCH indicates a microcytic, hypochromic anaemia, usually the result of iron deficiency or thalassaemia. A normal MCV and MCH indicate a normocytic, normochromic anaemia, usually the result of acute blood loss or the anaemia of chronic disease. A mild elevation of the MCV may result from an active bone marrow response to haemorrhage, the presence of liver disease, or, in the elderly, a disordered bone marrow (so-called myelodysplasia). A gross elevation of MCV may result from megaloblastic anaemia. The total white cell count and platelet count are also measured. The differential white cell count is measured automatically by some cell counters, but in the absence of this facility a manual white cell differential count of a stained blood film can be performed. Blood films are made by smearing a drop of blood on a glass slide and, after drying, the smear is fixed and stained with a Romanowsky dye, which stains the various cellular components 'differentially', depending on the chemical properties of the cellular constituents. Examination of a Romanowsky-stained film also allows visual inspection of the red cells and may provide further information regarding the possible cause of anaemia.

1.3 The coagulation and fibrinolytic systems

The coagulation and fibrinolytic systems are biological amplification mechanisms that work in unison to maintain the integrity of the vascular tree. Blood leakage is prevented by the coagulation system, and thrombotic occlusion is prevented by the naturally occurring anticoagulants, which prevent spontaneous coagulation, and the fibrinolytic system, which removes any fibrin that is formed within the circulation.

The coagulation system consists of a number of serine protease enzymes (that is, enzymes with the amino acid, serine, at the reactive site). These enzymes may be sequentially activated, in the presence of an adequate supply of cofactors and platelets, to generate thrombin. Thrombin, in turn, converts fibrinogen to fibrin monomer, which polymerizes, and clot stability is achieved through covalent cross-linking of fibrin strands and incorporation of platelets, white cells, and red cells in the fibrin meshwork.

The integrity of the serine protease enzymes and the cofactors can be evaluated in the laboratory by the prothrombin time (PT) and the partial thromboplastin time (PTT). These tests measure the time in seconds for a visible clot to form in a test tube after the addition of reagents that trigger the coagulation system. The PT results from rapid activation of the system by the addition of thromboplastin, thus bypassing the early 'contact-factor serine proteases' (historically known as the extrinsic pathway), whereas the PTT is a slower process, dependent on 'contact-factor' activation by a foreign substance such as kaolin (historically known as the intrinsic pathway). The amount of

fibrinogen can be determined by direct measurement or indirectly by the thrombin time (TT), which measures the time for a clot to form after the addition of a high concentration of thrombin to the plasma. The platelet count is measured directly by cell counting (see above).

The major anticoagulant effect of heparin is on the pathway measured by the partial thromboplastin time (PTT) and this is therefore used to monitor full-dose therapy with heparin, the PTT ratio indicating the degree of anticoagulation due to heparin. Low-molecular-weight heparins have no appreciable effect on the APTT and are usually given without monitoring or dose adjustment. The major anticoagulant effect of warfarin (and other vitamin K antagonists) is on the pathway measured by the prothrombin time (PT) and this is therefore used to monitor warfarin therapy. The PT ratio is greatly dependent on the reagents used as well the effect of warfarin, and so the PT ratio is adjusted to an international normalized ratio (INR) to allow for the reagents and thus give a standardized result. The INR therefore indicates the degree of anticoagulation due to warfarin.

Spontaneous coagulation is prevented by inhibition of the coagulation system by a complex physiological 'braking system', in which each component of the coagulation cascade is inhibited specifically. Antithrombin (previously known as antithrombin III) is a protein that specifically neutralizes the activated serine proteases; the protein C system inactivates the cofactors; and the platelets are inhibited by endothelial-derived prostacyclin and nitric oxide, as well as the natural anticoagulant properties of the endothelial surface. Any fibrin formed within the vasculature can be removed by plasmin, which is a protein that degrades fibrinogen and fibrin molecules. Plasmin is generated on the surface of fibrin clots from the circulating precursor molecule plasminogen, and thus fibrinolytic activity is relatively confined to the clot and there is no degradation of fibrinogen within the circulation. The most important physiological activator of plasminogen is endothelial-derived tissue plasminogen activator (tPA). While the integrity of these systems is contributory to the prevention of peri- and postoperative venous thromboembolic disease, laboratory evaluation of these systems is not used to influence venous thromboembolic prophylactic regimens and is not routinely warranted (see Section 6).

2 Preoperative assessment

2.1 Anaemia

Anaemia is one of the most common manifestations of illness. It is defined as a reduction in the circulating level of haemoglobin and it produces a reduction in the oxygen-carrying capacity of the blood.

The presence and severity of symptoms depends on the speed of onset of anaemia, the age of the patient, and his or her cardiorespiratory status. The clinical features of anaemia result from the increased demand on the cardiorespiratory system, with lassitude at rest and fatigue, muscle weakness, and dyspnoea on exertion. With increasing anaemia there may be dizziness and, in the elderly, angina, cardiac failure, and claudication may result from coexisting atherosclerotic vascular disease. As oxygen delivery to the tissues is dependent on haemoglobin concentration, the degree of oxygen saturation of the haemoglobin, and the cardiac output, with increasing anaemia there is a compensatory increase in cardiac output. In adults this is predominantly due to an increase in stroke volume but when anaemia is severe there is also a tachycardia. Systolic flow murmurs, maximal at the cardiac apex and in the pulmonary area are common and result from turbulence. With severe anaemia there is cardiac failure, with dilatation of the heart and the murmurs of valvular regurgitation.

Skin pallor is a poor indicator of the haemoglobin concentration. The mucous membranes give a better indication but the history is the most important aspect of the preoperative assessment, as it indicates the pathophysiological consequences of any degree of anaemia that may be present. The haemoglobin concentration can only be determined accurately by laboratory measurement (see laboratory investigation). In many instances the cause of anaemia will be apparent and may be related to the surgical condition being assessed. On the other hand, the cause may be obscure and it may not be apparent whether the anaemia is the result of a primary haematological condition or secondary to a systemic disorder. If time permits, a haematological opinion should be obtained so that appropriate management is planned and the prognostic significance of the anaemia considered.

Although anaemia is defined by the haemoglobin concentration (males, > 125 g/litre; females, > 120 g/litre; children, > 110 g/litre), this value is the result of both the circulating red cell mass and the plasma volume. With a gradual reduction in red cell mass there is a compensatory increase in plasma volume in order to maintain an adequate total blood volume, and thus anaemia occurs. In acute blood loss both the red cell mass and the plasma volume are reduced, consequently the haemoglobin concentration remains normal, and symptoms and signs result from the reduction in blood volume with progressively increasing degrees of shock. (It should be noted that the haematocrit is simply a cruder measurement of the haemoglobin level and does not provide any additional information, for example after acute blood loss both the haemoglobin concentration and the haematocrit remain normal, and as plasma expansion occurs both are reduced to the same degree.)

The severity of anaemia at which preoperative correction is required depends on the urgency of surgery, the age of the patient, and his or her cardiorespiratory status. Postoperative mortality and complication rates are inversely related to the preoperative haemoglobin concentration and the extent of blood loss at operation. It is common practice to attain a preoperative haemoglobin concentration above 100 g/litre, by blood transfusion if urgent surgery is required. However, this level is arbitrary and in a younger patient with normal cardiorespiratory function a level of 80 g/litre might be considered acceptable if the expected operative blood loss is less than 500 ml. In such an instance a red cell transfusion can be made available but deferred unless blood loss exceeds 500 ml. In some patients with chronic anaemia (e.g. renal failure), surgery may be safely performed with a level of 60–80 g/litre. Recent studies indicate that transfusion to critically ill patients to keep the haemoglobin above 80 g/litre may be associated with a higher mortality as compared to withholding transfusion.

2.2 Bleeding

It is imperative to determine whether a patient suffered excessive blood loss during or following any previous surgical or dental procedure. In addition a family history of bleeding or drug ingestion may also predict excessive operative blood loss. A complete history and examination are required to determine whether bleeding is already present, and also whether there is any evidence of organ dysfunction that may impair haemostasis (e.g. liver or renal disease). If excessive blood loss is anticipated, the potential cause of this must be determined so that appropriate management can be planned and correct blood components used effectively. Evaluation of the haemostatic system is mandatory in any patient with a bleeding history and a minimum clotting screen, consisting of a PT, APTT, and platelet count, should be performed (see above). Normal values exclude almost all severe bleeding disorders, but platelet function abnormalities and mild to moderate coagulation deficiencies may not be identified. Therefore, clinical assessment is crucial, as a comprehensive haematological opinion is required if there is a strong suspicion of a bleeding tendency, even if the clotting screen is normal. Clarification of any bleeding tendency and the strategic use of drugs and blood components is far more beneficial than the injudicious use of fresh, frozen plasma at the time of operative bleeding.

3 Blood component therapy

Transfusion therapy has progressed from protracted crossmatch procedures and the provision of whole donor units to the provision of rapidly available and compatible blood component therapy. Until recently whole blood was considered to be the ideal product for surgical patients requiring blood transfusion; however, it is now clear that whole blood is anything but 'whole', being deficient in functional coagulation factors, platelets, and white cells. The loss of functional forms of these components is so rapid on storage that there is no such thing as useful fresh whole blood. Therefore, whole blood ('fresh' or otherwise) is essentially a red cell transfusion in an inappropriately excessive volume. If correction of anaemia is required, then red cell components should be transfused (see Section 3.2). If replacement of whole blood is required (e.g. in the rapidly bleeding patient), then the individual components of the blood should be transfused in a fully functional form. Finally, blood products should not be administered unless there is a clinical requirement, as blood transfusion therapy is associated with a large number of potential complications (see below).

3.1 Complications of blood component therapy and prevention

Immunological complications

Immunological incompatibility between the recipient and the donor product can result from a variety of immunological mismatches. The most clinically relevant is incompatibility between the recipient antibody system and antigens on the surface of red cells.

Red cells

Antibodies to red cell antigens are most important for two reasons:

(1) the volume of red cells transfused is far greater than that of white cells or platelets so that the consequences of incompatible red cell transfusion are comparatively severe;

(2) red cell antibody formation following a transfusion to a woman in her reproductive years may subsequently cause haemolytic disease of the newborn.

Some red cell antibodies are always present, even without exposure to 'foreign' (allogeneic) red cells. These antibodies are termed 'naturally occurring' and include antibodies to the antigens of the ABO system. For most practical purposes, clinically relevant antibodies to antigens of the other red cell antigen systems only occur after exposure to foreign red cells and are therefore termed 'immune'. Even after exposure to foreign red cells, immune antibody formation may not necessarily occur. The 'D' antigen of the rhesus system is the most immunogenic of the non-ABO antigens and the majority of rhesus-D-negative patients who are exposed to rhesus-D-positive blood will develop anti-D. With other antigens, the risk is less; indeed, with some antigens the risk of antibody development is less than 5 per cent. However, when antibodies are present, whether natural or immune, it is essential to identify them and provide compatible red cells, that is red cells that do not express the antigens to which the antibodies are directed. Failure to provide compatible red cells will result in a haemolytic transfusion reaction. Provision of compatible red cells is achieved by red cell compatibility testing.

Red cell compatibility testing

Antibodies to the ABO system are naturally occurring and react at body temperature. Therefore, they may be responsible for an immediate haemolytic transfusion reaction and are thus clinically relevant. The ABO group of the recipient must therefore be determined and ABO compatible, preferably ABO identical, red cell components transfused. The classification of the ABO system and the naturally occurring antibodies are shown in Table 9.1.

In view of the high immunogenicity of the rhesus-D antigen it is of particular importance that rhesus-D-negative women of reproductive age should not be exposed to rhesus-D-positive red cells. Furthermore, anti-D formation may lead to difficulty in providing compatible red cells for further transfusions so all recipients should have their rhesus-D status determined in order to transfuse rhesus-D-negative patients with rhesus-D-negative red cells.

Having established the ABO and rhesus-D status of the patient, the presence of any atypical red cell antibodies (antibodies in the patient's serum to red cell antigens other than antigens of the ABO system) is established by antibody screening. The clinical relevance of these antibodies is established by incubating patient's serum, at body temperature (37 °C), with two or three selected cell types that express all the relevant red cell antigens. By this method any antibodies that are capable of reacting with transfused red cells are detected. The specificity of any antibodies that are present can then be determined and antigen-negative red cells selected.

Finally, a cross-match procedure may be performed to ensure red cell compatibility (see Section 3.2). Increasingly, it is recognized that traditional cross-matching is not required if the antibody screen is negative.

Haemolytic transfusion reactions

Transfusion of incompatible red cells may give rise to immediate or delayed haemolytic transfusion reactions. Symptoms and signs of an immediate reaction vary, depending on the potency, titre, and compliment activating ability of the antibody. When complement is activated, as is the case with naturally occurring antibodies to the ABO system, the patient may become unwell within a few minutes with apprehension and restlessness, fever, flushing, and malaise. Pain in the chest, loin, or abdomen may

Table 9.1 The ABO system and naturally occurring antibodies

A, B antigens on red cells	Assigned blood group	Frequency in UK	Naturally occurring antibody	ABO compatible groups[a]
None	O	47%	Anti-A, anti-B	O
A	A	42%	Anti-B	A, O
B	B	8%	Anti-A	B, O
A and B	AB	3%	None	AB, A, B, O

[a] Only ABO-identical red cells can be guaranteed ABO compatible as complications due to minor incompatibility may follow transfusion of compatible but non-identical red cell units. Therefore, ABO-identical red cells should be transfused if available.

ABO subgroups exist, which may give rise to unexpected ABO incompatibility and delays in obtaining compatible red cell units.

occur and anaphylaxis may rapidly follow. Due to a common activation pathway, the coagulation and fibrinolytic systems are activated and a consumptive coagulopathy can occur. In the unconscious patient hypotension and uncontrollable bleeding are the most important signs. Changes in renal blood flow and hypotension lead to oliguria and renal failure. Therefore, as soon as a transfusion of incompatible red cells is suspected the transfusion should be stopped and a saline infusion commenced to maintain renal perfusion. If oliguria occurs, the saline should be continued and 80 mg of frusemide (furosemide) given intravenously. The labels on the transfused units should be checked to ensure that the correct patient is receiving the correct transfusion and the bags and a blood sample from the patient should be returned to the blood transfusion laboratory, which should be notified immediately by telephone. Further advice on management should be obtained from a haematologist.

A delayed haemolytic transfusion reaction usually occurs in a patient who has been immunized to a foreign red cell antigen by a previous transfusion or pregnancy, but in whom the concentration of antibody is so low it cannot be detected by routine red cell compatibility testing. Following transfusion the antibody titre rises and destruction of the transfused red cell occurs, often 1 week after transfusion. Fever, a reduction in haemoglobin concentration, jaundice, and haemoglobinuria occur. Delayed reactions occur after about 1 in 500 red cell transfusions and, while rarely fatal, may debilitate an already ill patient.

It must never be forgotten that most fatal incompatible transfusions are not caused by serological errors in the blood transfusion laboratory but by clinical staff sending blood from the wrong patient to the laboratory or instituting a transfusion on the wrong patient. The former can be prevented by labelling samples immediately after taking blood, and not beforehand or after a delay when the sample may have been mixed up with another one. The latter can be prevented by double checking at the bedside that units for transfusion are going to be given to the correct patient.

White cells, platelets, and plasma proteins

Red cell components are inevitably contaminated with white cells and platelets as well as donor plasma, and febrile non-haemolytic transfusion reactions may occur when antibodies to plasma proteins or white cell or platelet antigens are present in the recipient. These febrile reactions are common in patients who have previously been pregnant or transfused. Most reactions are mild and can be managed simply by slowing the rate of transfusion. In patients with recurrent febrile non-haemolytic transfusion reactions haematological advice should be obtained.

Graft-versus-host disease

Graft-versus-host disease (GvHD) is uncommon after blood transfusion but may occur in the immunosuppressed patient or the HLA-heterozygous recipient of an HLA-homozygous donor unit. In both instances transfusion-associated GvHD is due to the establishment in the host of immunocompetent cells from the donor unit and the recognition of the host tissues by these cell as 'foreign'. In the immunosuppressed patient this is due to the incompetence of the host immune system which cannot destroy the 'donor immune cells' which are foreign. Patients undergoing transplantation and receiving immunosuppressive therapy are at risk. In the HLA-heterozygous recipient of an HLA-homozygous transfusion the 'donor immune cells' are not foreign to the host immune system, as they only express the same HLA antigens as the host, and hence are not destroyed. The host tissues, on the other hand, express some HLA antigens that are foreign to these donor immune cells and GvHD may occur. In certain ethnic groups (e.g. Japanese) such a transfusion may be given relatively frequently, and GvHD has been reported as a frequent occurrence in these patients after cardiac surgery. Transfusion-associated GvHD is usually fatal and there is no proven effective treatment. It can be prevented by irradiating blood products, but this approach is not possible for all blood products in all patients at risk. Therefore, once again, blood product transfusion should only be performed when there is a clinical need.

Infectious diseases

A large number of infectious diseases may be transmitted through administration of blood products (Table 9.2). Transmission of these diseases may be prevented in three ways:

(1) donor self-exclusion;

(2) laboratory screening tests;

(3) viral inactivation procedures.

Table 9.2 Infectious diseases transmitted through administration of blood products

	Transmission in UK
Viruses	
Hepatitis C[a]	Yes
HIV-1[a]	Yes
Hepatitis B[a]	Yes
Cytomegalovirus	Yes
EpsteinBarr virus	Yes
HIV-2	
HTLV-I/II	
Bacteria	
Bacterial contaminants	Yes
Treponema pallidum[a]	Yes
Brucellosis	Yes
Parasites	
Malaria	Yes
Toxoplasma	Yes
Trypanosomes	
Babesia	

[a] Testing is mandatory in United Kingdom.

In the United Kingdom donation of blood is on a voluntary basis and donor self-exclusion is a major factor in the prevention of disease transmission. This is particularly important when screening tests for infectious disease may be falsely negative (e.g. in the first 3 months after HIV infection). Thus, self-exclusion and laboratory testing are complementary. Donors must be in good health and not in a high-risk group for HIV or recently returned from an area of endemic malaria.

In the UK, laboratory screening for hepatitis B surface antigen, antibody to hepatitis C, antibody to HIV-1, and antibody to *Treponema pallidum* (syphilis) is mandatory. Treponemes are inactivated by storage at 4 °C and screening is essentially to identify donors at risk of infection with other sexually transmitted disease, notably HIV.

Viral inactivation procedures, such as heat treatment and washing in solvent–detergent, can only be applied to albumin and factor concentrates prepared from large donor plasma pools. Therefore, the majority of components, including all cellular components and fresh, frozen plasma, cannot be treated without destroying the product and so these products are potentially infectious.

Miscellaneous complications

In addition to immunological and infectious complications, blood transfusion therapy may cause circulatory overload when transfusion is too rapid for compensatory fluid redistribution. Phlebitis may develop if cannulas are left in place for more than 48 hours. Hyperkalaemia is possible as potassium leaks from red cells on storage but, in practice, clinical consequences are restricted to patients with renal failure and neonates. However, significant hyperkalaemia can result from red cell destruction if units of blood are heated before transfusion without the use of a clinical blood warmer.

Massive transfusion

Massive transfusion is defined arbitrarily as replacement of the patient's total blood volume by stored blood in less than 24 hours. This is usually the result of massive haemorrhage and acute hypovolaemic shock. Morbidity and mortality are high, due to the underlying condition, and routine unmonitored use of fresh, frozen plasma, platelets, alkalinizing agents, and calcium supplementation is dangerous and often unnecessary. Management should be directed by frequent clinical and laboratory measurement and appropriate replacement therapy.

The following strategy should be used to resuscitate the patient:

1. Replace and maintain blood volume, initially with plasma expanders and with red cell components once anaemia occurs.

2. Maintain oxygen-carrying capacity. The haematocrit should be maintained above 20 per cent and with modern preservative solutions the oxygen-carrying capacity of stored blood is normal.

3. Correct and maintain haemostasis with fresh, frozen plasma to keep prothrombin time within 5 seconds of normal, and platelet concentrates to keep platelet count greater than 50×10^9/litre. The empirical use of these products is common but is inferior to monitored use.

4. Correct metabolic disturbance. Hypocalcaemia rarely causes clinical problems and hyperkalaemia is usually transient. However, in combination with hypothermia, resulting from rapid transfusion of blood without a blood warmer, both may cause cardiac arrythmias. Citrate toxicity is rare as it is rapidly metabolized by the liver to produce alkalosis. Acidosis is usually the result of hypotension and hypoperfusion and attention should be directed to restoring tissue blood flow.

5. Maintain colloid osmotic pressure. Maintenance of albumin concentration above 20 g/litre is advisable as a reduction in plasma oncotic pressure may contribute to the acute respiratory distress syndrome.

3.2 Red cell transfusions

Red cell components

Correction of anaemia by transfusion should be by the use of red cell components rather than whole blood. Red cell components are either in the form of red cells suspended in a reduced amount of plasma (red cell concentrates or packed cells) or optimum additive solution. In either case, the platelets, a proportion of the white cells, and a variable amount of the plasma are removed, leaving a purer product with a higher haematocrit, which is more suitable for correction of anaemia. Optimum additive solutions (e.g. SAGM: saline, adenine, glucose, mannitol) permit removal of almost all the plasma, while its replacement with the additive solution maintains the integrity of the red cells. The plasma that is removed is used to make useful functional blood components, such as fresh, frozen plasma and factor concentrates.

Donor red cells

Testing

If ABO-identical red cell units are chosen for transfusion, then even if no further compatibility tests are performed, red cell compatibility will be achieved in 97 per cent of transfusions. Rhesus-D-negative units are selected for rhesus-D-negative recipients to prevent subsequent anti-D formation, but this procedure will also prevent incompatible transfusion to the 1 per cent of recipients who already have developed immune anti-D. Thus selection of ABO, rhesus-D-identical red cell units will result in red cell compatibility in 98 per cent of transfusions. To achieve compatibility in almost 100 per cent of transfusions an antibody screen is performed to detect atypical antibodies (see Section 3.1). Finally, a cross-match may be performed in which red cells from each donor unit are incubated with the patient's serum. In urgent situations an antibody screen will not have been previously performed and the cross-match not only confirms ABO compatibility but is the only means by which atypical antibodies will be detected. However, if an antibody screen has been performed, for example before elective surgery, the main purpose of the cross-match is simply to ensure ABO compatibility. The cross-match procedure has been refined so that with the use of 'enhancing agents' in the incubation mixture and 'spin techniques' the actual procedure may take only 15 minutes. Increasingly, the traditional cross-match is being replaced by computerized systems to ensure ABO compatibility when antibody screening has been performed.

Ordering

Most units of red cells are for patients undergoing elective surgical procedures. The majority of these patients do not require transfusion. It is therefore good practice to analyse red cell usage and establish which operative procedures routinely require transfusion. For those operations where more than 10 per cent of patients are transfused, a fixed number of units (previously agreed between haematologist, surgeon, and anaesthetist) are cross-matched. There should be a list of common operations for which blood is routinely cross-matched and the maximum number of units to be cross-matched for each procedure (this is termed a maximum ordering schedule). For operations where fewer than 10 per cent of patients are transfused, cross-matching need not be performed if an antibody screen is performed. If the screen is negative, no further action is taken as compatible blood can be provided rapidly as there are no atypical antibodies. If the screen is positive, specificity of the atypical antibody is determined and antigen-negative blood is selected and compatibility confirmed by cross-match, so that red cell units are available without delay in the unlikely event of a red cell transfusion being required. The development of antibody screening and a maximum ordering schedule minimizes unnecessary cross-matching, increases the efficiency of the blood transfusion department, and directs blood product usage, thus reducing wastage and permitting more surgery. It should be emphasized that such a policy cannot be rigid, and flexibility must be exercised for certain patients and procedures.

Autologous transfusion

The aims of autologous transfusion are to reduce the risks of transfusion therapy, and to permit more surgical procedures to be performed by conserving blood components and reducing requirements made of the blood transfusion laboratory. Avoiding homologous (allogeneic) blood transfusion prevents immunological and infectious complications, although clerical errors may still arise and the wrong blood may be given to the wrong patient. Autologous transfusion can be by predeposit, preoperative haemodilution, or blood salvage:

1. In predeposit programmes, up to 5 units of blood can be collected at weekly intervals. However, only 10 per cent of patients requiring surgery are eligible for predeposit autologous transfusion, as the majority are too old or unfit, or are suffering from infection, malignant disease, or anaemia, all of which preclude autologous transfusion.

2. Preoperative haemodilution has been used extensively in patients undergoing cardiac surgery but it may be extended to other types of surgery, depending on the health of the patient, the procedure being performed, and the likelihood of transfusion being required.

3. Blood salvage can be performed manually or by automated cell savers. Manual salvage is performed by collecting blood through drainage or suction into a reservoir containing anticoagulant. The blood is filtered, although particulate matter and partial coagulation are potential problems. Manual salvage has been used most frequently in orthopaedic surgery.

Automated cell savers are used when operative blood loss is high, for example in liver transplantation. The salvaged red cells are washed and reinfused in a packed cell volume of 50 per cent. Homologous blood transfusion is often also required but the procedure greatly reduces the number of donated units required during surgery.

Red cell substitutes

Disadvantages of blood transfusion include storage, transport, a shelf-life of 35 days, short supply, and compatibility. A fluid that has the same osmolarity of blood, transports oxygen from the lungs to the tissues, has a long shelf-life, and is non-antigenic would reduce the need for red cell transfusion. Polymerized haemoglobin solutions with a long circulation time and physiological oxygen affinity, microencapsulated haemoglobin contained in liposomes to prolong the circulation time, and perfluorochemicals are possible red cell substitutes. They are not in routine use and more human studies are required.

3.3 Plasma and plasma products

Unfractionated fresh, frozen plasma contains near normal amounts of all the clotting factors and other plasma proteins. It should be used to replace coagulation factors in patients shown to be deficient (e.g. in surgical patients with excessive haemorrhage resulting in abnormal coagulation). It is wasteful and dangerous to use it simply for volume replacement when alternative safer products are available.

Human albumin solutions

Human albumin solutions are produced by cold ethanol fractionation of large pools of human plasma, sterilized by filtration, and pasteurized at 60 °C for 10 hours to inactivate contaminating viruses. The sodium content is controlled. It is supplied in various forms: The protein in Albumin solution BP is 95 per cent human albumin and is available in 5 per cent and 20 per cent solutions, whereas the protein in Plasma Protein Solution (Plasma Protein Fraction, PPF) is 85 per cent human albumin. Albumin solutions were developed during the Second World War as alternatives to blood for treatment of casualties but have remained in clinical use despite few proper clinical studies comparing their efficacy with artificial colloids and cheaper crystalloid solutions. Albumin solutions are expensive (£25–40 for 400 ml 5 per cent albumin, compared with 50–80 pence for 500 ml of crystalloid) yet the clinical indications remain controversial. Adverse reactions are rare, although rapid infusions occasionally cause rapid falls in blood pressure due to the presence of prekallikrein activator.

Uses of human albumin solutions

Plasma volume replacement

There is no evidence from clinical trials that intravenous albumin therapy aimed at achieving target values for colloid osmotic pressure or albumin concentration have influenced important clinical outcomes. In trauma patients, and in older patients undergoing elective major surgery, albumin solutions have shown no advantage when compared with crystalloid solutions for volume replacement.

Burns

Burns cause a prolonged increase in microvascular permeability, with large losses of fluid and protein. However, there is no scientific evidence that albumin solutions are better than crystalloids for volume replacement.

Extracorporeal circulation during cardiac surgery

Again, no evidence that priming the bypass circuit and intraoperative volume replacement with albumin solutions is better than crystalloid.

Parenteral nutrition

In patients with albumin concentrations below 25 g/litre, a prospective study of total parenteral nutrition (TPN), with one group receiving 20–25 g albumin per day, showed no differences in complication, mortality, duration of ventilatory support, or length of stay.

Human albumin is of benefit in producing a diuresis in patients with nephrotic syndrome resistant to diuretics, and in preventing hypoalbuminaemia in patients with hepatic ascites undergoing repeated paracentesis. It is safe as a plasma expander but is not superior to alternative fluids and, in view of its high cost, needs to be critically evaluated. Albumin is now most frequently used in intensive care units where physiological monitoring can be used to rationalize therapy in critically ill patients with hypoproteinaemic oedema or respiratory distress syndrome.

Plasma fractions for therapeutic use

Donated plasma can also be fractionated into a variety of plasma derivatives for clinical use. As discussed above, human albumin is readily available although indications for its use for acute plasma volume replacement is controversial. Cryoprecipitate is the precipitate that forms after thawing frozen plasma. It is a rich source of some clotting factors, including fibrinogen. The only surgical indication for administration of cryoprecipitate is confirmed severe hypofibrinogenaemia (e.g. < 0.5 g/litre) causing bleeding. As there is a risk of disease transmission, this will soon be superseded by heat-treated fibrinogen concentrates. Factor concentrates are used exclusively for patients with severe specific coagulation factor deficits, and can only be used with the approval of a haematologist.

4 Modifying perioperative blood loss

Excessive blood loss can be due to surgical causes (suture deficiency) or defective haemostasis. Perioperative blood loss may be modified in two ways: first, blood can be conserved (i.e. autologous blood transfusion; see above); secondly, blood loss can be reduced by pharmacological manipulation of haemostasis. Obviously the latter assumes that the bleeding is not due to surgical failure, which must always be the first consideration.

Drugs that may reduce blood loss include fibrin sealants, antiplatelet agents, desmopressin (DDAVP®), tranexamic acid, and aprotinin.

1. Fibrin sealants are essentially fibrin glue, which can be added to patches and suture lines. Tisseel® is commercially available on a named-patient basis in the UK. Clinical experience is descriptive, mainly in cardiac surgery, and controlled studies are required to determine whether the use of Tisseel® reduces peri- and postoperative blood loss.

2. Paradoxically, antiplatelet agents may reduce postoperative blood loss in patients who have undergone cardiopulmonary bypass. Thrombocytopenia, platelet fragmentation, and platelet activation with resultant defective platelets results from interaction with the bypass circuit, and the degree of impairment of platelet function is proportional to the duration of bypass. Antiplatelet agents may theoretically 'preserve' platelets and, indeed, one study of dipyridamole in cardiac surgery using bypass reduced thrombocytopenia and significantly reduced the amount of perioperative blood loss. Prostacyclin has not yet been shown to be beneficial in this setting, but clearly more evaluation of drugs that affect platelet function is required in this area.

3. Desmopressin (DDAVP®) is a synthetic analogue of vasopressin with minimal vasoconstrictor activity. It has been shown to cause a massive release of von Willebrand protein from the endothelium, with a shortening of the bleeding time. Although this drug is unequivocally useful in reducing perioperative blood loss in patients with certain specific disorders of coagulation, it has not been shown convincingly to reduce preoperative blood loss in uncomplicated cardiac surgery. Furthermore, there is a risk of graft thrombosis and thromboembolic events, and its use cannot be recommended at the present time except in controlled clinical studies.

4. Tranexamic acid and aprotinin are antifibrinolytic agents, that is they reduce fibrinolytic activity and may theoretically reduce 'oozing' and hence blood loss. Tranexamic acid prevents binding of plasminogen/plasmin to fibrin clots and has been shown to reduce blood loss following transurethral

prostatectomy and cardiac bypass surgery. Aprotinin neutralizes plasmin and has produced the most dramatic reductions in perioperative blood loss in patients undergoing prostatectomy, cardiac surgery, and liver transplantation. However, the risk of graft thrombosis and venous thromboembolic disease has not been defined and these agents should be used cautiously and in a controlled manner.

5 Perioperative blood transfusion and tumour recurrence

Pretransplant blood transfusions have been shown to improve the survival of kidney allografts. With the use of cyclosporin, transfusion of blood products for this purpose cannot be advocated, but the effect highlights the potentially immunosuppressive effect of blood transfusion. This effect may be important in patients undergoing surgical removal of solid tumours. Increased relapse rates and reduced survival have been reported in patients with colonic, renal, lung, breast, cervical, and stomach cancer who were transfused at the time of surgery, compared to those who were not transfused. However, it is extremely difficult to control for all variables and it is not clear whether perioperative blood transfusion is an independent variable. Furthermore, results are conflicting as some studies have not shown any statistically different outcome in transfused patients. Whatever the effect, it is noteworthy that it is mediated through transfusion of components of blood other than red cells. The effect of transfusion on renal graft survival and any effect on cancer recurrence is greater after transfusion of whole blood rather than red cell components, although the reason for this is not clear. Possible mechanisms include transfer of anti-idiotypic antibodies, unspecified immunoregulatory molecules, or immunosuppression due to exposure to histocompatibility antigens on 'foreign' white cells. Whatever the mechanism, the available data emphasize the disadvantage of transfusion of whole blood compared to red cells.

6 Postoperative venous thromboembolic disease

Venous thromboembolic disease is a major cause of morbidity and, through pulmonary embolization, mortality. Patients suffering thromboembolic disease (TED) are usually in readily identifiable high-risk groups. In the community these are usually patients with medical conditions such as heart failure or terminal malignant disease. However, in a hospital environment they are often surgical patients who would enjoy a successful outcome from surgery if not for the complicating TED. There is now unequivocal evidence that surgery is associated with a high incidence of postoperative venous TED, and that the incidence of this can be reduced by a number of mechanical or pharmacological techniques.

6.1 Prevention

In general surgery, mechanical methods such as graduated pressure stockings, intermittent calf compression, or calf stimulation significantly reduce the incidence of postoperative venous thrombosis. It is likely that the incidence of fatal pulmonary embolization is also reduced, but this has not been shown statistically. Neither physiotherapy nor 'toe wriggling' have ever been shown to reduce the incidence of venous thrombosis. Anticoagulation with either oral warfarin or subcutaneous heparin also reduces the incidence of venous thrombosis. Of all the mechanical and pharmacological methods, fixed low-dose subcutaneous heparin has been shown to reduce the incidence of postoperative venous thrombosis most consistently and effectively, with a minimal risk of increased bleeding.

Many studies have used surrogate end points, such as radiolabelled fibrinogen leg scanning, which grossly overestimates the incidence of clinically significant venous TED, and some conclusions have been drawn from meta-analysis of combined studies. This has resulted in criticism of data and a reluctance by some surgeons to employ prophylactic heparin. However, large, complete, randomized studies, employing venography, lung scanning, and post-mortems, have shown that fixed low-dose subcutaneous heparin does reduce the incidence of clinically significant postoperative venous thrombosis and significantly reduces the incidence of fatal pulmonary embolization. A dose of 5000 units subcutaneously twice daily, commencing preoperatively, is effective and does not require any monitoring or dose adjustment. Administration three times daily is more effective, but there may be a slightly higher risk of bleeding. Low-molecular-weight heparins are at least as effective as standard heparin, but may be associated with less bleeding. The risk of heparin-induced thrombocytopenia and thrombosis (the most severe complication of heparin) is certainly much less. Furthermore, low-molecular-weight heparins only need to be given once a day. The combination of graduated pressure stockings with heparin is to be encouraged.

In orthopaedic surgery the benefit:risk ratio of heparin prophylaxis has recently been questioned, with an apparent reduction in the risk of pulmonary embolus in recent years.

6.2 Risk assessment

The risk of TED depends on the age of the patient, his or her general condition, and the nature of the operative procedure. The incidence of postoperative thrombosis rises exponentially with age and patients over the age of 40 years are at high risk. Conditions such as obesity, heart failure, and malignant disease greatly increase the incidence. Surgical procedures lasting more than 45 minutes are associated with an increasing risk, and the risk is particularly great with abdominal, pelvic, and orthopaedic surgery. In summary, all patients should be considered for some form of TED prevention and any patient satisfying any of the above criteria should be given prophylaxis unless there is a very good reason against it. If a decision not to give prophylaxis is made, the reasons for this should be documented in the case notes as there are likely to be an increasing number of litigation cases resulting from postoperative TED.

6.3 Treatment

No prophylactic method completely prevents postoperative TED. There may be few initial clinical manifestations and the first sign may be a fatal pulmonary embolus. Post-mortem studies have shown that 50 per cent of patients die of a fatal embolus in 1 hour and that many patients with more than one embolus were wrongly diagnosed as having a postoperative chest infection or heart failure. Therefore, clinical staff should have a high index of suspicion and suspected TED must be confirmed objectively, for example by venography or lung scanning, and effective treatment instituted immediately. On diagnosis, full-dose intravenous heparinization to maintain an APTT ratio of 1.5–2.5 times normal should be commenced, and continued with at least daily measurement of the APTT ratio and appropriate heparin dose adjustment until the patient is adequately anticoagulated with warfarin. Alternatively, once-daily subcutaneous low-molecular-weight heparin can be given. Once there is a low risk of postoperative bleeding, oral warfarin therapy can be commenced. A loading dose of 10 mg daily for 2 days should be followed by adjusted-dose warfarin to maintain an INR of 2.0–3.0. Once an INR of 2.0 has been achieved, the heparin infusion can be stopped. Anticoagulation with warfarin should be carefully controlled and continued for at least 3 months.

7   Arterial thromboembolic disease

Acute limb ischaemia may be due to either embolus or thrombosis. Immediate treatment is required when the limb is completely ischaemic, and embolectomy is indicated when embolic occlusion is responsible. If this fails, or if the occlusion is thrombotic, either arterial reconstruction or thrombolytic therapy is indicated. The relative and complementary roles of these approaches have not been defined, and while both may be effective, it is not clear which patients would benefit most from thrombolytic therapy followed by delayed definitive surgery. Furthermore, the most effective drug regimens have not been defined. Monitoring of therapy is performed to ensure that defibrination does not occur, but laboratory parameters have minimal predictive value for haemorrhage and any patient may suffer haemorrhage while receiving thrombolytic therapy. The risk is approximately 15 per cent for minor and 5 per cent for major haemorrhage, regardless of the drug used.

Traditionally, thrombolytic therapy has been by local infusion of low-dose streptokinase (e.g. 5000 units/hour) via the arteriography catheter. More recently, recombinant tissue plasminogen activator (rtPa) has been used at a dose of approximately 0.05 mg/kg by local infusion. At present, most patients are treated with surgery and thrombolytic therapy is reserved for poor-risk patients. The role of thrombolytic therapy in the management of limb ischaemia remains to be defined.

There are very few data on the effectiveness of secondary prevention with antithrombotic agents, including anticoagulants, in patients who have suffered limb ischaemia. Anticoagulation is clearly indicated for patients with a thromboembolic source, but these are a minority of patients. For the majority who have widespread vascular disease, anticoagulants have not yet been shown to alter the natural history of the process. In patients who receive an arterial graft there are some data suggesting that warfarin therapy may prolong graft patency. The importance of the relative roles of anticoagulants and antiplatelet agents requires urgent clarification.

For coronary artery bypass grafting, the incidence of early and late occlusion is reduced by warfarin but antiplatelet agents such as aspirin are as effective and are safer than anticoagulants.

8   Surgical management of the patient receiving anticoagulants

Patients receiving oral anticoagulants require careful monitoring and control of therapy in the perioperative period. The reason for anticoagulation and the risk of bleeding need to be considered and therapy adjusted accordingly. A preoperative review by a haematologist is preferable as management should be planned and control of this aspect of therapy by a clinician with a particular interest in haemostasis is advantageous. For most patients undergoing simple surgery, adjustment of warfarin dosage preoperatively to achieve an INR of 2.0–2.5 at the time of surgery is associated with a minimum risk of perioperative haemorrhage. For complex surgery or surgery with a significant risk of haemorrhage, the warfarin should be stopped. The requirement for conversion to heparin depends on the indication for warfarin therapy. Patients with mechanical prosthetic heart valves may require full anticoagulation, and continuous intravenous heparin to maintain a PTT ratio of 1.5–2.5 is essential. For most other patients, low-dose subcutaneous heparin is sufficient. Each patient requires a considered opinion and there cannot be a rigid protocol.

9   Surgery in the haemophiliac

Haemophilia is described classically as an inherited tendency to excessive bleeding. There are many forms of haemophilia, affecting either coagulant protein or platelet function. It is therefore essential that any patient undergoing elective surgery is assessed in the haematology outpatient clinic several weeks before scheduled surgery. This time is required to confirm, or indeed determine, the specific nature of the haemostatic defect. This may require repeated evaluation of the haemostatic system. It is necessary to determine whether any complications of the haemophilia are present that may influence the type of surgery or affect its outcome. If a patient has received replacement therapy in the past, it is mandatory to determine whether an 'inhibitor' has developed. This would render replacement therapy ineffective at the time of surgery.

The patient may have been infected through the use of blood products and could be an infection risk. This must be determined, and if a patient is, or is potentially, infectious, all staff involved in his or her care should be notified so that appropriate precautions can be taken to reduce the risk of infection to staff to an absolute minimum.

In many cases, restoration of normal haemostasis for surgery can only be achieved by a carefully planned regimen of therapy. It will often be necessary to measure 'levels' of factors immediately before surgery, and the timing on the operation list is therefore of primary importance and must be decided in advance between surgeon, anaesthetist, and haematologist. Haematological therapy will usually be required for at least 1 week postoperatively and in many cases this will be as an inpatient. Haemophiliacs must not be given drugs that impair haemostasis further (e.g. aspirin), and intramuscular injections must not be given because of the risk of severe muscle haematoma. Parenteral analgesia must be given intravenously or subcutaneously.

Surgical management of the haemophiliac is complicated for the haematologist but should not be complicated for the surgeon. However, this is only possible if the haematologist is given enough time to prepare the patient beforehand, and to plan and obtain the required drugs and blood components. With adequate preparation, haemostasis can be rendered normal in nearly all patients, allowing practically any surgical procedure to be performed.

When surgery is required urgently in a haemophiliac, the haematologist must be informed immediately in order to render haemostasis as near normal as possible. Most known haemophiliacs are registered with a haemophilia centre and carry a card with an emergency telephone number through which haematological advice and support can be obtained.

Bibliography

Chen, A.Y. and Carson, J.L. (1998). Perioperative management of anaemia. *Br. J. Anaesth.*, 81, (Suppl. 1), 20–4.

DiMichele, D. and Neufeld, E.J. (1998). Hemophilia. A new approach to an old disease. *Hemat. Oncol. Clin. North Am.*, **12**, (6), 1315–44.

Gitnick, G. (1998). Hepatitis C: controversies, strategies and challenges. *Europ. J. Surg., Suppl.* **582**, 65–70.

Goodnough, L.T., Brecher, M.E., Kanter, M.H., and AuBuchon, J.P. (1999). Transfusion medicine. First of two parts—blood transfusion. *NEJM*, **340**, (6), 438–47.

Malyon, D. (1998). Transfusion-free treatment of Jehovah's Witnesses: respecting the autonomous patient's motives. *J. Med. Ethics*, **24**, (6), 376–81.

Mercuriali, F. and Inghilleri, G. (1998) Management of pre-operative anaemia. *Br. J. Anaesth.*, **81**, (Suppl. 1), 56–61.

Moor, A.C., Dubbelman, T.M., VanSteveninck, J. and Brand, A. (1999). Transfusion-transmitted diseases: risks, prevention and perspectives. *Europ. J. Haematol.*, **62**, (1), 1–18.

Steinberg, M.H. (1999). Management of sickle cell disease. *NEJM*, **340**, (13), 1021–30.

Clinical Orthopaedics and Related Research, **357**, (December 1998) carried a range of review articles, including:

◆ Oxygen carriers as blood substitutes. Past, present, and future.

◆ Epoetin alfa. A bloodless approach for the treatment of perioperative anemia.

◆ Safety of the blood supply.

◆ Prospectus. Future trends in transfusion.

Vox Sanguinis, **74**, (Suppl. 2), 1998 carried a range of review articles, including:

◆ Donor selection: the exclusion of high risk donors?

◆ Haemovigilance: concept, Europe and UK initiatives.

◆ Replacement of massive blood loss.

◆ Alternatives to human blood and blood resources.

◆ Post-transfusion hepatitis: current risks and causes.

CHAPTER 10

Management of acute pain

Patrick Doyle and R. Munglani

1 Introduction

Pain is a subjective experience that can only be experienced directly by the sufferer. Nerve activation by noxious stimuli results in pain pathway activity that forms the central core of the perceived pain. However, emotional and behavioural dimensions to pain, for example suffering and anxiety, may also be experienced. This illustrates the complex nature of pain; the effective treatment of pain may require all these various levels to be addressed.

1.1 What is the extent of the problem?

The Royal Colleges of Anaesthetists and Surgeons examined the problems of postoperative pain management when they published the *Report of the working party on pain after surgery* in 1990 and suggested several ideas to improve the situation. Despite this recognition and suggested measures to alleviate pain after surgery, it is still a major problem world-wide, with 50–75 per cent of patients experiencing moderate to severe pain (Cousins and Mather 1989; Bruster *et al.* 1994; Warfield and Kahn 1995).

1.2 What is the attitude of health professionals?

Postoperative pain has been undertreated by health professionals for a number of reasons. These include patient and staff expectations, lack of knowledge, poor staffing levels, and concern about the side-effects of the drugs used. What is surprising is the lack of commitment to complete pain relief by health professionals, with less than 50 per cent expecting complete relief of pain after surgery (Kuhn *et al.* 1990). Despite the prevalence of significant pain, patients often report satisfaction with their pain relief. This is attributed to preconceived ideas, such as expecting there to be pain after surgery, finding that it was less than expected, knowing that it would eventually subside, and understanding the reasons behind their pain (Donovan 1983;Kuhn *et al.* 1990). A survey of newly qualified doctors on the intended management of acute postoperative pain, highlighted the continued failure to teach medical students and house staff the basics of pain management (Gould *et al.* 1994), with incorrect and dangerous prescription practised.

Timing of analgesia is also a major issue. Fung and Bentley (1994) identified lengthy delays in administration, and the failure of preoperative analgesia in those patients requiring it. Staff tend to underestimate the amount of analgesia required to maintain adequate pain relief and there is minimal early reassessment of the adequacy of the prescription. Medical and nursing staff also tend to overestimate the risk of addiction from opioids (Huskisson 1974;Cohen 1980;Kuhn *et al.* 1990). The real risk in this situation is estimated at 1 : 3000 (Porter and Jick 1980) and this should therefore not allow complacency in treating pain.

1.3 The effect of analgesia on outcome measures

There is a perception that pain is of secondary concern to the surgery itself. This has stemmed from the ill-formed belief that analgesia may mask surgical signs and that pain is a state that is expected to resolve itself in a reasonable period (Barrat 1997). The primary goal should be a basic humane principle of pain relief, and not directed purely by physiological outcome. The pain-free state can, however, be utilized to the patient's advantage.

Large numbers of morbidity outcome studies have been performed utilizing regional anaesthesia as the primary analgesic and anaesthetic component. Several studies have shown that neural blockade reduces endocrine stress responses to surgery, such as the catabolic hormonal response, hypermetabolism, and negative nitrogen balance. Spinal and epidural anaesthesia not only reduce intraoperative blood loss, but also result in a significant reduction in postoperative thromboembolic complications (Kehlet 1992). Regional anaesthesia, if continued postoperatively, has been shown to reduce cardiac morbidity in high-risk patients (Baron *et al.* 1991). It is not yet clear whether regional analgesia has any benefit on pulmonary function postoperatively, but from the available studies fewer pulmonary complications have been reported with extradural as opposed to parenteral analgesia (Bonnet and Delaunay 1992). It is suggested that regional analgesia may facilitate chest physiotherapy, which by itself could improve respiratory morbidity. Several studies on gastrointestinal function have shown that epidural analgesia with local anaesthetics alone, improves postoperative gastrointestinal function, with normalized gastric emptying and reduced paralytic ileus time (Wattwil 1992).

The final issue that should be considered is the prevention of chronicity (i.e. does treating acute pain efficiently prevent the potential for developing a chronic pain state?). Basic animal research has indicated that treatment before nerve injury will significantly reduce long-term consequences. However, the clinical evidence is less compelling;but there appears to be

enough evidence available to suggest that treating pain early, or before it starts, will result in less chronicity. Several risk factors have been identified, including age, the severity of the acute pain, concomitant treatment such as radiotherapy and chemotherapy, and the presence of depression and anxiety (Munglani and Hunt 1995;Munglani *et al.* 1996c;Kalso 1997).

Studies in the past decade have suggested that phantom pain can be significantly reduced if pre-amputation epidural pain relief was instituted (Bach *et al.* 1988;Jahangiri *et al.* 1994; Shug *et al.* 1995; Katsuly-Liapis *et al.* 1996). Only the first- and last-mentioned studies were randomized. However, a recent prospective randomized study of 60 patients (Nikolajsen *et al.* 1997) has shown no difference in those patients treated with pre-operative epidurals. The evidence for post-thoracotomy pain is also mixed, with the jury out on multimodal analgesia (see later). However, it does appear that early treatment of acute herpes zoster will reduce the incidence of chronic pain.

Having an understanding of the mechanisms of pain is important in order to appreciate its further management.

2 Understanding the pain system

2.1 What are the major components of postoperative pain?

There are three components to the mechanisms of pain, as shown in Table 10.1. These may all need to be addressed in its management.

2.2 How is pain first perceived?

Noxious stimuli will activate distinct nociceptors on the target organ involved. These are in fact naked nerve endings of fast-conducting myelinated A and slower-conducting unmyelinated C fibres. Skin, muscle, fasciae, joints, viscera, and other deeper somatic structures are supplied by a mixture of these nerve fibres. They may be activated by mechanical, thermal, and chemical noxious stimuli as well as disease, inflammation, contraction, ischaemia, and distension (Bonica 1990).

The resulting impulses then travel along their respective first-order nerve fibres to the dorsal horn of the spinal cord. Here the dorsal horn neurons synapse in the Rexed laminae, of which there are ten. The polymodal C fibres tend to synapse in laminae I, II (substantia gelatinosa), and V. The A fibres terminate in the same

Table 10.1 Major components of postoperative pain (Hayes and Molloy 1997)

1. Nociceptive	Tissue damage and inflammation in response to surgery, infection, haematoma, and recurrent tumour
2. Neuropathic	Direct nerve injury, entrapment neuropathies, complex regional pain syndromes (types 1 and 2)
3. Psychological	Cognitive and affective factors (e.g. catastrophizing, depression, and drug-seeking behaviour)

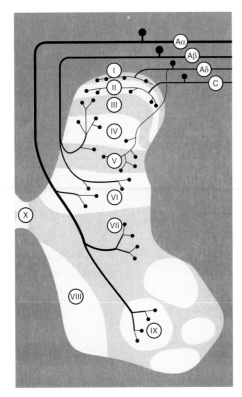

Figure 10.1 Dorsal root connections.

layers as well as in the deeper layers of X. In contrast, the A fibres that mediate light touch and proprioception synapse in laminae III and IV. A fibres do not normally mediate pain, but may do so after peripheral and central sensitization have occurred. Importantly, A fibres do not have opioid receptors and thus pain mediated by these fibres may not be opioid sensitive (see Fig. 10.1).

2.3 How is the dorsal horn involved?

The dorsal horn itself is a complex structure that includes numerous varieties of nerve fibres and synaptic arrangements. It has a rich biochemistry that allows reception and transmission of impulses and a high degree of processing that includes local abstraction, integration, selection, and appropriate dispersion of sensory impulses. In short, it is a central modulating unit. It is activated through central convergence and summation of impulses and modified by excitatory and inhibitory impulses from the periphery, local interneurons, and from the brainstem and cortex. It is here, within the dorsal horn, that the synapses occur between the primary afferent and second-order neurons.

2.4 The spinal and supraspinal pathways

The pathways for the transmission of nociceptive information occur in the spinothalamic tract (STT), the spinoreticular tract (SRT), and the spinomesencephalic tract (SMT). The lateral part of the STT, or neospinothalamic tract, courses to the ventro-posterolateral thalamic nuclei (VPL) and synapse with third-order neurons to the somatosensory cortex. The medial part of the STT, or paleo-STT, plus the SRT and SMT project to the reticular formation, the periaqueductal grey matter, the hypothalamus, and the medial and intralaminal thalamic nuclei. From here the fibres will connect to the limbic forebrain structures and other areas (Figs 10.2 and 10.3).

The supraspinal connections are related to the powerful autonomic responses concerned with ventilation, circulation, and neuroendocrine function, and the motivational drive and unpleasant affect that triggers behavioural responses to nociceptive input.

Each structure that sends fibres to the cortex can receive descending fibres that influence transmission. This can occur in the thalamus, the reticular system, the trigeminal system, and the spinal cord. Theses powerful descending inhibitory signals form part of the gate-control theory of pain and can modulate input before it is transmitted to the discriminative and motivational systems.

3 The neurophysiology of nociception

3.1 Physiological versus clinical pain

Nociception can be thought of as being physiological or clinical. Physiological pain involves noxious stimulation of the high-threshold A and C receptors. This is a well-localized, transient phenomenon, which has a stimulus–response relationship, and it is a fundamental warning and protective mechanism (Woolf and Chong 1993).

Clinical pain encompasses further inflammatory and neuropathic elements. It is the pain resulting from abnormal excitability in the peripheral and central nervous systems after injury. Continuing stimuli involve low-threshold receptors of the A type, resulting in amplification of the A and C fibre input into the spinal cord (Figs 10.4 and 10.5).

3.2 What is peripheral sensitization?

Under clinical conditions, trauma, including surgery, will result in the release of contents from damaged and inflammatory cells, causing a neurogenic inflammatory response. This results in an exaggerated response in the initial area of insult. This is due to a 'sensitizing soup' of inflammatory mediators such as potassium, serotonin, bradykinin, substance P, histamine, neuropeptides, nerve growth factor, and products from the arachidonic acid metabolic pathway. These sensitize nerve endings and modify their threshold from high- to low-threshold receptors (Breivik et al. 1996). Primary hyperalgesia, due to the above mechanism, is the tenderness or pain in the area of noxious stimulation, and is an accentuated response to the noxious stimulus. Secondary hyperalgesia is the pain perceived in the surrounding intact area (Campbell et al. 1988; Torebjork et al. 1992). Allodynia is the interpretation of non-noxious stimulation as if it was noxious (see Fig. 10.6).

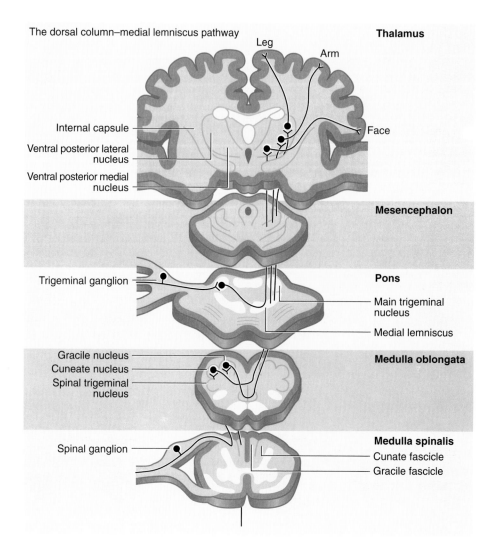

The dorsal column–medial lemniscus pathway

Thalamus

Leg
Arm
Face

Internal capsule

Ventral posterior lateral
nucleus

Ventral posterior medial
nucleus

Mesencephalon

Trigeminal ganglion

Pons

Main trigeminal
nucleus

Medial lemniscus

Gracile nucleus
Cuneate nucleus
Spinal trigeminal
nucleus

Medulla oblongata

Spinal ganglion

Medulla spinalis
Cunate fascicle
Gracile fascicle

Figure 10.2 The dorsal column and its connections.

3.3 What is central sensitization?

Within minutes of the spinal cord receiving noxious stimuli input, changes take place in spinal information processing. Neurotransmitter release from the A and C fibres in the dorsal horn causes postsynaptic excitatory potentials. These also result from release of neuropeptide tachykinins (substance P), neurokinin A and B, calcitonin gene related peptide (cGRP), vasoactive intestinal peptide (VIP), somatostatin, bombesin, and the excitatory amino acids (EAAs) glutamate and aspartate. The EAAs act at receptors, including N-methyl-D-aspartate (NMDA), 2-amino-3-hydroxy-5-methyl-4-isoxazole-propionic acid (AMPA), kainate, and metabotrophic receptors. Substance P, first isolated in 1931 by von Euler and Gadden, has been found to have prominent expression in the substance gelatinosa (Go and Yaksh 1987).

The result of this is central sensitization of the dorsal horn neurons with sprouting of the nerve ends into adjacent laminae and expansion of their receptive fields, as well as a decrease in the threshold and an increase in the magnitude and response to the suprathreshold stimuli of these cells (see Fig. 10.7).

It has been demonstrated that a repetitive painful stimulus progressively increases the activity and responsiveness of the spinal nerves throughout the duration of the stimulus. These phenomena such as 'wind-up' and long-term potentiation are components of central sensitization. Once a central sensitized state has been set up, abnormal or even normal input from the periphery can maintain it (e.g. inflamed tissue, sympathetic nerves, or even ordinary levels of nerve activity). The molecular basis of this sensitized state may exist into the long term, with processes such as activation of NMDA and tachykinin receptors causing calcium entry, activation of GTP-binding proteins, and change of secondary messengers. The increased calcium can also stimulate the production of protein oncogenes such as c-*fos* and c-*jun*. Thus protein kinase activity is altered, ion-channel proteins are phosphorylated, and immediate early gene expression is modified. These can all cause long-term changes in neurons (Munglani *et al.* 1995, 1996b, 1997;Munglani 1998).

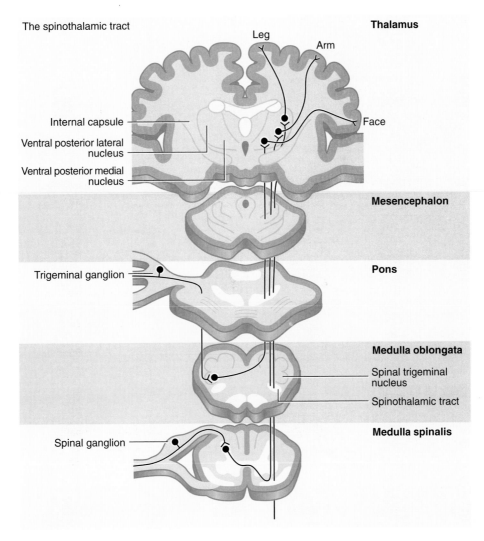

Figure 10.3 The spinothalamic tract and its connections.

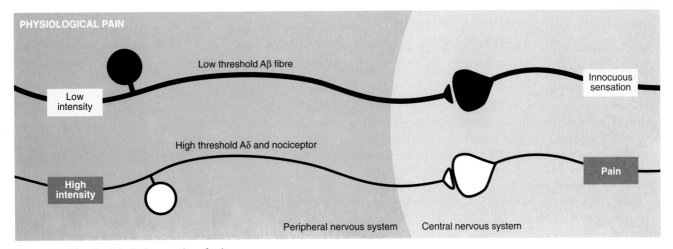

Figure 10.4 The physiological perception of pain.

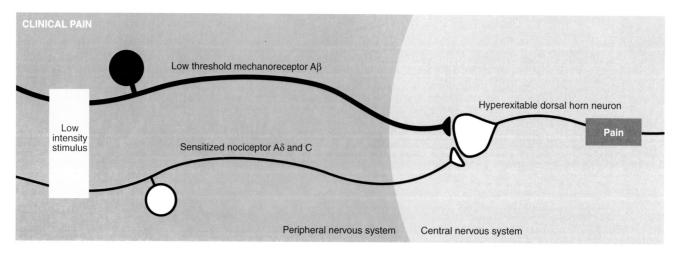

Figure 10.5 The clinical perception of pain.

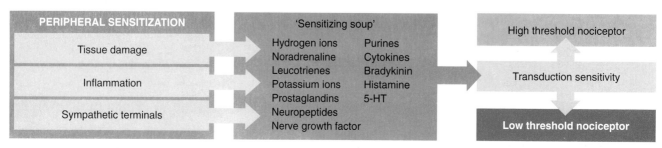

Figure 10.6 Peripheral sensitization of pain.

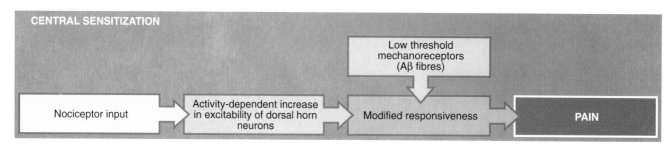

Figure 10.7 Central sensitization of pain.

3.4 How is the sympathetic nervous system involved in pain?

The sympathetic nervous system has a role in the generation and maintenance of chronic pain states. Minor trauma and nerve damage can result in disturbances of sympathetic activity. These can result in a sustained conditioned now known as 'complex regional pain syndrome' (CRPS), previously known as sympathetically maintained pain (SMP), or reflex sympathetic dystrophy (RSD) and causalgia. This condition is associated with trauma to a limb, but can arise spontaneously.

The exact mechanisms accounting for this condition are not known. However, it has been observed that peripheral nerve injury is associated with sprouting of sympathetic fibres into the cell bodies of the affected nerve. Nerve injury also causes the expression of adrenergic receptors on the peripheral nerves, which sensitizes them to peripheral sympathetic stimulation and circulating catecholeamines (Munglani and Hunt 1995; Munglani 1998).

4 Pharmacological agents for pain management

4.1 Opioids

For moderate to severe pain the opioids are still the mainstay of treatment. They are classically known as narcotic agents (from

Table 10.2 Principal pharmacological effects of the opioid agents

Desirable effects	Undesirable effects
Analgesia	Nausea and vomiting
Anxiolysis	Respiratory depression
Sedation	Constipation
Euphoria	Dysphoria
	Dependence
	Smooth-muscle spasm
	Depression of cough reflex
	Muscle rigidity
	Antanalgesia

the Greek word *narkoo*, meaning to benumb). Opium (Greek *opion* means poppy) was derived from the capsules of the unripe oriental poppy seed (*Papaver somniferum*) in the fourth century BC. By the sixteenth century, the actions of opium were well known in Europe. The principal active ingredient, morphine, was isolated in 1806 and named after Morpheus, the Greek god of dreams. It still remains the gold standard of opioids today. The words 'narcotic' and 'opiate' have now been superseded by 'opioids' as this covers both the naturally occurring and synthetic agents (Calvey and Williams 1991).

Opioid analgesics exert their action (Table 10.2) by modifying the complex emotional issues of pain as well as affecting the transmission as a sensory modality. Morphine is still the most commonly used postoperative opioid, despite the ongoing development of the synthetic phenylpiperidine class of drugs. Its principal pharmacological effects are mediated mainly by ? receptors, although there may be actions on the ? and ? receptors.

Pethidine is another commonly used opioid agent, particularly in obstetric practice. It was originally developed as an anticholinergic agent. There is no compelling evidence that one opioid is better than another, but there sufficient evidence that pethidine has a specific disadvantage and no advantage (Szeto *et al.* 1977; Hagmeyer *et al.* 1993). If given in multiple doses, the metabolite norpethidine can accumulate and act as a central nervous system irritant, ultimately causing convulsions, especially in patients with renal dysfunction. It should probably not be used when repeated injections are required (McQuay *et al.* 1997) and it is probably not true that pethidine is better for colicky spasmodic pain (Nagle and McQuay 1990). However, after equianalgesic doses, the rise in pressure in the common bile duct induced by pethidine is less than that caused by morphine, but greater than that caused by codeine (Reisine and Pasternak 1996).

It should be remembered that morphine has an active metabolite, morphine-6-glucuronide (M6G), and an antiopioid metabolite, M3G, which may accumulate in renal dysfunction. Thus vigilance is always required. A comparison of some common opioid analgesics is shown in Table 10.3.

Fentanyl, alfentanil, sufentanil, and remifentanil are all commonly used phenylpiperidine derivative drugs, especially in anaesthesia and intensive care. Tramadol is a newer synthetic agent. It is a useful analgesic with minimal sedation, respiratory depression, or abuse potential, although it is less potent than morphine (Minto 1997). It is a mixture of two enantiomers, (+) and (−) tramadol, which have low but preferential uptake at μ-opioid receptors. It also inhibits noradrenaline (norepinephrine) and 5-hydroxytryptamine (5-HT) reuptake and facilitates 5-HT release from nerve endings. It is available both orally and parenterally, and generally has fewer side-effects than pure opioid agonists, but still has an incidence of nausea of 30 per cent (Vickers *et al.* 1992). The different enantiomers may well have different potencies and this is an area of further research.

The most significant recent advance in the area of postoperative analgesia is the rediscovery of the oral route of administration (Barrat 1997). This is due to the slow-release morphine

Table 10.3 A comparison of common analgesics: dosage, interval of administration, and half-lives

Generic name	Dose (mg) 70 kg person	Route	Interval (hours)	Plasma half-life (hours)
Morphine	10 (5–20[a])	IM, SC, O	3–4 2	4–7
Pethidine	75 (50–150)	IM, SC, O	3–5 3–4	4–6
Heroin (diamorphine)	5 (5–10[a])	IM, SC, O	4–5 0.5	4–5
Codeine	60	IM, O	4–6 2–4	
Tramadol	50–150	IM, O	4	
Diclofenac	50–150/day	O, PR, IM, IV Divided doses	1–2	
Ketorolac	10	O, IM, IV	4–6	4–6

All dosages should be checked in the *British National Formulary*.

[a] Dose may be increased according to patient's needs.

preparations such as MST Continus® (Napp) and Oramorph® SR (Boehringer), which need only be given every 12 hours. It is important that the gut is functioning, as slow-release opioids can cause respiratory depression and arrest in the presence of an ileus.

The most effective method of opioid administration is to titrate the dose to a required effect, and the easiest short-term way of doing this is to observe the effect of small intravenous doses, for example every 5 minutes. If this is not possible due to time constraints or staffing levels, then intramuscular doses should be reassessed after a maximum of 1 hour has passed. Justins *et al.* (1997) give principles for the safe and effective use of opioids. If a patient requires further analgesia, then it is usually due to inadequate pain control. This may be due to:

♦ too little drug;

♦ too long between doses;

♦ too little attention paid to the patient;

♦ too much reliance on rigid regimens.

Added to this are the misconceptions due to poor staffing levels, poor knowledge, and fear of side-effects and addiction, as mentioned earlier in this chapter.

4.2 Non-steroidal anti-inflammatory drugs

Pharmacological management of mild to moderate pain should begin, unless there is a contra-indication, with an NSAID

Goudas and Carr (1996)

Non-steroidal anti-inflammatory drugs (NSAIDs) have now gained a definitive place in the management of acute post-operative pain. The main advantage that they infer is the reduction in opioid use and related side-effects, rather than an actual improvement in analgesia (Barrat 1997). In particular, with combination therapy there is more effective control of pain with less nausea and vomiting, ileus, pruritis, and respiratory depression (Dahl and Kehlet 1991; Parker *et al.* 1994; Fogarty *et al.* 1995). The NSAIDs are more effective for musculoskeletal forms of pain than visceral pain.

The main mechanism of action of aspirin and all the NSAIDs is the inhibition of the conversion of arachidonic acid to precursor prostaglandins by cyclo-oxygenase (COX) inhibition. COX is now known to exist in two forms:COX-1 and COX-2. COX-1 is expressed consitutively, and its inhibition underlies the gastrointestinal and renal side-effects of NSAIDs. COX-2 is expressed after tissue injury and it mediates inflammation. This is related to the sensitization of peripheral receptors to bradykinin. Thus the clinical application of COX-2 inhibition would appear to be attractive (Goudas and Carr 1996). NSAIDs also have a central mechanism of action on central pathways by enhancing descending inhibitory controls (McCormack 1996).

The introduction of parenteral ketorolac in 1990 changed clinical practice (Ballantyne and Dershwitz 1995). A powerful additional arm of analgesia was now available for those patients

Table 10.4 Side-effects shared by NSAIDs

Gastrointestinal ulceration and intolerance: prostaglandin inhibition and decreased mucosal barrier production (less with paracetamol)
Blockade of platelet aggregation (inhibition of thromboxane synthesis)
Inhibition of uterine motility (prolongation of gestation)
Inhibition of prostaglandin-mediated renal function
Hypersensitivity reactions (more so with aspirin)

who could not take medication orally or rectally. Since then diclofenac has also been licensed for IV use. There were initially some fatal reactions with ketorolac, which appeared to be related to the dose;lowering the initial dose from 30 to 10 mg has averted these problems.

The side-effects of the NSAIDs are now well known and include gastrointestinal ulceration, exacerbation of obstructive airway disease, platelet inhibition, and renal failure (Clive and Stoff 1984). These problems can be avoided with careful attention to patient selection and the avoidance of long-term use. In particular, patients who are elderly, have renal impairment, are dehydrated or hypotensive, have a history of peptic ulceration, and are receiving warfarin, should not receive NSAIDs. NSAIDs are one of the most common causes of renal failure seen by renal physicians, and it cannot be stressed enough that renal impairment is a contraindication for a NSAID. The mechanisms of action resulting in the side-effects are summarized in Table 10.4.

Paracetamol alone and in combination with agents such as codeine phosphate and dextropropoxyphene are available for use in mild to moderate pain. Purists would not prescribe combination agents, but they are an effective alternative to parenteral opioids.

4.3 *α*-2 agonists and NMDA antagonists

Clonidine and ketamine are the *α*-2 agonist and NMDA antagonist, respectively, that are in current use. The *α*-2 agonists have been shown to be effective for numerous surgical procedures (Eisenach *et al.* 1996; Sandler 1996), although they cannot provide sufficient pain relief alone. Although traditionally given via the spinal or epidural route, *α*-2 agonists have been given intrapleurally and in peripheral nerve blocks, but this application requires further research. The effect of clonidine is short lived after single doses and may be accompanied by side-effects such as sedation, bradycardia, or hypotension.

It is already known that the excitatory neurotransmitter glutamate is released with substance P in the dorsal horn of the spinal cord and mediates central sensitization. This acts via the NMDA receptor, which is now known to be blocked by ketamine. Its pre-emptive analgesic effects have been studied perioperatively (Woolf and Chong 1993), and recent combination trials suggest that it may be an effective therapy (Tverskoy *et al.* 1994). The side-effects of ketamine, such as salivation, dysphoria, and cardiac stimulation, preclude its use in high doses, and co-administration of medication to alleviate these may be required.

Further studies of these pain-modulating drugs, in cases where central sensitization and neuroplasticity occur, are needed to ascertain their clinical value.

Entonox®, a combination of inhaled 50 per cent oxygen and 50 per cent nitrous oxide, can be a very effective and efficient form of pain relief for quick procedures of medium intensity, such as dressing changes. It is used extensively in obstetrics. Its mechanism of action is central.

5 Management strategies

5.1 Pre-emptive analgesia

Pre-emptive analgesia consists of treatment with analgesic agents before the spinal cord receives nociceptive input. Extensive animal research (Woolf 1983; Woolf and Wall 1986) has shown that by blocking nociceptive stimuli from reaching the spinal cord, changes that are known to occur in the dorsal horn are prevented. The concept of pre-emptive analgesia in clinical practice was thus presented (Wall 1988); however, its clinical relevance still remains to be demonstrated (Munglani et al. 1996c; Munglani 1998). In an extensive review of the literature on the value of pre-emptive analgesia in the treatment of postoperative pain, Dahl and Kehlet (1993) found mixed evidence for this form of analgesia. A large number of the trials had methodological deficiencies and it was postulated that other mechanisms than the modulation of central hyperexcitability may have played a role.

However, the concept of preventing the neuroplastic and 'wind-up' type changes that are known to occur is still a plausible working hypothesis (Munglani et al. 1995, 1996). The strongest evidence for the efficacy of this practice comes from the animal experiments where a single nociceptive input of short duration and moderate intensity was studied. In the clinical intraoperative setting or other clinical scenarios, there are large, on-going stimuli and different modalities of intense pain. These therefore need to be compared to the duration of the given analgesia. To demonstrate clinically relevant effects, future studies will need to take into account that the extent and duration of the applied antinociceptive strategy needs to be counterbalanced against the extent and duration of the evoked pain.

Methods of pre-emptive analgesia include the application of non-steroidal anti-inflammatory drugs (Hudspith and Munglani 1996); systemic opioids; local, regional, and epidural/spinal local anaesthetics; and the modulator drugs such as NMDA antagonists and α-2 agonists. Breivik et al. (1996) have published an extensive review of the methods that are available. The NSAIDs affect the central processing of nociceptive input from injured tissue, as well as having a peripheral action on the cyclo-oxygenase system with reduction of prostaglandin formation. The pre-emptive effect of a single dose of NSAID has not been found to be sustained, highlighting the problem once again of continuing treatment for the duration of the stimulus.

Studies of opioids have, for the most part, been supportive (Dahl and Kehlet 1993; Kehlet 1994; Breivik and Breivik 1996), but study design and timing must be taken into account. Spinal and epidural anaesthesia with local anaesthetics do not have an effect beyond the duration of the block, although there may be a reduced need for analgesia when compared with general anaesthesia. As mentioned previously, there may be a beneficial effect on phantom limb pain if a regional local anaesthetic block occurs prior to amputation, although the latest study refutes this. Local anaesthetic techniques are known to be effective for reducing A or C fibre input to the dorsal horn and for reducing the need for other analgesic medication, but again this does not have an effect on central sensitization beyond the actual block if nociceptive input continues. It does, however, reduce primary and secondary hyperalgesia (Pederson et al. 1996) at the time of stimulus. If one takes into account the time course of applied analgesia with concordant stimulus then most studies are only partially or not supportive of pre-emptive analgesia.

NMDA antagonists such as ketamine may inhibit the central sensitization process, or in fact reverse the process (Woolf and Thompson 1991), and recent human work has shown that while there may not be abolition of postoperative pain, there is evidence that the same mechanisms are at work in the human spinal cord as in animals, which is encouraging for further evidence to be assembled (Ilkjaek et al. 1996).

5.2 Multimodal or balanced analgesia

All drugs have side-effects and different modes of action. Multimodal analgesia has therefore been the solution to balancing risk and benefit preferred by Kehlet and Dahl since the 1980s. They recommended combined analgesic regimes in the treatment of postoperative pain, as total or optimal pain relief cannot be achieved by a single drug or method without major strain on equipment and surveillance systems, or without significant side-effects (Kehlet 1989). The rationale behind this approach is the supply of sufficient analgesia due to additive or synergistic effects of different analgesics with the concomitant reduction in side-effects, due to a reduction in the doses of drugs and differences in side-effect profiles (Kehlet and Dahl 1993a).

Unfortunately the majority of the clinical work has dealt with conventional unimodal therapy, but the little available data on balanced analgesia suggest that it is important in postoperative pain (Kehlet 1994).

It is possible to use the pain-free state that may be attained to the patient's advantage, with early postoperative mobilization and the institution of early enteral feeding (Kehlet and Dahl 1993b), aimed at reducing postoperative venous thrombosis and protein wasting (by prevention of the catabolic state). Thus it is clear that although the primary outcome of pain relief is precisely that, from the viewpoint of the postoperative pain team, it is too simplistic to look analgesia without due consideration being given to other factors important in postoperative mobilization and recovery (Barrat 1997). The efficacy studies with respect to pain and secondary outcome data are controversial and further trials are still awaited (Braga *et al.* 1996).

There are a variety of different approaches to balanced analgesia. These include combinations of simple analgesics, opioids, local anaesthesia infiltration, regional nerve blocks, central neuraxial blockade, and dorsal horn-specific type drugs. Local anaesthetic infiltration by itself lasts for too short a time, and longer-acting agents are required. NSAIDs are well documented to be effective in postoperative pain of mild or moderate intensity, but in severe pain states their efficacy is too low for their use as the sole agent. They do represent an ideal alternative component in the balanced approach as they fulfil the ideal principles of the concept. Short periods (< 1 week) of NSAID treatment do not appear to have significant side-effects as long as high-risk patients are avoided (Dahl and Kehlet 1991; Kehlet and Mather 1992).

Clinical and animal experimental data agree on the additive and synergistic analgesic effects of combining epidural local anaesthetics, opioids, and α-2 agonists (Kehlet and Dahl 1993*a*). The studies of bupivacaine alone versus bupivacaine and opioid showed improved analgesia with the combination therapy. Epidural analgesia should be administered by infusion to prevent the risk of adverse side-effects such as muscle paralysis, hypotension, and bladder dysfunction. The choice of opioid for infusions is unclear, although fentanyl may give less nausea, vomiting, pruritis, and late respiratory depression than morphine. The logical choice of local anaesthetic is bupivacaine, due to its long action, but trials are still awaited on ropivacaine which has less motor block and cardiotoxic potential than bupivacaine.

The addition of clonidine (α-2 agonist) to epidural combination regimes appears to increase the analgesic power, but in high doses can result in hypotension and sedation, and further trials are thus required. Early results on the use of multimodal

pain therapy in combination with pre-emptive analgesia that is in accordance with the time frame of the stimulus, are encouraging, although further work is needed (Dahl *et al.* 1990).

5.3 Patient-controlled analgesia

To overcome the problems of interpatient variability, timing of analgesia, and side-effects, patient-controlled analgesia (PCA) was introduced into clinical practice. Originally designed for obstetric use in the 1960s (Scott 1970), it only gained prominence as an effective form of pain relief in the 1980s (Rowbotham 1992).

The technique involves the request for small intravenous boluses of opioids by the patient from a computer-driven syringe driver that is triggered by depressing a button. This is essentially independent of knowledge of the individual patient's pharmacokinetic profile and sensitivity to a given agent. Within the constraints of the programming of the syringe driver, the patient determines the timing and dose according to his or her own appreciation of the time course and intensity of the pain. The inherent principle is that of a 'closed-loop' titration based on the pharmacokinetics of the drug used (Nierhaus and Schulte 1997).

However, while PCA has been associated with superior pain relief, patient satisfaction, and less respiratory depression, there is no evidence that it changes postoperative outcome, nor does it attenuate the surgical stress response when compared to other methods of pain relief. It is important to realize that patients, on the whole, do not titrate themselves to complete pain relief and there is a lack of data to demonstrate that PCA opioid treatment provides sufficiently low pain scores during mobility (Kehlet 1994).

With regard to PCA, the point at which a patient is sufficiently uncomfortable to make a demand is known as the minimum

Table 10.5 One PCA method

Equipment required	Designated computerized PCA syringe driver	
	Dedicated IV line, or one valve should be used to prevent backflow of analgesia solution into the IV line	
Drugs	Morphine 60 mg	
	Cyclizine 50–100 mg or droperidol 2.5–5 mg can be added	
	Dilute to 60 ml with normal saline	
Pump settings	Bolus dose	1 mg (corresponds to 1 ml)
	Lockout time	4–10 minutes
	Dose duration	Stat
	Background	None
	Patient history	Reset
Monitor	Hourly for 12 hours then 2-hourly once stable	Pain score
		Sedation score
		Blood pressure
		Respiratory rate

This is a basic method; always become familiar with your own hospital policy on PCAs.

effective (blood) concentration (MEC). However, there appears to be a wide interpatient range of MECs and no direct relationship between individual MECs, opioid consumption, and analgesic efficacy (Gourlay *et al.* 1988; Owen *et al.* 1988; Mather and Woodhouse 1997). Different kinetic properties are insufficient to explain patient responses to PCA. Mather and Woodhouse added psychological factors to this problem, including fear, anxiety, pain history, personality, the meaning of pain, and the individual coping style. These may all, to a certain extent, be overcome by adequate patient education. In addition, both staff and patient concerns about drugs, addiction, and other anxieties surrounding hospitalization, are mentioned as reasons for poor patient demand from a PCA.

The PCA devices themselves require careful attention to programming, with adequate bolus doses and timing intervals. Patients do require vigilant attention to basic physiological parameters such as blood pressure and respiratory rate. Nevertheless, the technique remains an elegant solution to the problem of pain management. A method for setting up a PCA system is shown in Table 10.5.

5.4 Major neuraxial blockade

Epidural and spinal techniques are now an accepted of pain management for any major operative procedure below the neck and the technique is practised throughout Europe (Rawall and Alvin 1996). The literature has been well reviewed by Barrat (1997) and Nierhaus and Schulte (1997).

There is no doubt that epidural is an excellent, if not superior, form of pain relief compared to parenteral medication. The data on systemic outcome are, however, more variable. Most certainly there is a reduced incidence of deep venous thrombosis in lower-limb and pelvic surgery, and improved gut performance in abdominal surgery. The evidence for improved cardiac, pulmonary, and neurological outcome is less clear, with more non-beneficial studies than beneficial ones. However, there are beneficial effects on postoperative morbidity and overall cost in patients with an elevated preoperative risk due to underlying disease (Jayr *et al.* 1993).

5.5 What agents are in use?

A mixture of local anaesthetic and opioid is currently considered to be the optimal combination. Local anaesthetic as the basic analgesic, with added opioid, has shown improved analgesia as compared to situation in which opioid was the basic analgesic (Kehlet and Dahl 1993). The most common agents in use are bupivacaine and morphine. Epidural lipophilic agents, such as fentanyl, are less likely to cause nausea, vomiting, pruritis, and late respiratory depression than hydrophilic agents. However, no differences have been seen in the studies comparing intravenous versus epidural opioid administration. This may be explained by the hydrophilicity of the agent used. Before exerting their effects on the substantia gelatinosa in the dorsal horn, opioids must cross the dura. Lipophilic agents such as fentanyl will cross and be distributed rapidly in the CSF or be reabsorbed into the

epidural space. Hydrophilic morphine will cross slowly but will tend to stay in the subarachnoid space once there (Rauck 1994). This is manifested clinically by the reduced intraspinal to systemic dose ratio and the prolonged effect with this reduced dose.

Another synergistic effect is the combination of an α-2 agonist such as clonidine with epidural opioids. The analgesic effect of clonidine may be due to absorption and a systemic effect (Bonnet *et al.* 1990) as there appears to be no difference between oral, parenteral, or spinal routes of administration (Bonnet *et al.* 1989). Continuous administration of epidural clonidine can result in hypotension. Therefore further combination trials are awaited. The positive analgesic effects are nevertheless encouraging.

5.6 What risks are involved?

The risks of major regional analgesia are those of the epidural insertion itself (dural puncture, accidental venous or subarachnoid injection, infection, haematoma, and nerve damage), those of the local anaesthetic (hypotension, toxicity, motor block), and those of the opioid (nausea, vomiting, pruritis, respiratory depression, and urinary retention).

Of great concern to the anaesthetist is the risk of permanent neurological damage. From available studies, the risk appears to be about 1 in 10 000. Obstetric practice appears to have a lower risk, around 1 in 100 000, which may reflect a different patient population and anatomical differences from others. Deficits may be the result of needle damage, spontaneous haematomas, haematomas in the face of abnormal coagulation, lipomas, abscesses, meningeal tumours, redistribution of blood flow, and hysteria. The potential benefit is therefore always balanced against the risk involved. It is imperative that with the potential serious risk of paraplegia and respiratory depression, a continued high level of vigilance by trained medical and nursing staff should be guaranteed in patients with epidural analgesia.

6 An acute pain service

A solution to the problem of poorly managed pain is referral to an acute pain team with recourse to knowledge and advanced pain management skills. This should not take responsibility away from the primary physician looking after the patient, and one of the roles of the acute pain service would be the continuing education and training of staff. The brunt of pain relief must still, however, fall on the shoulders of the surgeons and anaesthetists looking after day-to-day management of the patient, and it is their responsibility to be aware of the benefits and risks of the techniques available for the management of postoperative pain.

References

Bach, S., Noreng, M.F., and Tjellden, N.U. (1988). Phantom limb pain in amputees during the first 12 months following limb amputation, after preoperative lumbar epidural blockade. *Pain*, **33**, 297–301.

Ballantyne, J.C. and Dershwitz, M. (1995). Nonsteroidal anti-inflammatory drugs for acute pain. *Curr. Opin. Anaesthesiol.,* **8**, 461–8.

Baron, J. *et al.* (1991). Thoracic epidural anaesthesia versus general anaesthesia for high risk surgical patients. *Anesthesiology,* **75**, 611.

Barrat, S. McG. (1997). Advances in acute pain management. *Internatl Anesth. Clin.,* **35**, (2), 27–47.

Bonica, J.J. (1990). Anatomic and physiologic basis of nociception and pain. In *The management of pain,* pp. 28–94. Lia and Febiger, London.

Bonnet, F. and Delaunay, L. (1992). Effects of regional anaesthesia on pulmonary complications. In *Practice in postoperative pain. Effect of regional anaesthesia and pain management on surgical outcome,* pp. 13–16.. Wells Medical, England.

Bonnet, F., Bioca, O., Rostaing, S., *et al.* (1989). Postoperative analgesia with extradural clonidine. *Br. J. Anaesth.,* **63**, 465–9.

Bonnet, F., Bioca, O., Rostaing, S., *et al.* (1990). Clonidine-induced analgesia in postoperative patients:epidural versus intramuscular administration. *Anesthesiology,* **72**, 423–7.

Braga, M., Vignali, A., Gianotti, L., *et al.* (1996). Immune and nutritional effects of early enteral nutrition after major abdominal operations. *Europ. J. Surg.,* **162**, 105–12.

Breivik, H., Breivik, E.K., and Stubhaug, A. (1996). Clinical aspects of pre-emptive analgesia:prevention of postoperative pain by pretreatment and continued optimal treatment. *Pain Rev.,* **3**, 63–78.

Bruster, S., Jarman, B., Bosanquet, N., Weston, D., Erens, R., and Delbanco, T.L. (1994). National Survey of Hospital Patients. *BMJ,* **309**, 1542–6.

Calvey, T.N. and Williams, N.E. (1991). *Principles and practices of pharmacology for anaesthetists,* (2nd edn), pp. 299–353. Blackwell Scientific Publications, Oxford.

Campbell, J.N., Raja, S.N., Meyer, R.A., and MacKinnon, S.E. (1988). Myelinated afferents signal the hyperalgesia associated with nerve injury. *Pain,* **32**, 89–94.

Clive, D.M. and Stoff, J.S. (1984). Renal syndromes associated with non-steroidal anti-inflammatory drugs. *NEJM* **310**, 563–72.

Cohen, F.L. (1980). Post surgical pain relief:patient's status and nurses' medication choice. *Pain,* **9**, 265–74.

Cousins, M.J. and Mather, L.E. (1989). Relief of postoperative pain:advances awaiting application (editorial). *Med. J. Aust.,* **150**, 354–6.

Dahl, J.B. and Kehlet, H. (1991). Non-steroidal anti-inflammatory drugs:rationale for use in severe post-operative pain. Review. *Br. J. Anaesth.,* **66**, 703–12.

Dahl, J.B. and Kehlet, H. (1993). The value of pre-emptive analgesia in the treatment of postoperative pain. *Br. J. Anaesth.,* **70**, 434–9.

Dahl, J.B., Rosenberg, J., Dirkes, W., *et al.* (1990). Prevention of postoperative pain by balanced analgesia. *Br. J. Anaesth.,* **64**, 518–20.

Donovan, B.D. (1983). Patient attitudes to postoperative pain relief. *Anesth. Inten. Care,* **11**, 125–9.

Eisenach, J.C., De Kock, M., and Klimscha, W. (1996). Alpha 2-agonists for regional anesthesia—a clinical review of clonidine. *Anesthesiology,* **85**, 655–74.

Fogarty, D.J., Ohanlon, J.J., and Milligan, K.R. (1995). Intramuscular ketorolac following total hip replacement with spinal anaesthesia and intrathecal morphine. *Acta Anaesthesiol Scand.* **39**, 191–4.

Fung, A.S.Y. and Bentley, T.M. (1994). Preoperative analgesia for acute surgical patients. No place for complacency. *Ann. R. Coll. Surg. Engl.,* **76**, 11–12.

Go, V.L.W. and Yaksh, T.L. (1987). Release of substance P from the cat spinal cord. *J. Physiol.,* **391**, 141–67.

Goudas, L.C. and Carr, D.B. (1996). Postoperative pain control:a survey of promising drugs and pharma-coeconomic criteria for purchasing them. In *Pain 1996. An updated review,* pp. 189–94. IASP, ?.

Gould, T.H., Upton, P.M., and Collins, P. (1994). A survey of the intended management of acute postoperative pain by newly qualified doctors in the South West Region of England. *Anaesthesia,* **49**, 807–10.

Gourlay, G.K., Kowalski, S.R., Plummer, J.L., *et al.* (1988). Fentanyl blood concentration—analgesic response in the treatment of postoperative pain. *Anesth. Analg.,* **67**, 324–8.

Hagmeyer, K.O., Mauro, L.S., and Mauro, V.F. (1993). Meperidine related seizures associated with patient controlled analgesia pumps (review). *Ann. Pharmacother.,* **27**, 29–32.

Hayes, C. and Molloy, A. (1997). Neuropathic pain in the perioperative period. *Internatl Anesth. Clin.,* **35**, (2), 67–81.

Hudspith, M. and Munglani, R. (1996). Pre-emptive analgesia with NSAIDS, what do we achieve? *Br. J. Anaesth.,* **77**, 128–32.

Huskisson, E.C. (1974). Measurement of pain. *Lancet,* ii, 1127–34.

Iljaek, S., Petersen, K.L., Brennum, J., Wernberg, M., and Dahl, J.B. (1996). Effect of systemic *N*-methyl-D-aspartate receptor antagonists (ketamine) on primary and secondary analgesia in humans. *Br. J. Anaesth.,* **76**, 829–34.

Jahangiri, M., Bradley, J.W.P., Jayatunga, A.P., and Dark, C.H. (1994). Prevention of phantom pain after major lower limb amputation by epidural infusion of diamorphine, clonidine and bupivacaine. *Ann. R. Coll. Surg. Engl.*, **76**, 324–6.

Jayr, C., Thomas, H., Rey, A., *et al.* (1993). Postoperative pulmonary complications. Epidural analgesia using bupivacaine and opioids versus parenteral opioids. *Anesthesiology*, **78**, 666–76.

Kalso, E. (1997). Prevention of chronicity. Proceedings of the 8th World Congress on Pain. *Progr. Pain Res. Management*, **8**, 215–30.

Katsuly-Liapis, I., Georgeakis, P., and Tierry, C. (1996). Pre-emptive extradural analgesia reduces the incidence of phantom limb pain in lower limb amputees. *Br. J. Anaesth.*, **76**, 125 (abstract).

Kehlet, H. (1989). Surgical stress:the role of pain and analgesia. *Br. J. Anaesth.*, **63**, 189–95.

Kehlet, H. (1992). The rationale for regional anaesthesia—effects on stress, blood loss, thromboembolism and mental function. *Practice in postoperative pain. Effect of regional anaesthesia and pain management on surgical outcome*, pp. 5–8. Wells Medical, England.

Kehlet, H. (1994). Postoperative pain relief—what is the issue? (editorial). *Br. J. Anaesth.*, **72**, (4), 375–8.

Kehlet, H. and Dahl, J.B. (1993a). The value of 'multimodal' or 'balanced analgesia' in postoperative pain treatment. *Anesth. Analg.*, **77**, 1048–56.

Kehlet, H. and Dahl, J.B. (1993b). Postoperative pain (review). *World J. Surg.*, **17**, 215–19.

Kehlet, K. and Mather, L.E. (1992). The value of NSAIDs in the management of postoperative pain. *Drugs*, **44**, (Suppl. 5), 1–63.

Kuhn, S., Cooke, K., Collins, M., Jones, J.M., and Mucklow, J. (1990). Perceptions of pain relief after surgery. *BMJ*, **300**, 1687–990.

McCormack, K. (1994). The spinal actions of non-steroidal anti-inflammatory drugs and the dissociation between their anti-inflammatory and analgesic effects (review). *Drugs*, **47**, (Suppl. 5), 28–45.

McQuay, H., Moore, A., and Justins, D. (1997). Treating acute pain in hospital. Review. *BMJ*, **314**, 1531–5.

Mather, L.E. and Woodhouse, A. (1997). Pharmacokinetics of opioids in the context of patient controlled analgesia. *Pain Rev.*, **4**, 20–32.

Minto, C.F., Power, I. (1997). New opioid analgesics: an update. *Int. Anesthesiol. Clin.*, **35**, 49–65.

Munglani, R. (1998). Advances in chronic pain therapy with special reference to back pain. *Anaesth. Rev.* **14**, in press.

Munglani, R. and Hunt, S.P. (1995). Molecular biology of pain. *Br. J. Anaesth.*, **75**, (2), 186–92.

Munglani, R., Bond, A., Smith, G., Harrison, S., Elliot, P.J., Birch, P.J., and Hunt, S.P. (1995). Changes in neuronal markers in a mononeuropathic rat model:relationship between Neuropeptide Y, pre-emptive drug treatment and long term mechanical hyperalgesia. *Pain*, **63**, 21–31.

Munglani, R., Fleming, B., and Hunt, S.P. (1996a). General anaesthesia-what do we achieve?' *Br. J. Anaesth.*, **77**, 300–1.

Munglani, R., Fleming, B., and Hunt, S.P. (1996b). Remembrance of times past:the role of c-*fos* in pain. *Br. J. Anaesth.*, **76**, 1–4.

Munglani, R., Hunt, S., and Jones, J.G. (1996c). Spinal cord and chronic pain. *Anaesth. Rev.*, **12**, 53–76.

Nagle, C.J. and McQuay, H.J. (1990). Opiate receptors; their role in effect and side effect. *Curr. Anesth. Crit. Care*, **1**, 247–52.

Nierhaus, A. and Schulte, J. (1997). Postoperative pain management. *Pain Rev.*, **4**, 149–57.

Nikolajsen, L., Ilkjaer, S., Christensen, J.H., *et al.* (1997). Randomised trial of epidural bupivacaine and morphine in prevention of stump and phantom pain in lower-limb amputation. *Lancet*, **350**, 1353–7.

Owen, H., Currie, J.C., and Plummer, J.L. (1991). Variation in the blood concentration/analgesic response relationship during patient controlled analgesia with alfentanil. *Anesth. Inten. Care*, **19**, 550–60.

Parker, R.K., Haltmann, B., Smith, I., and White, P.F. (1994). Use of ketorolac after lower abdominal surgery. Effect on analgesic treatment and surgical outcome. *Anesthesiology*, **80**, 6–12.

Pederson, J.L., Crawford, M.E., Dahl, J.B., Brennum, J., and Kehlet, H. (1996). Effect of pre-emptive nerve block on inflammation and hyperalgesia after human thermal injury. *Anesthesiology*, **84**, 1020–6.

Porter, J. and Jick, H. (1980). Addiction rate in patients treated with narcotics. *NEJM*, **302**, 123.

Rauck, L.R. (1994). Management of postoperative pain. In *Current review of pain*, (ed. Raj P. Prithvi), pp. 47–60. Current Medicine Phil.

Rawall, N. and Allvin, R. (1996). Euro Pain Study Group on Acute Pain. Epidural and intrathecal opioids for post-operative pain management in Europe. A 17—Patient questionnaire study of selected hospitals. *Acta Anaesthesiol. Scand.*, **40**, 1119–26.

Reisine, T. and Pasternak, G. (1996). Opioid analgesics and antagonists. In *Goodman and Gillman's The pharmacological basis of therapeutics*, (ed. Hardman *et al.*), pp. 521–55. McGraw-Hill,

Rowbotham, D.J. (1992). The development and safe use of patient-controlled analgesia. *Br. J. Anaesth.*, **68**, 331–2.

Royal College of Surgeons of England and the College of Anaesthetists (1990). *Report of the Working Party on Pain after Surgery.* Commission on the Provision of Surgical Services. RCSE, London.

Sandler, A.N. (1996). The role of clonidine and alpha (2) agonists for postoperative analgesia. *Can. J. Anesth.,* **43**, 1191–4.

Scott, J.S. (1970). Obstetric analgesia. A consideration of labour pain and a patient-controlled technique for its relief with meperidine. *Am. J. Obstet. Gynecol.,* **106**, 959–78.

Shug, S.A., Burrel, R., Payne, J., and Tester, T. (1995). Pre-emptive epidural analgesia may prevent phantom limb pain. *Reg. Anesth.,* **20**, 256.

Szeto, H.H., Inturrisi, C.E., Houde, R., *et al.* (1977). Accumulation of norperidine, an active metabolite of meperidine, in patients with renal failure or cancer. *Ann. Intern. Med.,* **86**, 738–41.

Torebjork, H.E., Lundberg, L.E.R., and La Matte, R.H. (1992). Central changes in processing of mechanoreceptive input in capsaicin-induced secondary hyperalgesia in humans. *J. Physiol.,* **448**, 765–80.

Tverskoy, M., Oz, Y., Isakson, A., *et al.* (1994). Pre-emptive effect of fentanyl and ketamine on postoperative pain and wound hyperalgesia. *Anesth. Analg.,* **78**, 205–9.

Vickers, M.D., O'Flaherty, D., Szekely, S.M., *et al.* (1992). Tramadol:pain relief by an opioid without depression of respiration. *Anaesthesia,* **47**, 291–6.

Wall, P.D. (1988). the prevention of postoperative pain. *Pain,* **33**, 289–90.

Warfield, C.A. and Kahn, C.H. (1995). Acute pain management—programmmes in U.S. hospitals and experiences and attitudes among U.S. adults. *Anesthesiology,* **83**, 1090–4.

Wattwil, M. (1992). Effect of epidural analgesia on gastrointestinal function. In *Practice in postoperative pain. Effect of regional anaesthesia and pain management on surgical outcome,* pp. 17–20. Wells Medical, England.

Woolf, C.J. (1983). Evidence for a central component of post injury pain hypersensitivity. *Nature,* **306**, 686–8.

Woolf, C.J. and Chong, M.S. (1993). Pre-emptive analgesia—treating post-operative pain by preventing the establishment of central sensitisation. *Anesth. Analg.,* **77**, 362–79.

Woolf, C.J. and Thompson, S.W.N. (1991). The induction and maintenance of central sensitisation is dependent on *N*-methyl-D-aspartic acid receptor activation; implications for the treatment of post-injury pain hypersensitivity states. *Pain,* **44**, 293–9.

Woolf, C.J. and Wall, P.D. (1986). Morphine sensitive and morphine insensitive actions of C-fibre input on the rat spinal cord. *Neurosci. Lett.,* **64**, 221–5.

CHAPTER 11

Critical care of the surgical patient

*V.J. Pappachan, M.M. Jonas,
A. Oduro, and H.S. Smith*

1 Indications for the admission of postoperative surgical patients to an intensive care unit

A. Oduro

The availability of adequately equipped and staffed recovery units and the lowering of the threshold for the admission of these patients to ITU are important advances in the management of postoperative surgical patients which have contributed towards improved quality of patient care.

The perioperative mortality rate for elective surgery as a whole is between 0.5 and 1.9 per cent. However, this increases substantially when factors such as urgent and emergency operations, heart failure, chronic lung disease, and age over 75 years are involved. The most common complications contributing to this increased morbidity and mortality are those of the circulatory and respiratory systems.

In order to minimize this risk, patients with conditions considered to be reversible and who could benefit from more extensive care than is available on the standard surgical ward should be admitted to an area with enhanced physical and nursing facilities for monitoring and care. In many cases, a high-dependency unit (HDU) will fit the bill. In general, these units have higher staffing ratios but are not equipped for prolonged stay or mechanical ventilation. Indeed, the need for ventilation is often the deciding factor as to which unit a patient is best suited. HDUs are not yet universal and, in this case, patients are more readily transferred to an intensive care unit. In this chapter, we largely consider ITUs but much of the discussion is also relevant to HDUs.

1.1 Factors influencing admission to the ITU

1. Preoperative condition of patient (e.g. patients in poor medical condition requiring extensive surgery; trauma patients requiring surgery but with compromised conscious level).

2. Postoperative condition of patient (e.g. unstable haemodynamic state as a result of haemorrhage, heart failure, or other causes; compromised airway as a result of surgery (e.g. maxillofacial) or anaesthetic difficulty; respiratory distress; need for circulatory support).

3. Duration of surgery. Particular factors as a result of long operations are: hypothermia, fluid losses, and accumulating analgesia.

4. Extent of surgery (e.g. surgery on the abdominal aorta; oesophagogastrectomy; cystectomy).

5. Serious unanticipated complications (surgical or anaesthetic) (e.g. haemorrhage; cardiac arrest from both surgical and anaesthetic causes).

6. Advanced age, particularly with medical comorbidity.

Although patients in the above categories should ideally be considered for ITU or high-dependency care, the relative unavailability of beds in these units means that the situation is not always optimal. The decision to admit a surgical patient to an ITU should be made following consultation between the surgeon, the anaesthetist, and the ITU consultant.

2 Management of surgical patients on the intensive care unit

H.S. Smith

2.1 Introduction

The ICU is an environment in which the physiology of the severely ill patient can be supported until recovery takes place. It involves a multidisciplinary approach to medical care. Those health care professionals likely to be involved are intensivists, anaesthetists, surgeons, physicians, clinical chemical pathologists and bacteriologist, physiotherapists, dietitians, pharmacists, and intensive care nursing staff. It is usually necessary for the intensive care physician to take overall charge on the understanding that pertinent decisions will be made in consultation with the admitting team. An effective ICU is one where good inter-personal relations exist.

2.2 General ICU care

Analgesia and sedation

ICU patients find the following distressing: therapeutic paralysis, anxiety, pain, lack of rest and REM sleep, thirst, intubation, face masks, NG tubes, physiotherapy, urinary catheterization, and nausea. Septic patients in particular often have vivid hallucinations.

The aims of analgesia and sedation on ICU are to produce a comfortable, cooperative, intermittently asleep but easily rousable patient. This can be achieved by:

- reducing stress or fear by talking to and reassuring the patient wherever possible;

- continually assessing the sedation. The critically ill may have profound changes in their ability to eliminate drugs and/or their metabolites and drug accumulation often occurs especially where infusions are employed. Sudden emergence from sedation can be life-threatening, e.g. with the patient self-extubating or pulling indwelling vascular lines out;

- minimizing side effects of the drugs such as hypotension and respiratory depression;

- using several drugs in combination to achieve the desired effect and minimize the side effects of each;

- considering other analgesic techniques such as regional analgesia or non-steroidal anti-inflammatories;

- ensuring sedations is adequate if paralysis is necessary.

Bacteriological principles

Adequate infection control consists of clinical and bacteriological surveillance and strictly adhered to antibiotic policies, as well as strict hand washing in between touching patients.

Seriously ill patients are at risk of developing oropharyngeal and upper gut colonization with aerobic gram negative bacilli such as Klebsiella, Proteus, Enterobacter etc., and this is often the process that precedes an infection such as nosocomial (hospital acquired) pneumonia.

Stomach acid is an important agent in preventing such colonization. Routine stress ulcer prophylaxis with H_2 blockers such as ranitidine may predispose to colonization, but the benefits usually outweigh the risks.

Any indwelling artificial structure in the body breaks down normal host defences and can lead to ingress of bacteria. Other ICU nosocomial infections therefore commonly occur in wounds, blood, and urine. Professional bacteriological advice is essential where infection and antibiotics are concerned, as antibiotic restriction is the main method of minimizing bacterial resistance.

Fungal infections, especially with the Candida species, have become an increasing cause of nosocomial ICU infections and may occur with any breach in gut integrity or peritonitis. Candidaemia carries a high mortality, and resistance to antifungal antibiotics has now begun to emerge.

Fluid and electrolyte balance

Critically ill surgical patients display the signs of neuro-endocrine response to stress, with excess sodium and water retention, potassium loss, and hyperglycaemia. These changes are mediated through increased ADH, glucocorticoid, thyroxine, growth hormone, renin-angiotensin-aldosterone release, and increased sympathetic activity. These patients often display interstitial oedema, oliguria, hypovolaemia, hypokalaemia, anaemia, hypothermia and metabolic acidosis, and septic patients show endothelial leakage of capillary fluids with widespread interstitial ('third space') oedema and reduced perfusion of multiple organs. In addition, fluid and electrolyte imbalance can have iatrogenic causes, so constant meticulous attention to fluid and electrolyte balance is required.

The types of fluid administered will depend on what has been lost and in what the patient is deficient. Restoration of a good blood volume and blood pressure are the most important factors for sustaining organ function. Colloids stay mainly intravascularly whereas 5% dextrose is redistributed throughout all body fluid compartments and only about 12% stays in the circulation. Available colloidal solutions include albumin, gelatin, starch, and dextrans. The use of albumin to restore blood volume is now felt to be unjustifiable on cost/benefit grounds.

2.3 Respiratory care

Ventilation

Respiratory failure associated with surgery is usually treated by intubation and positive pressure ventilation or support. Other methods such as high frequency jet ventilation or external high frequency oscillation are available, and these can reduce the incidence of pulmonary barotrauma and air leaks.

If the patients is well enough, continuous positive airway pressure (CPAP) can be given via a face or nose mask. If gas exchange can be improved before respiratory exhaustion has occurred, this alone may be successful. However, the majority of ICU patients require full ventilation followed by a progressive weaning process as lung pathology and strength improve. The weaning process follows the sequence of controlled mandatory ventilation (CMV), synchronized intermittent mandatory ventilation (SIMV) with pressure support, CPAP, and then spontaneous ventilation via a T-piece.

Positive pressure ventilation can have adverse effects on blood pressure, lung dynamics, and regional organ and tissue perfusion. There is marked variability in how patients respond to ventilation, and this depends on their individual anatomy, the pathophysiology, the depth of sedation and the psychological make up of the patient. Optimum inspired oxygen tension, positive end expiratory pressure (PEEP), and ventilator parameters need to be checked every day.

Tracheostomy

This has become an indispensable part of airway care on ICU. Early surgical or percutaneous tracheostomy has facilitated weaning from ventilation by allowing cessation of sedative drugs and mobilization, together with more accessible lung toilet. Percutaneous tracheostomy is now performed on most intensive care units using a single or sequential dilatational technique. The average time to tracheostomy is 7 days (though this is likely to become progressively shorter) and surgical patients likely to undergo it are those in respiratory failure as a result of sepsis or acute respiratory distress syndrome (ARDS), and those with chronic respiratory disorders. Serious morbidity from the tracheostomy procedure is rare.

2.4 Cardiovascular care

Circulatory failure

Surgery in the presence of poor cardiac contractility carries a substantial mortality. Such patients may have co-existing carotid or coronary arterial disease, both of which predispose to coronary artery occlusive complications during surgery. Preventing regional hypoperfusion of vital organs must be the aim in both the perioperative period and the ICU stay. Optimum oxygen delivery to tissues is determined by cardiac output and the oxygen content of the blood. Cardiac output itself is determined by the filling pressures of the heart, the heart rate and the contractility of the ventricles. Oxygen content depends on haemoglobin concentration and the percentage oxygen saturation of the haemoglobin in the blood. Many perioperative factors affect these variables, including hypovolemia, bradycardia, hypothermia and acidosis.

Circulatory support

A period of cardiovascular support is often necessary after operations involving intraperitoneal sepsis, massive blood transfusion and major organ dysfunction. The first aim is to achieve good blood volume. Invasive venous monitoring is essential. The second aim is to achieve good cardiac contractility. Correction of underlying electrolytic and acid-base abnormalities is important here, and may have to be achieved by haemofiltration. Then chronotropic and inotropic support of the heart can be instituted with drugs:

- **adrenaline** affects α-1, β-1 and β-2 adrenoceptors. Cardiac output is increased together with peripheral vasoconstriction, bronchial smooth muscle relaxation and pulmonary vasodilatation. Side effects are tachydysrythmias and hyperglycaemia.

- **noadrenaline** affects α-1 (weakly β-1) adrenoceptors, and is useful in low systemic vascular resistance/high cardiac output states due to sepsis. It causes vasoconstriction and redistributes blood volume to vital organs;

- **dobutamine** affects mainly β-1 and β-2 (weak α 1) so it has positive inotropic and vasodilator properties, increasing cardiac output. It is mainly of use in low cardiac output states, although can be administered with noradrenaline in septic patients;

- **dopamine** has α-1, β-1, β-2 and dopamine receptor DA1 effects which are dose dependent. It is a useful inotrope but has not been shown to have a renoprotective effect in elective major surgery. It may have however do so in sepsis;

◆ **dopexamine** has β-1, β-2 and DA1 effects and was first introduced to aid myocardial contractility following cardiac surgery by reducing systemic vascular resistance. It increases mesenteric regional blood flow and may thus have a benefit in sepsis;

◆ **phosphodiesterase** inhibitors block intracellular cyclic adenosine monophosphate (cCMP) breakdown and increase myocardial contractility, cause coronary vasodilatation, but are contraindicated in sepsis because of potential hypotension;

◆ **vasodilators** such as nitrates cause reduction in venous tone and reduced myocardial preload, whereas sodium nitroprusside reduces myocardial afterload. Nitrates are mainly used in preventing perioperative myocardial ischaemia, and nitroprusside in controlling perioperative hypertension;

◆ **ACE inhibitors** are useful in established poor left ventricular function, especially when it causes failure to wean off ventilation. They exert their effect through blockade of production of angiotensin 2

Seriously ill ICU patients often need simultaneous infusions of several of the above drugs.

2.5 Renal problems

Introduction

Acute renal failure (ARF) develops in 0.017 per cent of the population every year. Causes include complications of obstetrics or surgery, cardiovascular insufficiency, prostatic obstruction, and medical disorders, but ARF is often multifactorial in origin. Sepsis and cardiovascular complications are the leading causes of death in patients with ARF. The overall mortality of the condition is 50 per cent, and this has not varied over many years, despite the appearance of new causative factors. In ICU patients mortality due to renal failure is 70–80 per cent, usually because of concomitant multiorgan failure.

The most common underlying cause of ARF in intensive care patients is acute tubular necrosis (ATN). ATN affects 1 per cent of all hospital patients and is caused by a combination of renal ischaemia and circulating nephrotoxins. This occurs in a range of conditions, including shock, haemorrhage, burns, crush injuries, septicaemia, acute pancreatitis, haemoglobinuria, hepatorenal failure, antibiotic intoxication, or the presence of other renal poisons. Renal histology in ATN shows normal glomeruli with loss of cell nuclei, vacuolation of the cytoplasm and absence of brush borders in the proximal tubules, tubular dilatation, cell necrosis, and interstitial oedema. However, unlike in animals, there is very little intratubular obstruction.

Why does ischaemic damage occur so easily?

Most of the work of the kidney is carried out in reabsorbing glomerular filtrate, and this entails a high oxygen consumption. This renal concentrating ability is present only in mammals and birds, both of which possess loops of Henle, but susceptibility to ARF is the price we pay for this capability. Any process that increases active transport will increase the cell damage (e.g.

amphotericin, high protein feeding, partial renal ablation, or indomethacin (a PGE_2 inhibitor)). Renal oxygen consumption (related mainly to the concentrating function of the tubular cells) falls if sodium transport is decreased and renal blood flow (RBF) is maintained or increased. This can result from ureteric occlusion, osmotic diuresis, or a decreased GFR. Thus, the proximal tubule (which descends into the renal medulla) and the thick ascending limb of the loop of Henle are the sites most commonly damaged in ischaemic acute renal failure.

The normal Pao_2 of 8–10 mmHg in the renal medulla is also the critical level at which the supply of oxygen begins to limit the rate of mitochondrial electron flow in intact cells, which, in this position, live on the brink of anoxia. Hypovolaemia causes activation of the renin–angiotensinogen–angiotensin I–angiotensin II mechanism, which increases Na^+ and H_2O reabsorption. This process puts a further oxygen demand on the kidney.

Protective mechanisms in the kidney depend largely on renal arachidonic acid metabolism. The kidney is one of the most active prostaglandin-producing organs. The major cyclo-oxygenase products PGE_2 and PGI_2 act as local tissue hormones to maintain blood flow, regulate tubular processes involving electrolytes, and modulate the effect of other renal hormones. Frusemide and mannitol also stimulate renal production of prostaglandins. PGE_2 also reduces O_2 demand by decreasing Na^+ reabsorption in the ascending loop of Henle. Vasoconstrictor hormones, including renin, angiotensin, noradrenaline (nor epinephrine), and vasopressin, produce a compensatory increase in the renal synthesis of vasodilator prostaglandins.

Cyclo-oxygenase inhibitors (e.g. indomethacin) cause marked decreases in RBF and GFR. Patients on regular non-steroidal anti-inflammatory drugs (NSAIDs) are very susceptible to ARF if they suffer hypovolaemia, even up to 2 weeks after the drugs have been stopped. Thus NSAIDs are contraindicated if there is hypovolaemia causing decreased RBF and GFR, septic shock, reduced cardiac output, pre-eclampsia, sodium depletion, renal artery stenosis, glomerulonephritis, toxic injury, advanced age, or chronic renal failure.

Preventing the establishment of ARF

Volume replacement

Volume repletion is by far the most important renal protective therapy. It can be more difficult in sepsis owing to third-space sequestration of fluid. It is important to give enough fluid to elevate depressed atrial pressures as this improves renal blood flow by 50–100 per cent at any given blood pressure. This is because atrial hypotension is a potent stimulus for renal vasoconstriction.

Mannitol

Mannitol is an alcohol that does not undergo metabolism in the body. It has negligible tubular reabsorption and reduces Na^+ and H_2O reabsorption in the proximal and distal tubules. Its sole route of excretion is via the kidneys. Mannitol is an oxygen free-radical scavenger and helps maintain glomerular pressure and prevent tubular obstruction.

Many studies have found mannitol to be no better for renal protection than simple hydration in non-septic or jaundiced patients, but it has been shown to be better in post-transplant renal protection.

Loop diuretics

These act by inhibiting the Na/K/Cl co-transporter mechanism in the thick ascending loop of Henle, so reducing Na$^+$ reabsorption and the high medullary energy requirements. Frusemide (furosemide) is usually given as an infusion of approximately 1–5 mg/hour to avoid vestibulotoxic and nephrotoxic peaks. Loop diuretics also cause renal vasodilatation, apparently by promoting renal prostaglandin production. This effect can be blocked by prostaglandin synthetase inhibitors (e.g. indomethacin).

Dopamine

Dopamine is the immediate precursor to noradrenaline (norepinephrine). It improves renal function by increasing the cardiac output and systolic blood pressures at even less than the so-called renal dose of 5 μg/kg/min. Dopamine also inhibits Na$^+$,K$^+$-ATPase on the tubular cell membrane, so reducing sodium reabsorption and renal O$_2$ demand. Despite claims, dopamine has not been shown to have additional renoprotective effects in obstructive jaundice or elective aortic aneurysm surgery in non-oliguric patients. However, there is some evidence that the drug can reverse renal dysfunction secondary to sepsis and anticancer therapy.

Noradrenaline

In humans, careful use of noradrenaline (norepinephrine) without dopamine has been shown to markedly reduce the incidence of ICU-acquired renal failure. In a fluid-resuscitated septic patient, it increases blood pressure, renal blood flow, and glomerular filtrate. GFR also increases because efferent glomerular vasoconstriction is greater than afferent.

Nutrition

The renal medulla uses glucose as its obligatory energy substrate. If enteral feeding is not possible, it is important to provide energy as an intravenous glucose solution. In an adult, intravenous glucose can be started at a rate of 25 ml/hour of 50 per cent dextrose until total parenteral nutrition is available.

Summary of measures to prevent ATN in patients at risk

- Maintain good hydration, cardiac filling pressures, blood pressure, oxygenation, and renal nutrition.

- Measure urine output and 24-hour urine urea and electrolytes.

- Avoid NSAIDs.

- Decrease medullary work with mannitol or frusemide (furosemide).

- Monitor nephrotoxics (e.g. gentamicin) with serum levels.

Treatment of established acute renal failure

Peritoneal dialysis

This is no longer practised in adult intensive care units. However, it is still useful in neonates and infants. Its disadvantages are low clearance rates with poor metabolic control, poor fluid removal, the risk of peritonitis, a high technical failure rate, hyperglycaemia, protein loss, fluid leakage, and a potentially compromised respiration. It is also contraindicated if there has been previous abdominal surgery.

Intermittent haemodialysis

Intermittent haemodialysis involves treatment several times a week, and requires specialized renal facilities and staff. It is not usually available 24 hours a day and so is of little use in intensive care. Haemodialysis gives the highest urea clearance per unit time (150 ml/min) but causes cardiovascular instability, and can cause a rapid onset of cerebral oedema. Solutes are lost mainly by diffusion across the semipermeable membranes of the dialyser.

Continual renal replacement therapies

Continual renal replacement therapy (CRRT) is the modern title for all modalities of haemofiltration. The techniques have taken over as the preferred methods of treating acute renal failure in intensive care. The most commonly used varieties nowadays are **continuous veno-venous haemofiltration** (CVVH) and **continuous veno-venous haemodiafiltration** (CVVHDF). Haemofiltration utilizes a convective loss of solutes across a semipermeable membrane, as against dialysis which gives a diffusive loss. Both techniques are combined in haemodiafiltration. They are much better tolerated than haemodialysis by very sick patients. Both methods use sophisticated blood safety modules to remove blood from the patient, pass it through a semipermeable filter, expose it to a dialysate if necessary, and return it to the patient. These machines have safety devices to prevent air embolism, and to provide warning of the imminent failure of the filter or blood flow through it. Blood flow is maintained through the filters at a rate of 50–200 ml/minute, and this is sufficient to provide a urea clearance rate of 14–24 ml/minute.

Newer membranes have been developed and are now used in all CRRT modalities. They consist of synthetic polyacrylonitriles or polysulphones with pore sizes of less than 30 000 Da; all have good biocompatibility.

Once extracellular fluid has been filtered from the patient's blood it has to be replaced with a commercial preparation with an electrolyte content similar to that of normal blood. This is usually pumped back via the same blood safety module. Commercial replacement fluids contain a buffer in the form of lactate, which is well metabolized by the liver even in ARF, sepsis, or circulatory shock. However, bicarbonate solutions can be used instead where there is established hyperlactataemia or impaired lactate metabolism (e.g. in liver failure).

Mediators of the inflammatory response in sepsis can be measured in high-flux dialyser ultrafiltrates of ICU patients. However, it is still uncertain whether the clearance rates available with current filters are high enough to remove enough of these mediators to improve the outcome of affected patients.

2.6 Nutritional care

Parenteral nutrition has always been useful in complete gut failure. It is recognized, however, that early postoperative return to enteral feeding is more physiological and less hazardous. Addition of certain immune enhancing nutrients to either type of feed is now felt to be beneficial. Such substances are arginine, glutamine, omega 3 fatty acids, and nucleotides and their addition to enteral feed post-operatively has been shown to reduce hospital length of stay and infection rates. Other advantages of enteral feeding are in protecting gut mucosal integrity and immune function. (see Chapter 8).

3 Multiple organ dysfunction syndrome

V.J. Pappachan, M.M. Jonas, and A.Oduro

When fever is persistent the external surface of the body is cold and internally great heat is perceived with thirst, the affliction is mortal

Hippocrates (400 BC)

Multiple organ failure or multiple organ dysfunction syndrome (MODS) was first recognized in the early 1970s. Since then, progress in the management of critically ill patients has revealed more about the pathophysiology involved in this potentially lethal cocktail of sequential organ dysfunction. The pattern of progressive organ impairment and eventual failure can complicate illnesses with a range of diverse aetiologies and still carries a high mortality despite progress in understanding it.

MODS is the organ-specific manifestation of a systemic process, namely a severe, uncontrolled systemic inflammatory response initiated by one or more of an array of triggering events such as infection, inflammation, ischaemia–reperfusion injury, or trauma. In simple terms, it represents the deregulation of the host immune system and inflammatory response.

MODS has become the most common reason for surgical patients to stay in ITU for more than 5 days and, in these patients, is the most frequent cause of death. MODS, which is a pan-endothelial, multisystem disease, needs to be distinguished from isolated organ dysfunction occurring after operation or trauma, as the pathogenesis and outcomes are markedly different.

3.1 Epidemiology of MODS

Organ failure can be defined using either measures of physiological derangement (e.g. hypotension, acidosis, plasma creati-

Table 11.3 Approximate mortality versus number of organ systems failed

Number of organs failing	Mortality
1	40%
2	60%
3	>90%

nine) or on treatment methods (e.g. dialysis, ventilation). Controversies have frequently arisen about the definition of organ failure and the mechanisms involved, partly because of the wide range of dysfunction that can occur in each organ (from minimal physiological impairment to overt failure) and partly because of the difficulty of monitoring the function of all the organs involved. This lack of a codified diagnostic system has hampered epidemiological surveys and the assessment of treatment outcomes. Thus, the true incidence of MODS is unknown, as published studies have used differing clinical and temporal definitions of organ failure. However, an approximation can be obtained by reviewing published studies: depending on the case-mix of ICU patients studied and the diagnostic criteria used, MODS appears to develop in 5–15 per cent of patients requiring ICU admission. The outcome of MODS is remarkably consistent between studies, with mortality linked to the number of organs failing (Table 11.3).

3.2 The emergence of MODS

The emergence of MODS broadly follows one of two clinical courses, differing in the time of onset relative to the initial event, the time course, and the sequence of organ failure.

◆ **Primary MODS** is a fulminant process following an insult such as major tissue injury involving either one or more organs. For example, primary MODS may follow a direct pulmonary insult such as trauma or aspiration of gastric contents. In this form, the course of the disease may be short, with MODS becoming evident just before death.

◆ **Secondary MODS** is more common and has a more insidious onset. This pattern of organ dysfunction is often seen in severe sepsis and septic shock. Covert or subclinical MODS is present early in the illness, and is followed by signs of a continuing **systemic inflammatory response syndrome** (SIRS). After 7–10 days, the process progresses with manifestations of pulmonary failure (ARDS) and hepatic and renal failure. During the evolution of MODS, gastrointestinal (GI) failure in the form of increased mucosal permeability and a paralytic ileus is often seen. This has led to speculation that the intestine becomes the 'motor' or driving force of MODS, either as a consequence of bacterial translocation from the intestine or immunomodulation in the splanchnic circulation (Fig. 11.1).

Animal models of sepsis clearly demonstrate that bacterial translocation occurs. The situation in humans is less clear. It is

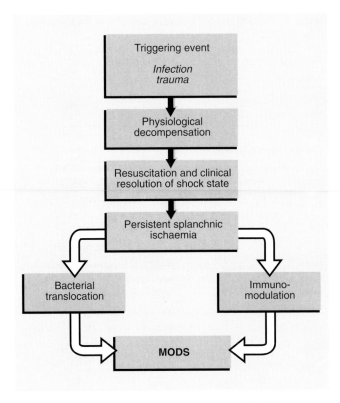

Figure 11.1 Covert splanchnic ischaemia can persist despite apparently adequate haemodynamic resuscitation. Mucosal integrity can be impaired, resulting in bacterial translocation and the activation of neutrophils passing through the splanchnic circulation. In this way an inflammatory state can be propagated and the intestine can act as the 'motor' of MODS.

improbable that bacteraemia as a consequence of increased mucosal permeability is the fuel for the gastrointestinal 'motor' in MODS. If the intestine has a pathogenic role to play in the development of MODS, the concept of the activation of both the mesenteric vascular endothelium and the hepatic Kupffer and stellate cells is far more attractive. Translocation of bacterial endotoxins and exotoxins could then stimulate a systemic response, by local activation of white cells within the splanchnic circulation. Moreover, such translocation and activation may impair the usual role that Kupffer and other hepatic reticuloendothelial cells play in clearing toxins and pathogens from the portal circulation, allowing overspill into the systemic circulation.

Within the range of initiating events for MODS, by far the most common association is with severe sepsis and ARDS. The likelihood of MODS occurring and progressing is dependent on the severity of the initiating event but also the pre-morbid physiological reserve of the patient and any co-morbid conditions; for example, cardiovascular, pulmonary, renal, hepatic, or malignant disease.

3.3 The aetiology of MODS

MODS is now recognized as a systemic disorder that occurs as a consequence of widespread endothelial injury and activation,

Table 11.4 Recognized initiating events for MODS

Severe infection: peritonitis
Trauma: chest injuries, multiple injuries, burns
Shock: cardiogenic, haemorrhagic
Surgery: major vascular surgery, abdominal surgery (particularly involving large bowel anastomoses)
Medical: pancreatitis, aspiration pneumonitis
Other: massive transfusion

disordered haemodynamics, and impaired tissue oxygen extraction. Most of the initiating events can be characterized as infective, traumatic, or ischaemic (Table 11.4).

Mechanistically, MODS represents exaggeration and loss of control of host defence so that it becomes a disorder itself. There is an unregulated and exaggerated immune response, which initiates an excessive release of inflammatory mediators. These circulating mediators produce the widespread microvascular, haemodynamic, and mitochondrial changes that lead to organ failure.

3.4 Progression of MODS

It has been proposed that MODS in its classical form progresses through four clinically distinct phases:

1. **Hypoxic or mitochondrial electron transport chain dysfunction.** Periods of cellular hypoxia are common to all of the diverse initiating events associated with MODS. There is either an episode of relative or total ischaemia or a defect of oxygen extraction at the level of the mitochondrial electron transport chain. Either of these may be clinically silent. The severity of the triggering event, the lag time to resuscitation, and the initial functional reserves of the organs concerned appear to determine the course of the condition and its outcome: either organ dysfunction with recovery or progressive organ failure.

Table 11.5 Definition of the systemic inflammatory response syndrome (SIRS) and its relationship to sepsis and septic shock

SIRS is manifested by two or more of the following:

· Temperature >38 °C or <36 °C

· Heart rate >90 beats/min

· Respiratory rate >20 breaths/min or $Paco_2 < 4.3$ kPa

· White cell count >12 000 cells/mm³, <4000 cells/mm³, or more than 10% immature forms

Sepsis is present if SIRS is associated with culture-proven infection

Severe sepsis is present if it is associated with signs of end-organ dysfunction:

1. Oliguria or anuria

2. Disordered mentation

3. Hypoxia

Septic shock is present if SIRS is associated with hypotension which is refractory to volume replacement alone and requires the use of vasopressors

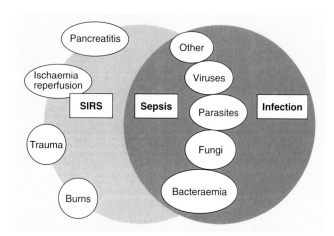

Figure 11.2 The relationship between SIRS and sepsis and a brief outline of the triggering mechanisms involved in the induction of the inflammatory response.

2. **Active resuscitation.** If resuscitation is rapid and effective, the sequence of events that precipitates MODS may be aborted. However, despite apparently adequate resuscitation to achieve conventional clinical goals, the syndrome often progresses because cellular hypoxia persists. Covert shock states can persist even when traditional end points have been reached and, furthermore, we currently have no reliable non-invasive methods of assessing the adequacy of regional oxygenation.

3. **Systemic inflammatory response syndrome.** SIRS (defined in Table 11.5) is the systemic manifestation of the generalized inflammatory response to a variety of triggers and often occurs in the absence of proven sepsis. The relationship between SIRS and sepsis is described in Fig. 11.2. Inadequate or delayed resuscitation at the cellular or at specific organ level may result in further progression of the disease towards MODS. Factors determining the progression from SIRS to MODS or otherwise are poorly understood, but one factor may be a genetic predisposition.

4. **MODS.** The original hypoxic or mitochondrial insult may lead, through poorly identified but self-amplifying pathways, to the multisystem failure characteristic of MODS. The appearance of clinically overt organ failure is an important prognostic event. With one- and two-organ system failure, mortality increases to 40–60 per cent and, as the disease progresses, if three or more organs fail, mortality reaches 90–100 per cent. The number of organ system failures and their duration are both directly related to the risk of hospital mortality.

3.5 Mediators of SIRS and MODS

Experimental and clinical studies have shown that the metabolic and physiological alterations found in SIRS/sepsis and subsequent cellular damage are caused by complex interactions of endogenous and exogenous mediators (Table 11.6). **Chemo-**

Table 11.6 Humoral and cell-mediated systems implicated in the pathogenesis of MODS

- Endotoxin
- Complement
- Leucocytes
- Macrophages
- Cytokines
    Tumour necrosis factor
    Interleukins
    Platelet activating factor
    Interferon
- Hormones
    Triiodothyronine
    Growth hormone
    Insulin
    Glucocorticoids
- Eicosanoids
    Prostaglandins
    Thromboxanes
    Leukotrienes
- Free-radicals of oxygen
- Nitric oxide
- Enzymes
    Proteases
    Lysozymes
- Amines
    Histamine
    Serotonin
    Adrenaline (epinephrine)
    Noradrenaline (norepinephrine)

kines (cytokines) are released from the host endothelial and reticuloendothelial cells, principally from neutrophils. These cells respond to provocation by a variety of stimuli, including ischaemia–reperfusion injury, bacterial, viral, and fungal products and membrane constituents. Experimental administration of mediators that are normally produced either endogenously (e.g. tumour necrosis factor (TNF), interleukins IL-1, IL-2, IL-6, platelet activating factor (PAF)) or exogenously (e.g. lipopolysaccharide) give rise to physiological responses similar to those found in SIRS and invoke a clinical syndrome indistinguishable from MODS.

A growing number of chemokines are thought to be involved in the pathogenesis of the SIRS/sepsis syndrome. Plasma levels of these mediators change with time, making it difficult to correlate any individual chemokine plasma levels with outcome. In addition, these molecules exert their destructive or protective effects at the cellular level and their plasma concentrations correlate poorly with concentrations found in end organs. Effector systems involved in translating the trigger for the condition into MODS include not only the cellular and humoral

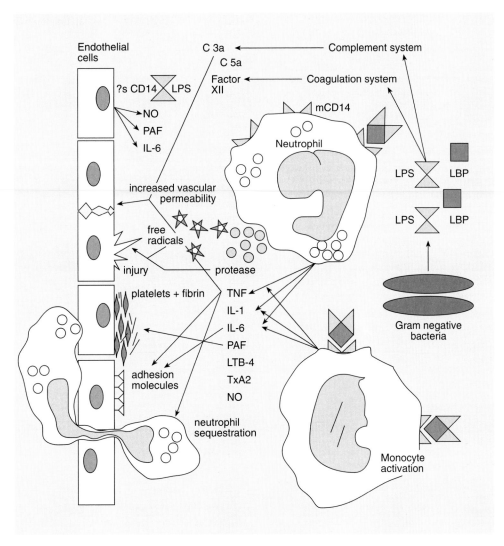

Figure 11.3 Mediators involved in the pathogenesis of sepsis and MODS.

components of the inflammatory response but also the endocrine and central nervous systems. Following injury, a local inflammatory response occurs. The primary response to chemokine induction is endothelial activation and expression of intercellular adhesion molecules (ICAMs). Later, neutrophils begin to roll along endothelial surfaces, adhere, and then diapedese into tissues. Subsequent activation of complement, coagulation, and other components of the inflammatory system occurs and the primary response is amplified. If the injury is severe or persistent, this localized reaction may spill over into the systemic circulation, producing the systemic inflammatory response or, if identified with infection, produce the sepsis syndrome. MODS may develop subsequently (Fig. 11.3).

3.6 Mediators involved in the pathogenesis of sepsis and MODS

The trigger in this case is the lipopolysaccharide (LPS) moiety of Gram-negative organisms. LPS is bound to a binding protein

(LBP) and directly activates neutrophils and components of the coagulation and complement pathways. Activated neutrophils produce a large number of chemokines, including tumour necrosis factor (TNF), the interleukins (IL-1, IL-6), platelet activating factor (PAF), the leukotriene family (LTBs), thromboxane (TxA$_2$), and nitric oxide. These chemokines result in endothelial activation, the expression of adhesion molecules (ICAMs, selectins, CD11/18, CD14), an increase in vascular permeability, vasoparesis, and neutrophil–endothelial interaction. The final common pathway is thought to involve the migration of activated neutrophils into the interstitial space of the affected organ and the development of tissue hypoxia and MODS.

3.7 The role of chemokines (cytokines) in MODS

In health, chemokines are produced by immune cells following activation by foreign particles (e.g. bacteria) and inappropriate activation is strongly repressed. As with many biological

Table 11.7 A summary of some of the chemokines involved in the pathogenesis of sepsis and MODS that have been targeted in phase III clinical trials

Target	Actions	Drugs	Outcome
LPS	The lipid A moiety of LPS is an inner-core cell-wall constituent ubiquitous to all Gram-negative organisms. It acts as the trigger for the inflammatory cascade that these organism can originate	2 MCAs XOMA HA-1A	Phase III multicentre randomized controlled trials No significant survival benefit Suggestion of increased mortality in Gram-positive sepsis with HA-1A
TNF	Levels peak early in sepsis; widespread effects on neutrophils and endothelium. Trigger–independent release makes it one of the primary targets for pharmacotherapy	MCA Bay X 1351	NORASEPT trial: no overall improvement in 28-day mortality, but a non-significant 17% reduction in shocked patients INTERSEPT trial: increased mortality in sepsis suggested
Adhesion molecules	Neutrophil/endothelial interaction is dependent on the expression of intracellular adhesion molecules (CD11/18, E- and P-selectin, etc.). The expression of these molecules is greatly upregulated in sepsis and may play a pivotal role in the migration of neutrophils into tissues and the development of MODS	MCAs	Data only from animal studies, co-clinical trials in progress to date
IL-1 receptor antagonists	IL-ra binds to both IL-1 receptor subgroups but has no agonist activity. Plasma levels of IL-ra are 100–1000 times that of IL-1. This is important as binding of only 5% of receptors will lead to clinical effects	Recombinant IL-ra	Two phase III trials failed to show any improvement in 28-day mortality

Most of the therapeutic agents are specifically designed monoclonal antibodies. These drugs represent a huge potential cost burden and so far none of the trials has shown a significant survival benefit except when *post hoc* analysis has been used to select specific subgroups of patients.

LPS, lipopolysaccharide; TNF, tumour necrosis factor; MCA, monoclonal antibody; RCT, randomized controlled trial.

systems, chemokine induction and production are closely regulated so that the host benefits from localization and destruction of the invading organisms. However, in certain situations, the control systems fail and chemokine production becomes both inappropriate and excessive, leading to destruction of normal cells with a generalized inflammatory response.

A decade of study has underlined the role of the immune system, the endothelium, and the chemokines they produce in the sequence of events ultimately producing SIRS and MODS. The precise roles and hierarchy of importance of these mediators in the pathogenesis of SIRS, sepsis, and MODS have not yet been clearly defined. A rational approach therefore is to describe one possible set of interactions schematically (Fig. 11.3) and to describe those chemokines whose genetically designed and produced antagonists have been the topic of clinical research in the ICU setting (Table 11.7).

3.8 Specific organ involvement in MODS

Respiratory system

In the majority of critically ill patients who develop MODS, the lung is the first organ to fail, with the other organs following in a sequential fashion. The respiratory system may be pivotal in the development of MODS, either by generating inflammatory mediators and aggravating endothelial dysfunction or by causing an increase in the circulatory half-life of chemokines as a result of a decreased metabolic capacity. As with other organs, a spectrum of dysfunction exists, and lung injury is a continuum ranging from minor defects in gas exchange to life-threatening hypoxia despite maximal ventilatory support. Acute lung injury (ALI) is a term that has been coined to describe this spectrum of disease. The acute respiratory distress syndrome (ARDS) has replaced the 'adult' respiratory distress syndrome in the nomenclature describing the most severe form of acute lung injury seen in critically ill patients. The American–European consensus conference defined ARDS as being present when the PaO_2/FiO_2 ratio falls below 26.7 kPa, there are three or more segments of intra-alveolar infiltrates on chest X-ray (CXR), and clinical evidence to suggest that the pulmonary artery occlusion pressure is less than 18 mmHg. These clinical and radiological features must be acute and associated with a diagnosis that is recognized to predispose to ARDS.

ALI/ARDS can be initiated either by a direct alveolar epithelial insult, such as aspiration, or by alveolar capillary endothelial activation (direct or indirect). Subsequently leucocyte adhesion, diapedesis, chemoattraction, and oxygen free-radical formation occurs. In ARDS, damage to the pulmonary capillary endothelial–epithelial interface causes low-pressure alveolar flooding with protein-rich fluid. Secondary surfactant deficiencies may occur, but surfactant replacement therapy is not associated

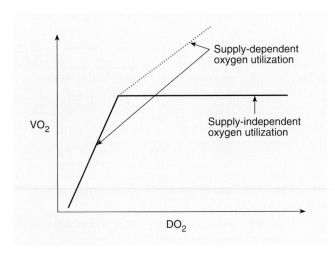

Figure 11.4 The oxygen flux equation:

$$Do_2 = \{\text{cardiac output Hb } 1.39 \, Sao_2\} + \{0.003 \, Pao_2\}$$

represents the factors that influence oxygen transport from the cardiorespiratory complex to peripheral tissues. Although it defines the oxygen content of arterial blood ejected from the left ventricle, it does not necessarily reflect regional oxygen delivery, as not all of the ejected blood will be available for regional utilization. The graph of oxygen delivery (Do_2) plotted against oxygen consumption (Vo_2) shows the normal situation, in which as long as Do_2 remains above a very low level (critical Do_2), Vo_2 remains independent of any changes in oxygen delivery. This is achieved by organs changing their oxygen extraction ratio (OER). In sepsis it is postulated that the ability of tissues to alter their OER is impaired, so that reductions in Do_2 are followed by reductions in oxygen utilization. The corollary is that increasing Do_2 to supranormal levels will augment Vo_2 and improve outcome. Neither pathological supply dependency nor the usefulness of supranormalization of Do_2 has been proven in humans.

with improved outcome. This damage to pulmonary architecture causes a reduction in functional residual capacity and increased ventilation–perfusion mismatching. Initially pulmonary arterial hypertension is reactive and is mediated by hypoxia. Failure of gaseous exchange with hypoxia and hypercarbia occurs and a subsequent exacerbation of peripheral tissue dysoxia ensues. This so-called exudative phase of ARDS can proceed to either resolution or fibrosis. An appropriate balance of neutrophil apoptosis, fibroblast proliferation, and parenchymal regeneration is required in order that resolution occurs.

Cardiovascular system

Under normal physiological conditions, tissue oxygen utilization (Vo_2) is closely linked to oxygen delivery (Do_2)—see Fig. 11.4. The total body oxygen extraction ratio (OER) is 25 per cent and oxygen uptake by cells is dictated by need. Cardiac output, minute ventilation, and regional blood flow in the microcirculation are regulated to prevent cellular dysoxia. If stressed in this situation, cells cope with increasing metabolic demands by increasing their OER. However, under pathological conditions, as found in patients with MODS, the normal linkage mechanisms between Do_2 and Vo_2 appear to fail and cellular dysoxia results. Animal models of sepsis, in which oxygen

delivery is progressively reduced by haemorrhage or pericardial balloon tamponade, confirm that the usual maximum OER is reduced and that the rate of oxygen utilization is directly proportional to the oxygen delivery. This results in a 'pathological **supply-dependent** oxygen utilization'. Pathological supply dependency of Vo_2 upon Do_2 has not, however, been demonstrated consistently in septic humans. Strategies to improve Vo_2 by increasing Do_2 to supranormal levels have similarly failed to produce a consistent survival benefit in critically ill patients with or without MODS. Cellular hypoxia is undoubtedly the cause of MODS, but whether this is as a consequence of regional failure of Do_2 or of an intracellular oxygen utilization defect is unclear.

Some studies have suggested that Vo_2 is impaired at the microcirculatory level, as a consequence of sludging of activated leucocytes de-recruiting nutrient capillaries. This would increase diffusion path lengths for oxygen and potentially exacerbate cellular dysoxia. Other investigators have suggested that a state of 'luxury perfusion' exists in which tissues are hyperoxic but unable to utilize oxygen owing to a defect of mitochondrial electron transport, possibly at the level of cytochrome aa_3.

Whatever the cause, the response to increased metabolic demands coupled with less effective utilization or delivery of oxygen, must be met by increases in cardiac output. This, together with mediator-induced systemic vasodilatation, gives rise to the hyperdynamic state characteristic of the SIRS/sepsis syndrome.

Impaired myocardial performance may also contribute to the oxygen supply and utilization disequilibrium. Pig models of sepsis have demonstrated a myocardial depressant factor in sepsis. Ultrafiltrate from septic pigs significantly decreases cardiac output when infused into non-septic animals. Investigators in Vancouver have also clearly shown both diastolic and systolic ventricular dysfunction in septic pig models. Furthermore, if pre-existing coronary artery disease coexists with this hyperdynamic state, myocardial ischaemia and failure may ensue progressively. Do_2 may thus be further impaired.

The gastrointestinal tract

The gastrointestinal tract is particularly vulnerable in critically ill patients who develop MODS. There is a growing body of evidence to suggest that the persistence of the SIRS/sepsis syndrome may be driven by abnormal colonization of the normally sterile upper gastrointestinal tract with pathogenic enteric bacteria. Some investigators believe that the development of MODS in the absence of a recognized focus of infection is caused by intestine failure with translocation of bacteria and toxins from the intestine which eventually reach the systemic circulation.

The theory that the intestine acts as the 'motor' of MODS is based upon this concept. There is no consistent evidence that bacterial translocation occurs in septic humans, but it is likely that the conditions that predispose to MODS do result in a deficiency of intestinal mucosal epithelial integrity. It is certainly accepted that the countercurrent pattern of flow present in the mucosal circulation predisposes to villous hypoxia and that small-intestinal villous shedding occurs in septic humans. This in turn could lead to the exposure of the mesenteric microcirculation to immunomodulatory influences in the absence of bacterial translocation. Leucocyte, endothelial, and hepatic Kupffer and stellate cell activation could then occur.

The kidney

Renal dysfunction and failure is a common feature of MODS and is traditionally associated with a large increase in mortality. In terms of function and danger to the host, failure of renal glomerular filtration and tubular function are straightforward to support. Continuous methods for both ultrafiltration and dialysis are widely available. Patients rarely die as a consequence of renal failure: they die instead of the pan-endothelial and cellular hypoxic insult that accompanies the failure of this organ. Problems relating to haemodynamic instability and bio-incompatible membranes have been largely solved with continuous techniques and non-cellulose-based membranes.

3.9 Management of MODS

Despite major advances in our understanding of the inflammatory processes involved, the mortality associated with MODS is high. Prevention is best because management of the established syndrome remains almost entirely supportive. This is corroborated by recent research that has demonstrated a significant negative correlation between late referral, suboptimal ward care, and survival in patients admitted to ICU.

ICU mortality is currently 19 per cent and hospital mortality 28 per cent and it has often been stated that intensive care mortality has not changed over the past decade. However, crude mortality figures do not reflect the increasingly severe case-mix that ICU caters for. Complex surgical procedures, both elective and emergency, are now performed which would not have been considered a decade ago. This increasing surgical sophistication has encouraged improvements in the range of ICU support, so the scope of surgical activity and the severity of illness of patients treated have greatly increased. This perhaps explains why crude mortality figures remain unchanged.

Early circulatory resuscitation is of paramount importance. Whether this should be guided by pulmonary artery catheterization with calculation of peripheral oxygen flux and oxygen consumption is disputed. It may be appropriate to increase oxygen delivery to a point where oxygen consumption no longer rises, or else to a level where markers of anaerobic metabolism such as plasma lactate fall. It does appear that the use of less-invasive clinical markers for the adequacy of the circulation, such as mean arterial pressure, temperature gradients, and urine output, may not entirely reflect the success of microcirculatory resuscitation. However, recent work suggests that pulmonary artery catheterization may be associated with an increase in length of hospital stay as well as mortality. Unfortunately, this work concentrated on data from an era when continuous cardiac output data were unavailable.

Goal-directed therapy in terms of attaining a set target for oxygen delivery and consumption has attracted criticism. No prospective randomized trial has shown that such a strategy produces survival benefit in patients once MODS is established. Trials looking at pre-emptive oxygen supply optimization in at-risk surgical patients have shown short-term benefits in terms of mortality and morbidity, but these do not translate into long-term survival. The inherent problem in the trial of optimization of global indices of D_{O_2} is that it tells us nothing about what happens at the cellular- or organ-specific level. This is where MODS begins and is perpetuated, and it is therefore unlikely that therapies targeted at global indices of oxygen delivery will ever have an influence on outcome.

More recently the impetus has changed towards measuring and titrating therapy to regional indices of the adequacy of oxygen delivery. Gastric mucosal tonometry is a method by which an air-or saline-filled balloon is introduced into the stomach at the tip of a nasogastric tube. Changes in the Pa_{CO_2} in the balloon are thought to directly reflect intramucosal Pa_{CO_2}. Substitution into the Henderson–Hasselbalch equation can then be used to calculate intramucosal pH (pH_i), acidosis being a surrogate marker for mucosal ischaemia. Attractive in concept when married to the idea of the intestine being the motor of MODS, such monitoring should then allow one to titrate therapy to mucosal blood flow. Although a low pH_i correlates with subsequent morbidity and mortality, prospective trials using the restoration of pH_i to the normal range as a therapeutic target, have not produced survival benefits. This may be due to measurement error, the influence of systemic acidaemia, or the fact that regional oxygenation is difficult to control selectively with available therapies.

Once the sequence of MODS is established, early and appropriate institution of basic and advanced organ support (e.g. endotracheal intubation and ventilation) are essential.

Malnutrition is a common and major contributing factor to MODS. Nutritional starvation combined with hypermetabolism leads to structural catabolism. Unlike ordinary starvation, the metabolized substrates are mixed, with a significant increase in amino-acid oxidation. With the temporal progression of MODS, direct amino-acid oxidation becomes increasingly prevalent, with rapid destruction of skeletal muscle. Balanced nutritional support to provide adequate calories and maintain nitrogen balance is fundamental if lean body mass is to be preserved and 'auto-cannibalism' slowed. This has led to recommendations for early parenteral feeding.

A balanced calorie source has to be given to prevent adding iatrogenic problems to the metabolic mayhem already occurring. While it is known that glucose has a protein-sparing effect, excessive amounts confer no additive advantages and may cause complications. These include fatty liver, hyperosmolarity, hyperglycaemia, and increased CO_2 production. The latter increases the excretory load on the lungs and can potentially exacerbate respiratory failure. The glucose load should not therefore exceed 4–5 mg/kg/minute, with a non-protein calorific load of 25–30 kcal/kg/day and 0.5–1.0 g/kg/day of lipids. Protein requirements run at 1–2 g/kg/day. Modified amino acids appear to be the most efficient protein source, producing less urea and better nitrogen retention.

Compared with the parenteral route, enteral feeding is safer, cheaper, has a lower complication rate, and probably has an important trophic effect on intestinal mucosa. There is a growing body of evidence to suggest that supplementation of feed with either specific essential amino acids such as glutamine or immunomodulatory mixtures of fish-oil extracts may confer additional survival benefit.

At present early referral, rapid and controlled resuscitation, and rigorous attention to the areas highlighted earlier are the main determinants of outcome once MODS has become established. Newer treatment strategies remain largely un-proven. For example, selective decontamination of the intestine by administration of non-absorbable antimicrobial agents may reduce the incidence of nosocomial pneumonia by re-sterilizing the upper gastrointestinal tract. However, trials have yet to demonstrate that the lower infection rate that this strategy produces translates into reduced mortality. Conversely, the use of aggressive early enteral feeding in patients without an ileus may not only reduce the effects of catabolism, but also, by stimulating the secretion of bactericidal gastric acid, prevent upper-intestinal colonization by bacteria. Recent studies appear to suggest that this may have a positive effect on outcome.

Perhaps the most recent advances in treatment of MODS have been attempts at modification of the inflammatory response by specific agents. These include monoclonal antibodies against endotoxin and TNF, inhibitors of nitric oxide synthase, and receptor antagonists for interleukin-1. As yet, no prospective trial of any of these agents has proved their efficacy. Indeed the trial of HA-1A—the monoclonal antibody against endotoxin—demonstrated an excess mortality in patients with proven Gram-positive sepsis. These novel therapies are prohibitively expensive and, in the absence of evidence produced by randomized controlled trials, their use cannot be recommended. Consider-ing the complexity of the inflammatory cascade involved in sepsis and MODS, it is extremely unlikely that any monotherapy is likely to succeed. More recently attention has focused on the molecular biology of sepsis and MODS, and in particular the genotypic predisposition to these disease processes.

MODS is a major cause of mortality in ICU and it cannot be overstated that prevention is better than attempted cure. The emphasis should be on surveillance, identification of patients at risk, reduction of suboptimal ward care, and a consultant-based referral and treatment system.

Bibliography

ACCP/SCCM (1992). Consensus conference on definitions of sepsis and multiple organ failure, 1991. *Crit. Med.*, **20**, (6), 864.

Baue, A.E. (1975). Multiple, progressive or sequential systems failure: A syndrome of the 1970s. *Arch. Surg.*, 110, 779–81.

Bihari, D., Cerra, F.B. (1989). *Multiple organ failure.* Society of critical care medicine, Fullerton, California.

Decamp, M.M. and Demling, R.H. (1988). Post-traumatic multisystem organ failure. *JAMA*, **260**, 530.

Dinarello, J. (1984). Interleukin-1 and the pathogenesis of the acute-phase response. *NEJM*, **311**, 341

Dobb, (1991). Multiple organ failure: Words mean what I say they mean. *Inten. Care World*, **8**, (3), 157.

Fry, D.E., Pearlstein, L., Fulton, R.L., *et al.* (1980). Multiple systems organ failure. The role of uncontrolled infection. *Arch. Surg.*, **115**, 136.

Marshall, J.C. (1992). Multiple organ failure and infection; cause, consequence, or coincidence. In *Yearbook of Intensive Care and Emergency Medicine*, (ed. J.L. Vincent), p. 3. Springer-Verlag, Berlin.

Michie, H.R., Manogue, K.R., Spriggs, D.R., *et al.* (1988). Detection of circulating tumour necrosis factor after endotoxin administration. *NEJM*, **318**, 1481.

Petty, T.L., Ausbaugh, D.G. (1971). The adult respiratory distress sybdrome. Clinical features, factors influencing prognosis and principles of management. *Chest* **60**, 233–9.

Shoemaker, W.C., Appel, P.L., Kram, H.B., *et al.* (1988). Prospective trial of supranormal values of survivors as therapeutic goals in high risk surgical patients. *Chest*, **94**, 1176.

CHAPTER 12

Soft-tissue surgery and wound management

*K. Simon Cross, Michael J. Earley,
Jane McCue, and Clive R. Quick*

1 Soft-tissue surgery

K. Simon Croft

1.1 Introduction

Surgery of the superficial tissues requires care and attention to ensure that a good functional and cosmetic outcome is achieved. Skin operations are often regarded as 'minor' and are often performed by general practitioners or assigned to the most junior member of the hospital surgical team. However, disasters can occur if assessment is not carried out adequately and an appropriate level of surgical expertise employed. The principles of asepsis/antisepsis pioneered by Semmelweis (1847) and Lister (1867) must also be observed. The underlying principles have changed little during the twentieth century, but the practice has evolved markedly, with new methods of sterilization, disposable items, and single-use packs improving the chances of maintaining sterility.

The criteria used by patients to judge their surgeon differ from those that would be used by another surgeon. Aspects of particular importance to the patient include:

◆ communication skills—the intelligibility of the explanation and preparation for the operation and the understanding with which the patient's concerns are handled;

◆ how soon the operation can be performed after the assessment;

◆ the degree of discomfort endured during the operation;

◆ the end result in terms of scarring, deformity, and neurological damage;

◆ whether the condition recurs (e.g. ingrowing toenail).

1.2 Benign tumours and cysts of skin and subcutaneous tissues

Epidermal proliferative lesions

Seborrhoeic keratoses are the most common epidermal proliferative lesion. They are benign and occur in later life, mainly on the trunk, hands, and face (especially the temporal areas or cheeks). Seborrhoeic keratoses are normally coloured light brown but are occasionally black and resemble a malignant melanoma. Keratoses range from a few millimetres to several centimetres across, and the surface may be smooth or verrucous. Histologically, they consist of proliferations of epidermal keratinocytes. Excision biopsy or curettage, usually under local anaesthesia, is indicated when there is doubt about the diagnosis or for cosmetic purposes.

Keratoacanthoma is a benign cutaneous lesion believed to arise from hair follicles. The lesion is probably initiated by a local virus infection. It is characterized by rapid growth initially, then spontaneous resolution after a few weeks if left untreated. Keratoacanthoma most commonly occurs on exposed areas of skin in white, middle-aged males. The differential diagnosis includes squamous or basal cell carcinoma, nodular malignant melanoma, and pyogenic granuloma. Excision biopsy is indicated if there is doubt about the diagnosis.

Epidermal cyst (sebaceous cyst)

Epidermal cysts are the most common cysts of skin. They are often, but inaccurately, referred to as sebaceous cysts. They can occur on any hair-bearing skin, particularly on the scalp and back, and range from 0.5 to 5.0 cm across. They are most common in early adulthood and are rare in children. Cysts are often single but can be multiple; the presence of multiple epidermal cysts should raise the possibility of Gardner syndrome.

A dilated follicular orifice is usually visible near the dome of the cyst and the cyst is attached to the skin at this point. Epidermal cysts arise from the epithelium of the hair follicle. The cyst wall is composed of epithelium and contains desquamated keratinocytes shed into the cyst, producing a white cheesy and often smelly material.

Patients often present acutely with an inflamed epidermal cyst. Clinically, there has usually been a small cyst present for years which has recently expanded rapidly and become red, tense, and painful. The likely initiating event is rupture of the cyst wall, invoking a foreign body inflammatory response. Antibiotic therapy is usually inappropriate although infection may supervene. Incision and drainage is often required but attempts to remove the lesion at this stage are likely to be unsuccessful. It is better to await resolution and to electively remove the small residual cyst a few weeks or months later.

Pilar cysts (synonym: tricholemmal cysts) are clinically indistinguishable from epidermal cysts but differ in distribution and frequency. Ninety per cent of pilar cysts occur on the scalp and 70 per cent are multiple, either at the outset or else appear sequentially in different parts of the scalp.

Benign dermal tumours

Lipomas

Lipomas are the most common benign neoplasm of soft tissues and are composed of mature adipose tissue. The peak incidence is in the fourth and fifth decades and they most often arise in the subcutaneous regions of the back, shoulder, and neck. They often occur singly and grow slowly but inexorably over many years. Some patients have multiple subcutaneous lipomas. In one type, there may be 100 or more lesions, mostly less than 1 cm in diameter. In another variant, there are multiple lesions, particularly on the forearms. Trauma may be the initiating factor in these cases.

The clinical significance of subcutaneous lipomas is their cosmetic effect and the occasional need to differentiate them from more serious lesions (e.g. liposarcomas). At operation, most are obviously encapsulated and easily distinguished from the surrounding adipose tissue. However, on the back of the neck, a profusion of fibrous tissue strands intersperses the lesion, making excision difficult. General anaesthesia is wise in these cases. Lipomas may be lobulated with a delicate encapsulation, requiring care to ensure that the whole lesion has been excised. The blood supply of small lesions is minuscule and haemostasis is not usually required. Larger lesions, particularly on the back, often have a larger blood supply, often entering from the deep surface. It is wise to have diathermy available for these. Lipomas may occur within muscle, bone, or organs, but these are beyond the scope of this description, except to alert the surgeon to the possibility that a superficial lipoma may in fact lie deeper and require a different approach.

Neurofibromas and schwannomas

Neurofibromas usually occur as solitary, innocent flesh-coloured tumours which protrude from the skin. Patients with a neurofibroma should be examined for other similar lesions and for *café-au-lait* spots, in case of von Recklinghausen syndrome.

Schwannomas occur singly on cutaneous nerves. They are often exquisitely tender when pressed. Standard excision results in loss of function of the appropriate nerve but function can be preserved if the lesion is excised using an operating microscope. This makes it possible to separate the lesion from the nerve trunk.

Dermatofibromas

Dermatofibromas, also known as histiocytomas, result from proliferation of dermal fibroblasts. They present clinically as intradermal, dark-pink, firm nodules on the trunk or extremities. Simple excision is performed if there is doubt about the diagnosis or for cosmetic reasons.

1.3 Benign pigmented lesions of the skin

Lesion types

Benign pigmented lesions are mainly of significance because they need to be distinguished from malignant melanomas; in certain cases they may be markers of increased risk of malignant

Table 12.1 Types of pigmented skin lesion

Lentigo	Flat brown lesions with sharp borders. Often on sites of chronic solar exposure, such as the face or back of the hand
Seborrhoeic keratoses	Lesions that appear rough and 'stuck on' and with clearly demarcated margins. Lesions range in colour from flesh-coloured to dark brown
Junctional naevus	Brown, well-defined lesions which may be flat or slightly elevated
Compound naevus	Papillomatous or dome-shaped lesions which vary in colour from flesh coloured to dark brown. Usually well defined
Blue naevus	Blue/blue-grey in colour. Occur in pre-pubescent subjects. Resembles nodular melanoma and must be distinguished from them
Subungual haematoma	Red-brown discoloration of the nail. It is important to ascertain a clear history of trauma and to check that the lesion expands from the nail fold. If not, consider the sinister possibility of a subungual melanoma
Haemangioma	Raised lesions that may be blue, red, or purple. The lesion blanches if compressed with a glass slide. Lack of blanching raises the possibility of nodular malignant melanoma

change. In addition, some skin lesions may represent cutaneous markers of underlying syndromes. Clinical examination alone is often insufficient to clearly identify one lesion from another. Nevertheless a basic knowledge of the features of the common lesions will allow the surgeon to correctly determine the significance of the pathology reports (Table 12.1).

Risk factors for malignant melanoma

Various factors are associated with an increased risk of malignant melanoma. These include:

◆ Previous history of malignant melanoma: 10 per cent of patients who develop a malignant melanoma later develop a second primary melanoma (McKie 1992).

◆ Family history of malignant melanoma: when a history of malignant melanoma is combined with the presence of dysplastic naevi in the **familial dysplastic naevus syndrome**, there is a 500-fold increase in risk for malignant melanoma (Greene *et al.* 1985).

◆ Large numbers of pigmented skin lesions or lesions of large size in an individual. Holman and Armstrong (1984) and Swerdlow *et al.* (1986), in separate studies, have shown that the presence of increased numbers of naevi greatly increases the risk of development of malignant melanoma.

◆ Dysplasia of benign lesions. Dysplastic features include variable mixtures of pigment with each naevus, irregular borders, and size larger than 6 mm. Any change is suspicious.

◆ Previous extreme sun exposure. Naevi of all kinds are associated with sun exposure. Patients who have suffered blistering sunburn in childhood have larger and more irregular moles compared with those who did not.

◆ Fair skin is a risk factor and combinations of the above factors greatly increase the likelihood of malignant melanoma (MacKie 1992).

1.4 Premalignant and malignant tumours of the skin

Risk factors

Sunlight

The evidence for sunlight as an important aetiological factor in malignant tumours of the skin is as follows (Gordon and Silverstone 1976):

◆ 90 per cent of skin malignancy occurs on exposed skin sites;

◆ 'outdoor people' have a higher incidence of skin malignancy;

◆ local incidence increases steadily the closer the location is to the equator;

◆ the less the skin pigmentation, the greater the incidence of skin cancer.

Other risk factors

1. In transplant patients, immunosuppressive therapy increases the risk of skin malignancy. Such lesions may arise *de novo* or as a result of accelerated progression of solar keratoses via in situ carcinoma to invasive carcinoma.

2. Many chemicals have been recognized as being involved in the initiation or promotion of skin cancers. These include creosote oil, paraffin oil, coal tar, and hydrocarbons.

3. Skin cancer developing in chronic ulcerated tissue due to burns was first described by Marjolin in the nineteenth century, but is rare nowadays in developed countries.

Premalignant lesions

Solar keratoses

Solar keratoses are also known as **actinic keratoses**. They are common premalignant tumours of the epidermis, occurring in sun-exposed skin. Histologically, solar keratoses represent the earliest recognizable phase of malignant transformation of the epidermis. Anaplasia and disorderly proliferation of keratinocytes are seen in the deepest parts of the epidermis. Clinically, the lesion often starts as a collection of dilated capillaries and later an adherent skin scale develops. Removal of this scale usually reveals a hyperaemic base with multiple bleeding points. Ultimately the scale may become thick and develop into a cutaneous horn. These lesions can treated by cryosurgery with liquid nitrogen or by curettage under local anaesthesia. If, however, there is doubt regarding the histological nature, excision biopsy should be performed.

Bowen's disease

Bowen's disease (squamous carcinoma in situ) is probably the most common premalignant skin lesion excised by the trainee surgeon. Clinically these lesions begin as small, slightly scaly, red areas. The lesion gradually enlarges to form a slightly raised red plaque with sharp margins. Surgical excision is usually the most appropriate therapy. The lesion is common on the anterior aspects of the lower leg, and in this position it may be difficult or impossible to close the wound edge primarily. In this situation consideration should be given to use of cryotherapy or allowing the wound to heal by secondary intention after excision.

Malignant skin lesions

Basal cell carcinoma

Basal cell carcinoma (BCC; rodent ulcer) is a malignant epithelial tumour of the skin that arises from the basal cells of the epidermis. It is the most common form of skin cancer. BCC arises mainly in late middle life and men and women are equally affected. Electromagnetic radiation is thought to be a major aetiological factor because basal cell carcinoma occurs mainly on sun-exposed sites. More than 90 per cent of basal cell tumours arise on the face between the boundaries of the palpebral fissure and the mouth. The common sites are on the nose, near the inner canthus of the eye, and on the cheek near the nasolabial fold. The macroscopic appearance varies from a small nodule with a pearly edge to an ulcerating lesion surrounded by crusting and irregular scarring. If the diagnosis is uncertain, a punch biopsy may be performed. However, the best therapy is skilled surgical excision which produces a histological specimen that can be examined to ensure that the margins are free of tumour. Adequate excision should never be compromised simply to make closure easy. Other treatment modalities include cryotherapy for small lesions, and radiotherapy, which has a role in the elderly patient for whom surgery is undesirable or unsafe. If recurrence happens, it does so locally since basal cell carcinomas never metastasize.

Squamous cell carcinoma

Squamous cell carcinoma (SCC) is a malignancy of epidermal keratinocytes. It is the second most common skin malignancy. It occurs in later life and is twice as common in men than women. Chronic sunlight exposure is the most important aetiological factor and, as might be expected, squamous cancers in Caucasians are usually found on the hands, head, and neck. Amongst dark-skinned populations, SCCs are most commonly found on the lower limbs, occasionally developing in a chronic wound sinus or ulcer. Although these tumours are locally invasive and do not usually metastasize, it is important to remember that squamous cell carcinoma arising at mucocutaneous borders (i.e. anal margin) are much more aggressive and frequently metastasize. Patients who are immunosuppressed, having undergone organ transplantation, are at increased risk of developing SCC. Clinically, squamous cell carcinomas present as exophytic nodules or plaques which often ulcerate. Aberrant keratinization may occur and produce a scale or cutaneous horn.

In general, surgical excision is the optimum method of treating cutaneous squamous cell carcinoma. There should be a 1–2 cm clearance of the edge of the tumour. Involved underlying tissues and regional lymph nodes should be excised *en bloc*. When dealing with a large and deeply invasive tumour, neoadjuvant radiotherapy (i.e. before surgery) may allow the surgeon to preserve underlying structures.

Malignant melanoma

This is a tumour of the pigment-producing cell, the melanocyte, normally located in the basal layer of the epidermis. A malignant melanoma may arise in a previously benign naevus or it may arise *de novo* in an apparently normal area of skin. The incidence of malignant melanoma has been rising inexorably in all countries for which data are available (Holman *et al.* 1980; Schreiber *et al.* 1981; MacKie *et al.* 1985). Because of these disturbing trends, many countries have organized major public information programmes aimed at modifying risk behaviour patterns and detecting lesions earlier. It is crucial that malignant melanoma is treated early because it can be eradicated in the early stages but is universally fatal if neglected. The aetiological risk factors have been discussed earlier.

Malignant melanoma can be divided into four types:

- **Hutchison's melanotic freckle** (HMF or lentigo maligna, LM);
- **acro-lentiginous melanoma** (ALM) and subungual melanoma;
- **superficial spreading melanoma** (SSM);
- **nodular melanoma** (NM).

Clinical features in a pigmented skin lesion which suggest malignancy include:

- change in colour—particularly increased pigmentation or variation in pigmentation across the lesion;
- increase in size;
- bleeding;
- itching;
- development of satellite lesions near the primary lesion.

The diagnosis is best established by excision biopsy of the whole lesion. This allows the pathologist to select the thickest part to measure. The thickness of the primary tumour in millimetres (**Breslow scale**) is the single most important prognostic feature for malignant melanoma patients with no clinical evidence of disease elsewhere. Thin lesions (<0.76 mm) have an excellent outlook, with 95 per cent survival at 5 years. Thick lesions (> 3.5 mm) have a poor outlook, with less than 40 per cent 5-year survival (MacKie 1992).

Superficial spreading melanomas are the most common form of presentation. The excision margins should be related to the tumour thickness, 1 cm all round per millimetre thickness. Controversy continues to exist over the benefit derived from excision of non-palpable regional lymph nodes. Patients with melanomas thinner than 1 mm rarely have nodal metastases, making the value of elective nodal dissection in this group low. In contrast, most patients with melanomas thicker than 4 mm will die from systemic metastases and elective nodal dissection does not improve their prognosis. Currently it seem appropriate to offer *en bloc* node excision to those who have good prognosis tumours after excision but who develop nodal involvement later. Limb perfusion and chemotherapy can be helpful in advanced disease, but the overall long-term results of these modalities are poor. Malignant melanoma seems to respond to some aspect of immunomodulation and the future may include developments in this area, such as specific vaccines.

1.5 Miscellaneous lesions of superficial tissues

Ganglion

Ganglia are common and consist of a cystic swelling with a fibrous tissue wall occurring adjacent to tendon sheaths and joint capsules. The pathophysiology of these lesions is unclear but is thought to be a degenerative process. Ganglia most commonly occur on the dorsum of the wrist but may also occur on the flexor aspect of the wrist and dorsum of the foot and ankle. The indications for excision include pain, limitation of movement, and cosmesis. The operation should ideally be performed in a bloodless field secured by a pneumatic cuff. This necessitates general or regional anaesthesia and the patient must be made aware that this is not a minor procedure as ganglia often extend deep into the tissues and meticulous dissection is required to minimize recurrence rates. There is also a substantial recurrence rate.

Verruca (synonym: warts)

Warts result from infection of the skin by a papillomavirus. This virus infects epidermal cells by direct inoculation. Susceptibility to infection by the papillomavirus and the rate of resolution of the resultant wart depends on the patient's immune response. Thus it is not surprising that the incidence increases in immuno-suppressed patients and in patients with certain myeloproliferative disorders. Warts can occur on any part of the body, but the surgeon is most commonly asked to see patients with plantar warts.

Pain is a common but not universal symptom. Plantar warts are often confused with simple callosities and the two may occur together. Callosities have a uniformly smooth surface across which the epidermal ridges continue without interruption; these ridges are interrupted over the surface of the wart. Surgical treatment of warts is appropriate only after medical therapy has been tried and failed. Diathermy excision is effective but requires regional or general anaesthesia. Scarring is inevitable and wart recurrences in the scar are frequent.

Ingrowing toenail

Ingrowing toenail is a painful condition that commonly affects adolescents. Although traditionally chiropody offers many different treatment options, the best results and the lowest recurrence rates are given by combined wedge resection and segmental phenolization so that the nail is permanently narrowed by about 25 per cent (Issa and Tanner 1988). It is important to expose the lateral or medial extent of the nail bed adequately otherwise phenolization may be inadequate and the patient likely to develop a troublesome 'nail spike'.

Hidradenitis suppurativa

Hidradenitis suppurativa arises because of an abnormality of the apocrine (scent) sweat glands located in the axillae, groin, perineum, and around the nipples. Affected patients suffer from repeated attacks of pain and inflammation. The abscesses may resolve or burst spontaneously to form chronic discharging sinuses. The disorder is most common in the second and third decades and is three times more common in women than in men. The axilla is the most commonly affected region. The aetiology of this progressive chronic process is duct obstruction by keratin plugging followed by rupture of the apocrine glands into the dermis and hypodermis, with superimposed infection. Wide excision is the surgical treatment of choice.

1.6 Surgical techniques for superficial skin lesions

Anaesthetic techniques for surgery of superficial tissues

Introduction

It is important to take sufficient time to fully anaesthetize the area to be operated upon. Too often the local anaesthetic injection is followed immediately by the surgical procedure, which proves painful for the patient, with full anaesthesia reached only after the procedure is completed. The surgeon must also know the maximum safe dose of local anaesthetic for each individual patient (Table 12.2).

Local anaesthetic infiltration

Local anaesthetic infiltration is particularly suited for surgery of the superficial tissues and is therefore widely used. Local anaesthetics work by reversibly blocking membrane depolarization, preventing the initiation and propagation of nerve action potentials. The most commonly used agents are lignocaine (lidocaine; Xylocaine®) and bupivacaine (Marcain®).

If larger volumes of lignocaine (lidocaine) are required, the volumes listed in the table can be approximately doubled if the preparation contains adrenaline (epinephrine). However, it must be remembered that dosages should be reduced

Table 12.2 Dosage of local anaesthetic agents (maximum doses for a 70 kg adult)

Anaesthetic agent	Concentration (%)	Dose (mg)	Volume (ml)
Lignocaine (lidocaine)	1	200	20
	0.5	200	40
Bupivacaine	0.5	140	28
	0.25	140	56

Table 12.3 Complications of local anaesthesia

At the injection site	Pain, haematoma, delayed recovery of sensation (direct nerve trauma), infection
Vasoconstrictor effect	Ischaemic necrosis (digits, penis, or nose)
Systemic effects	Idiosyncratic or allergic reactions (very rare)
	Toxicity due to excessive dosage or inadvertent intravenous injection, including vomiting, fits, CNS depression, cardiac arrhythmias

proportionately in the elderly, debilitated, or young and that adrenaline-containing preparations should not be used for the digits, penis, or nose, in case prolonged vasoconstriction causes ischaemia and gangrene (Table 12.3). Remember that the correct dose is the smallest dose required to produce the desired anaesthesia.

Infiltration technique

1. The finer the needle, the less the discomfort. Use a 25G needle to raise a small bleb of local anaesthetic in the skin initially before advancing the needle to deeper tissues. Once there is 'surface' anaesthesia, use a larger-bore needle to inject larger volumes more deeply.

2. Sudden injections of large volumes cause pain—therefore inject slowly.

3. Remember, wait long enough for anaesthesia to develop before initiating surgery.

4. Use an aseptic technique.

How to excise the lesion

Skin preparation

Commonly used skin antiseptics include chlorhexidine 4 per cent w/v (Hibiscrub™, Zeneca), or povidone-iodine 0.75 per cent w/v (e.g. Videne™, DePuy). Coloured solutions allow the surgeon to see clearly where the antiseptic has been applied but may not be appropriate in some areas (i.e. the face). Removal of hair from the immediate area to be operated on is helpful to the surgeon but may produce a poor cosmetic appearance. Moreover, an increased incidence of wound infection has been reported in patients who were shaved. Superficial skin abrasions can easily occur during shaving and provide routes of entry for endogenous staphylococci.

Skin incisions

Patients judge their surgeons on the end result, and the most obvious manifestation is the scar. Therefore a little forethought is important. Skin crease or wrinkle lines generally run perpendicular to the action of underlying muscles and are orientated along the line of dermal collagen. Incisions made in these lines give the neatest scars. The following points should be borne in mind:

1. Look for the natural skin creases and follow these lines wherever possible.

2. In areas of the body where the traditional Langer's lines (Fig. 12.1) are at variance with natural wrinkle lines, it is better to use the skin creases.

3. In skin overlying a joint, the incision should be placed transversely as this results in less distraction of the wound edges and a better cosmetic result.

4. If there are no skin creases, gently compress the skin in different directions to determine the most likely line of crease development.

Wound closure

Ideally the wound should be closed by primary intention, using suture material that is as fine as possible and then covered by an optimal dressing. The choice of whether to use an absorbable or non-absorbable suture depends on the location of the wound and the distracting forces that are expected on the wound. Some synthetic absorbable suture materials may be associated with increased scarring and some surgeons believe that fine (5/0, 6/0) nylon sutures give best results. 'Cross-hatching' of wounds following the use of interrupted or continuous non-absorbable sutures can be minimized by keeping the needle puncture site as close to the wound edges as possible, and, in the face, removing the sutures after 3–5 days. However, newer materials such as Vicryl Rapide (Ethicon™), designed to be absorbed rapidly, may give good results even in critical areas such as the face, particularly when used in a subcuticular technique. If the wound is small and there is no tension on the wound edges, then self-adhesive tape (i.e. Steristrips 3-M®) alone may be the best way to close the wound. Extra adhesion can be obtained by first coating the skin around the wound with Nobecutane spray or benzoin tincture, compound.

The optimum dressing should be sterile, impermeable to bacteria, allow gaseous exchange, and remove excess exudate (see Section 2.5).

1.7 Techniques of plastic and reconstructive surgery

Michael J. Earley

Introduction

Wounds associated with skin loss include leg ulcers, pressure sores, and wounds following excision of large skin lesions. Healing of these wounds depends on natural mechanisms (i.e. epithelial migration over granulation tissue and eventually fibrosis, together with wound contraction), or else on surgical intervention, such as skin grafting or flap transfer.

The epithelium that migrates from the wound edges is fragile and does not possess the rete pegs that normally assure union between the epidermis and the dermis, and new epithelium is

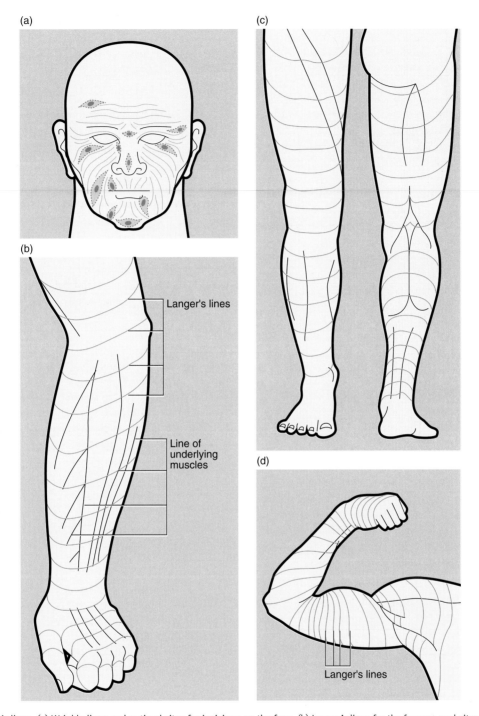

Figure 12.1 Langer's lines. (a) Wrinkle lines and optimal sites for incisions on the face. (b) Langer's lines for the forearm and sites for incisions across underlying muscles. (c) Langer's lines for the lower limb, crossing the direction of the underlying muscles. (d) Langer's lines for the upper limb.

easily avulsed by shearing forces. This migratory epithelium can be recognized clinically as the blue–grey border encircling the granulating wound.

Surgeons intervene with skin grafts or flaps in order to limit deformity and disability. The process of grafting is defined as tissue transfer without maintaining an intact blood supply, whereas flaps have a vascular supply. Skin grafts require a

recipient surface consisting of living regenerative tissue for successful neovascularization, and vascular union must develop quickly for the graft to survive the transfer.

Methods of skin cover

Extensive skin loss can be reconstructed using either grafts or flaps. Grafts do not have their own inherent blood supply but are dependent upon the recipient site for nutrition. They are autografts, composed of the patient's own **split skin** taken from a donor area such as the thigh, or else **full-thickness** skin (Wolfe grafts) taken from the upper forearm or from behind the ear for use in small, specific areas such as the fingertip. Pinch grafts are a variety of full-thickness graft and these have occasionally been employed for treatment of leg ulcers. They give a poor cosmetic result at both donor and recipient sites and have been largely replaced by meshed skin grafts.

Flaps carry their own blood supply. They are therefore of use in unfavourable situations for skin grafts (e.g. over bare bone or tendon and over body cavities).

There have been major developments in recent years in both grafting and in flap design. In grafting, the use of a tool to mesh the skin graft has allowed skin to be stretched to a much greater area and has also ensured that grafts can 'take' over a surface with substantial exudation. When a mesh graft has taken, the epithelial cells migrate rapidly from all of the skin edges to cover the bare areas in between. Advances are currently occurring in the use of **cultured epithelial cells** from the patient's own skin and in the use of artificial dermis. Although in their infancy, these techniques show great promise for the future, particularly where large areas of skin have been lost as a result of burns.

In the field of flaps, the advent of the free flap in the 1980s opened a new era in reconstructive plastic surgery and rendered the use of the staged tubed pedicle flap largely redundant. Careful study of the vascular anatomy of many areas revealed that large areas of skin could remain viable when supplied and drained by a single artery and vein. This led to an ever-increasing range of donor sites for reconstruction and enabled other tissues, such as muscle and bone, to be moved in combinations as **composite flaps**. In parallel with this, the same micro-surgical techniques enabled replantation of digits and even limbs. This field continues to develop.

Problems with grafts and flaps

Split-skin grafts

Split-skin grafts have the advantages of a high 'take' (revascularization) rate. In addition, the donor areas heal spontaneously and the same area can be reused as a harvest site in the future. The best donor sites for spit-skin grafts are the buttock and the thigh. The disadvantage of the split-skin graft is that the skin is not durable and that shrinkage and contraction occur owing to the lack of dermis.

Success with split-skin grafts depends on:

◆ A good recipient site, for example muscle or healthy granulation tissue (grafts will not take over bare bone or tendon or in the presence of substantial infection; streptococcal infection, in particular, is fatal to grafts).

◆ Thin grafts take better than thick ones.

◆ Good haemostasis at the recipient site is essential to prevent the graft being lifted by haematoma.

◆ The graft should be immobile. Various techniques are used: quilting (i.e. stitching down in squares); gluing; tie-over dressings or foam coverings to exert gentle pressure; and splintage of body parts.

◆ The graft should be left undisturbed for 5 days or more.

◆ Grafts should be **perforated** to allow drainage of serum and, if fluid production is likely to be excessive, meshed.

◆ Care needs to be taken when a graft site is inspected as the desiccated dressings may avulse the graft. This can be avoided by using dressings that do not dry out and which provide a good protective physical barrier to the graft.

Management of the donor site

The donor site should be undisturbed for at least 10 days. Dressings should be either non-adherent or composed of alginate (e.g. Kaltostat®) to maintain the site in a moist state conducive to rapid healing and to minimize pain.

Flaps

A flap is defined as a vascularized block of tissue. It may be cutaneous, fasciocutaneous, myocutaneous, muscle only, bone only, or osteomyocutaneous. All flaps have a pedicle through which the flap receives its arterial input and effects its venous drainage. There is no such thing as a 'flap graft'. Tubed pedicled flaps are now seldom employed but are occasionally used in reconstruction of the pinna and for flaps to the hand. In these, the flap is mobilized at its donor site and rolled into a tube, leaving both ends attached. After a period, one end is divided and sutured to one edge of its new location. After a further period to allow it to develop a new blood supply at the new site, the other end of the donor site is divided and the pedicle unrolled and placed in its new location. It is a lengthy and tedious process and, in most situations, cosmesis is poor. This type of flap has been largely replaced by the free flap or by better designed axial flaps.

The blood supply of a flap can be classified either as **random** or **axial**. For all random flaps, the base needs to be broader than the length of the flap in order to maintain its blood supply. Most flaps used nowadays are axial flaps, where a known blood supply enters the flap through its pedicle.

Flaps can also be described as **rotation** or **advancement** flaps. This is a purely descriptive term, referring only to the way in which the flap is moved to the recipient site and has nothing to do with the blood supply. In any flap surgery, the donor site of the flap may require split-skin grafting in order to achieve healing.

A **free flap** is a block of tissue that is entirely removed from its donor area after being isolated on its pedicle, which usually consists of a single artery and vein. It is then moved to a different part of the body and the artery and vein are anastomosed using microsurgical techniques to a local artery and vein. The process requires much less time in hospital and fewer procedures than the old-style pedicle flap, although the operations may take a very long time.

Many eponymous flaps have been described, based on the anatomy of the blood supply and the ability of the body to function without the part removed. In addition, flaps are classified according to the types of tissue included. The blood supply of each type is different (Fig. 12.2):

1. **Cutaneous.** In the cutaneous flap, the blood supply is in the subcutaneous tissue, an example being the forehead flap which is supplied and drained by the superficial temporal artery and vein.

2. **Fasciocutaneous.** The fasciocutaneous flap depends upon the fascial vessels that run over the muscles inside the deep fascia. In the lower limb, these vessels are usually longitudinally placed, radiating between the muscle septa. The popular radial forearm flap (the '**Chinese flap**') is supplied in a ladder-like fashion via the fascial vessels from the radial artery.

3. **Myocutaneous.** A myocutaneous flap consists of skin depending upon the muscle blood supply deep to it. It can, therefore, be **islanded** (i.e. isolated from the adjoining skin while receiving its blood supply from the muscle's own pedicle). Frequently used examples are the latissimus dorsi flap (supplied by the thoraco-dorsal artery); the TRAM (transverse rectus abdominis muscle) flap, depending on the superior epigastric vessels; and the pectoralis major flap (supplied by the pectoral branches of the thoraco-acromial trunk).

4. **Osteocutaneous and osteo-fascio-cutaneous.** An osseous flap (usually referred to as a **vascularized bone transfer**) is supplied either through the periosteum (e.g. rib on a serratus anterior muscle flap) or via its own nutrient artery. Examples are vascularized fibula, radius, spine of scapula, and iliac crest flaps.

Success and failure in skin cover using flaps

1. Most important is the choice of flap (i.e. one with a reliable blood supply and best suited for the purpose).

2. The vascular pedicle needs to be protected from the dangers of kinking.

3. There should be no tension.

4. Haematoma formation should be avoided.

Microsurgery

Principles

Microsurgery in this context relates largely to the methods of forming the vascular and nerve anastomoses. Magnification is essential and most surgeons use an operating microscope. Technique needs to be meticulous and this is impossible without appropriately designed microsurgical instruments and a comfortable posture for the surgeon.

Applications of microsurgery in plastic and reconstructive surgery

Trauma

1. Early—for the primary or delayed primary repair of defects. For example, in lower-limb defects to preserve as much bone as possible or to cover neurovascular bundles.

2. Intermediate reconstruction after loss or surgical ablation of tissue.

3. Late reconstruction of deformities (e.g. contractures following burns).

Cancer surgery

1. After excision of cancers of the head and neck—for example using the radial forearm flap to reconstruct the floor of the mouth, the fibula to reconstruct the mandible, or the rectus abdominis muscle to fill defects at the skull base.

2. For breast reconstruction, either primary at the time of cancer surgery or delayed (e.g. TRAM or gluteal flaps).

Replantation

Severed digits and limbs can often be replanted (i.e. put back in their original position) or transplanted (e.g. a big toe transplanted to replace a lost thumb). Where replantation is to be considered, amputated parts should be transported in saline-

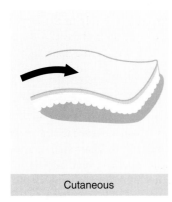
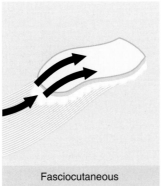
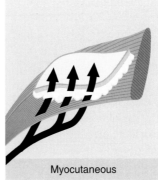
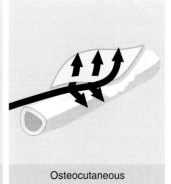

| Cutaneous | Fasciocutaneous | Myocutaneous | Osteocutaneous |

Figure 12.2 Blood supply of different types of flap.

soaked gauze then placed in a plastic bag surrounded with ice in another plastic bag in order to achieve cooling rather than risking frostbite.

While it is often possible to replant freshly and cleanly severed digits, it is not good practice to always replant because of the technical failure rate and the prolonged convalescence while sensation is regained. In addition, a replanted part is never as good functionally as the original, and function may be better without it. Thus, if practicable, thumbs and hands are always replanted, multiple fingers are often replanted, and single digits seldom.

If an upper limb is severed proximal to the nerve supply of the forearm muscles, then the results of replantation are often poor despite a viable limb. Replantation is seldom indicated in the lower limb, owing to the difficulty of regaining sensory and motor function. Children are the exception, and replantation of lower limbs should virtually always be attempted. Other replants such as ears, nose, scalp, or genitalia are often worth attempting.

Free-tissue transfer

This is so called because it is at some stage during the operation rendered 'free' from its blood supply (i.e. the pedicle consisting of artery and vein is divided). It is by definition both a flap and axial.

The flap is raised, pedicle divided, and its artery and vein sutured to a recipient artery and vein at the site required. An example is the radial arterialized fasciocutaneous forearm flap being transferred to the floor of the mouth after ablative cancer surgery, where the radial artery is anastomosed to a branch of the external carotid, and a vein (usually cephalic) to the jugular system.

This technique has been a major advance in reconstruction, enabling large defects to be filled at a one-stage operation.

Potential problems:

◆ poor technical anastomoses;

◆ poor choice of vessels or flap;

◆ kinked anastomosis;

◆ poor flap blood flow if the patient is cold or poorly perfused (e.g. by undertransfusion), leading to anastomotic sludging and clotting;

◆ postoperative monitoring is vital.

Tissue expanders

Skin and subcutaneous tissues and other soft tissues near wounds can be expanded or stretched to enable wound closure, or prior to placement of, for example, a permanent breast prosthesis. To achieve tissue expansion, a special inflatable silicone implant is placed subcutaneously and the pressure within it gradually increased by injecting increments of saline. With expansion, the dermis and skin become thinned, but the rate of mitosis in the epidermal layer increases, thus gradually expanding the amount of epidermal tissue. Tissue expanders have proved particularly useful in scalp reconstruction (as the expanded skin continues to grow hair), and in breast reconstruction (where colour match and sensitivity can be maintained). In the extremities, blood supply is less tolerant of expansion and the usefulness of tissue expanders is limited.

1.8 Infections of superficial tissues

Introduction

The skin is an efficient antimicrobial barrier. It normally harbours a resident population of bacteria (e.g. *Staphylococcus epidermidis* and corynebacteria), which do no harm as long as there is no break in the continuity of the skin, and the ducts of the skin and its accessory structures remain patent.

Cellulitis

Acute cellulitis is a spreading subcutaneous infection caused by *Strep. pyogenes* or *Staph. aureus*. It is characterized clinically by tender, swollen, and diffusely erythematous skin with no distinct border. Once recognized, antibiotic therapy should be initiated immediately, usually parenterally, and designed to cover both streptococci and staphylococci. A common combination is penicillin G and flucloxacillin. It is important to consider the possibility of **necrotizing fasciitis** (see below) when the cellulitis does not appear to be resolving sufficiently rapidly and in patients who become inappropriately toxic.

A less serious form of cellulitis occurs in the lower limb. The origin is sometimes obscure but the limb is often affected by chronic venous insufficiency or lymphatic oedema (primary or secondary). In these cases, the process is more indolent and carries little systemic risk to the patient. Treatment includes appropriate antibiotics (often tetracyclines), elevation, compression bandaging, and, if appropriate, attention to the underlying condition.

Abscess formation

Apparently superficial 'abscesses' commonly presenting to the surgeon include inflamed epidermal (sebaceous) cysts, furuncles, perianal or pilonidal abscesses, and breast abscesses. For an established abscess, the appropriate therapy is almost always incision and drainage, performed urgently. In a few cases, where the abscess is small, needle aspiration is sufficient. If the abscess has not yet 'pointed' and is still at the cellulitic stage, antibiotic therapy may abort the process. However, it is sometimes difficult to determine clinically whether pus is present. The most common organism cultured from superficial abscesses is *Staph. aureus*. The exception is abscesses in the anal region, where *E. coli* is most common.

Candidiasis

This is a common hospital infection, especially amongst frail or debilitated patients. Other predisposing factors include broad-spectrum antibiotic therapy and obesity. Clinically one sees an erythematous macerated eruption in intertriginous areas.

Attention to skin care, topical application of antifungal agents, and, occasionally, appropriate antibiotics are employed.

Bacterial synergistic gangrene

This is a life-threatening condition with a 20–30 per cent mortality rate. It occurs in relation to recent surgical incisions or traumatic wounds. The condition is also known as **necrotizing fasciitis** because of its propensity to cause necrosis of subcutaneous fascia. Necrotizing fasciitis has given rise to several scare stories in the popular press in recent years because of the rapidity of its spread, high mortality, and the need for mutilating surgery to treat it effectively. However, there has been no evidence of an epidemic as such. Cases have occurred sporadically with little change in frequency or any increased clustering over the years. Various media names have been given to the condition, including 'flesh-eating bug' and 'killer virus'. In general, prejudicial reporting of this nature has been unhelpful in coping locally with affected cases.

The initial presentation may be as a simple wound infection but it spreads with frightening rapidity and with severe toxic signs and symptoms. If found on the abdominal wall, it is known as **Meleney's gangrene**. **Fournier's gangrene** is a variant found in the scrotum which often arises in a chronic hydrocoele with no wound. The infection in this case is probably blood-borne.

The most characteristic clinical feature of synergistic gangrene is the woody-hard texture of the subcutaneous tissues. As the name suggests, an array of organisms, both anaerobic and aerobic, can be found in various combinations acting together to induce gangrene, as shown in Table 12.4.

Treatment requires high-dose antibiotic therapy combined with early and complete surgical excision of all infected tissue, and drainage of abscesses. Surgical intervention often has to be repeated several times, with loss of huge areas of skin. Reconstruction after elimination of all infection often requires complex reconstructive surgical techniques.

Infected ulcers

The aetiology of any skin ulcer needs to be determined. Common causes are arterial insufficiency, venous insufficiency (or both), trauma, and malignancy. Whatever the aetiology, ulcers are always colonized by bacteria and are sometimes infected. It is useful to know what organisms are currently present in the ulcer. Parenteral antibiotics are indicated only in patients with cellulitis or with systemic signs of toxicity. Pressure (decubitus) ulcers are the end result of chronic pressure on skin over a bony prominence. Friction and prolonged contact with faeces or urine are important

Table 12.4 Organisms involved in bacterial synergistic gangrene (necrotizing fasciitis)

Anaerobes	Aerobes
Bacteroides spp.	*E. coli*
Clostridium spp.	*Klebsiella* spp.
Peptococcus spp.	*Pseudomonas* spp.
Peptostreptococcus spp.	*Citrobacter* spp.

predisposing factors. The common sites for pressure ulcers are the sacrum, ischial tuberosities, heels, and malleoli. Prevention is the best approach to pressure sores. This includes protection of areas at risk with special beds and padding, frequent repositioning of the patient, and maintaining good nutrition.

Methicillin-resistant *Staphylococcus aureus*

Methicillin-resistant *Staphylococcus aureus* (MRSA) was recognized 30 years ago, shortly after the introduction of methicillin into clinical use. It is almost invariably resistant to all penicillins and is now one of the most intractable problems in hospital, particularly in surgical practice. All patients in hospital are at risk of developing carrier status and some, particularly the debilitated, develop severe invasive infection. Carriers, both staff and patients, can now be treated effectively with topical mupirocin, which represents an important advance in the prevention of spread. Other precautions are covered in Chapter 7.

Vancomycin remains the treatment of choice for severe wound infection with MRSA. However, teicoplanin (a glycopeptide) has several potential advantages over vancomycin, including ease of administration, low toxicity and a long half-life. The drug is likely to become more widely utilized.

2 Wound management

Jane McCue and Clive R. Quick

2.1 Introduction

This section deals with the management of wounds in the broadest sense, including breaks in the integrity of the skin surface which would only loosely be classified as wounds. Many of the principles of management considered here can be applied to a wide range of conditions involving skin loss. These include:

- surgical wounds—planning, performing, closing, dressing, and wound complications;
- traumatic wounds—early care, surgical cleansing, dressings, secondary, and reconstructive procedures;
- burns;
- sinuses and fistulas;
- chronic skin ulcers.

2.2 Classification of wounds

Many different wound classifications are in common usage (e.g. by wound type, by causative agent, by involvement of adjacent structures, or by degree of contamination or infection). Traumatic wounds also have their own classifications.

Types of wound

Mechanical wounds of skin or mucosa

Surgical wounds are deliberately inflicted for access or excision of superficial lesions. These may be simple wounds which heal by primary intention or may become complicated by necrosis, infection, or sinus or fistula formation.

Traumatic wounds may be **superficial** (e.g. abrasions, lacerations, and bites), or **penetrating** wounds caused by knives, guns, blast injury, or impalement. In either group, compromising tissue loss may occur which precipitates the need for special treatment. In the latter group, actual or potential injury to deep structures is the main factor in deciding the treatment required.

Burns and scalds

Thermal, chemical, electrical, and ionizing radiation burns affect skin, leading to partial or complete skin loss. It is important to note that burns can also affect deeper tissues to an extent governed by the intensity of the burning agent.

Chronic ulcers

The leg below knee is the site most commonly afflicted by chronic ulceration. The most common cause is chronic venous insufficiency. For further details of management see Chapters 22 and 23. Pressure sores usually occur in skin overlying bony prominences such as the sacrum or heel in bed-ridden patients, particularly those with diminished intellectual function.

Areas of skin treated by radiotherapy, particularly the early low kilovoltage and often poorly planned treatment which led to occasional overdosage of superficial tissues with consequent necrosis due to endarteritis obliterans. Wounds in such areas, even years later, fail to heal because of local ischaemia. Only a new blood supply brought by an axial flap or omental mobilization can persuade these wounds to heal.

Systemic disorders such as scleroderma or pyoderma gangrenosum and certain skin disorders such as pemphigus, cause breakdown of skin in apparently random fashion. Sclerodermal ulceration of fingertips usually heals normally if calcific deposits are removed. In dermatological disorders, successful treatment of the underlying disorder usually allows healing.

Fistulas and sinuses

A sinus is a blind track leading to an epithelial surface, whereas a fistula is an abnormal communication between two epithelial-lined surfaces. Examples of these different types include pilonidal sinus, fistula in ano, and enterocutaneous fistula. The classical teaching is that fistulas (or sinuses) will heal spontaneously unless one of the following is present:

◆ distal obstruction;

◆ an implanted foreign body;

◆ incomplete drainage; or

◆ the track has become epithelialized or involved by malignancy.

Ineffective drainage via a fistula predisposes to wound infection or cellulitis; furthermore, the effluent from an enterocutaneous fistula may excoriate the surrounding skin.

2.3 Wound healing

Types of wound healing

Wound healing may take place by **primary intention** after surgical closure, by **secondary intention** (open granulation), by **delayed surgical primary closure** of a contaminated wound, or by **reconstructive surgery** such as skin grafting or flap creation.

Biology of wound healing

Normal wound healing is a complex process, mediated by the interplay of many cellular and biochemical factors. Using DNA recombinant technology and other modern biochemical purification techniques, a number of polypeptide growth factors have recently been identified. These **growth factors**, in addition to promoting cellular proliferation, encompass a wide range of non-mitogenic activities in wound healing and should more properly be called **cytokines**. Identified cytokines involved in wound healing include: transforming growth factor-β, platelet-derived growth factor, and epidermal growth factor. Cytokine functions include chemotaxis, induction and inhibition of cellular differentiation, and control of protein synthesis.

The main sources of wound cytokines are the various cells that accumulate during the acute phase of tissue injury, namely platelets, macrophages, and lymphocytes. Initially, cytokines promote the inflow of cells (such as fibroblasts) involved in wound healing and later they control the synthesis of collagen.

Healing of clean surgical wounds by primary intention

Phase of acute inflammation

After surgical closure, there is a period of acute inflammation that, if uncomplicated, lasts about 3 days. The initiating factor appears to originate from platelets activated by contact with mature collagen exposed in the wound. Platelets first aggregate then release a variety of active agents including lysosomal enzymes, ATP, serotonin, and wound cytokines. At the same time, a fibrin clot develops, which completes haemostasis and provides strength and support to the wound. The surface dries to form a scab. Platelets and macrophage factors cause local vasodilatation which produces warmth and increases capillary permeability, allowing serum and white blood cells to accumulate and causing swelling. It should be noted that neutrophils are not essential to healing of an uninfected wound and are concerned primarily with defence against bacteria.

Phase of demolition

After the initial acute inflammation, macrophages become active as the main agents of demolition, removing unwanted fibrin, dead cells and dead bacteria, and creating fluid-filled spaces for granulation tissue. Macrophages also release factors that stimulate formation of new capillary buds during this phase and later initiate and control fibroblast activity during repair.

Phase of healing

Within the connective tissue, randomly orientated collagen begins to form after a few days, reaching a peak of activity after

5–7 days. Epithelial cells at the edge of the wound start to proliferate after 24 hours and slide over each other and over the dermis and beneath the scab. This proliferative phase lasts for about 3 weeks.

Phase of maturation and remodelling

This phase continues for up to a year. During this period, the wound tensile strength increases and the random collagen is replaced by a more stable form orientated along lines of stress. The parallel fibres gradually form cross-linkages for increased strength. Thickened areas flatten out and excess vascularity diminishes, causing the skin wound to fade from red towards normal by approximately 1 year.

Healing by secondary intention (open granulation)

Introduction

The term '**dirty wound**' implies that there has been loss or destruction of epithelium, leaving an ulcer or cavity containing necrotic tissue, slough (fibrin, leucocytes, cellular debris), bacteria, or pus. Inflammatory mediators appearing in the wound promote inflammation around the wound, and if pathogenic organisms predominate, spreading cellulitis with systemic signs of infection may supervene. Devitalized tissue and slough inhibit local defences against infection, including the capacity of leucocytes to kill organisms. Experiments have shown that different devitalized tissues suppress leucocyte phagocytosis and killing of bacteria to different extents. One of the most powerful suppressors is devitalized fat.

The normal processes by which the body heals 'dirty' wounds act slowly and relatively ineffectively. If contamination is too great, infection spreads and may kill the patient. Thus effective wound cleansing by surgery or wound dressings is an important step in setting the scene for healing.

When there has been substantial loss or destruction of surface tissue, healing takes place by filling in of the defect with granulation tissue (and later fibrosis) and gradual migration of skin cover from the edges. The process is aided by wound contraction. Healing by granulation is a slow process which is further retarded by dead tissue in the wound. However, it is relatively safe because granulation tissue is very resistant to bacterial contamination. Allowing healing to take place by granulation avoids the infective risks of suturing contaminated wounds. Neglected wounds in undeveloped countries or remote areas usually heal by secondary intention. None the less, there are substantial disadvantages if the process is not supervised:

◆ infection can spread before it is isolated by body defences;

◆ disability occurs during the prolonged healing process;

◆ deformity results from wound contraction (particularly across joints);

◆ poor cosmesis is caused by scarring;

◆ healing is slow.

The process of healing by secondary intention

Much of the process of healing by secondary intention is similar to healing by primary intention, with early neutrophil predominance, replaced after a few days by macrophages and fibroblasts. Capillary endothelial buds start to form after 2–3 days and the new vessels remain permeable to fluid and cells from the blood. At the same time, macrophages clear debris and liberate growth factors and other cytokines. This carpet of new capillaries and the developing collagen network with its proteoglycan gel-like matrix is known as **granulation tissue**. It provides a healthy base for epithelial growth or skin grafting which, even if contaminated with micro-organisms, resists their invasion. Granulation tissue continues to proliferate and collagen is laid down in the wound so that the defect gradually fills until almost level with the surface. Epithelial cells at the periphery proliferate vigorously and slide over one another towards the centre. The process is accelerated if the wound surface is moist and viable, and is impeded if it is dry, covered with eschar, or is infected.

Healing by secondary intention as deliberate policy

Allowing healing by granulation is a deliberate policy in certain cases. These include wounds where it is impossible or undesirable to bring the wound edges together, where there is a high risk of infection, when wound dehiscence associated with infection has occurred, where there is relative ischaemia of the wound environs, and sometimes in areas of irradiated tissue. However, after all the dead tissue has been removed and the initial phase of granulation is well established, secondary procedures can be performed to accelerate healing. These may involve direct wound closure (delayed primary closure) or reconstructive surgery using skin grafts or axial flaps.

Optimal conditions for wound healing

For optimum wound healing the following criteria should be fulfilled (see Table 12.5). The wound should be moist but not macerated (waterlogged) and free of infection. It should look clinically clean and be devoid of *Strep. pyogenes* on bacterial culture. However, even apparently clean wounds may have significant infection or colonization which may impair healing. Research studies suggest that this occurs where quantitative bacterial culture exceeds 100 000 organisms/gram of tissue.

The wound must also be free of dead tissue or slough, foreign bodies, harmful chemicals, and particles or fibres from dressings. Foreign material may provoke an inflammatory

Table 12.5 Conditions required for optimal wound healing

Moist but not macerated
Uninfected
Viable tissue without ischaemia
No foreign bodies
Near body temperature
Optimum pH
Atraumatic dressing changes

foreign-body reaction which persists as long as the foreign body remains, causing consequent chronic infection. Foreign material may also conceal micro-organisms, which body defences and systemic antibiotics are often unable to eradicate.

The wound surface should be near body temperature for optimum metabolic function. Certain dressings are poor insulators and changing dressings lowers the temperature for prolonged periods. Traumatic dressing changes should also be avoided. Dressing changes can lift off delicate new epithelium, tear new capillaries, and allow new bacterial contamination and potential secondary infection.

Optimum wound pH is required. An acid environment is generally more favourable as it encourages collagen synthesis, whereas an alkaline environment promotes growth of certain bacteria such as *Pseudomonas* spp.

2.4 Wound-cleansing agents

For cleansing clean, non-infected wounds, sterile normal saline solution is all that is required. Antiseptics and other topical agents are likely to do more harm than good. Wounds that are not clean heal most quickly when dead tissue and slough are removed. Surgical cleansing (excision, débridement) is most effective but may be inappropriate where slough is not too tough, in small wounds, or in patients unfit for anaesthesia. However, local applications are not a panacea and should be used with a distinct purpose in mind:

◆ Is there a dry necrotic eschar covering the wound which needs surgical excision before dressings are employed, or can the eschar be rehydrated, allowing natural autolysis?

◆ Is there a modicum of slough that can realistically be removed by wound applications or dressings?

◆ Is this a recently drained abscess cavity which merely needs its superficial aperture kept open while the cavity either fills in or while awaiting further surgical curettage or excision of dead tissue?

Hypochlorite solutions

Hypochlorite solutions have been in use for combating infection since about 1820 and were used effectively by Semmelweis to prevent spread of puerperal sepsis. Hypochlorites are highly reactive solutions, combining rapidly with proteins to cause chlorination, oxidation, and hydrolysis of nitrogenous material. Because of this reactivity, these agents are rapidly inactivated by pus, serum, and other organic matter. Sodium hypochlorite solution is alkaline (pH 11) and is too irritant for use on tissues. Various buffered solutions have been devised to overcome this. **Dakin solution**, described in 1915, was the first. It contains 0.5 per cent available chlorine and is buffered with boric acid to a pH of 9.5. It needs to be freshly prepared as it remains stable for only 2 weeks. **EUSOL** (Edinburgh University solution of lime) is similar with 0.25 per cent available chlorine and is buffered to pH 7.5–8.5. **Milton solution** contains 1 per cent sodium hypochlorite and 16.5 per cent sodium chloride and is a stable solution often used at a 1 : 80 dilution to sterilize babies' feeding bottles. For wound management, a 1 : 4 dilution (0.25 per cent available chlorine) is often supplied as a EUSOL equivalent but has a pH of about 11 and cannot be recommended. Chlorasol® is unbuffered hypochlorite and chloramine is an organic chlorine compound said to be relatively non-irritant.

Hypochlorites were introduced for treating infected wounds before antibiotics became available and had dramatic effects in minimizing wound infection during the First World War. Wounds were irrigated with large quantities of Dakin solution which was noted to rapidly dissolve necrotic tissue. Later, this was shown to be dependent on the alkaline pH and was associated with a rapid fall in the chlorine content which occurred in wounds but not in contact with intact skin. Experimentally, 100 ml EUSOL is needed to dissolve 1 g soft, yellow slough and it is wholly ineffective against dehydrated black necrotic skin. Hydrocolloids and hydrogels have been shown to aid in removing slough by rehydration, which assists autolysis. It is likely that any benefit from hypochlorites is by this mechanism.

In recent years, experimental work has shown that hypochlorites can have markedly adverse effects on wound healing when compared with saline and chlorhexidine, including disruption of capillary circulation in granulation tissue, increased inflammation, and retardation of collagen formation. In addition, very low concentrations inhibit neutrophil migration. For these reasons, hypochlorite solutions have fallen from favour as more effective agents have become available.

Hydrogen peroxide

Six per cent hydrogen peroxide solution liberates 20 times its own volume of oxygen on dissociation. The enzyme catalase, present in all living tissue, causes the solution to dissociate rapidly. It is relatively non-toxic but any beneficial effect is produced solely by the mechanical action of the rapid liberation of bubbles of oxygen. The solution must *never* be used to irrigate wounds under pressure or be placed in closed wound cavities as liberated oxygen can enter the bloodstream, causing life-threatening oxygen embolism.

Proflavine

Proflavine is an acridine derivative that is mildly bacteriostatic against Gram-positive bacteria but ineffective against Gram-negative organisms. It is usually supplied as an emulsion in which the proflavine is concentrated in the aqueous phase of the cream, rendering it unavailable for antibacterial activity. Alternative formulations based on polyethylene glycol permit release of the active ingredient. It is a useful agent to prevent dressings sticking to cavities and has a certain aesthetic appeal out of proportion to its effectiveness.

Cetrimide

This quarternary ammonium compound has pronounced emulsifying and detergent properties as well as bactericidal activity against Gram-positive and some Gram-negative organisms. Even in low concentrations it has marked cytotoxic or cytostatic effects, restricting its use to dirty wounds alone.

Chlorhexidine

In the gluconate form, this is a widely used antiseptic active against a wide range of Gram-positive and Gram-negative organisms. Savlon® is a combination of cetrimide and chlorhexidine which is useful for cleaning contaminated skin wounds.

Povidone-iodine

This is a potent antibacterial agent effective against a wide range of organisms but with activity much reduced by contact with pus or wound exudate. It is available as aqueous or alcoholic lotions, a paint, and as dry-powder spray. A few patients may develop sensitivity to iodine even though it is organically bound. In experimental studies, 1 per cent povidone-iodine showed marked cytotoxic properties against human fibroblasts in tissue culture (a similar but more marked effect than 0.5 per cent hypochlorite and 3 per cent hydrogen peroxide).

Enzyme preparations

Tryptar® and Trypure Novo® contain stabilized trypsin and Varidase® contains a mixture of streptokinase and streptodornase. Streptokinase reacts with plasminogen to produce plasmin, a proteolytic enzyme that degrades fibrin. It also activates peptidases. Streptodornase liquefies DNA derived from cellular nuclei, which constitutes 30–70 per cent of the solid component of purulent exudate and is responsible for its stickiness. Experimental work has shown that Varidase® is more effective than trypsin-containing products and is better tolerated by patients. Direct injections of Varidase® into an eschar can be used when toughness prevents penetration. There is little clinical work on the effectiveness of Varidase® but one study on infected wounds found dextranomer beads to be more effective; another comparing Varidase® with Betadine® solution in leg ulcers found that it produced a more rapid appearance of granulation tissue.

Other wound-cleansing agents

Other wound-cleansing agents include Aserbine® and Malatex® creams and lotions containing benzoic acid, malic acid, salicylic acid, and propylene glycol. When used as creams applied thickly to mummified skin, rehydration may be effected, allowing autolysis or later surgical removal.

Acetic acid 5 per cent eliminates *Pseudomonas* from infected wounds but promotes *Staph. aureus* and *Proteus* overgrowth; furthermore, application is painful.

Azo dyes such as brilliant green and gentian (crystal) violet have antibacterial effects and have been used in skin disorders and minor wound infections for many years. However, they cause skin staining which may be cosmetically unacceptable. More alarmingly, the Department of Health has suggested that crystal violet may be toxic if applied to broken skin or mucous membranes. Mercurochrome is another dye, formerly applied to skin grazes and minor burns, but in quantity, this can cause mercury intoxication.

2.5 Wound dressings

History

In former times, dressing materials were often made from clothing and were frequently contaminated with microorganisms. Dedicated wound dressings were developed only with recognition of the needs of asepsis. In the 1880s, **Gamgee** devised a dressing consisting of cotton wadding covered with a woven cotton sleeve. The dressing was often soaked in iodine or phenol. In the early 1900s, **tulle gras** was developed as a non-stick dressing. This is an open-weave cotton or linen gauze coated in paraffin jelly, which is still widely used today (e.g. for burns).

Until the early 1970s, open wounds were managed with the intention of keeping them dry. This was believed to be the best way of encouraging wounds to heal. Dressings used were mainly simple woven fabrics such as cotton gauze, absorbent cotton wool, or viscose wool.

However, the work of Winter (1962) signalled a radical departure from this practice which is now the accepted norm. He found that experimental wounds in animals healed faster and more successfully when they were kept moist. These ideas gradually became accepted and this has led to the development of a range of new products designed to keep wounds moist.

Desirable properties of wound dressings

Absorbance

Dry cotton dressings are highly absorbent and are useful as temporary dressings after excision of dead tissue where absorbance of blood and exudate is important. They are also useful as backing pads for certain modern dressings, or alone to cover a dry wound that is nearly healed. For most wounds, however, dry dressings tend to encourage scab formation. A scab or eschar is made up of dried serous exudate, devitalized debris and, often, fibres released from dressings. It may be firmly entangled with collagen fibres at the wound surface. Although a scab provides mechanical protection for a wound, it retards epithelial migration from the wound edges and probably destroys healthy tissue while this process takes place.

If dry dressings are used in burns, dehydration of the skin in the peripheral, partially damaged 'zone of stasis' may cause avoidable necrosis of the remaining epithelial elements, thus extending the area of full thickness loss.

If occlusive or semipermeable dressings are used, this prevents secondary dehydration of wounds and avoids eschar formation. These dressings may also be used to rehydrate existing eschar and allow its removal after autolysis.

Bacterial permeability

If micro-organisms contaminate the external surface of a dressing, they may infect the wound unless the dressing prevents their transit. Similarly, organisms from an infected wound may pass out through the dressing to be shed into the locality, risking nosocomial or cross-infection—'strike through'.

A dry pad on a wound prevents both forms of bacterial penetration by acting as a depth filter, which eliminates most airborne bacteria attached to dust particles as well as drying any wound exudate before it reaches the surface. However, this property is lost if the dressing becomes wet or if there is 'strike through' of blood or serum. In either case, there is a potential two-way passage of bacteria through the dressing.

Non-motile organisms take about 48 hours to pass through a dressing whereas motile bacteria like *Pseudomonas* or *Proteus* can pass through in a few hours. Bacterial transit can be arrested if the dressing incorporates cellulose spreader layers or a layer impermeable to bacteria. Polyurethane film dressings (e.g. Opsite®) are impermeable to bacteria but organisms can disseminate around the edge if skin adhesion is incomplete.

Adverse chemical or physical factors

Dressings must be free of harmful chemicals, particles, and fibres. Residual chemicals from manufacturing processes can interfere with wound healing, and foreign particles or fibres remaining in a wound dramatically reduce the number of bacteria needed to establish clinical infection.

Adherence to wounds

Material in contact with wounds should not adhere to the wound. Furthermore, the dressing should be sufficiently porous to prevent maceration. Other layers of padding may be applied over the wound-contact material to absorb excess exudate. If dry dressings are applied directly to wounds, blood and plasma may soak into the dressing, where it forms a clot. When the dressing is removed, delicate granulation tissue and new epithelium forming at the surface would be stripped off and would need to regenerate under the next clean dressing. If this process were repeated frequently delayed healing would result.

Low-adherence dressings have a facing layer of non-absorbent material with pores of small size to allow gas and water vapour to permeate but to prevent clot penetration. These include perforated plastic films (such as Melolin®) and heat-treated knitted viscose apertured cloth (N-A Dressing®, Johnson and Johnson). A similar effect is achieved by open cell foams such as Synthaderm® or Lyofoam®. However, the small apertures in these materials may become clogged by viscous exudate which accumulates on the wound beneath the dressing.

Gas permeability

Permeability of dressings to oxygen and carbon dioxide is a subject of much research but with conflicting conclusions. There is little evidence that differences in gas permeability of dressings materially affect healing. Attention to systemic factors affecting local perfusion is probably more important. These include hypovolaemia, hypoxaemia, and increased sympathetic nervous system activity caused by pain and anxiety.

Molecular oxygen is a vital component of wound healing, required for energy-dependent processes such as cell replication and proline hydroxylation during collagen synthesis. In resisting infection, oxygen is required to produce superoxide radicals that kill phagocytosed bacteria. When oxygen tension is low, as in most wounds, production of superoxide radicals is reduced proportionately to local oxygen tension.

Increased metabolic activity during the acute phase of healing increases demand for molecular oxygen, causing a fall in local wound oxygen tension, a rise in lactate level, and a fall in pH, all of which seem to stimulate aspects of the healing process. In the initial stages, hypoxia stimulates macrophages to release an angiogenesis factor that causes endothelial cell chemotaxis. In addition, raised lactate levels stimulate fibroblasts to produce collagen. These processes are impaired only at unusually low oxygen tensions and are turned off when capillary ingrowth to the central portion of the wound is complete.

Loss of carbon dioxide from a wound surface produces a local alkalosis, as does the production of ammonia by bacterial urease. Reduced acidity impairs the release of oxygen from haemoglobin as much as fivefold.

In summary, the role of gas permeability in dressings is uncertain but it is likely that allowing free exchange of oxygen, carbon dioxide, and water vapour at the wound surface is desirable.

Temperature control

Wounds heal best at or near body temperature. After exposure of a wound for dressing, it takes about 40 minutes for the local temperature to be regained and about 3 hours for mitotic and leucocytic activity to return to normal. Both of these processes are greatly retarded below 28 °C, which is an argument in favour of infrequent dressing changes where circumstances allow. Hypothermia also reduces oxygen dissociation from haemoglobin. An exposed wound is virtually at ambient temperature; a gauze dressed wound is between 25 and 27 °C, similar to a hydrogel-dressed wound which loses heat by evaporation. Polyurethane films and foams and hydrocolloid dressings effectively insulate the wound, keeping it above 30 °C. In theory at least, this should be beneficial.

The ideal properties of wound dressings are summarized in Table 12.6

Table 12.6 Properties of an ideal wound dressing

Acts as a physical barrier
Absorbs inflammatory exudate
Prevents bacterial flux
Moistens not macerates
Protects delicate healing tissue
Prevents sutures snagging
Conceals the wound from the patient
Helps arrest wound bleeding

Types of wound contact material

Dry dressings

These simple dressings, usually of sterile cotton gauze, are suitable for dressing new wounds that are expected to lose fluid or blood, as absorbent dressings for new wounds to be closed later by delayed primary closure, or for dry wounds and ulcers where a scab or crust has formed. Dry dressings have the advantage of availability and low cost but, if left in place for more than a few hours, suffer from the major disadvantage of incorporation into fibrin clot and adherence to the wound. Removal may thus be difficult, requiring soaking, and the process may damage delicate healing granulation tissue or new epithelium. For most wounds, therefore, dry dressings are used as a temporary measure until the wound has stabilized and more suitable dressings can be substituted.

Tulle gras (paraffin gauze)

The first widely used non-stick wound dressing was tulle gras, developed in the First World War by Lumière. This is an open-weave cloth soaked in soft paraffin jelly and is still widely used today. Modern tulle gras are made of cotton or viscose with either a high or low paraffin load. Tulle gras may be impregnated with antibiotics (e.g. framycetin, Fucidin®) or antiseptics (e.g. chlorhexidine, povidone-iodine). However, there is little evidence that these agents have any advantage over non-medicated tulle gras.

Tulle gras suffers from several drawbacks. First, the weave is so open that blood clot easily penetrates and becomes incorporated into the dressing. Secondly, soft paraffin evaporates fairly rapidly, so it loses its non-stick properties after about 24 hours. Together, these properties mean that removing the dressing is painful and it often damages the delicate healing tissue. In addition, the dressing is greasy and tends to produce maceration of the wound surface. A further, perhaps theoretical disadvantage, is that soft paraffin is released into the wound. This probably has little effect on wound healing.

Despite its disadvantages, tulle gras is still widely used for covering raw areas (e.g. skin-graft donor sites and chronic ulcers) although many believe that better materials are available (e.g. alginate-based dressings).

Semipermeable film dressings

Collodion was developed in the mid-1800s. It is a clear, sticky fluid which when applied to wounds dries to form a flexible, adherent skin. It is made from gun cotton (cotton dissolved in nitric and sulphuric acids), which is dried and dissolved in an ether and spirit mixture. It is a cheap and effective material but has been largely supplanted by expensive acrylic sprays such as Nobecutane® with little apparent advantage but convenience.

In 1945, cellophane film was used successfully on burns and was shown to reduce pain and accelerate healing. All of these early materials are essentially impermeable and may produce maceration.

Little improvement took place in this field until the emergence of transparent Opsite® film dressing for wounds in 1971. This is a polyurethane film with multiple tiny perforations and a vinyl ether adhesive. It is permeable to water vapour and oxygen but impermeable to bacteria and water. Other similar materials have since appeared with similar characteristics. The main variables are in the type of adhesive and method of application.

Film dressings reduce water loss from an open wound fivefold. All are biocompatible and Tegaderm® even supports growth of cells in tissue culture. Skin-graft donor sites heal more quickly under these dressings and are ready for further harvesting after 5 days compared with 12 days for conventional dressings. When compared with gauze dressings, film-dressed wounds are more comfortable, make the wound easily visible without redressing, permit bathing, and are cleaner. Film dressings are not suitable for heavily exuding wounds.

Indications for film dressings include surgical wounds, superficial burns, split-skin donor sites, and intravenous catheter sites.

Solvent-based film dressings (Opsite® spray dressing, Nobecutane®)

These are variations on the old established collodion, described above. They consist of acrylic polymers or resins dissolved in solvents and are used mainly to provide tough, protective, bacteria-impervious dressings to minor, clean, surgical wounds.

Simple non-adherent dressings and composite pre-packed dressings

These convenient dressings are widely used. The structure includes a perforated plastic film in contact with the wound, an absorbent pad, and an adhesive backing layer on synthetic non-woven cloth. Examples include Mepore®. They have the advantages of sterility, non-adherence, absorbency, and depth filtration but suffer from the disadvantages of high cost, zero wound visibility, and bacterial penetration if wet.

Foam dressings

Silastic foam dressings first appeared in the early 1970s and have been increasing in popularity since. They are intended to provide a non-stick filling for a cavity (e.g. pilonidal sinus or perianal abscess wound) which is intended to heal over a period by secondary intention. It has the dual purpose of maintaining the cavity open to encourage infilling from the base and of absorbing exudate. Dressings are made *in situ* by mixing two components and pouring the foaming mixture into the wound to form a cast. The result is a soft, flexible, open-celled foam that is able to absorb exudate and conforms to the wound shape. It is comfortable to wear, does not damage delicate tissue and can be washed in chlorhexidine by the patient and replaced. New dressings are made at intervals as the wound shrinks.

Lyofoam® is a hydrophobic, open-cell polyurethane, supplied in the form of an 8-mm-thick sheet with a heat-modified surface. It draws up exudate and loses water by evaporation from the exposed surface. Wounds are maintained more dry than moist, so this dressing is unsuitable for rehydrating eschar. No secondary backing dressing is required and the dressing is effective beneath compression for leg ulcers. Compared with Melolin® for skin wounds, it produced less pain and less adherence.

Alginate dressings

Alginates are polysaccharides derived from kelp seaweed. The wound dressing material is manufactured in the form of fibres of insoluble calcium sodium alginate. Alginates depend for their activity on absorbing exudate to form a hydrophilic gel that encourages wound healing and is atraumatic when dressings are changed. Alginate dressings (e.g. Sorbsan®, Kaltostat®) absorb three times more exudate than gauze, weight for weight. They are therefore particularly indicated for exudative wounds but inappropriate for use on dry wounds. Dressing change is indicated when maximum absorbency has been reached. A composite dressing of alginate with an occlusive backing prevents inhibition of healing caused by drying out.

Alginates also accelerate haemostasis, rendering the dressing ideally suited in the management of bleeding cavity wounds. Blood loss is reduced by 50 per cent when used on skin-graft donor sites. The haemostatic action probably results from its local provision of excess calcium ions.

When used appropriately, alginates have many of the properties of an ideal dressing discussed earlier. Some anti-bacterial effect has also been shown, possibly by bacterial entrapment.

In use, sheets of the material are applied directly to the wound. For heavily exudative wounds, a gauze backing pad is taped in place, but for most wounds, a composite type of dressing with an occlusive backing is preferred. The frequency of dressing change depends on the needs of the individual wound. Infected or heavily exudative wounds need dressing daily, gradually reducing the frequency of change until dressings can be left in place for several days. There is a particular advantage of alginate dressings here as they can be washed away with saline with no danger of irritant fibres becoming embedded. Clean, uninfected wounds do best if disturbed little, but infected wounds usually need daily dressing changes.

To remove the dressing, it is first irrigated with saline. This causes insoluble calcium alginate to transform into soluble sodium alginate, which washes away painlessly and without damaging newly formed tissue. Any scale or crust that accumulates around the wound edge is removed with forceps.

Alginate dressings are comfortable in use and no sensitivity has been shown. Skin-donor sites heal in 50 per cent less time than under paraffin tulle and the quality of healing and patient comfort is reportedly improved. Other studies have shown more effective healing of chronic leg ulcers using these dressings than with paraffin tulle treated ulcers.

Hydrogel dressings

Hydrogel dressings are composed of insoluble polymers with hydrophilic sites which absorb and retain substantial volumes of water. The polymers are synthetic or semisynthetic materials and the properties can be varied by changing the monomer used and its cross-linking. There are two main types used for wound dressings: sheets with stable dimensional structure, and amorphous hydrogels.

Stable sheets

These swell as they absorb water to saturation point but retain their general shape (e.g. Geliperm®, Vigilon®). Geliperm® sheet is a composite of a weak agar gel and polyacrylamide to provide strength. In experimental implantation studies, it provokes virtually no reaction. The material is usually supplied as a hydrated sheet containing 96 per cent water. The material is strong, flexible, moist, and transparent, but will dry out in warm, dry conditions. Geliperm® is also available as a dry sheet containing glycerol as a humectant, and as a hydrated gel, a minced up version of the hydrated sheet, which can be injected into cavities. It is impermeable to bacteria and fungi and does not support their proliferation. It is permeable to water vapour and gases as well as solutes with molecular weights up to 10^6 Da. It may absorb toxins and other bacterial products from infected wounds. This property also suggests that the material might be effective as a carrier agent, for example for growth factors, to the surface of wounds.

Sheet hydrogels can be applied and removed without causing pain or damage to delicate tissues, provided they are not allowed to dry out. They reduce pain from wounds and can be best held in place using self-adhesive dressing retention sheet (e.g. Mefix® or Hypafix®). Their main application is for wide areas of partial epithelial loss as in donor sites, abrasions, and partial thickness burns.

Disadvantages of sheet hydrogels largely outweigh their potential advantages. These include the difficulty of retaining them in place, the difficulty of maintaining the correct level of hydration without drying or maceration, and the need for frequent dressing changes. Wounds infected with *Pseudomonas* deteriorate rapidly under these dressings. They are also expensive.

Amorphous hydrogels

These decrease their viscosity as they absorb fluid and flow to take up the shape of the wound (e.g. Scherisorb Intrasite®). As water absorption continues, the amorphous hydrogels eventually become simply a dispersion of polymer in water. Scherisorb® is a transparent aqueous gel based on corn starch, chemically modified by adding hydrophilic side-chains. The dressing is supplied in sachets consisting of 2 per cent copolymer, 78 per cent water, and 20 per cent propylene glycol as preservative and humectant. It can be left in wounds for up to 3 days. It appears particularly useful for wounds containing dry slough or necrotic tissue, which it rehydrates, allowing autolysis to take place.

Hydrocolloid dressings

These are relatively new materials based on gel-forming agents, primarily carboxymethylcellulose. They are usually presented in sheet form, usually with a film or foam backing, but the base material is also available as granules and paste.

The first agent of this type, Orabase® (ConvaTec) was a viscous paste designed to adhere to the moist surface of mouth ulcers. Here it slowly absorbs water, to form a protective gel. This was modified in the early 1970s into a sheet or wafer form, Stomahesive®, to protect excoriated skin around intestinal stomas. The pliable sheet contained carboxymethylcellulose, pectin, and gelatin, and was backed by a sheet of polyethylene. Excoriated skin is protected and heals under Stomahesive® and the polyethylene sheet provides sound attachment for stoma appliances. The material was modified again as Varihesive® (which later became Granuflex®) which consists of a semipermeable polyurethane film/foam backing attached to hydrocolloid base dispersed as granules in an adhesive sheet. Several similar agents are now marketed, including Comfeel® (Coloplast®) and Tegasorb® (3M).

Hydrocolloid dressings adhere to dry skin by virtue of the adhesive sheet. The hydrophilic granules of the base slowly absorb water from ulcerated areas to form a semisolid gel in contact with the wound (which, disconcertingly, resembles pus). Certain hydrocolloids (e.g. Comfeel®) retain exudate in a more stable structure. Fluid migrates only slowly across the dressing so its base is moist and easily removed. Conversely, for exudative wounds, maceration occurs easily. The dressings have been shown to effectively isolate infected ulcers from the environment and may be of value in MRSA-infected ulcers. Very low oxygen tensions occur under hydrocolloid dressings that may overstimulate the formation of granulation tissue. However, the acidic nature of the liquefying dressing may be beneficial in inhibiting some bacteria, particularly *Pseudomonas*. Granuflex® also has fibrinolytic effects, perhaps due to pectin, but any real benefit has yet to be demonstrated.

Hydrocolloid dressings have frequently been shown to reduce pain and to accelerate healing. Nevertheless, they are best used in non-infected minimally exudative wounds. These dressings have been used successfully in burns (similar results to silver sulfadiazine and human allografts) and split-skin donor sites (more rapid healing and less pain than tulle gras or saline gauze). They are useful as occlusive dressings for rehydrating heel pressure sores, but careful observation is required to prevent maceration or spreading infection. Hydrocolloids have their devotees for venous ulcer dressing, but the characteristic odour of the liquefying dressing and the leakage of liquefied gel from beneath are disadvantages, as is the occasional overgrowth of granulation tissue. However, when the correct treatment for venous ulceration, effective compression bandaging, has been used, no advantage in healing rate has been shown for hydrocolloids over simple non-adherent dressings. When these dressings have been used for fresh surgical wounds, healing and pain have been reported as beneficial.

Pastes and beads

Honey and sugar

Honey has been used for over 3000 years as a dressing for wounds. It consists principally of glucose and fructose—which exert a high osmotic pressure—and has a low pH; both these properties are unfavourable for bacterial growth. Modern studies have shown it to kill or inhibit the growth of a broad range of pathogenic bacteria, although it does not prevent the growth of *Candida* species. When applied to wounds, sterility can develop in 3–6 days. Granulated sugar has been used alone or in combination with povidone-iodine in a number of trials that lacked scientific rigour. However, results suggest that further work might be justified.

Polysaccharide beads

Debrisan®

Debrisan is based on a derivative of dextran known as dextranomer in which dextran is cross-linked to render it insoluble. It is biologically inert and has not been shown to cause sensitivity reactions. In implantation experiments, unchanged beads become enclosed in fibrous capsules but without granuloma formation.

It is supplied as highly hydrophilic granules, 0.1–0.3 mm in diameter, capable of holding four times their weight in fluid. They absorb molecules up to a molecular weight of 1000 Da freely, 1000–5000 Da slowly, and larger molecules not at all. When placed in a wound, exudate (containing bacteria and cellular debris) is progressively drawn away from the surface of the wound. Provided it is changed before saturation, this physical action of extracting bacteria is potentially useful. The granules also have a marked fibrinolytic activity, preventing clotting in the wound and keeping it soft and supple. Debrisan® has been shown to reduce inflammation and increase rates of healing in discharging burns compared with saline dressings.

Debrisan® is recommended for wounds containing pus, debris, and soft yellow slough, changing to an alternative dressing when this has been achieved. After cleansing with saline, the granules are poured into a wound to a depth at least 3 mm. A covering with a dressing pad or semipermeable film is then applied. Dressings are changed once or twice daily by saline irrigation. For shallow wounds, Debrisan® paste or pads are recommended, although much of the fluid-absorbing ability of the beads is lost.

Infected abdominal wounds heal faster than when dressed with EUSOL and paraffin, but at a comparable rate compared with silicone foam dressing (although Debrisan® was reported as being much more expensive).

Iodosorb® (cadexomer iodine)

This is similar to Debrisan® but contains 0.9 per cent elemental iodine (demonstrated to improve on the bactericidal effect) and is biodegradable. Studies have shown it improves the healing rate in leg ulcers as well as giving better wound débridement, odour reduction, pain relief, and reduction in inflammation than simple dressings.

Indications are not clear-cut but the material is one possible choice for the early stages of cleaning sloughy or infected wounds.

Enzymatic agents

Odour-absorbing dressings

Infected wounds may produce unpleasant odours, distressing to patient and hospital staff. The odour of necrotic wounds is largely caused by diamines such as cadaverine and putrescine produced, in particular, in wounds infected with *Clostridia*, *Bacteroides*, and mixed growths of Enterobacteriaceae. Odour is best treated by effective treatment of the infected wound, but if this is impossible, dressings incorporating activated charcoal cloth may be useful. Activation produces many small pores on the carbon fibres, effectively enlarging the surface area many fold. Examples include Actisorb Plus® (which is a wound contact dressing containing silver as an antibacterial agent), Kaltocarb®, and Lyofoam C®. There is little published scientific data on the use of these products and, at present, they can be recommended only for malodorous wounds.

Choice of dressing

Introduction

There is a great deal of mythology and confusion attached to surgical dressings. Most surgical trainees learn whatever they know from their seniors and from observing nurses dress wounds. However, the reasons why one type of dressing is preferred to another are often illogical and may be out of date. Traditional dressings had simple absorptive or protective functions, whereas newer dressings are often of a more interactive type, designed to bring about changes in the local environment of a specific type of wound. For example, the dressing may form

Table 12.7 Contact dressings: appraisal and indications

Type of dressing	Advantages	Disadvantages	Indications
Dry gauze	Cheap Absorbent	Sticks to wound	Temporary dressing
Wet dressings, e.g. saline gauze, proflavine gauze	Simple Cheap May be antiseptic	Sticks when dries out	Temporary dressing if infection present
Non-stick dressing			
(a) Tulle gras	Cheap Convenient	Sticks when dries out Macerates	Temporary dressing
(b) Composite, e.g. Mepore®; Melolin®	Stays non-stick Convenient	Conceals wound	Standard post-op. dressing
(c) Silastic® foam	Stays non-stick Moistens Absorbent	Fiddly	Cavity dressing
(d) Surgicel®	Haemostatic Easy to remove	Expensive	Anal wounds
Film dressings			
(a) Semipermeable, e.g. Opsite®	Reduces water loss Can see wound	Not for exudative wounds	Superficial burn Cannula sites Split-skin donor sites
(b) Solvent based, e.g. Nobecutane® Hydrophilic dressings	Impervious to bacteria	Patient can see wound	Minor clean wounds
(a) Alginates	Absorbent Haemostatic Atraumatic	Not for dry wounds	Exuding wounds Bleeding cavities Skin graft donor sites
(b) Hydrogels Stable, e.g. Geliperm®	Comfortable	Tend to dry out Expensive Frequent changes	Wide areas of partial loss of epithelium
Amorphous, e.g. Scherisorb®, Intrasite® gel	Rehydrates slough	No benefit to clean wounds	Wounds with necrosis or slough
(c) Hydrocolloids, e.g. Granuflex®	Reduce pain Accelerate healing	May macerate wound or permit spreading infection	Skin excoriation around stomas Uninfected, minimally exudative wounds
Other			
Polysaccharide beads, e.g. Debrisan®; Iodosorb®	Bacteriostatic Highly absorbent Effective cleansing of infected wounds	Difficult to retain in shallow wounds Needs frequent changes	Exudative, sloughy, or infected wounds
Odour absorbing, e.g. Actisorb Plus®	Contains activated charcoal cloth which reduces smell	Usually unnecessary	Malodorous wounds when no other treatment possible

a **gel** to cover the wound, or enable rehydration of eschar, or draw exudate from the wound.

Most people who use dressings use a limited range of products, sometimes inappropriately. Dressings cannot cure chronic infected wounds by local medication, nor can they magically deslough a wound that needs surgical cleansing. However, appropriate dressing selection for a particular stage in the evolution and progress of a healing wound, and attention to the frequency of dressing change, can undoubtedly shorten hospital stay and duration of healing (Table 12.7).

In order to determine what is the most suitable dressing for a given wound, taking into account the cost, the availability, and any known patient sensitivities, the wound should be considered under the following headings:

◆ Is this a clean surgical wound expected to heal primarily? (Simple dressings only are required.)

◆ Is this a clean, granulating wound with substantial skin and other tissue loss?

◆ Is this a superficial partial skin loss (graze or burn)?

◆ In a dirty wound, does it need early surgical treatment (i.e. surgical cleansing to remove contamination, yellow slough, or dead tissue) or, if the wound is infected, are there collections of pus that need drainage? (Choice of dressing is made after surgical treatment.) If surgery is not needed, how can the choice of dressing facilitate removal of slough, scabs, etc.?

◆ Is the wound superficially infected? (Dressings should prevent dissemination of infection. They need changing frequently and the wound should be inspected regularly to see whether surgical treatment is needed.)

◆ Is the wound covered with a hard, dry, black necrotic layer of dehydrated eschar?

◆ Is the wound bleeding, discharging, or exuding serous fluid? (An absorbent dressing will be needed, at least initially.)

◆ Is the wound or skin break long standing and, if so, what are the underlying factors that need attention? For example, chronic venous hypertension in leg ulcers, intestinal fistulas, Crohn's disease in a non-healing perineal wound after rectal resection.

◆ In a deep wound, is packing required to maintain the surface opening?

◆ Does the site require a particular type of dressing (e.g. to keep it in place or because the wound is visible)? Such sites may include the head and neck and perianal area.

2.6 Wound problems and complications

Although wound healing is generally uncomplicated, numerous complications may arise (Tables 12.8 and 12.9). Numerous factors may impair wound healing; these are illustrated in Table 12.10.

Table 12.8 Wound problems—early

Wound haematoma	Swelling, pain
Wound dehiscence	
	Superficial
	Complete (burst abdomen)
Wound infection	
	Wound abscess
	Cellulitis
Other wound discharge	
	Liquefying haematoma
	Lymphatic leak
	Fistula

Table 12.9 Wound problems—late

Delayed wound infection
Deep infection (suppressed by antibiotics)
Wound pain
'Neuroma'
Nerve entrapment
Incisional hernia
Stitch sinus

Table 12.10 Factors that impair wound healing

Poor closure technique
Wound infection
Patient factors causing retarded healing
Intestinal fistulas
Foreign bodies
Chronic infection with tuberculosis
Malignant wound invasion—peritoneal seedlings of e.g. colonic carcinoma

Wound haemorrhage or haematoma

Wound haemorrhage or haematoma formation most commonly occurs when primary haemorrhage at operation has not been fully controlled, or else reactionary haemorrhage has taken place during the ensuing 24 hours. There is little substitute for effecting careful haemostasis in a patient who has been restored to normal blood pressure by the conclusion of surgery. However, in areas where there is substantial dead space or extensive raw surfaces, suction drains or pressure dressings may help to prevent accumulation of haematoma.

Continuing haemorrhage from a wound in the immediate postoperative period warrants either re-exploration or pressure dressing. The choice depends on the severity and site of bleeding.

Wound haematomas often develop slowly over several days after operation and patients may present up to a week or two after discharge with swelling beneath the wound and 'bleeding' from a small area of the wound. On inspection, there is often bruising around the wound and the swelling may be fluctuant. The apparent bleeding is usually liquefying haematoma; the fluid is deeper red and rather watery. Blood is an excellent culture medium and a wound haematoma places the patient at risk of wound infection. Small haematomas resorb spontaneously but larger ones usually require surgical evacuation. Sometimes needle aspiration under aseptic conditions can be performed after liquefaction has occurred.

Wound infection

Introduction to wound infection

Infection is the most common factor that delays or prevents healing of surgical wounds. The presence of bacteria alone in a wound is not the major component, but whether the balance between host resistance (local and systemic) and the size and virulence of the bacterial population is tipped against the host. Quantitative culture has been used to demonstrate that the presence of more than 100 000 bacteria/gram of tissue prevents wound healing. For split-skin grafts, the 'take' rate is 94 per cent if the bacterial count is less than this figure, but only 19 per cent if it is greater.

Similar proportions of wound breakdown have been shown when primary closure of contaminated wounds has been attempted. The mechanism seems to be secretion of proteases by the organisms as well as production of virulence factors such as haemolysins and inhibitors of leucocyte chemotaxis. It has been demonstrated that the bacterial concentration in a traumatic wound steadily increases with time following wounding. Even after a 'clean' laceration of the hand, the critical level of bacterial concentration is reached after 5–6 hours. Quantitative culture is not yet a standard part of wound management but may have a role to play in the future, as more than 100 000 organisms/gram have been shown to be present in one-third of wounds that appear to be ready for closure.

A further specific factor is the presence of β-haemolytic streptococci. Regardless of the concentration, the presence of this organism nearly always prevents wound healing.

Superficial wound infection leads to separation of the opposed edges and retards the formation of granulation tissue. Mild cellulitis caused by non-pyogenic bacteria may resolve spontaneously or with antibiotic treatment and cause minimal delay in healing. However, if local necrosis and pus formation occurs (typically in staphylococcal infection), healing cannot begin until drainage of the wound abscess has been achieved, either spontaneously or by surgical drainage.

Many apparently superficial wound infections appear to heal satisfactorily after treatment, only to present as an incisional hernia months or years later. Deep wound infections involving the abdominal wall probably destroy the tissues encircled by sutures, leading to partial or complete dehiscence of the wound.

The role of antibiotics in wound infection

Antibiotics should be employed in wound infections only as follows:

- prophylactically, if given within 4 hours of traumatic injury to prevent bacterial infection becoming established;

- to treat spreading cellulitis or systemic infection.

Surgical intervention in wound infection is necessary to drain abscesses or remove dead tissue or foreign bodies. Healing then occurs by secondary intention or after delayed primary closure.

Definitions of wound infection

The features that constitute different severities of wound infection need to be defined precisely if reported rates of wound infection are to be relied upon. Validated figures for wound infection should be part of the quality control mechanisms of any surgical unit. This information is also used to assess the effectiveness of prophylactic measures against wound infection, particularly when comparing results from different units.

Describing a wound as regards infection is straightforward if it is obviously not infected (i.e. the wound edges are in contact, it is dry, painless and not red or inflamed, and the patient has no systemic signs of infection). Description is also non-controversial if the wound is obviously infected (i.e. it has broken down and discharges pus or is red, swollen, hot and tender, or pathogens have been cultured from fluid discharging from the wound, often in a patient with an elevated temperature and tachycardia).

However, intermediate stages can be difficult to assess. These include wounds that become slightly red but do not break down or discharge fluid and which resolve without intervention. Provided healing is not delayed and complications such as delayed infection after discharge from hospital or incisional hernia are absent, the wound is usually regarded as not infected.

Another difficulty is when the wound looks uninfected but where the patient has local or systemic signs of deep infection. This can usually be resolved only by observing the eventual outcome.

For clinical trials, a coherent approach can best be brought if all wounds are inspected by a single, obsessional observer, using a local protocol. This helps avoid doubtful definitions in an individual study, but the problem of comparing studies in different units remains.

Wound infections are usually labelled **major** if they cause systemic signs of infection and delay the patient's discharge from hospital, and **minor** if they do not. However, it is important to recognize that about half of all wound infections present late, so the evaluation period must be at least 6 weeks, and longer if a sinus or fistula is present. Incisional hernias usually present at least 6 months after operation.

Rate of infection related to initial level of contamination

When describing surgical or traumatic wounds with regard to the potential risk of later infection, it is useful to break them down according to the level of initial contamination. This is particularly useful when analysing groups of cases for the frequency of wound infection. Using risk groups, the expected rates of infection can be compared with the observed rates. A widely used method of classification is as follows:

◆ **Clean**: where no viscus is opened (e.g. inguinal herniorrhaphy). Anticipated wound infection rate 1–2 per cent.

◆ **Clean-contaminated**: where a viscus is opened with no spillage or with minimal spillage. Anticipated wound infection rate with antibiotic prophylaxis is less than 10 per cent.

◆ **Contaminated**: when a viscus is opened and there is obvious spillage, or in the presence of obvious inflammatory disease such as Crohn's disease. Anticipated wound infection rate with antibiotic prophylaxis 15–20 per cent.

◆ **Dirty**: in the presence of frank pus or when there has been gross soiling resulting from intestinal perforation. Anticipated wound infection rate with antibiotic prophylaxis up to 40 per cent.

Gas gangrene and necrotizing fasciitis

The most sinister wound complication is gas gangrene. Fortunately it is rare and, when it does occur, is usually seen in contaminated accidental wounds. The causative bacteria are clostridia, the most common being *Cl. perfringens* (formerly known as *Cl. welchii*), often in association with other anaerobes such as bacteroides and peptostreptococci. *Clostridium perfringens* is found in soil that has been manured and in the normal human intestine. In gas gangrene, there is rapidly spreading gangrene and profound systemic disturbance. Gas in the tissues may be detectable clinically as crepitus or be visible on plain X-rays, and a foul, brownish exudate is seen. The management of this condition involves intensive care resuscitation and support, together with large doses of benzylpenicillin and early and radical excision of all affected muscle and overlying skin. Hyperbaric oxygen may be used as an adjunct if available.

Patients with substantially contaminated traumatic wounds should be given prophylactic antibiotics to minimize the risk of this dread complication.

Necrotizing fasciitis is a related condition in which infection spreads along fascial planes but does not directly affect muscle. Extensive surgical excision of dead tissue is required but is restricted to the subcutaneous fat and skin; otherwise the management is similar to that of gas gangrene (see earlier). This is a synergistic infection caused by mixed bacteria, including anaerobic and micro-aerophilic streptococci, bacteroides, and *Staph. aureus*.

Incisional hernia

Incisional hernias usually become evident months or years after an operation. They occur most commonly in abdominal incisions, with the lower abdomen more at risk. Numerous publications have reached the same conclusion, namely that poor closure technique and unsuitable suture materials are responsible for most incisional hernias. However, major wound infections, particularly if associated with anastomotic leakage of bowel contents or bile, strongly predispose to herniation.

The choice of abdominal incision is of lesser importance but does have a bearing on hernia development. Of abdominal incisions, the vertical lateral rectus incision has, somewhat surprisingly, been shown to give the lowest rate of incisional hernia. However, it gives relatively poor access to many areas of the abdomen and is not popular. Midline incisions closed properly are the next most reliable, and paramedian incisions least satisfactory. Transverse muscle-cutting incisions are of intermediate security.

Optimum closure technique employs mass closure of the abdominal wall utilizing a continuous monofilament suture (which must persist in the wound for at least 6 months). Bites are placed at least 1 cm from the wound edge and 1 cm apart. Incisional hernias rarely occur in chest wounds, probably because of the relative rigidity of the thoracic wall and the generous layers of muscle overlying it.

If an incisional hernia is left untreated, it gradually enlarges and its contents become progressively more irreducible. If the sac has a narrow neck, strangulation or bowel obstruction becomes a particular concern.

If the patient is infirm and the hernia is freely reducible and painless, control of the hernia with a surgical belt may be considered. This may be preferred to surgical reduction of a sizeable and long-standing hernia which may compromise respiratory function by splinting the diaphragms.

Repair of the defect follows the principles of all hernia surgery (i.e. reduction of the contents of the sac, excision of the sac, and repair of the defects). Many different methods of repair have been proposed but all of them fail on occasions. This is often caused by the poor quality of the remaining abdominal wall or because of tension in the wound. The recurrence rate is particularly high in obese patients where muscle is weakened by the interposition of adipose tissue. Currently, mesh repair techniques utilizing Prolene® mesh are popular. Whichever technique is used, the important principles are: to define the edges of the hernial defect clearly; to perform a tension-free repair, taking good bites of healthy surrounding fascia and muscle with a permanent monofilament suture; and to ensure meticulous haemostasis. Transient suction drainage is useful for the hernia dead-space.

Other wound complications

Late **wound sinuses** may present days, weeks, or months after a wound has healed. Often, there is a history of infection of the original wound which appeared to heal. Later, a small abscess develops and discharges spontaneously, leaving a characteristic sinus opening. In nearly all cases, the sinus is related to a deep, non-absorbable suture. Treatment consists of an operation, usually under general anaesthesia, to probe the sinus, enlarge the opening and extract the offending suture. The wound is left open and will usually heal rapidly without complication or recurrence.

Scar hypertrophy may occur during the first few months after an operation to produce a red and widened scar. Spontaneous improvement occurs within the year, in contrast to **keloid scars** where deterioration continues. Keloid occurs predominantly in pigmented races, particularly in children and on the anterior chest wall. It is thought to arise as a result of faulty collagen maturation and it is a difficult condition to treat. Excision of the wound is invariably followed by recurrence, but intralesional steroids, silicone dressings or low-dose radiotherapy immediately after excision can be effective.

Patients with cosmetically unsightly scars should be considered for referred to a plastic surgical colleague for revision.

Delayed healing and wound breakdown

Poor closure technique

Faulty closure of body cavity wounds is the most common cause of early wound breakdown, although general conditions that predispose to poor wound healing are also of relevance (see below). Complete dehiscence with parting of the abdominal wall and skin and the bursting forth of abdominal contents into the wound sometimes occurs. This is an alarming condition for the inexperienced but is remarkably painless. In complete dehiscence, the bowel should be covered temporarily with saline-soaked swabs and early resuturing arranged. A **contained dehiscence** may occur if the skin remains intact. Here, the skin sutures should be left in place to allow the patient to recover from the primary operation and arrange for secondary repair of the incisional hernia at a later date.

The most common errors in body-wall closure are:

♦ Excessively tight placement of sutures, which leads to ischaemic necrosis of the wound edges with cutting out of the sutures. Taking bites of abdominal wall too close to the edge may have a similar effect, and placing sutures too far apart may allow intestinal contents to herniate between the sutures. Thus there is a mechanical failure of the closure, together with the presence of necrotic tissue providing a culture medium for bacteria, which itself may contribute to the wound breakdown.

♦ Inadequate haemostasis during closure may lead to accumulation of a wound haematoma. This prevents the wound edges coming into contact, causes pain and delayed mobilization, and the haematoma may become secondarily infected.

♦ Unrecognized bowel trauma during closure, particularly suture-needle perforation of bowel. If this causes leakage of bowel contents, wound infection is inevitable, wound breakdown is likely, and fistulation possible.

♦ Ill-advised attempts at primary closure of the superficial tissues when the wound is contaminated or if there is obvious infection. This usually results in superficial wound infection and breakdown. Delaying primary closure should be the treatment of choice for wounds like these.

Patient factors causing retarded healing

Introduction

It is remarkable that most patients with disorders that are potential causes of delayed wound healing manage to heal wounds normally. Advanced age, often blamed for retarding wound healing, is rarely a factor on its own.

Immunosuppression and collagen disorders

Patients may be immunocompromised by immunosuppressive treatment such as chemotherapy and radiotherapy, or by sepsis, malnutrition, advanced age, or the acquired immunodeficiency syndrome (AIDS). Chemotherapy for cancer has not been shown to interfere with wound healing, provided it is not given within the immediate perioperative period.

Patients with rheumatoid arthritis have a bad reputation for healing. The disease itself affects healing rate and may affect maturation of collagen. Furthermore, these patients are often on long-term corticosteroid therapy or non-steroidal anti-inflammatory agents, which retard healing. Corticosteroid therapy is likely to have a significant effect on healing only if doses are high (more than 10 mg prednisolone equivalent/day) or treatment is prolonged for more than a few weeks. It is probable, however, that maturation of collagen is affected and wounds may take longer to reach full strength.

Patients on immunosuppressive treatment heal for the most part as well as normal people, unless infection occurs or the wound is relatively ischaemic. Under these circumstances, there is no reserve to overcome these problems and wound healing does not take place.

Irradiation therapy

Irradiation therapy, particularly older treatments using low kilovoltage therapy, causes obliterative endarteritis and relative ischaemia. Wounds in these patients should be placed remotely from the irradiated area or else there is a risk of catastrophic wound breakdown. An example is the broad-field radiotherapy that used to be used for bladder carcinoma. If surgery is needed subsequently, an 'inverted U' incision should be used to avoid the lower abdomen.

Malnutrition

Malnutrition and malignant cachexia may be implicated in wound complications, although in most cases, wounds heal surprisingly well. Malnutrition is known to affect hydroxyproline synthesis as well as the inflammatory reaction and immune functions. Surgical patients may become nutritionally depleted by lack of oral intake, malabsorption, the catabolic effects of illness, or by drug–nutrient interactions. Physiological processes begin to be impaired when a patient has lost approximately 10 per cent of normal body weight. In addition to glucose (energy), protein (amino acids for repair and synthesis of tissues), fat (for cell membranes), vitamins, and trace elements are important elements of wound healing. In particular, vitamin C is required for fibroblast proliferation, collagen synthesis, and for production of neutrophil free-oxygen radicals. Wound dehiscence is up to eight times more likely in vitamin C-depleted patients. Vitamins A and E and pantothenic acid are believed to be associated with improved strength in wounds, but the effects of deficiency are poorly understood. Zinc plays an important role in cell mitosis and proliferation during the fibroblastic phase of wound healing. Serum levels lower than 100 μg/dl are associated with poor healing. Zinc sulphate supplements are probably appropriate in patients with sepsis, prolonged diarrhoea, an ileostomy or fistula, where zinc loss is excessive.

Unfortunately, supplemental nutrition in advance of surgery seems to provide little additional benefit over meticulous technique.

Ischaemia

Ischaemic impairs healing. Thus amputation through a profoundly ischaemic segment of a lower limb will be unsuccessful. However, many amputation wounds heal satisfactorily even in the presence of relative ischaemia. Unfortunately, there are no tests that can reliably distinguish between a limb that will heal and one that will not. Experience and good technique are the best guides, but if the modern belief is employed that 70 per cent or more of patients can undergo a below-knee amputation, 10 per cent will require reamputation at a higher level and another 10 per cent will require other secondary surgical procedures before healing.

When local ischaemia caused by trauma to the local blood supply prevents healing, revascularization can often be accomplished using a free musculocutaneous or fasciocutaneous flap, with its axial vessels anastomosed to a nearby artery and vein. This solution is not appropriate in wounds or ulcers failing to heal because of generalized limb ischaemia due to atherosclerosis or embolism. Here, arterial reconstruction may solve the problem of ischaemia.

Oxygen tension

Increased metabolic activity during the acute phase of healing results in increased local oxygen consumption and a fall in wound oxygen tension. Moderate hypoxia stimulates angiogenesis, and this is impaired only at unusually low oxygen tensions.

Molecular oxygen is required for energy-dependent processes and for the production of superoxide radicals used to kill phagocytosed bacteria. Attention should be paid to factors affecting local perfusion such as hypovolaemia, elevated sympathetic nervous system activity (anxiety, pain, avoiding smoking), and central hypoxaemia.

Diabetes

Diabetic patients heal normally unless blood sugar control is awry or infection supervenes. Diabetics experience a slightly elevated risk of wound infection and the infection may be more virulent. This is probably caused by a combination of cellular nutrition, mild immunosuppression, and, in those affected, small-vessel disease.

Unusual factors causing delayed healing

Intestinal fistulas

Persistent leakage of bowel contents or digestive juices into a wound via an enterocutaneous fistula will interfere with wound healing. Fistulas usually follow anastomotic dehiscence after surgical reconstruction of bowel, the biliary system, or the pancreas, but may also occur as a result of unrecognized trauma to bowel at operation or after penetrating trauma by knife or gunshot.

Minimal-output fistulas can be controlled with simple gauze dressings, but those with higher output are better controlled by a stoma bag or device designed for the purpose (e.g. Wound Manager®) with Stomahesive® to protect the surrounding skin.

Foreign bodies

Foreign bodies in wounds prevent full healing unless they are sterile and biologically inert. Certain foreign materials that the body cannot remove excite a frustrated inflammatory response, thus entering the recurring cycle of chronic inflammation. This involves inflammation, and often pus formation, combined with persistent but frustrated attempts at healing.

Arterial or joint prostheses are routinely employed and, luckily, are rarely complicated by delayed healing. However, infection around a prosthesis causes local tissue destruction, sinus formation, and septicaemia. An infected prosthesis must generally be removed (or otherwise sterilized) if healing is to occur. Non-absorbable sutures may also form a nidus for chronic infection, often with recurrent local abscesses, discharge to the surface forming a sinus, and healing over. Such sutures must be removed before healing can occur.

Rarely, a surgical instrument or swab is inadvertently left within a patient. Great efforts are taken by theatre nurses to account for every instrument and swab used during surgery and when the count is deficient it is a good maxim that the nurse is always right! Retained surgical instruments rarely cause symptoms and are usually discovered accidentally on X-ray years later. Cotton swabs, however, excite a marked foreign-body response and eventually form an abscess.

Other chronic infections with tuberculosis and other undrained chronic abscesses

Pre-existing chronic infections with specific disorders such as tuberculosis may cause primary failure of wound healing. If suspected, appropriate bacteriological examinations should be performed on biopsy material. If body cavities are explored for peritonitis or multilocular abscesses are found, entry wounds are likely to heal poorly unless all infection is eliminated. If other undrained chronic abscesses persist, wound healing is impaired.

Invasion of a wound or drain site by intracavity malignancy

A rare cause for failure of a body-cavity wound or drain site to heal is spreading of malignant cells along the track (e.g. peritoneal seedlings of colonic carcinoma). If suspected, the wound edge should be biopsied.

2.7 Management of individual types of wound

The aims of wound management are to establish a favourable local (and systemic) environment to facilitate normal healing mechanisms and discourage disorganized attempts at healing (e.g. excess granulation tissue, premature closure of a cavity opening, or sinus formation) (Table 12.11).

Table 12.11 Principles of wound management

Correct any systemic factors that may impair wound healing

Plan appropriate surgical incision

Prevent perioperative wound contamination and subsequent cross-infection

Optimize wound-closure technique

Choose appropriate dressing

Monitor the healing process

Well-timed suture removal

Once a wound has been closed, the doctor has three main responsibilities: choosing the dressing, monitoring the progress of healing, and deciding when to remove the sutures. Wound management must be flexible according to changing circumstances, which may require secondary surgical procedures. Complications must be managed expeditiously. If a wound is already infected, adequate and thorough drainage should be carried out at the appropriate time, all dead material removed, and primary wound closure avoided, at least until later when the wound is granulating.

If skin and other tissues have been lost, secondary procedures may be required to prevent contractures and to obtain skin and 'padding' cover.

Principles of surgical wounds

Many factors need to be considered when planning the optimum wound incision (Table 12.12).

Principles of skin closure

The objective of skin closure is to approximate the cut edges so they heal rapidly without complication and leave a minimal scar. Edges to be apposed should have been cut in a clean line and at right angles to the skin surface; ragged or angled edges should be trimmed. The cut edges should be able to be brought neatly together and without tension, otherwise the wound may break down or the scar slowly stretch, giving an ugly result. To achieve this, it may be necessary to place a layer of subcutaneous sutures or to mobilize the skin by undercutting in the fatty layer. Undue laxity should also be avoided by trimming excess skin.

Table 12.12 Factors in planning surgical wounds

Access to the relevant anatomical structures

Smallest size consistent with above

Permit wound extension or later re-use

Minimal tissue trauma

Meticulous haemostasis

Minimal postoperative pain and interference with function

Rapid and complete healing with minimal deformity

Ease of closure

Cosmetic (Langer's lines, etc.)

Consider local factors likely to impair healing

There are many techniques of skin closure, the choice being governed by the nature and site of the operation and by the surgeon's personal preference. In general, facial wounds are closed with multiple fine, interrupted sutures which are removed after 4 or 5 days. Subcuticular sutures are used for longer wounds in cosmetically sensitive areas, provided the risk of infection is low. Elsewhere, the choice is between interrupted and continuous suture techniques. Interrupted sutures or skin staples are indicated if there is a particular risk of infection, in which case some of the sutures can be removed early to facilitate drainage.

Principles of body cavity closure

The aim here is to secure the wound so that it will not break down, while preserving the cavity wall function including muscles and nerves. Further aims are to cause minimal pain, minimize infection risk, and obtain an acceptable cosmetic appearance.

Changing or removal of dressings

Provided the dressing remains clean and dry and the patient afebrile and generally well, there is no need to inspect the wound until the time of suture removal. If wound complications are suspected, the dressing should be removed and the wound checked and redressed as appropriate. If infection is apparent, a wound swab should be taken for culture and sensitivity; spreading cellulitis requires antibiotic therapy, whereas localized abscess formation requires suture removal and probing to effect drainage.

Suture removal

Skin sutures should be removed as soon as the wound is strong enough to remain intact without support. In the abdomen, this takes about 7–10 days (longer in the presence of steroid therapy or infection), but in the face and neck healing is more rapid and is less influenced by functional stresses. Here, sutures can be safely removed after 4–5 days, giving a better cosmetic result. Sutures on the back or legs are best left *in situ* for around 14 days, or longer in the case of peripheral vascular disease.

Postoperative wound management

Most surgical wounds heal by primary intention without complication so that skin sutures may safely be removed at the anticipated time. It should be noted that healing is not complete at this stage, but the wound is unlikely to part unless unusual stresses are applied. If, for example, an uncomplicated abdominal wound has to be reopened after a week, the skin incision can easily be reopened by finger pressure. Similarly, the abdominal wall incision can be parted readily once the deep sutures have been removed. After 2 weeks, however, healing is further advanced and a scalpel is usually needed to divide healing tissue. Virtually full strength is reached by 6–9 weeks, but complete healing of fibrous and muscular tissue with maturation of collagen takes 3–6 months.

The clean surgical wound

Dressings are traditionally applied to most surgical wounds but most wound problems originate during surgery. The main causes are contamination with micro-organisms or problems with blood supply. Closed, minimally contaminated wounds rarely become newly infected in the postoperative period, even if left exposed. This is because a fibrin seal develops within 24 hours. However, these wounds need protection from external infection sources, such as a colostomy or a drain site, by appropriate impermeable dressings. Overfrequent dressing changes may cause secondary wound infection, particularly if the patient has acquired methicillin-resistant *Staph. aureus* (MRSA) or a multiply resistant coagulase-negative staphylococcal infection.

Head and neck wounds usually have an excellent blood supply and are particularly resistant to infection. For this reason, small head or neck wounds are often left without a dressing or with a simple acrylic wound spray, and larger wounds are often dressed only for the first 24 hours, when oozing of blood from the wound edges may occur.

Wounds elsewhere in the body are usually covered at the end of the operation before removing sterile towels. Prepacked sterile dressings are most commonly used. These are of two main types: the **composite type** with a non-adherent perforated film which lies on the wound, backed by an absorbent pad and covered with adhesive backing, and **microperforated film dressings**.

Wound dressings should be left in place until sutures are due to be removed unless a wound problem is suspected. Minimal disturbance of the wound avoids damage to newly healing tissues and reduces the chances of wound contamination from the patient's own body fluids or by cross-infection. Transparent films allow the wound to be inspected without removing the dressing but the composite type needs to be removed if clinical features suggest infection. These include wound pain, purulent discharge soaking through the dressing, unexplained fever, or spreading cellulitis in the wound area.

The contaminated wound

In the head and neck, wounds contaminated by road dirt should be cleaned vigorously. This may require general anaesthesia and scrubbing with a sterile scrubbing brush, or high-flow irrigation with saline and careful exploration to remove foreign bodies. It is tempting to use hydrogen peroxide solution, which is seen to bubble satisfyingly and removes dirt easily and it is certainly safe to use on superficial open wounds. However, its use in deep wounds is to be condemned because of the risk of potentially fatal oxygen embolism when its oxygen is released under pressure in a closed compartment. Once cleaned, facial wounds can be safely closed primarily.

During emergency operations for intra-abdominal infection (abscesses, peritonitis, or faecal contamination), the abdominal wall incision must be assumed to be contaminated. In these cases, the abdominal wall should be closed in the usual way but the superficial fat and skin should be left open initially and packed with a saline swab. The wound can then be closed safely by delayed primary closure 2–3 days later. In some cases (e.g. after appendicectomy), skin sutures can be loosely placed at the original operation and tightened later without the need for further anaesthesia.

If an abdominal wound is inadvertently contaminated during elective bowel surgery, the above procedure can be adopted, but many surgeons would prefer to place a wound drain. This usually consists of a narrow length of corrugated drain material placed superficial to the abdominal wall closure and beneath skin closure. This is removed after 24–48 hours. However, the efficacy of this is somewhat controversial. The use of abdominal drains during surgical treatment of abdominal infection (whether primary or secondary) is controversial, but there is little evidence for their value in widespread intra-abdominal infection. The main indication is probably where a single abscess cavity with a mature fibrous wall exists. Where widespread infection is present, peritoneal toilet is performed to remove pus, infected fibrin and clot, and necrotic tissue. Elective second-look laparotomy should be planned after 48 hours and the same process gone through. Several laparotomies may be required at intervals to clear all infection.

The infected wound

The principles of management of dirty and infected wounds are illustrated in Table 12.13. Wounds resulting from trauma require thorough cleaning to remove devitalized tissue and foreign bodies. Prophylactic antibiotics should be given early and the wound closed.

If a wound becomes infected, systemic treatment with antibiotics is necessary only if there are signs of cellulitis or signs of systemic infection. Patients with implanted materials, particularly if recent, should be treated with systemic antibiotics on suspicion of wound infection because of the serious consequences of prosthetic infection. The infected wound may require local surgical treatment if pus or necrotic tissue is present.

Mild wound infections may resolve spontaneously. Small superficial abscesses may drain spontaneously, whereas deeper superficial abscesses can often be drained by removing a few sutures and gently probing the wound with a sterile probe or sinus forceps, usually without need for anaesthesia. More extensive superficial infections are better explored formally under general anaesthesia. Necrotic tissue can be excised, all abscesses explored and drained, and deep layers inspected. If there are no deep extensions, the wound should be packed with

Table 12.13 Principles of management of dirty and infected wounds

Prevent spreading infection
Remove all dead and foreign material
Prevent further contamination
Protect healing surface until epithelialized
Prepare base for secondary suture or grafting
Get rapid healing, minimizing interference to patient's life

a wet dressing to permit free drainage of pus. Medication of the wound packing was once favoured, but there is little evidence of benefit over a simple saline-soaked sterile gauze. Favoured agents for wound packing have included proflavine emulsion, a mild antiseptic mixed with liquid paraffin to prevent adhesion, or Betadine® solution (although any antibacterial activity is immediately neutralized by contact with body fluids). Formerly, an emulsion of EUSOL and liquid paraffin was employed widely but is rarely used nowadays because of controversies (probably exaggerated) about its adverse effect on granulation tissue.

In most instances, healing by secondary intention is then allowed to proceed. The patient may often leave hospital before full healing and the dressings changed safely by the district nurse. The patient should be warned that healing may take many weeks or even months. However, this process can often be truncated, once the wound is clean and uninfected, by secondary suture. This is only indicated providing it does not place undue tension on the wound.

Often, an extensive superficial infection of an abdominal wound communicates deeply with intra-abdominal collections of pus or with an intestinal fistula. If deep problems exist, the whole wound requires exploration to enable drainage of the deep collection.

Traumatic wounds

The management of traumatic wounds can be considered in four stages: first aid, definitive surgery, reconstructive surgery, and rehabilitation.

Simple clean wounds are without tissue loss. All are contaminated by micro-organisms, but irrigation and closure within 6 hours usually forestalls infection. Cleanly divided muscle should not be sutured but fascial wounds should be closed without tension.

Simple infected wounds have no tissue loss attributable to the trauma but infection will destroy tissue if untreated. They often present late with signs of bacterial invasion with pus and slough covering raw surfaces and surrounding cellulitis. These wounds should never be closed immediately. The wound should be explored for foreign material, devitalized tissue, and pockets of infection, then packed open with saline-soaked gauze. Systemic antibiotics are used if appropriate and the dressing changed daily until the wound is granulating, no longer discharging. and the surrounding skin is neither oedematous nor red. The wound can then be closed by delayed primary closure, usually after 3–7 days.

Complicated, clean wounds result when there is damage or destruction to skin, muscle, blood vessels, nerve, or bone, or when foreign bodies are present in the wound. Low-velocity missile wounds fall into this category since dirt and clothing are not drawn into the wound.

All devitalized tissue should be removed and partial repair carried out. Damaged major blood vessels should be reconstructed, using vein interposition grafting if necessary. Bony, tendon, or nerve damage will necessitate orthopaedic involvement. Foreign material should be removed, except for low-velocity missiles placed deeply. Tracks of these missiles do not need to be laid open. Superficial shotgun pellets should be removed. Damaged skin should be excised and closure effected by making relaxing incisions nearby. Doubtful specialized skin from the hands should be left and excised later if necessary.

Complicated, dirty wounds are seen when there is tissue destruction or foreign bodies and heavy contamination, for example by bowel perforation. If such a wound is not seen until more than 18 hours after injury, it is particularly likely to fall into this category. These wounds require excision of devitalized tissues and removal of foreign material. Major blood vessels should be repaired and nerves and tendons marked for later repair. Primary skin closure must not be performed but skin cover achieved later when the wound is clean, if necessary after further excisions. Only when skin cover is healed can secondary repair of damaged structures be attempted.

High-velocity missile wounds impart enormous kinetic energy which dissipates on impact. The entry wound is often small, but the missile causes a cavity to open within the body, the walls of which oscillate, destroying nearby structures and devitalizing tissue. The cavity then collapses, drawing in fragments of clothing and dirt which contaminate the wound. If bone is struck, many secondary missiles are created, doing further damage. These wounds must be widely opened and all foreign matter, missile fragments, clothing, and dirt removed from deep in the wound. The track should be explored and the devitalized walls excised. All pulped and damaged muscle should be excised. Divided tendons and nerves are marked and bone fragments removed. The wound is packed with saline gauze that is changed daily. Further wound inspections and excisions are likely to be necessary. Only when infection is controlled and all dead tissue removed can skin cover be attempted.

Exuding wounds

Wounds that exude large quantities of fluid need an absorbent dressing during the early stages. One method is to use simple absorbent pads (e.g. Gamgee® or a pad with a non-woven cover containing cellulose fibre or wood pulp powder, similar to infant nappies). Non-absorbent but water-permeable films or foams, which transfer water from wound to the outer surface where it evaporates, may also be used. The rate of fluid transfer must be at least equal to the rate of production. Finally, alginates and hydrocolloids absorb exudate but change their physical form into an aqueous gel on the wound surface, which is particularly conducive to healing.

Burns

The general surgeon becomes involved in the management of burns at the resuscitation stage or where the injury is too severe for management on an Accident and Emergency outpatient basis and yet not extensive enough to warrant plastic surgical input. What follows is an outline of burn management principles (Table 12.14). For more details the reader is referred to specialist burn textbooks.

Table 12.14 The principles of burn management

Fluid resuscitation

Prevent pain

Minimize risk of infection

Non-stick

Painless changing of dressing

Satisfactory preparation for skin cover

Ease of management at home or hospital

Reduce risk of scar formation

Burn severity is proportional to temperature of heat source, thermal inertia of source (a function of thermal conductivity and density), and duration of contact or exposure. Burns are classified into **superficial**, **deep dermal**, and **full thickness**. With superficial burns, skin cover is generated from epithelial elements in the residual dermis. In deep dermal burns there are few epithelial remnants which, if undisturbed, may be capable of regeneration, but may be destroyed by infection. Full-thickness burns result in loss of both dermis and epidermis as well as loss of pain sensation. Mortality rises both with rising percentage of body area burned and increasing patient age.

The mainstays of early management are adequate fluid replacement, analgesia, and oxygen. As a rule of thumb, initial fluid administration (either colloid or plasma) should be at a rate of 60 ml/per cent burn area over 8 hours. More precise calculations can be performed according to formulae such as that of Muir and Barcley. Subsequent fluid administration depends on pathophysiological responses. Blood transfusion is likely to be required for full-thickness burns over 10 per cent of body surface area.

Escharotomy is needed when there are circumferential burns on the limbs or thorax, in order to counteract the constricting effect of contracting scar tissue.

Local treatment of the burn should aim to expedite healing and prevent extension of tissue loss. Options include relatively sterile exposure techniques, dressings (see above), early or late skin grafting, and the use of heterotopic skin. Later management involves rehabilitation and attention to cosmetic deformity.

Pressure sores

Pressure sores involve an area of skin necrosis that extends for a variable depth. Once the skin has died, it rapidly dehydrates and becomes leathery, inhibiting the normal process of autolysis that would allow it to separate. In areas such as the heel, which contain much collagen, this process of separation rarely happens naturally. When surgically removed, the cavity beneath the eschar may be superficial or may be deep, extending to the underlying bone. If underlying infection causes local infection or systemic sepsis, surgical excision of all dead tissue should not be delayed. If surgery is not indicated, dehydrated eschar can be rehydrated with occlusive dressings designed to prevent vapour loss. Suitable dressings include hydrocolloids and semi-permeable films. Thick layers of eschar once softened should be removed with scissors or scalpel; this does not usually require anaesthesia. Superficial layers may separate spontaneously.

Once débridement has been effected, healing of small pressure sores should occur, provided care is taken to avoid further pressure and, if appropriate, the patient's general state can be improved. Larger pressure wounds require complex reconstructive techniques, including flap procedures.

Bibliography

Soft-tissue surgery

Gordon, D.and Silverstone, G. (1976). World-wide epidemiology of premalignant and malignant cutaneous lesions. In *Cancer of the skin*, (ed. R. Adrade, S. Gumport, and G. Popkins), p. 405. Saunders, Philadelphia.

Green, M.H., Clark, W.H., and Tucker, M.A. (1985). High risk of malignant melanoma in melanoma prone families with dysplastic naevi. *Ann. Intern. Med.*, **102**, 458–65.

Holman, C.D.J. and Armstrong, B.K. (1984). Pigmentary traits, ethnic origin, benign naevi and family history as risk factors for cutaneous malignant melanoma. *JNCI*, **72**, 257–66.

Issa, M.M. and Tanner, W.A. (1988). Approach to ingrowing toenails: the wedge resection/segmental phenolization combination treatment. *Br. J. Surg.*, **75**, 181–3.

MacKie, R.M. (1992). In *Rook, Wilkinson, Ebling Textbook of Dermatology*, (5th edn), (ed. R.H. Champion, J.L. Burton, and F.J.G. Ebling), pp. 1545–60.

MacKie, R.M., Smyth J.F., Soutar D.S., Calman K.C., Watson A.C.H., and Hunter J.A.A. (1985). Malignant melanoma in Scotland 1979–83. *Lancet*, **ii**, 859–62.

Schreiber, M.M., Bozzo, P.D., and Moon, T.E. (1981). Malignant melanoma in Southern Arizona. *Arch. Dermatol.*, **117**, 6–11.

Swerdlow, A.J., English J., and MacKie R.M. (1986). Benign naevi as a risk factor for malignant melanoma. BMJ, **292**, 1555–9.

Wound management

Winter, G.D. (1962). Formation of the scab and the rate of epithelization of superficial wounds in the skin of the young domestic pig. *Nature*, **193**, 293–4.

CHAPTER 13

Recovery from surgery

Briony Ackroyd and Clive R. Quick

1 Introduction

During the Second World War a British Army order decreed that patients must be kept in bed for 21 days after inguinal herniorrhaphy, and up until recently, it was usual for patients to stay in hospital for 6 days after a hernia repair. Now day-case surgery or overnight stay for hernia repair is the norm. Established notions about the rate of recovery after any surgical operation have undergone gradual evolution towards shorter hospital stays and more rapid return to normal activities, in line with improved surgical techniques and, particularly, improved anaesthetic techniques. However, there are still large differences between one surgeon's practice and another's with regard to the same operation. Each firmly held but often conflicting view is often based purely on tradition or intuition rather than scientific evidence, and in any case, scientific evidence is often lacking. Economic arguments for shorter stays are often pressed by healthcare purchasers and providers, but there is often little rationale for any of particular practices other than 'experience' and tradition.

Few meaningful investigations have been published about any aspect of recovery, but there has been a recent kindling of interest in these issues, driven by several factors:

- the development of cash-limitation of healthcare systems and the rising emphasis on 'value-for money';

- an increased awareness of the issues among patient groups and consequent publicity disseminated by them;

- a genuine recognition by surgeons of the perceived and objective well-being of their patients;

- the increasing importance and penetration of surgical audit.

Some hard data are now becoming available concerning recovery from surgery, from both a practical point of view and from a psychosocial point of view; each of these will be explored in this chapter.

The critical evaluation of perceived advances in surgery is becoming more structured because of the increasing use of protocols or guidelines for care, and these often include the recovery period. There are many thought of but rarely answered questions, such as 'When should this drain come out?'; 'How long do I need to leave that nasogastric tube in place?'; 'How can I help my patients to feel better more quickly after this operation?'; 'When is it safe to let that patient get out of bed?'; or 'When should I let this patient go home?'. With such questions in mind, the aim of this chapter is to help readers analyse their own practice and to generate their own guidelines about recovery from surgery.

2 Practical aspects

2.1 Immediate postoperative care: the first 24 hours

Recovery from anaesthesia

After operation, there are well-understood procedures to be undertaken which are established practice amongst recovery staff (Freidin and Marshall 1984). Patients are handed over to recovery nurses by the anaesthetist and surgeon, with information about the anaesthetic, a record of drugs given, current vascular access, and monitoring in progress, together with a record of the perioperative progress of the patient, a record of the operative procedure, and whether drains and catheters are *in situ*. The recovery team is given any necessary specific instructions about the patient. Their task is to monitor the immediate postoperative phase of the patient and to carry out the specific instructions.

Destination of patients after the theatre recovery area

A patient's destination after theatre depends on the preoperative condition of the patient, the diagnosis, the operation performed, and the facilities of the hospital. Uncomplicated patients return to the general surgical ward (or the day ward) from whence they came. Patients with organ failure, or incipient or potential organ failure, are likely to be admitted to an intensive care unit (ICU).

Patients who fall between these groups may be cared for in a high-dependency unit (HDU). These patients might have serious pre-existing medical conditions or become clinically unstable during or after surgery. The role of the HDU is to provide a higher level of monitoring and nursing care than is readily available on a general ward, short of the ventilatory support characteristic of an ICU.

Recent publications, in particular the NCEPOD report of 1995, have found that provision of HDU care is deficient in many UK districts. A major expansion of this service was advocated to overcome inadequate levels of care on surgical wards and, at the same time, prevent unnecessary use of scarce and expensive ITU resources.

The importance of early postoperative care can be appreciated by analysing the complications arising during this period. Gamil and Fanning (1991) analysed data obtained during the first 24 hours after over 2000 consecutive operations. Many of the findings would be expected intuitively, but the quantitative results are likely to prove invaluable for planning and justifying future levels of care. This study showed that 5 per cent of patients developed major complications which were potentially life-threatening. Three-quarters of this 5 per cent began deteriorating within 24 hours of surgery, and one-third were considered likely to have achieved a better outcome if the initial deterioration had been managed more aggressively. Patients most at risk of early deterioration are those undergoing complex major operations, particularly for multiple injuries, arterial disease, emergency conditions, major urological disorders, or fractured neck of the femur. Older patients are more at risk. This report produced the alarming claim that 17 per cent of the deaths in the series, and all of the permanent disabilities, might have been prevented if HDU facilities had been readily available.

2.2 Pain

Introduction

The management of postoperative pain should begin before the end of anaesthesia and continues well beyond the immediate postoperative period. No patient should be allowed to suffer substantial postoperative pain and, to this end, all should receive analgesia appropriate to the surgery carried out. However, this does not always happen. When doctors themselves undergo surgery, they often discover that pain management is inadequate.

There is good evidence that adequate analgesia is not only an act of kindness, but is associated with fewer cardiovascular, respiratory, locomotor, and gastrointestinal complications of surgery. Thromboembolism is less likely, convalescence is faster, and stays in hospital are shorter (Justins and Richardson 1991).

The management of perioperative pain is increasingly seen as the province of a specialized **acute pain team**. The team may include nurses, surgeons, and anaesthetists. With this enlightened approach, patients are visited preoperatively by the pain team to assess likely problems and explain procedures. An individual perioperative plan for analgesia is then drawn up. This may include a range of options, including preoperative measures such as analgesic premedication, nerve blocks, and non-steroidal anti-inflammatory analgesics (NSAIDs), all of which can reduce postoperative analgesic needs (Kehlet and Jørgen 1993). During the operation, the anaesthetist can combine peroperative and postoperative analgesia, and may use an epidural infusion of local anaesthetic with or without opiates, for example, to cover both. Preoperative and peroperative analgesia may be given **pre-emptively** (i.e. to anticipate pain and to treat it before it becomes established). The patient is visited regularly by the pain team during the postoperative period and treatment is modified according to clinical need. More detailed pain management options are described in Chapter 10.

Patient-controlled analgesia (PCA) is a popular choice for preventing and treating postoperative pain. PCA allows the patient to self-administer small bolus doses of analgesic by means of a programmable pump, and so avoids the problems of intermittent prescriptions or fixed infusions. PCA pumps have the unique advantage of providing powerful analgesia in appropriate dosage as soon as it is needed, for example when the patient needs to move, and the advantage that none is given when none is needed.

Intermittent intramuscular injections of opiates have proved inadequate for all but the mildest of pain. This is partly because of the difficulty of maintaining adequate blood levels, as injections are nearly always given after the pain has become established. In addition, nurses often fear overdosage and are concerned about the drug's addictive potential.

Automatically monitored **continuous intravenous infusions** can maintain blood levels, but fine control is difficult. These are most useful for patients unable to control their own analgesic administration.

The prime consideration in managing postoperative pain is that relief should be reliably effective. To be maximally effective, the mechanisms of delivery and the dosage must be individually tailored for each patient, ideally by a specialist team (Justins and Richardson 1991).

Perioperative analgesia for day cases

Day-case patients require special postoperative analgesia because their needs have to be considered in the light of early discharge. It must be both safe and effective. There is evidence that considerable morbidity after discharge is due to uncontrolled postoperative pain. This is a drain on the patient's resources, leading to prolonged convalescence and a delayed return to work on the one hand, and presents a call on community and GP services on the other, if they are called in acutely to treat the pain. Careful attention to postoperative analgesia should minimize these problems. Nausea and vomiting or hypotension associated with opioid analgesia often delays discharge, and the judicious use of local anaesthetics for analgesia avoids the need for large doses, allowing pain to be controlled by oral analgesia. Patients operated on under local anaesthesia or peripheral nerve block can often be discharged sooner than after general anaesthesia because of persisting analgesia.

2.3 Postoperative nausea and vomiting

In the 'ether era' of anaesthesia, at least three-quarters of patients experienced postoperative nausea and vomiting. The surprising conclusion of some recent large studies is that even now the incidence remains at 20–30 per cent. Vomiting is not only an unpleasant experience, but it may also result in potentially serious complications such as fluid depletion, electrolyte imbalance, disruption of suture lines, haematoma formation, and pulmonary aspiration. It is a particular problem after day-case surgery, when it may delay discharge and enforce an unplanned admission. After discharge, vomiting may cause serious distress and make additional demands on community services (Hirsch 1994). There is therefore good reason to study its causes and management in an effort to make the bedside vomit bowl redundant.

Many factors influence postoperative nausea and vomiting:

1. Patient factors—including age (worse in children, particularly in pre-adolescents); gender (worse in women, and varies with the menstrual cycle and other hormonal factors); obesity; susceptibility to motion sickness; anxiety; patients with delayed gastric emptying for whatever reason.

2. The operative procedure—more likely after laparoscopic procedures, head and neck surgery, and upper gastrointestinal and biliary surgery. The longer the duration of the procedure, the higher the incidence.

3. Drugs used in anaesthesia—some of these, particularly opioids, are potent causes of postoperative emesis. Regional anaesthesia generally causes less postoperative nausea and vomiting than general anaesthesia, but epidural morphine often causes vomiting.

4. Postoperative factors—pain is important, particularly visceral and pelvic pain. Adequate analgesia can thus relieve nausea and vomiting. Postoperative dizziness, which may be due to postural hypotension or to increased vagal tone, is also associated with an increase in nausea and vomiting. Changes in position, sudden motion, or ambulation may cause nausea and vomiting, presumably by a mechanism similar to motion sickness. Early introduction of oral fluids may not increase the overall incidence of emesis but it does advance the first episode of vomiting, and there is evidence that it increases the incidence *per se*. Finally, the use of opioids for analgesia is a potent cause of increased postoperative nausea and vomiting. This is the reason for the widespread practice of automatic prescribing of an antiemetic with this type of analgesia.

The multifactorial nature of postoperative nausea and vomiting requires a multifactorial approach to its management. Routine prophylaxis is not appropriate, as less than 30 per cent of patients suffer from it, and many of these will only have transient nausea, or vomit no more than once. In addition, antiemetic drugs have their own adverse effects, including sedation and extrapyramidal symptoms. If, however, a patient falls into one of the high-risk groups described above, prophylaxis should be considered. In addition to pharmacological manoeuvres, every effort should be made to reduce anxiety by appropriate preoperative counselling.

Peroperative manipulations may also have a place. In a fascinating well-controlled randomized study, trial patients were played a soothing tape assuring them that the surgery would progress smoothly and reassuring them they would not experience postoperative sickness. The effect was to more than halve the incidence of vomiting (Williams *et al.* 1994). There have also been some reports of the successful use of acupuncture in this context.

Several neurotransmitter systems play key roles in mediating the emetic response and this allows a range of therapeutic approaches to the problem, so that the appropriate drug, or a combination of the many drugs available with antiemetic action, may be employed. A detailed discussion of these agents is not appropriate here, but a valuable survey of available agents may be consulted (Watcha and White 1992).

2.4 Early postoperative care

Psychosomatic recovery

During the first 24 hours after major surgery, high levels of analgesic drugs are often employed and the patient's consciousness is often obtunded. Thus, the patient is usually comfortable, somewhat sedated, and not feeling anxious. Over the next 24 hours, analgesia may be reduced and pain often breaks through. The patient becomes more aware of what has been done but is often most concerned with simple achievements such as moving about and readjusting to the immediate environment rather than about what was done at the operation and what the histology might be. Many major complications are unlikely to have presented yet.

On the third day, normal awareness and concerns have usually returned. Pain relief may be suboptimal and the patient's concerns about the operation, as well as anxiety about future difficulties of returning to normal life loom large. Complications such as anastomotic leakage, pulmonary collapse, retention of urine, failure of intravenous infusions, and others may now begin to emerge. Even in uncomplicated major surgery, the low point is often the third day, known as the 'third day blues'. This low point is often over after the next day or two as mobility improves and the patient becomes resigned to his or her new (even though temporary) status.

Telling the patient about the diagnosis

Prior preparation of the patient by way of discussion and explanation is indispensable before major surgery is undertaken. Most patients nowadays want to know the surgical options for treatment as well as any other options and the consequences of all these options. Good information also helps the patient to come to terms with disfigurement and loss of function afterwards. This is most in evidence with mastectomy, major limb amputations, and operations involving intestinal stomas.

If the diagnosis proves to be malignant, this fact may confirm a proven preoperative diagnosis, it may be a histological resolution of a suspected diagnosis or, occasionally, a completely unexpected diagnosis. Patients have a right to know the full extent of the disease, the likely prognosis, and whether any further treatment is likely to be recommended. However, it is unwise to be too precise until a definitive histological diagnosis and sometimes full staging of the disease are available. Furthermore, it should be remembered that most patients are not ready to take in the details for 3 or 4 days after surgery. A dilemma arises if a spouse or close relative is told the diagnosis of malignancy before the patient and then asks that the patient

should not be told. In almost every case, the clinician should try to persuade the relative that the patient should be informed. It is far easier for a couple to face the diagnosis together than for one to know and the patient to suspect but not be told or, worse still, to be lied to. If and when recurrences or metastases occur, the diagnosis becomes more distressing to break to the patient and treatment becomes difficult to initiate. If the surgeon suspects that a relative is likely to keep a diagnosis of malignancy from a patient against the surgeon's better advice, some surgeons deliberately tell the patient first to avoid this predicament.

It is worth asking the patient first what he or she thinks the problem might be. Often cancer has been suspected and finding out the truth is sometimes (and paradoxically) a relief. The patient will always seek signs of optimism in the clinician and it is important not to mislead by transmitting false optimism. A realistic approach is best, tempered by kindness and confidence that treatment will help or relieve symptoms. Even anticipation of future developments in medical research gives some cause for hope. Taking away all hope is unwise and unkind. If the illness is likely to become terminal, the mode of deterioration can be discussed at later visits, together with assurances that the patient will be looked after. It is important to take cues from the patient and to allow a friend or relative to be present, setting aside enough time for the process not to be rushed and then ensuring that a nurse talks to the patient afterwards to help ensure that misunderstandings don't arise. Patients take in only a small percentage of bad news under these stressful conditions and reinforcement and checking the patient's understanding later is important.

Drains

The management of drains after surgery tends to be an individual one for each surgeon, and the trainee must relearn the local rules for each firm. This variation is largely due to the lack of scientific evidence on the outcomes of various drainage procedures. The questions at issue are:

◆ Do drains prolong or accelerate recovery from surgery?

◆ Do drains reduce or increase complication rates?

◆ How should drains be managed after operation?

Whether drains cause or prevent morbidity depends on the circumstances. Some indications for drainage are so incontrovertible that a trial would not be considered ethical. For example, drainage of the pleural cavity in tension pneumothorax. Other less clear-cut indications have been put to the test. One such, after elective cholecystectomy, showed that patients who had the gallbladder bed drained had longer average postoperative stays and a higher incidence of postoperative fever, wound infections, and other postoperative complications than undrained patients (Mittelman and Doberneck 1982) . Yet it was virtually standard practice until laparoscopic cholecystectomy became the norm, after which it rapidly declined. A similar study after thyroidectomy (Wihlborg et al. 1988) showed no difference in outcome or complications between the drained and the undrained group, and concluded (somewhat controversially) there was no reason to drain routinely after uncomplicated thyroidectomy. In other operation sites, the balance of evidence shows that drainage, for example after axillary lymph node dissection, results in reduced seroma formation and fewer wound infections (Somers *et al.* 1972; Terrell and Singer 1992). However, grouped studies of this nature are somewhat ingenuous for the reason that even if only one case suffers severe adverse consequences preventable by a drain, the advantage of having used a drain may more than offset the minor nuisance a drain causes in those that turned out not to have needed drainage. A policy of selective drainage in cholecystectomy, thyroidectomy, and mastectomy thus seems appropriate.

The question of how drains should be managed postoperatively again depends on circumstances. Most surgeons drain the axilla after lymph node dissection, in an attempt to minimize haematoma and seroma formation. Reports in the literature do not give a clear answer of how long drains should be left, nor indeed, agree on whether they should be used at all. In the light of the increasing emphasis on cost containment, one study randomly compared axillary drain removal after mastectomy at 3 days and 6 days. No differences were found in total number or volume of drainage of seromas formed after drain removal, nor any other differences in wound complications. It was calculated that early drain removal with discharge the following day could save 43 per cent on bed costs, with no detriment to the patient (Parikh *et al.* 1992). A recent report suggests that low-pressure suction drainage of the axilla is better than high-vacuum drainage (van Heurn and Brink 1995), on the grounds that it allows earlier drain removal. Seroma formation was not significantly different in the two groups.

Table 13.1 Management of skin closure

Absorbable sutures, interrupted	Generally do not require removal. If persistent after 10 days, cut off flush with skin
Absorbable sutures, subcuticular	Do not require removal. Catgut has been superceded by short-lived polyglactin (Vicryl Rapide™) as it causes no inflammation
Non-absorbable sutures, subcuticular	Most are removed after 7 days by cutting the retaining device at one end and pulling the suture through. If it breaks and is incompletely removed, the suture may often be left *in situ* and may eventually work itself out. The patient must be warned of this
Non-absorbable sutures, continuous or interrupted	Face: 3–5 days Chest and abdomen: 7–10 days Limbs: 7 days Back and limbs where subject to stretching: 14 days
Michel clips	Neck: 1–3 days Abdomen: 7–10 days
Skin staples	As for non-absorbable sutures

Sutures and other forms of skin closure

Removal of skin-closure devices is subject to personal idiosyncrasies, but there are generally observed broad rules (Table 13.1).

Wound dehiscence

Now that catgut is obsolete for abdominal wall closure and mass closure is the norm, wound dehiscence is unusual. However, this calamity still occurs. If the risk is high, as in a generally debilitated patient, or if there are warning signs, such as a sudden discharge of sero-sanguinous fluid from the wound, the closure should be carefully assessed. In normally healing wounds, a 'healing ridge', formed by collagen repair in the deeper tissues, is palpable deep to the wound as a zone of induration about 2 cm wide. When there is dehiscence of the deep layers, this ridge is absent. If the area of dehiscence is small and the patient is a poor risk, the situation may be salvaged by leaving the skin closure in place for up to 3 weeks. An incisional hernia is inevitable and may or may not require repair later. In major disruptions, the patient should be returned to theatre within a few hours for resuturing to prevent complete abdominal wound dehiscence.

Supplemental nutrition after abdominal surgery

The role of supplemental nutrition, both intravenous and enteral, is covered in Chapter 8.

Gastric decompression

Operations on the abdominal cavity often cause disruption of gastrointestinal function and some degree of paralytic ileus, during which normal peristalsis is disturbed or uncoordinated. If the surgery is relatively minor, as in appendicectomy for early appendicitis, nasogastric tube drainage is unnecessary. Operations on the small and large bowel are often performed without postoperative nasogastric drainage, but this becomes necessary if vomiting occurs or acute gastric dilatation threatens. Many surgeons choose to use a nasogastric tube on free drainage as a matter of routine for this type of operation in the early postoperative period as prophylaxis against vomiting and particularly against acute gastric dilatation. If the latter occurs, massive vomiting may occur and carries a high mortality. Most surgeons, on the other hand, use postoperative gastric drainage selectively, restricting it to certain types of upper gastrointestinal surgery and after surgery for intestinal obstruction.

Gastric drainage may be via a nasal or a percutaneous route (gastrostomy). In either case, the tube should be firmly secured to prevent it becoming displaced. The need for gastric decompression has been challenged for many years, because of unwanted effects such as discomfort, irritation, pressure effects, and disturbance of function of the cardia, and there is much discussion in the literature regarding the issue. In 1972 Miller *et al.* compared the randomized use of nasogastric tubes, gastrostomy tubes, or no gastric decompression after vagotomy and drainage. Chest infections and dysphagia were more common when a nasogastric tube was used, wound infections were more common when gastrostomies were used. Nasogastric tubes were judged unpleasant or distressing by the majority of the patients, gastrostomies less so. Only one patient out of the 43 without decompression later required a nasogastric tube because of paralytic ileus. This study was discussed in a leader in the *British Medical Journal* (Anon. 1973) which conceded the superiority of the 'tubeless routine', but cautioned that 'whenever a surgeon has the slightest doubt about the soundness of a gastrointestinal suture line, he will be well advised to leave in a nasogastric or gastrostomy tube for suction as a precaution against leakage'. Interesting light was shed on this assumption from a study in 1977 (Burg *et al.*, 1977) which compared a group of patients after small- or large-intestinal surgery who were decompressed with a group that was not. No adverse effects occurred from the lack of a tube, although 4 per cent needed a tube later to relieve distension. The rates of complications thought to be related to lack of gastric drainage (e.g. prolonged ileus, anastomotic leak, wound disruption) were the same in each group. The authors recommended that elective abdominal surgery should be performed expectantly without postoperative gastric decompression, thus sparing a majority of patients the discomfort and minor problems associated with tubes.

The same issue was studied after upper abdominal surgery (Argov *et al.* 1980), with regard to respiratory complications. These were 10 times more frequent in the drained group than the undrained, and the incidence increased with the duration of the tube *in situ*. Another randomized study of 200 patients again failed to demonstrate any benefit in a drained group after gastrointestinal surgery (Bauer *et al.* 1985). Five per cent of the drained patients needed tubes replacing after removal, whereas only 6 per cent of the undrained group needed a nasogastric tube at any stage. With the wealth of published opinion against postoperative gastric decompression and no experimental study (as opposed to unsubstantiated assertion) to support its use, the continued use of routine postoperative decompression must be seriously questioned.

If a nasogastric tube is employed, it should usually be removed at an early stage in the return of gastrointestinal function. In clinical terms, this is usually when the aspirate diminishes to below 30 ml/hour, when oral fluids above 30 ml hourly are tolerated and when bowel sounds return or flatus is passed.

Introduction of oral fluids and food

After abdominal surgery, the question of when and how to reintroduce oral fluids and food needs to be considered. As with so many issues dealt with in this chapter, tradition abounds and there is no consensus across the surgical world. One important publication was a randomized comparison of two postoperative fluid regimens carried out in Leicester (Cook *et al.* 1989). Recognizing that the variable duration of postoperative paralytic ileus that follows substantial gastrointestinal surgery had led to a variety of empirical and time-consuming oral fluid regimens, the authors set out to compare a traditional method of fluid administration with an unstructured, simpler, patient-

determined approach. The 'regulated' group received hourly aliquots of oral fluid, determined twice daily on ward rounds. Patients in the 'unregulated' group were given a jug of water and instructed to drink as they desired. There were no significant differences in mean durations of intravenous therapy, nasogastric intubation, or hospital stay, and postoperative complication and mortality rates were similar. Even patients who underwent gastric or duodenal procedures showed similar results. It was concluded that 'patient-determined' regulation of postoperative oral fluid intake after abdominal surgery is safe and effective and may greatly simplify ward management. Despite this convincing publication, most units still employ the traditional approach.

Urinary considerations

Bladder function and micturition

The rate of urine output is one of the most useful guides to a patient's fluid homeostasis and is thus one of the most useful ward measurements to make in patients with fluid-balance problems. Urine output should be measured hourly in the early stages after any major surgery with a potential for profound fluid-balance derangements, and this requires bladder catheterization. When interpreting the urine output, the normal responses to the surgical insult should be borne in mind. These include fluid retention and catabolism. Thus, urine output is reduced early on, and later increases as diuresis returns towards normal.

Use of a urinary catheter after operation

Apart from specific indications in urological surgery, there are two main reasons for using a urinary catheter after surgery: one is to monitor urine output and the other is to relieve postoperative acute retention of urine.

In acute retention, each patient must be assessed individually. Failure to pass urine after surgery is common and only a small proportion of patients ultimately need a catheter. There is usually no cause for concern until 12 hours after operation. After that, the state of hydration should be assessed. The patient may have fasted for many hours preoperatively, may not have received sufficient volume of fluid intraoperatively, and may have drunk little postoperatively because of the effects of the anaesthetic and the type of surgery. Sometimes a fluid challenge is all that is required, simply giving the patient more to drink or increasing the intravenous infusion rate. If hydration is adequate, and the patient is unable to void, or there is a palpable bladder, every effort should be made to allow the patient to void spontaneously. A male patient should be encouraged to sit on the edge of the bed or to stand, and a female patient to sit on a commode. Privacy is important, and success may result simply by wheeling the patients to the bathroom and running the water taps. If these simple methods fail, it may be possible to put the patient in a bath and let him or her pass urine into the warm water. A catheter should be passed only if these conservative methods fail.

Techniques of catheterization are not covered here except to advocate consideration of a suprapubic rather than a urethral catheter. Suprapubic catheters have the advantage of reducing the risk of urinary tract infection as well as being easily clamped to test for normal voiding. If it fails, the catheter can easily be unclamped.

Once a catheter is in place, consideration will have to be given to its removal. When fluid balance is stable and renal function satisfactory, a catheter inserted for monitoring can be removed. If a catheter has been inserted for acute retention, removal is influenced by other factors such as pre-existing urinary outflow tract malfunction (which may only come to light on postoperative questioning), or whether extensive pelvic dissection has taken place (for example after abdomino-perineal excision of rectum). Either of these would encourage conservatism and invite delay in catheter removal until a day or two after the patient returns to normal mobility. A catheter placed for uncomplicated postoperative retention may often be removed after 24 hours or less. A suprapubic catheter should be clamped to test voiding before removal.

The time of day of removal of urethral catheters is another matter of contention, where different surgeons have strongly held opinions, not always based on available evidence. Removal in the early morning is popular, in the belief that retention would become apparent at a more social hour. However, there has been discussion of this issue in the urological literature. The findings from most trials are that catheters should be removed whenever the decision to remove them is made (Wyman 1987) or else at midnight. This is more convenient for nursing staff, gives a more rapid return to a normal voiding pattern, and allows earlier recognition of post-catheterization retention and earlier discharge from hospital (Noble *et al.* 1990; Crowe *et al.* 1993).

Mobilization

In general, a patient is confined to bed during the early postoperative period after major surgery. This period is prolonged if admission to a high-dependency unit or to an intensive care unit is needed. However, immobilization is of significant risk to the patient and steps must be taken to prevent its attendant complications of pressure necrosis, deep vein thrombosis, pulmonary collapse, urinary retention, and faecal impaction. Because of the risks of bed rest, early mobilization is now the rule in all patients capable of doing so. After laparotomy, patients may sit out of bed on the first postoperative day, thus improving ventilation by reducing pressure on the diaphragm caused by abdominal flexion. The following day they should be able to take their first steps and walk around the bed and perhaps sit for a period in a chair. Even patients with drains and drips in place should be able to walk to the toilet with assistance soon after this.

The surgical literature reveals that passions have been raised throughout history against the classical practice of prolonged bed rest after surgical operations. An author from Chicago made a challenge before the turn of the twentieth century, indicating by the title of his paper that he knew he was being controversial: 'Some radical changes in the after-treatment of celiotomy cases'. Yet the changes advocated by him hardly seem radical to us:

Many of my patients with ventral, inguinal or lumbar incisions have sat up as early as three days after their operations; others I have kept in bed until after removal of the stitches on the sixth to the eighth day … the patients, however, are permitted to turn over and move about in bed as soon as and as often as they want to. The consequence … is discharge from the hospital about twelve days after the operation.

Surgical tradition has long fought against the radical ideas of early mobilization and discharge but there has been a very gradual reduction in lengths of bed rest and stay. In the past few years, economic forces have prompted rapidly increasing proportions of surgery to be performed on a day-case basis and has drastically cut preoperative hospitalization and to a lesser extent, postoperative stay. Farquharson took up the issue in 1955, pointing out that 'early' ambulation is a relative term, but then put current interpretation as: ' … walking, not 5 or 6 days after the operation, but if possible within 24 hours, and certainly within three days'.

Time of discharge from hospital

Farquharson's contribution was radical, challenging not only the moment to begin mobilization but, even more radically, the timing of hospital discharge. For example, he advocated herniorrhaphy as an outpatient procedure, performed under local anaesthesia, after which the patient: ' … climbs down from the operating theatre, dresses in his lounge suit, walks out of the theatre, and then walks out to the ambulance in which he is then taken home'. This was perhaps the beginning of the modern era of day surgery.

In 1960, the median duration of stay for inguinal herniorrhaphy was 10.2 days. During the 1960s, the problem of long waiting lists for elective surgery came to prominence in the UK, and this prompted a surge of interest in shortening hospital stays. In 1961, in a *Lancet* article, day-case surgery was advocated for varicose veins and inguinal hernias under general anaesthesia, and in 1968, a randomized controlled trial was published, comparing discharge 1 day and 6 days after hernia repair which demonstrated no difference between the groups as regards postoperative progress. Another randomized study came from the USA, in which patients were randomly assigned to home care or to hospital care after herniorrhaphy, vaginal hysterectomy, or varicose vein ligation and stripping. In practice, patients went home by ambulance or back to the ward after 3–5 hours in the recovery room. The complication rate in each group was identical, the costs in the home-care group were a quarter of those in the inpatient group, and patient satisfaction was greater in the home-care group.

A frequently cited reason for delaying discharge after herniorrhaphy is that recurrence rates were thought to be greater with earlier discharge. This, among other variables, was addressed by a study from St Thomas's in which patients with inguinal hernias were randomized to spend either 48 hours or 6–7 days in hospital. There proved to be no difference in recurrence rates between the two groups.

In crude terms, days spent in hospital as inpatients are expensive. This is usually calculated on the costs involved in a fully staffed ward, with a relatively high intensity of nursing, and assuming full occupancy. Further factors are the inevitable overheads of hospital care, such as hospital maintenance, new equipment, medical staff salaries, radiology and laboratory costs, and operating theatres. The economics are complex but it seems logical that the most efficient use of facilities is to use them to the full. The only way to save substantial quantities of money is to close an entire department or ward. With many patients, particularly those with disorders unsuitable for day surgery, there is a variable period between them requiring full medical and nursing care and being able to cope at home. This period has shortened, and in some cases disappeared, with improvements in surgical and anaesthetic techniques, better analgesia, improved rehabilitation, and better care in the community and general practice, but there is still an occasional need for a period of convalescence. This can take place in a unit with lower staffing levels and with lower overheads than a hospital ward. Convalescent hospitals and GP units were common 20–30 years ago, but most have been closed in an attempt to save money. Some hospitals retain convalescent units, but most make use of local private facilities, with a greater or lesser degree of satisfaction. The introduction of **patient hotels or hostels** has proved popular in parts of Scandinavia and USA. These are usually privately funded units located near the acute unit and taking uncomplicated patients early after surgery. Claims have been made for their efficiency and effectiveness, but their greatest value is perhaps for units such as cardiac surgery rather than coloproctology for example, because of the rapid recovery and minimal nursing care required when all goes well.

Factors affecting speed of recovery

The metabolic response to surgery

The metabolic response to the surgical insult was first described by D.P. Cuthbertson in the 1930s. Since then, its mechanisms have gradually been unravelled, allowing improved control and mitigation of its effects.

Cuthbertson observed that the body reacts to any injury, including surgery, in two phases. The first phase is characterized by sodium and water retention, aimed at preservation of extracellular fluid volume and hence cardiovascular efficiency. The second follows about 36–48 hours after the insult (provided recovery is uncomplicated). This is a catabolic phase in which water, electrolytes, and nitrogen are lost from the body.

Respiratory effects of surgery and anaesthesia

Respiratory compromise after general anaesthetic is to be expected. If the anaesthetic and surgical procedure have been short, the patient is reasonably young and fit, and a non-smoker, recovery should be rapid and uncomplicated. The patient needs only adequate analgesia, explanation, and encouragement to self-ventilate effectively. In contrast, a patient with pre-existing pulmonary compromise as a result of lung disease or extreme age, or when surgery has been prolonged and involved opening

body cavities, a more active programme is required. The patient should ideally be visited before operation by a physiotherapist to teach him or her how to optimize ventilation and help prevent sputum retention, atelectasis, and superadded infection. Effective analgesia is fundamental, and immediately after recovery from the anaesthetic the patient should be encouraged to breathe deeply and to cough, with reassurance that coughing is beneficial rather than harmful. Chest physiotherapy may be necessary, often several times a day, pneumonias should be treated promptly, and bronchospasm treated with appropriate bronchodilators. It should be recalled that lying flat compromises pulmonary function, and should be avoided as far as possible. If pulmonary collapse occurs, fibre-optic bronchoscopy may be needed to remove sputum plugs.

3 Psychosocial aspects of postoperative care

3.1 Introduction

It has been understood for many years that improved outcomes from medical conditions result from better doctor–patient relationships (Balint 1972). The effects of improved communication on recovery form surgery have been reviewed and categorized by several authors. Ley (1977), in a review of 13 studies, found that good communication resulted in reduced hospital stay and reduced need for analgesia. He classified the interventions as **information giving**, **instruction** (for example on how to cough or turn in bed), and **quasi-therapeutic** (for example, discussion of the patient's worries and providing reassurance), but observed that in practice the three components are combined. A later review by Anderson and Masur (1983) also showed the beneficial effects of enhanced information provision on surgical outcomes, confirming Ley's conclusions.

There is evidence that personality is related to surgical outcome. Anxiety prior to operation impedes recovery (Wallace 1987), and the anxiety may be mitigated by preoperative intervention (Anderson and Masur 1983). Information-giving preoperatively has been shown to be of value, and sensory information has been demonstrated to be superior to procedural information.

3.2 Psychological aspects of postoperative pain

The experience of postoperative pain and the anxiety resulting from it are potent causes of postoperative morbidity and delayed recovery from surgery. The physical management of postoperative pain has already been discussed, but there is also a psychological aspect. In an early study (Egbert et al. 1964), patients about to undergo abdominal surgery were visited by an anaesthetist who informed and reassured them about postoperative pain, and gave them suggestions about how it could be controlled by such techniques as relaxation and breathing exercises. The results were striking. Requests for opioids were half those in non-visited controls, independent observers rated the experimental group as experiencing significantly less pain, and members of the intervention group were discharged 2.7 days earlier from hospital.

Preparatory procedures that mitigate the adverse effects of pain and distress

Four principal categories of preparatory procedure have been identified which mitigate the adverse effects of pain and distress (Johnston 1990):

◆ Provision of information that provides sensory preparation for the feelings the patient will experience, including pain, as well as details of the procedure the patient will undergo.

◆ Behavioural instructions, such as how to turn over in bed, how to cough, how to relax.

◆ Cognitive methods to encourage constructive thinking about the condition. These may include instruction in techniques designed to alter the perception of pain, such as somatization and imaginative transformation.

◆ Psychotherapeutic approaches, exploring the patient's emotional responses, either individually or in groups.

These approaches have been extensively studied, and have all been shown to reduce analgesic consumption, although via different mechanisms.

3.3 Summary of effects

An impressive meta-analysis of a range of preoperative interventions, ranging from psychotherapeutic to educational methods, showed consistent effects on a range of variables (Mumford 1982), including drug administration, pain, postoperative complications, and speed of recovery. A mean overall effect size of 0.49 suggested that intervention patients were improved by 67 per cent compared with controls, with psychotherapeutic methods being most effective.

3.4 Learning communications skills

The evidence is incontrovertible that good communication skills and concern for the psychosocial welfare of patients improves outcomes and aids recovery. However, these issues are not, in general, well handled by surgeons. Nine out of ten complaints and litigation by patients result from poor communication by clinicians. Some teaching of these skills is now integrated into most medical undergraduate curricula, and education is improving. The earlier qualified clinician may not have been exposed to such course elements. It has been shown that clinical communication skills do not reliably improve with experience alone. Active development of skills is needed as clinicians encounter more complex situations, and interpersonal skills, like other skills, benefit from reinforcement.

Psychosocial skills can be taught successfully. Helpful attitudes include a belief that they are important, and an unprejudiced positive regard for patients. More effective programmes are those that are highly structured, in which specific skills are identified, demonstrated, practised, and evaluated, with multiple opportunities for feedback. Role play, video- and audiotape reviews, and standardized patients are effective teaching techniques. Since, like technical skill, it improves the surgical outcome for patients, and is highly cost-effective, such training should be an integral part of higher surgical training and continuing medical education.

4 Optimizing recovery from surgery

4.1 Clinical audit

Economic perspective

In an increasingly cost-conscious world, where escalating healthcare costs and an increasingly informed and critical public are enforcing appraisal of medical practices, all aspects of treatment and recovery are coming under scrutiny. Increasingly, it is important to know the total 'cost of an illness'. This includes the direct costs of the episode of intervention, but also the indirect costs, such as the loss of income for the patient, the loss of support for his family, and the community implications, such as lost working time and need for community support during recovery. For these reasons as well as the human, personal reasons, it is important to optimize the recovery of each surgical patient, and to evaluate recovery continually so that improvements can be made and the audit cycle is completed.

4.2 When is a patient fit to drive?

Very few objective studies have been performed to assess when a patient is likely to be safe to begin driving again after an operation. One study (Wilson *et al.* 1995) examined the methodology of such testing by constructing a driving simulator that measured aspects of a patient's ability to use a brake pedal effectively. The device measured the reaction time taken to depress the pedal in an emergency stop and also the time take to achieve maximum depression of the pedal. A subsequent paper used the simulator to test the effects of different types of hernia repair on the ability to brake and compared these groups with others after varicose vein surgery. The latter group showed no alteration in response times as a result of surgery. After hernia repair, only 33 per cent of Bassini repair patients had returned to normal by the seventh postoperative day, whereas 64 per cent of those after Lichtenstein repair and 82 per cent after laparoscopic repair had returned to normal in the same period (personal communication, W. Brough).

Bibliography

Anderson, K.O. and Masur, F.T. (1983). Psychological preparation for invasive medical and dental procedures. *J. Behavioural Med.*, **6**, 1–40.

Anon (1973). Gastric decompression after abdominal surgery, *BMJ*, **1**, 189–90.

Argov, S., Goldstein, I. and Barzilai, A. (1980). Is routine use of the nasogastric tube justified in upper abdominal surgery? *Am. J. Surg.*, **139**, 849–50.

Balint, M. (1972). *The doctor, his patient and the illness.* New York, International University Press.

Bauer, J.J., Gelernt, I.M., Salky, B.A. and Kreel, I. (1985), Is routine gastric decompression really necessary? *Ann. Surg.*, **201**, 233–6.

Bridenbaugh, P.O., (1988). Postoperative analgesia. *Acta. Chir. Scand. Suppl.*, **550**, 177–81.

Burg, R., Geigle, C.F., Fasco, J.M. and Theuerkauf, F.J. (1977). Omission of routine gastric decompression. *Dis. Col. Rect.*, **21**, 98–100.

Cook, J.A., Fraser, I.A., Sandhu, D., Everson, N.W., Fossard, D.P. (1989). A randomised comparison of two postoperative fluid regimens. *Ann. R. Coll. Surg. Engl.*, **71**, 67–9.

Crosby, D.L. and Rees, G.A.D. (1994). Provision of post-operative care in UK hospitals. *Ann. R. Coll. Surg. Engl.*, **76**, 14–18.

Crowe, H., Clift, R., Dunggan, G., Bolton, D.M. and Castello, A.J. (1993). Randomized study of the effect of midnight versus 0600 removal of urinary catheters. *Brit. J. Urol.*, **71**, 306–8.

Freidin, J. and Marshall, V. (1984). *Illustrated guide to surgical practice.* Chapter 5, Normal progress after surgery. Churchill Livingstone, Edinburgh.

Gamil, M. and Fanning, A. (1991). The first 24 hours after surgery. *Anaesthesia*, **46**, 712–15.

Hirsch, J. (1994). Impact of postoperative nausea and vomiting in the surgical setting. *Anaesthesia*, **49**, 30–3.

Johnston, M. (1990). Counselling and psychological methods with postoperative pain: a brief review. *Health Psychology Update*, **5**, 8–14.

Justins, D.M. and Richardson, P.H. (1991). Clinical management of acute pain, *Br. Med. Bull.*, **47**, 561–83.

Kehlet, H. and Jørgen, B.D. (1993). Postoperative pain. *World J. Surg.*, **17**, 215–19.

Miller, D.F., Mason, J.R., McArthur, J. and Gordon, I. (1972). A randomized prospective trial comparing three established methods of gastric decompression after vagotomy. *Br. J. Surg.*, **59**, 605–8.

Mittelman, J.S. and Doberneck, R.C. (1982). Drains and antibiotics perioperatively for elective cholecystectomy. *Surg. Gynaec. Obstet.*, **155**, 653–4.

Mumford, E., Schlesinger, H.J. and Glass, G.V. (1982). The effect of psychological intervention on recovery from surgery and heart attacks: an analysis of the literature. *Am. J. Publ. Health*, **72**, 141–51.

NCEPOD Report (1995).

Noble, J.G., Menzies, D., Cox, P.J. and Edwards, L. (1990). Midnight removal: an improved approach to removal of catheters. *Br. J. Urol.*, **65**, 616–17.

Parikh, H.K., Badwe, R.A., Ash, C.M., Hamed, H., Frietas, R., Chaudary, M.A. and Fentiman, I.S. (1992). Early drain removal following modified radical mastectomy: a randomized trial. *J. Surg. Oncol.*, **51**, 266–9.

Somers, R.G., Jablon, L.K., Kaplan, M.J., Sandler, G.L. and Rosenblatt, N.K. (1972). The use of closed suction drainage after lumpectomy and axillary node dissection for breast cancer. *Ann. Surg.*, **215**, 146–9.

Terrell, G.S. and Singer, J.A. (1992). Axillary versus combined axillary and pectoral drainage after modified radical mastectomy. *Surg. Gynaecol. Obstet.*, **175**, 437–40.

van Heurn, L.W.E. and Brink, P.R.G. (1995). Prospective randomized trial of high *versus* low vacuum suction drainage after axillary lymphadenectomy. *Br. J. Surg.*, **82**, 931–2.

Wallace, L.M. (1987). Trait anxiety as a predictor of adjustment to and recovery from surgery. *Brit. J. Clin. Psychol.*, **26**, 73–4.

Watcha, M.F. and White, P.F. (1992). Postoperative nausea and vomiting: its etiology, treatment and prevention. *Anaesthesiol.*, **77**, 162–84.

Wihlborg, O., Bergijung, L. and Mårtensson, H. (1988). To drain or not to drain in thyroid surgery: a controlled clinical study. *Arch. Surg.*, **123**, 40–1.

Williams, A.R., Hind, M. and Sweeney, B.P. (1994). The incidence and severity of postoperative nausea and vomiting in patients exposed to positive intraoperative suggestions. *Anaesthesia*, **49**, 340–2.

Wilson, M.S., Deans, G.T., Williams, J.P., Bose, R., Brough, W.A. (1995). A method of objective measurement of rehabilitation after inguinal hernia repair. *Minimally Invasive Therapy*, **4**, 115–16.

Wyman, A. (1987). What time of day should a urethral catheter be removed? *J. Roy. Soc. Med.*, **80**, 755–6.

CHAPTER 14

Minimal access surgery

Ali Majeed and Matthew J. Carmody

1 Introduction

Minimal access surgery (MAS) is a term introduced relatively recently into the surgical literature to indicate techniques where there is a substantial reduction in the size of the access wounds through which a surgical procedure is performed. Initially, this type of procedure was called 'minimally invasive' until it was realized that it was only the trauma of access that was reduced; the procedure and the 'invasion' into the patient remained the same. The old adage that 'big surgeons make big incisions' has been superseded by the rapid pace of development of sophisticated instruments and techniques. It must be remembered that whatever the route of access, the procedure performed remains the same and that the safety of the patient is paramount. If an attempt at minimal access surgery is found to give inadequate access, then it is prudent to make a standard incision to help achieve a safe resolution. Persisting with inadequate access is indefensible.

Minimal access surgery is not necessarily performed endoscopically; the introduction of 'mini' cholecystectomy is a prime example of non-endoscopic MAS. Since the advent of laparoscopic surgery, surgeons have sometimes attempted to resurrect procedures already proven to be ineffective by the open route (e.g. ligamentum teres gastropexy for gastro-oesophageal reflux) and this type of practice cannot be ethically justified, however technically interesting it may be.

2 'Open' minimal access surgery

2.1 Small-incision ('mini') cholecystectomy

Open cholecystectomy through a small incision has been shown to lead to a shortened period of postoperative recovery and may combine the advantages of laparoscopic cholecystectomy (in terms of reduced wound-related morbidity) while retaining the inherent advantages of the open procedure (i.e. direct three-dimensional vision, 'feel', instant access to the operative field, and a much reduced incidence of remote injuries, e.g. vascular and visceral). There is, however, considerable confusion about what is meant by a 'small incision' and some anxiety about the adequacy of exposure. For cholecystectomy, incisions have traditionally been made over the surface marking of the gallbladder fundus, the part which is of least concern during cholecystectomy. Access to the junction of the cystic duct and common duct (**Calot's triangle**) is difficult with traditional approaches; a small, laterally placed subcostal incision is probably the worst option.

Procedure

The patient is placed supine on the operating table and prepared and draped as for a standard open cholecystectomy. It is preferable to extend the right arm as this allows the surgeon to stand closer to the patient and to view the operative field directly from above. An operating headlight may be used, but is not essential.

Incision

Positioning of the incision is critical to the operation. A transverse 5 cm skin incision (± 2 cm, depending on the size of the patient) is commonly employed, extending from the midline across to the right costal margin. The incision should be placed at the junction of the upper one-third and lower two-thirds of a line joining the xiphisternum to the umbilicus. In patients with wide costal arches, it is best to place the incision at the junction of the upper quarter and lower three-quarters of this line (i.e. as high as possible). This incision is much higher than described in standard texts but has the advantage of being sited directly over the junction of the cystic and common bile ducts. This is in contrast to subcostal or laparoscopic approaches, which view the junction obliquely from below.

The skin edges are retracted with Langenbeck retractors and the anterior rectus sheath is divided in the line of the skin incision. The rectus muscle may be divided with diathermy in the same line (or in very thin patients may be retracted laterally) or split longitudinally. The combined posterior rectus sheath and peritoneum are picked up with haemostats and incised. These structures are divided to the full extent of the skin incision.

A Deaver retractor (standard or narrow) is used to retract the liver edge and a small abdominal gauze pack is then inserted over the surface of this retractor into the peritoneal cavity. A Kelly retractor (or narrow Deaver retractor) is placed over the gauze pack (which may need to be adjusted) to retract the colon and duodenum inferiorly. It is helpful to deflate the stomach with a nasogastric tube as a matter of routine; this is removed at the end of the operation. The gallbladder neck is identified and grasped with forceps. Retraction of the gallbladder neck to the patient's right stretches the peritoneal covering of the cystic– common hepatic duct junction, which is then carefully cleared. Pledget dissection reveals the cystic duct, which is cleared anteriorly and posteriorly with the help of a Lahey dissector; the cystic–common hepatic duct junction must be clearly demonstrated at this stage. A medium–large Ligaclip™ on a clip applier is used to place a clip on the cystic duct at its junction with the gallbladder. It is helpful if the clip appliers are angled at the tip to allow the clip to be

applied at right angles to the cystic duct and later to the artery. If a cholangiogram is to be performed (we believe operative cholangiography should be performed routinely), the cystic duct can be cannulated at this stage. If not, two further clips are applied to the cystic duct which is then divided.

Further blunt dissection reveals the cystic artery, which is similarly clipped. The gallbladder is usually dissected from the liver bed with diathermy as in the laparoscopic approach. Removal of the abdominal pack requires caution if accidental avulsion of the metal clips from the ducts is to be prevented. The Deaver retractor is positioned to protect these clips and the pack can be gently removed over its surface. The rectus sheath is closed in two layers with a continuous suture.

If cholangiography reveals common-duct calculi, common bile duct exploration or even choledocho-duodenostomy can be performed, often without the need to extend the incision. Occasionally, an intrahepatic, densely adherent gallbladder may require extension of the incision laterally and downwards along the costal margin.

Evidence of effectiveness

Evidence of the effectiveness of mini-cholecystectomy was published in the American literature as early as 1983 and subsequently by Dubois in France who quoted the results of over 1500 cases. Randomized trials between 'mini' and 'standard' open cholecystectomy were never performed because laparoscopic cholecystectomy rapidly became popular as the method of choice for cholecystectomy. Subsequent randomized trials between mini-cholecystectomy and laparoscopic cholecystectomy have not shown a clear advantage for either procedure, and an important review by the Royal College of Surgeons of England concluded that surgeons should not be encouraged to replace mini-cholecystectomy with laparoscopic cholecystectomy.

3 Laparoscopic surgery

When you have a new hammer, suddenly every problem seems like a nail.

3.1 Introduction

Soon after its introduction in 1987, laparoscopic surgery was billed as the greatest revolution in surgery since the invention of general anaesthesia. Indeed, it was predicted that over 80 per cent of abdominal surgical procedures would be conducted laparoscopically by the turn of the century. While this may have been an overstatement, it is true to say that laparoscopic surgery has induced a fundamental change in the attitudes of surgeons towards operative outcomes, postoperative recovery, postoperative pain, and cost effectiveness of surgical procedures.

3.2 The current scope of laparoscopic surgery

To a greater or lesser degree, laparoscopic surgery has been responsible for a resurgence in the specialty of general surgery, and trainees now seek it as keenly as other specialties. It has also been responsible for much harm, but the phase of using outdated operations to allow the procedure to be accomplished laparoscopically should now have passed. Critical assessment of indications, operations, and results is now the norm rather than the exception.

3.3 Historical perspective

The Arabian physician Abul Kasim (AD 936–1013) is credited as being the first to use reflected light to inspect an internal organ, in this case the cervix. Centuries later, this was followed by the development of a cystoscope, which included a light bulb at the tip. In 1901, Kelling reported using such a cystoscope to inspect the peritoneal cavity of a dog after insufflation with air, and the term **coelioscopy** was coined. The Swedish physician Jacobaeus performed the first coelioscopy in a human in 1910. These examinations were performed by introducing the cystoscopes directly into the peritoneal cavity without pneumoperitoneum; this was not introduced for another 30 years. Veress later developed an insufflation needle for the (relatively) safe introduction of gas into the abdomen.

Professor Kurt Semm in Kiel, Germany, was one of the pioneers of diagnostic and interventional laparoscopy. He is credited with the development of an automatic insufflation device for monitoring abdominal pressure and gas flow and for popularizing the technique of laparoscopy, especially in gynaecology. The development of the rod-lens system in 1966 by the British physicist, Hopkins, was a revolution in rigid endoscopy. His designs resulted in vastly improved image brightness and clarity, and these principles are still utilized in modern laparoscopes. Until this time, laparoscopy was usually considered a diagnostic procedure because it was impracticable to perform surgical procedures while maintaining eye contact with the laparoscope in the abdomen. The development of the miniaturized video camera revolutionized interventional laparoscopy.

Mouret, in Lyon, France, is generally credited with performing the first laparoscopic cholecystectomy in a human in 1987. The technique was rapidly popularized after these initial reports, appealing to the technical side of surgeons and being pushed onwards by media hype.

3.4 Common procedures

Laparoscopic cholecystectomy is the most commonly performed laparoscopic operation by general surgeons. Most candidates approaching the end of their training would expect to be confident with it. However, there is no doubt that the risk of bile-duct injury is higher than at open surgery. While this has dropped from the devastating Southern Surgeons' Club figures (Moore and Bennett 1995), this damage remains about twice as common as at open cholecystectomy. The precise rate of injury varies widely. If one assumes the average (although high) rate of bile-duct injury to be 0.4 per cent, a surgeon doing one laparo-

scopic cholecystectomy per week may go 5 years without causing one injury.

Laparoscopic fundoplication is probably the operation of choice for gastro-oesophageal reflux but it demands greater skill than laparoscopic cholecystectomy. The operation may be accomplished by many routes, but the same tenets remain: meticulous patient selection, anatomical dissection of the hiatus, crural re-approximation, and a tension-free and durable wrap are the mainstays of this operation. A wrap performed in the Nissen style accounts for around three-quarters of the antireflux surgery performed around the world, although this varies widely on a geographic basis.

Laparoscopic appendicectomy would seem to be a natural extension of laparoscopy for right iliac fossa pain. In some institutions, over 95 per cent of cases of appendicitis are managed this way. Critical evidence in favour of this technique is less apparent, however. Criticisms include increased cost and increased operating time. In favour of it are a significantly shorter admission time, lower wound infection rates, and an earlier return to work. It is an ideal operation for the teaching of laparoscopic skills.

Laparoscopic inguinal hernia repair is the most controversial of the common procedures. It is the most susceptible to technical failures, and when difficult can be the least satisfying to complete. On the other hand, many surgeons would agree, an open hernia is an enjoyable operation to perform and to teach. To supplant open inguinal hernia, laparoscopic repair will need to endure the scrutiny that the myriad of open techniques have undergone, to test both claim and counterclaim. At present, a multicentre study with surgeons experienced in laparoscopic hernia repair has shown a lower recurrence rate than traditional anterior darned repairs, and patients have earlier return to work. The laparoscopic technique requires general anaesthesia and is currently regarded as most suitable for bilateral and recurrent hernias.

Within a specialized unit, advanced laparoscopic procedures can be undertaken. Unlike many equivalent open operations, these cases require investment in equipment, skills, and patience. An example might be laparoscopic anterior resection. This requires skills, time, and staff that an open procedure does not. The optimal setting for advanced laparoscopic techniques is within a unit that is prepared to make the appropriate investment.

3.5 Research and experimental procedures

The literature contains numerous case reports, retrospective analyses, personal series, and unusual cases (Table 14.1). Laparoscopic retrieval of an ingested padlock from the stomach of a child was a personal favourite of the authors. In the culture of evidence-based medicine, such scenarios do not add to the esteem of laparoscopic surgery. Progress needs to be made through meticulous research, not thinly veiled experimental series. This should take place in centres where advances will be made the most of, rather than in places where the next 5 years

Table 14.1 Less commonly performed laparoscopic procedures

Gastrointestinal bypass procedures (e.g. gastrojejunostomy)

Gastrostomy

Gastric banding for morbid obesity

Heller's cardiomyotomy

Perforated duodenal ulcer repair

Common bile duct exploration

Splenectomy

Liver cyst fenestration

Adrenalectomy

Pelvic lymphadenectomy

Colonic resection

Rectopexy

Adhesiolysis

Laparoscopic procedures not commonly performed but reported in the literature
    Vagotomy (truncal and highly selective)
    Pyloroplasty
    Gastropexy
    Pylorus-preserving pancreatico-duodenectomy
    Gastrectomy (Billroth I and II)
    Hepatic resection
    Ligation of bleeding duodenal ulcer
    Cholecysto-jejunostomy
    Drainage of pancreatic abscesses
    Drainage of pancreatic pseudocyst
    Enterolithotomy for gallstone ileus
    Caecopexy
    Ileostomy and colostomy (and closure)

Laparoscopically assisted operations
    Devascularization of oesophageal varices
    Repair of ruptured diaphragm
    Anterior resection of rectal villous adenoma
    Abdomino-perineal resection of rectum
    Continent catheterizable cutaneous appendico-vesicostomy
    Meckel's diverticulectomy
    Ileocolectomy for Crohn's disease

are spent undoing the damage caused by improperly monitored procedures.

3.6 Principles of laparoscopic surgery

Basics

In any medical field, familiarity with standard equipment is fundamental and this applies especially in laparoscopic surgery. A trainee is expected to be able to check the equipment as well as troubleshoot common problems. The 10 seconds spent fixing the video image is worth more to a pupil than the 6 months of encouraging camera banter!

Electronics

A good-quality video screen is essential. It should be mounted on a mobile trolley along with the other essential laparoscopic equipment. It should be stationed at around eye level. In most cases, one screen is sufficient. A facility to lock the controls for adjusting the screen brightness, contrast, and colour is useful. A video recorder is often included, but without a machine of broadcast quality, the images obtained at surgery are often disappointing. Developments in digital image storage are promising in this respect.

A three-chip CCD camera is a necessity. The quality of image is vastly superior to that of one-chip models, especially with respect to colour representation, colour bleed, and sensitivity at low light levels. The camera should connect to a camera control unit that allows automatic iris setting, white balance, and gain. The use of a sterile camera sleeve obviates the need for repeated camera disinfection and improves turnaround times. Other systems available on the market and in various stages of development include three-dimensional cameras. The technology in three-dimensional imaging is evolving, but most laparoscopic surgeons would agree that two-dimensional views are adequate for most procedures.

The light source should be a dedicated to laparoscopic use and regular bulb changes are important. A poorly performing light source detracts considerably from the view. Regular checks of the integrity of the light cables are also important: breaches of the outer coat may allow solution ingress, and cables with broken light fibres will not transmit light well. A light lead with an uncovered end will burn theatre drapes if left on them while at full power. The use of paper drapes adds to this risk. For safety, always connect the light lead to the source last, or to the eyepiece first.

Setting up for laparoscopic surgery

It is important to be mindful of the setting in which any form of surgery is undertaken. The specialized unit with the resources—in both skill and equipment—can undertake an array of procedures that a smaller department cannot. If safe and successful procedures are to be undertaken, the occasional laparoscopic operator needs to consider carefully his or her abilities and the backup available. Remember that the average American general surgeon (doing laparoscopic surgery) performs two laparoscopic cholecystectomies per month. Opportunities to hone one's skill under these circumstances are therefore limited.

Basic hardware

Optics

Eyepieces vary in diameter, angle, and field of view. The larger the diameter, the larger the light-carrying elements can be. A 10 mm eyepiece gives a brighter and more detailed picture than its 5 mm brother. In addition, the 5 mm eyepiece is less robust, less tolerant of fogging, and much more susceptible to physical bending. The instrument's angle describes the relationship between the visual axis and the light axis. The 25° eyepiece allows a sensation of perspective using shadowing effects, and rotation of the camera with respect to the light axis allows corners to be looked around. It does, however, carry less light than a 0° eyepiece. For most situations a 25–30° is most useful and is recommended for beginners. Some proprietary eyepieces have an enlarged field of vision, much like a wide-angle lens in a camera. The greater benefit of these is their greater depth of field, obviating much of the need for refocusing.

Diathermy

Diathermy equipment is usually the standard monopolar diathermy available in most theatres; however, sophisticated diathermy machines with safety cut-outs to prevent capacitance coupling or arcing are available but are expensive.

Insufflator

The basic hardware required for any laparoscopic procedure includes a machine for delivering high-flow carbon dioxide to establish and maintain a pneumoperitoneum. The minimum standard should be a pressure-alarmed, single-channel CO_2 insufflator. The use of volume-limited insufflators is unsafe, as they have no way of alarming when intra-abdominal pressure escalates. Modern devices measure the pressure via the insufflation tubing (single-channel) as opposed to a separate channel (dual-channel). The latter system has been shown to be unsafe as the pressure-measuring tubing can inadvertently become occluded or disconnected.

The optimum intra-abdominal pressure is 12 mmHg, which allows adequate visibility for most situations in adults. There is some evidence that this low pressure of pneumoperitoneum lowers the incidence of venous stasis and deep vein thrombosis. For pelvic laparoscopy, pressures even less than 12 mmHg are often adequate. A pressure-alarmed insufflator will autoregulate when this preselected pressure is reached and give an audible signal above this level. A flow rate of 6 litres/minute is a minimum; newer technologies allow rates of up to 25 litres/minute to be delivered under controlled circumstances. Other options include gas warming and humidification.

Hand instruments

Basic concepts

Laparoscopic instruments that are commonly used include dissectors, scissors, and various grasping devices. For advanced procedures, retractors made of 'memory metal' are available which return to a preformed shape once they are inserted into the abdomen and reach body temperature. Most laparoscopic instruments are available as: disposable after a single use, completely reusable, or reusable–disposable.

Opinion varies as to the best instruments for dissection: some surgeons prefer to use an electrocautery hook while others prefer straightforward dissectors to minimize the risk of inadvertent injury. Various suction–irrigation devices are also available. Needle-holders and automatic suturing devices are available for more advanced procedures, although the automatic devices are disposable and can be expensive.

Many instruments are available in a range of sizes. Early in the evolution of laparoscopic surgery, only a limited range of instruments was available at 5 mm diameter and these were particularly prone to failure. This no longer the case, and for most situations there is now an adequate 5 mm instrument. Further design improvements have produced 'needlescopic' instruments of 3 mm diameter, which can be used without a port.

Heavy graspers, stone scoops, and clip appliers are, by their nature, invariably 10 mm in diameter. Graspers come in a bewildering array of jaw designs, and some incorporate ratchet locks. Graspers are typically straight, although angled tips do exist. All should be insulated, and a selection that allow the use of monopolar diathermy are an advantage. Few of these instruments are suitable for grasping bowel. This is principally because of the great mechanical advantage afforded by a long instrument, so that tearing of bowel occurs long before there is any tactile appreciation of it. Other essential instruments include cholangiogram forceps.

Ports

Ports are sophisticated sleeves which traverse the abdominal wall and allow instruments to be placed and replaced without trauma and without losing pressure. Ports begin at 5 mm diameter and go up to no less than 40 mm. They broadly divide into disposable, reusable, and a combination of the two. Disposable ports can add markedly to the cost of a procedure but, in most cases, excellent-quality reusable ports exist. Concerns have been raised regarding the adequacy of sterility inside the valve and seal mechanisms of reusable ports, and this mechanism often exacts a high toll on the barrel insulation of instruments as they are passed through. Hybrid ports combining a reusable shaft/trocar assembly, with a small, disposable multiadapter seal, offer the best of both worlds. Ports must have a self-retaining mechanism; this may be crude as in the style of suture and stanchion, through to special alloy, non-slip surfaces, or threaded barrels which 'screw' into the abdominal wall.

Reusable versus disposable

Certainly in recent years, the gulf between reusable versus disposable instruments has narrowed considerably. Reusable–disposable instruments have recently been introduced which can be discarded after a certain number of uses. Disposable instruments that enjoy advantages over comparable reusables are restricted to combined sucker–irrigators and scissors. Disposable sucker–irrigators, using battery-driven pumps, can irrigate litres through an abdomen in minutes, allowing management of peritonitis and haemoperitoneum. Disposable scissors, by their nature, are sharp and cut well from the onset. They might be a luxury for short procedures, but represent a better option for operations requiring substantial dissection.

Staplers, clippers, guns, and tackers

Control of ducts, bowel, and vessels in laparoscopic surgery requires a range of devices. The simplest is the reusable 10 mm clip applier for control of cystic artery and duct in cholecystectomy. Reloading requires removal from the abdomen. Common problems include the clip falling out, and the clip 'scissoring', where the clip legs cross and fail to occlude the structure; both are often caused by loose applier jaws. Disposable 10 mm clip appliers typically hold 20 clips and add to the overall cost, but in situations where close to this number of clips is necessary, this may represent an efficient use of resources. A 5 mm clip applier is available, but is not in regular use in the United Kingdom.

Tackers and staplers may be necessary for hernia repairs where prosthetic mesh is inserted. Staplers apply a staple similar in appearance to a skin staple, and are available in 10 mm straight and flexible-head models. A 5 mm tacker is available and uses a corkscrew arrangement to spiral a small wire coil to hold prosthetic mesh in place. It may be preferable to staples owing to its greater strength and the fact that it causes less local tissue damage. Staple guns are 10 mm or larger in diameter and are multiload (i.e. they allow reloading after firing). They are typically manually operated, with an optimum 30–35 mm staple line with a single grip squeeze. The longest staple line is 60 mm and firing is gas-assisted. Some machines offer angled firing via a flexible head. Cartridges come in different staple lengths and spacing, reflecting their suitability for thick tissue, normal tissue, and vascular purposes. Instruments are colour-coded for this, and different cartridges of one brand are interchangeable in their own stapler. All work on the principle of an initial action to approximate the jaws, and a second action to activate the staple anvil and the blade. Note that none of these instruments staples all the way to the limit of the jaws—the limit of the knife and anvil travel is marked on the jaws. Insertion of the instrument through the port requires closure of the jaws. In general, these instruments are neither cheap nor foolproof, and require a ready stock of replacement cartridges. Before opening a stapling device, a supply of cartridges for that brand must be at hand.

Specimen retrieval

Once the tissue or organ has been resected, its retrieval should not be overlooked. If a gallbladder is intact, it is simple to deliver it carefully, but for a spleen, appendix, or colon, delivery may present major problems. In the case of the appendix, delivery into the port intracorporeally may be all that is needed. This allows it to be removed without contacting the abdominal wall. A colon specimen should be delivered through a small muscle-splitting incision via a plastic wound protector. This device consists of a semirigid plastic ring and flange that is placed across the abdominal wall, and its use excludes the specimen from contact with the abdominal wall. In the case of solid organs or a punctured gallbladder, a specimen retrieval bag can be inserted intracorporeally and the specimen placed within. These may be found in 10 mm or 15 mm diameter. In the case of splenectomy, the spleen is fragmented or 'morselized' within the bag prior to delivery through the port incision.

Cost

All the necessary equipment adds substantially to the cost of an operation. If capital purchases and the cost of disposables are taken into account, the cost of a laparoscopic cholecystectomy compares unfavourably with the cost of an open cholecystectomy. In defence of minimally invasive surgery, the larger picture, which includes length of hospital stay and time off work, may draw the issue into sharper focus. Length-of-stay is a major issue in American and Australian hospitals and in many situations has fuelled the laparoscopic fire. When it is realised that the cost of a stapler is equivalent to 10 hours in a post-operative surgical ward, the overall cost of treatment of a disorder with a particular technique can be scrutinized equitably.

Theatre set-up

Lighting

The theatre lights need to be dimmed and, importantly, all natural light should be capable of being excluded.

Sister, surgeon, and screen

The surgeon should try to achieve the most familiar view of the operative field. This means standing by the right iliac fossa, facing the left upper quadrant for a splenectomy, and standing by the right iliac fossa, facing the left flank for left-sided colonic operations. Cholecystectomy can be performed from left or right sides. Appendicectomy is best done from the left flank, looking towards the right flank. The camera should be between the surgeon's hands, and the screen should be within a field of 30° either side of the surgeon–camera–field axis. Exceptions do exist, but spatial relationships are most evident in these positions, particularly so in the lower half of the abdomen.

The positioning of the staff and cables should allow the surgeon and assistants free access towards and away from the table. This is best achieved by laying all cables, tubing, and equipment across the patient's upper body, leaving the lower body free.

The scrub nurse should set up in such a position that instruments can be passed without the surgeon having to look away from the field. The scrub nurse must also have an un-restricted view of the screen, which is essential for anticipation of the surgeon's requirements. The camera operator should, in general, be positioned on the side of the patient opposite to the surgeon. In certain circumstances, the camera operator may stand behind the surgeon, particularly for teaching purposes.

Pneumoperitoneum

This is the single most dangerous step in laparoscopic surgery. More fatalities and major morbidity arise from the establishment of the pneumoperitoneum than from any other step.

Veress needle cannulation

Closed cannulation by **Veress puncture** causes a large proportion of the complications of laparoscopy. Pneumoperitoneum established with a Veress needle is a blind procedure and may, in inexperienced hands, cause serious complications. Injury to bowel, bladder, and large vessels (aorta and vena cava) have all been reported in the literature. Complications include vessel injury with haemorrhage, gas embolism, and tissue infarction, as well as organ injury, which is potentially catastrophic if it goes unrecognized. Veress cannulation requires blind insertion of sharp instruments twice, and insufflation without visual confirmation of satisfactory placement. Logic dictates that open cannulation should avoid all of this and it is therefore recommended that all trainee surgeons should be trained only in the open insertion technique, to prevent these mostly avoidable and potentially serious complications.

Open cannulation

Open cannulation allows establishment of the pneumoperitoneum under vision, using blunt insertion, and permits immediate full insufflation rates. Veress puncture can be done safely, but open cannulation is simple once taught, and excludes manoeuvres that cannot be accepted as safe surgical practice.

For the right-handed surgeon, open cannulation via the **Hasson technique** is best performed from the patient's right side. The umbilicus is elevated with tissue graspers and a vertical or semilunar infra-umbilical incision is made. This is deepened so that the inferior limit of the umbilical cicatrix is seen. With umbilical elevation using the left hand, the cicatrix is incised vertically in the midline for a distance of around 10 mm. Note that a longer incision will cause gas leakage. While maintaining the elevation, a closed pair of blunt-pointed artery forceps is inserted to the plane superficial to the peritoneum and is opened with the curve pointing downward. The largest artery forceps on the instrument set usually has the most blunt tip and lends itself best to this task. This manoeuvre occasionally needs to be repeated, but in most cases the peritoneum can now be opened and the viscera will have fallen away. The situation is checked by relaxing the left hand, and allowing the abdominal wall to descend until the viscera can be seen easily though the defect. Now the cannula is inserted using a blunt obturator, and the pneumoperitoneum can be established at normal flow rates.

The technique allows easy establishment of the pneumoperitoneum, with a mean period of 40 seconds taken to insert the cannula and start normal gas flow. Previous surgery renders any method of cannulation difficult, but performing it under vision is the safest method. Open cannulation can also be performed easily through a small incision in either flank if a midline scar influences the surgeon not to use the umbilicus.

Port insertion and placement

Port insertion should be performed under direct vision, using the camera to check the trajectory. A small stab incision is made in the most suitable location and the port inserted. Should any resistance be encountered, the skin incision should be enlarged first, as this is the most common cause of increased entry resistance. If parietal adhesions are found which prevent use of a favoured port site, then alternative port sites can be used to clear adhesions from the favoured site.

Port placement must avoid the inferior epigastric arteries, and placement in the lower abdomen must avoid bladder and iliac vessels. In thin patients, the abdominal wall should be transilluminated from the inside to demonstrate large vessels, which can thus be avoided. These are general rules which govern port placement, and specific operations have a variety of well-founded port positions.

Working and visual space

Ideal port sites should allow the surgeon to work within an arc of 120°; this can be thought of as 'the visual space'. When instruments enter and leave the space via the ports, a good camera operator will keep the instrument tip constantly in view. Most of the operation takes place with the two working instruments at a 90° angle; this can be thought of as 'the working space'—where movements are most precisely controlled in the visual 'fairway'. The visual or camera axis should bisect this space. This is particularly important when advanced laparoscopic skills, such as suturing, are needed.

3.7 Laparoscopic skills

Ligating, knotting, and suturing

Ligation can be by suture transfixion, loop ligation, clip application, or stapling devices. **Loop ligation** can be via pre-tied suture loops or via hand-tied loops slipped in with a knot pusher. A common example is a suture loop around the appendix base. **Clips** may be applied to a structure either in continuity or following division. **Staple guns** allow the control of larger structures, for example, they are the method of choice for dividing bowel and its vascular pedicles. The correct cartridge is essential: attempts to control the splenic pedicle with a bowel cartridge are doomed to fail.

The **endoloop ligature** is a preformed loop supplied with an introducer. This is useful for ligating pedicles where one end is free. A grasping instrument is passed through the endoloop and the pedicle is grasped and the endoloop can then be tightened over the pedicle. Endoloops are most useful for ligating appendicular stumps and large cystic ducts. They are rarely employed for ligating blood vessels, which would need to be divided before the endoloop could be passed over them.

Suturing can be achieved by extracorporeal or intracorporeal methods. The former allows the knot to be thrown outside the port and, by way of a **knot-pusher**, slid down the port. Intracorporeal suturing requires the suture to be brought into the abdomen. Most laparoscopic suturing follows the general principles of open suturing. The needle with its suture material is passed into the abdomen via a port, with care taken to grasp the thread rather than the needle as it passes through the port. This is to prevent the thread being pulled off the needle if it becomes trapped in the valve mechanism of the port. Standard 4/0 sutures require a 10 mm port because of the curve of the needle, but less-curved 'ski' needles can be passed through a 5 mm port.

Laparoscopic suturing is usually carried out with two needle-holders, one in each hand, to allow safe and secure passage of the needle through the tissue. After passing the needle through the tissue with the right-hand instrument, the needle can be grasped with the left hand and then transferred back to the right hand to place the next suture. Knots can be made extracorporeally, employing a long suture, one end of which remains outside the body. The needle is passed through the port, the suture inserted, and the needle is brought back through the port and a knot

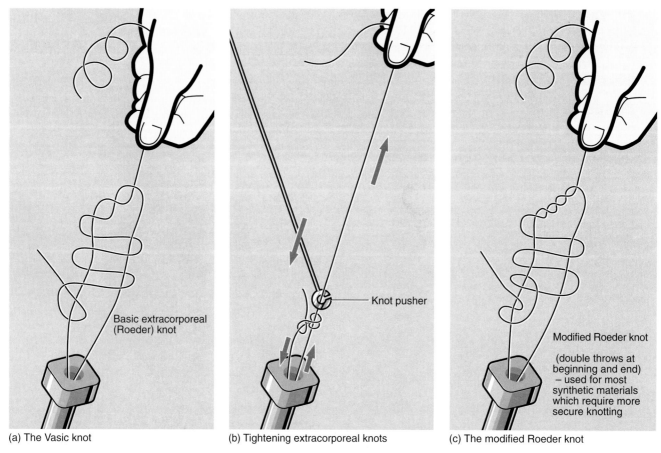

(a) The Vasic knot

Basic extracorporeal
(Roeder) knot

(b) Tightening extracorporeal knots

Knot pusher

(c) The modified Roeder knot

Modified Roeder knot

(double throws at
beginning and end)
– used for most
synthetic materials
which require more
secure knotting

Figure 14.1 Extracorporeal knotting.

formed outside. The knot needs to be a lockable slip-knot which is carried into the abdomen with a knot-pusher and tightened to prevent it slipping. The basic extracorporeal knot is shown in Fig. 14.1. There are several variations, which follow the same general principle.

Intracorporeal knots are more difficult to perform and require more practice, but are recommended for surgeons conducting laparoscopic suturing. The curved needle is passed using a needle-holder and the knot tied *in situ*. This requires skill, but allows better knot placement; it also permits a surgeon's knot to be used, rather than having to use slip knots. A needle for 4/0 sutures usually passes easily through a 10 mm port. There are several techniques for intracorporeal knots, but the simplest one is to form a slip knot which can be tightened to the desired tension. A reverse throw is then made to create a reef knot which locks the first knot in place (see Fig. 14.2).

A disposable suturing device is available which uses a small, straight needle attached to a thread. The needle is passed between the right and left jaws of the instrument using a lever and it is then automatically grasped on the other side after passing through the tissue. A potential drawback of this instrument is that the tissues have to be in close approximation and one cannot 'feel' the needle passing through the tissue to ensure that a substantial bite has been taken.

Retraction

Expert retraction requires the best choice of grasper, applied to the most suitable part of the viscus, with traction in the optimum direction, maintained, and appropriately repositioned. It is therefore crucial to the successful completion of an operation.

Diathermy

Diathermy in laparoscopy must be employed using strict safety measures to prevent inadvertent burns, which can lead to delayed perforation of hollow organs. The phenomena of capacitance coupling and arcing are well recognized and it is a surgeon's responsibility to ensure that the insulation on instruments is intact before connecting them to diathermy. It is advisable that metal ports should not be used in conjunction with plastic instruments and vice versa, to avoid capacitance coupling.

Most laparoscopic dissection is achieved with a monopolar hook. Bipolar diathermy does not lend itself well to dissection, but does offer certain advantages laparoscopically. In particular, it avoids current spreading outwards from the point of application. For example, it is preferred for control and coagulation of the mesoappendix, thus avoiding current conduction across the thin-walled caecum. It is also beneficial for sympathectomy,

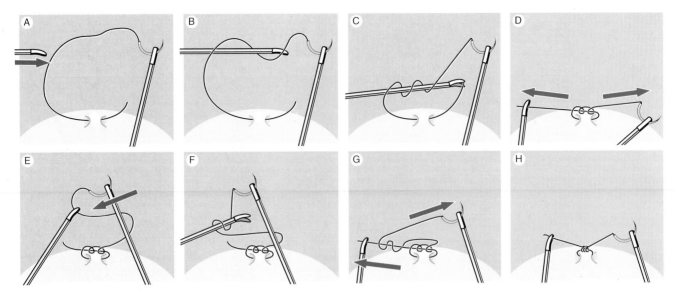

Figure 14.2 Intracorporeal knotting.

where conduction of a monopolar current along the sympathetic chain can give unpredictable results. Bipolar diathermy does not need a large, indifferent electrode applied to the body surface.

Dissection

Once the pneumoperitoneum is established, the ports are in place, and the diagnosis confirmed, dissection can proceed. Dissection may be performed with a diathermy hook or scissors, but it cannot be emphasized too strongly that the working tip of the instrument should always be in view. Removal and reinsertion of instruments via the ports should be conducted under direct vision to prevent inadvertent injury to other organs. This is especially important if instruments are connected to diathermy.

If diathermy is used for hook dissection, the minimal amount of 'collateral damage' should be caused. This is achieved by the pulling up the hook in order to 'tent' the tissue to be diathermized, away from the other tissues. Heating of adjacent tissues will thus be kept to a minimum and the 'current of injury' avoided. This is of crucial importance in dissecting ductal structures. The diathermy should be activated for the shortest possible time in these areas; short, carefully directed bursts also help to minimize local heating. In areas where structures can safely be cleared, the heel of the hook can be swept in a gentle arc across the tissues. Spot bleeding points can be dealt with using the flat side of the hook.

Cannulation

Cannulation of ducts is a necessary skill and should become routine. For example, the cystic duct can readily be cannulated whenever cholangiography is important. Purpose-made cholangiogram forceps (e.g. Olsen–Reddick forceps) make this a simple step.

Maintaining vision

Laparoscopes tend to fog. There is no entirely satisfactory answer, but it is preventable, and several small steps can minimize this frustrating problem. A prewarmed eyepiece fogs less, and the use of minimal amounts of irrigation fluid, or delaying irrigation until the last step of the procedure, also helps. Coating the lens in peritoneal fluid allows a phospholipid bilayer to form and thus minimize condensation. Proprietary solutions exist which achieve a similar end.

The appearance of blood in the field absorbs light and leads to picture degradation. It is best to prevent bleeding, use appropriate suction to clear blood should it appear, and control it early. The picture quality can often be improved by increasing light output to maximum and opening the camera aperture to maximum. Irrigation merely disperses the blood and seldom alleviates the situation.

Organ manipulation

Appropriate traction on structures is difficult to gauge. The leverage of the long instrument can allow considerable force to be applied inadvertently to a viscus, and the limited feedback may allow damage to the viscus before it is detected. Control of a structure should be through the use of a wide-jawed grasper applied to the most robust part of the structure. The use of toothed graspers, while adding to the purchase on a structure, also lead to significant local trauma. Inappropriate grasping can lead to damage to the specimen so that it becomes unrecognizable histologically. Bowel can be damaged with even minimal manipulation.

Advanced techniques
Resection

In order to carry out laparoscopic resection, it is essential to appreciate the 'dynamic viewpoint'. The camera allows the picture to be appreciated from different angles, magnified to different degrees. When combined with retraction in various directions, there are many variables in the way the field appears. For example, a view of the splenic flexure can be obtained from the left paracolic gutter, from above the greater omentum, and from the transverse colon. This has inherent benefits but also may cause disorientation. Anatomical landmarks, as is the case in all forms of surgery, are important, but predicting, for example, the direction in which the ureter will cross the operative field depends entirely on the camera angle and position. It is important at all times to recognize where the camera is situated and its direction.

Anastomoses

Anastomoses are usually achieved with a combination of stapling and suturing. A side-to-side anastomosis can be created with a linear stapler, with the remaining defect closed by sutures, typically using a continuous absorbable monofilament suture. Triangulation of instruments and an ergonomic working position are essential.

Stone retrieval

Laparoscopic exploration of the common bile duct requires skills additional to basic cholecystectomy. With appropriate equipment, the duct can be trawled via the cystic stump, allowing retrieval of common bile duct stones using a flat, wire basket. Success requires visualization of the calculus, and this can be via X-ray image intensification or flexible choledocho-scopy. In the first, the stone is localized after contrast injection and delivered via the cystic stump under fluoroscopy. The choledochoscopic technique requires the introduction of the endoscope into the cystic stump and visualization of the calculus and 'basketing' under vision. This can be done via a 'buddy system' in which the basket is slid alongside the endoscope, or by using a very small-calibre basket down the endoscope working port. This allows the stone to be basketed under direct vision.

Anaesthetic considerations

For most laparoscopic procedures an abdominal insufflation pressure of 12 mmHg is adequate, although recently it has been shown that lower abdominal insufflation pressure causes reduced venous stasis and hence reduces the risk of deep venous thrombosis. Hypercarbia resulting from carbon dioxide absorption may require increased ventilation, and anaesthetists have to be aware of this. Rarely, a patent pleuroperitoneal canal exists, which causes a pneumothorax as soon as the abdomen is insufflated. Difficulties with ventilation before any dissection has begun should alert the surgeon and anaesthetist to this possibility. Procedures that require dissection of the diaphragmatic hiatus (e.g. laparoscopic fundoplication) may cause an iatrogenic breach of the pleura and lead to a pneumothorax. It is important to be aware of this potential complication. However, only very infrequently will the patient require insertion of a chest drain; most resolve spontaneously or can be aspirated with a needle.

It was considered previously that minimal access surgery is also 'minimally invasive'. It must be remembered that the inva-siveness of a procedure depends not upon the route of access, because the procedure within the abdomen is exactly the same whether open or laparoscopic access is used. General anaesthesia is invariably required and a complete risk assessment must be carried out before embarking on these procedures in patients who are elderly or have significant co-morbidity.

3.8 Commonly performed procedures

Laparoscopic cholecystectomy

Introduction

Laparoscopic cholecystectomy is the most commonly performed laparoscopic procedure. It is essential that the trainee surgeon is adequately supervised until he or she is completely familiar with the anatomy and potential pitfalls. Major complications have too commonly been associated with this procedure and the incidence of common bile duct is statistically higher than that for open cholecystectomy. This feared complication can lead to a prolonged and troublesome period of illness for the patient and there are reports in the literature of patients even requiring liver transplantation as a consequence. The following is a general description of the procedure, recognizing that there are many variations in individual technique.

Preoperative preparation

Preoperatively, subcutaneous heparin is administered, and antithrombotic stockings fitted. After informed consent is obtained, the procedure commences with administration of a prophylactic antibiotic, typically a cephalosporin, and the patient is anaesthetized, paralysed, and intubated. The patient's and surgeon's position is variable: the essential features of each position are the same. In most situations the technique of 'fundal traction' is used. This involves lifting the gallbladder fundus above the liver, and allows the surgeon to stand on the patient's left or right. The surgeon may prefer the 'French' technique, which uses a different style of retraction.

Patient position

The patient is positioned supine on the table. The arms may be extended on sideboards to facilitate access to intravenous sites for the anaesthetist. Emptying the bladder with a urinary catheter is no longer recommended, but it is advisable to ask the patient to void the bladder before coming to theatre.

Cannulation and port placement

The abdomen is prepared in the usual way, an open can-nulation of the abdomen performed and a 10 mm trocar with a blunt obturator is inserted under vision into the abdomen. The anaesthetist is informed that insufflation is to begin, and the gas flow can then commence. If cannulation of the peritoneal space is not certain, simply introducing the eyepiece into the cannula will confirm this. Ports are then introduced under direct vision after appropriate skin incisions. The

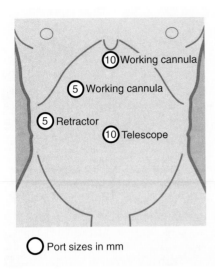

Port sizes in mm

Figure 14.3 Common port layout for laparoscopic cholecystectomy.

positions and sizes of ports employed vary considerably between individual surgeons, and the following are only suggestions (Fig. 14.3). If the surgeon prefers to stand on the right, the epigastric port should be as high as possible; if the surgeon stands on the left, the ports should be equidistant along the costal margin. A small degree of head-up tilt assists the dissection. If the stomach is distended with gas from the mask ventilation, a nasogastric tube, in position for the duration of the case, allows decompression.

Initial laparoscopic inspection and gallbladder retraction

Once the laparoscope is in place, a view of the whole abdomen should be obtained. Any obvious pathology should be noted, although with adequate preoperative workup the occurrence of surprise findings should be reduced to a minimum. At this point it is advisable to tilt the operating table so that the patient is 30° head-up. The operating table should next be tilted towards the surgeon who stands on the left of the patient. These tilts are very helpful in displacing bowel away from the operating field and bringing the liver down for better access, especially in obese patients. Positioning of assistants depends on the number of assistants available. If there is one assistant, he or she can stand across the table from the surgeon on the patient's right-hand side and manipulate the camera with one hand while holding the gallbladder retractor with the other hand. If two assistants are available, the camera operator can stand alongside the surgeon on the patient's left, while the assistant holding the gallbladder retractor stands on the patient's right.

Clearing the gallbladder

A locking grasper is placed on the fundus of the gallbladder and it is retracted upwards towards the right shoulder. This can be performed by the camera operator. The surgeon's left hand holds a non-locking, non-toothed grasper to control Hartmann's pouch. The surgeon's left hand should control the diathermy

hook at this stage. The omentum may be adherent to the right lobe of the liver; adhesions should be divided with diathermy. Adhesions around the gallbladder should be tackled next, but beware the duodenum which may be tented up and become vulnerable to diathermy. At this point the inferior surface of the gallbladder should be free in its entirety. If there is a tense mucocoele of the gallbladder, it is then advisable to aspirate it first using a long, wide-bore spinal needle attached to a 50 mm syringe. The needle is passed directly through the abdominal wall under vision into the fundus of the gallbladder. This allows a tense gallbladder to become flaccid and permits the grasping instrument to be applied.

Dissection

It is critical that dissection be kept as close to the gallbladder as possible; no structures must be ligated or divided until the anatomy is unambiguously defined. The dissection proceeds as follows. The peritoneum on the posterior surface of the gallbladder can be divided first. This is performed on the surface of the gallbladder rather than the liver, with the left hand retracting the pouch firmly over towards the patient's left shoulder. This is a frequently neglected but important step. This is continued for about two-thirds of the gallbladder length. Attention is then turned to the opposite aspect, where it is essential to commence the dissection in the correct operator position. With firm traction directed to the right, the hook is used to divide the peritoneum along the gallbladder, parallel to its hepatic edge. The hook is used in a lifting fashion to divide only the peritoneum at this stage, so structures in the deeper plane remain undisturbed.

Traction to the right should now clearly display the contents of Calot's triangle. The cystic node is a good landmark for Calot's triangle. At this point the lowermost boundary of the dissection should be the cystic duct, and above this, crossing the triangle, should be the cystic artery. Anatomical variations abound, and familiarity with the variations is essential. Dissection parallel with the cystic duct allows the fat of the mesentery to be cleared, but the use of indiscriminate diathermy is forbidden in this angle. Each structure must first be identified. The key structure to be identified is the junction of the cystic duct and the gallbladder neck and not the cystic duct and common bile duct (in contrast to open cholecystectomy). The hook allows upward traction, pulling the contents of the triangle out piece by piece, to allowing unequivocal identification. Alternatively, blunt dissection may be used with a grasper opened little by little in the triangle to isolate the structures.

At this point the triangle has been opened to reveal a 'double-windowed flag', with the cystic duct–cystic artery space, and the cystic artery–triangle apex cleared. A grasper must be able to be passed behind the two structures traversing the triangle, and when this is achieved, the cystic duct may be ligated close to the gallbladder. At this stage an operative cholangiogram should be performed. Operative cholangiography is recommended by many surgeons in as many cases as possible because this has the advantage of defining the anatomy clearly. If a major bile duct is inadvertently ligated, the damage becomes evident immediately and can be repaired. Performing routine intraoperative cholangiography also keeps the surgeon in practice and ready to employ the technique for a particularly difficult cholecystectomy when cholangiography would be most useful.

Operative cholangiography

After application of a Ligaclip™ between the cystic duct and gallbladder neck, a small incision is made in the cystic duct close to the clip, not more than half the diameter of the cystic duct. A cholangiography catheter is then introduced into the cystic duct, secured with purpose-made cholangiogram forceps (e.g. Olsen– Reddick forceps). Many gadgets are available for facilitating laparoscopic cholangiography, but they all add to the expense of the technique. A ureteric catheter passed down a large intravenous cannula is a simple way of low-cost cholangiography. Once cholangiography is completed, the retaining forceps are removed, the cholangiography catheter pulled out, and the cystic duct then doubly clipped. It is important that both the jaws of the Ligaclip™ applicator should be in view when the clip is applied. This ensures circumferential application of the Ligaclip™, preventing bile leakage from the cystic-duct stump. Occasionally a very wide cystic duct requires placement of an endoloop ligature. Hard-film copies of the cholangiogram are saved, and the anatomy confirmed before proceeding.

Ligation of cystic artery and duct

Ligation of artery and duct can be accomplished in quick succession. Dissection further along the medial side of Hartmann's pouch will identify the cystic artery. Manipulation in this area can sometimes send the cystic artery into spasm so that pulsation may not be clearly visible. Ligaclips™ should be applied to the cystic artery as close to the gallbladder wall as possible, and the artery divided between clips. While the structures remain in continuity and dissected, they will be at risk of diathermy conduction, and so the use of diathermy at this point is forbidden. Scissors are used to divide the structures after clipping, and the hook may be then used to complete the dissection of the gallbladder bed.

Completing the operation

Traction and dynamic positioning of the fundal retractor are important at this stage. Repositioning of the fundal retractor and swinging the gallbladder from side to side allows dissection to continue in the correct plane. This plane is usually avascular; should any blood appear, either the gallbladder wall or liver bed has been strayed on to. A diathermy hook or spatula can be used to divide adhesions between the gallbladder and the liver. Traction on the surgeon's left-hand instrument will display fibrous strands and small veins which can be diathermized to allow separation of the gallbladder from the liver bed. Care must be taken to remain in the plane between the liver and the gallbladder as it is easy to wander either into the liver substance (which causes bleeding) or into the gallbladder lumen (which causes spillage of bile and stones from the gallbladder). Both of these obscure the view and can be a potential source of infection.

Once the gallbladder is detached from the liver, it should be kept in place with the ratcheted grasper on the gallbladder fundus. The surgeon's left-handed instrument should also keep hold of it to prevent inadvertent loss of the gallbladder into the abdomen. Removal of the dissected gallbladder from the abdominal cavity should be performed under direct vision. The exact mode of removal varies between surgeons, and can be either via either the umbilical or the epigastric port. It is not uncommon for extraction to be complicated by a thickened gallbladder wall or the presence of large calculi. The simplest manoeuvre is to enlarge the incision in the umbilicus to allow delivery of the gallbladder. Endoscopic retrieval bags can be used to prevent stone spillage if gallbladder perforation has occurred during dissection. The gallbladder is retrieved intact, and delivered via a 10 mm port. The umbilicus appears to be the less painful of the two to extend, but necessitates a change of camera position.

Irrigation and final check

Once the gallbladder has been removed, the ports are replaced in the umbilicus or epigastric incisions and the abdomen reinsufflated with carbon dioxide. The patient is tilted back to head-down and towards the right; this allows any collection of bile or blood to accumulate in the right subphrenic space. A suction–irrigation cannula is inserted through a 5 mm port, and a thorough washout of the right subphrenic space is carried out until the returning fluid is clear.

If there is evidence of bleeding, the liver can be retracted with an instrument in the epigastric port and the bleeding point identified and dealt with. According to the preference of the surgeon, at this stage a drainage tube connected to a closed suction drain can be inserted. This is placed through one of the 5 mm ports and the surgeon grasps it with a grasper inserted through the epigastric port and keeps the drain in place while the port is removed over it. Spilled stones must be retrieved, and to this end a specimen bag may be helpful. Once the final-check laparoscopy has shown that there is no evidence of bleeding and all the irrigating fluid has been sucked out, the pneumoperitoneum machine is switched off and all ports are withdrawn.

Closure of the subumbilical port with non-absorbable sutures is recommended to prevent postoperative umbilical hernias, which are an avoidable complication. The use of a J-shaped needle mounted on a non-absorbable suture makes umbilical closure very simple. The skin is then closed with subcuticular non-absorbable suture. Infiltration of the laparoscopic incisions with 1 per cent bupivacaine helps reduce postoperative discomfort.

The difficult case

Obesity

The obese patient makes for a difficult laparoscopic cholecystectomy, but an open approach is often no easier. The solution is to employ a fifth port in the right mid-clavicular line a hand's breadth below the costal margin. The omentum can then be retracted gently down and away, without grasping it. The patient is placed head-up, and rolled slightly to the left. Obese patients frequently have a bulky mesentery to the gallbladder, and this requires careful dissection, as the structures in Calot's triangle may be a little less obvious.

Chronic cholecystitis

Repeated attacks of cholecystitis render the gallbladder thick-walled and tough, and typically contract the mesentery, closing up Calot's triangle. It is in these situations that the overlying peritoneum should be widely divided to ensure maximal opening of the triangle. Fibrosis is always greatest in the region of Hartmann's pouch, and dissection should proceed parallel to the cystic duct, from the gallbladder first. Once the fibrosis at this point has been divided, the triangle will open often, allowing the cystic artery and duct to uncoil several millimetres. An impacted stone in the pouch can make dissection here difficult but dislocation of the stone into the gallbladder fundus is simple and creates more room in the triangle.

Obstructed cystic duct

Gallbladder decompression may help in an obstructed cystic duct, and is best done by reinserting the sharp trocar into the right upper quadrant port and puncturing the fundus. The sucker is then placed down the port directly into the gallbladder and the bile or mucus aspirated. The fundal grasper is then reapplied over the defect.

Other problems

Abscesses around the gallbladder or an intrahepatic component may make dissection of the bed of the gallbladder difficult, but careful repositioning of the fundal traction, and swinging from side to side allows the dissection to be accomplished piecemeal.

Excess bleeding

The issue of bleeding from the gallbladder bed is usually dealt with relatively easily using diathermy. If the bleeding is issuing from the posterior surface of the original mesentery position, a small posterior branch of the cystic artery may be responsible. In the same way, any other bleeding should be sought meticulously, and controlled under vision. The blind application of clips into the region that was Calot's triangle or, worse still, diathermy, places vital structures at great risk. Excessive bleeding from this region may be one of the first signs of bile-duct injury. Local pressure with a grasper or a pledget often allows the situation to be controlled and then recovered. However, surgeons should be aware that clips may become caught in gauze squares introduced to apply pressure, and make the situation worse.

Bile-duct leakage

It is rare to see a bile leak intraoperatively without major damage. Occasionally a small duct of Luschka may be transsected in the bed of the gallbladder, but without distal obstruction, seldom leads to problems. If it is identified convincingly, and a cholangiogram has been normal, suture transfixion with drainage may be indicated. If any other injury is suspected, repeat cholangiography via the cystic stump usually elucidates the problem. At completion of their training, all trainees should be familiar with the types of bile-duct injuries and be acquainted with general principles of management. Suffice to say that the amount of damage is frequently underestimated by the original surgeon, excessive bleeding is a more common sign than an intraoperative bile leak, and adequate delineation of the damage is seldom possible by laparoscopy alone.

Complications of laparoscopic cholecystectomy

Inadvertent injury to the common bile duct

Inadvertent injury to the common bile duct is the most feared complication of laparoscopic cholecystectomy; unfortunately the incidence of this complication remains statistically higher than that for open cholecystectomy. It was envisaged that with better training the incidence of common bile duct damage would be reduced, but unfortunately this has not been borne out in recent publications of large series of patients from relatively experienced units. The apparently inevitable slightly increased risk of this complication must be explained to patients when obtaining their consent.

Various types of injury to the common bile duct have been described. The most common is that the common bile duct is mistaken for the cystic duct and clips are applied across it. Occasionally long segments of the common bile duct have been excised, requiring high hepatico-jejunostomies.

If a common bile duct injury is recognized during laparoscopic cholecystectomy, the procedure must immediately be converted to an open operation and the exact nature and extent of the damage carefully assessed. If local biliary expertise is available, this should be called upon. Repair of the damage depends on its nature and the availability of an experienced biliary surgeon.

The following are recommendations if common bile duct injury is recognized at operation:

1. If a Ligaclip™ has been applied across the common bile duct this should be removed. The common bile duct should be carefully inspected and if bile leakage is noticed a small-calibre T-tube should be inserted into the common bile duct. These patients are at increased risk of stricture formation at the site of injury and should be followed up with this in mind.

2. If damage to the common bile duct is not circumferential, but a part of its wall has been excised, a large-bore T-tube should be inserted into the opening in the common bile duct, which is then closed over the T-tube with interrupted sutures. If this produces undue tension, sutures should not be inserted as a stricture will certainly ensue. If the common bile duct damage is in its lower part, a side-to-side choledocho-duodenostomy should be performed. Where the damage is higher, a side-to-side hepatico-jejunostomy is the procedure of choice.

3. If a segment of the common bile duct has been resected, the treatment of choice is to perform a hepatico-jejunostomy.

This requires specialist biliary expertise and if an experienced biliary surgeon is not available, the best treatment is to insert a drainage tube into the proximal cut end of the common bile duct and retain it in place with a ligature. This should be brought out as an external drain. The distal cut end of the common bile duct should be ligated. The patient should then be referred to a specialist biliary centre for secondary repair.

It cannot be emphasized too strongly that a surgeon who does not regularly perform biliary surgery must not attempt to repair a damaged common bile duct.

Postoperative bile leakage

Postoperative leakage of bile may present as generalized biliary peritonitis, which generally necessitates an emergency laparotomy. At laparotomy, a clear delineation of the anatomy of the biliary tract must be made and the site of bile leakage identified. An intraoperative cholangiogram should be performed to exclude damage to a major bile duct. A T-tube should be inserted into the point of bile leakage and brought out externally.

If the postoperative bile leakage is contained within the subhepatic space, the patient may present with a tender swelling in the right hypochondrium. Ultrasound scanning confirms the presence of a fluid collection and needle aspiration is performed to confirm that it is a collection of bile. A pigtail catheter can then be inserted into the collection. If drainage persists from the pigtail catheter, the patient should have an ERCP or a PTC to delineate the biliary anatomy and ensure there is no obstruction to the biliary tree, as well as to confirm the site of the leakage. Bile leakage occasionally presents in the postoperative period, with excessive amounts of bile appearing in a suction drain placed at the completion of cholecystectomy. Often the cause is displacement of the Ligaclips™ on the cystic-duct stump. If this is confirmed by ERCP, and providing there is no distal obstruction, the patient can be allowed to settle with a period of drainage and stenting.

Evidence for the effectiveness of laparoscopic cholecystectomy

When laparoscopic cholecystectomy was newly introduced in the late 1980s, it was stated that a randomized trial of laparoscopic versus open cholecystectomy would be 'impossible to conduct' because the new procedure was clearly superior to open cholecystectomy. This was partly driven by media enthusiasm and the belief that 'keyhole' surgery was an unqualified advance. This statement was lamented 2 years later, after it became evident that the incidence of common bile duct and other visceral damage had risen steeply, causing a furore in American surgical and legal circles. Since that time, various randomized controlled trials between laparoscopic and open cholecystectomy have been reported. Most of the trials show only a small advantage for laparoscopic cholecystectomy in terms of hospital stay and time back to work, but there are wide variations, and most trials do not control for observer bias. Laparoscopic cholecystectomy may be associated with a better cosmetic result and reduced postoperative pain, but open cholecystectomy (small incision) is certainly quicker to perform in most hands. Unfortunately, the laparoscopic approach continues to be associated with a higher risk of bile-duct damage and patients must be clearly informed of this risk when explaining the procedures available.

Clinical problems

Asymptomatic gallstones

Indications for cholecystectomy have changed. Older patients are now considered, and in certain circumstances, asymptomatic gallstones may be treated by laparoscopic cholecystectomy. In this regard, diabetics, the porcelain gallbladder, and the barrel calculus are more traditional indications. Young women with small stones contemplating a family may represent a more recent indication, avoiding the situation of the jaundiced pregnant patient.

Gallstone pancreatitis

The timing of laparoscopic cholecystectomy in the patient with gallstone pancreatitis is controversial. The operation is technically difficult in the acute phase, with the hepatoduodenal ligament frequently oedematous, structures in Calot's triangle poorly defined, and delineation of the most distal part of the common bile duct to the ampulla difficult because of local oedema. Often in the acute situation the swollen peripancreatic tissues obscure visibility. If the operation is delayed until convalescence, there is the risk of a second attack. A suitable compromise time may be just prior to discharge from the acute attack. However, should diagnostic scanning show significant persisting peripancreatic swelling, further deferment may make completion of the case laparoscopically more certain. In any case, plans must be in hand for possible duct exploration.

Acute cholecystitis

Laparoscopic cholecystectomy in acute cholecystitis is a demanding and potentially difficult operation. The patient is frequently unwell, the timing less than optimal, and inflammation and oedema render the dissection difficult. Mirizzi syndrome is one of the most testing situations. When completed, cholecystectomy for acute cholecystitis allows rapid resolution of the disease, and the rapid improvement is gratifying. Important points for the acute case are the use of a good sucker, minimizing the use of irrigation until the gallbladder is removed, the best light source and camera available, selective decompression of the gallbladder and disimpaction of the stone to make the dissection easier. An experienced anaesthetist is essential. If the sick patient is on minimal muscle relaxants, it makes the working space small and any coughing causes instruments to move unpredictably.

Laparoscopic common bile duct exploration

The trend to deal with all stones in one procedure was usual with open cholecystectomy. This changed when laparoscopic cholecystectomy emerged, but the trend has now swung back. With a simple extension in technique, most calculi can be retrieved transcystically. Referring all patients for preoperative ERCP would swamp most gastroenterology units and expose a great number of people to an excessive risk from ERCP. Young women in particular are at risk of iatrogenic pancreatitis.

Laparoscopic common bile duct exploration, however, is an advanced laparoscopic procedure and should only be undertaken by experienced biliary surgeons who have the necessary laparoscopic expertise to perform this procedure. Exploration techniques depend on the anatomy. A long common segment with a low cystic–common bile duct confluence is not suitable for a laparoscopic approach by any means. A large stone in a dilated common bile duct, with a small cystic duct is not best treated by stone retrieval alone, and a formal drainage procedure may be indicated. In most cases, a small mobile calculus is seen in the distal common bile duct, and transcystic exploration can be effected. If need be, the cystic stump can be dilated with an embolectomy balloon to improve access. Transcystic exploration can then be achieved by either fluoroscopic guidance or under direct vision. The former requires less equipment. For the latter, a 4.5 Fr. flat-wire stone basket is delivered via the cystic stump either down a ureteric catheter as a sheath, or alone into the common bile duct, and using cholangiogram contrast material to outline the stone, it is basketed under fluoroscopy and retrieved. A completion cholangiogram is then obtained. If the surgeon is skilled in the use of a flexible choledochoscope, this obviates the need for continued X-ray screening, which is particularly contraindicated in the management of common bile duct stones in pregnancy. Choledochoscopy necessitates dilating the cystic stump to a greater degree, so that a flexible choledochoscope can be passed. These have a small working channel, and an ERCP stone basket can be introduced via the endoscope to basket the stone directly. Alternatively, the basket can be passed in a 'buddy' system beside the endoscope, and the stone basketed under vision. This allows the basket to be larger and to be moved independently of the endoscope.

Evidence of effectiveness of laparoscopic common bile duct exploration

Laparoscopic common bile duct exploration is a technically demanding procedure and remains in the domain of specialized centres or individual enthusiasts. Randomized studies of its effectiveness in comparison to open common bile duct exploration have not yet been reported.

Laparoscopic antireflux surgery

Gastro-oesophageal reflux disease (GORD) is one of the most common disorders affecting the upper gastrointestinal tract. The introduction of powerful acid inhibitors may allow healing of the oesophagitis which is associated with GORD, it is often a chronic or recurrent problem requiring costly long-term medical management in a high proportion of patients. Conventional open surgery for selected patients has been shown to be effective at curing reflux; however, this requires a laparotomy through a relatively long midline incision, because the oesophageal hiatus lies along the posterior abdominal wall and can be deeply situated. Moreover, the surgeons' hands need to be introduced into the incision to allow retro-oesophageal dissection and construction of the gastric wrap. Laparoscopic fundoplication is thus the treatment of choice for significant gastro-oesophageal reflux judged to require surgical intervention. However, it is a difficult operation, combining a three-dimensional dissection of the hiatus around a vulnerable structure, organ dissection, manipulation, and intracorporeal suturing.

Selection of procedure

Several laparoscopic antireflux procedures have been introduced, and improved results have been claimed for each of these individual variations. The wide variety of techniques available is testimony to the fact that none is clearly superior. Nissen fundoplication is the most commonly performed and involves wrapping a portion of the gastric fundus 360° degrees around the lower portion of the oesophagus. The aim of the operation is to augment the resting lower oesophageal sphincter pressure by reconstituting a length of intra-abdominal oesophagus. This, combined with crural repair, allows for an effective antireflux mechanism. Dysphagia is unfortunately quite common after any type of fundoplication and the 'floppy' Nissen wrap was introduced to reduce the incidence of this unpleasant complication. Similarly, the advocates of partial (less than 360°) fundoplication claim that this is associated with a lower incidence of postoperative dysphasia.

Preoperative assessment

All patients in whom antireflux surgery is being considered must be carefully assessed, both subjectively and objectively, and must undergo the following investigations:

1. **Endoscopy:** this is essential to assess the degree of oesophagitis and the size of the hiatus hernia, if present. Endoscopy would also reveal the presence of Barrett's oesophagus and biopsies must be taken to establish whether there is dysplasia.

2. **Oesophageal manometry:** this is important to exclude problems with oesophageal motility which cause problems with oesophageal emptying in the postoperative phase after fundoplication and result in a poor outcome.

3. **pH monitoring:** 24-hour pH monitoring is a useful investigation, especially in patients with symptoms of reflux but no endoscopic evidence of oesophagitis. It is also useful to assess any benefit objectively if the test is repeated postoperatively.

4. **Oesophageal motility:** this should also be assessed, ideally including pressure studies.

The operation

General anaesthesia is administered and the patient placed in a slightly sitting-up position with a small amount of hip flexion (a modified Lloyd-Davies position); with a significant degree of head-up tilt, the bowel is displaced distally and allows a better view of the operative field. Some surgeons like sequential com-

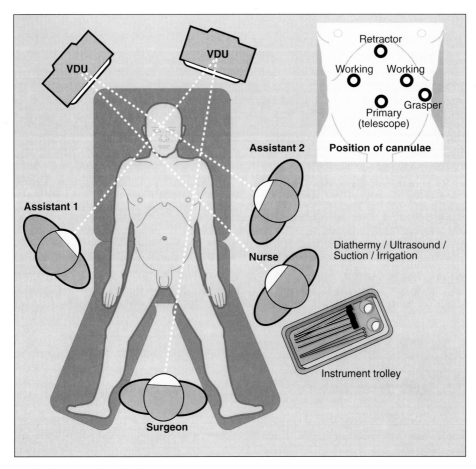

Figure 14.4 Theatre setup for laparoscopic anti-reflux surgery.

pression pneumatic stockings to have been fitted in the ward. Two monitors should be used, one on each side of the patient's head, so that the assistants can have an uninterrupted view. The operating surgeon stands between the patient's legs, the camera operator stands on the patient's right and the second assistant stands on the patient's left Fig. 14.4). After induction of anaesthesia, an orogastric tube is inserted, which will be removed on completion of the procedure. Whilst the operation is usually performed from between the legs using the umbilicus as the camera port, in an obese male this gives a poor view. For such patients, a left upper paramedian port gives a better view and allows more precise attention to be given to the splenic vessels. Ports are placed in an arc around the camera port, and all may be 5 mm diameter if a small clip applier is available. An epigastric stab incision is made for insertion of the liver retractor. It is helpful to have a rigid table-fixed device to hold this instrument and this also frees the assistant's hand. In addition, a monofilament suture is passed through the omentum laterally, gathering it up with repeated throws. In this way, it can be controlled with lateral traction on artery forceps outside the body to pull it away from the operative field. An atraumatic grasper is next introduced into the leftmost port. The fundus of the stomach is grasped as high as possible and pulled inferiorly and laterally by the assistant's left hand to retract the stomach away from the operating field. The phreno-oesophageal 'ligament' is next dissected. At no stage should the oesophagus be grasped.

A hook is used to carefully mobilize the distal oesophagus and any hernial sac is dealt with. The nerve of Latarjet is spared, and the diaphragmatic crus is dissected anatomically and displayed with particular reference to its posterior limit. A nylon or Teflon tape is passed around the oesophagus, brought out via the left port and traction applied. The oesophageal dissection is checked, and the short gastric vessels are divided in their upper half with a multifire clip applier. The vessels are carefully traced and divided progressively to reach the left side of the retro-oesophageal window.

Crural repair

Note that crural repair is now regarded as an essential component of this operation. Upward retraction of the oesophageal sling displays the lower part of the crura. These are repaired with two interrupted non-absorbable sutures. The knots placed can be constructed extracorporeally or intracorporeally, depending on the surgeon's expertise.

The crural repair is then evaluated and a phreno-oesophageal repair is fashioned.

Construction of wrap

Once crural repair has been performed and a satisfactory window behind the oesophagus created, the anaesthetist is requested to pass a 52–60 French gauge bougie into the patient's oesophagus and this is led under vision into the stomach. The presence of a large intra-oesophageal bougie is essential to allow the formation of a 'floppy wrap' to minimize the risk of post-operative dysphagia. An atraumatic grasper is passed through the right port behind the oesophagus, through the oesophageal window, and an appropriate part of the gastric fundus is fed into the atraumatic grasper. The grasper is pulled towards the right, bringing the gastric fundus along with it. The grasper holding the oesophageal sling can now be transferred to the portion of stomach behind the oesophagus and manipulated to the patient's right to keep it in place.

Three non-absorbable sutures (for a 2 cm wrap) are then placed between the portions of gastric fundus to the left and right of the oesophagus, and tightened over the bougie.

Completion

The bougie is removed and a final inspection made to ensure there is no undue tension on the wrap. Once a satisfactory inspection has been made, saline washout of the perihiatal area is recommended to remove blood spilled in the procedure. The omental stay suture is pulled through, the abdomen deflated, trocars removed, and the incisions closed with absorbable subcuticular stitches. Drainage is not necessary. A twice-daily dose of ondansetron is prescribed for the first 24 hours, to prevent all retching.

Postoperative care

The patient can be started on fluids the day after surgery and built up to a soft diet if tolerating fluids satisfactorily. If the dissection has been particularly traumatic, it might be wise to be cautious with oral intake in the early postoperative period.

Complications of laparoscopic fundoplication

- **Bleeding** from port sites may be troublesome. If this occurs, and does not stop with tamponade, it is best to underrun the vessel with a suture. An aberrant branch of the right hepatic artery running in the free edge of the lesser omentum is prone to inadvertent damage. This should be identified and be clipped and divided to prevent it bleeding. Some surgeons do not divide the short gastric arteries and they can occasionally bleed if the gastric fundus is insufficiently mobile to go round the oesophagus. It is a simple manoeuvre to divide the short gastric arteries, although there have been many large series where this has not proved to be necessary. Bleeding may also occur from inadvertent injury to the spleen or liver. Splenic injury is uncommon during laparoscopic fundoplication, but has to be borne in mind. It cannot be overemphasized that instruments should be passed in and out of the abdomen under direct vision to prevent inadvertent damage to viscera.

- **Pneumothorax**: dissecting the oesophageal hiatus risks damage to the pleura and a pneumothorax. This is evidenced by increased ventilatory pressures. The anaesthetist must be aware of this before operation. If a pneumothorax occurs, insertion of a chest drain may be necessary, although some reports suggest that conservative management may be successful.

- **Injury to vagus nerves**: the posterior vagus can be encountered during posterior dissection of the oesophagus. This should be identified and dissection should proceed posterior to the posterior vagus so that it can be included in the wrap. If the oesophagus is included in the suture that secures the wrap, the anterior vagus may be at risk and it is important to ensure that it is not damaged.

- **Gastric or oesophageal perforation**: the gastric fundus is liable to perforation if sharp instruments are used to grasp it or excessive traction is employed. This injury is avoidable if atraumatic instruments are used and the stomach wall handled with care. If perforation occurs and expertise is available, this can be sutured laparoscopically. Injury to the lower oesophagus is more serious and usually occurs during oesophageal dissection or passage of the bougie by the anaesthetist. Bougie placement should be performed under direct vision, because the tapered tip of the bougie can easily perforate a friable oesophagus.

- **Early wrap migration**: this is a serious postoperative complication and usually occurs if an adequate crural repair has not been performed. Occasionally the body of the stomach is inadvertently wrapped around the oesophagus and this can predispose to wrap migration. Excessive postoperative vomiting is another important risk factor.

- **Dysphagia**: this is unfortunately a common complication after fundoplication. The incidence of postoperative dysphagia is minimized by proper use of the bougie and ensuring that the wrap is loose. If there is any doubt about the tightness of the wrap, the sutures must be taken down and the wrap performed again.

Other serious complications reported in the literature include transsection of the oesophagus, and mistaking the vena cava for the oesophagus, resulting in massive haemorrhage, However, with adequate training and care these complications should not occur.

Evidence of effectiveness

Randomized trials between open and laparoscopic fundoplication are in progress but none has been published in full. Large prospective series show good results and these clearly improve with experience. Unfortunately, even in experienced hands there remains a significant (10 per cent) reoperation rate and this must be explained to patients when obtaining their consent.

Laparoscopic hernia repairs

Laparoscopic repair of inguinal hernia has not gained widespread acceptance despite early enthusiasm. Randomized trials have failed to show substantial benefits for this technique over conventional open hernia repairs in first-time hernia repairs.

However, the technique may be of benefit in patients with recurrent hernias, particularly multiple recurrences, because the surgeon operates in a virgin field and the risk to cord structures is minimized and the effectiveness of the repair is good. The method may also be indicated for bilateral hernias, which can easily be accomplished at a single operation, using a single piece of mesh, with little increase in operating time over that for a unilateral hernia.

Commonly used laparoscopic methods are the trans-abdominal preperitoneal technique, the intraperitoneal onlay mesh technique, and the extraperitoneal technique. The port site placement for the transperitoneal techniques is similar: a sub-umbilical 10 mm port is used for the telescope. Two further ports are inserted in the right and left iliac fossae, midway between the umbilicus and the anterior superior iliac spines. A 12 mm trocar is inserted on the side of the hernia being repaired and a 5 mm trocar on the contralateral side.

Transabdominal preperitoneal herniorrhaphy

An intra-abdominal peritoneal flap is created by incising and reflecting the peritoneum from the medial umbilical ligament to the anterior superior iliac spine 2 cm above the hernial defect. The flap is then mobilized downwards using sharp and blunt dissection. The inferior epigastric vessels and cord structure are thus exposed. For direct hernias, the sac is reduced from the hernial orifice using gentle traction. This leaves the preperito-neal fat behind. As the dissection continues inferiorly, Cooper's ligament and the iliopubic tract are exposed. The dissection is completed by mobilizing the cord structures away from the peritoneal flap. Direct hernias are much easier to manage than indirect hernias because of the much reduced risk to the vas and vessels passing through the internal inguinal ring.

For direct hernias, a large piece of mesh is placed directly over the defect, partly covering the internal inguinal ring. For indirect hernias, a slit has to be constructed in the mesh which is then wrapped round the cord structures as they pass through the internal ring. In the early days, the mesh was stapled into position but there is a trend to avoid stapling because of its potential for injury. This requires careful placement of a mesh external to the peritoneum. There has also been a trend towards larger and larger meshes which have been shown to minimize recurrences.

Intraperitoneal onlay mesh technique

In this technique, a mesh is placed directly over the defect without reflecting the peritoneum. This carries an increased risk of bowel adhesions to the mesh and bowel obstruction. Although results have not been as poor as might be anticipated, this now probably represents an outdated technique.

Extraperitoneal laparoscopic herniorrhaphy

Extraperitoneal inguinal hernia repair can be accomplished laparoscopically and this avoids the potential complications of entering the peritoneal cavity. However, if the peritoneum is likely to be adherent to the inguinal canal, as in recurrent hernias, the extraperitoneal route may not be appropriate. The technique requires dissection of the space of Bogros in the extra-peritoneal plane and dissecting out of the indirect sac if present. Dissecting the space is facilitated by using a proprietary distension balloon or a hydro-dissector. Some surgeons use the laparoscope to sweep the peritoneum away from the under-surface of the abdominal wall. A piece of tailored prosthetic mesh is then inserted and tacked into position, covering the deep ring and Hesselbach's triangle on its deep surface.

Evidence of efficacy of laparoscopic hernia repair

Randomized trials between open (mesh/darn) and laparoscopic hernia repairs have shown no clear benefit for the laparoscopic procedure, which is significantly (25–40 per cent) more expensive than the open method. However, evidence is emerging that postoperative analgesic requirements are lower and that the force required to safely operate a car brake pedal can be reached earlier after operation. Further trials are in progress but on current evidence laparoscopic hernia repair cannot be recom-mended as a substitute for Lichtenstein repair of primary inguinal hernias. Recurrences (especially those with multiple attempts at repair) and bilateral hernias may be more suitable for a laparoscopic approach but there is no scientifically controlled evidence for this at present.

Laparoscopic appendicectomy

Laparoscopy for the diagnosis of right iliac fossa pain has been performed for at least two decades, especially in continental Europe. It can be a valuable investigation in young women, particularly when the diagnosis of acute appendicitis is in doubt and the alternative diagnosis is pelvic inflammatory disease. If, however, the preoperative diagnosis is not in doubt then an open appendicectomy should be performed, as randomized trials of open versus laparoscopic appendicectomy have not revealed any advantage in favour of the laparoscopic technique. Unlike in open appendicectomy, it is not yet certain whether the finding of a normal appendix at diagnostic laparoscopy should be followed by laparoscopic appendicectomy in an attempt to prevent future problems.

Laparoscopic appendicectomy can be achieved using a variety of methods and port positions. The following technique has proved easy to teach, uses minimal disposable equipment, and is, above all, safe. The patient is placed flat, the bladder emptied, and prophylactic antibiotics are administered. The surgeon and assistant stand on the left side, facing a screen on the right. The umbilicus is cannulated in an open fashion and this port is used for insertion of the laparoscope. A pneumoperitoneum is created and the pelvic organs inspected. Substantial head-down tilt of the operating table helps to display the pelvic organs. The appendix is usually easily identified, especially if the inflam-mation is not too severe. If appendicectomy is to be proceeded with, then two 5 mm ports are placed under vision. The first port is in the midline at the upper border of the pubic hair and the second in the left iliac fossa. Through the midline port, bowel-grasping forceps are introduced with the left hand, and these remain as a static retractor. A commonly used alternative arrangement is to use a 5 mm port in the right hypochondrium and a 10 mm port between the subumbilical port and the anterior superior iliac spine.

The tip or midpoint of the appendix is grasped and elevated towards the right shoulder. Adhesions are mobilized either bluntly (if friable and acute), or with reusable bipolar diathermy forceps. A window is then created between the base of the appendix and the mesoappendix. The mesoappendix is ligated, usually with 2–3 ligatures, or coagulated carefully with bipolar forceps. The appendix base can be dealt with by ligature or, if an endostapler is available, the appendix and its mesentery can be stapled and cut in a single manoeuvre, making the procedure simple and quick. If ligation is to be used, a pre-tied endoloop is passed around the base and a further loop placed distally, leaving an appropriate cuff of appendix to divide. The appendix is then divided and removed. A 5 mm eyepiece is passed through the iliac fossa or suprapubic port and the appendix delivered into the 10 mm camera port without touching other structures. Irrigation can be performed under direct vision provided by the 5 mm eyepiece, and the operative site checked. Alternatively, the appendix can be delivered directly into the 10 mm port, removing the 10 mm eyepiece ahead of it, thus obviating the need for a 5 mm eyepiece.

An important point is the fixed retraction on the appendix, avoiding grasping and regrasping which potentially leads to trauma and soilage. Bipolar diathermy avoids the high concentration of current of monopolar diathermy through the thin wall of the caecum.

Finally, the umbilical port is closed, and the patient can return rapidly to a selective diet.

Evidence of efficacy of appendicectomy

Various trials of laparoscopic appendicectomy versus open appendicectomy have been reported but none has shown a clear benefit for the laparoscopic approach. In particular, the laparoscopic procedure has consistently longer operating times than the open method. On present evidence, laparoscopic appendicectomy cannot be recommended routinely as an alternative to open appendicectomy. Its main indication is where the preoperative diagnosis in female patients is uncertain and a diagnostic laparoscopy shows an inflamed appendix.

Splenectomy

Splenectomy for many haematological disorders can be accomplished laparoscopically. Laparoscopic splenectomy requires the spleen to be 'morselized' for delivery through a 12 mm port incision; thus, in the rare situation of a splenic tumour (where the splenic architecture needs to be preserved for pathological examination, requiring the spleen to be delivered intact) this technique is inappropriate.

The upper limit of splenic weight suitable for the laparoscopic technique has not been established clearly, although a good rule of thumb is that if the spleen is clearly palpable, the case is likely to be technically difficult. Disorders ideally suited to laparoscopic splenectomy are hereditary spherocytosis (where it may be combined with cholecystectomy), idiopathic thrombocytopenic purpura, and hereditary anaemias. The technique has the advantage of causing minimal disruption of tissue planes, and wound complications such as haematomas or infections in these patients appear to be uncommon.

Laparoscopic splenectomy requires the usual preoperative preparation. With the head of the table elevated and the surgeon standing on the right, access is gained via the umbilicus. The spleen is elevated using the left hand via an epigastric post and this allows the lower pole to be approached with a multifire stapler loaded with a vascular cartridge which is introduced via the left flank. The short gastric vessels and the splenic pedicle are taken in a stepwise manner, after clearly visualizing the pancreatic tail. The pedicle requires 5–7 fires and it is important to have this number of cartridges available. This technique does not require the use of a clip applier.

An alternative technique employs individual dissection of the short gastric vessels and their control with clips. After this, the spleen is elevated to reveal the splenic vessels. Laparoscopic dissection of the short gastric vessels is fraught with hazard, and simple stapling of the pedicle as described earlier, with the pancreatic tail under direct vision, avoids this.

Once dissected, the spleen is placed in a large specimen retrieval bag within the abdomen and morselized. The larger port sites are closed. Diet is usually recommenced immediately on recovery. The patient may be discharged when fit, to have appropriate platelet counts carried out by their haematologist.

Pericardial fenestration

This is a dramatic operation which can be performed quickly for certain indications and is a boon for medical teaching. In the less urgent case, malignant pericardial effusions may be treated with transabdominal laparoscopic pericardial fenestration. The typical patient is beyond cure, and frequently in extremis. An open laparoscopy is performed under general anaesthesia, using minimal insufflation pressure. A 20 mm square window is cut in the diaphragmatic central tendon with a diathermy hook. The effusion protects the heart from direct instrument trauma, but a pulling motion with the hook adds an extra level of safety. Once the tendon is breached, a torrent of typically bloodstained fluid emerges and the entire theatre fears the worst. The recovery of normal haemodynamics is already under way by the time the patient reaches the recovery room and the rate of clinical improvement seldom fails to impress.

Hepato-biliary surgery other than cholecystectomy
Biliary bypass

The situation of the jaundiced patient with an advanced pancreatic tumour is all too common. These patients can be well palliated using a laparoscopic bypass. This consists of a stapled cholecysto-jejunostomy, and a side-to-side stapled gastro-jejunostomy. Using the gallbladder has drawbacks, however, not least because the patency of the cystic duct must be confirmed by intraoperative cholangiography. The life expectancy in these patients is so short, however, that the long-term reliability of the new conduit seldom reaches significance. Most patients die at home, anicteric and with no more vomiting. For the patient who has had a previous cholecystectomy, a laparoscopic Roux-en-Y loop drainage is achievable but technically demanding.

Laparoscopic ultrasonography

Intraoperative ultrasound can give high-resolution imaging of the biliary tree, the intrahepatic anatomy, and the upper abdominal viscera. In the realm of hepatobiliary surgery, it allows high-resolution delineation of hepatic lesions and is particularly useful in planning liver resections. Pancreatic lesions can be sought and visualized and endocrine tumours can sometimes be localized. The relationship between the portal vein and the pancreatic tumour can be examined using contact alone, avoiding the radical 'trial dissection' phase of the standard Whipple's procedure.

Liver cyst marsupialization

Non-parasitic hepatic cysts are a tertiary referral condition, but can be effectively deroofed and marsupialized laparoscopically. Recurrence has been reported, but repeat treatment is feasible.

Upper gastrointestinal surgery

Perforated ulcer

Closure of the perforated peptic ulcer laparoscopically is well described. Important stages are the confident closure or patching of the defect laparoscopically, ruling out of malignant pathology in gastric ulcers, and above all, a thorough peritoneal toilet. A pressure irrigator allows several litres of warm irrigant to clear the peritoneal cavity of contamination under direct vision, to a degree not possible through a conventional small upper midline incision.

Heller's procedure for achalasia

Laparoscopic management of achalasia is a logical extension of fundoplication. A longitudinal myotomy is performed along the anterior of the oesophagus, and is continued beyond the angle of His. The procedure should include a fundoplication, or else troublesome postoperative gastro-oesophageal reflux is the norm. An anterior partial wrap is the preferred technique.

Highly selective vagotomy

The operation of vagotomy has almost disappeared, but there remain a few patients with recalcitrant ulcer disease, or intolerance of acid-suppression medication. Laparoscopic highly selective vagotomy can be achieved by a variety of techniques, including diathermy, argon-beam diathermy, cryoablation and laser ablation.

Bleeding peptic ulcer

Control of upper gastrointestinal tract bleeding using laparoscopic techniques requires accurate endoscopic localization, and a favourable ulcer site. A bulbar source on the posterior surface lends itself well, but an intragastric source is difficult to find unless a totally intragastric procedure is planned. This involves making a pneumogastrium, using a hernia balloon structural trocar. The source is controlled in the stomach or, if this fails, a resection is performed. None of these techniques is in common use: they are occasionally seen in centres where surgical intervention for upper gastrointestinal bleeding is common.

Oesophageal surgery

Preoperative laparoscopy allows staging and exclusion of inoperable abdominal disease. Involved paracrural nodes, easily missed on CT scanning, can be visualized, and subtle tumour dissemination clearly seen.

Staging laparoscopy

This allows accurate staging for upper GI malignancy and selection for neo-adjuvant treatment.

Gastric resection

Symptomatic benign gastric tumours can be well excised laparoscopically. A Polya-type anastomosis is preferred and is effected with a stapler.

Laparoscopic biopsy

An ideal indication for laparoscopy is staging and biopsy of intra-abdominal tumours of unknown origin or type. Haematological malignancies lend themselves well to biopsy, and lymph-node biopsy is reasonably straightforward. Accurate localization of lymph nodes with a recent CT scan avoids a haphazard search. Mesenteric deposits of lymphoma and metastases can yield tissue that allows confident diagnosis and staging beyond that of fine-needle biopsy. However, biopsy of resectable tumours is not encouraged.

Laparoscopy in trauma cases

In certain situations, laparoscopy for trauma may yield more information than CT scanning or peritoneal lavage. A breach of the peritoneum can be easily diagnosed, but hollow-viscus perforations can be difficult to exclude. A combination of an unknown missile trajectory, positive intra-abdominal pressure limiting small bowel effluent leakage, and difficulty in confidently examining the entire bowel make these difficult injuries to rule out with confidence.

Adhesiolysis

Elective

A small proportion of patients with well-localized abdominal pain in relation to scars benefits from laparoscopy and division of these adhesions. These must be divided with scissors, not monopolar diathermy, as the risk of conductive damage to the attached viscus is high.

Small bowel obstruction

This can be one of the most rewarding procedures to complete laparoscopically. Such obstruction is often due to a peritoneal band which can be easily divided laparoscopically, and in this situation the procedure can be completed quickly. The choice of port sites is made allowing the greatest distance possible between the scar or likely site of obstruction and the working ports. Note, however, that handling of the bowel itself has a high rate of perforation, and manipulation by the mesentery is far safer. As in open surgery, the principles are based on identifying collapsed bowel and tracing it proximally to the obstructing point.

Colorectal surgery

Stoma formation

Laparoscopic stoma formation is well suited to palliative situations, and formation of a loop ileostomy or colostomy can alleviate obstruction or control rectal effluent.

Resections

Colorectal resections for malignant disease should currently be undertaken only as part of randomized controlled trials. Concern over port site recurrence has dampened enthusiasm towards management of malignant disease in this way. Laparoscopic anterior resection of diverticular disease, however, can be accomplished with excellent results.

Incontinence and prolapse

Laparoscopic resection rectopexy can be used to manage prolapse and incontinence via an abdominal approach.

Endocrine and breast surgery

Adrenalectomy

Adrenalectomy can be accomplished via a transabdominal or a retroperitoneal approach. In many centres, it is the operation of choice for the management of non-malignant adrenal pathology, including phaeochromocytoma.

Axillary dissection

This has been reported laparoscopically for breast cancer staging but remains experimental.

Endoscopically assisted muscle-flap transfer

This has allowed mobilization of muscle flaps on vascular pedicles via a subcutaneous approach in reconstruction of the breast.

Vascular surgery

Sympathectomy

Cervical (thoraco-dorsal) sympathectomy is best performed thoracoscopically. It is the approach of choice for management of upper-limb hyperhidrosis and reflex sympathetic dystrophy, and can be used for temporary relief of Raynaud syndrome. Lumbar sympathectomy has also been reported.

Other procedures

Laparoscopic equipment has been used to good effect in endoscopic perforator ligation ('SEPS') and in endoscopically assisted saphenous vein harvest.

Bibliography

Bailey, I.S., Rhodes, M., O'Rourke, N., Nathanson, L., and Fielding, G. (1998). Laparoscopic management of acute small bowel obstruction. *Br. J. Surg.*, **85**, (1), 84–7.

Burke, E.C., Karpeh, M.S., Conlon, K.C., and Brennan, M.F. (1997). Laparoscopy in the management of gastric adenocarcinoma. *Ann. Surg.*, **225**, (3), 262–7.

Gotley, D.C., Smithers, B.M., Rhodes, M., Menzies, B., Branicki, F.J., and Nathanson, L. (1996). Laparoscopic Nissen fundoplication—200 consecutive cases. *Gut*, **38**, (4), 487–91.

Hansen, J.B., Smithers, B.M., Schache, D., Wall, D.R., Miller, B.J., and Menzies, B.L. (1996). Laparoscopic versus open appendectomy: prospective randomized trial. *World J. Surg.*, **20**, (1), 17–20.

Hollyoak, M.A., Lumley, J., and Stitz, R.W. (1998). Laparoscopic stoma formation for faecal diversion. *Br. J. Surg.*, **85**, (2), 226–8.

Korman, J.E., Ho, T., Hiatt, J.R., and Phillips, E.H. (1997). Comparison of laparoscopic and open adrenalectomy. *Am. Surg.*, **63**, (10), 908–12.

Moore, M.J. and Bennett, C.L. (1995). The learning curve for laparoscopic cholecystectomy. The Southern Surgeons' Club. *Am. J. Surg.*, **170**, (1), 55–9.

Stevenson, A.R., Stitz, R.W., Lumley, J.W., and Fielding, G.A. (1998). Laparoscopically assisted anterior resection for diverticular disease. *Ann. Surg.*, **227**, (3), 335–42.

Vittimberga, F.J. Jr, Foley, D.P., Meyers, W.C., and Callery, M.P. (1998). Laparoscopic surgery and the systemic immune response. *Ann. Surg.*, **227**, (3), 326–34.

CHAPTER 15

Organ transplantation

Nial Ahmad and Peter J. Friend

1 Introduction

Whilst the clinical practice of organ transplantation is comparatively recent, its potential has been appreciated for a great deal longer. In 1902 the French surgeon Alexis Carrell published his pioneering work on vascular anastomosis which became the basis of the current practice of solid organ transplantation (Carrel 1902). In the same year Emerich Ullmann, a Viennese surgeon first described experimental kidney transplantation (Ullmann 1902). It was also Carrel who observed the phenomena responsible for the failure of allografts and called these 'biological factors' (Carrel 1910). Williamson built on Carrel's work and in 1926 gave a description of transplant rejection along with its microscopic features. He also suggested the need for blood grouping for experimental animal transplantation. Between 1933 and 1946, Yu Yu Voronoy in the former USSR performed six human allograft kidney transplants, all with primary non function and subsequent loss of the grafts due largely to several hours of warm ischaemia and blood group mismatch (Hamilton 1984). In 1946, Hufnagel in Boston performed the first functioning renal allograft which was lost after three days probably due to rejection (Moore 1964). The principles of immunosuppression and organ preservation, the two fundamental arms of organ transplantation, remained largely unknown. The groundwork for transplantation immunology was established by Medawar and Gibson who in 1943 demonstrated the principles of the immune response to foreign tissue (Gibson 1943). However, at that stage, it was thought to be of only theoretical interest since no effective means existed to control the immune response. In 1953, Billingham, Brent, and Medawar described the experimental 'actively acquired tolerance' (Billingham 1953). Much experimental work followed in search of means to manipulate transplant rejection which would bring transplantation out of the laboratories and into regular clinical practice.

Seven years after Hufnagel's earlier attempt at the same hospital, the first successful human kidney transplant took place in Boston in 1953 (Hume 1955). A cadaveric kidney was transplanted into a 26 year old doctor with end stage renal disease. The kidney worked for six months after which the patient died suddenly of uncontrolled hypertension and recurrent renal failure. The discovery that identical twins share tolerance of each others antigens led to a series of successful 'twin' kidney transplants, mainly in Boston during the 1950s (Murray 1958). The pioneering work of Kolff in developing the artificial kidney 1947 and its further refinement, retarded the advancement of renal transplantation in the late 1950s (Kolff 1947).

Transplants were performed in the 1950s without immuno-suppression and there was no real success except in identical twins. In 1958, whole body irradiation was first used to suppress the immune response (Murray 1960). Despite success in preventing rejection, this was soon abandoned because of life threatening complications including bleeding and infection. The modern era of chemical immunosuppressive therapy started following the demonstration of the immunosuppressive effects of azathioprine in 1959 (Schwartz 1959). Roy Calne showed aza-thioprine to be effective in dog kidney transplantation (Calne 1960) and it was first used in human kidney transplantation in 1961 (Murray 1962). In 1962, the combination of azathioprine and steroids was shown to be beneficial and was rapidly adopted by most centres (Murray 1963). This combination remained the mainstay of clinical immunosuppression throughout the 1960s and 1970s and this period saw the rapid development of kidney transplantation in many centres across the world. A smaller number of centres pioneered the development of heart and liver transplantation; however the results in these groups remained poor because of the technical complexies of the procedures and the inadequacies of available immunosuppression. The first clinical liver transplant was carried out in 1963 by Starzl (Starzl 1969) and the first heart transplant in 1966 by Barnard (Barnard 1967).

The development and first clinical use of cyclosporine in 1978 by Calne in Cambridge (Calne 1979) marked a milestone in the development of transplantation. This drug was shown to be a highly effective immunosuppressant and was responsible for a substantial improvement in the results of renal transplantation. During the ensuing two decades, cyclosporine also facilitated successful heart, lung, and liver transplantation.

The increasing success and availability of transplantation has fuelled the demand as the therapeutic potential has become more widely recognized and facilities more available. As a result, the demand for transplantation exceeds the number of donors available and long waiting lists exist in most units. This has emphasized the need for careful recipient selection to ensure that the limited numbers of available organs are offered to patients most likely to benefit from them.

2   Organ donation

The clinical practice of organ transplantation depends upon the provision of human organs in good condition. The majority of transplanted organs are from cadaver donors the great majority of whom are donors who are brain-dead and have an intact circulation. A smaller number of donors for kidney transplantation are 'non-heart-beating'—this necessitating rapid removal of the kidneys from the donor after the cessation of the circulation. Increasingly, in kidney transplantation, donor organs from living donors are used; this practice is now being extended into liver transplantation. Many of the ethical and legal debates that have surrounded transplantation over the years have been centred on organ donation issues.

2.1 Brain death

Heart-beating, ventilated donors have to have fulfilled the criteria for brain death. The two most important sets of criteria for this purpose are the *Harvard criteria* (Ad hoc Committee 1968) and the *UK Code* (Conference of the Royal Colleges 1976). The UK code, agreed upon by the Royal Colleges in 1976, is more widely employed and is simpler because the diagnosis of brain stem death can be made on clinical tests alone (Table 15.1), whereas the Harvard criteria require an EEG to confirm brain stem death.

The concept and diagnosis of brain death has been closely linked with the development of clinical transplantation, but it is important to note that the need to define death as an irreversible loss of brain function is a consequence of the development of modern intensive care and mechanical ventilation rather than the requirements of transplant surgeons. In the days before artificial ventilation, a massive injury to the brain would inevitably lead to cessation of respiration followed shortly by cardiac arrest, such patients are now ventilated. With respiratory function supported artificially, cardiac output is maintained in the absence of any neurological input from higher centres.

The UK code for the diagnosis of brain stem death is summarized as follows:

Preconditions for testing:

a. A positive clinical diagnosis of the cause of irreversible brain injury

b. Patient must be deeply unconscious and ventilated

c. Exclusion of other causes for the neurological state

- ◆ CNS depressant drugs
- ◆ Hypothermia ($< 35°C$)
- ◆ Neuromuscular paralysing drugs
- ◆ Metabolic or endocrine disturbance
- ◆ Other reversible cause

Absent brain stem reflexes

a. Pupils fixed and unresponsive to light

b. Absence of vestibulo-ocular reflex (eye movement in response to ice cold water applied to each ear)

c. Absence of corneal reflex

d. Absence of motor response within the cranial nerve distribution in response to stimulation of appropriate somatic areas

e. Absence of gag reflex or response to bronchial stimulation by endotracheal suction catheter

Apnoea

Absence of respiratory movements when patient is disconnected from the ventilator for long enough for pCO_2 to rise above the threshold for respiratory stimulation (6.65 kPa)

Other considerations

a. Doctors carrying out the tests: The tests are carried out by two doctors clinically independent, and specialists in the areas of neurology, neurosurgery, anaesthesia and intensive care or general medicine

b. Repetition of testing: The tests are repeated by the same specialists after an undefined interval

The diagnosis of brain death based upon these criteria, as practised in the UK, has been shown to be reliable and, because it does not rely upon complex special investigations, can be applied to patients in any hospital. In some other countries, the use of electroencephalography or cerebral blood flow studies is practised; there is no evidence that these investigations are helpful in the diagnosis of brain death—indeed false positive and false negative results can occur.

2.2 Management of the heart-beating donor

The majority of organs for kidney transplantation, almost all livers and all donor hearts are from brain dead, heart-beating donors. Until the diagnosis of brain death has been made, the management of the brain-injured patient is wholly directed to an attempt to minimize the injury to the brain with maintenance of cerebral perfusion by reduction in brain swelling. This usually necessitates powerful diuretic treatment and fluid restriction; this often leads to hypovolaemia and may compromise the perfusion of potentially transplantable organs.

As soon as the diagnosis of brain death is confirmed, the management of the donor is redirected towards the optimization of the function of the transplantable organs. In general this requires replacement of fluid, with concomitant attention to electrolyte balance; treatment with inotropic agents is also frequently required. Brain death is associated with marked haemodynamic changes, partly as a consequence of the massive overactivity of the sympathetic nervous system—the 'sympathetic storm'—and partly due to hormonal and other changes. Donors may be difficult to manage for this reason. However, careful attention to the management of the circulation of the donor is critical to the function of transplanted organs. Indeed, by using invasive monitoring and correction of cardiovascular parameters, it is now clear that viable organs can be

retrieved from donors that would otherwise be deemed unsuitable.

2.3 Non-heart-beating donors

The success of transplantation has increased the demand for the treatment of end stage organ failure. During the same time the availability of suitable donors has not kept pace and, in recent years, there is evidence of a reduction in donor numbers. Waiting lists for all types of transplantation have increased. For this reason there is renewed interest in expanding the number of transplants by the use of organs from donors who have died following circulatory arrest. This implies an inevitable period of warm ischaemia of the organs and consequent damage. This precludes the use of non-heart-beating donor organs for heart, lung and liver transplantation, in which immediate function of the transplanted organ is essential to patient survival. However, renal transplantation can be carried out successfully because the patient can be maintained on dialysis whilst awaiting recovery of the transplanted kidney.

Such patients may be those suffering from an irreversible neurological disease (for example a cerebral tumour) in which case death may be predictable. Alternatively, many patients are admitted to Accident and Emergency centres having died suddenly and unexpectedly. The duration of warm ischaemia is critical to the success of transplantation—if this extends beyond 60 minutes the likelihood of long-term success is greatly diminished. The logistic aspects of this procedure are, therefore, considerable, requiring a very rapid response and cooling of the organs (usually by cannulation of the aorta via the femoral artery) before transferring the donor from the Accident Department to the operating theatre.

2.4 Living donation

Living donors have played a major role in kidney transplantation in several countries, especially in those where cadaveric donation is difficult for cultural or legal reasons but also in a number of Western countries including the USA and Scandinavia. In recent years living donation has played an increasing role in kidney transplantation in the UK, with some units now obtaining 25% of donor kidneys in this way. Living donors are usually genetically related to the recipient, although there is a recent trend towards the use of donors who have a strong emotional relationship but who are genetically unrelated (usually between spouses). The results are better following living donor transplantation, particularly if the donor and recipient are HLA identical. Much of the benefit is related to using an organ removed under ideal conditions and transplanted with minimal delay; even when transplanted across a substantial HLA mismatch between genetically unrelated patients, the long-term outcome of this procedure is better than that of comparable cadaveric grafts.

There are important considerations in relation to the donor. It is essential that all attempts be made to reduce the risk to the donor who therefore requires a very full medical assessment. It is important to ensure that the decision of the donor to proceed is not the result of coercion and that the donor is fully informed of the nature and risk of the procedure. Although the risks of the operation are small, deaths have occurred and less severe complications are not uncommon. There are probably few nephrological implications following the removal of one kidney from a healthy donor; the long-term follow-up studies which have been carried out do not suggest a significant risk of hypertension, proteinuria, or renal failure.

In recent years, living donors have been used for other organ transplants. Considerable experience now exists in the transplantation of part of the liver of a living donor; initially this procedure was developed to enable the transplantation of paediatric patients, usually from parental donors. This has now been extended to the transplantation of adults, requiring removal of a larger proportion of the liver, often the right lobe. The greatest experience of this procedure is in Japan where, for legal reasons, cadaveric transplantation has not developed. The risks to the donor are greater than in kidney donation and a number of deaths have been reported.

Living donors have also been used for lung transplantation and pancreatic transplantation, both in small numbers.

2.5 Legal and ethical aspects of organ donation

Consent

The increasing success of organ transplantation has widened the spectrum of diseases for which such treatment is appropriate. There is a considerable disparity now between the requirement for donor organs and the supply. Despite much publicity over the years, it appears likely that a large number of potential organ donors are not referred to transplant centres. Different policies have been adopted in various countries in an attempt to improve this situation. In the UK, organ donation is based upon an 'opt in' system. People are encouraged to carry a donor card which states their willingness to become an organ donor in the event of their death. Even if a card is carried, the next of kin of a potential organ donor is always asked for consent before organ donation. Elsewhere in the world, a system of 'opting out' has been tried. All citizens are regarded as potential donors unless they have stated their objection to this during their lifetime. In certain parts of the USA, a system of 'required request' exists. Under this system any doctor who is looking after a potential donor is required to ask the next of kin for their consent for organ donation.

There is no good evidence that any one of these systems is superior to the others in terms of maximizing the available number of organs. Evidence would suggest that increasing education of the general public and, most importantly, other members of the health care professions is likely to be of greatest benefit. The highest donor rates in Europe are in Spain, where it is agreed that a highly effective system of local, hospital-based transplant coordinators has led to a very large proportion of donors being identified.

Commercial aspects

The long waiting lists for transplantation have led to some concern over the possibility of a trade in human organs, either cadaveric or from living donors. It has been agreed by the members of the International Transplantation Society that organ donation should not be carried out with the intention of financial benefit.

Allocation

Organ transplantation is unusual among medical therapies in the developed world in that it is an effective treatment that is limited by a factor other than funding. Transplant surgeons and physicians have to decide which of many possible patients should receive a transplant. Increasingly it is agreed that scarce organs should, in general, be allocated in such a way as to provide the maximum net benefit. Although this is a logical principle, in effect it leads to very difficult choices and clearly has to be modified according to circumstances at the time.

3   The donor procedure

The criteria governing suitability for organ donation vary according to the organ to be transplanted and, to some extent, by the clinical urgency of an individual recipient (this applying particularly to extra-renal organs). The majority of organ donors are suitable for multi-organ donation with removal of kidneys, liver, heart, and lungs. In addition, pancreas transplantation is carried out on a limited basis and, most recently, there is considerable interest in small intestinal transplantation. It is possible for all these organs to be removed from an individual donor without significant compromise to the function of any of them.

Maintenance of the donor is of critical importance in the period between the diagnosis of brain death and removal of the organs. Heart beating organ donors have usually suffered a major intracranial catastrophe such as haemorrhage, trauma, ischaemia or tumour, and their management will, up to the time of certification of brain death, usually have involved fluid restriction and diuresis in order to reduce cerebral oedema. Many donors develop diabetes insipidus which may exacerbate the negative fluid balance. The management of an organ donor preoperatively is primarily to optimize the perfusion of all organs. This may require intensive management of fluid and electrolyte status and the careful use of inotropic agents.

The donor operation is usually carried out via a long incision opening both sternum and abdominal cavity. The liver is fully skeletonized so that it remains attached only by its vascular connections. The kidneys may be mobilized in a similar way although many units now prefer to remove the kidneys after *in situ* perfusion. Heparin is given, the heart mobilized, and cardioplegia infused into the aortic root. If the lungs are to be removed, this is usually carried out *en bloc* with the heart. The intra abdominal organs are perfused via cannulae placed into the abdominal aorta and the portal vein (via the inferior mesenteric vein). Once the heart has stopped, the intra abdominal organs are perfused with cold preservation solution. All organs are excised rapidly to avoid warming *in situ* and packed in preservation solution on ice.

4 Organ preservation

Hypothermic storage of organs is a well established method of organ preservation. The aim of transplant preservation is to protect the organ during the cold ischaemic period and to provide viable and functional tissue upon reperfusion. In the early 1960s, Belzer described continuous hypothermic machine perfusion of kidneys for transplantation (Belzer 1967). Later Collins described successful 'cold flush preservation' without the need for machine perfusion (Collins 1969). Although the former method is still used in some centres in the USA, flush preservation and static storage is most widely practised worldwide. University of Wisconsin solution developed in the late 1980s is widely used for multi organ procurement and is accepted as the most effective preservation solution to date (Ploeg 1988). Other solutions in clinical use are Eurocollins (EC), Hyperosmolar citrate (HOC), Phosphate buffered sucrose (PBS) and Histidine-Tryptophan-Ketoglutarate (HTK)

A harvested organ is subjected to two types of ischaemia; *cold ischaemia* during its storage and *warm ischaemia* during transplantation. An inadvertent period of warm ischaemia may occur during organ procurement if the heart stops before perfusion or if prolong dissection is needed after perfusion. A transplant organ is particularly vulnerable to injury at the time of reperfusion, a complex phenomenon mediated partly by formation of oxygen free radicals. Attempts to prevent this injury by manipulation of preservation solutions and donor and recipient pre-treatment has been only partly successful.

There is a considerable discrepancy between different organs as regards maximum acceptable preservation times. The function of a transplanted heart or lung appears to deteriorate rapidly after 4–6 hours of cold ischaemia, but recent developments in liver preservation enable cold ischaemia times of 18 hours or more. In kidney transplantation, it is common for cold ischaemia times to range between 24 and 36 hours.

4.1 Matching of donor and recipient

Recipients of organ transplants are matched to the available donor organ and this is one of the keys to the success of the transplant.

Age and size

Kidneys from donors at extremes of age do less well. For example, there is a 10% lower graft survival at one year when the donor is below the age of 5 and many centres do not use kidneys from donors under 2 years. Although there is no strict upper age limit owing to the shortage of donors, most centres do not use kidneys from donors over 75 years. Although there is no proven advantage in matching the ages of donor and recipient, as a general rule, kidneys from older donors are transplanted into older recipients. Size matching is much more important in liver, heart, and lung transplantation and there is no absolute lower age limit for these organs. Recently, the practice of reduced or split liver grafts, as well as living donor liver grafts has partly helped to overcome the donor shortage especially for paediatric recipients.

Blood group

ABO blood group compatibility is a prerequisite for solid organ transplants. On occasions this is over-ruled in emergency liver transplantation, but with generally poor results.

Tissue type

Tissue typing to match donor and recipient for histocompatibility antigens has greatly improved graft survival. For example, long-term kidney transplant graft survival is increased by 20% with a 6 antigen match as compared to a 6 antigen mismatch.

Antigen expression on the surface of cells is genetically controlled by the major histocompatibility complex (MHC), located on chromosome 6. Six major loci, A, C, B, D, DR, and DQ have been defined; in addition a number of minor antigens exist. The practice of matching donors and recipients on the basis of HLA typing at A, B, and DR loci is well established in renal transplantation. Although there is good evidence for improved long-term graft survival in well matched grafts, the advantages of tissue typing are partly offset by the logistic complexities involved. The best match between donor and recipient can be achieved if the most suitable recipient can be chosen from a large pool of potential candidates. For this reason a national organ sharing network ensures that kidneys can be transferred to the transplant centre with the appropriate recipient on their waiting list. Tissue typing, patient selection, and transport of the organ adds considerably to the ischaemia time of the graft.

Tissue typing is practicable only in kidney transplantation for several reasons. Firstly, the constraints of organ preservation are more demanding in transplantation of liver, heart, and lungs and little time is available for tissue typing before selecting the most suitable recipient. Secondly, there is no long term maintenance support for patients requiring liver, heart, or lung transplants equivalent to renal dialysis. Dialysis enables large numbers of potential kidney transplant recipients to be maintained in relatively good health, often for years. The waiting lists for other organs are therefore much smaller, substantially reducing the likelihood of achieving a good HLA match, even in the absence of other constraints. Thirdly, the survival advantage for well matched liver, heart, or lung transplants is not as well established as for kidney transplants. Indeed, recent studies have shown that there is no advantage for tissue typing in liver transplantation.

Thus, although tissue typing is carried out in most solid organ transplants, it is of direct practical significance mainly for kidney transplants.

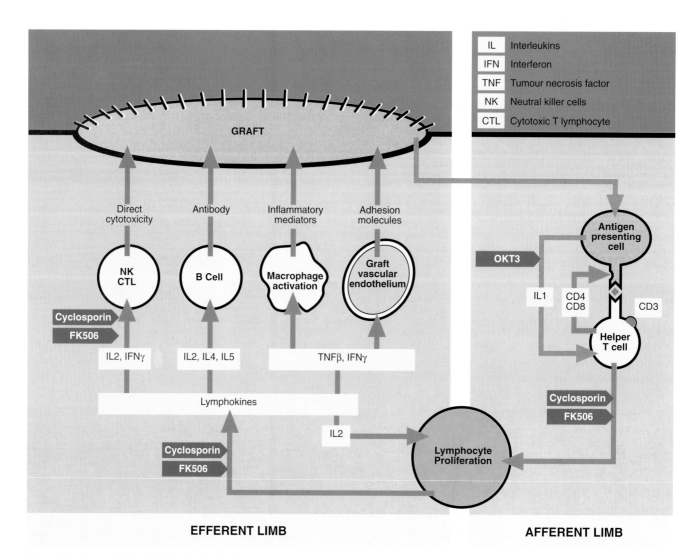

Figure 15.1 Immunological Mechanism involved in rejection.

Cytotoxic crossmatch

A lymphocytotoxic crossmatch is usually performed immediately prior to renal transplantation in order to demonstrate preformed antibodies in the recipient against donor lymphocytes. A complement-dependent lymphocytotoxic assay is routinely used to demonstrate anti-HLA antibodies in transplantation.

The immune response

Rejection of a vascularized organ transplant is conventionally classified into three groups:

◆ *Hyperacute rejection* is manifest by rapid destruction of graft tissue, usually within minutes or hours of transplantation. This occurs in recipients with preformed antibodies to donor antigens and is the result of complement activation, platelet aggregation, and thrombosis leading to ischaemic necrosis. Hyperacute rejection can be prevented by screening recipients for lymphocytotoxic antibodies before transplantation. Liver

grafts, however, can be successfully transplanted despite the presence of preformed cytotoxic antibodies against the donor.

◆ *Acute rejection* typically occurs within six to eight days of transplantation in the absence of effective immunosuppression. This is a cell mediated immune response initiated by the recognition of foreign histocompatibility antigens within the graft. The 'afferent arc' involves presentation of graft antigens by antigen-presenting cells to the appropriate T-cells of the recipient. This induces proliferation and activation of the relevant clones of lymphocytes. The 'efferent limb' of the rejection response involves destruction of the graft. This requires cytotoxic T-cell lysis as well as non-specific mechanisms such as activation of macrophages and neutrophils which induce an inflammatory response (Figure 15.1).

◆ *Chronic rejection* usually occurs months or years after transplantation. It is characterized by progressive ischaemic atrophy of the graft as a result of arterial lesions. The presentation of chronic rejection varies with different organs. In kidney transplantation, it is manifest by progressive arteriolar obliteration together with tubular atrophy and interstitial fibrosis. With passage of time, the kidney contracts and distinction between cortex and medulla is lost. In liver transplantation, chronic rejection is commonly manifest by the 'vanishing bile duct syndrome' together with arteriolar wall thickening. In heart transplants chronic rejection presents as accelerated coronary artery disease and in lung transplantation as obliterative bronchiolitis. The aetiology of chronic rejection is almost certainly multifactorial and the end-product of a number of different injuries to the organ including preservation injury, ischaemia-reperfusion injury, acute rejection and viral infection.

Immunosuppression

The immunosuppressive agents available at present produce a relatively non-specific effect and render the patient susceptible not only to infection but also to malignancy. The infection risk is both from common pathogens and from organisms that do not normally cause pathology in immunocompetent individuals—'opportunist' infections including cytomegalovirus and pneumocystis. The risk of malignancy is restricted to certain tumours; in particular transplant patients are at greatly increased risk of skin tumours and lymphoma. The objective of immunosuppressive treatment after transplantation is to titrate the total dose of immunosuppression to prevent rejection but to avoid these adverse effects.

4.2 Azathioprine

The first chemical agent demonstrated to have effective immunosuppressive properties was 6-mercaptopurine which could prevent rejection of renal allograft in dogs. Subsequently, azathioprine was shown to have a higher therapeutic index. Azathioprine is converted in the body to 6-mercaptopurine and becomes incorporated into DNA where it interferes with nucleotide synthesis. Use of this drug alone is limited by its myelotoxicity and it is normally used in combination with other agents.

4.3 Corticosteroids

Shortly after the discovery of azathioprine in the early 1960s, it was shown that a combination of azathioprine and corticosteroids both provided effective immunosuppression and reduced the myelotoxic effect of azathioprine.

The pharmacological effects of steroids are very complex and this class of drugs interacts with the immune system in many ways. Steroids are very widely used in both long-term immunosuppressive maintenance and the treatment. However, steroids have many unwanted side effects. Acute side effects include impaired wound healing, peptic ulceration, sodium and water retention, impaired carbohydrate metabolism, and psychosis. Chronic side effects include skin changes, characteristic redistribution of fat (Cushing's syndrome), growth retardation, cataracts, myopathy, osteoporosis,and avascular necrosis, particularly of the femoral head.

Although highly effective in suppressing the immune response, the side effects of steroids are life threatening and disfiguring and limit the usefulness of this class of drug.

4.4 Cyclosporine

Cyclosporine is a lipophilic cyclic endecapeptide extracted from the fungus *Tolypocladiun inflatum*. It was identified in 1972 during a search for antifungal agents. It blocks the action of calcineurin and inhibits the activation cascade involved in lymphokine synthesis by activated T-cells. The drug was first used in clinical practice in Cambridge in 1978 and is now a major component of most immunosuppressive protocols world wide (Calne 1979). Its introduction led to improved renal graft survival at one year of 20%. Many trials comparing cyclosporine with steroids and azathioprine have since confirmed its benefit in both graft and patient survival. Cyclosporine facilitated the development of heart, lung, liver, and pancreas transplantation during the 1980s.

Cyclosporine has major toxic side effects which are compounded by its narrow therapeutic index and wide individual pharmacokinetic variations. Regular monitoring of plasma levels is needed, at least in the early phase of treatment, to establish a safe and effective dose. The most serious side effect is nephrotoxicity. This effect may be acute, with reduced glomerular filtration and renal plasma flow during the first week of treatment. Chronic toxicity is characterized by interstitial fibrosis and vascular lesions involving glomerular and arteriolar vessels. Early cyclosporine nephrotoxicity is reversible by dose reduction but chronic toxicity is irreversible and often progressive. It may be difficult to distinguish chronic cyclosporine toxicity from chronic rejection of a renal allograft. However, cyclosporine toxicity has been well documented in patients with non renal disease, as has progression to chronic renal failure in such patients.

Neurological side effects are common in cyclosporine treated transplant recipients. The most common manifestations are seizures, tremors, paraesthesia, headaches, visual disorders, and peripheral neuropathy. Other common side effects of cyclosporine therapy include hypertension, hypercholesterolaemia, hirsutism, gingival hyperplasia and, less commonly, hepatotoxicity.

When cyclosporine was first used, it was seen as an opportunity to avoid steroid treatment and patients were treated with cyclosporine alone. In recent years, however, there has been a trend towards the use of multiple drug therapy, with a combination of two or three drugs, including cyclosporine. This enables lower doses of each drug to be used, thereby reducing the risk of the side effects associated with each drug. There is no consistent evidence as to which of the various drug combinations is the most effective.

4.5 Tacrolimus

Tacrolimus (FK506) was developed in the 1980s (Kino 1987). It is a naturally occurring antibiotic derived from the fungus

Streptomyces tsukubaensis. It was first used clinically in Pittsburgh (Starzl 1989), followed by multicentre trials in USA and Europe with encouraging results (US Multicentre Liver Study Group 1993; European Multicentre Liver Study Group 1994). Many centres now use tacrolimus routinely for liver transplant recipients and selectively for renal transplant recipients, especially those with refractory rejection. The drug remains the agent of choice in small bowel transplantation.

Although tacrolimus is structurally different from cyclosporine, its mechanism of action is similar. Like cyclosporine, it is a calcineurin antagonist and inhibits T-cell activation and proliferation. In early studies in liver transplantation, tacrolimus was shown to have some advantages over cyclosporine in terms of rejection rate. Serum levels of the drug are closely monitored, as with cyclosporine. Tacrolimus also has serious toxic effects including nephrotoxicity, neurotoxicity, and hyperglycaemia (leading to insulin requirement in some cases)

4.6 Mycophenolate

Mycophenolate mofetil is a further immunosuppressive drug which has recently become available and is used as part of multidrug combinations. It inhibits the 'de novo' pathway of purine synthesis in lymphocytes and has been shown to be an effective inhibitor of both t and B cell function. Clinical trials in kidney transplantation showed a reduction in the incidence of acute rejection when used in combination with cyclosporine and steroids. Gastrointestinal side effects may limit the use of this drug in some patients.

4.7 Polyclonal antilymphocyte globulin

The potential advantages of using a 'biological' rather than a 'chemical' system were recognized many years ago when it was shown that polyclonal antilymphocyte serum (ALS) has a powerful immunosuppressive effect. ALS is prepared by immunizing an animal (horse, rabbit) with human lymphoid cells or purified thymocytes. For clinical use, the IgG fraction is isolated from the serum (antilymphocyte globulin, ALG and antithymocyte globulin, ATG). Purified ALG and ATG contain high levels of antibodies directed against human lymphocyte antigens, thus eliminating T-lymphocytes from the circulation. These preparations have been have been in use since the 1960s and been shown to be effective in preventing and reversing cellular rejection.

The effectiveness of treatment with ALG or ATG depends on their ability to induce lymphopenia, a state which is reversible after stopping treatment. The main and potentially most serious adverse reaction is hypersensitivity effects and serum sickness due to administration of foreign proteins. A test dose (intravenous or subcutaneous) and administration of steroids and antihistamines with the first dose prevent such reactions. Peripheral administration is likely to cause phlebitis and the agents should be given via a central venous catheter. The limitations of polyclonal antilymphocyte globulin include variability between manufacturers and batches, reactivity with

cells other than lymphocytes, the risk of serum sickness, lymphoproliferative disorders on prolonged use and the high cost of these preparations.

4.8 Monoclonal antilymphocyte antibodies

A monoclonal antibody is secreted by a *hybridoma*, a cell line produced by the fusion of a myeloma cell line and spleen cells from an animal which has been immunized with the appropriate antigen. From the variety of hybridomas produced from a single fusion, the appropriate cell line is identified and isolated. A hybridoma secretes only one antibody; and growth of that cell line therefore results in a continuous production of that particular antibody.

A monoclonal antilymphocyte preparation avoids most of the limitations of the polyclonal preparations described earlier. Until recently, the only commercially available monoclonal antilymphocytic antibody was OKT3 (Ortho Cilag). This antibody recognizes the CD3 antigen on the surface of T lymphocytes which is intimately linked to the T-cell receptor (Figure 15.1). The antibody exerts its immunosuppressive effect in two ways: first, the interaction of OKT3 with its target leads to modulation of the CD3/T-cell receptor complex on the surface of the lymphocyte, rendering the cell unable to respond to its corresponding antigen. Second, OKT3 causes cell lysis through the process of opsonization. However, this agent is not free from adverse effects. In 90% cases, the first dose is followed by fever, chills, and malaise. Fortunately, severe complications are rare but can include acute pulmonary oedema and aseptic meningitis. The former can be mitigated by ensuring that the patient is not fluid overloaded prior to treatment.

OKT3 has been widely used to reverse steroid resistant allograft rejection. More recently, it has been employed as an 'induction' agent. For this, the antibody is given for 10–14 days after transplantation to prevent early allograft rejection and to reduce the immediate requirement for other agents

Recently two new monoclonal antibodies have been registered, both of which recognize the interleukin-2 receptor, which is present on the surface of t-cells only when activated. These antibodies, which have been engineered to contain largely human protein in order to reduce the risk of immunization, have been shown to reduce the incidence of acute rejection when given as a short 'induction' course after transplantation.

4.9 Complications of immunosuppression

Several effective immunosuppressive agents are available but their use is constrained by the consequent risks of infection. As a result, the dose of immunosuppression has to be carefully titrated to suppress rejection adequately without increasing the risk of infection to unacceptable levels. When rejection episodes occur, these are usually treated with short courses of very high dose steroids or an antilymphocyte preparation (polyclonal or monoclonal).

Infections in immunosuppressed patients may be caused by organisms similar to those seen in other branches of surgery.

However, 'opportunistic' infections tend to occur in immuno-suppressed patients. These include protozoal (e.g. pneumocystis carinii), viral (e.g. cytomegalovirus, Epstein-Barr virus), fungal (e.g. cryptococcus, Aspergillus) and yeast (e.g. candida) infections.

Patients receiving long-term immunosuppression also have a greater risk of malignancy than a normal age matched population. The pattern does not follow the usual distribution of malignancy; many common malignancies (lung, colon, breast, prostate) are no more common than in the normal population but lymphomas and squamous cell carcinomas of skin occur much more frequently in transplant patients.

Several potential mechanisms for this have been postulated, including impaired immune surveillance, susceptibility to oncogenic viruses (e.g. Epstein Barr virus), chronic low grade immune stimulation and direct carcinogenic effects of the drugs.

5 Kidney transplantation

Kidney transplantation is carried out for patients in chronic renal failure. Patients have nearly always been established on a programme of haemodialysis or peritoneal dialysis and have been maintained in a stable condition for as long as required to obtain a suitable donor organ. The main groups of primary renal disease for which transplantation is commonly offered include pyelonephritis, glomerulonephritis, diabetes mellitus, hypertension, and adult polycystic kidney. Advanced age is a relative contraindication. As a general rule, transplant is not offered if the chance of patient survival is less than that of the graft. Primary diseases with a high incidence of recurrence in the transplanted kidney, such as Goodpasture's syndrome, focal and segmental glomerulosclerosis (FSGS), and primary oxalosis also constitute strong contraindications. Many patients with end stage renal disease have associated cardiac and vascular problems which need to be assessed and treated prior to transplant

As mentioned earlier, a significant minority of kidney transplants are carried out using a living donor. In the UK, this is nearly always a relative who has been shown to have two kidneys with normal function and anatomy and with a tissue type which is either identical or a very close match. In other countries, donation between, for example, husband and wife is considered acceptable. However any practice which includes the payment of money in exchange for a donor organ is considered unethical and has been banned in the UK.

The requirements for a cadaver donor include a maximum age of 70 years, normal renal function, and no strong evidence of hypertension or arterial disease. As with all organ donors, a history is taken for hepatitis B and HIV and serological examination performed.

The technical aspects of renal transplantation have been well established for many years (Figure 15.2). An extraperitoneal approach is used in the iliac fossa, exposing the iliac vessels and bladder. The renal vessels are anastomosed end to side to the iliac vessels. Usually both vein and artery are anastomosed to the external iliac vessels, though it is possible to carry out an end to end anastomosis between the internal iliac artery of the recipient and the renal artery of the donor. After carrying out the vascular anastomoses the kidney is re-perfused. The ureter is then implanted into the bladder. Several techniques are used for this: the simplest is direct suture of the spatulated end of the ureter into the dome of the bladder using interrupted absorbable sutures. Various anti-reflux techniques have been used but there is little evidence of benefit.

An initial diuresis is encouraged by giving high doses of diuretic agents at the time of reperfusion. Some centres also use renal dose dopamine routinely for the first 48 hours to support

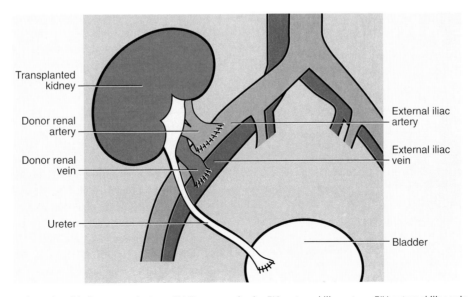

Figure 15.2 Kidney transplantation. RA, Donor renal artery; RV, Donor renal vein; EIA, external iliac artery; EIV, external iliac vein;

renal function. Most transplanted kidneys function immediately but a proportion fail to do so (delayed graft function), usually as a consequence of preservation-induced acute tubular necrosis. These patients require regular dialysis until adequate kidney function is established. Maintenance immunosuppression therapy is started at the time of surgery or immediately afterwards. Heparin prophylaxis is started to prevent DVT and graft thrombosis.

Patients are closely monitored in the early postoperative period. Good hydration is vital and monitoring of CVP is ideal for this purpose. Most transplanted kidneys produce large quantities of dilute urine in the immediate postoperative period before the concentrating power returns. At that point a reducing fluid regimen is instituted. Early graft dysfunction can have several causes (see Table 15.1), the most common ones being dehydration, rejection, drug toxicity (cyclosporine), infection and obstruction. Any deterioration in graft function is manifest by a drop in urine output and should be promptly and adequately investigated. An ultrasound scan combined with either Doppler or DTPA scan (for perfusion) and a percutaneous biopsy of the graft are usually performed. Cyclosporine levels are regularly monitored and doses adjusted accordingly. The usual time for first rejection is at the end of first week but a rejection episode within the first five days may be due to preformed antibodies in the recipient. Rejection episodes are first treated with pulses of high dose steroids, usually intravenous methyl prednisolone. Steroid resistant rejection can be treated with polyclonal or monoclonal globulin or changing cyclosporine to tacrolimus . Patients are also monitored closely for the development of infection, either bacterial infections in the early postoperative phase such as UTI or chest infection, or opportunist infections later. Most units routinely treat patients with low dose co-trimoxazole in order to prevent development of pneumocystis. In the event of active CMV infection, the agent gancyclovir has proved to be of considerable benefit. This drug is currently under trial for prophylaxis against CMV in recipients of a CMV positive organ. After an uncomplicated kidney transplant, the patient is likely to be able to leave hospital in approximately ten days.

The one year graft survival rate following kidney transplantation depends upon several factors including the quality of the donor organs and the proportion of medically high risk recipients transplanted. Most centres in the UK achieve 85–90% graft survival at one year.

Approximately 1600 kidneys are transplanted in the UK each year, but this is much less than the demand, with over 4000 patients waiting for kidney transplantation.

6 Liver transplantation

The first clinical liver transplant was carried out in 1963 by Starzl but the technical complexities of the operation and the problems inherent in operating on patients with liver failure meant that the first medium term success was not achieved until 1967 (Starzl 1969). During the 1970s liver transplantation was carried out in a small number of centres, notably by Thomas Starzl in Denver, Colorado and Roy Calne in Cambridge. The advent of cyclosporine as the major immunosuppressive agent led to a rapid expansion of liver transplantation throughout the world during the 1980s.

Contraindications for liver transplantation may be absolute, including extra-hepatic malignancy, active alcohol abuse and AIDS or relative including cardiac or pulmonary disease, advanced age, past malignancy, psychiatric disorders, HIV infection, and hepatitis B DNA positivity.

From merely an experimental procedure in the 1960s and 1970s, liver transplant has now become the established treatment for end stage liver disease. In 1983, the National Institute of Health declared liver transplant as a therapeutic modality for end stage liver disease with calls for its broader application (National Institute of Health 1984).

There are four major categories of patient who are potential liver transplant recipients: chronic liver failure, acute liver failure, primary liver tumours, and inborn errors of metabolism.

6.1 Chronic liver failure

This is the largest group of potential liver graft recipients. Chronic liver failure can be due to a wide variety of causes, particularly post hepatitic, auto-immune, primary biliary cirrhosis, sclerosing cholangitis, and alcohol induced liver damage. The indication for transplantation is determined by the development of life threatening complications of liver disease, particularly recurrent variceal haemorrhage, encephalopathy, spontaneous bacterial peritonitis, and diuretic resistant ascites.

The issue of disease recurrence is particularly important in patients with chronic hepatitis secondary to hepatitis B infection. This is the commonest cause of chronic liver disease world wide but, unfortunately, the majority of patients develop recurrent hepatitis B in the transplanted liver with resultant recurrent liver failure within a few years. The issue of transplantation for patients with alcohol induced liver disease remains controversial. It is however, generally agreed that there is a small but important subgroup of these patients who are abstinent, have insight into the nature of their alcohol addiction and who are deemed psychologically acceptable. Such patients,

Table 15.1 Causes of early renal graft failure

Prerenal	Dehydration
	Renal artery thrombosis
	Renal vein thrombosis
Renal	Acute tubular necrosis (preservation induced)
	Rejection
	Drug nephrotoxicity (cyclosporine)
	Infection (Pyelonephritis, CMV)
Post-renal	Ureteric (Clot, kink, leak, anastomotic stricture)
	Pre-existing disease (Prostatic hyperplasia, urethral stricture)

after successful transplantation, do remain at risk from recurrent alcohol addiction but, nevertheless, have proved to be a highly successful group of liver transplant patients.

The timing of liver transplantation in chronic liver failure may be difficult to judge. Clearly it is important that the operation should be carried out before the patient is so sick that the morbidity and mortality of the procedure rises. On the other hand it is difficult to justify an operation for a patient who, without surgery, is likely to live for several years. As a general rule transplantation is offered if the patient has a survival chance of less than one year or an intolerable quality of life or both. Most of these patients have advanced portal hypertension and abnormal coagulation presenting particular problems for surgery.

6.2 Acute liver failure

Patients with acute liver failure may require emergency liver transplantation. The most common causes of acute liver failure are viral hepatitis, ingestion of hepatotoxic substances (e.g. paracetamol poisoning), and idiosyncratic drug reactions. A number of clinical and biochemical features have been identified to define patients who will die without transplantation. These include the degree of encephalopathy, metabolic acidosis, coagulopathy, raised bilirubin, low serum albumin, raised intracranial pressure and degree of renal impairment. As a rule transplantation is not offered to patients with grade I and II encephalopathy. A significant proportion of these patients will recover spontaneously, but there are no prognostic criteria to predict which patients will deteriorate. Many patients in grade IV encephalopathy already have secondary organ damage (brain, kidney). It is therefore important that the decision to proceed to emergency transplantation is made before the patient has suffered irreparable brain damage secondary to liver failure

and to enable as much time as possible to obtain a suitable organ for transplantation.

6.3 Primary liver tumours

Patients with primary liver tumours may be suitable candidates for liver transplantation. These patients tend to have a lower morbidity from the operation as liver function is usually normal and portal hypertension rare. However, despite every attempt to exclude patients with extra hepatic malignancy, the incidence of tumour recurrence remains high. Patients with liver tumours in excess of 4 cm in diameter or which are multifocal are at a very high risk of recurrence. For the same reason, patients with secondary liver tumours with very rare exceptions are no longer regarded as suitable candidates for transplantation.

6.4 Inborn errors of metabolism

Liver transplantation may be indicated in a wide variety of inborn errors of metabolism in which a normal liver enzyme system is deficient with potentially lethal consequences. Conditions successfully treated by liver transplantation include primary hyperoxaluria (in which combined liver and kidney transplantation is usually performed), alpha-1 anti-trypsin deficiency, Wilson's disease, glycogen storage disease, and hypercholesterolaemia. The indication for transplantation in such patients depends upon the specific complications of the condition.

6.5 Budd-Chiari disease (hepatic vein thrombosis)

Most patients with acute Budd-Chiari disease are candidates for emergency liver transplantation. Indications for transplantation

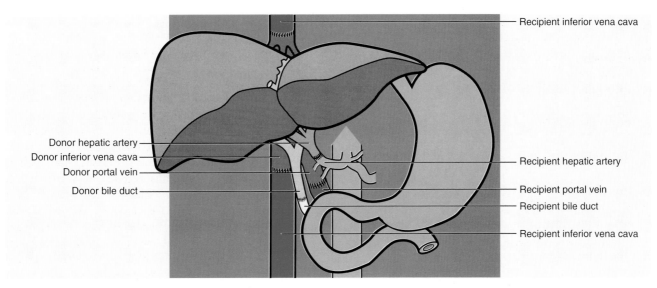

Figure 15.3 Liver transplantation. In a standard liver transplant operation donor hepatic artery, portal vein and bile duct are anastomosed end to end to that of the recipient. Inferior vena cava (IVC) is anastomosed in continuity with the recipient's IVC. HA$_d$, Donor hepatic artery; HA$_r$, Recipient hepatic artery; PV$_d$, Donor portal vein; PV$_r$, Recipient portal vein; CBD$_d$, Donor bile duct; CBD$_r$, Recipient bile duct.

in acute Budd-Chiari are encephalopathy, jaundice, ascites, abdominal pain, and portal hypertension. Half the patients with chronic Budd-Chiari will need transplantation, the main indication being intractable ascites and portal hypertension. Aetiology of acute Budd-Chiari remains unknown in most cases and these patients will remain at risk of developing further thrombotic episodes even after transplantation.

6.6 Techniques of liver transplantation

Almost all liver transplants are orthotopic. Heterotopic auxiliary liver transplants have been performed for certain conditions with claims of benefit (Terpstra 1988); but the indications for this are uncertain and there are major technical difficulties. Orthotopic liver transplant operations involve complete mobilization of the liver leaving its vascular connections intact. These are then clamped and the liver excised. The donor liver is transplanted by anastomosing the suprahepatic inferior vena cava, the infrahepatic inferior vena cava, the portal vein, the hepatic artery and the common bile duct. The bile duct anastomosis is usually between donor and recipient common bile ducts; if the recipient bile duct is diseased (as in sclerosing cholangitis in adults or biliary atresia in children) a Roux loop of jejunum is constructed with a choledochojejunostomy (Figure 15.3).

The use of veno-venous bypass during transplantation remains somewhat controversial. The standard bypass system involves venous drainage from the inferior vena cava (approached from the groin) and portal vein, and inflow via the axillary or internal jugular vein. This system uses heparin bonded tubing and a centrifugal pump to avoid the need for heparinization. In some units this system is used for all adult patients. However, some patients are able to tolerate clamping of the inferior vena cava without a catastrophic fall in cardiac output and surgeons in some centres prefer to carry out the operation without bypass. Bypass is not generally used in paediatric liver transplantation.

Immunosuppression therapy is started at or after transplantation. Common regimens in use are cyclosporine, azathioprine, and steroids. Some centres have recently started using tacrolimus (FK506) as the standard drug in place of cyclosporine. All patients are given prophylactic antibiotics.

Postoperatively, patients are monitored closely in an Intensive Care Unit. Immediate graft function is essential to the survival of the patient. In recipients with primary graft non function, emergency re-transplantation is necessary within one or two days if the patient is to survive. Liver function tests are followed closely. Common causes of early graft dysfunction include preservation injury, rejection, cholangitis, and cholestasis. Any derangement in liver function is investigated, usually by means of an ultrasound scan and percutaneous needle biopsy of the graft.

Biliary complications are common after liver transplantation (5–15%). Early anastomotic leaks may be related to bile duct ischaemia. Biliary strictures may develop later from ischaemia or immunological factors. Management of these complications involves either stenting or surgical biliary reconstruction.

Infections, particularly cholangitis, should be promptly treated with antibiotics. Some centres routinely use co-trimoxazole prophylaxis against pneumocystis and gancyclovir against cytomegalovirus (if the donor is CMV positive and recipient CMV negative). Fungal sepsis is also common and should be vigorously treated.

Vascular complications, particularly hepatic arterial thrombosis (2–5%), are significant causes of morbidity and have a higher incidence in children. Hepatic artery thrombosis usually presents as acute graft failure or, when occurring later, with biliary complications. Although arterial thrombectomy may be successful, treatment usually requires emergency re-transplantation.

Rejection is common and most patients are treated for an episode of acute cellular rejection during the early postoperative weeks, usually successfully. Some refractory rejection episodes respond to switching of cyclosporine to tacrolimus (Starzl 1989) or vice versa. Chronic rejection in liver transplantation is manifest as obliteration of bile ducts in the portal tracts and obliterative arteriolitis. This does not respond to increased immunosuppression and usually requires re-transplantation.

The risk of recurrent disease is high in three groups of patients: chronic active hepatitis secondary to hepatitis B, alcoholic liver disease and liver tumours. As the indication for transplantation in these patients not clearly defined, the only means to circumvent the problem is careful patient selection.

6.7 Results of liver transplantation

The long term results of liver transplantation are very satisfactory, with an 80% graft survival at one year now being achieved by most major centres. There is a low attrition rate beyond one year with most complications which lead to graft loss or patient death occurring within months of surgery. There is relatively little evidence of the long-term graft loss that continues to plague both renal and heart transplantation.

6.8 Paediatric liver transplantation

The indications for paediatric liver transplantation have quite a different pattern from adults: nearly half are for congenital biliary atresia with other main indications including inborn errors of metabolism, hepatitis, cholestatic liver diseases, and liver tumours.

The outcome following paediatric liver transplantation is as good as for adults. A major advance has been the use first of reduced adult grafts and, later, the use of liver splitting. This has enabled the use of a liver from an adult to be transplanted into a small (less than 10 kg) child. As a result, the waiting list for paediatric liver transplantation has been substantially reduced. More recently, segmental grafts from parental donors has further improved the access to transplantation for very small children, although this has not been carried out widely in the UK.

7 Heart transplantation

In 1964 Hardy transplanted a chimpanzee's heart into a 68 year old man (Hardy 1964). The patient died after one hour due to poor cardiac output. The first human allograft heart transplant was carried out by Barnard in 1967 and led to an initial period of enthusiasm which soon waned as the immunological problems became apparent (Barnard 1967). Since the advent of cyclosporine, the results of cardiac transplantation have greatly improved and the procedure is now widely practised across the world.

The main indications for cardiac transplantation are end-stage cardiac failure secondary to cardiomyopathies, ischaemic heart disease, and congenital heart disease.

With the improving success of heart transplantation, the indications expanded rapidly such that transplant activity is now greatly constrained by donor availability. Donor criteria are more stringent than for kidney or liver donors, particularly in respect of age and previous medical history.

The recipient operation requires a median sternotomy, cardiopulmonary bypass and cooling. Implantation is carried out by anastomosing both the atria, the pulmonary artery, and the aorta.

Cellular rejection is a common postoperative complication which is diagnosed by endomyocardial biopsy. Endomyocardial biopsy is carried out on a regular basis during the first three months after surgery. The requirement for immunosuppression is relatively higher than that for kidney and liver transplantation and infection constitutes one of the major postoperative risks. The most important cause of later postoperative death is accelerated coronary artery disease in the transplanted heart. This is manifest as progressive narrowing of the coronary vessels and is thought to represent chronic rejection. The incidence of this complication appears related to the severity of early graft rejection. The condition may be diagnosed by annual cardiac angiography but it may present as sudden death from myocardial infarction. This usually presents without chest pain because the heart is denervated by the surgery.

8 Lung transplantation

Initial attempts to transplant the lung alone encountered many problems, in particular with bronchial healing. The earliest clinical success was in 1981 with a combined heart and lung graft. More recently techniques have been developed to enable successful single or double lung transplantation.

Patients who may be suitable for lung transplantation fall into four groups:

1. Patients with chronic fibrotic lung disease, for example idiopathic pulmonary fibrosis, may be treated successfully by single lung transplantation. The graft is more compliant and has a lower vascular resistance than the remaining lung and therefore receives preferential perfusion and ventilation

2. Patients with obstructive lung disease, for example emphysema, may be treated with single lung transplantation

3. Patients with infective lung disease, particularly cystic fibrosis and intractable bronchiectasis, require removal of both diseased lung because of the risk of infection. Either heart-lung transplantation or bilateral lung transplantation has been used successfully in these patients. In the event of an essentially normal heart being removed from the recipient, this can be transplanted into a second recipient ('domino transplantation').

4. Patients with pulmonary vascular disease, particularly primary pulmonary hypertension, have usually been treated by combined heart-lung transplantation. Right ventricular function sometimes, however, recovers after transplantation in some of these patients who undergo single lung transplantation

Donor selection criteria are even more restrictive for lung than for heart transplantation. Donors who have been ventilated for a prolonged period are likely to develop pulmonary oedema and infection and are generally unsuitable. Size matching of donor and recipient is critical; it is judged from chest X-rays, employing a formula based on the donor's height and weight. Lung donor procurement is usually carried out as part of multi-organ retrieval. In addition to pre-donation heparinization, prostacyclin is given to dilate the pulmonary vascular bed. A pulmonary artery cannula is inserted for pulmonary perfusion in addition to the usual aortic cannula. After cessation of the circulation, the trachea is cross-stapled with the lungs inflated.

For combined heart-lung transplantation, the recipient operation is carried out via a median sternotomy. The heart and lungs are removed with the donor on cardiopulmonary bypass. The pericardium is incised, taking care to preserve the parts of the pericardium containing the phrenic nerves. The donor heart-lung block is placed in the recipient thoracic cavity and the tracheal anastomosis carried out before the right atrial and aortic anastomoses.

Single lung transplantation can be carried out without cardiopulmonary bypass although this may become necessary and must therefore be available. The operation is carried out through a posterolateral thoracotomy. Double lung transplantation is carried out through a bilateral anterior thoracotomy, crossing the midline as a sternotomy. The lungs are transplanted sequentially.

Postoperatively, patients are monitored closely for evidence of infection or rejection. Rejection is diagnosed by observing deteriorating pulmonary function and by transbronchial biopsy. Patients use their own spirometer daily to measure FEV_1 and FVC; a decrease of 5–10% indicates infection or rejection. Chronic rejection is manifest by obliterative bronchiolitis and presents as progressively reducing pulmonary function. Transbronchial biopsy demonstrates a peribronchial infiltrate of mononuclear cells. Lymphoproliferative disease is a major cause of morbidity and mortality in lung transplant recipients. This may be related to the Epstein Barr virus and sometimes responds to lowering the level of immunosuppression.

9 Pancreas and islet cell transplantation

Combined kidney and pancreas transplantation is offered at some centres to carefully selected patients with type I diabetes mellitus and nephropathy. Pancreas-only transplantation is offered in some centres to diabetic patients with severe progressive neuropathy, insulin resistance, and frequent hypoglycaemia. Pancreas-only transplantation is not a treatment for uncomplicated diabetes mellitus for two main reasons: first, there are insufficient suitable donors and second, replacement of a relatively simple routine of insulin therapy by more complicated and hazardous immunosuppressive treatment cannot be justified. The survival of vascularized pancreas graft at one year is about 85%.

The pancreas is retrieved usually from a young multiorgan donor, with the entire pancreas removed en bloc with the second part of the duodenum. The superior mesenteric and splenic arteries are joined on table using an iliac bifurcation graft. The most common technique of implantation involves vascular anastomosis to the external iliac vessels, usually on the right side and anastomosis of the duodenum to the dome of the urinary bladder (Figure 15.4). Postoperatively, progress is monitored by blood glucose estimation, urinary and serum amylase levels, duplex Doppler scanning and percutaneous renal biopsy or DTPA radionuclide scanning. A cystoscopic transduodenal biopsy of pancreas is helpful in some cases. The initial drainage of the pancreas into the urinary bladder can be electively converted to enteric drainage after few months once the transplant function is fully established. There is now a trend towards draining the pancreas into the intestine as a primary procedure.

Pancreatic islet cell transplantation remains an experimental procedure rather than established treatment for diabetes mellitus. The main limiting factors at present are technical difficulties in isolating pancreatic islet cells and problems of rejection.

10 Small bowel transplantation

Small intestinal transplantation is performed in few centres around the world in highly selective patients with intestinal failure (Abu-Elmagd 1992). Causes of irreversible intestinal failure range from congenital atresia, volvulus, gastroschisis, and necrotizing enterocolitis in neonates to massive resections in Crohn's disease, desmoid tumours, and mesenteric vessel thrombosis. The limiting factors are mainly organ specific: first, the small bowel is highly immunogenic and responsible for a high incidence of rejection; second, the intestinal mucosa is highly sensitive to hypoxia which makes preservation difficult; third, the bacterial content of bowel combined with mucosal sensitivity to ischaemia and rejection render infection a major problem.

Most small bowel transplantation has been from cadaveric donors, although live donors have been used. Implantation is performed by anastomosing the superior mesenteric artery to the aorta and the superior mesenteric vein (SMV) to the inferior vena cava. Venous drainage into the portal system is technically difficult and does not provide any proven benefit. The proximal end of the donor intestine is anastomosed to native jejunum and the distal end is brought out as a stoma. This helps in maintaining mucosal nutrition and conditioning. High dose Tacrolimus-based immunosuppression is maintained

Postoperatively, the patient is started on enteral feeding as soon as there is evidence of intestinal motility. The mark of success of small bowel transplantation is the ability to maintain

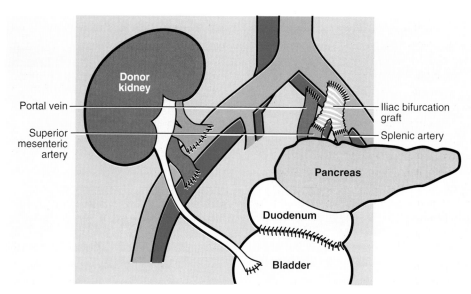

Figure 15.4 Combined kidney and pancreas transplant. SMA, superior mesenteric artery; SA, splenic artery; IBG, iliac bifurcation graft; PV, portal vein.

the patient off TPN. The distal end may be anastomosed in continuity with the residual bowel at a later date.

The demand for intestinal transplantation is small. If the outcome of the procedure were at the same level as kidney or liver transplantation, it would become the treatment of choice for intestinal failure. At present, however, approximately 40% of patients can expect to benefit from this procedure in the medium to long-term and the treatment of choice for uncomplicated intestinal failure, therefore, remains carefully managed total parenteral nutrition. In the UK, experience with small bowel transplants has been limited to a relatively small number of transplants at Cambridge, Birmingham, and Leeds

11 Multivisceral and cluster grafts

Complete multivisceral transplantation and upper abdominal cluster transplantation for malignancies involving liver and pancreas have been performed in a handful of patients with some success (Starzl 1989a, 1989b). The indications for this very radical procedure are rare.

12 General issues in organ transplantation

Transplantation is seen as an expensive, high technology form of medical therapy that benefits a few patients and has faced criticism from those who feel that limited health care resources should be allocated elsewhere. The early developments in transplantation were focused upon achieving biological survival and overcoming the major technical and immunological barriers to success, but with widespread introduction of this form of therapy, more fundamental issues now have to be addressed.

Although transplantation as a single procedure is relatively expensive, the benefits that can be achieved are relatively great. A successful transplant can free a young and otherwise productive individual from either a life of chronic disability or premature death. A huge proportion of health care resources are expended on people who are older but the majority of transplant patients are middle aged or young. Analyses of the true benefits of transplantation are now being carried out, using such measures as Quality Adjusted Life Years (QALYs) gained in order to achieve some measure of the real benefit and not only the biological survival.

The need for organ donation is fundamental to transplantation and has raised a number of ethical issues. The concept of brain death in an individual with an intact circulation is widely accepted and no fundamental objections are raised by the major religions of the world. Of the developed countries, only Japan did not (until recently) accept the legal concept of brain death.

The potential for transplantation is likely to increase as the results improve. Of fundamental importance is the development of better methods of immunosuppression. If the long term goal of donor-specific immunological tolerance were achievable, it would free recipients from the long-term complications of immunosuppression, which is the major cause of morbidity and mortality in the late postoperative phase. If this occurs, it will further broaden the spectrum of conditions for which transplantation may be appropriate.

There is a resurgence of interest in the concept of xenografting, by utilizing animals that have been genetically engineered in such a way as to circumvent the xenograft response. This would clearly remove the restriction of donor availability but would raise new ethical issues. However, a number of scientific obstacles need to be overcome before this becomes a reality.

Further reading

Allen, R.D.M., Chapman, J.R. (1994). *A manual of renal transplantation*. Edward Arnold, London.

Calne, R. (ed). (1987). *Liver transplantation*. Grune and Stratton,

Morris, P.J. (1994). *Kidney transplantation,* 4th edition. WB Saunders, London.

Neuberger, J., and Lucey, M.R. (1994). *Liver transplantation: practice and management*. BMJ Publishers, London.

Wallwork, J. (ed.). (1989). *Heart and heart-lung transplantation*. WB Saunders, London.

References

Abu-Elmagd, K., Fung, J.J., Reyes, J. *et al.* (1992). Management of intestinal transplantation in humans. *Transplant Proc.*, **24**, 1243–4.

Ad hoc Committee of the Harvard Medical School. (1968). A definition of irreversible coma. *JAMA.*, **205**, 337–40.

Barnard, C.N. (1967). The operation. *S. Afr. Med. J.*, **41**, 1271–4.

Belzer, F.O., Ashby, B.S., Dunphy, J.E. (1967). 24 hours and 72 hours preservation of canine kidneys. *Lancet*, **2**, 536–9.

Billingham, R.E., Brent, L., Medawar, P.B. (1953). 'Actively acquired tolerance' of foreign cells. *Nature*, **172**, 603.

Calne, R.Y. (1960). The rejection of renal homograft inhibition in dogs by 6-mercaptopurine. *Lancet*, **1**, 417.

Calne, R.Y., Rolles, K., White, D.J.G. *et al.* (1979). Cyclosporine A initially as the only immunosuppressant in 36 recipients of cadaveric organs: 32 kidneys, two pancreas and two livers. *Lancet*, **2**, 1033–6.

Carrel, A. (1902). La technique operatoire des anastomoses vasculaires et la transplantation des visceres. *Lyon Med.*, **98**, 859–64

Carrel, A. (1910). Remote results of transplantation of kidney and spleen. *J. Exp. Med.*, **12**, 146.

Collins, G.M., Bravo-Shugarman, M., and Terasaki, P.I. (1969). Kidney preservation for transplantation. Initial perfusion and 30 hours ice storage. *Lancet*, **2**, 1219–22.

Conference of Medical Royal Colleges and their Faculties in the UK. (1976). Diagnosis of brain death. *BMJ.*, **2**, 1187–8.

European FK506 Multicentre Liver Study Group. (1994). Randomized trial comparing tacrolimus (FK506) and cyclosporine in the prevention of liver allograft rejection. *Lancet*, **344**, 423–8.

Gibson, T.M., Medawar, P.B. (1943). The fate of skin homograft in man. *J. Anatomy*, **77**, 299–310.

Hamilton, D., Reid, W.A. (1984). Yu Yu Voronoy and the first human kidney allograft. *Surg. Gynecol. Obstet.*, **159**: 289–94.

Hardy, J.D., Kurrus, F.D., Chavez, C.M. *et al.* (1964). Heart transplantation in man. Developmental studies and report of a case. *JAMA*, **188**, 1132–40.

Hume, D.M., Merrill, J.P., Miller, B.F., and Thorn, G W. (1955). Experience with renal homotransplantation in humans: report of nine cases. *J. Clin. Invest.*, **34**, 327–81.

Kino, T., Hatanaka, H., Hashimoto, H. *et al.* (1987). FK506, a novel immunosuppressant isolated from Streptomyces. I. Fermentation, isolation and physicochemical and biological characteristics. II. Immunosuppressive effects of FK506 in vitro. *J. Antibiot.*, **40**, 1249–65.

Kolff, W. J. (1947). *New ways of treating uraemia: the artificial kidney, peritoneal lavage, intestinal lavage.* Churchill Livingstone, London.

Moore, F. D. (1964). *Give and take: the development of tissue transplantation.* WB Saunders, Philadelphia, p. 1.

Murray, J.E., Merrill, J.P., Harrison, J.H. (1958). Kidney transplantation between seven pairs of identical twins. *Ann. Surg.*, **148**, 343

Murray, J.E., Merrill, J.P. *et al.* (1960). Study of transplant immunity after total body irradiation: clinical and experimental investigation. *Surgery*, **48**, 272.

Murray, J.E., Merrill, J.P., Damin, G.J., Dealy, J.B., Alexander, G.P.J., and Harrison, J.H. (1962). Kidney transplant in modified recipients. *Ann. Surg.*, **156**, 337–55.

Murray, J.E., Merrill, J.P., Harrison, J.H., Wilson, R.E., and Damin, G.J. (1963). Prolonged survival of human kidney allograft by immunosuppressive drug therapy. *N. Eng. J. Med.*, **268**, 1315–23.

National Institute of Health Consensus conference. (1984). *Hepatology*, **4**, 107–10(suppl).

Ploeg, R.J., Goosens, D., McAnulty, J.F., Southard, J.H., Belzer, F.O. (1988). Successful 72 hour storage of dog kidneys with UW solution. *Transplantation*, **46**, 191–6.

Schwartz, R.S. and Damashek, W. (1959). Drug induced immunological tolerance. *Nature*, **183**, 1682–83.

Starzl, T.E. (1969). *Experience in hepatic transplantation.* WB Saunders,

Starzl, T.E., Todo, S., Fung, J., Demetris, A.J., Venkattramman, R., Jani, A. (1989). FK506 for liver, kidney and pancreas transplantation. *Lancet*, **2**, 1000–4.

Terpstra, O.T., Reuvers, C.B., Schalm, S.W. (1988). Auxiliary heterotopic liver transplantation. *Transplantation*, **45**, 1003–7.

Starzl, T.E., Rowe, M., Todo, S., *et al.* (1989). Transplantation of multiple abdominal viscera. *JAMA*, **261**, 1449–57

Starzl, T.E., Todo, S., Tzakis, A., *et al.* (1989). Abdominal organ cluster transplantation for treatment of upper abdominal malignancies. *Ann. Surg.*, **210**, 374–86.

Ullmann, E. (1902). Experimentelle Nientransplantation. *Wien. Clin. Wsch.r*, **15**, 281.

U S Multicentre FK506 Liver Study Group. (1993). Multicentre prospective randomized trial comparing FK506 to cyclosporine after liver transplantation: Primary outcome analysis. *Am. Soc. Transplant Surg. Ann. Meet.*, p. 33.

Williamson, C.S. (1926). Further studies on the transplantation of the kidney. *J. Urol.*, **10**, 275.

CHAPTER 16

Principles of management of malignant disease

Rachel Hargest

1 Whose responsibility is cancer treatment?

In Western societies, cancer is an increasingly important cause of death and imposes a substantial burden of morbidity on the community. In the UK, approximately 160 000 cancer deaths are recorded annually and it is estimated that the known prevalence of cancer is approximately 1 per cent of the population. Therefore at any one time, over half a million people in the UK have a history of cancer. The incidence figures show that over 270 000 new cancers are registered annually. These statistics translate into a lifetime risk of 1 in 3 for developing cancer and a 1 in 4 risk of dying from it. However, it is important to note that 70 per cent of all new cases are diagnosed in people over 60 years of age.

Cancer is not a single disease but a range of diseases which share common features but differ according to their anatomical site and biological activity. In the UK, one-third of all male cancer deaths are due to lung cancer, which is also the second most common cancer threat to women. In Scotland, lung cancer has overtaken breast cancer as the leading cause of cancer deaths in women. The results of treatment vary for different cancer types and depend on the stage of presentation and the nature of the cancer.

1.1 Responsibilities of the medical profession

The UK *Health of the Nation* White Paper identified the potential for reducing deaths from certain cancers by prevention and screening. Thereafter an Expert Advisory Group was convened which produced a report—*A policy framework for commissioning cancer services* (1995). This report, often referred to as the **Calman–Hine proposals**, provides guidance for purchasers and providers of cancer services. It includes recommendations as to the way in which cancer services are to be provided, the standard of care that patients can expect, and monitoring of treatment and outcomes. The general principles laid down in the report are as follows.

1. All patients should have access to a uniformly high quality of care in the community or hospital, wherever they may live, to ensure the maximum possible cure rates and best quality of life. Care should be provided as close to the patient's home as is compatible with high quality, safe, and effective treatment.

2. Public and professional education to help early recognition of symptoms of cancer and the availability of national screening programmes are vital parts of any comprehensive programme for cancer care.

3. Patients, families, and carers should be given clear information and assistance in a form they can understand about treatment options and outcomes available to them at all stages of treatment from diagnosis onwards.

4. The development of cancer services should be patient centred and should take account of patients', families', and carers' views and preferences, as well as those of professionals involved in cancer care. Individuals' perceptions of their needs may differ from those of the professional. Good communication between professionals and patients is especially important.

5. The primary-care team is a central and continuing element in cancer care for both the patient and his or her family from primary prevention, pre-symptomatic screening, initial diagnosis, through to care and follow-up or, in some cases, death and bereavement. Effective communication between sectors is imperative in achieving the best possible care.

6. In recognition of the impact that screening, diagnosis, and treatment of cancer have on patients, families, and their carers, psychological aspects of cancer care should be considered at all stages.

7. Cancer registration and careful monitoring of treatment and outcomes are essential.

Many of these general principles are already in widespread practice and are not controversial. However, the specific recommendations in the Calman–Hine report with regard to the future organization of, and responsibility for, cancer services have generated much debate and controversy. The main recommendation of the report with regard to organization of cancer services, is that cancer care should be organized at three levels:

1. **Primary care**—this level is seen as the focus of care, with primary-care teams able to determine referral patterns and to ensure integration of services.

2. **Designated cancer units**—these units should be created in many district general hospitals and will support clinical teams with sufficient expertise and facilities to manage the more common cancers.

3. **Designated cancer centres**—these centres will provide expertise in the management of all cancers in their geographical locality along with less common cancers by referral from cancer units. They will provide specialist diagnostic and therapeutic services, including radiotherapy.

The importance of good communication between primary care and specialist services is repeatedly emphasized in the Calman–Hine recommendations. Local factors will determine the exact arrangements for diagnosis and treatment. The extent to which general practitioners wish to be involved in the initial diagnosis will vary, but all doctors are obliged to have a high index of suspicion with regard to symptoms which may suggest malignancy and to refer for appropriate investigation.

Surgeons undertake and coordinate the initial management of most common cancers, and it is unlikely that this will change in the foreseeable future. Therefore both the Calman–Hine report and guidelines produced by organizations such as the British Association of Surgical Oncology seek to recommend standards of practice to which surgeons should adhere. Surgeons therefore have a duty to investigate promptly patients with clinical symptoms or signs causing suspicion of malignancy, and to reach a diagnosis. Treatment for most solid-organ tumours should be planned jointly by surgeon and oncologist. Other appropriate specialists, such as radiologists or pathologists, will often need to be involved in the management plan for treatment and follow-up, and surgical practice should be organized in such a way as to facilitate liaison between all relevant disciplines. Surgeons will continue to be responsible for liaison with primary-care services on behalf of their cancer patients. Communication with general practitioners and palliative-care specialists and the voluntary sector must be an integral part of the administration of a surgical practice.

1.2 Responsibilities of patients

Although cancer treatment is primarily the responsibility of the medical and allied professions, there are issues relating to compliance with treatment and particularly relating to cancer prevention which rest with patients themselves. Cigarette smoking causes lung cancer, which is a major killer in Western societies. Certain dietary habits are implicated in the development of colorectal cancers and tobacco and alcohol are related to head and neck malignancies. Although the general public is more aware of the dangers of smoking, this has not been translated into a decrease in tobacco consumption and the number of new smokers is rising, particularly among teenage girls.

Although the recent Patients' Charters have placed great emphasis on patients' rights, there are certain responsibilities which, although not legally binding, do fall on patients. If treatment plans have been discussed and agreed between patient and clinician, it is then assumed that the patient will comply with that course of treatment unless circumstances change or side-effects supervene. Participation in clinical trials is also an area where patients have voluntarily participated in treatments of unproved benefit in order to advance scientific or medical research. Many of these trials offer no obvious advantage to individual patients and have been supported by altruistic participants who hope that improved cancer therapies may be developed in the future.

1.3 Responsibilities of politicians

Public health policy is the responsibility of local and national governments. Public health covers many aspects of daily life, from the quality of the water supply to health education initiatives. Laws relating to working conditions and the safety and disposal of industrial waste are all within the remit of politicians. Certain toxic carcinogens, such as asbestos and ethidium, are strictly controlled by environmental health regulations and there are severe penalties for flouting these rules. With regard to lifestyle carcinogens, such as alcohol, cigarette smoking, and diet, the government can only act in an educational and advisory capacity. However, the relationship between government and industry, particularly with regard to advertising and sponsorship, has recently raised the profile of these arguments.

2 Tumour biology

2.1 Cell cycle and apoptosis

Cancer develops when cell growth and differentiation occur in an uncontrolled manner and the balance between cell production and loss found in healthy tissues is disturbed. The normal cell cycle was described in the early 1950s by Howard and Pelc and consists of a stepwise progression between stages. Figure 16.1 shows a diagrammatic representation of the cell cycle, which can be seen to consist of four consecutive phases between one mitosis and the next.

After one complete cycle, G_2 cells (Table 16.1) then proceed to mitosis again to produce the next generation of cells. Progression of cells from one phase to the next is influenced by numerous factors in both healthy and diseased cells. From studies of different cell types it is now recognized that in some cell populations, the number of G_1 cells vastly exceeds the number of G_2 cells. In other words, during G_1 phase, cells either become committed to continued cell cycling or withdraw from the cell division cycle. This population of non-proliferating cells is known as the G_0 phase. The problem with Howard and Pelc's work was that they chose to study a cell type in which all the cells were dividing, namely the nuclei of bean roots, and hence the G_1 and G_2 populations were equal.

In normal tissues, cells with significant damage to their DNA do not progress through the cell cycle. These cells are arrested at the G_1 phase and either undergo repair of their DNA before proceeding to cell division or else are directed to **apoptosis** or programmed cell death. This mechanism ensures that cells

Table 16.1 Phases of mitosis in the cell cycle

M	Mitotic phase	Cells undergo mitosis
G_1	Gap phase	
S	Synthetic phase	Pre-mitotic DNA synthesis
G_2	Gap phase	Cells contain twice as much DNA as non-dividing cells

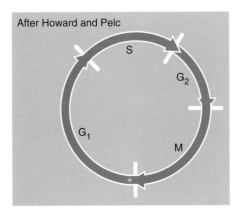
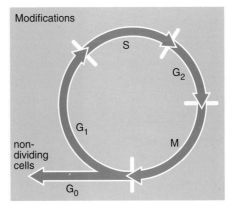

Figure 16.1 Cell cycle: after Howard and Pelc.

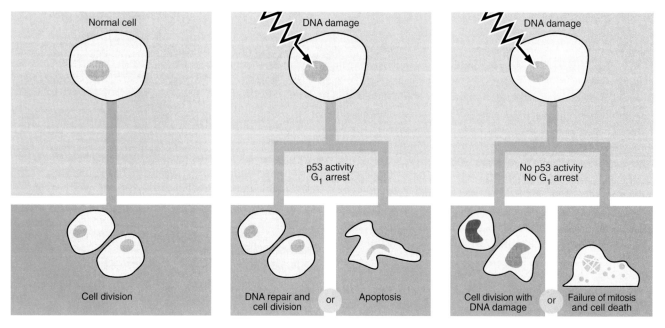

Figure 16.2 Regulation of the cell cycle by p53.

carrying abnormal amounts of DNA, or mutations in their DNA, do not replicate in healthy tissues. DNA 'proof reading' and repair, or diversion to apoptosis, are controlled by numerous genes, but the most important appears to be *p53*. This tumour-suppressor gene appears to control G₁ arrest and prevents a cell continuing to DNA synthesis with 'mistakes' in its DNA. Cells in which the DNA cannot be repaired are then redirected to apoptosis. Inactivating mutations in *p53* are an almost universal feature of human cancers. It has been shown experimentally that in the absence of *p53*, cells containing abnormal amounts or copies of DNA are able to progress to cell division, and hence uncontrolled growth and proliferation occur (Fig. 16.2). P53 knockout mice (transgenic mice which produce no p53 protein) are born looking normal but begin to develop tumours during infancy. All have tumours or are dead by the age of 6 months. A wide range of tumours occurs in p53 knockout mice and other genes are involved in the cascade of changes that leads to specific tumour types.

2.2 Genetic changes in malignant cells

Over the past 15 years, our understanding of the genetic basis of malignancy has increased exponentially. Cancer develops due to an accumulation of genetic changes in a cell which lead to uncontrolled growth. Two main groups of genes are responsible for such changes:

◆ proto-oncogenes are dominantly acting genes which induce or maintain cell proliferation when activated;

◆ tumour-suppressor genes are inactivated in a recessive manner and release cells from growth suppression.

In normal cells, these two groups of genes act in a balanced manner to ensure normal growth and division of the cell, and to prevent uncontrolled growth and entry to cell division of cells bearing major genetic abnormalities. However, if there is activation of proto-oncogenes or loss or malfunctioning of tumour-suppressor genes, this equilibrium is disturbed, leading to a relative overactivity of the proto-oncogenes and uncontrolled

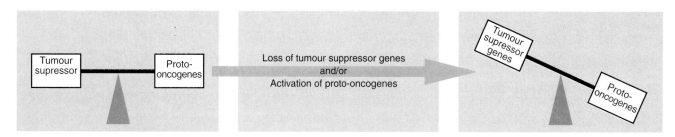

Figure 16.3 The genetic control of cell proliferation.

growth and proliferation (Fig. 16.3). Most of the common solid-organ cancers are associated with mutations or other abnormalities in several genes, so that the balance between proto-oncogenes and tumour-suppressor genes is disturbed.

Retinoblastoma

Retinoblastoma provides the model par excellence to illustrate the effect of loss of tumour-suppressor genes. This rare disorder of childhood eye tumours can arise sporadically or as a dominantly inherited condition. Sporadic tumours arise because of loss of both copies of the *Rb* gene within a single cell or mutations in both copies. However, in the inherited form there is already a germline mutation in one copy of the *Rb* gene so that tumours develop when only one allele is lost or a somatic mutation occurs in it. Therefore at a cellular level, mutations in *Rb* act in a recessive manner but the disease appears to be inherited in a dominant manner in affected families (Fig. 16.4). Retinoblastoma and other inherited cancer syndromes, such as familial adenomatous polyposis (FAP) provide classic examples of Knudson's 'two hit' hypothesis, which explains why loss or mutation of both alleles of a recessively acting tumour suppressor gene are required to produce the tumour phenotype.

Colorectal cancer

Colorectal cancer has been studied extensively at a genetic level. Sporadic tumours are thought to arise from pre-existing polyps, the so-called adenoma–carcinoma sequence (see Chapter 20). The evidence for this progression comes from the observations:

(1) that hereditary polyposis syndromes such as FAP predispose to the development of cancer; and

(2) that certain types of sporadic colorectal adenoma are more likely to turn malignant; these include polyps over 2 cm in diameter, those with a villous component, those with a degree of cellular atypia, and multiple polyps.

The phenotypic progression from adenoma to carcinoma has been shown to be associated with the accumulation of multiple genetic changes in both tumour-suppressor genes and proto-oncogenes. This association was first described by Vogelstein *et al.* in 1988 and numerous further studies have provided detailed analyses of the mutations found in various stages of premalignant adenomas and malignant lesions. Approximately

60 per cent of colorectal adenomas and colorectal carcinomas contain a mutated adenomatous polyposis coli (*APC*) gene and a similar rate of *APC* mutation has been found in all sizes of adenomas from 0.5 cm diameter. The similar frequency of *APC* mutations as lesions progress from benign to malignant suggests that *APC* is one of the earliest genes involved in the sequence of events that leads to colorectal neoplasia. Vogelstein's study and other work has also confirmed the finding that small adenomas that contain *APC* mutations are less likely to carry *ras* gene mutations (only 9–20 per cent of adenomas under 1 cm diameter). This indicates that *ras* gene mutations occur later during colorectal carcinogenesis than *APC* mutations. Similarly inactivation of the *p53* tumour-suppressor gene increases in frequency as the lesions advance, both for sporadic colorectal adenomas and those arising in patients with FAP.

These and other genetic changes were summarized in Fearon and Vogelstein's seminal paper in 1990, which presented a model for the genetic basis of colorectal carcinogenesis (Fig. 16.5). They concluded that colorectal neoplasia occurred as a result of the accumulation of multiple changes, including inactivating mutations in tumour-suppressor genes and activation of proto-oncogenes. Although there appears to be a preferred order in which these changes accumulate, as borne out by the above studies, the total mutation load rather than the exact order of changes appears to be important. At least five or six genes appear to be involved in the development of malignant tumours. These include tumour-suppressor genes such as *APC*, *p53*, *DCC* ('deleted in colorectal cancer') and putative tumour-suppressor genes located at 1q, 4p, 6p, 6q, 8p, 9q and/or 22q. Loss of heterozygosity at these loci has been observed in 25–50 per cent of colorectal cancers. Most individual cancers exhibit loss of heterozygosity at a total of four or five sites.

Proto-oncogenes such as the *ras* family are mutated with increasing frequency as lesions progress from early adenomas to full-blown cancers, as described above. Other genetic changes, such as hypomethylation of DNA, appear to occur early during tumorigenesis. Such a widespread change is thought to contribute to instability in the tumour cell genome, allowing an increased rate of accumulation of other genetic changes. The genetic changes that allow the subsequent development of metastases were not defined in Vogelstein's original hypothesis but are thought to involve genes coding for cell adhesion molecules and intercellular proteins.

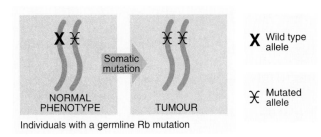

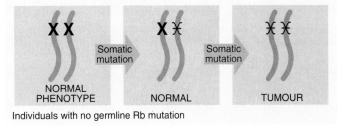

Figure 16.4 Germline and somatic mutations causing retinoblastoma.

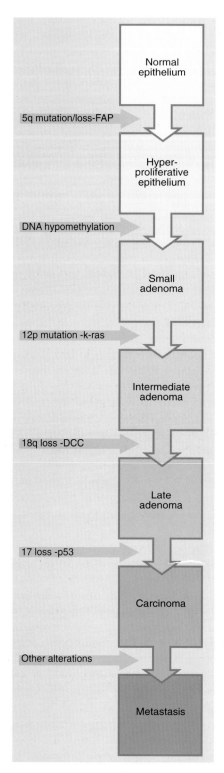

Figure 16.5 A genetic model for colorectal carcinogenesis (after Fearon and Vogelstein 1990).

Hereditary non-polyposis colorectal cancer

Over the past few years, great advances have been made in understanding the genetic basis of hereditary non-polyposis colorectal cancer (HNPCC) and these findings have implications for the ways in which families are counselled and treated.

HNPCC is defined as an inherited condition in which at least three relatives in two generations have colorectal cancer, with one of the cases diagnosed at less than 50 years of age. These cases are thought to account for 4–13 per cent of all colorectal cancers in industrial nations. Two groups of HNPCC patients can be distinguished: **Lynch syndrome I**, which is restricted to a site-specific predisposition to colon cancer inherited in an autosomal dominant manner; and **Lynch syndrome II**, which shows all the features of Lynch syndrome I accompanied by an increased risk of extracolonic carcinomas, particularly of the ovary and endometrium. Colonic tumours in these families exhibit a range of clinicopathological features which, in combination, help to identify such lesions and correlate them with the recently discovered genetic abnormalities. These features include a higher proportion of right-sided cancers, multiple lesions, villous-type tumours with increased mucin production, exophytic growth, inflammatory infiltrate, and improved prognosis.

At present six genes implicated in the development of HNPCC have been identified by linkage studies, cloning, and mutation analysis: *hMSH2, hMLH1, hPMS1, hPMS2, hMSH6* and *hMSH3* (Table 16.2). All six genes are concerned with DNA mismatch repair and maintaining the integrity of the genome at each cell division. Mismatch repair (MMR) is a highly conserved cellular function in which gene products recognize mismatched base pairs, excise them, and replace them with the correct base before cell division can proceed.

The mechanism of pathogenesis in these familial cancers appears to be different to that of the sporadic type. Most of the familial cancers show widespread alterations in short, repeated DNA sequences or microsatellites. These observations suggest that numerous replication errors occur during carcinogenesis, and tumours can therefore be defined as being replication error positive (RER+) or replication error negative (RER−). Table 16.3 shows the proportion of RER+ tumours in different groups of patients. The phenomenon of RER+ findings at a genetic level has confirmed the hypothesis that generalized genetic instability is a component of HNPCC. The term 'mutator phenotype' is

Table 16.2 Genes implicated in the development of HNPCC

Gene	Locus	% HNPCC
hMSH2	2p16	30–50
hMLH1	3p21	30
hPMS1	2q31–33	
hPMS2	7p22	
hMSH3, hMSH6	2p16	

Table 16.3 Incidence of replication error positive tumours

Sporadic colorectal cancer	15%
HNPCC cancers	±100%
Sporadic adenomas	3%
HNPCC adenomas	75%

sometimes used to describe the phenomenon of microsatellite instability exhibited by these patients.

Patients with HNPCC tumours carry a germline mutation in one of the MMR genes in every cell. However, only the cells that make up their tumours exhibit microsatellite instability; the microsatellites in the rest of their tissues are normal. Therefore one mutated copy of an MMR gene is not by itself sufficient to cause the mutator phenotype, even though the syndrome is inherited in an autosomal dominant manner. There are conflicting opinions as to what constitutes the 'second genetic event' which allows the development of a tumour. Loss of the remaining normal wild-type allele of the particular MMR gene would fit in with Knudson's 'two hit' hypothesis for the functioning of tumour-suppressor genes. However, there is conflicting evidence as to whether this occurs. It has been shown that patients with mutations in one of the MMR genes accumulate multiple mutations in other tumour-suppressor genes, such as *APC* and *p53*, which are known to be involved in the pathogenesis of colorectal cancer.

The work on DNA repair and microsatellite instability has important implications for as yet unaffected members of families with HNPCC. Germline mutations in one of the known DNA mismatch repair genes can be identified in affected members. The inheritance of such a mutation can be used to predict the future development of a colorectal neoplasm in other family members. In other words, the recent advances in molecular genetics have provided a parameter that can predict the development of cancer in a young person from a HNPCC family, in the same way that the presence of adenomas in the colon predict the development of cancer in a young person from a family with FAP. Genetic testing of as yet unaffected family members therefore offers the possibility of surgical intervention at an early stage to prevent the development of colorectal cancer.

Breast cancer

Breast cancer is predominantly a sporadic disease which affects approximately 10 per cent of women in Western societies. However between 5 and 10 per cent of cases occur in families with an inherited predisposition to the disease, sometimes in conjunction with familial ovarian cancer. These families have been studied extensively leading, in 1990, to the localization of the *BRCA1* gene by linkage analysis to chromosome 17q21. This gene was cloned in 1994 and has been shown to contain disease-causing mutations in approximately 30 per cent of breast/ovarian cancer families. A second locus, *BRCA2*, has been identified on chromosome 13q12–13: this gene appears to be linked to the development of up to 45 per cent of cases in families with breast cancer but not ovarian cancer. Familial male breast cancer is also linked to this *BRCA2* gene. Further familial breast cancer genes are under investigation but have not been published outside the scientific community as yet.

Descriptive genetics has identified a myriad genetic changes in tumours of all types over the past few years but as yet no unifying feature has been elucidated. The challenge of the next 10 years for basic science is whether these genetic abnormalities can be utilized as a basis for interventional genetics to prevent or treat cancer.

2.3 Environmental carcinogens

Certain environmental agents that damage DNA and lead to specific types of tumours have been identified. The interaction between environmental and genetic factors has only recently been addressed at a basic science level, but this area is likely to provide opportunities for novel approaches to cancer treatment in the future.

Chemical carcinogens

Chemical carcinogens have long been recognized to cause certain malignancies: these include vinyl chloride and angiosarcoma of the liver, β-naphthylamine dyes and bladder cancers, polycyclic aromatic hydrocarbons and lung cancer, and asbestos and bronchial carcinoma and mesothelioma. These chemicals are known as indirect carcinogens because they cause a degree of DNA damage known as 'initiation' but a further 'promotion' event, such as exposure to a drug or hormone, is required for malignant transformation. Direct carcinogens are typified by the alkylating agents, which cause direct DNA damage and carcinogenesis.

Hormones are implicated in the causation and growth of cancers, particularly of the genital organs. Diethylstilbestrol has been shown to cause adenocarcinoma of the vagina, and oestrogens are necessary for the development of endometrial carcinoma. Other tumours, such as those of the breast and prostate, may depend on appropriate hormonal environment for growth, and hence hormonal intervention can be used as treatment in these conditions.

Oncogenic organisms

Oncogenic viruses have been recognized to cause both human and animal malignancies. Some of the most common human cancers world-wide appear to be caused by oncogenic viruses. For instance human papillomavirus is thought to cause cervical carcinoma, hepatitis B virus is associated with hepatocellular carcinoma, Epstein–Barr virus appears to cause several malignancies including nasopharyngeal carcinoma and Burkitt's lymphoma, and the human T-lymphocyte virus I (HTLV-I) is associated with the development of leukaemia.

Other organisms have been implicated more rarely in the development of tumours. *Clonorchis sinensis* is associated with cholangiocarcinoma, *Schistosoma* is associated with squamous carcinoma of the bladder, and *Aspergillus fumigatus* is associated with hepatocellular carcinoma.

Radiation

Radiation is known to induce DNA damage and one of the unfortunate late sequelae of therapeutic radiotherapy is the development of second malignancies. Many different tumours, including haematological and solid-organ cancers, have been described after both therapeutic and accidental exposure to ionizing radiation. Ultraviolet light, particularly UVB, is associated with the development of skin cancers of both squamous and melanocytic origin.

All of the above environmental agents act to damage DNA in some way and may therefore act alone or in combination with pre-existing genetic changes to cause malignant transformation of affected cells. The classical example of the interaction between genetic and environmental agents is provided by the rare condition xeroderma pigmentosum, in which affected individuals have a DNA repair defect and are hypersensitive to ultraviolet light and prone to the early development of skin cancers.

2.4   Mechanism of metastasis

Most cancer-related deaths occur as a result of metastases rather than the primary tumour itself. The genetic and cellular events that control the development of metastases are less well understood than the changes that cause primary tumours. One particular conundrum is the differing metastatic potential of different tumour types. However, certain mechanisms have been identified that seem to be important in the spread of tumours.

Neovascularization

Tumours need to acquire a new blood supply in order to grow and spread, since the passive diffusion of nutrients can only supply tumours of less than 2 mm diameter. This phenomenon of tumour angiogenesis or neovascularization is well documented in many tumour types and appears to occur in response to the release of angiogenic peptides by the tumour itself or by the host inflammatory cells. The new vessels that supply the tumour are derived from endothelial cells arising from surrounding capillaries and venules in the host tissue. These new vessels are not identical to the vessels from which they originate in that they are more 'leaky', they do not possess a smooth muscle layer and do not have the neural innervation usually associated with vessels of similar size. There is a direct correlation between the number of new vessels at the margin of a tumour and subsequent metastasis and prognosis for many solid tumours. Novel treatments aimed at preventing or destroying neovascularization are therefore being explored.

Loss of cell to cell adhesion

One of the cardinal features of malignant tumours is the loss of cell to cell cohesion that occurs in normal tissues. Numerous cell adhesion molecules (CAMs) have been identified, of which one important group are the cadherins, a family of transmembrane glycoproteins that mediate calcium-dependent cell aggregation. Carcinomas that have reduced or absent expression of the epithelial cadherin (E-cadherin) are associated with a propensity to metastasize and a significantly reduced survival rate for primary colorectal and prostate tumours. The matrix metalloproteinase (MMP) family of molecules have been shown to be associated with the metastatic potential of tumours of the stomach, pancreas, and colon.

At present, histopathological reports concentrate on the degree of differentiation and the resection margins of the excised tumour in order to provide prognostic information to the clinician. Guidelines on the pathological reporting of specific tumours such as breast and colorectal carcinomas recommend that the presence or absence of features such as lymphovascular invasion and lymphocytic infiltration should also be identified. It may be that tumour angiogenesis and reduced CAM expression will also prove to be useful prognostic features and may indicate the need for adjuvant treatment.

2.5   Immune response

Although tumour cells are recognized as being abnormal by the host, tumours are not 'rejected' and destroyed in the same manner as allogeneic grafts. The relationship between the tumour and the host's immune system is complex and varies between different tumour types and between individuals with the same primary tumour. Immune phenomena in relation to malignant tumours have long been recognized: for example, spontaneous regression of both solid cancers and acute leukaemias has been observed. Such examples are too rare to draw meaningful conclusions in terms of cancer treatment but do point to the importance of the host's immune system in recovery from or survival with cancer. Conversely, individuals who are immunosuppressed, either as a result of congenital disorders or pharmacologically after organ transplantation, show a higher incidence of many types of cancers. Histopathologists have long reported the presence of varying degrees of inflammatory cell infiltrate in certain types of solid tumours. The presence of tumour infiltrating lymphocytes (TILs) in primary tumours is recognized as a good prognostic factor.

Advances in immunology have defined some of the mechanisms by which tumours interact with the host's immune system:

1. Some tumours express antigens which can elicit an immune response in the host. These may be tumour-specific antigens (TSAs) or tumour-associated antigens (TAAs). TSAs are neoantigens which are expressed by tumour cells but not by the corresponding normal tissue. Therefore they can induce a strong immune response by the host. TSAs are found in experimental tumours but rarely in naturally occurring human malignancies. One example is the MAGE antigen in human melanoma, which is being studied with a view to vaccination. TAAs occur more commonly—these antigens are expressed at low levels by normal tissues but become overexpressed after malignant transformation (Table 16.4). Examples include CEA (carcinoembryonic antigen), which is expressed by colonic adenocarcinoma cells, and p97 (melanotransferrin), which is expressed at high levels by most malignant melanomas. Overexpression of TAAs can be measured and may be useful in the diagnosis and monitoring of the associated tumours. However, it is the extent to which a TAA is able to stimulate an immune response which will determine whether anti-TAA strategies can be developed.

Table 16.4 Tumour-associated antigens

Antigen	Associated tumour
AFP (alphafetoprotein)	Hepatocellular carcinoma
	Hepatoblastoma
	Testicular teratoma
	Yolk sac tumours
	(Carcinoma lung)
	(Carcinoma pancreas)
ALP (alkaline phosphatase)	Prostatic adenocarcinoma
BCM	Breast cancer
CA125	Ovarian epithelial cancers
	(Endometrial cancer)
	(Cervical cancer)
	(Breast cancer)
	(Colorectal cancer)
	(Gastric cancers)
	(Lung cancer)
	(Pancreatic cancer)
CA15-3	Breast cancer
	(Ovarian cancer)
	(Endometrial cancer)
	(Cervical cancer)
CA19-9	Pancreatic cancer
	Colorectal cancer
CA50	Colorectal cancer
	Pancreatic adenocarcinoma
	(Other gastrointestinal cancers)
CA242	Pancreatic adencarcinoma
CA549	Breast cancer
CA-M26	Breast cancer
CA-M29	Breast cancer
CEA (carcinoembryonic antigen)	Colonic adenocarcinoma
	Head and neck cancers
	Hepatocellular carcinoma
	Lung cancer
	Pancreatic adenocarcinoma
	Prostatic adenocarcinoma
HCG (human chorionic gonadotrophin)	Testicular teratoma
	Testicular seminoma
	Germ cell ovarian tumours
	Choriocarcinoma
	(Carcinoma pancreas)
	(Carcinoma breast)
	(Carcinoma kidney)
	(Carcinoma lung)
LDH (lactate dehydrogenase)	Testicular seminoma
	Mixed germ cell tumours
MCA	Breast cancer
MSA	Breast cancer
Neurotensin	Fibrolamellar hepatocellular carcinoma
PIVKA-II des-g-carboxyprothrombin	Hepatocellular carcinoma
PLAP (placental alkaline phosphatase)	Testicular seminoma
	(Breast cancer)
	(Ovarian cancer)
PSA (prostate-specific antigen)	Prostatic adenocarcinoma
	(G-seminoprotein)
p97 (melanotransferrin)	Malignant melanoma
Vitamin B_{12}-binding proteins	Fibrolamellar hepatocellular carcinoma
14C1	Ovarian epithelial tumours
	(Colonic adenocarcinoma)

2. Human tumours express class I and II major histocompatibility (MHC) antigens to varying extents. The immune response to a tumour requires the expression of MHC antigens by the tumour cells in order for immune recognition to occur. The loss of class I MHC antigens has been observed in colorectal cancers and correlates with a poor prognosis. Similarly class II antigen-positive tumour cells can present TAAs directly to the immune system, thus improving the immune response against the tumour. Cytokines such as γ-interferon (γ-IFN) have been used to try to augment class II antigen expression and hence the immune response to experimental tumours. The specific cytotoxic T-lymphocyte (CTL) response appears to be increased under these conditions. Conversely, tumour cell lysis by non-specific mechanisms is reduced when MHC expression is increased.

3. Infiltration of tumours by lymphocytes is recognized to indicate an inflammatory or immune response to the tumour, and for many tumour types correlates with prognosis. Such infiltrates consist of a heterogeneous population of cells, including TILs and other cell types. TILs include CTLs, non-MHC-restricted T lymphocytes, and natural killer (NK) cells. Monocytes, macrophages, and granulocytes also form part of the tumour infiltrate. B lymphocytes occur rarely as part of tumour inflammatory infiltrates, but do occur in melanoma. The cellular infiltrate is recruited due to the local release of chemotactic factors within the tumour microenvironment. Such factors may be secreted by the tumour cells or by the cells of the infiltrate; NK cells, in particular, produce a number of cytokines, including interleukins-4 and -6 (IL-4, IL-6) that reduce the proliferation of malignant cells, and γ-IFN, IL-2, and tumour necrosis factor (TNF) which cause direct lysis of tumour cells. Many of these cytokines are chemotactic for other cells of the inflammatory cell infiltrate and thus the local immune response to the tumour is augmented.

4. Paradoxically, there are individuals who fail to mount an immune response to tumours bearing TSAs or TAAs which would normally be expected to elicit such a response. The CD4+ population of T lymphocytes is capable of suppressing the specific CD8+ T-lymphocyte-mediated tumour-cell killing. The ratio of CD4+ to CD8+ T lymphocytes varies in different tumour infiltrates. A subgroup of T cells which are CD3+, CD8+ can suppress both specific and non-specific T-lymphocyte responses. The tumour immunosuppressive effect is a complex phenomenon which appears to result from the interaction of immunosuppressive T lymphocytes, tumour, and lymphocyte-derived cytokines and tumour antigens.

2.6 Therapeutic immunology

Numerous attempts have been made to harness immune mechanisms in anticancer treatments. These include non-specific treatment with cytokines and similar mediators, specific monoclonal antibody therapies, and the use of gene therapy to enhance the immune response against a tumour.

Active immunotherapy

The host's immune system may be stimulated to produce a response using a variety of specific cancer cell components or non-specific adjuvants.

Tumour-cell vaccines

The ideal anticancer treatment would, of course, be a cancer vaccine. However, at present this is still a goal to be achieved. The cancer vaccines that are under investigation have limited clinical use within the constraints of clinical trials, or for patients who have exhausted other treatment options. Certain tumours, such as melanoma, soft-tissue sarcoma, and some haematological malignancies, express antigens which are recognized by the immune system. Trials using modified tumour cells have shown variable antitumour response.

Antigen presentation

Many tumour cells lack MHC class I and II antigens, which are necessary for the presentation of 'foreign' antigens to the immune system, and therefore tumour cells may escape immune surveillance. The expression of class I and II antigens can be modified by cytokines and chemicals such as swainsonine, but it is the newer gene therapy techniques that have revived interest in this approach. Gene transfer of sequences encoding γ-interferon have been used to augment class I and II expression and enhance antigen presentation.

Non-specific adjuvants

The best-known non-specific adjuvant is BCG (bacille Calmette–Guérin), which stimulates macrophages and has been used in several trials of immunotherapy. It appears to be of some effect in certain of the leukaemias but has very little benefit in solid tumours.

Cytokines

The most promising area of immunotherapy is the use of cytokines to act as antitumour agents and to stimulate other parts of the immune system to produce an antitumour response. Interferon-α has been used in clinical trials and shows some benefit in hairy cell leukaemia, non-Hodgkin's lymphoma and chronic myelogenous leukaemia. The early promising results in trials of α-interferon in melanoma and renal cell carcinoma have not been reliably reproduced. Studies of β- and γ-interferons have proved disappointing. Currently the interferons are being studied in combination with cytotoxic drugs, such as 5-fluorouracil, in order to try to produce a synergistic effect.

Other cytokines, such as the interleukins, have been explored alone and in combination for their antitumour effect. IL-4 is a promising molecule since it can induce IgE and IgG1 responses, it causes T-cell growth *in vitro*, and appears to play a role in the development of T-cell memory. This latter characteristic is particularly interesting since the ideal immunotherapy would be a once-only treatment which provided the patient with lasting protection against a given tumour. IL-4, alone and in combination with IL-2, has shown the ability to produce tumour regression in animal tumours, such as mouse melanoma, and has passed into the stage of human clinical trials.

Other cytokines such as TNF-α and granulocyte–macrophage colony-stimulating factor (GM-CSF) also have antitumour effects *in vitro* and in animal models, and the therapeutic benefits of these observations continue to be explored.

Passive immunotherapy

Monoclonal antibodies

Antibodies can be produced which target tumour-specific or tumour-associated antigens and can theoretically destroy cancer cells with preservation of the normal surrounding tissue. Many of the tumour antigens listed in Table 16.4 have been studied as potential targets for monoclonal antibodies. However, as yet, monoclonal antibody therapy has not been very successful in clinical practice. One of the major problems is that although specific antibodies can be generated that bind to the antigen of interest, binding does not translate to cell destruction. One strategy to try to overcome this problem is the generation of bispecific antibodies which link target and immune cells due to their dual specificity for tumour-associated antigens and immune effector cells. These bispecific antibodies have shown effective cancer-cell killing in animal tumours.

Advances in gene therapy have recently rekindled the interest in tumour-associated antigens and monoclonal antibodies as the basis of cancer treatment. Plasmids encoding antigens such as CEA have been developed and have been shown, in animal models, to function as a tumour vaccine and induce dose-dependent antibody and cell-mediated immune responses. A clinical trial of CEA polynucleotide vaccination in advanced colorectal cancer is now in progress.

Adoptive immunotherapy

A further immunological approach to cancer treatment is the transfer of lymphocytes or macrophages between individuals. These cells are usually modified in culture with a number of factors collectively known as lymphokines. These include T-cell growth factor (TCGF) and interleukin-2 (IL-2). Cells which have been transduced with lymphokines exhibit cell killing properties that are not restricted by MHC compatibility or antigen–antibody interaction. This lymphokine activated killer (LAK) activity is a useful independent immune mechanism for the destruction of tumour cells. The first LAK cells described were peripheral blood lymphocytes derived from cancer patients, which were shown to be effective in the destruction of both autologous and allogeneic tumour cells following culture with TCGF. It is now possible to generate LAK cells from the lymphocytes of normal, healthy individuals by using a combination of lymphokines to transduce the cells. A number of clinical trials of LAK cells, alone or in combination with IL-2, are in progress. The patients involved in these trials predominantly have metastatic tumours which have progressed despite all other conventional treatments. Melanoma and renal cell tumours are two of the primary tumour sites which are being studied, since preclinical studies have shown effective LAK cell-mediated destruction of these tumour types.

The complex interaction between malignant cells and the host's immune system determines the prognosis for an individual tumour. As our understanding of immune phenomena increases, the potential for therapeutic strategies also improves. Recent advances in molecular genetics have allowed the development of vectors that can transfect cells with immune components in order to produce a response which is not complicated by immune phenomena provoked by preformed proteins. It is likely that immunotherapy will play an adjuvant role in cancer treatment in the future.

3 Diagnosis and staging

The term 'cancer' includes a spectrum of diseases which vary greatly in their presentation, pathology, response to treatment, and outcome. Therefore accurate diagnosis is essential for patients in order that treatment options can be discussed and a realistic assessment of prognosis made. The diagnosis of cancer may be made in the course of investigating symptoms or signs exhibited by a patient, or incidentally during other medical interventions, or as part of a screening protocol. In general, the earlier in its natural course a cancer is diagnosed, the better the outcome, and therefore screening and other programmes aimed at early detection have been instituted in many developed countries.

Once the diagnosis of cancer is made, the most important determinant of outcome is the stage of the tumour. Staging systems have been devised for most tumour types and describe the characteristics of the local tumour and the extent of spread, if any. Where the same staging systems are used by all interested parties, collaboration between professionals is facilitated and results of different treatments can be compared. The most widely accepted staging system for solid tumours is the Tumour Node Metastasis (TNM) system, which was originally developed by Pierre Denoix in France. In this system 'T' describes the size of the primary tumour and its relation to adjacent structures, 'N' refers to nodal status, and 'M' to the presence or absence of metastases. Staging is initially based on the findings of clinical examination and preoperative imaging techniques. However, when histopathological evidence is available staging may be modified to provide a more accurate assessment of the disease. The TNM system has been modified for individual tumour types and is now accepted by national and international bodies, such as the World Health Organization, the Union Internationale Contre le Cancer, and the American Joint Committee for Cancer Staging, as a versatile system that allows comparison of epidemiology, treatment, and outcome in different parts of the world.

Diagnosis of symptomatic tumours is a major part of the workload of most general surgeons since many of the common solid tumours present with symptoms which are traditionally 'surgical'. It is unlikely that referral patterns for the investigation and treatment of conditions such as 'lump in breast', 'change in bowel habit', 'rectal bleeding', or emergencies such as 'intestinal obstruction' will change in the foreseeable future. Therefore surgeons need to have an understanding of the many and varied presentations of malignancy and to have a high index of suspicion in those presenting with atypical clinical features. Diagnosis commences with the clinical assessment of the patient and the initial history and examination cannot be over-emphasized. The symptoms reported in the history will give indications not only to the diagnosis but to the extent of spread in many instances. The presence or absence of features such as back pain, weight loss, and breathlessness should be recorded. Examination findings are notoriously unreliable since the assessment of the size of palpable masses and the presence and extent of lymphadenopathy vary between individual observers.

Investigations are therefore necessary for the confirmation of the diagnosis and staging of cancer. A balance has to be drawn between making an accurate diagnosis with enough information to advise on treatment, and subjecting the patient to a plethora of unpleasant, time-consuming, and expensive tests, which do not influence the subsequent management of the patient. In order to confirm the diagnosis of cancer, a tissue sample must be obtained for histological or cytological examination. The ease with which this can be achieved varies with the primary site of the tumour. 'One-stop' cytology is available in many breast clinics, since breast cancers may be easily palpable and adequate information obtained on the basis of a fine-needle aspirate from a breast lump. For many tumours, however, tissue samples can only be achieved by more invasive procedures such as endoscopy, ultrasound- or CT-guided biopsy, laparoscopy, or surgical biopsy. These modalities do, however, offer advantages in that assessment of the extent of local, nodal, or metastatic tumour spread can often be made at the time of obtaining a tissue sample.

For solid tumours, the most important decision is whether the tumour is locally contained and therefore potentially curable by surgery, or whether there is extensive locoregional disease or metastases so that surgery and adjuvant therapy will be palliative. Defining the primary tumour type allows the likely sites of spread to be identified and the prognosis assessed.

General investigations such as full blood count, renal and liver function tests, and chest radiography should be performed in virtually all cancer patients. The full blood count may demonstrate a normochromic anaemia in advanced malignancy, an iron-deficient anaemia in any cancer where blood loss is a feature, or a leucoerythroblastic picture where bone-marrow infiltration has occurred so that immature red and white cells spill over into the peripheral blood. Bone-marrow aspiration is only necessary for the diagnosis and staging of specific tumour types—haematological malignancies and myeloma routinely require examination of the bone marrow for diagnosis, and the staging of small-cell lung cancer requires bone-marrow aspiration since 5 per cent of cases show marrow involvement when no other evidence of spread can be detected. Various research protocols have looked for micrometastases within the bone marrow for tumours such as breast cancer, but there is no indication for routine examination of the bone marrow since treatment decisions are not influenced by such information. Liver function tests often remain normal despite extensive metastatic disease within the liver, because of the enormous reserve of this organ. Derangement of liver function due to metastatic disease is a poor prognostic indicator. Renal function may be impaired in cancer patients due to a number of mechanisms. These include prerenal failure due to dehydration as a result of poor fluid intake, vomiting, or intestinal obstruction, or postrenal failure due to obstruction of the urinary tract due to pelvic or abdominal masses. Some tumours, classically small-cell lung cancer, have paraneoplastic effects that cause derangement of salt and water balance, leading to abnormal urea and electrolyte measurements. A plain chest radiograph will show the presence of extensive metastatic disease within the lungs or mediastinum, which, if present, obviates the need for more expensive imaging, such as computed tomography.

Specialized imaging techniques such as ultrasound (US), computed tomography (CT), magnetic resonance imaging (MRI), and isotope scanning each have their own indications and limitations in the diagnosis and staging of malignant disease. As a general principle, as few investigations as possible should be performed in order to obtain the information necessary to make clinical decisions. If a patient has obvious extensive metastatic disease, invasive expensive investigations should not be performed.

Ultrasound is quick, cheap and non-invasive and is widely used in the assessment of the liver for the presence or absence of metastases. Its main drawback is that it is operator dependent and therefore results are not reproducible. Where appropriate expertise exists, the role of ultrasound in diagnosis and staging has been expanded to include endoluminal ultrasound for the assessment of gastrointestinal, pancreatic, and prostatic tumours, and intraoperative ultrasound performed at laparoscopy or open surgery. With the most technically satisfactory probes and highly skilled operators, the accuracy of endoluminal and intraoperative ultrasound in assessing nodal involvement of oesophageal or gastric cancers exceeds that of any other method of assessment. At present such techniques are confined to specialized centres but may become more widespread with the dissemination of knowledge and expertise in the future.

CT and MRI have found more favour with most British surgeons because they provide an anatomical picture of the area of interest. The quality of the images produced is improving continuously as each new generation of machines develops. CT is particularly useful in assessing lesions in the thorax or abdomen. It is more sensitive than plain radiography for detecting pulmonary metastases because its greater resolution can demonstrate small parenchymal lesions and also because lesions hidden by the heart are revealed. CT is very reliable in assessing retroperitoneal structures, particularly renal tumours, and can demonstrate tumour extension into the renal vein or inferior vena cava. Modern spiral CT is playing an increasing role in the assessment of resectability of hepatic and pancreatic tumours. MRI is less widely available but is superior to CT in several areas. Spinal tumours are particularly well demonstrated on MRI and there is no requirement for intrathecal contrast which is necessary for CT or myelography. Intracranial tumours, particularly those in the posterior cranial fossa, are better demonstrated by MRI, especially if the intravenous contrast agent gadolinium–diethylenetriaminepentaacetic acid (Gd–DTPA) is used. MRI has also replaced CT in the assessment of musculoskeletal tumours since the extent of soft-tissue involvement is better delineated by MRI. More recently the development of appropriately shaped coils has allowed MRI to be used for the assessment of breast cancer. Although confined to a small number of specialist institutions, MRI appears to be more sensitive than mammography at detecting recurrent disease after radiotherapy and breast-conserving surgery and in the assessment of axillary lymph-node involvement.

Isotope scanning uses small doses of radioactive substances which are attached to a suitable vehicle that is taken up by the target organ or tissue. For example technetium-labelled phosphate compounds are preferentially taken up by bone and the degree of uptake is related to the blood flow and the amount of new bone formation. Bony metastases appear as 'hot spots' due to the increased blood flow and bone formation in these areas. A hot spot can also be produced by trauma and infection, and therefore the results of isotope bone scans should be interpreted in conjunction with the clinical situation and the findings on plain radiography. Radiolabelled monoclonal antibodies to tumour-associated antigens have been generated and several research studies have reported promising results in detecting occult and recurrent disease. Anti-CEA antibodies for the detection of colorectal metastases are the most commonly used at present, and such an approach opens up the possibility of combining tumour identification with targeted treatment.

3.1 The unknown primary

Approximately 5 per cent of cancer patients present with metastatic disease as their principal problem. Common presentations include pleural effusion, ascites, lymphadenopathy, liver, or cerebral metastases. The median survival of these patients is only 6 months and therefore investigation should be reserved for those whose tumours or symptoms may be amenable to treatment rather than subjecting all patients to expensive, uncomfortable, and time-consuming tests for tumours where the outcome is invariably poor. The history and clinical findings at presentation may give a clue to the primary source, particularly if the relevant areas are examined when lymphadenopathy is the presenting feature. Baseline investigations, such as full blood count, renal and liver function tests, and chest radiography should be performed in conjunction with tumour markers, such as CEA along with PSA for men and CA125 for women.

There are certain tumours which respond to treatment even when disseminated at presentation; the most common are the lymphomas. Approximately 70 per cent of patients with poorly differentiated or anaplastic tumours have lymphomas, and therefore lymph-node biopsy for histological assessment and immunocytochemistry should be performed if lymphadenopathy is a presenting feature. Germ-cell tumours are particularly chemosensitive and therefore should be sought by clinical examination, testicular ultrasound scanning or pelvic ultrasound, or CT and measurement of tumour markers such as AFP, β-HCG, or PLAP (Table 16.4). The overall cure rate for germ-cell tumours is approximately 85 per cent and since these tumours generally occur in young adults they should be sought and treated aggressively. Tumours which are hormone sensitive, such as breast or prostate, should also be sought since fairly simple hormonal manipulation can cause tumour regression and provide symptomatic relief. Small-cell cancers have a neuroendocrine origin and may be chemosensitive and have a relatively good prognosis. Immunocytochemical staining for chromgranin or neuron-specific enolase and electron microscopy may be useful in diagnosing these tumours if the clinical picture suggests such a diagnosis. Thyroid tumours can be identified by the presence of thyroxine synthesis, and even widespread disease may be treated with radioactive iodine with significant improvement in survival. If a poorly differentiated adenocarcinoma is identified at the metastatic site, there is no indication for invasive procedures such as colonoscopy, bronchoscopy, and laparoscopy unless there are symptoms from the primary tumour which need to be controlled. 'Blind' chemotherapy for poorly differentiated tumours of unknown primary site has been attempted using cisplatin, vinblastine, and bleomycin. Variable responses have been reported but only anecdotal patients derive any long-term benefit.

3.2 Screening

In general, the earlier in its natural history that malignancy is detected and treated the better the outcome. Screening programmes have therefore been instituted on the basis that early detection is possible and will improve outcome. Screening can be defined as the examination of an asymptomatic population in order to detect and treat a disease at an early stage. Screening may be population-based or targeted at those groups of individuals at increased risk. Population screening occurs, mainly in neonates, for diseases such as hypothyroidism and phenylketonuria, where simple biochemical tests are available that can detect these disorders at a stage before mental and physical retardation has occurred. For most cancer-screening programmes, only selected groups are targeted, such as women aged 50–65 years for breast screening or those in high-risk families for ovarian cancer screening. In order for screening programmes to be clinically and financially justified, certain conditions have to be fulfilled:

◆ the disease must be a significant cause of morbidity or mortality in the screened population;

◆ effective treatment for early disease must be available;

◆ the screening procedure should be acceptable to patients;

◆ the screening procedure must be reliable (low false-positive and false-negative rates);

◆ screening should not provoke excessive anxiety in patients;

◆ the cost of a screening programme must be justified by the yield of cases detected and the effectiveness of early treatment.

Of course no screening programme fulfils all these criteria perfectly and the value of any particular project is the source of much debate in both healthcare and political circles. In the UK, national programmes to screen for breast and cervical cancer are in operation, while screening for colorectal and ovarian cancer is currently offered only to high-risk groups.

Cervical cancer screening

Invasive cervical cancer is usually preceded by the condition described as cervical intraepithelial neoplasia, which is not life threatening in its own right and can be treated locally to prevent progression to invasive cancer. Cervical smear tests are relatively cheap and easy to perform and acceptable to patients. The fact that mortality from cervical cancer has remained at the same level despite an increase in promiscuity and in other sexually transmitted diseases is taken as evidence that this programme has been effective. All sexually active women between the ages of approximately 20 and 65 years are eligible for screening and the current arrangement is for the service to be arranged by the individual's general practitioner. The main problems with this programme relate to the technical proficiency with which the smears are performed and the expertise with which the smears are read. Cervical screening is currently very labour intensive and recent, well-publicized instances of misreporting of smears have rekindled interest in quality-control issues. The development of automated slide readers is likely to occur in the near future, but whether such technical advances can improve on current systems remains to be evaluated.

Breast cancer screening

Women in developed countries have a lifetime risk of approximately 1 in 15 of developing breast cancer, and the cure rate for symptomatic disease is relatively low—at best 25 per cent. Therefore screening programmes have been instituted in order to try to detect early asymptomatic disease, in an effort to improve response to treatment and survival. The Swedish two-counties trial showed that there is an overall reduction in mortality of approximately 25 per cent in the mammographically screened population. Similar results were obtained from the HIP trial in New York during the early 1980s. These studies provided impetus to the Forrest Report in the UK (Forrest Committee 1986) on the basis of which the national screening programme was commenced in August 1988. All women aged 50–65 years are currently invited triennially for single oblique-view mammography. More frequent examinations or performing two views instead of one would obviously raise the cost of this programme considerably and has yet to be justified in terms of number of extra cases detected in small pilot studies of different protocols. Results from the first rounds of screening show that there is a trend towards decreased overall mortality in the screened population, but as yet no significant reduction in breast cancer deaths. Screen detected cancers are of significantly smaller size and earlier stage than symptomatic presentations. Furthermore, approximately 30 per cent of screened detected cancers are carcinoma *in situ* with no invasive component and only 20 per cent have positive axillary nodes, compared with 40 per cent of symptomatic cancers. Although this evidence looks encouraging, it is clear that longer-term follow-up is required in order to determine whether there is a true improvement in outcome or whether screen-detected cancers just exhibit lead-time bias and there is no improvement in overall survival. The breast cancer screening programme has enormous costs—in terms of finance, personnel, and the psychological effects on women of the screening process. Mammography itself can be physically uncomfortable and engenders anxiety, up to 10 per cent of women are recalled for further assessment, which leads to further worries, and approximately 1–2 per cent will require a biopsy. Less than half of these women will have cancer and so there is a large cohort of women for whom uncomfortable invasive procedures have been performed unnecessarily. The risks of repeated exposure to ionising radiation are low but have been taken into account when the current protocols for the programme were devised. Younger women may be screened if there is a family history of breast cancer or any other high-risk features, but extending this programme to younger women on a population basis would considerably increase the costs.

Colorectal cancer screening

Colorectal cancer is one of the most common malignancies in Western societies, accounting for over 20 000 deaths per annum in the UK. It is thought that most colorectal cancers develop from a pre-existing adenomatous polyp—the so-called adenoma–carcinoma sequence—and that if these lesions could be detected at a premalignant stage, or when the cancer is still relatively small and localized, then curative resection could be performed. Although there is good molecular and biological evidence for the adenoma–carcinoma sequence, the speed with which cancers develop varies. Paradoxically, patients reporting longer duration of symptoms have been shown in some small studies to actually have earlier stage tumours, suggesting inherent differences in the biology of colorectal cancer between individuals.

Screening programmes for colorectal cancer use a variety of procedures, including faecal occult blood (FOB) testing, rigid sigmoidoscopy, flexible sigmoidoscopy, and colonoscopy. FOB testing is cheap and easy to perform but has a high false-positive rate and is not acceptable to a significant minority of patients. Endoscopic examinations are more reliable but are more invasive and labour intensive. Their added advantage is that small adenomas can be removed at the same time, reducing the risks of progression. Although all the local and regional population screening programmes have shown that they can detect small lesions and that compliance is good, none has been able to demonstrate a reduction in the death rate from colorectal cancer. Therefore the economic case for a national colorectal cancer screening programme is still under debate.

Targeted screening, however, has long been accepted as worthwhile and is financed by health service purchasers for those at high risk. The example par excellence is familial adenomatous polyposis (FAP), an autosomal dominantly inherited condition in which affected individuals develop numerous intestinal polyps during adolescence, one or more of which invariably progresses to colorectal cancer. Individuals from affected families have therefore been offered colonoscopy from approximately 12 years of age and, if polyps develop, then colectomy is performed, usually during the late teens or early twenties. This aggressive screening programme and drastic intervention is justified in these high-risk individuals because the natural history of FAP is well described and colectomy is the only way to prevent early death. More recently, targeted screening for those with family histories of colorectal cancer, particularly those with hereditary non-polyposis colorectal cancer (HNPCC), has been instituted. Colonoscopy is usually the method of choice, but there is much debate as to the frequency of examinations, and because HNPCC individuals do not develop adenomatous polyps, the best that can be achieved is early detection of established cancer. Genetic testing may supersede colonoscopy in HNPCC families in the future.

Ovarian cancer screening

Although ovarian cancer is relatively uncommon, it is a major cause of cancer deaths in women because of its advanced stage at presentation. Targeted screening programmes for first-degree relatives of women who have, or have had, ovarian cancer are available in many regions. Ultrasound, CA125 testing, or a combination of the two are the common methods used. However, the advice as to when to intervene varies in different centres. Prophylactic bilateral salpingo-oophorectomy (BSO) and total abdominal hysterectomy (TAH) is offered by some centres to women with a family history of dominantly inherited ovarian cancer when they have completed their families. There is still a small risk (approximately 6 per cent) of developing a malignancy histologically identical to ovarian cancer within the pelvis or retroperitoneum even after TAH and BSO in these individuals. Some centres therefore advise a watch and wait policy, with repeated CA125 measurements and ultrasound or CT scanning, and only offer surgery if lesions within the ovaries are detected. This diversity of opinion indicates that there is as yet no hard evidence that prophylactic surgery achieves an overall improvement in survival.

Gastric cancer screening

Gastric cancer has been a major cause of death in Japan and therefore a national screening programme has been established. Double-contrast barium meals are performed on a population basis and suspicious cases are referred for endoscopy. This programme is expensive and highly labour intensive and detects approximately 4000 new cases per year, at a rate of about 1 per 1000 screened. However, the proportion of cases of early gastric cancer (EGC) detected has increased. Surgery for EGC is potentially curative and the overall probability of dying from gastric cancer has been shown to be reduced by more than 50 per cent in the screened population. However, gastric cancer is more than twice as common in Japan than in Europe and there is some evidence that the results of Japanese surgeons are superior to those in the West; therefore it would be difficult to prove a case for establishing a national gastric cancer screening programme in the UK.

Genetic testing

Advances in molecular genetics are likely to allow genetic tests to replace other methods of screening. At present genetic abnormalities are relatively easy to detect but the implications of such defects are not necessarily understood. In the USA, over-the-counter gene testing is available for a small fee. A classical problem is the individual who has undergone such a gene screen and is told that he or she has a defective *p53* gene; this gives no indication of whether he or she is likely to develop any particular cancer and, if so, when. Such a finding has enormous psychological and financial effects on the individual without any possible therapeutic intervention. In the UK, genetic testing is strictly regulated and proper genetic counselling must occur before testing is performed.

One area where genetic testing is already starting to replace conventional techniques is FAP, where the causative mutation in the adenomatous polyposis coli (*APC*) gene has been determined for about two-thirds of affected families. Genetic testing can now replace the first colonoscopy at around 12 or 13 years of age. Individuals who do not carry the *APC* mutation found in their families will not develop FAP and therefore no longer need to undergo regular colonoscopy. One interesting problem that has arisen recently is that some individuals who have 'enjoyed' annual colonoscopies since their teenage years are reluctant to forego these examinations, even when genetic testing has shown that they do not carry an *APC* mutation.

HNPCC is now becoming amenable to genetic testing with the identification of the mismatch repair (MMR) genes. Individuals from HNPCC families may now be offered prophylactic colectomy without colonoscopy if they carry the same MMR gene mutation as affected family members. Some individuals prefer not to undergo prophylactic surgery and therefore screening colonoscopy can be targeted at those with MMR gene mutations, and family members with no MMR mutations can be removed from screening programmes.

Genetic screening for breast cancer has been the source of much debate and media interest. The coding sequence of the *BRCA1* gene was the first DNA sequence to be patented, which has major financial implications for research and therapeutic developments. At the time it was thought that this gene may account for the majority of familial breast cancers, but in fact *BRCA1* only accounts for a small proportion of familial cancers, which themselves comprise less than 5 per cent of all breast cancer. At present our knowledge of disease-causing *BRCA1* mutations is evolving and genetic testing is currently more of a research tool than a useful clinical service.

Virtually every week new papers describing genetic changes in various cancers are published. Which, if any, of these can be translated into a useful diagnostic or screening test remains to be seen. It is important that the legal and ethical restrictions which currently regulate genetic testing in the UK remain in place in order to protect the public. Unfounded claims as to the accuracy and predictive implications of specific tests are seized eagerly by the media and publicized, so that ill-informed individuals may undergo tests which do not improve their chances of avoiding cancer and may seriously damage their financial or employment prospects.

4 Principles of treatment

Approximately 1 in 3 of the population of Western societies will eventually develop cancer, and this imposes an enormous burden on healthcare resources. Although public awareness regarding suspicious symptoms is rising and screening programmes concentrate on early diagnosis, it must be remembered that cancer is predominantly a disease of the elderly. These individuals are likely to have concomitant non-malignant disorders which will influence the treatments that can be offered and the likely recovery period from the major surgery which is often necessary for solid tumours. Because of increasing life expectancy in developed countries, the total number of cancer patients is rising in these regions. Table 16.5 lists the incidence of the 10 most common cancers in each sex in the UK. Most of the solid tumours present in the first instance to surgeons and at any given time approximately 40 per cent of general surgical inpatient beds are occupied by cancer patients. Therefore most surgeons will need to be familiar with the general principles of cancer treatment along with the specifics of treatment of those tumours within the remit of their subspecialty.

Once a diagnosis of cancer has been made, the most important treatment decision is whether there is any possibility of achieving a 'cure' or whether treatment will be palliative. The choice depends on the tumour type, the extent of locoregional spread, the presence or absence of metastases, and the patient's age and general state of health. Staging investigations appropriate to each tumour type will usually indicate whether an attempt at cure is possible. Staging also allows a reasonable estimation of prognosis and allows comparison of different treatment protocols.

The definition of 'cure' varies with different tumour types. For many of the solid tumours, such as colorectal cancer or testicular tumours, 5-year survival is taken as being equivalent to cure. However, it is well known that late recurrences do occur and for some tumours, such as melanoma or breast cancer, recurrences after 20 or even 30 years are not uncommon. Five-year survival, however, is a useful measurement of outcome for many adult tumours, and is used as the method of assessment of efficacy in many trials of adjuvant treatment. For paediatric

Table 16.5 Cancer incidence and deaths in the UK (source: *Cancer Research Campaign Year Book 1996–97*, figures from UK cancer registries for 1991)

Cancer type	Incidence	Deaths	5-year survival
Men			
Lung	28420 (21%)	23470 (28%)	8%
Skin[a]	16930 (13%)		97%
Prostate	15550 (12%)	9840 (12%)	43%
Bladder	9260 (7%)	3650 (4%)	62%
Colon	9220 (7%)	5840 (7%)	38%
Stomach	6920 (5%)	4810 (6%)	11%
Rectum	6510 (5%)	3180 (4%)	36%
Non-Hodgkin's lymphoma	3890 (3%)	2120 (3%)	44%
Oesophagus	3540 (3%)	4040 (5%)	7%
Pancreas	3410 (3%)	3080 (4%)	4%
Women			
Breast	34590 (25%)	14080 (18%)	62%
Skin[a]	15390 (11%)		97%
Lung	13760 (10%)	12990 (17%)	7%
Colon	10730 (8%)	6440 (8%)	37%
Ovary	5940 (4%)	4350 (6%)	28%
Rectum	4990 (4%)	2420 (3%)	36%
Stomach	4480 (3%)	3190 (4%)	10%
Cervix	4340 (3%)	±2000	58%
Uterus	4210 (3%)	±2000	70%
Bladder	3650 (3%)	1760 (2%)	±60%

[a] Excludes melanoma.

malignancies, however, 5-year survival is not such a useful measure of outcome because of the young age of these patients at presentation, and because second primary cancers as a result of treatment can themselves cause premature death. When assessing the effectiveness of new treatments, it is important to understand the various measures of outcome which may be scientifically significant but have little or no effect on patients' survival or well being. Disease-free interval, tumour response rate, and tumour regression rate are all used to report observed response to treatment but do not necessarily translate into improved survival.

4.1 Treatment options

The mainstays of treatment for cancer are surgery, radiotherapy, and chemotherapy, alone or in combination. Hormonal manipulation, immunotherapy, laser therapy, and novel interventions have a limited role in certain tumour types. For those patients who have advanced disease at presentation or whose disease progresses despite treatment, palliative care should be given instead of, or alongside, active treatment. Patients and their relatives should be involved in the decision-making process as to the aims and likely outcomes of treatment.

For patients undergoing potentially curative treatment, surgery, radiotherapy, and chemotherapy all carry the risk of significant side-effects and even, in rare cases, the risk of death as a result of treatment. Patients should be given a realistic assessment of side-effects and risks, preferably before treatment is commenced. One added advantage of early diagnosis and screening programmes is that patients are able to take time to discuss their diagnosis and treatment options with their surgeon or oncologist and can therefore be more involved in decision making. A significant minority of cancer patients present as emergencies with haemorrhage, intestinal obstruction, or perforation of various parts of the gastrointestinal tract. For these patients diagnosis and treatment often occur simultaneously at surgery. These patients usually give open-ended consent for 'laparotomy and proceed' or at best 'laparotomy ± bowel resection ± stoma formation'. They are often extremely ill at presentation and have a stormy postoperative course. Because their tumours are usually more advanced, their long-term prognosis is significantly worse for most primary tumour types.

Some basic principles apply to the surgery of malignant disease whatever the primary site. As a result of staging investigations it should be possible to decide preoperatively whether the intention of surgery is cure or palliation. Curative surgery aims to remove all macroscopic and microscopic cancer. This may be a realistic proposition for non-melanoma skin cancers, or for very early gastrointestinal tumours but many cancers (e.g. breast) exhibit micrometastases at an early stage and therefore local surgery and lymphadenectomy does not render the patient disease free. Findings at surgery may alter the surgeon's opinion as to whether a resection is curative or palliative—this is particularly true for colorectal cancer and is important in terms of comparing results between different centres.

Other modalities of treatment may also be used with curative or palliative intent, as discussed in the sections which follow. The inherent radio- or chemosensitivity of particular tumour types will determine which approach is used. Many patients nowadays are treated with a combination of therapies in order to address the unseen problem of micrometastases and to reduce the risk of relapse. Agents that enhance the effects of radiotherapy or certain chemotherapeutic drugs are being developed.

5 Surgery

Most of the common solid cancers present to surgeons in the first instance, and for many localized tumours surgery is the only potentially curative treatment. The Calman–Hine report recognizes the role of surgeons in cancer management and places responsibility on surgeons to ensure that their practice corresponds with acceptable standards. The importance of auditing results is emphasized. In order to compare results between centres it is important that preoperative staging is accurate, since outcome is usually reported in relation to stage at presentation. Pathological reporting should be performed in a standard manner so that tumours of similar biological activity can be compared.

5.1 Surgery for diagnosis and staging

A significant part of any general surgical practice is the technical service of obtaining tissue specimens for histological analysis. The subgroups of haematological malignancies can only be differentiated on the basis of tissue architecture rather than cytology and so excision biopsies of lymph nodes are frequently performed. Occasionally, splenectomy may be required in such patients, either for staging or treatment.

Small skin lesions, such as basal cell carcinoma, can be excised with a margin of normal skin so that diagnosis and treatment occur simultaneously. Incision or excision biopsy of larger lesions may be required when cytological analysis is inadequate.

Abdominal or pelvic masses which are not amenable to ultrasound or CT-guided biopsy may require surgical biopsy to make a diagnosis. Laparoscopy is an ideal tool for obtaining biopsies from intra-abdominal malignancies and for assessing the abdomen for signs of intraperitoneal dissemination or involvement of adjacent or distant organs. Prior to resection for pancreatic, gastric, or oesophageal cancers, laparoscopy is recommended as the staging investigation of choice. Its major advantage over all other imaging modalities is its ability to detect small peritoneal seedlings which will contraindicate resectional surgery. The addition of ultrasound to laparoscopy may provide further information, particularly regarding intraparenchymal liver metastases.

5.2 Curative surgery

The ideal result of cancer surgery is the complete eradication of the malignant disease, but this is only achieved in about one-third of patients. It is assumed that when the primary tumour is small, with no evidence of lymph node or distant metastases, surgery can provide a cure. This is a rather simplistic view but does underpin some important principles of cancer surgery. It is assumed that cancers spread predominantly by local extension and by lymphatic spread. Therefore curative resectional surgery should include a margin of normal tissue and the draining lymph nodes from the tumour. This principle underlies the choice of surgical technique for most localized cancers.

Breast cancer

Breast cancer that appears to be confined locoregionally at presentation is treated by resectional surgery for the primary cancer and either resectional surgery or radiotherapy for the draining lymph nodes in the axilla. The extent of resectional surgery varies, but the importance of tumour-free margins of approximately 1 cm is understood by all. Multifocal disease, involved margins, and large tumours are all indications for further treatment, which may necessitate a mastectomy. Radiotherapy to the breast is given after conservational surgery in order to reduce the risk of local recurrence, but it is not the ideal treatment for residual local disease. Axillary dissection is a contentious issue but its undoubted advantage is that it allows accurate staging of the axillary nodes, which is the single most important prognostic indicator in breast cancer. In expert hands the morbidity of axillary dissection should be very low (2–3 per cent) and a level III axillary clearance will treat a positive axilla simultaneously with staging. There are two disastrous situations with regard to the management of the axilla which should be avoided if possible. Combined surgery and radiotherapy to the axilla carries a 20 per cent risk of lymphoedema and this is an argument against incomplete axillary dissection which yields positive nodes which are subsequently treated with radiotherapy. Uncontrolled axillary disease is very difficult to control and is very distressing for patients, due to problems with arm function. A formal axillary clearance in good hands currently offers the lowest risk of axillary recurrence and least interference with function. There is now some evidence that node-negative patients have improved survival if given adjuvant chemotherapy, and therefore the importance of axillary dissection for staging is less important, but the axilla still needs to be treated in its own right in order to prevent local problems. It may be that the recently described technique of sentinel node biopsy will indicate which patients will benefit from axillary clearance.

Colorectal cancer

Guidelines from the Royal College of Surgeons of England and the Association of Coloproctology of Great Britain and Ireland have emphasized the importance of surgical technique in potentially curative colorectal resection. The importance of removing adequate local tissue along with the draining lymphatic channels is emphasized. The area that has generated most debate over the past 10 years is the rectum, where the local recurrence rate has been shown to be reduced significantly if a total mesorectal excision is performed. The important principle behind this observation is that longitudinal tumour spread can occur distally as well as proximally within the mesorectum and therefore the whole area should be removed without breaching the lateral margins of the mesorectum. Radiotherapy can be used as an adjuvant therapy to reduce the risk of local recurrence but it cannot compensate for inadequate resectional surgery.

Gastric cancer

The 5-year survival after resection for gastric cancer is of the order of 20–25 per cent in Western series. Many patients present at a relatively late stage, which may account for these somewhat poor results, but there have been efforts to try to improve results, based on the Japanese series which report much better survival figures. The Japanese have popularized more extensive surgery —the so-called D2 gastrectomy. 'D' refers to the lymph-node resection performed in continuity with the gastrectomy. Lymph nodes around the stomach are classified as D1 if they are applied to the stomach wall and D2 if they are related to the branches of the coeliac axis. A D2 gastrectomy is significantly more time consuming and technically demanding than a D1 resection. Recent trials in the UK and The Netherlands comparing D1 and D2 resections for similar lesions have encountered numerous difficulties. Standardization of surgical techniques has proved virtually impossible and pathological examination has shown that the actual resections performed did not always correspond to the procedure to which the patient was randomized. Some firm conclusions have been drawn from these studies, which include the recognition of a learning curve for performing a D2 gastrectomy, and the association of significant morbidity with resection of adjacent organs such as the spleen or tail of the pancreas.

Debulking surgery

Surgery may be used to reduce tumour load prior to chemotherapy. This approach is used for germ-cell testicular tumours which are reasonably chemosensitive and appear to respond well if they have been debulked by surgery prior to treatment.

5.3 Palliative surgery

A wide variety of surgical procedures are performed for palliation of malignant disease. For many gastrointestinal cancers resection performed with curative intent is in fact palliative, as evidenced by the low 5-year survival figures for pancreatic, oesophageal, gastric, or Dukes C colorectal cancer after resection. However, resection is often the best form of palliation, especially for colonic tumours which cause obstruction or bleeding.

Gastrointestinal cancers which are not amenable to resection may need to be bypassed. This particular surgical workload has reduced over recent years as the skills of endoscopists and radiologists have improved. Most oesophageal and pancreatic or biliary cancers can be stented endoscopically with good palliation of symptoms during the relatively short survival time of these patients. Duodenal stents to overcome obstruction at that level are in use in some specialist centres and may well reduce the need for gastroenterostomy formation in the future. Although a gastroenterostomy is a relatively straightforward procedure, it often fails to provide symptomatic relief because the dilated, chronically obstructed stomach may not empty well or bile reflux may occur.

It is sometimes necessary to defunction colonic or rectal tumours which are very advanced at presentation, or in patients who are extremely frail or ill. If possible, resection is a better option for palliation. Stoma formation may occasionally be needed to aid nursing care in terminally ill patients with incontinence and diarrhoea causing skin excoriation and distress.

Advanced presentation of breast cancer still occurs. Most surgeons have seen anecdotal women who appear in the outpatient clinic with a fungating carcinoma of the breast which has been kept hidden for months or years. Although some of these women will respond to tamoxifen or radiotherapy, for many the best option is a toilet simple mastectomy to remove the unsightly smelly mass.

5.4 Emergency surgery

Malignant disease often presents as an emergency, usually with obstruction, perforation, or haemorrhage. These patients are often elderly and very unwell at presentation. The first priority is to resuscitate the patient and then to decide whether surgery can be performed to deal with the emergency and, if possible, with the underlying tumour at the same time. The classic example is the elderly patient who presents with peritonitis from a perforated caecum secondary to an obstructing carcinoma in the left colon. Resuscitation with attention to fluid balance and antibiotics should be administered on admission, and then a decision to operate can be made in conjunction with the patient and relatives. Operative options include caecostomy, Hartmann's procedure, and subtotal colectomy and ileorectal anastomosis with or without covering ileostomy. The final decision may be made at the time of surgery when the degree of peritoneal contamination can be assessed.

5.5 Conclusion

For most general surgeons emergency and elective cancer surgery comprise a significant proportion of their total workload. The most important decision for the surgeon is whether the cancer is potentially curable or not. Curative surgery must include adequate local clearance and lymphadenectomy for some solid cancers. If palliation is required, the non-surgical options to deal with specific symptoms should be considered.

Heroic resectional surgery is not indicated in patients with metastatic or terminal disease.

6 Adjuvant treatment

Many tumours are not amenable to surgical cure due to their primary site, multifocal nature, or extent of spread, and therefore other modalities of treatment are used in combination with surgery (or each other) to attempt to effect a cure. In the case of malignancies such as carcinoma of the breast, colon, or rectum adjuvant treatment has been shown to improve 5-year survival and disease-free interval. Radiotherapy and chemotherapy are the mainstays of adjuvant treatment, but hormonal manipulation has an important role in specific tumours. Novel therapies such as laser treatment, immunomodulation, and gene therapy are currently only available within clinical trials or research protocols.

6.1 Radiotherapy

About 25 per cent of the population of developed countries will develop cancer, about half of whom will be treated with radiotherapy. Most radiotherapeutic treatment is directed towards the primary tumour with additional treatment often given to draining regional lymph nodes. Over the past decade systemic radiotherapy has been employed for certain multifocal tumours, such as multiple myeloma, aiming to ablate malignant cells throughout the body. This often requires bone-marrow transplantation later to replace the bone marrow destroyed by radiotherapy.

Cellular effects of radiotherapy

X-rays lie at the most energetic end of the electromagnetic spectrum and have a short wave length and a high oscillating frequency. These properties explain the molecular ionization that takes place when X-rays penetrate human cells. The cytotoxic activity of X-ray therapy is largely mediated by producing ions in the cellular water which then attacks DNA. These ions are probably largely oxygen free-radicals. A proportion of the effect of radiotherapy is caused by direct ionization of DNA. Cells are able to repair single-strand breaks in DNA and these have little adverse consequence. However, if the dose of X-rays is high enough, two single-strand breaks will be close enough to cause a double-strand break, thus losing the intact template for repair and disrupting the integrity of the chromosome. These chromosomal aberrations do not normally affect the survival or function of cells until they attempt to replicate, but cell death usually occurs at the first or early subsequent mitotic divisions.

Both normal tissues and tumours demonstrate a radiation response proportional to their rate of proliferation. Cells that turn over rapidly, such as bone marrow, may demonstrate a rapid effect with falls in platelet and white cell counts within a few days of exposure. The mucosa of the digestive and respiratory tracts develop a reaction within 2–3 weeks of exposure. Similarly skin, when it is deliberately irradiated, develops desquamation and hair loss, or both, within about 3 weeks. Slowly proliferating tissues, such as connective tissue, kidney, cartilage, bone, lung, and oligodendrocytes, respond slowly to X-irradiation and demonstrate signs of damage only months or years after exposure.

Principles of radiotherapeutic treatment

The basic action of radiotherapy is to kill cells *in situ* and then allow the body to remove the dead cells. Radiotherapy is carefully planned and targeted to give maximum local control and minimum local and systemic toxicity. This therapeutic differential between damaging malignant cells but avoiding damage to normal cells is the mechanism by which radiotherapy can cure or palliate cancer.

Successful radiotherapeutic treatment depends on the following factors, which are discussed in detail below:

- the inherent radiosensitivity of the tumour;
- the size and extent of the tumour;
- biological differences in response between tumour cells and normal cells;
- effective planning and delivery of radiotherapy;
- any supplementary or adjuvant treatments, including surgery and chemotherapy.

The inherent radiosensitivity of the tumour

Certain tumours are inherently radioresistant—these include malignant melanoma, anaplastic thyroid carcinoma, ovarian carcinoma, most bone sarcomas, and renal carcinomas. Radiotherapy is rarely employed in treating these. Other tumours are very radiosensitive, including squamous-cell carcinomas, small-cell lung carcinoma (which, however, is rarely cured), well-differentiated thyroid carcinoma, germ-cell tumours, and lymphomas. Most other tumours fall somewhere between these extreme sensitivities. However, radiosensitivity alone is not the only factor determining cure rate. Tumours with a high proliferative activity and a high rate of cell loss shrink rapidly with radiotherapy but may also recur quickly. Other more indolent tumours may take months to respond yet ultimately disappear and never recur. Thus, when monitoring a patient for the effectiveness of radiotherapy, repeat biopsies are counterproductive as long as the tumour continues to regress clinically.

The size and extent of the tumour

Radiotherapy can be delivered in three ways—as an external beam, by local application of radioactive isotopes or brachytherapy, and systemically by radioactive isotopes or antibodies. Each of these modes of delivery has advantages in delivering radiotherapy to tumours of different size and extent. External-beam radiotherapy can be focused on localized tumours but its efficacy depends on many factors, including the size of the tumour and the degree of hypoxia within the centre of the tumour, since hypoxic cells are less radiosensitive. External-beam total-body irradiation is used to treat bone-marrow micrometastases after chemotherapy in certain haematological malignancies prior to bone-marrow transplant. Brachytherapy is useful for the treatment of solid-tumour deposits which are amenable to wire insertion, and for the treatment of malignancies within a hollow organ. Targeting of radioisotopes to specific tumour cells has been well described for ^{131}I but is still at the stage of clinical trials for the many antibodies and targeting compounds that have been proposed as the 'magic bullet' of cancer treatment.

Biological differences in response between tumour cells and normal cells

The therapeutic differential between normal tissues and tumour can be amplified by giving radiotherapy in a series of fractionated doses, usually 5 days a week for 3–8 weeks. The reasons can be thought of as the four Rs:

Repair of cellular injury

Repair of DNA damage is completed over a few hours. In general, slowly responding normal tissues are capable of greater repair than malignant tissues. Thus by spacing dose fractions by at least 6 hours, the recovery of slowly responding normal tissues is relatively greater than of tumour tissue. The effectiveness of cell killing by fractionation is logarithmic rather than linear and thus the difference in each dose effect between normal and tumour tissue is amplified exponentially. For example, if 60 per cent of normal cells survive each dose fraction compared with only 50 per cent of cancer cells, then after 30 dose fractions the relative survival of normal cells will produce a therapeutic differential of 237.

Repopulation by surviving viable cells

The rate of repopulation after cell damage of the average tumour is less than of acutely responding normal tissues. In rapidly proliferating normal tissues, repopulation by surviving cells allows normal cells treated incidentally (such as mucosa) to tolerate a high dose given to the tumour. By extending treatment over several weeks, this regenerative response is allowed to take greatest effect. However, some cancers demonstrate treatment–induced acceleration of growth, and for these treatment needs to be completed in as short a time as possible. Balancing these two aspects means that the exact pattern of dose fractionation for a given patient must be calculated individually.

Redistribution within the division cycle

As cells progress through the mitotic cycle they demonstrate large changes in their radiosensitivity. Thus cells irradiated in their most sensitive phase are killed, leaving the surviving cell population partly synchronized in the more radioresistant phases after each dose. By fractionation of treatment, cells in radioresistant phases are likely to progress into radiosensitive phases. In addition, in contrast to normal tissues, most malignant tumours exhibit a wide range of cell division cycle times, so the tumour as a whole gradually returns to an asynchronously dividing population. Thus, again, a therapeutic differential develops between normal and tumour cells.

Reoxygenation of cells after treatment

As solid tumours grow, they often outstrip their blood supply and develop areas of hypoxia and necrosis. Hypoxic cells are two to three times more radioresistant than normally oxygenated cells and even a small proportion of hypoxic cells could limit the radiocurability of a tumour. With fractionated treatment, normally oxygenated cells, being more sensitive, are killed selectively and are eliminated and previously hypoxic cells gain better access to oxygen and become vulnerable to treatment.

Effective planning and delivery of radiotherapy

Finally, it is important to recognize that a planned course of radiotherapy must be completed if there is to be hope of killing every malignant cell. If only 80 per cent of the calculated dose is given, it will not achieve an 80 per cent cure rate. If a tumour contains 10^{10} malignant cells capable of indefinite proliferation, then 80 per cent of the dose calculated to be curative would reduce malignant cells by only about 10^8 leaving 10^2 malignant cells capable of causing a recurrence. Effective planning and delivery of radiotherapy aims to treat target areas while minimizing unwanted damage to normal tissues.

Imaging improvements

Advances in imaging, including computed tomography and magnetic resonance imaging, enables radiotherapy to be given more safely and effectively to patients with low-grade tumours because treatment can be delivered precisely to a more restricted area.

Advances in radiotherapeutic equipment

The quality and penetrating power of radiotherapy equipment can now produce well-localized radiation beams capable of being delivered anywhere in the body with homogeneous energy deposition across the tumour and a satisfactory fall off outside the target volume. This enables a much lower dose to be given to surrounding sensitive tissues and usually completely spares the skin.

Individual treatment plans

Individual treatment plans are now usually developed with radiation fields shaped by shielding blocks, computerized planning, and automatic tracking techniques. This allows larger areas to be treated continuously (such as pelvic and para–aortic lymph-node fields) with sparing of local tissues despite a high dose to the target volume. This form of treatment, although not yet fully assessed in randomized studies, is likely to cause fewer side-effects in patients requiring large-volume irradiation.

Brachytherapy and systemic radiotherapy

Improved planning in three dimensions permits localization and treatment of irregular fields. There is renewed interest in brachytherapy, which is the positioning of sealed radioactive sources close to or within malignant tissue. These are modern variations on much older techniques, with improved choice of radionuclides, systems of delivery, and protection of staff and patients. These treatments are now employed in cancers of head and neck, breast, cervix, and oesophagus, which require high local doses of irradiation. If necessary, external-beam irradiation can be added. Brachytherapy can sometimes be used in patients with recurrences after external-beam treatment untreatable by other means (e.g. recurrent carcinoma of the oesophagus or bronchus). In other cases, highly specific radioisotope treatment is important, for example ^{131}I treatment of well-differentiated thyroid carcinoma.

Other types of radiation and particle therapy

Progress has been slow in other types of radiation and particle therapy. Neutron-beam therapy has not fulfilled its early promise. No consistent role has yet been found for drugs that radiosensitize tumours, mainly because of severe side-effects.

Hyperfractionation

Reducing the radiation dose per fraction and increasing the frequency to twice a day is under investigation. This is intended to enhance self-sensitization of the tumour through division cell redistribution at the same time as sparing late-responding normal tissues. A randomized trial of head and neck cancer showed a 15 per cent gain in local control rate with no increase in side-effects.

Accelerated treatment

Accelerated repopulation as a response to radiotherapy (discussed earlier), takes place in head and neck cancers and may occur in cancers of the cervix, bladder, skin, lung, and some lymphomas. Shorter treatment courses but with more frequent treatments—up to three times a day—are the subject of clinical trials. It may be that tumours with a rapid doubling time, as demonstrated by flow cytometry, may be the most likely to escape a standard regimen lasting 6–8 weeks. Other predictive assays are under investigation to endeavour to predict the radiation response of a tumour to allow a more carefully planned approach. Suitable tumour variable characteristics include the proportion of cells that survive a dose of 2 cGy, the potential doubling time, tumour ploidy, tumour hypoxia, and the degree of expression of oncogenes.

Supplementary or adjuvant treatments, including surgery and chemotherapy

Combining surgery and radiotherapy has distinct advantages in certain cases with a large tumour mass. Daily fractions of radiotherapy treatment (usually 200 cGy) reduce tumour cell survival to about 50 per cent. The larger the number of tumour cells to be eradicated, the higher the dose required and the higher the risk of complications. Radiotherapy is thus best at eradicating small tumours and subclinical tumour deposits. Surgery, on the other hand, is excellent for removing large masses but its therapeutic value in subclinical disease is low.

Combining surgery and radiotherapy in certain cases increases the chances of eliminating locoregional cancer and at the same time reduces morbidity. In many settings chemotherapy and radiotherapy combine to consolidate the cytotoxic achievements of the other, for example in lymphomas, leukaemias, and testicular cancers. This type of combined therapy is currently under investigation for lung, oesophageal, anal, and rectal cancers. Other supplementary treatments such as cytokine therapy, immunotherapy, hyperthermia, or the use of drugs to modify the biological behaviour of malignant cells are at various stages of clinical investigation but are not yet a regular part of the oncologist's armamentarium.

Radiotherapy in clinical practice

Indications for radiotherapy in clinical practice are given in Table 16.6.

Potentially curative radiotherapy

Radiotherapy has an important role in treating most common solid cancers and in Hodgkin's and non-Hodgkin's lymphomas. It also has a role in the treatment of non-malignant neoplasms, such as benign adenomas of the pituitary and parotids. Widening indications for radiotherapy have led to a progressive decrease in major surgery for many common cancers.

In squamous head and neck cancer radical radiotherapy, with or without chemotherapy, is often the treatment of choice to avoid mutilating surgery and does not preclude surgical salvage procedures for later recurrences. In bladder cancer radical irradiation has been shown in a randomized trial to produce results little different from preoperative irradiation followed by total cystectomy, with the advantage that the bladder can be retained and an ileal conduit avoided. In cancer of the cervix, radical irradiation (usually with combined external-beam irradiation and brachytherapy) has replaced surgery entirely for patients in stages 2B to 4, and cure can be achieved in up to 50 per cent of even advanced cases. For early stage cancer of the cervix, radiotherapy and surgery are equally effective. Surgery may be preferred for younger women in order to spare the ovaries. For inoperable non-small-cell lung cancer radiotherapy remains the most useful non-surgical method of palliation.

On the other hand, radiotherapy has been abandoned for most childhood tumours because of growth retardation. Chemotherapy has replaced it for the treatment of, for example, non-Hodgkin's lymphoma and Wilm's tumour. However, irradiation has become increasingly important for craniospinal tumour treatment in children and has improved the overall cure rate to about 40 per cent. In adults, radiotherapy has been largely replaced by chemotherapy in treating testicular germ-cell tumours and non-Hodgkin's lymphoma.

In multiple myeloma, the poor efficacy of second-line chemotherapy has led to increasing use of systemic irradiation. Hemibody irradiation, treating the upper or lower half of the body, or both, can provide long-term symptomatic benefit, even in drug-resistant cases. Total body irradiation in conjunction with bone-marrow transplantation is being used in multiple

Table 16.6 Indications for radiotherapy in clinical practice

Tumour type	Treatment	Five-year survival	Complications
Skin: BCC, SCC	Highly curable by radiotherapy	Over 95%	Cosmetic results excellent
Kaposi's sarcoma	Usually treatment of choice	Depends on HIV status	–
Head and neck (squamous cell)	Treatment of choice for early carcinomas	Over 90% if localized	Dryness of all mucosae Radionecrosis of bone
Laryngeal and all nasopharyngeal carcinomas	Often avoids need for surgery in other cases	About 35% for advanced cases	Spinal cord damage
Lung: non-small-cell carcinoma	Good palliative treatment for younger patients with inoperable disease; probably no place in attempted cure	Combined with surgery, gives about 50% cure in stage I cases. Lower survival in later cases	Pneumonitis, oesophagitis, spinal cord damage
Small-cell carcinoma of lung	Radiotherapy and chemotherapy better than chemotherapy alone	Under 10%	Pneumonitis, oesophagitis, spinal cord damage
Thyroid	Well-differentiated cases usually treated by surgery alone if localized and by systemic radioiodine if metastasized and metastases pick up iodine	Well differentiated, 75–95%; poorly differentiated, less than 25%	–
Breast	Radiotherapy usually combined with surgery; radiotherapy alone may be used for advanced fungating tumours, sometimes with toilet mastectomy later	About 70% in operable cases (but 5-year survival is not cure in breast cancer)	Pneumonitis, brachial plexus damage, lymphoedema of arm, skin changes, and chest wall damage
Genitourinary tract—bladder	Often definitive therapy	Dependent on stage and grades: between 75% for T1 to 10% for advanced disease	Small bladder syndrome, large bowel damage
Testis	Radiotherapy largely being supplanted by chemotherapy, particularly for non-seminoma germ-cell tumours	Excellent (almost 100%) with early tumours and over 50% even with very advanced cases	Abdominal wall and small bowel damage. Myocardial damage and pneumonitis
Soft-tissue sarcoma	Wide surgical excision plus adjuvant radiotherapy and sometimes chemotherapy is most useful treatment if localized tumour	Varies with stage and site, up to 80%	Limb sites tolerate radiotherapy well, although may cause joint ankylosis and residual oedema
Bone sarcoma	Usually treated with limb-preserving surgery and chemotherapy	–	–
Gastrointestinal tract—rectum	Increasingly used as adjuvant postoperative treatment for locally extensive tumours as well as for palliative treatment of recurrences	Depends on Dukes stage	Small and large bowel damage, rectal bleeding, strictures
Anus	Increasingly replacing surgery as definitive treatment	Relates to age of patient and grade of tumour; 60% for tumours of anal verge. Chemotherapy may improve local control further	Local fibrosis and stricturing, perineal erythema, and soreness
Hodgkin's disease	Usually curative and treatment of choice in more advanced cases	Very good in asymptomatic supradiaphragmatic disease. Greater than 85% in localized cases and about 60% in more advanced (stages I to IIA). Often used with chemotherapy	Pneumonitis, pericarditis, thyroid dysfunction
Non-Hodgkin's lymphoma	Chemotherapy more important but radiotherapy often more valuable than systemic radiotherapy in relapsed cases	Variable; depends on cell type, localization or dissemination, and cellular architecture	–

myeloma, acute leukaemias, and high-grade lymphomas, and can prove curative.

Adjuvant radiotherapy

The principle underlying adjuvant therapy is that clinically undetectable micrometastases are often present in tissue surrounding a primary lesion, in regional nodes, and in remote locations. These are believed to be responsible for local, regional, and systemic recurrence after a primary lesion has apparently been completely removed. Adjuvant radiotherapy can be applied to local tissue and regional nodes after (or occasionally before) surgery to try to eliminate micrometastases. The technique is most widely employed for cancer of the breast after removing the primary lesion locally or by mastectomy. There is still controversy as to the best management of the axilla in breast cancer. Formal axillary clearance without radiotherapy is preferred by most surgeons, as the combined morbidity of the two modalities is considerably greater than either alone. If axillary nodes are involved, radiotherapy can be used as an alternative to radical lymph-node clearance; survival rates are comparable to those achieved after more extensive surgery. However, the trend of opinion favours radical lymph-node clearance for the improved diagnostic accuracy it provides and the prognostic value of knowing the number of nodes involved. The preference for surgery or radiotherapy remains one of local choice.

Radiotherapy has been shown to improve the local recurrence rate after surgery for rectal cancer. Because of the difficulties in standardizing surgical technique, the relative contribution of the radiotherapy is difficult to quantitate. However, most surgeons and oncologists would agree that adjuvant radiotherapy is beneficial in rectal cancer. Preoperative radiotherapy has been shown to downstage rectal tumours and may make some locally advanced cancers operable.

Palliative radiotherapy

For patients with widespread cancer in whom cure is unrealistic, palliative radiotherapy is often a most valuable treatment. In recent years palliative fractionation has become simpler, shorter, and more effective. Radiotherapy is particularly effective in controlling metastatic deposits in bone and brain. The pain of bone metastases can often be completely relieved by radiotherapy, as can some of the neurological manifestations of brain secondaries. In ulcerating breast cancer, radiotherapy can shrink the primary lesion, controlling exudation and bleeding and permitting healing of overlying skin. Similarly, the distressing symptoms of cough, haemoptysis, and pleuritic pain from advanced lung cancer can be eased by palliative radiotherapy. Symptoms associated with local tumour recurrence can often be controlled (e.g. haematuria from advanced bladder cancer or pain from rectal carcinoma). In abdominal malignancy the main factor limiting the use of radiotherapy is incidental radiation injury to normal bowel. This can cause stricture formation, obstruction, and continual bleeding, often years later.

Combined modality treatment

For certain tumours there is a move towards combined treatment. For example, premenopausal women with node-positive breast cancer may be offered local surgical resection, post-operative radiotherapy and adjuvant chemotherapy, and hormonal manipulation thereafter. In Hodgkin's disease with a large mediastinal mass, or small-cell lung cancer, combined radiation and chemotherapy has emerged as the standard treatment. In recent years squamous-cell carcinomas previously thought to be chemoresistant are now demonstrating response rates above 50 per cent with modern combination chemotherapy. When applied to the head and neck, combined radical irradiation and neoadjuvant chemotherapy has demonstrated improved local

control and overall survival in randomized trials. In rectal carcinoma, surgery plus adjuvant pelvic irradiation has given improved results over surgery alone in certain studies from the USA, particularly in patients who have also been given chemotherapy. In recent years limb-bone sarcomas have undergone transformation in their treatment. It was previously thought essential to perform amputation, but combined radiotherapy and limb-preserving surgery with the use of endoprostheses has been demonstrated to be effective in many cases. Similarly, soft-tissue sarcomas of limbs have been treated effectively with radiotherapy.

Obstructed hollow viscera

Combining laser and radiation treatment has been demonstrated as an attractive option for the treatment of tumour-obstructed hollow viscera, for example oesophagus or bronchus. When critical obstruction has taken place, the obstruction can be cleared rapidly by laser destruction, allowing palliative radiotherapy to be given safely.

Conclusion

There have been rapid changes in the treatment of cancer over the past decade. Radiotherapy has emerged as the primary treatment for many formally surgically treated tumours, and treatment with combined modalities is becoming more commonplace. Technical developments will continue in both radiological imaging and computer-assisted radiation targeting techniques, to allow safer delivery of high doses of radiation with greater precision, effecting better local control. Improving chemotherapy regimens hold out hope of eliminating clinical or even subclinical metastatic disease.

6.2 Chemotherapy

In 1943 a ship carrying sulphur mustard gas exploded accidentally, exposing the crew to the effects of the gas. It was noted that most of these individuals subsequently had a low white blood cell count and it was thought that this type of agent could be applied to the treatment of leukaemias and lymphomas. From this observation the first anticancer drugs were developed. The first nitrogen mustard compounds were used to treat haematological malignancies in the late 1940s and produced tumour shrinkage, but the effects were short lived.

Over the following 50 years understanding of the kinetics of tumour growth has improved, allowing the development of anticancer agents which attack malignant cells by different mechanisms. The ideal chemotherapeutic agent should be active against malignant cells but not damaging to normal cells. Therefore strategies to exploit the differences between normal and malignant cells have been explored. As yet no ideal chemotherapeutic agent exists and therefore most chemotherapy regimes are associated with side-effects due to damage to normal cells, particularly those of the bone marrow and gastrointestinal tract, which undergo rapid cell division.

Certain basic concepts are important in the understanding of tumour growth and anticancer treatment. Dividing cells under-

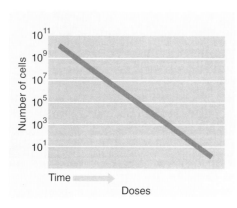

Figure 16.6 The effect of chemotherapy on tumour cell growth according to Skipper's laws.

go a cycle consisting of four phases: M (mitotic), G_1 (gap phase), S (synthesis of DNA), and G_2 (premitotic phase)—as described above (Fig. 16.1). Rates of tumour growth and response to chemotherapy have been studied in various animal models, from which certain principles can be derived.

Skipper's laws

Using a mouse leukaemia model, Skipper described the growth rates and cell killing effects of chemotherapeutic drugs. The animal tumour in this model contains cells which are all dividing and therefore exponential growth occurs. A plot of cell number against time is therefore a straight line on a semi-log scale. In this model the drugs used exhibited first-order kinetics, killing a fixed proportion of the tumour cells with each dose. Therefore if the original number of cells in the tumour is estimated and the proportion killed by each dose is known, then the number of cycles of chemotherapy required to destroy the tumour can be calculated (Fig. 16.6).

Gompertzian growth

It is only in experimental tumours that all cells are dividing; in the clinical situation only a proportion of the cells within a tumour are actively dividing. Similarly, if tumours exhibit central necrosis due to outgrowing their blood supply, these central cells will not undergo division. Therefore tumour growth will not be exponential and a plot of cell number against time

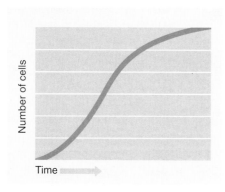

Figure 16.7 Sigmoidal Gompertzian growth curve.

will be sigmoid shaped when plotted on a semi-log scale (Fig. 16.7). This is known as a Gompertzian growth curve.

Goldie–Coldman hypothesis

Spontaneous mutations within tumours can result in the development of clones of cells resistant to one or more groups of chemotherapeutic agents. These cells are therefore able to grow selectively and therefore overall tumour growth may continue despite cytotoxic treatment which is killing a fixed proportion of the appropriately sensitive tumour cells with each dose. The rate at which tumours develop drug resistance depends on the frequency at which mutations occur, which itself depends on the size of the tumour and the inherent instability of its cells.

Cytotoxic agents

Most cytotoxic agents damage DNA or interfere with DNA synthesis and therefore are most toxic to dividing cells which are unable to repair their DNA prior to cell division. Side-effects of chemotherapy therefore occur mainly in relation to tissues with a high proportion of dividing cells. Bone-marrow suppression; mucositis of the gastrointestinal tract, causing ulceration, vomiting, and diarrhoea; alopecia; and infertility are common problems.

Alkylating agents

These drugs react with DNA to form covalent bonds between an alkyl group on the drug molecule and nitrogen atoms within the bases in the DNA, resulting in single- or double-strand DNA breaks and cross-linking of adjacent DNA molecules. Therefore normal replication, repair and transcription of DNA are inhibited. Alkylating agents are used in the treatment of many haematological and solid tumours and are useful for dose intensification strategies because of their steep dose–response curve. Their common side-effects include alopecia, gastrointestinal disturbances, bone-marrow suppression, and infertility.

Nitrogen mustards

- **Melphalan.** Commonly used in myeloma and chemotherapy regimes prior to bone-marrow transplantation.

- **Chlorambucil.** Used in chronic lymphoid leukaemia, well tolerated, orally active.

- **Mustine (chlormethine).** Occasionally still used in Hodgkin's disease but superseded by newer drugs due to its toxic side-effects—profuse vomiting, tissue necrosis following extravasation.

Oxazaphosphorines

- **Cyclophosphamide.** This compound is inactive as given but is metabolized in the liver into two active molecules—phosphoramide mustard and acrolein. The former appears to be the active cytotoxic agent and the latter accounts for some of the side-effects, such as bladder toxicity. Cyclophosphamide is widely used in the treatment of haematological malignancies and other cancers, such as carcinoma of the breast, and for treatment prior to bone-marrow transplantation. It may be given orally or intravenously and has a moderate degree of toxicity, causing emesis, marrow suppression, and alopecia. Acrolein causes haemorrhagic cystitis but this can be prevented by pretreatment hydration and administration of mesna, which binds to and inactivates acrolein.

◆ **Ifosfamide.** This compound is similar to cyclophosphamide and requires activation in the liver. It is useful in a similar range of tumours to cyclophosphamide but also has a role in the treatment of sarcomas. It is administered intravenously in conjunction with mesna to reduce bladder toxicity. Its profile of side-effects is similar to that of cyclophosphamide but, in addition, it may cause encephalopathy.

Alkyl aziridines

◆ **Thiotepa.** Its major use is for intracavity administration to treat malignant effusions or bladder cancer. It is occasionally used as a second- or third-line agent in the treatment of breast cancer.

Alkyl alkane sulphonates

◆ **Busulfan.** Its major role is in the treatment of chronic myeloid leukaemia. It is well tolerated and orally active.

Bioreductive agents

◆ **Mitomycin C.** This highly toxic agent is an antibiotic which acts by alkylation of DNA. It is used widely in the treatment of upper gastrointestinal malignances, breast cancer, and non-small-cell lung tumours. It is myelosuppressive with delayed onset typically 4–6 weeks after treatment. Prolonged use can cause permanent marrow damage. It can also cause pulmonary fibrosis and renal toxicity. It is administered intravenously or instilled into the bladder.

Nitrosureas

◆ **Lomustine (CCNU).** A lipid-soluble nitrosurea given orally in the treatment of Hodgkin's disease. It causes moderately severe emesis and delayed marrow suppression which can be permanent.

◆ **Carmustine (BCNU).** A non-lipid soluble nitrosurea given intravenously for the treatment of myeloma, lymphoma, and brain tumours. Side-effects include renal failure and delayed pulmonary fibrosis.

Antimetabolites

These are cytotoxic agents which have a similar structure to naturally occurring purines, pyrimidines, or nucleic acids. They therefore can either inhibit enzymes involved in DNA synthesis or can become incorporated into DNA or RNA causing strand breaks or premature chain termination. They generally act during the synthetic (S) phase of the cell cycle and therefore they usually need to be delivered over a relatively long period of time and are mostly administered by continuous intravenous infusion.

Antifolates

◆ **Methotrexate (MTX).** This commonly used antimetabolite is structurally related to folic acid and therefore inhibits the enzyme dihydrofolate reductase (DHFR) for which it has a greater affinity than the normal substrate folic acid. MTX is metabolized to a polyglutamated form which has an even greater affinity for DHFR and leads to further enzyme inhibition. MTX and its metabolites also inhibit thymidine synthetase. Because MTX and its metabolites are preferentially bound by DHFR, its effects cannot be reversed by folic acid. However, restoration of cellular reduced folic acid administered as folinic acid or leucovorin can ameliorate some of the toxic effects of MTX. Oral, intravenous, or intrathecal routes are all used for the administration of MTX. It is used in a wide spectrum of malignancies, including leukaemias, lymphomas, breast, and gastric cancer. Combination chemotherapy includes MTX in several of the commonly used regimes (e.g. CMF: cyclophosphamide, methotrexate, and 5-fluorouracil) is current first-line treatment for adjuvant chemotherapy for breast cancer. Side-effects of MTX include myelosuppression and gastrointestinal disturbances.

Antipyrimidines

◆ **5-fluorouracil (5FU).** This fluoropyrimidine is metabolized intracellularly to 5-fluoro, 2-deoxyuridylate monophosphate (FdUMP) and fluorouridine triphosphate (FUTP). In the presence of reduced folates, FdUMP forms a covalent bond with and inhibits thymidylate synthetase. FUTP becomes incorporated into RNA, leading to strand breaks and malfunction. Folinic acid can be administered to increase the cytotoxic effects of 5FU because it potentiates the inhibition of thymidylate synthetase. 5FU and leucovorin are therefore usually given together. One of its major uses is in the treatment of colorectal cancer, both as adjuvant treatment and for metastatic disease. 5FU is also used as part of the CMF regime for breast cancer and in other advanced gastrointestinal malignancies. Side-effects include vomiting, diarrhoea, marrow suppression, and plantar-palmar erythema.

◆ **Cytosine arabinoside.** This pyrimidine analogue is derived from the sponge *Cryptothethya crypta*. It is phosphorylated intracellularly to a triphosphate which inhibits the enzyme DNA polymerase and therefore interferes with DNA synthesis. Cytosine arabinoside is administered by intravenous infusion because of its relatively short half-life, due to inactivation by cytidine deaminase. Its main use is in the treatment of acute myeloid leukaemia, but it must be monitored carefully because of its profound myelotoxicity.

Antipurines

◆ **6-Mercaptopurine.** This adenine analogue is used in the maintenance therapy of acute leukaemias. It is useful because it can be administered orally.

- **6-Thioguanine.** Similarly this guanine analogue is given orally to maintain remission in acute myeloid leukaemia.

- **Fludarabine.** This relatively new antipurine is given intravenously for the treatment of B-cell chronic lymphocytic leukaemia which has failed to respond to alkylating agents. It can cause myelosuppression and neurological and renal problems and needs to be monitored carefully.

Heavy metals

Platinum compounds bind to DNA to produce DNA adducts which form intrastrand DNA links and inhibit DNA replication and function.

- **Cisplatin.** This highly toxic compound is very active against germ-cell testicular tumours and has revolutionized their treatment. It causes renal damage, severe emesis, and is neurotoxic and ototoxic.

- **Carboplatin.** This is a newer analogue of cisplatin and retains the potent cytotoxic effects of its parent. It causes less renal, gastrointestinal, and neurological damage, but does produce some myelosuppression, particularly thrombocytopenia.

Antitumour antibiotics

A variety of antimicrobial agents have cytotoxic activity and all cause a degree of myelosuppression, alopecia, mucositis, and emesis. Several mechanisms of action have been ascribed to this class of antitumour agents:

- intercalation between DNA strands;
- inhibition of topoisomerase II;
- free-radical formation;
- covalent binding to DNA;
- cell-membrane interactions.

Anthracyclines

- **Doxorubicin/Adriamycin®.** This useful drug acts by intercalation between DNA strands and interferes with DNA replication. It is administered intravenously and is used in a variety of solid tumours, both carcinomas and sarcomas.

- **Daunorubicin.** Used in the treatment of acute leukaemias.

- **Epirubicin.** A newer drug with similar spectrum of activity to doxorubicin.

- **Idarubicin.** Used recently in the treatment of haematological malignancies.

- **Bleomycin.** This agent causes DNA strand breaks and is used to treat lymphomas, germ-cell tumours, and squamous-cell carcinomas. It can be given systemically by intravenous or intramuscular injection, or instilled into the pleural cavity after drainage of a malignant effusion. Its particular side-effect is pulmonary fibrosis.

Topoisomerase inhibitors

These agents inhibit the topoisomerase enzymes, which are a group of enzymes that allow unwinding and uncoiling of supercoiled DNA.

Topoisomerase I inhibitors

This is a relatively new group of drugs used for salvage treatment of metastatic cancers. These drugs cause myelosuppression which may be dose limiting, along with diarrhoea, alopecia, and anorexia.

- **Irinotecan.** Used for the treatment of colorectal cancer which progresses on 5FU.

- **Toptecan.** This compound is used for the treatment of metastatic ovarian cancer when first-line or subsequent therapy has failed.

Topoisomerase II inhibitors

- **Etoposide (VP16).** An epiphyllotoxin extracted from the mandrake plant which is active against a variety of tumour types, including lymphomas, leukaemias, and small-cell lung cancer. It can be given orally or intravenously and is excreted via the kidney. Myelotoxicity, emesis, and alopecia are the major side-effects.

- **Teniposide.** Not licensed for clinical practice but shows some promising activity in research protocols.

Tubulin-binding drugs

Tubulin is the basic subunit of microtubules which are essential for maintenance of cell structure and spindle formation during mitosis.

Inhibitors of assembly—vinca alkaloids

These agents bind to tubulin dimers and prevent their assembly into microtubules. They are used in the treatment of acute leukaemias, lymphomas, breast, and lung cancer. They are all administered intravenously and must never be given intrathecally because of severe, potentially fatal, neurotoxicity.

- **Vinblastine.** Also shows activity against germ-cell tumours. More myelosuppressive but less neurotoxic than vincristine

- **Vincristine.** Its uses also include treatment of myeloma, Ewing's sarcoma, Wilm's tumour, and rhabdomyosarcoma. Its major limiting side-effect is peripheral neuropathy.

- **Vindesine.** Similar range of activity and toxicity profile to vinblastine.

Inhibitors of disassembly—taxanes

This relatively new group of compounds promote microtubule assembly, resulting in abnormally long microtubules which cannot function normally and therefore cell division is inhibited. Their major side-effects are neutropenia, neurotoxicity, alopecia, gastrointestinal disturbances, and hypersensitivity, including anaphylaxis.

◆ **Paclitaxel**. This compound is derived from the bark of the Pacific yew tree and is showing great promise in the treatment of primary and metastatic ovarian cancer. It is also licensed for use in metastatic breast cancer which has relapsed or progressed on anthracycline-containing chemotherapy. This drug is expensive and has enormous resource implications for oncology services if it becomes accepted as first-line treatment in ovarian cancer. Debate about limiting the use of new drugs to specialist centres and arguments about rationing have focused on this particular agent.

◆ **Docetaxel**. This agent is used for the treatment of metastatic breast cancer which has failed to respond to conventional chemotherapy. It is toxic and causes hypersensitivity reactions and peripheral oedema which can be resistant to treatment.

Cytotoxic chemotherapy protocols

Single agents

It is rare to use single agents nowadays but Adriamycin® is still used occasionally in the treatment of a range of solid tumours.

Combination chemotherapy

According to the Goldie–Coldman hypothesis, clones of cells resistant to cytotoxic agents develop within tumours and by the time a tumour is large enough to be clinically apparent it is likely to contain one or more of such clones. Therefore single-agent chemotherapy would exert a selective growth pressure on the resistant clones, allowing tumour growth to increase. In order to combat this problem, combination chemotherapy aims to give drugs that act in different ways and enhance each other's cell killing activity. Most combinations contain at least three drugs and must be selected for both their activity and for their side-effects. Common combinations include CMF (cyclophosphamide, methotrexate, and 5-fluorouracil) for the adjuvant treatment of breast cancer and FAMTX (5-fluorouracil, Adriamycin®, and methotrexate) for gastric cancer.

Indications for chemotherapy

As the armamentarium of cytotoxic drugs increases so the indications for their use expand. Some tumours, particularly haematological malignancies, are very chemosensitive and cure may be possible. So-called curative chemotherapy is the mainstay of treatment of germ-cell tumours and choriocarcinoma.

Table 16.7 lists tumours of differing chemosensitivity. For many of the 'surgical' cancers, such as breast and colon, adjuvant chemotherapy has been shown to be of some benefit in reducing relapse. More recently, neo-adjuvant chemotherapy administered before surgery has been shown to improve outcome in young women with advanced breast cancer at presentation.

Future developments

Chemotherapy plays an important role in the multidisciplinary approach to cancer treatment. Current cytotoxic drugs are limited by their side-effects on normal tissues. New agents, which can target malignant cells while sparing normal dividing

Table 16.7 Indications for chemotherapy in clinical practice

Highly chemosensitive tumours, 'curative' chemotherapy possible

Hodgkin's lymphoma

Intermediate and high-grade non-Hodgkin's lymphoma

Testicular teratoma

Testicular seminoma

Choriocarcinoma

Ovarian cancer

Acute lymphoblastic leukaemia

Acute myeloid leukaemia

Small-cell carcinoma of bronchus (early stage)

Chemosensitive tumours, adjuvant chemotherapy useful

Breast cancer

Colorectal cancer (Dukes C)

Ovarian cancer

Chemosensitive tumours, neoadjuvant chemotherapy useful

Breast cancer

Osteosarcoma

Non-small-cell lung cancer

Chemosensitive tumours, chemotherapy used for advanced/metastatic disease

Breast cancer

Ovarian cancer

Small-cell carcinoma of bronchus (advanced stage)

Soft-tissue sarcomas

Anal cancer

Tumours unresponsive to chemotherapy

Melanoma

Hypernephroma

cells, are continually being sought. An alternative approach is to use gene therapy to protect the normal tissues by transducing them with the MDR (multiple drug resistance) gene. This strategy has been used in advanced breast cancer where the combination of cytotoxic drugs used is likely to result in marrow failure. Therefore bone-marrow stem cells are harvested prior to treatment and transduced with the MDR gene, so that when the patient is treated with aggressive combination chemotherapy a proportion of the bone-marrow stem cells are resistant to these agents and will therefore be able to proliferate and repopulate the bone marrow. This type of novel strategy may allow currently available cytotoxic drugs to be used with greater efficacy and safety.

6.3 Hormonal therapy

A number of cancers, particularly of the genital tract or secondary sexual organs, are hormone sensitive for their development and growth, and therefore hormonal manipulation plays a role in their management. These tumours express receptors for specific hormones and so therapeutic intervention based on receptor blockade or reducing supply of a given hormone can be beneficial.

Prostatic cancer

It has long been recognized that prostatic cancer is androgen dependent, and for many years orchidectomy was the treatment of choice. This is a very effective way of preventing progression of prostatic cancer and is associated with good medium-term survival. Because of the psychological side-effects of orchidectomy, pharmacological agents are used more commonly nowadays.

LHRH agonists

The hypothalamic hormone, luteinizing hormone-releasing hormone (LHRH) causes transient stimulation of pituitary luteinizing hormone (LH) followed by downregulation and a fall in testosterone levels within 4 weeks. The transient stimulation of LH may cause a surge of testosterone and a 'flare' of bone pain on commencing treatment. Therefore an anti-androgen should be administered during the first 2 weeks of treatment.

A variety of these hypothalamic hormones is available, including gonadorelin and its analogues buserelin, goserelin, leuprorelin, and triptorelin. Goserelin is currently the most commonly used and is well tolerated by patients since it can be administered as a subcutaneous injection monthly (or three-monthly for the newer long-acting preparations). Side-effects can include impotence, gynaecomastia, and hot flushes. LHRH agonists are first-line treatment for many patients.

Antiandrogens

Cyproterone acetate and flutamide inhibit androgens by competing for binding to androgen receptors and are effective in reducing tumour size and symptoms. However, they appear to be less effective than orchidectomy in terms of long-term survival. This group of drugs is associated with a number of cardiovascular and gastrointestinal side-effects, and they are poorly tolerated by many patients. Their use is mainly restricted to covering the first 2 weeks of LHRH agonist treatment in order to prevent tumour 'flare'.

Combination androgen blockade

Orchidectomy combined with an LHRH agonist to block adrenal androgens has been recommended as a way of removing all androgen stimulation to prostatic tumours. However, a survival advantage has yet to be demonstrated.

Breast cancer

The response of breast cancer to hormonal manipulation is extremely variable and is difficult to correlate with the presence or absence of hormone receptors as they can be detected by current techniques. In premenopausal women oestradiol is synthesized from androgens in the ovarian follicles. The pituitary hormones, follicle stimulating hormone (FSH) and luteinizing hormone (LH), stimulate oestradiol production. For oestrogen-

Table 16.8 Hormonal manipulation in the treatment of breast cancer

Class	Drug	Side-effects
Anti-oestrogens	Tamoxifen	Hot flushes, depression, menstrual irregularities
Aromatase inhibitors	Aminoglutethide	Lethargy, rash, nausea, ataxia, depression
	4-Hydroxy-androstenedione	Rash, flushes
Progestins	Megestrol	Weight gain, tremor, sweats, hypertension, vaginal spotting
LHRH agonists	Goserelin	Menopausal symptoms

dependent tumours, removal of oestrogens by either oophorectomy or oestrogen-receptor blockade can be very effective. Tamoxifen is the most common anti-oestrogen in current use; it binds to oestrogen receptors and appears to cause tumour regression in about 30 per cent of premenopausal women with breast cancer. In those with oestrogen-receptor-positive tumours, regression occurs in approximately 50 per cent. A greater proportion of postmenopausal women respond to tamoxifen, which is currently recommended as adjuvant treatment for all postmenopausal women, regardless of receptor status. There is debate as to the optimum length of treatment, but there is evidence from large series that 5 years is better than 2 years in preventing recurrent disease. For tamoxifen usage longer than 5 years there is some risk of increased side-effects for little or no added benefit. In the very elderly, over 80 years, the response to tamoxifen can be dramatic. Primary tamoxifen therapy is a valid treatment choice in these individuals and approximately 50 per cent of these women will never need any other treatment for their tumours. Tamoxifen is generally well tolerated but its mechanism of action is not fully understood because it has partial agonist activity. Attempts to produce a safe, effective pure oestrogen antagonist have, as yet, proved unsuccessful.

Table 16.8 lists second-line hormonal agents used in the treatment of breast cancer. The aromatase inhibitors act to block conversion of adrenal androgens to oestrogens and cause tumour regression in approximately 30 per cent of patients. However, side-effects are more troublesome than for tamoxifen. LHRH agonists tend to be used only in refractory cases.

Pancreatic cancer

Tamoxifen has been used in the treatment of advanced pancreatic cancer. There is some experimental evidence that the growth of pancreatic cancer cells is retarded by tamoxifen, but no significant clinical benefit has been obtained by this approach.

6.4 Immunological and genetic interventions for cancer treatment

Therapeutic immunology has been discussed in detail above and is undergoing a resurgence of interest due to the use of molecular genetic techniques to enhance immunological treatments.

Gene therapy is the term used to describe any type of treatment strategy that involves the transfer of genetic material into cancer cells. There are over 100 clinical trials of cancer gene therapy in progress world-wide. The most promising genetic approach to treatment at present is VDEPT (virally directed enzyme prodrug therapy). This strategy uses a virus vector to transfect a gene encoding an enzyme into cancer cells. The enzyme chosen is one that can catalyse the conversion of a non-toxic prodrug into an active cytotoxic compound. When the tumour is subsequently exposed to the inactive prodrug the cells containing the transfected gene produce the enzyme necessary to metabolize the drug to its active form and are therefore destroyed selectively. Various combinations of enzyme and prodrug are in use, but the most commonly used pair is the herpes simplex virus thymidine kinase (HSVtk) enzyme with ganciclovir. Ganciclovir is used in the treatment of herpes virus infections, since HSVtk converts inactive ganciclovir to its active triphosphate metabolite in infected cells which are destroyed, while non-infected mammalian cells survive because they do not contain the appropriate enzyme and inactive ganciclovir is harmless. Several gene therapy trials have introduced the HSVtk gene on a retroviral vector into malignant brain tumours. Retroviruses target dividing cells and therefore only the malignant tumour cells take up the retroviral vector and when the patient is subsequently treated with ganciclovir only the cells containing HSVtk are destroyed while the non-dividing surrounding normal brain cells are spared. A series of children with recurrent glioblastomas have been treated by this method and have shown tumour regression, and improvement in disease-free interval and survival time.

An alternative gene therapy approach is the introduction of the MDR gene into bone-marrow stem cells prior to myelosuppressive chemotherapy for advanced cancers, as described above.

The ideal genetic intervention would be some form of corrective gene therapy so that the balance between proto-oncogenes and tumour suppressor genes in the control of cell growth and division could be restored. Antisense blockade of proto-oncogenes has shown some promise *in vitro* but has not proved useful *in vivo*. Transfection with normal copies of defective tumour suppressor genes has long been dismissed as unworkable, but recently a small number of trials of this approach have commenced. The *p53* gene has been used in trials of gene therapy for advanced lung cancer and hepatoma, with interesting observations of reduced tumour growth and some regression. Whether there will be any long-term benefit from such treatment is a matter for further study.

Advances in diagnostic and interventional genetics are likely to continue apace over the next 10 years and genetic therapy will have an increasing role in the adjuvant treatment of cancer. The breakthrough in the development of a mammalian artificial chromosome in 1997 has paved the way towards a future human artificial chromosome (HAC). Such a vector would allow stable introduction of large pieces of genomic DNA along with their controlling sequences into somatic cells. A HAC would therefore allow once-only treatment of cancer cells with the gene or genes of choice.

7 Counselling and support

There is strong evidence that professional counselling for patients with cancer can be helpful in relieving anxiety and depression and in improving fighting spirit and quality of life. This need not be prolonged—a recent study showed an average of 6 hours of counselling was extremely helpful. There is even a possibility that group therapy for patients with cancer may improve survival. Unfortunately, although most patients with cancer undoubtedly experience severe psychological stress, only a very small proportion accept counselling, and it is perhaps to be hoped that counselling should become part of the standard package of patients treated with palliative intent.

7.1 Psychological support of patients undergoing breast surgery

All treatment requires explanation, but in the surgical care of a patient with a breast problem this is doubly important. The emotional aspects of care are important and it is necessary to explain to the patient exactly what is happening right from the first consultation. There is now more openness about discussion of the diagnosis, and patients are far more knowledgeable as a result of media and newspaper publicity. This often means that patients may express a preference for a particular form of treatment, and as long as this does not prejudice the aims and likely success of the proposed therapy then it may be possible to accommodate these wishes.

Patient support is facilitated by the development of multidisciplinary teams who cooperate in the management of cancer patients. One of the problems of such a team approach, however, is that slight differences in emphasis between clinicians or other team members may be exploited by patients to suit their perceptions. It is therefore essential that regular team meetings are held so that management plans are agreed and any changes in treatment discussed.

The clinician

Both general practitioners and specialist clinicians have a responsibility to support their breast cancer patients. It is essential that there is good communication between hospital and community-based services, particularly in relation to patients who are terminally ill and wish to be cared for at home. Surgeons are responsible for coordinating the care of most breast cancer patients in the first instance and therefore they have a particular duty to ensure that patient diagnosis and management is in line with accepted professional guidelines and that their patients are well informed in order to participate in treatment decisions. Surgeons, of course, have a responsibility to ensure the technical skill with which surgery is performed and to refer appropriately for adjuvant treatment.

Breast counselling

Additional support for patients with malignant breast disease should be provided by nurse counsellors. Nurses with special experience of the worries and the practicalities of living with a diagnosis of breast cancer are now an integral part of most breast surgical departments. They provide a cross-boundary service and support the patient within hospital and also in the community. Close liaison with the surgical team is essential if confusion is to be avoided in explaining the details of treatment.

7.2 Maintaining the body image after breast surgery

The absence of a breast carries with it a double burden—it is a constant reminder of the underlying disease as well as being a major disfigurement. Attempts to compensate for the loss have always formed a part of the scheme of treatment in breast disease. The move towards more limited surgery was stimulated by the realization of the deep psychological effects of mastectomy. Although most patients after mastectomy maintain the cosmetic appearance of a breast by wearing a prosthesis, some are less inclined to accept this form of compensation and require breast reconstruction.

Prostheses

Immediately after surgery a lightweight pad filled with foam or fibre and covered with cotton can be used to fit within the bra. This is not suitable for the rigours of everyday life and needs to be replaced by a silicone prosthesis. The softer prosthesis can still be retained for nightwear. Silicone prostheses are covered with an outer polyurethane skin which is waterproof and hence can be used with swimwear. The fitting of a permanent prosthesis usually occurs 6 weeks from surgery and this allows time for the wound to settle. It is important that the fitter is skilled in advising patients on the correct shape and size because a badly fitted prosthesis is worse than not having one at all.

Breast reconstruction by tissue expansion

Placing a subpectoral silicone prosthesis is the easiest form of breast reconstruction. It is useful for women with small breasts and can be performed late after mastectomy. The prosthesis can be made of silicone gel, an inflatable silicone envelope which is filled with saline, or a combination prosthesis which is a centre of gel surrounded by a saline-filled envelope. It is placed beneath pectoralis major muscle by splitting the muscle along its length, creating a cavity in the subpectoral space and implanting the prosthesis. The volume of the saline-filled prosthesis can be gradually increased to allow the overlying tissues and skin to expand.

Breast reconstruction by myocutaneous flaps, for example latissimus dorsi or rectus abdominis

The principle with these techniques is to move a segment of muscle with its overlying skin to the mastectomy site. It is a technique that allows compensation for the removal of a large breast. The creation of the latissimus dorsi flap also allows a prosthesis to be placed under the muscle to equate the breast sizes (see Fig. 25.10). A nipple can be reconstructed from skin taken from the opposite nipple, the labia, or the inner aspect of the thigh. There is sometimes a need to consider the other breast, particularly if there is inequality of size, when a reduction mammoplasty could help.

7.3 Stoma care

Treatment of intra-abdominal malignancies is often marred by the necessity to form a stoma as either a temporary or a permanent measure. Stoma-care nurses play a vital role in helping patients cope with the physical and psychological aspects of having a stoma. Most patients, except for those with severe limitation of upper limb function or mental incapacity, have the physical ability to change their stoma appliance and maintain cleanliness. However, even the most dextrous patient may have significant psychological problems in coming to terms with a stoma. There are practical issues to be addressed in order to restore the patient's confidence for daily activities, particularly for young people in employment. Ideally, stoma-care nurses meet patients in hospital prior to, or just after, surgery and can then continue to see them at home after discharge and give practical advice when patients have resumed their normal diet and meal frequency. Stoma-care nurses also provide psychological support for patients during the almost inevitable problems with self-confidence and body image that occur after formation of a stoma. It is a tribute to the improvements in appliance manufacture and the stoma support services that so many individuals are able to lead independent and fulfilled lives without having noticeable hygiene problems or social stigma.

8 Palliation and palliative care

In recent years dramatic improvements have taken place in the treatment of many less common cancers, and adjuvant chemotherapy has improved the cure rate for several common cancers when these are diagnosed and treated in the early stages. However, most advanced common cancers remain incurable. In treating incurable cancer, the aim is to provide the maximum prolongation of good-quality life. This may involve palliative treatment (surgical, radiotherapeutic, or chemotherapeutic), symptomatic treatment, for example for vomiting or pain, and psychological support. When potentially toxic anticancer treatment is to be employed for palliative treatment, it is particularly important that the side-effects should not outweigh any actual or perceived benefit.

8.1 Effects on a patient's life of a diagnosis of incurable cancer

Cancer and its treatment often create havoc among the lives of patients and their families, to a much greater extent than other potentially fatal conditions like myocardial ischaemia. This is made up of several features:

- fear of the effects of cancer and its inexorable progress towards death—a sort of suspended sentence;
- lack of understanding about expectations of the disease and its treatment;
- fear of the effects of treatment and the fact that treatment may be ineffective and that further, perhaps more radical, treatments may be required later.

Patients with metastatic cancer may have only minor symptoms and yet have to cope with the realization that something is 'growing inside them' while they are still feeling well. The lack of symptoms perhaps makes the disease more frightening unless it is clearly controllable, particularly when the cause of the illness cannot be explained. If patients are told by doctors '… there is nothing more we can do for you' or they are given an inaccurate prediction that they have say 6 months or a year to live, it is not surprising that patients can feel miserable, anxious, and despondent.

8.2 Measuring quality of life

There have been moves towards measuring the quality of life as an integral component of most cancer trials and many attempts have been made to produce systematic mechanisms for doing so. None is wholly satisfactory in terms of clinical usefulness, simplicity of collecting information, scoring of results, or overall reliability and validity.

It has been demonstrated that patients who are given appropriate tools are more reliable at estimating their own quality of life than are doctors or nurses. Two instruments that use self-assessment have proved useful. These are the Rotterdam Symptom Check List, which comprises 30 items each rated on a four-point scale measuring physical and psychological elements of quality of life, and the Hospital Anxiety and Depression Scale, which is designed to measure anxiety and depression in patients who are physically ill. This scale deliberately excludes somatic symptoms of depression, such as weight loss or constipation. It is a self-rating scale, it is short and easy to understand and has a simple scoring system, and has proved valid in several studies. These two scales together currently represent the most practical and reliable measures for assessing quality of life in cancer patients.

8.3 The balance of benefit versus toxicity for palliative treatment

The overall balance of benefit versus toxicity in patients treated with palliative intent can only be obtained by careful documentation of quality of life. The results of several studies have sometimes produced surprising and unexpected results. For example, total gastrectomy was shown to be superior to proximal gastric resection in terms of quality of life and has the potential advantage of a greater cure rate.

A further study in comparing mastectomy with breast-conserving treatment for carcinoma of the breast showed no solid proof in favour of better psychological adjustment after breast-conserving treatment. However, these patients had a better body image and sexual functioning as compared with mastectomy patients. Surprisingly, fear of recurrence seemed to be more intense in patients after mastectomy than after breast-conserving treatment. As regards adjuvant chemotherapy for breast cancer, at present the results suggest there is approximately a 10 per cent improvement in survival in premenopausal patients. This might be considered to be too small to recommend chemotherapy in these patients but in a group of women who had received adjuvant chemotherapy, who were asked what improvement in survival would justify 6 months of adjuvant chemotherapy, almost half judged that 1 per cent improvement in a 5-year survival would justify treatment, and 80 per cent would find a 10 per cent improvement in 5-year survival sufficient to justify treatment.

8.4 Factors that influence the quality of life perceived by the patient with metastatic disease

Several disparate factors influence the quality of life as perceived by the patient. Clearly, a response in the state of metastatic disease is likely to make the patient feel better, but in a group of patients with advanced colorectal cancer treated with low-toxicity chemotherapy and with very few objective responses, most felt they had benefited from the treatment. Some benefit might arise merely from increased medical attention associated with being in a study, in addition to any placebo effect providing the patient with hope. In another study of chemotherapy in advanced symptomatic colorectal cancer, which compared a group treated with single-agent 5–fluorouracil with a group combining two other agents, the response rate in both groups was small, although slightly better in the more intensively treated group, which suffered more side-effects. Despite this, more than half the patients in the intensively treated group rated themselves as having improved quality of life, compared with only 9 per cent in the single-agent group. This and other studies suggests that side-effects are not the major determinants of quality of life. After response of metastatic disease, perceived benefits must be related to optimism and support provided by close medical supervision.

8.5 Alternative medicine

Many specialist alternative medicine clinics have set up to help treat cancer patients and it is often thought that they provide improved quality of life for patients. However, in a study from the United States comparing carefully matched patients, both receiving conventional treatment but one also receiving alternative therapy (including injections of BCG, strict vegetarian diet, etc.), found that quality of life scores were consistently better among patients treated only with conventional therapy.

Thus alternative therapies cannot be assumed necessarily to enhance the quality of life of patients with advanced cancer.

8.6 Symptom control

Symptom control is an important facet in quality of life estimation. This may be related to effectiveness of therapy, degree of emotional support, the extent to which the patient feels hopeful and optimistic, and their ability to function socially. Maximum symptom control must therefore be the first priority in trying to improve quality of life in incurable disease. Specialists in treating advanced incurable cancer have a full range of expertise in symptom control at their fingertips, but control of the disease may be an important aspect of symptom control even when the effect of treatment on survival is minimal.

Pain control

One of the symptoms that most frightens patients with incurable cancer is the fear of uncontrolled pain. With modern analgesics and other non-pharmacological approaches patients and their relatives should be able to be reassured that there will be no undue suffering no matter how advanced the cancer. It is important to understand that there are both physical and psychological aspects to pain perception and both should be addressed. If there is a remediable underlying physical cause for a specific pain, then appropriate surgery or radiotherapy should be employed to remove the source of the pain. Short courses of radiotherapy for isolated, painful skeletal metastases are particularly useful.

Analgesic drugs should be chosen on the basis of pain severity. The World Health Organization has produced an 'analgesic ladder', which aims to allow patients to be free from pain by using increasing potency and amounts of analgesic drugs in response to increasing or persisting pain (Fig. 16.8). Non-opioids such as paracetamol- and aspirin-based preparations are the mainstay of treatment for mild pains. These drugs are inexpensive and well tolerated orally and therefore should be used regularly in adequate doses to control pain and prevent breakthrough pains. For moderate pains, opioid drugs such as codeine or dextropropoxyphene should be introduced. Regular administration of adequate doses of these drugs should be added to the non-opioid analgesics already in use. If pain persists or increases, stronger opioids should be introduced, and fears about addiction and dependence should be dismissed. Morphine is the most commonly used strong opioid and is available in numerous preparations. Initially, rapid-release oral preparations, such as Oramorph®, should be administered as often as required in order to calculate the total daily dose required. Thereafter slow-release preparations, such as MST Continus®, can be given on a regular basis, with supplementation for breakthrough pain as required. Dosages should be reappraised frequently so that as few breakthrough episodes occur as possible. When the oral route is not tolerated, or dose frequency becomes excessive, opiates such as morphine,

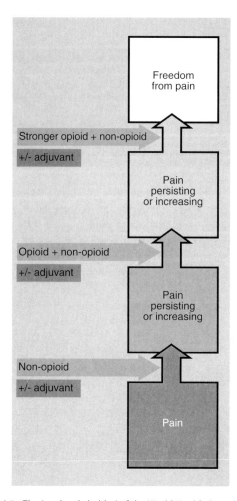

Figure 16.8 The 'analgesic ladder' of the World Health Organization.

diamorphine, or pethidine can be administered as a continuous subcutaneous infusion via a small syringe driver. Antiemetics, sedatives, and anticholinergic drugs can be added to the 'cocktail' in such a pump if necessary. Opiates are also available as rectal preparations, such as morphine suppositories, and transcutaneous fentanyl patches have proved useful in some patients. Buprenorphine can be administered sublingually and can be used in patients requiring relatively small doses of opioids.

There are numerous drugs that reduce pain in terminal cancer, even though they are not primarily analgesic in action. For instance, steroids such as dexamethasone are useful to reduce oedema and hence pain in patients with widespread hepatic or cerebral metastases. Tricyclic antidepressants and carbamazepine reduce certain neuralgic-type pains, and the former have a mood-altering effect. Some of the antiarrhythmic drugs are useful for cramps and muscle spasms. The latter may also be alleviated by diazepam or baclofen.

Non-pharmacological methods such as nerve blocks should not be overlooked. An effective coeliac plexus block can transform the day-to-day existence of a patient with inoperable pancreatic cancer. Transcutaneous electrical nerve stimulation (TENS) uses surface electrodes to stimulate large-diameter nerves in the skin and reduce pain perception. For some patients this is extremely effective, but it is difficult to predict which particular individuals will benefit.

Physiotherapy, ultrasound treatment, and acupuncture can help those with musculoskeletal pains and help to restore useful function. Individual patients may find pain relief from a multitude of alternative therapies alone or in conjunction with conventional medicine.

Nausea and vomiting

Gastrointestinal disturbances such as nausea and vomiting are common both due to cancer progression and due to treatments such as chemotherapy, radiotherapy, or analgesics. The mechanisms by which nausea and vomiting occur may be classified as central (those mediated via the brain) or peripheral (those mediated by the gastrointestinal tract) (Fig. 16.9). Central pathways from the cerebral cortex and vestibular system act directly on the vomiting centre and peripheral input is via afferent vagal neurons to the vomiting centre in the brainstem.

Treatment of nausea and vomiting depends on the underlying cause. For instance, hypercalcaemia can be reversed by rehydration and biphosphonates, and oesophageal or gastric outlet obstruction may be relieved by stenting or surgery. For many patients, however, there is no single cause of vomiting but numerous factors, as both the disease and its treatment contribute to feelings of nausea and vomiting. Therefore antiemetics will be required as a mainstay of treatment. Oral preparations are available but may not be tolerated if gastric stasis is a prominent feature or if profuse vomiting occurs. Therefore rectal and intramuscular or subcutaneous routes of administration should be used.

Prokinetic agents such as metoclopramide or cisapride are effective against opioid-induced vomiting and should be used prophylactically in order that beneficial analgesic effects of the opioids are not sacrificed due to unacceptable nausea and vomiting. Cytotoxic treatment carries a significant risk of producing vomiting as a side-effect, but the new 5HT3 antagonists, such as ondansetron or granisetron, have proved effective in the reduction of chemotherapy-induced vomiting, even that due to cisplatin. Dexamethasone may be used in conjunction with ondansetron and an anxiolytic such as lorazepam when chemotherapy is given. Eventually intestinal obstruction may supervene and may not be amenable to stenting or surgery. In such cases steroids can be used to reduce oedema if the obstruction is partial, but thereafter octreotide may be required to decrease the volume of intestinal secretions. Anticholinergic drugs such as hyoscine can also be used to reduce gastrointestinal secretions and motility. Both octreotide and hyoscine can be given by continuous subcutaneous infusion as well as bolus administration.

Chlorpromazine and haloperidol have proved useful in some groups of patients, particularly those with renal failure, severe hiccups, or intestinal obstruction. Such drugs may also have a sedative and anxiolytic effect and hence reduce distress and enhance general well being.

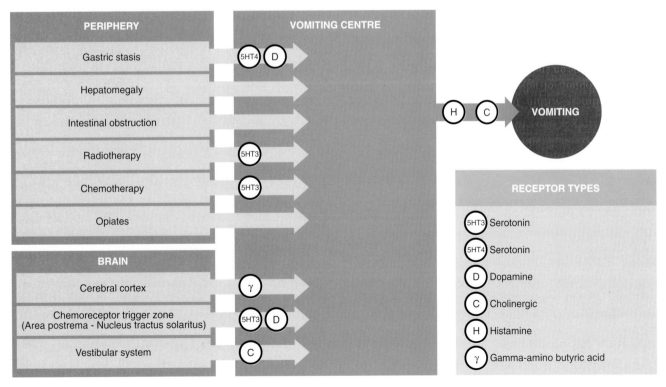

Figure 16.9 Control of the vomiting centre.

Bowel disturbances

Constipation is extremely common in cancer patients, either as a result of the disease itself or their treatment. In terminally ill patients admitted to hospices over 80 per cent will require laxatives. The aetiology of constipation is usually multifactorial in an individual patient, due to reduction in food intake, impaired intestinal motility, poor mobility, and opioid usage. It is important to note that in extreme cases overflow diarrhoea may occur and faecal impaction may also lead to urinary retention.

In managing constipation, simple measures such as attention to diet, fluid intake, and general mobility should not be overlooked. When pharmacological measures are necessary, stool softeners, peristaltic agents, or a combination of the two may be used. Stool softeners, such as sodium docusate or lactulose, are commonly used and can be used regularly to maintain a comfortable bowel habit. Flatulence and bloating may limit their use in some patients. Laxatives, such as senna or bisacodyl, stimulate the myenteric plexus to enhance peristalsis and are useful in opioid-induced constipation. Care should be exercised that intestinal colic and severe purgation do not occur with these drugs. Most patients can be managed with oral laxatives but occasionally rectal preparations may be necessary. A distended rectum or colon can be a source of pain and agitation in a terminally ill patient and administration of an enema to evacuate the bowel may help such as patient to settle and reduce terminal distress.

Diarrhoea is most commonly caused by overuse of laxatives to treat constipation, and polypharmacy should be avoided. 'Spurious' diarrhoea due to faecal impaction and overflow should be diagnosed and treated appropriately. Diarrhoea is also seen in patients undergoing potent chemotherapy or radiotherapy to the pelvis or abdomen. Because intestinal epithelial cells are turning over fairly rapidly, they are susceptible to damage by chemotherapy and radiation and hence diarrhoea ensues. Opioids being given for pain relief may counteract some of this effect, but antidiarrhoeals such as loperamide may be required. Usually diarrhoea ceases after chemotherapy but radiation enteritis may continue to provoke symptoms for many years.

Nutrition

Cancer cachexia is seen in approximately 80 per cent of patients before death and comprises a complex syndrome of anorexia, weight loss, muscle wasting, and fatigue. Clinical assessment is usually all that is required to confirm the presence of cancer cachexia—there is a history of substantial weight loss and the patient appears malnourished with reduced skin-fold thickness. Muscle wasting is usually evident. Biochemical parameters such as reduced serum albumin may be more useful for monitoring progress than for diagnosis.

Anorexia is almost universal in cancer cachexia and may be due to organic dysphagia in patients with pharyngeal or oesophageal malignancies, but is more commonly due to a combination of reduced taste sensation, depression, nausea, and drug side-effects. Metabolic abnormalities such as hypercalcaemia may impair appetite and it is thought that certain cytokines, such as interleukins 1 and 6 and cachectin-tumour necrosis factor, also reduce appetite. It seems likely that anorexia is the effect and not the cause of cancer cachexia and may explain why hyperalimentation has failed to influence survival or symptoms in patients with advanced malignancy. In the UK aggressive enteral and parenteral nutrition regimes are rarely used in terminally ill patients, but in continental Europe and the USA advanced cancer is the single most common indication for home nutritional support. There is no scientific rationale for this approach and it may have more to do with cultural reactions to terminal disease and palliative care.

There are, however, measures that can be taken to improve nutrition and a sense of well being, even in terminally ill patients. Dietary advice and the presentation and timing of meals are obviously important. In the busy schedule of hospital life it is easy to overlook simple measures such as liquidizing food or providing meals away from the noise and odours of the open ward. Alcohol can be usefully employed as an appetite stimulant. Drugs such as corticosteroids can enhance both appetite and well being, and prokinetic drugs such as cisapride may be useful if taken regularly before meals. Progesterone derivatives such as medroxyprogesterone and megestrol acetate can improve appetite, enhance calorific intake and well being, and increase deposition of fat.

In patients undergoing potentially curative treatment, aggressive nutritional support is indicated and therefore percutaneous gastrostomy or jejunostomy feeding can be used with great efficacy in patients with head and neck tumours or following oesophageal or gastric resection. Similarly, platinum-based chemotherapy and toxic regimens which include intrathecal methotrexate or cranial irradiation may cause such severe vomiting that enteral nutrition is impossible. Therefore parenteral nutrition for a limited time to support the patient through the anticancer treatment may be useful. Young patients with haematological malignancies, especially those undergoing bone-marrow transplant, are particularly helped by such intervention.

Depression and anxiety

Psychological reactions to the diagnosis of cancer and the subsequent course of the disease and its treatment almost invariably include both depression and anxiety. Therefore participation in treatment decisions and counselling, both formally and informally, by members of the multidisciplinary team are important in helping patients to rationalize their circumstances. However, up to 20 per cent of patients exhibit such extreme psychological reactions that formal psychiatric disorders may be diagnosed. Confusion can cause worsening of psychological symptoms and may be due to reversible or iatrogenic causes. The elderly and those with impaired hearing or vision are particularly at risk. Organic causes of confusion such as opiate intoxication, hypercalcaemia, uraemia, and infection should be treated appropriately.

Depression may present both somatic and psychological symptoms. Fatigue, sleep disturbances, poor appetite, and psychomotor retardation may be out of proportion to the physical pathology and respond poorly to conventional physical treatments. The psychological features of depression include low mood, particularly in the morning, reduced concentration, feelings of guilt, and hopeless and suicidal thoughts. These features are particularly common in those who have a pre-existing personality disorder or a history of drug or alcohol abuse and those without support from family or friends.

Anxiety may manifest with physical symptoms such as anorexia, agitation, palpitations, and sleep disturbances, or with psychological features such apprehension, constant need for reassurance, and panic attacks. In general, support from family, friends, and professionals can help to ameliorate symptoms in some patients, but a small minority will require formal psychiatric treatment. It is particularly important that those with suicidal thoughts are not overlooked as occasionally compulsory measures under the Mental Health Act 1983 may be necessary.

If supportive measures and counselling do not relieve symptoms, then drug treatment is indicated. The tricyclic antidepressants, such as amitriptyline or lofepramine, are well established for their sedative, anxiolytic, analgesic, and antidepressant properties. They produce a worthwhile response in 80 per cent of patients but are not without hazard, particularly in overdose. The newer specific serotonin reuptake inhibitors, such as sertralin or paroxetine, are also effective antidepressants but are less sedative and have less anticholinergic side-effects and are safer in overdose. Lithium, monoamine oxidase inhibitors, and electroconvulsive therapy may be used in individual patients with refractory depression or pre-existing psychiatric problems.

Anxiety requiring pharmacological intervention is best treated by a short, intermittent course of benzodiazepines. Prolonged administration can lead to tolerance, dependence, and psychomotor retardation. Midazolam and diazepam are the drugs of choice. If confusion is a feature, then a neuroleptic drug such as haloperidol is indicated. Where palpitations, tremor, and other physical symptoms predominate, a beta-blocker may be useful. It is essential that drug treatment does not replace family and professional support for patients, and that religious and cultural factors are taken into account.

Mouth and skin care

Oral problems are some of the most distressing symptoms for terminally ill patients. Simple measures with regard to hydration and cleaning of the teeth or dentures can transform the patient's existence. Dry mouth is a common complaint and can be ameliorated by regular sips of cold fluids or water sprays. Semifrozen tonic water, fruit juice, or gin can help restore the sensation of hydration. Petroleum jelly rubbed on the lips is also beneficial. Regular mouthwashes and dental cleaning can remove dirt and oral debris. Numerous mouthwashes have been advocated, but cider and soda is a particularly palatable remedy. Pineapple chunks are useful since the proteolytic enzyme annanase,

present in both fresh and tinned fruit, acts to clear a coated tongue. Painful oral conditions may impair fluid and dietary intake, and therefore should be addressed promptly. Coating agents such as sucralfate or carbenoxolone may be used but topical anaesthetics may be required. Mouthwashes and lozenges containing benzocaine and similar agents are available. Oral infections need specific treatment—candidiasis is probably the most common infection and responds to nystatin suspension or ketoconazole. Aphthous ulcers are also common and respond to topical corticosteroids or tetracycline mouthwash. Herpes infection requires specific treatment with aciclovir for 5 days. Malignant mouth ulcers are particularly distressing as they can be extensive, malodorous, and prone to secondary infection. Metronidazole, given systemically or applied topically as a gel, is the most useful remedy in this situation.

Skin problems are common in terminally ill patients due to their poor nutrition, reduced mobility, and often prolonged hospitalization. Pressure area care to prevent the development of pressure sores should be a core part of nursing any hospital inpatient. Pressure-reducing mattresses and lifting devices should be employed in both a preventative and therapeutic capacity. Attention should be paid to hydration, nutrition, and the avoidance of contamination by urine or faeces.

Skin problems related to malignant ulcers are also common and a variety of dressings are available. There are, however, certain general principles of care, and simple dressings are often as effective and more convenient, particularly for patients in the community. Pain relief is essential since cutaneous pain from malignant ulcers can be severe. All ulcers should be kept clean, and for shallow ulcers a simple moisture-retaining dressing, such as a hydrocolloid preparation, should be applied. Deeper ulcers should, if possible, be encouraged to granulate with dressings such as calcium alginate hydrogel or cavity foam preparations. If the ulcer is dirty or covered in slough, débridement may be achieved with hydrogel or hydrocolloid dressings, or surgically if the patient can tolerate such a procedure. Infected malodorous ulcers (and pressure sores) are best treated with metronidazole paste and dressings. Radiotherapy can be used to treat bleeding ulcers and has a more prolonged effect than adrenaline (epinephrine) or other vasoconstrictors.

Enterocutaneous fistulas may produce excessive volumes of secretions which have a damaging effect on the surrounding skin. Octreotide can reduce the volume of such secretions and custom-made stoma bags are essential for managing such patients.

Breathlessness and terminal restlessness

Breathlessness is a frightening symptom and is made worse by the panic that it engenders in patient and family. Over 70 per cent of cancer patients are likely to experience breathlessness in their last few weeks of life. General supportive measures such as reassurance, positioning of the bed, and relaxation techniques may be important, particularly if there is no easily remediable cause. In specific situations breathlessness can be abolished or improved by specific medical intervention. Drainage of pleural effusions or gross ascites is associated with marked improvement in symptoms and can be repeated as necessary. Similarly pericardial aspiration with or without fenestration may be required. Oxygen can provide both physical and psychological relief of breathlessness and can be administered at home. Corticosteroids have a useful role in both lymphangitis carcinomatosis and endobronchial disease to reduce oedema and improve air flow.

Paradoxically low doses of benzodiazepines and opioids are useful in the management of breathlessness since they help to break the vicious cycle between panic attacks and the sensation of breathlessness. In the last few days of life, when it is obvious that the patient is slipping away, heroic measures are counter-productive and if opioids are required for pain relief or benzodiazepines required to alleviate agitation and distress, some sedation must be accepted. In the terminal stages hyoscine is often administered in the same syringe driver as morphine and antiemetics, and can reduce the upper airway secretions and 'rattle', which are so distressing to patients and their carers.

8.7 Providing hope

Providing hope is vitally important for all patients with cancer. Patients may grasp any glimmer of hope, however small, which might explain why many patients enter trials of experimental therapy despite understanding that the chance of benefit is small. When asked, most patients appear to gain most emotional support from their doctors, and more senior doctors are seen as capable of giving more support. Thus patients seem most supported when they believe the information they are given is authoritative as well as accurate. This is probably the most important means of overcoming panic and restoring to the patient a sense of control over his or her life.

It is almost always counter-productive to tell people they have a fixed life expectancy; to do so removes hope and provokes depression and despondency. The average survival for a particular condition derived from published data applies only to populations and should not be used for individuals. It is more appropriate and helpful to indicate that while life might be short if things go badly, the length of life could still be long if things go well, and its duration cannot be estimated.

8.8 The hospice movement and the interface with primary care

Dame Cecily Saunders founded the St Christopher's Hospice in 1967 and since then palliative care has emerged as a speciality in its own right. The hospice movement is funded partly by the National Health Service and partly by charitable funds and is dedicated to the care of terminally ill patients. Traditionally, these have been cancer patients, but in recent years AIDS patients have required similar care. Hospices are able to take patients for inpatient admission and outpatient treatment and generally provide a far more relaxed and sympathetic environment than a busy hospital ward. Some hospices employ dedicated palliative care physicians who supervise treatment,

but others rely on local general practitioners. Since, in many areas, general practitioners no longer provide 24-hour care, terminally ill patients are often admitted from home, or even from a hospice, inappropriately to acute medical or surgical teams, since these are the only options 'out of hours'. The Calman–Hine proposals suggest that patients and their families can expect palliative care in the community, at home or in a hospice, if desired, but manpower issues will need to be addressed if this is to become a reality.

8.9 Conclusion

Therapists are now in a better position than ever before to treat patients with palliative chemotherapy and radiotherapy, with minimal side-effects. Using modern single agents for palliative chemotherapy with low side-effects, together with symptom control with powerful drugs, offers the patients a chance to benefit without excessive cost. The current reality is that most advanced cancers are treated with palliative intent and quality of life issues must be of prime concern. Treatments should aim to reduce the physical effects of cancer where possible. In addition, the doctor who understands what information the patient needs, will help the patient regain a sense of control while not removing all hope for the future.

Bibliography

Carmichael, J. and Woll, P.J. (Eds.) (1995) Oncology, parts 1 & 2. *Medicine*, **23**, 10–11.

Expert Advisory Group on Cancer to the Chief Medical Officers of England and Wales (1995). *A Policy Framework for Commissioning Cancer Services*. Department of Health, London.

Fallon, M. and O'Neill, B. (ed.) (1998). *The ABC of palliative care*. BMJ, London.

Fearon, E. and Vogelstein, B. (1990). A genetic model for colorectal carcinogenesis. *Cell*, **61**, 759–67.

Forrest Committee (1986). *Breast cancer screening*. Report to the Health Ministers of England, Wales, Scotland and Northern Ireland by a working group chaired by Professor Sir Patrick Forrest. Department of Health and Social Security. HMSO, London

Heald, R.J. and Ryall, R.D.H. (1986). Recurrence and survival after total mesorectal excision for rectal cancer. *Lancet*, i, 1479–82.

Miki, Y., Swensen, J., Shattuck-Eidens, D. *et al*. (1994). A strong candidate for the breast and ovarian cancer susceptibility gene *BRCA1. Science*, **266**, 66–71.

Royal College of Surgeons of England and Association of Coloproctology of Great Britain and Ireland (1996). *Guidelines for the management of colorectal cancer*. RCSE, London.

Taylor *et al.* (ed.) (1996). *Essential general surgical oncology*. Churchill Livingstone, New York.

Vile, R. and Russell, S. (1994). Gene transfer technologies for the gene therapy of cancer. *Gene Therapy*, 1, 88–98.

Vogelstein, B. and Kinzler, K.W. (1992). p53 function and dysfunction. *Cell*, 70, 523–6.

Vogelstein, B., Fearon, E., Hamilton, S., *et al.* (1988). Genetic alterations during colorectal tumour development. *New England Journal of Medicine*, 319, 525–32.

Trauma

Iain D. Anderson

1 Introduction

1.1 The scale of the problem

Accidental injury is a major yet neglected health problem. Trauma is the principle cause of hospital admission in males aged less than 35 years and is the most common cause of death in males and females between 1 and 34 years of age. In Britain, 40 deaths a day occur from accidents of all kinds and 100 deaths per week result from road traffic accidents alone. Trauma results in the loss of more economically productive years than cancer and heart disease combined. Trauma patients over 65 years of age are twice as likely to die and cost twice as much as young patients to treat. Deaths, however, are only the tip of the iceberg, with more than half a million patients surviving hospital admission as a result of trauma each year. Unlike other serious illnesses, some 80 per cent of trauma patients can be returned to full productive and unrestricted life if high-quality care can be provided.

1.2 The provision of trauma services

It is completely accepted that the provision of organized trauma services is essential if unnecessary death and complications are to be prevented. Debate continues about the method by which this organization should be achieved. Over the past 20 years numerous studies from around the world have shown that some 1 in 3 deaths occurring from injury in the absence of an organized system of trauma care, will be potentially preventable. This was the position in England and Wales in the mid 1980s and the problem has been tackled on several fronts.

First, the response in hospitals of all sizes to the arrival of a multiply injured patient has become more organized with the creation of **trauma teams**. Experienced staff from surgical, anaesthetic, and critical care disciplines are scrambled to the resuscitation room, preferably in advance of the patient's arrival. Hand in hand with this, the equipment required for the immediate management of injured patients of all ages is prepared for instant readiness within that defined area. Secondly, the wholesale adoption of advanced trauma life support (ATLS) training has made an enormous impact on the standard of care. Although this system deals only with the initial resuscitation of injured patients, the organization of a coordinated team approach, where specialists now share common rather than divergent goals, cannot be underestimated. Resuscitation is faster, better prioritized, and immediate outcome is improved.

Thirdly, the question of trauma centres arises. A trauma centre is a hospital that acts as a tertiary referral centre for injured patients. It will offer the full range of specialties round-the-clock. The development of trauma centres has been associated with improved outcome in other countries, but not to date in Britain. At least as important as the question of individual outcome is the role these large hospitals play in allowing a body of expertise in trauma management to accumulate, leading to advances in trauma training, research, and case management.

The success of implementing these measures is slowly being realized. Formerly, three peaks of death from injury were identified. The first was virtually immediate and usually resulted from irretrievable laceration of the central nervous system or great vessels. The second peak occurred within the first hour or two of injury, usually from haemorrhage or hypoxia, and recent initiatives have been directed primarily towards these patients. The third peak occurred days or weeks after injury and was usually due to sepsis and multiple organ failure. Again the perception is that expert resuscitation in the early phase, together with timely definitive surgery, serves to minimize this last peak. It is of interest that in centres that have adopted recent changes wholeheartedly, the second peak of 'golden-hour' deaths has been enormously reduced.

Simultaneously, paramedics have undergone specific trauma training. Debate continues about the relative merits of a 'scoop and run' policy—where the patient is immediately transferred to hospital—and the merits of paramedic or medic-directed treatment at the scene. No clear evidence of benefit of the latter approach has been demonstrated. Likewise, helicopter transport has specific advantages in certain cases, but data do not exist to support widespread adoption.

1.3 Immediate hospital management of the injured patient

The aim is to identify and treat injuries in the order of priority determined by the greatest threat to the well-being of the patient, and to do this as quickly and as safely as possible. To achieve this successfully and thereby prevent unnecessary deaths from injury, tardy or uncoordinated treatment, haemorrhage, or hypoxia, it is vital that these patients are managed by a multidisciplinary team that follows an established and commonly taught system of injury management.

Airway

The first step is to secure a patent airway through which high-flow oxygen (12 litres/minute) should be delivered, using a reservoir mask. A hierarchy of interventions may be necessary to secure the airway and the surgeon should be familiar with all of these. These begin with chin lift or jaw thrust to open the airway, suction aspiration to remove debris, and insertion of a pharyngeal airway by the oral or nasal route to maintain patency. If an airway is inadequate, a cuffed endotracheal tube is inserted, again by oral or nasal route, depending on circumstance. When these measures are unsuccessful it will occasionally be necessary to create a surgical airway. The method of choice is **needle cricothyroidotomy with jet ventilation** while preparations are made for early surgical cricothyroidotomy or formal tracheostomy. Throughout the airway manoeuvres discussed, the cervical spine must be protected by the technique known as manual in-line immobilization or else by application of a semirigid collar, sandbags, and forehead tape. This is necessary to prevent aggravation or creation of a spinal-cord injury consequent upon an unrecognized fracture or dislocation of the cervical spine.

Breathing and ventilation

The patient must be assessed and treated to ensure that adequate ventilation is taking place. Any hindrance to this must be diagnosed and treated directly at this stage. For example, a **tension pneumothorax** will require needle decompression followed by formal chest drainage. The management of other immediately life-threatening chest injuries is discussed below.

Circulation and haemorrhage

The third priority is to establish adequate circulation. External haemorrhage must be controlled immediately with pressure. Intravenous access must be obtained at two peripheral sites with large-bore (14–16 g) cannulae and blood sent for cross-matching and biochemical analysis. Peripheral access is the priority and if prompt access cannot be obtained in the arms, the surgeon should be prepared to cut down on the long saphenous vein at the ankle. Central venous access is less favoured because of the likelihood of failing to cannulate relatively collapsed central veins, as well as the risk of causing a pneumothorax; its principal use lies in monitoring at a later stage. The circulation should be assessed clinically and if not promptly restored by immediate administration (in an adult) of 2 litres of warm crystalloid solution, then the source of internal haemorrhage should be identified and treated forthwith. Thus during this stage of the assessment, the surgeon may be called upon to take the patient to the operating theatre immediately to deal with major haemorrhage. It has recently been shown that following penetrating torso trauma in young patients, fluid resuscitation before induction of anaesthesia may be associated with worsened outcome. The reason may be that restoring blood pressure precipitates further haemorrhage. Clearly, young patients with penetrating injury constitute only a small minority of cases in the UK, but the findings at least stress the importance of early surgery. It is important to avoid the temptation to remove impaled weapons and objects other than in the operating theatre! The role of emergency department thoracotomy and laparotomy is discussed below, but the outcomes of these procedures is generally poor. It is perhaps better to emphasize that the profoundly shocked patient is likely to need immediate definitive surgery before reaching the stage of asystole or electromechanical dissociation.

The importance of stopping haemorrhage, usually by surgical means, has been emphasized earlier. Most shocked trauma patients have hypovolaemia as the only, or the major, contributing factor, and the relative roles of fluid replacement and surgery in this must be considered carefully. With certain injuries it is important to remember that shock may be arising from a tension pneumothorax, cardiac tamponade, neurogenic shock, septic shock, or myocardial contusion and dysfunction. These are all less common and their specific features are discussed elsewhere. Following injury, patients with these conditions usually exhibit a hypovolaemic element in addition.

The choice of intravenous fluid for resuscitation has excited some debate. Crystalloids (normal saline, Hartmann's solution) are free from the potential side-effects of colloids. A larger volume of crystalloid will be required initially to bring the same benefit as colloid, but there is no risk of interfering with cross-matching or causing anaphylaxis. Whatever non-blood fluid is used, it is important to continually remain aware of the volume infused. Once 1500 ml of infusion is approaching, very active consideration should be given to infusing blood and to surgical arrest of haemorrhage.

Neurological disability

When the circulation has been stabilized rapidly, the degree of neurological disability should be assessed. At this stage all that is required is to record the pupillary state and the degree of alertness or the type of stimuli to which the patient responds. The patient should then be undressed to permit a top-to-toe assessment. Throughout this stage, thought should be given to preventing hypothermia and preserving dignity. It is worth re-emphasizing that any life-threatening problems identified during the initial rapid assessment should be treated immediately they are discovered and that each system should be stabilized before progressing to the next.

Monitoring

Once this stage has been completed, it is appropriate to begin basic ECG and pulse oximetry monitoring, to insert a urinary catheter and nasogastric tube (unless contraindicated by suspicion of urethral injury or skull fracture, respectively) and to plan radiography of the cervical spine, chest, and pelvis. A full history of the accident and the scene should now be obtained from the paramedic crew. The aim of this is to bring to mind potential injuries typically associated with certain types of accident but which may not be evident or which might be overlooked on examination.

The patient should now undergo a secondary head-to-toe assessment and every injury should be identified and documented. If the patient becomes unstable during the course of this, a prompt re-assessment of the ABCs (with appropriate intervention) should be carried out. By the end of this assessment, a definitive treatment plan under the care of appropriate specialists should be emerging. In many cases, joint care is necessary for injured patients as a substantial proportion cannot easily be allocated to one or other specialties. The patient remains at risk during the hours where involved radiological investigations are undertaken and it is essential that patients are not abandoned to the care of a single junior doctor while investigation is proceeding. At this stage all involved specialists must maintain some responsibility for continuing assessment and care of the trauma victim.

2 Common major injuries

Common injuries are discussed systematically below. In all cases a system of management such as the advanced trauma life support system should be pursued initially and re-deployed whenever the patient becomes unstable. The management discussed assumes that appropriate care of airway, cervical spine, breathing, and circulation are being employed in all patients. The importance of this care cannot be overemphasized as failure to do so contributes to the phenomenon of secondary injury (further tissue damage caused by slow or in-appropriate management), which is still a depressingly common occurrence.

Table 17.1 Cricothyroidotomy

Indication	Failure to intubate the trachea
Position	Supine with neck slightly extended. Protect against cervical spine damage
Technique	Palpate the cricothyroid membrane between thyroid and cricoid cartilages. Use a 14-gauge cannula and puncture the skin in the midline directly over the cricothyroid membrane, directing the cannula caudally 45°. Aspirate continuously with an attached syringe as the cannula is inserted. Free aspiration of air indicates entry to the trachea. Remove the stylet and advance the cannula. Attach Y piece with oxygen at 15 litres/minute. Occlude the other limb of the Y piece for 1 second and observe for bilateral lung inflation. Release the thumb to permit passive deflation for 4 seconds. Exhalation is inefficient with this technique, causing CO_2 retention. This limits its use to 30–45 minutes
Surgical cricothyroidotomy	With appropriate anaesthesia and asepsis, a transverse incision is made over and down to the cricothyroid membrane and the airway entered. The stoma should be spread with a tracheal dilator and a size 6 tracheostomy tube inserted and secured. Check for adequate bilateral ventilation

2.1 Head injuries

Introduction

Head injuries are common. About 1 in 400 of the population require hospital admission following head injury each year and 70 per cent of all road traffic accidents result in head injuries. One-quarter of all multiply injured patients who die do so as a result of head injury. Appropriate early resuscitative treatment can prevent unnecessary morbidity and mortality and a low threshold for neurosurgical referral and definitive care should be maintained.

Classification and pathophysiology

Head injuries may be classified simply into penetrating (open) injuries and concussional (closed) injuries:

1. Penetrating injuries traverse the layers of the skull and require neurosurgical referral.

2a. Concussional injuries are caused by the continued movement of intracranial contents relative to the skull, and brain injury occurs at the principal point of impact as well as at remote sites (*contrecoup*). Contusions of the cortical surface are usually multiple and often affect the under surfaces of the frontal and temporal lobes. Laceration may result near sharp, bony edges (e.g. sphenoid wing) and contusion and laceration together may cause a 'burst lobe'.

2b. Diffuse axonal injury is caused by shearing resulting from rotational acceleration or deceleration. It is associated with cerebral oedema and raised intracranial pressure and occurs in approximately half of all severe head injuries. Focal contusions or haematomas are absent but, despite this, mortality is as high as 30 per cent and specialized care is needed.

Brainstem injury and unconsciousness

The causes of unconsciousness are poorly understood but coma may result from bilateral cortical injury or from a functional disconnection between the cortex and the reticular activating system in the upper brainstem. Duration and depth of unconsciousness and amnesia depend upon the severity of injury sustained.

Physiology of brain injury

The primary brain injury is that which occurs at the accident scene as a result of the forces applied. Secondary injury denotes damage that results from the responses to this injury as a result of hypoxia, hypovolaemia, or raised intracranial pressure, sometimes as a consequence of delayed surgery. An understanding of cerebral physiology and the principles of treatment is necessary to prevent secondary injury. The brain is essentially fluid and therefore incompressible and its biological response to injuries is swelling. As the skull is rigid, brain swelling or intracranial haemorrhage leads to elevation of intracranial pressure (ICP). The only possible compensatory mechanisms are reduction in cerebral blood volume (and usually perfusion), diminution of CSF volume, or displacement of the brain (herniation and

Table 17.2 Factors contributing to raised intracranial pressure

Oedema from primary or secondary injury
Intracerebral haemorrhage or intracranial haematoma
Hypoxia (airway/breathing difficulty, chest injury)
CO_2 retention and cerebral vasodilatation
Hypovolaemia (untreated other injuries)

coning), the last being rapidly fatal. Adequate cerebral perfusion is vital: cerebral perfusion pressure (CPP) is the blood pressure minus the intracranial pressure, and brain death occurs when CPP becomes inadequate and falls towards zero.

Following closed injury, the brain becomes progressively swollen. This occurs diffusely as well as at the site of injury. Intracranial haemorrhage may further increase the volume of intracranial contents, sometimes extremely rapidly. Oedema is aggravated by episodes of hypoxaemia or hypovolaemia early on. Airway obstruction or inadequate ventilation results in hypercarbia, which causes cerebral vasodilatation and a further rise in ICP (Table 17.2).

A net increase in intracranial volume within a fixed skull capacity causes rising intracerebral pressure, which is likely to impair cerebral perfusion. In the early stages, swelling can be accommodated by reduction in the volume of blood in the dural sinuses and by absorption and displacement of CSF as ventricles are compressed. Later, perfusion can be maintained only by a rising systemic arterial blood pressure (Cushing's reflex). Further rises in intracranial pressure, particularly if localized, cause shifts of brain tissue and herniation of brain tissue between left and right sides or through the tentorial opening and foramen magnum. These herniations may obstruct venous outflow from the brain or the CSF pathways, removing compensatory mechanisms and causing a further rapid rise in ICP.

Herniation of the uncus of the temporal lobe downwards through the tentorial hiatus causes deterioration in the patient's clinical condition by secondary compression of the brainstem. This is the classical result of a temporo-parietal haematoma. The effects include disturbances of consciousness, respiration, and contralateral motor movement. The ipsilateral third nerve may be compressed, causing pupillary dilatation. Once pupils are dilated and fixed, brainstem injury is usually calamitous and terminal infarction is likely.

Closed head injuries

Introduction

Closed blunt head injuries present a spectrum from the trivial to the inevitably fatal.

Minor closed head injuries

This group comprises the vast majority of head-injury patients seen at hospital and admission is not always required. After a blow to the head, which may be quite trivial, there may be a transient period of loss of consciousness. Particularly in children, it may not be clear whether consciousness has been lost

Table 17.3 Criteria for hospital admission after head injury

Loss of consciousness >5 min

Confusion or depressed level of consciousness at the time of examination

Post-traumatic amnesia longer than 5 minutes

Neurological symptoms or signs

Persisting headache or vomiting

Patient under influence of alcohol or drugs

Complicating co-morbid conditions: epilepsy, diabetes, haemophilia

Skull or facial fractures or suspected fractures (i.e. periorbital or subconjunctival haematoma, mastoid bruising)

Large scalp lacerations or scalp lacerations suspected of communicating with a skull fracture or penetrating injury

Cerebrospinal fluid leakage from nose or ear

Poor social conditions or lack of a responsible adult at home

In children, loss of consciousness or amnesia at any time

Table 17.4 Indications for CT scan in closed head injury

Severe head injury: Glasgow Coma Score < 8

Focal neurological signs

Epileptic fit

Fractured skull

Penetrating injury

Prolonged depression of conscious level (> 6 hours)

and the child may appear dazed and may vomit. If consciousness recovers quickly, only a tiny proportion of patients develops potentially lethal complications. The key is to recognize patients at particular risk of deterioration (Table 17.3).

If an adult has returned to normal consciousness and is asymptomatic, then subsequent deterioration is very unlikely and admission is not necessary unless there are other risk factors (Table 17.3). Since most complications manifest within 24 hours of injury, this is a suitable duration for admission for the large number of patients with moderate or minor head injuries who recover quickly and have no other reason for continued admission. Thus, the general indications for admission to hospital after transient loss of consciousness are: all patients with persisting signs or symptoms, all patients under the influence of drugs or alcohol where consciousness may be clouded, and all children.

The place of skull radiographs is debated: anyone with scalp bruising or swelling should have skull radiographs. Fractures are certainly associated with a higher risk (1 in 32) of intracranial complication, including haemorrhage. This risk rises to 1 in 4 if the patient is also disoriented, but patients at risk of developing complications after a fracture are likely to have other indications for a CT scan. If local policies determine that patients with a fracture are to be observed routinely for a longer period (e.g. 5 days), then a policy of subjecting all patients to be admitted to skull radiography is appropriate. When patients are discharged, it should be to the care of a responsible adult who should be warned about signs and symptoms of concern, both verbally and on a printed card.

Management of closed head injuries

Immediate management should follow ATLS guidelines. The aim is to prevent secondary injury, diagnose the nature and severity of the primary injury, and transport those requiring neurosurgery to a specialist safely and as quickly as possible. Initially, secondary injury is prevented by managing the ABCs

well and this will often include artificial ventilation and treatment of other injuries. At a later stage, ICP monitoring may be needed.

The severity of primary injury is assessed by neurological examination, including assessment of the Glasgow Coma Score (GCS), while the nature of the primary injury is diagnosed by CT scan. This is immediately required in a patient with a GCS of less than 8 and focal neurological signs, and in any patient who meets any criterion shown in Table 17.4. The primary aim is to diagnose and treat intracranial bleeding as quickly as possible. Intracranial haematomas occur in only 7 per cent of all head injuries but in 50 per cent of severe head injuries (GCS < 8), particularly those with neurological signs.

The level of consciousness is the most important clinical sign in assessing the severity of a head injury. In mild head injury, disturbance of consciousness is transient but may be followed by a period of mild confusion and drowsiness. In severe head injury, coma with complete unresponsiveness may occur and last for months (or even permanently).

The Glasgow Coma Scale (GCS) (Table 17.5) is the most widely used method of quantifying conscious level and has the advantages of simplicity of observation, consistency between

Table 17.5 Glasgow Coma Scale

GCS is the sum of the best score achievable in each of three domains of response:

Eye-opening response (E)
4. spontaneous
3. to speech
2. to pain
1. none

Motor response (M)
6. spontaneous
5. localizes pain
4. withdraws from painful stimulus
3. abnormal flexion (decorticate)
2. abnormal extension (decerebrate)
1. none

Verbal response (V)
5. appropriate
4. confused
3. inappropriate speech
2. incomprehensible—grunts, etc.
1. none

When discussing a case with a neurosurgeon it is useful to have the component E, M, and V scores to hand different observers and the fact that the practical significance of a changing score has been clearly established. It should be employed routinely and recorded serially on the patient's charts at the end of the bed.

Intracranial haemorrhage is one of the main causes of deterioration in patients admitted conscious after head injury. Deterioration may be rapid and may transform an apparent minor injury into one with serious and permanent neurological injury or death. Many of these consequences are avoidable and much of the thrust of management is aimed at diagnosing and treating them. Intracranial haemorrhage may be arterial or venous. It may occur as a result of damage to the middle meningeal artery or its branches (typically with a squamous temporal bone fracture), to one of the dural venous sinuses, or to veins bridging between brain and skull.

Extradural (epidural) haematoma

These occur in 1–2 per cent of severe head injuries and may be arterial or venous. Temporal or parietal extradural haematomas result from middle meningeal damage, whereas frontal or occipital extradural haematoma is more likely to result from a dural sinus laceration. The typical course is a minor head injury from which the patient rapidly regains consciousness (and starts talking again) before deteriorating into coma, perhaps with ipsilateral pupillary dilatation and contralateral limb weakness, before succumbing ('talk and die'). The prognosis is excellent if treatment is begun when the patient is well. This involves evacuation of the clot and control of the bleeding vessel. Once coma is established, mortality rises sharply.

Acute subdural haematoma

This usually results from rupture of bridging veins that traverse the subdural space between cortex and dural sinuses. Unlike epidural haematomas, it is usually associated with a severe primary injury. Consequently, the outcome is much worse, with a typical mortality of 50–60 per cent. Sometimes, subdural and intracerebral haematoma occur together as a result of laceration or contusion of brain substance.

Subarachnoid blood may be seen on CT scan but requires no treatment. Occasionally an intracerebral haematoma or pulped lobe will require removal if it is responsible for an excessive mass effect.

Skull fracture

A skull fracture indicates that a substantial blow to the head has occurred and represents an independent risk factor for intracranial haemorrhage. Patients with skull fractures are usually observed in hospital for 5 days or so. Fractures may predispose to infection and a missed skull fracture can be medicolegally negligent. Clinical signs suspicious of fracture are scalp lacerations, CSF leakage, periorbital haematoma, and subconjunctival haematoma with no visible posterior border or mastoid haematoma (**Battle's sign**). Most fractures can be diagnosed if high-quality skull radiographs are taken and interpreted correctly. Fluid levels in the paranasal sinuses are suspicious of skull fracture even if a fracture line is not visible.

CSF leakage

CSF leakage from the ear (CSF otorrhoea) or nose (CSF rhinorrhoea) indicates the presence of a skull fracture with an associated dural tear (i.e. a compound fracture). CSF rhinorrhoea is more common and occurs in about 25 per cent of anterior fossa fractures (including the frontal, ethmoid, and sphenoid sinuses), particularly if the cribriform plate is involved. Occasionally it occurs in petrous temporal fractures with CSF leakage from the middle ear via the Eustachian tube. CSF otorrhoea is uncommon, occurring in about 7 per cent of basal skull fractures. It requires an associated laceration or perforation of the ear drum. When there is CSF leakage, there is about a 20 per cent risk of meningitis and prophylactic antibiotics should be given. As the most common infecting organism is pneumococcus, penicillin is the most effective drug, and should be given until a week after leakage has ceased. Most skull-base leaks cease spontaneously but anterior fossa leaks are more likely to persist and to require dural repair. There is a risk of delayed meningitis after spontaneous cessation of CSF leakage. Dural repair is indicated if leakage persists or if meningitis has developed.

Cranial nerve injury

This occurs in about 30 per cent of major head injury patients. Anosmia is the most common abnormality. Less commonly, pupil dilatation may occur as a result of traumatic mydriasis. Facial nerve palsy and deafness result from fractures of the petrous temporal bone. Neurosurgical referral is needed in this case.

Scalp injury

Closed head injuries rarely cause hypovolaemia. The only and rare exception to this rule is when subgaleal haemorrhage occurs in very small children. Tangential blows may partially avulse the scalp and cause little brain damage but the absence of scalp damage does not exclude serious brain injury. Scalp flaps should be restored to their normal position and pressure dressings applied. Obvious bleeding vessels can be directly undersewn.

Associated problems affecting management

Alcohol intoxication is usually apparent at blood concentrations of 10 mg/100 ml, whereas coma is likely with levels greater than 400 mg/100 ml. Intoxicated patients may underventilate or inhale vomitus or their disruptive behaviour may be wrongly blamed on intoxication and a serious head injury missed. If the patient has pinpoint pupils suspicious of opiate use, naloxone 4 mg intravenously should be given to attempt reversal. Hypoglycaemia must be excluded in all patients and treated with intravenous glucose as necessary. It is unwise to attribute neurological or mental state abnormalities to factors other than head injury except by exclusion.

Managing deterioration

Deterioration after admission needs urgent action to trace the cause. Actively re-exclude hypoxia, hypercarbia, or hypovolaemia, and treat appropriately. A (repeat) CT scan should be performed and the neurosurgeon contacted. Performing blind burr holes is no longer acceptable in areas with accessible CT scanning facilities: significant haematomas can be easily missed and the time taken for the non-specialist to carry these out is often more than that needed to transfer to a neurosurgeon.

Outcome of severe closed head injuries

Without definitive care, the mortality for major head injuries is around 50 per cent, reducing to 30 per cent if comprehensive neurosurgical care is provided—a very clear message. Patients with severe head injuries with very low scores on the Glasgow Coma Scale rarely survive beyond 24 hours. The need to transfer a patient with a haematoma is self-evident. Although operative decompression is not indicated in severe diffuse bilateral brain swelling, the prognosis can be correlated with the intracranial pressure. If pressure is persistently above 40 mmHg, there is a very high mortality, whereas below 20 mmHg, the mortality is about 20 per cent. Young patients fare better than elderly patients with similar injuries and children are capable of surviving and overcoming the most severe injuries.

Managing brain swelling

In the absence of haematoma, deterioration may be attributable to contusion and developing swelling, partly due to loss of vasomotor control. Simple early measures include elective ventilation, the administration of intravenous mannitol, and the search for intracranial haemorrhage. Hyperventilation to induce hypocapnia is no longer used, because it has no proven benefit, but avoiding hypercapnia and hypoxia is essential; ventilatory maintenance reduces metabolic demand of the brain and assists in maintaining temperature control. Osmotic diuretics such as mannitol may give temporary relief during investigation or prior to surgery, but if given to undiagnosed head injury patients, may precipitate further haemorrhage or result in rebound swelling. It should be used only after neurosurgical consultation. Dexamethasone has no useful function in diffuse brain swelling following injury. In patients with significant brain swelling, intracerebral pressure (ICP) should be monitored invasively; the chance of survival can be directly correlated with level of intracranial pressure and techniques exist to modify ICP. Alternatively, methods exist for monitoring cerebral perfusion pressure directly.

Neurosurgical referral

Given the documented benefit of expert care of head injuries with regard to outcome, prompt referral of cases likely to benefit from neurosurgery or ICP monitoring should be made (Table 17.6).

Systemic abnormalities after head injury

In addition to the problem of ventilatory inadequacy and secondary injury, patients with severe head injury may exhibit respiratory abnormalities such as hyperventilation. Abnormalities of temperature control are also seen and hyperpyrexia increases the metabolic demand of the damaged brain and may increase swelling; extreme hyperpyrexia may be fatal. Most head-injured patients vomit; intestinal absorption is impaired

Table 17.6 Criteria for obtaining a neurosurgical opinion after head injury

Abnormal CT scan

Fractured skull with any of the following:
    confusion or persistent headache or vomiting
    focal neurological signs
    fits

CSF leakage from nose or ear, even if not persistent

Suspected fracture of the skull base

Penetrating or compound fracture of the skull

Coma or altered consciousness persisting for more than 6 hours

Deterioration in a previously well patient—depression of consciousness, pupillary changes, meningism, headache, and vomiting

Any doubts

and ulceration of upper gastrointestinal mucosa may occur, leading to haemorrhage or perforation (Cushing's ulcer). Endocrine disorders include diabetes insipidus and inappropriate ADH secretion.

Late outcome

Patients with intermediate Glasgow Coma Scores, particularly with predominant brainstem signs, may take weeks to recover. The most basic functions tend to recover first, usually within 1–2 weeks of injury. These include control of blood pressure, respiration, and body temperature. This is usually followed by gradual return of consciousness, after which assessment of cerebral cortical functions can be performed. Disturbances of memory, concentration, deductive powers, mood and patterns of behaviour, as well as permanent focal neurological disorders, such as anosmia, paralyses, and sensory loss can occur and these may be permanent. Patients suffering severe diffuse shearing injury may be rendered effectively decorticate. The patient appears alert but is incapable of responding to speech and of initiating any movement or other activity. This 'semi-vegetative' state may persist for years and raises profound ethical dilemmas. The general surgeon may become involved with delivery of enteral nutrition at this stage.

Penetrating (open) head injuries

Penetrating injuries are less common and result from a 'blunt' injury against a sharp corner or from weapons of assault or missiles. Gunshot wounds to the head are usually catastrophic, unless the injury is peripheral. Brain penetration should be suspected in any injury of the above types and the scalp carefully examined for entry wounds. Any scalp laceration should be suspected of lying over a skull fracture which, if present, would inevitably be compound. Penetrating injuries rarely cause loss of consciousness but may cause a focal neurological deficit if a sensitive area of the brain is damaged. These deficits are likely to be permanent. Compound, depressed skull fractures come into this category. When the brain coverings are penetrated, the cranial cavity is open to the exterior. Foreign bodies, dirt, and fragments of scalp and skull bone may be carried into the brain substance with an attendant serious risk of infection, such as meningitis or brain abscess. Penetrating injuries may also cause epilepsy, early or late, in 12–20 per cent of cases. There is a greatly increased risk of late epilepsy (as high as 70 per cent) if there has been post-traumatic amnesia for longer than 24 hours, early epilepsy, or a dural tear. These cases should be given long-term prophylactic anticonvulsants.

Managing penetrating head injuries

These patients should be referred to a neurosurgeon after initial stabilization. Formal surgical cleaning of the wound and skin closure should be performed under general anaesthesia as soon as practicable and certainly within 24 hours. Devitalized tissue, including brain and bone, should be removed together with accessible foreign bodies, exercising great care near the venous sinuses. Prophylactic antibiotics should be given. Closed depressed skull fractures need elevating only if the depression is greater than the thickness of the skull or if there is a marked cosmetic disturbance.

Factors associated with a poor prognosis are listed in Table 17.7.

Facial injuries

The surgeon may be called upon to manage facial injuries in a number of circumstances, for example to perform a cricothyroidotomy to secure the airway, as bleeding and distortion of the oropharynx are common with maxillofacial trauma. Major haemorrhage may require emergency control. Balloon catheters can arrest nasopalatine haemorrhage, while, very occasionally, immediate direct control of major vessels will be needed.

Severe facial injuries are often associated with other severe injuries of the head, neck, or chest. About 15 per cent of patients with facial fractures have significant cervical spine injuries. Thus the patient's neck should be immobilized, the patient should be evaluated neurologically, and the cervical spine carefully X-rayed. In addition, about 70 per cent of patients with facial fractures are likely to have sustained ocular injuries. Facial fractures are common and should be referred to a maxillofacial surgeon. The presence of facial injury should be sought in head-injured patients following overnight observation, as new facial injuries may come to light (and require radiography and treatment) once aggression and alcohol have dissipated.

Table 17.7 Factors associated with poor prognosis after head injury

Multiple injuries associated with head injury

Massive areas of skull or brain damage

Advanced age

Abnormal motor signs

Pupil abnormalities

Diffuse bilateral lesions on CT scan

Increasing intracerebral pressure

Soft-tissue injuries of the face

Road dirt, glass, and other foreign bodies must be removed to ensure aesthetic healing. Bleeding can be arrested with local anaesthetic injections containing adrenaline (epinephrine) and by local pressure, but not by using artery forceps to clip the artery proximally as the facial nerves may be damaged. In repairing soft tissues, the goal is exact anatomical alignment with minimal débridement because of the good blood supply of the face, which allows even quite damaged tissue to heal. The facial nerve must be tested for injury. Facial nerve branches should be repaired if divided lateral to an imaginary vertical line at the lateral canthus of the eye. Medial to this line, cross-over branching usually allows good regeneration of function without repair. Parotid duct injuries should be sought and repaired if possible, although the duct may be ligated with minimal adverse effects. Eyelid injuries should be repaired by an ophthalmologist, as it is vital to repair a damaged levator palpebrae superioris to prevent ptosis. Skin sutures in the eyelid should be removed after 2–3 days to prevent early epithelialization of the suture tracks.

Skeletal injuries

Recognizing bony injuries to the face depends on careful clinical examination, as facial fractures are not always obvious. Surgical emphysema may indicate paranasal sinus fractures, and subconjunctival haemorrhage with no visible posterior margin is usually a sign of orbital or skull-base fracture. Eye movements should be examined to reveal diplopia or **ocular entrapment** after a blow-out fracture of the orbit. The latter is manifest by a loss of upward gaze. Entrapment is an indication for surgery but diplopia alone may be a result of muscle contusion. Loss of sensation in the cheek may be caused by compression or laceration of the infraorbital nerve associated with a zygomatic fracture. Mandibular movements should be checked, as these may be restricted by mandibular fractures or by a zygomatic fracture. The occlusion of the teeth should be checked, as this is a very sensitive indicator of distortion. Diagnosis is confirmed by plain radiography and CT. The three patterns of fracture described by Le Fort in 1901 are of historical interest only as CT scanning has demonstrated that individual injuries deviate to varying degrees from the classical Le Fort patterns, with asymmetry common. Nasal fractures may cause septal haematomas, which obstruct nasal breathing, as well as ugly deformity and haemorrhage. Teeth are often damaged in facial injuries, they maybe displaced, fractured, or dislodged. Displaced, loose teeth should be collected, put in milk, and sent with the patient for possible later replantation. If the tooth is only partially displaced, it should be pushed back into its socket.

2.2 Spinal injuries

Introduction

The price paid by the patient for a missed spinal injury is high, hence the presence of spinal injury is best assumed until it has been actively excluded. This will require almost all injured patients to be managed with semirigid collar, sand bags, tape, and often a spine board as well, until a specialist is satisfied that no spinal injury exists. The major problems are due to spinal cord injury, causing major paralysis or death. Cord injury is usually, but by no means always, associated with spinal fracture or dislocation.

Aetiology

Spinal injuries occur chiefly as a result of forced flexion, extension, or lateral flexion of the spine. Most occur following motor vehicle accidents and motor cyclists are particularly vulnerable. In cars, ejection from the vehicle or trauma caused by another unrestrained passenger colliding with the victim may result in spinal injury. Spinal injuries are commonly found in patients with chest injuries and sternal injuries. Falls from a height on to the feet or head, often under the influence of alcohol or as a suicide attempt, or accidental falls down stairs, are other causes of spinal injury. Sporting injuries may also lead to spinal damage, particularly trampolining, rugby football with scrum collapse, horse riding, skiing (particularly collision between skiers), hang gliding, and diving into shallow pools (especially under the influence of alcohol). Industrial injury with a weight falling onto the back, or following ejection from a military aircraft, may also cause spinal damage.

Pathophysiology

Bony injury

Different forces cause differing bony injuries, each with a different likelihood of cord damage. Certain bony injuries are unstable, in that major ligaments are torn and the propensity for further damage is high. The general surgeon should assume that all bony injuries are unstable and immobilize the patient until expert help is summoned to take over care.

Spinal cord injury

Partial or complete transsection of the cord may occur because of abnormal movement of one component of the spinal column in relation to another. This causes impaired distal motor function, sensation, and autonomic function. The higher up the spinal cord the lesion, the greater the resulting disability and the risk to life. Secondary injury may occur: this may be mechanical, with movement of the victim causing bony fragments to impinge on the cord, or as a result of hypoxia (due to airway obstruction or ventilatory problems), or underperfusion caused by hypovolaemia resulting from multiple injuries. Hypoperfusion may be aggravated by orthostatic hypotension resulting from cord injury causing a loss of sympathetically mediated vascular tone (neurogenic shock).

Symptoms and signs of spinal cord injury

Symptoms following spinal cord injury may be bizarre and include sensation that the body is still in the position that it was at the time of the accident, paraesthesia, and burning pains. It is important to assess whether the cord lesion is complete or incomplete and to try to find a level of motor and sensory change. Incomplete lesions are more likely to recover. Classical signs of spinal injury include local tenderness and boggy swelling or a step at the site of the spinal fracture, and complete sensory loss below the injury. In unconscious patients, up to 15 per cent are likely to have a spinal injury. This may be indicated by differential pain responses in different parts of the body, loss of flaccidity, priapism, loss of anal tone, hypotension and bradycardia, or pure diaphragmatic ventilation. Loss of sensation may compromise diagnosis of an abdominal injury.

Cervical spine injury

The cervical spine is the most vulnerable to injury and therefore is the most commonly injured. It also causes the most severe disability. Injuries are usually caused by an indirect force such as occurs when the head strikes the ground or a heavy object.

It is safest to assume that all significantly injured patients (Table 17.8) have a cervical spine injury and immobilize them appropriately until this is disproved at an appropriate point in management by at least a full lateral cervical spine film (showing top of T1) or preferably, a full three-film series. In establishing an airway the cervical spine should be moved the minimum amount necessary to achieve a clear airway (no more than 10°) and only a jaw thrust should be used. Oxygen should be given and if ventilation is ineffective or the patient is in danger of aspirating, then intubation should be performed, preferably by an expert. Specialist help should be obtained immediately when injury is highly likely or confirmed. Fluid replacement should be kept to the minimum necessary for other injuries.

Thoracic and lumbar spine injuries

Thoracic and lumbar spine injuries are relatively uncommon but are easily overlooked. There is an increasing trend to manage those at risk on full spine boards until clinical and radiological assessment can be undertaken. Again, immediate expert help should be obtained with any spinal fracture. There is little room around the thoracic cord and displaced fractures here commonly result in total cord transsection. The spinal cord itself ends at the level of L1. Below this it becomes the cauda equina and only lower motor neuron or visceral (bladder) signs will be found. Injuries to the cauda equina carry a better prognosis than injury to the spinal cord because recovery can take place.

Management

Successful management depends upon identifying the injury before further damage is done, specialist referral, immobilization until necessary surgery can be undertaken, attention to coexisting injuries and their systemic effects, and specialist support and rehabilitation. Associated injuries are common and

Table 17.8 Patients at particular risk of cervical spine injury

Unconscious patient
Blunt injury above the clavicles
Local neck symptoms or signs
Neurological symptoms or signs

often severe. Loss of vasomotor tone causes vasodilatation and shock. Fluid therapy is needed, initially with crystalloids and blood, as indicated by other injuries, but once haemorrhage is controlled, colloid solutions or even controlled vasopressor therapy may be required.

Penetrating injuries of the neck

Introduction

Penetrating injuries of the neck are among the most difficult forms of trauma to manage because many vital structures are concentrated in a small area and because exposure of deep-seated structures, such as the subclavian or vertebral vessels, is difficult. Most penetrating injuries are caused by knife or low-velocity missiles and the crucial decision is whether surgical exploration is needed. The degree of aggression needed in investigating and exploring these patients has been debated at length. Clinical examination may be only 60–80 per cent accurate but it appears that selective exploration is a safe method of handling these difficult cases, provided certain criteria that indicate the need for urgent surgery are accepted (Table 17.9). For example, from a recent South African experience of 335 patients, 80 per cent were managed conservatively without death or major complication and only two of these required elective surgery (Demetriades *et al.* 1993).

Superficial wounds (platysma intact) constitute the majority and can be cleaned and sutured. Avoid probing wounds: they should be explored digitally by an experienced surgeon to determine whether the track leads towards the midline structures (in which case endoscopy or contrast swallow is needed) or away from them (no investigation needed). Concomitant thoracic injury should be searched for and an early chest radiograph will be standard. Patients with a bruit in the neck, a widened mediastinum, or diminished peripheral pulses can undergo angiography if stable. Subcutaneous emphysema should be investigated by bronchoscopy and water-soluble contrast swallow, as should those with other symptoms or signs suspicious of tracheo-oesophageal injury. In general, nerve injuries alone are not thought to be an indication for urgent surgery, although brachial plexus injuries should be repaired within 24–72 hours.

Management

General principles

The immediate management follows the principles already outlined with attention to the airway, breathing, and cardio-vascular system, an assessment of the neurological status, as well as a systematic survey for other injuries. Airway obstruction can be a particular problem in these patients because of neck haematoma or extensive laryngotracheal injury, and immediate endotracheal intubation or tracheostomy may be needed.

Active bleeding from the neck wound requires external pressure to control haemorrhage and the patient put into the Trendelenburg (head-down) position to prevent air embolism. Air embolism is a preventable cause of death when there is laceration of major veins. The neck is then explored urgently in the operating theatre.

Pneumothorax

This is common in penetrating neck injuries: an intrapleural drain must be inserted.

Cardiac arrest

Cardiac arrest following penetrating neck trauma requires endotracheal intubation and an immediate thoracotomy. Bleeding is controlled from inside the chest in cases of subclavian vessel injury and open cardiac resuscitation is carried out. The right ventricle should be aspirated of air if the arrest may be caused by air embolism.

The stable patient

If the patient is stable on admission, general examination and detailed examination of neck structures can be carried out (Table 17.10). Erect chest and neck radiographs are inspected for pneumothorax, mediastinal or subcutaneous emphysema, and widening of the upper mediastinum. Subcutaneous emphysema may result from a perforation of the pharynx, oesophagus, larynx, and trachea, or may originate from a pneumothorax. A widened mediastinum may indicate an injury to the aorta or its major branches and an aortogram should be performed if the patient is stable. If no major injuries are discovered, the patient should be admitted for observation. It is wise to re-examine patients a few weeks after a neck injury to exclude the development of a traumatic arteriovenous fistula, often not evident on presentation.

Table 17.9 Signs indicating the need for urgent surgery in penetrating neck injuries

Active bleeding from the neck

Shock, not responding to resuscitation and with no other causative injury

An expanding or pulsatile haematoma in the neck

Lost peripheral pulse

Air escaping through the neck wound

Major haemoptysis (or other evidence of airway penetration)

Haematemesis (or other evidence of oesophageal perforation)

Table 17.10 Assessing the stable patient with penetrating neck injury

1. Cranial nerve examination
2. Examination for cervical and brachial plexus injury
3. The sympathetic chain in the presence of Horner's syndrome
4. Peripheral pulses
5. Bruits
6. Sputum containing blood
7. Subcutaneous emphysema
8. Loss of air through the wound on coughing

Operative management of neck wounds

Anaesthetic induction is often difficult because of the neck wound. If a haematoma makes intubation difficult, an urgent cricothyroidotomy may be needed. Thoracotomy is likely to be needed for wounds at the base of the neck and the operation site should be prepared for a median sternotomy. An incision along the anterior boarder of the sternomastoid gives good exposure of the carotid sheath, pharynx, oesophagus, larynx, trachea, and vertebral artery. If subclavian or brachial plexus injury is likely, the neck may be exposed along the clavicle, dislocating the sternoclavicular joint.

Major arterial injuries are best managed by repair with vein grafts. Synthetic materials carry the risk of sepsis. Major veins can usually be ligated without serious consequence but bilateral ligation of the internal jugular is contraindicated. Major nerve injuries are repaired at the same time.

Specific injuries

Carotid sheath structures

Ten per cent of patients admitted with neck wounds have injuries to the carotid neurovascular bundle. The mortality of carotid artery injury is high and most are dead on arrival at hospital. Survivors should undergo repair of the artery, although it may be ligated to save life in a patient where a stroke has already occurred. In general, internal jugular injuries should be repaired but ligated if wounds are extensive or the patient cardiovascularly unstable.

Subclavian and innominate vessels

Venous injuries have a higher mortality than arterial injuries in this site because of the combined effects of haemorrhage and air embolism. The approach is either by dislocating the clavicle or via a median sternotomy. Arteries and veins are best repaired except to save life, when ligation of both can be carried out.

Vertebral artery injury

This is infrequent but dangerous because haemorrhage cannot be controlled by pressure. Diagnosis is made at operation. An anterior sternomastoid incision is made and the track of the penetrating injury probed with a finger. If there is persistent bleeding and the track passes to the area between the transverse processes, this strongly suggests vertebral artery damage.

Thoracic duct injury

Thoracic duct injury is rare. Diagnosis is made if chyle leaks from a left-sided wound. The duct should be ligated if recognized. If it is not recognized, a fistula will probably develop but most will close spontaneously within about 2 weeks.

Pharynx and oesophagus

Dysphagia, haematemesis, or surgical emphysema suggest injury to the pharynx or oesophagus. Injury is confirmed by contrast swallow and early operative repair is indicated.

Larynx and trachea

Haemoptysis, subcutaneous emphysema, or air bubbling through the skin wound suggest laryngotracheal injury. Primary

Table 17.11 Pathophysiological insults threatening life from thoracic trauma

1. Haemorrhage and shock from cardiac or major vessel injury
2. Hypoxia and acidosis resulting from obstruction of major airways or diaphragmatic injury
3. Cardiac tamponade or contusion

surgical repair is indicated and a tracheostomy performed to protect the repair from coughing during the healing phase. If the defect is difficult to close, a flap of muscle or facial skin can be used.

2.3 Thoracic injuries

Introduction

Twenty five percent of trauma deaths are due to thoracic trauma alone and half of all trauma deaths have chest injuries. Major injury to the heart, aorta, or tracheobronchial tree often cause death at the accident site, but if patients with these injuries reach the Accident Department alive, they can survive if they receive rapid and appropriate care (see Table 17.11). This includes resuscitation and recognition and treatment of the immediately life-threatening injuries such as tension pneumothorax and a search for occult but equally life-threatening injuries such as aortic arch rupture and oesophageal perforation.

Most chest injuries can be managed successfully by no greater surgical intervention than insertion of a chest drain, together with attention to oxygenation and the circulation. The exceptions to this rule require very rapid identification and definitive surgery, preferably with the involvement of a cardiothoracic surgeon. In such cases of penetrating vascular injury, blood loss may be exacerbated during resuscitation as the blood volume expands. If the injuries are not recognized and treated, the patient may exsanguinate. Unnecessary administration of excess colloid and crystalloid has been associated with a reduced survival rate and stresses again the importance of early surgery.

Types of injury

Blunt trauma

High-velocity impact (deceleration)

This is a highly dangerous type of injury, commonly occurring in road traffic accidents and falls. Usually, the victim is travelling fast and comes to a sudden stop on impact with another vehicle. The chest wall may be intact, particularly in young people, and conceal serious intrathoracic injuries. However, there may be a fractured sternum or bilateral rib fractures caused by direct impact with a steering wheel or with a restraining seat belt. Potential injuries include ruptured aorta, cardiac contusion, major airways injuries, and ruptured diaphragm (Fig. 17.1). All of these need early recognition if life is to be saved.

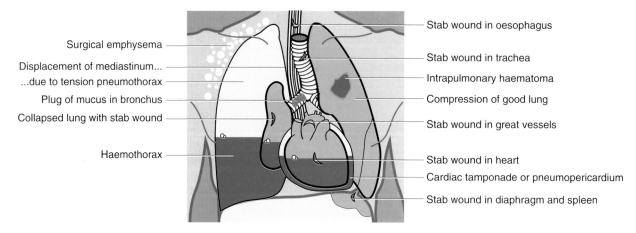

Figure 17.1 Common types of penetrating and blunt thoracic injury.

Crush injury

This type of injury may produce bilateral rib fractures with a flail chest, cardiac and pulmonary contusion, and bronchial rupture. Liver and spleen damage may be associated with the crushed lower thoracic cavity.

Penetrating trauma

This includes stab wounds and gunshot and missile injuries as well as secondary penetrating injuries from fragments of fractured sternum or rib (Fig. 17.1). The location of knife wounds gives some indication of the likely visceral injury but the same does not hold for missile injuries—their courses are unpredictable.

Management

Initial management follows standard guidelines (Table 17.12) but the comments made above concerning necessary surgical intervention and fluid therapy should be considered. As ever, the history of injury is important in helping identify injuries that are not immediately obvious.

Blood gas analysis and chest radiography should follow immediately after the initial assessment and resuscitation is completed.

The chest X-ray in thoracic trauma

Chest X-rays are taken only after immediate life-threatening chest injuries have been excluded on clinical examination or treated. Figure 17.2 illustrates common abnormalities found on chest X-rays and Table 17.13 describes the X-ray changes of particular conditions.

Chest wall injuries

Nearly all injuries to the heart, lungs, and great vessels have associated chest wall injuries. Each side of the thoracic cavity is airtight and maintains a negative pressure relative to atmospheric (–5 to –10 cmH$_2$O) to assist in lung expansion. Downward movement of the diaphragm and elevation of ribs produces a negative inspiratory pressure. Any damage to the thoracic cavity can disrupt the pressure gradients, interfering with respiration and threatening life.

Rib fractures

Rib fractures resulting from blunt trauma are the most common thoracic injury. Attention needs to be paid to the pain from the fracture and to the potential for injury of underlying structures by the injuring force or by a fractured rib end. Ribs in the middle

Table 17.12 Initial management of immediately life-threatening chest injuries

Potential problem	Clinical signs	Action
Persistent airway obstruction	Absent breath sounds and cyanosis	Oral/nasal endotracheal intubation or cricothyroidotomy
Tension pneumothorax	Absent breath sounds, hypotension, hyper-resonant chest	Needle then chest drain
Haemothorax	Absent breath sounds, hypotension, chest dull to percussion	Chest drain; if unstable, urgent thoracotomy
Open pneumothorax	Sucking chest wound	Three-sided occlusion dressing, chest drain
Cardiac tamponade (usually penetrating injury)	Hypotension with or without distended neck vein. Difficult to diagnose—maintain high index of suspicion	Difficult—if suspected pericardiocentesis, thoracotomy

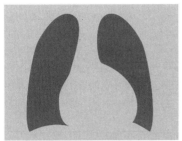

Distended heart from cardiac tamponade

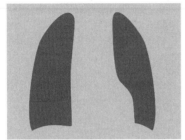

Widened mediastinum - aortic transection

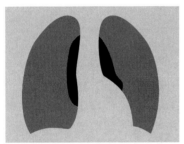

Bilateral free air - ruptured trachea

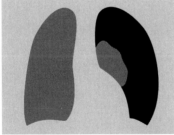

Unilateral free air - pneumothorax

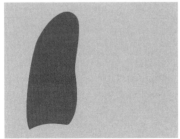

Opaque mediastinum from blood or ruptured diaphragm

Figure 17.2 Findings on chest X-rays after thoracic trauma.

area of the thorax are most commonly fractured. The upper ribs are short and thick and deep in the neck, rendering them difficult to fracture. If these ribs or the scapula is fractured, great force is likely to have occurred and subclavian or aortic damage is likely. Fractures of the tenth to twelfth ribs may indicate liver or splenic injury. In young people, these ribs are pliable and organ injury can occur without fracture. If the patient is conscious, careful palpation of the chest wall for tenderness and crepitus will reveal fractures. A plain chest X-ray may show gross rib fractures, lung contusion, pneumothorax, or pleural fluid. Young, healthy adults with isolated rib fractures can generally be treated as outpatients. Elderly or unfit patients and those with multiple rib fractures should be admitted to hospital and managed with good analgesia, humidified oxygen, and physiotherapy. In patients with limited cardiopulmonary reserve, multiple rib fractures may be life-threatening, with rapid deterioration after an apparently stable presentation. These patients are often best managed in an intensive care unit with careful monitoring. Pain relief may be obtained with intercostal blocks with bupivacaine but thoracic epidural analgesia is most effective in permitting full respiratory excursion and coughing.

Flail chest

Flail chest occurs when three or more ribs are fractured in more than one place, usually anteriorly (fracture or costochondral separation, not visible on X-ray) and laterally. The condition occurs commonly in unrestrained car drivers propelled into the steering wheel. During inspiration, the mobile or flail segment is pulled inwards by negative intrathoracic pressure. On expiration, it is pushed outwards, impairing ventilation. In the past, attempts at fixation of flail segments by bone wiring have been made, but results were disappointing because the main problem is the underlying lung injury and associated hypoxia. Current management is aggressive non-operative treatment aimed at maintaining adequate spontaneous ventilation. The patient should be managed in the ITU with good analgesia and bronchial toilet measures as indicated above. Intubation and mechanical ventilation is not mandatory but is often required for large flail segments or associated injuries.

Open pneumothorax

Penetrating injuries disrupt the airtightness of the pleura. A chest wall defect two-thirds the diameter of the trachea allows air to enter the wound in preference to the trachea during ventilatory movements, causing profound impairment of gas transfer. First aid of a sucking chest wound is to cover the defect with a dressing taped on three sides to create a flutter valve which closes on inspiration. A tube drain should be inserted remote from the wound. The chest wound should never be occluded completely with a dressing without first placing a chest drain, or a tension pneumothorax will result. Definitive treatment of these wounds is by formal operative cleansing, closure, and chest drainage.

Table 17.13 Common types of abnormality on chest X-ray after thoracic trauma

Rib fractures	Fractures of any of the first three ribs (indicates severe trauma and may be associated with spinal or blood-vessel damage)
	Multiple fractures in ribs 4–9 suggest a flail chest
	Fractures of the lower three ribs may be associated with damage to the liver or spleen
Pneumothorax	Best seen on an erect film. On a supine chest radiograph, suspicious signs are: sharp mediastinal contours diaphragmatic border of the heart is seen to a greater extent than usual
Haemothorax	Supine—blood collects in the paravertebral gutter causing a diffuse haze over one lung without a fluid level
	Erect—fluid in costophrenic angle
Diaphragmatic rupture	Indistinct diaphragm (most common), viscera or nasogastric tube in chest (rare)
Oesophageal rupture	Mediastinal air with surgical emphysema of neck
Aortic or innominate artery rupture	First or second rib fractures
	Mediastinum 8 cm or more wide at level of carina or more than 25 per cent of width of chest
	Blurring of contours of aortic arch
	Left apical pleural 'cap' or pleural effusion
	Deviation of trachea or nasogastric tube to right
	Depression of the left main stem bronchus
Aortic branch injury	Suspect if first or second rib fracture or 'apical cap' (haematoma)
Pulmonary injury	Blunt thoracic trauma can cause contusion and bleeding into alveoli, which shows as patchy, ill-defined infiltrates. These may not be immediately evident
Major airways trauma—rupture of the trachea or one of the major bronchi	Pneumomediastinum with non-expanding lung
	Pneumothorax—may be large and fail to respond adequately to a chest drain
	The 'fallen lung' sign. Due to complete disruption of a main tube
Foreign bodies	Teeth (real and false) may be aspirated, leading to pulmonary collapse
	Position of tubes
Indirect effects of trauma on the lungs	Fat embolism produces widespread pulmonary infiltrations
	Pulmonary oedema in the traumatized patient may be due to cardiac trauma, inhalation of gastric contents, or from excessive intravenous fluids
	Acute respiratory distress syndrome (ARDS) Radiological features (fluffy, ill-defined shadows) difficult to differentiate from pulmonary oedema, infection, or fat embolism. X-ray changes often appear only 24–48 hours later

Ruptured diaphragm

Diaphragmatic injuries result from both blunt and penetrating trauma. In the UK, rupture is usually caused by a compression injury of the chest or abdomen. In 10 per cent of diaphragmatic injuries, evisceration occurs of intra-abdominal organs, such as stomach and colon, into the left thoracic cavity. Two-thirds of diaphragmatic ruptures occur on the left side, mainly through the central tendinous portion; the liver provides some protection for the right side. These injuries can be overlooked easily because there are no fail-safe physical signs or chest X-ray appearances. Thus maintaining a high index of suspicion is necessary. The patient may suffer respiratory distress or have bowel sounds audible in the left chest. The chest radiograph usually shows an obscure hemidiaphragm, a gas bubble in the chest, or a curled nasogastric tube in the thorax. Diaphragmatic rupture can be diagnosed with confidence if investigation (below) reveals herniation of abdominal viscera through the diaphragm, or if air or fluid can be shown to pass from one side of the diaphragm to the other during imaging. Herniation of stomach or bowel can be detected by giving oral contrast, and herniation of solid viscera by ultrasound or CT scanning. Laparoscopy gives a good view of the left hemi-diaphragm and the diaphragm must always be examined during a laparotomy for trauma. Treatment is operative because of the risk of strangulation of displaced organs. In the acute injury, the approach is via a laparotomy unless thoracotomy is otherwise indicated. Any prolapsed abdominal contents are returned to the peritoneal cavity and the diaphragm repaired in two layers. Diaphragmatic ruptures may go undiagnosed for years but should still be

Table 17.14 Technique of chest drain (tube thoracostomy)

1. Select appropriate interspace—usually fourth or fifth in mid-axillary line
2. Infiltrate skin and pleura with local anaesthetic
3. Incise at upper border of rib with scalpel
4. Blunt dissection with artery forceps at upper border of rib until pleura opened
5. Palpate with gloved finger to ensure free entry to chest and to separate lung adhesions
6. Advance thoracostomy tube *without* rod
7. Attach to underwater seal
8. Secure chest drain to skin with purse-string suture around skin wound and drain
9. Attach drainage tube to chest wall with secure adhesive strapping
10. Do not clamp drainage tube but ensure underwater seal bottle is always below level of chest
11. Give a dose of prophylactic antibiotics to cover the procedure
12. Applying suction to the system may reinflate a stubborn lung or assist in the temporary management of a major air leak

repaired when recognized. In these cases, repair should be via a posterolateral thoracotomy to allow freeing of intrathoracic adhesions.

Pulmonary injuries

Introduction

These include trauma to the pulmonary parenchyma, the major airways, and the pulmonary arteries and veins. Injuries to these structures have interrelated effects. For example, a stab wound may cause a pneumothorax and bleeding from a pulmonary vessel. The haemopneumothorax may compress the mediastinum, restricting venous return and causing hypotension, which is aggravated by the blood loss. Thus oxygenation and ventilation, cardiac output, and circulating volume are all impaired by the one traumatic event.

Tension pneumothorax

Tension pneumothorax is a highly dangerous condition which must be recognized clinically and treated immediately. It should be suspected in any penetrating injuries of the neck, chest, or upper abdomen, but may occur with rib fractures caused by blunt trauma, which penetrate the visceral pleura. Pleural air accumulates on account of a valve-like effect of the injury. This causes lung collapse and mediastinal compression. This impairs venous return, causing a fall in cardiac output and hypotension. The diagnosis is clinical, with decreased breath sounds, hyper-resonant percussion note and tachypnoea and often hypotension. Before collapse occurs, the patient is often distressed and agitated. Treatment is by urgent needle thoracostomy, inserting a large-bore needle anteriorly into the second intercostal space. This should release a rush of air. Definitive treatment is by chest drainage in the fourth or fifth intercostal space in the mid-axillary line. If the lung fails to re-expand

promptly, a major air leak probably exists. This suggests tracheobronchial injury (see below). If the lung has re-expanded, then the tube can usually be withdrawn after 48–72 hours as most lung leaks will have sealed by then.

Simple pneumothorax

All traumatic pneumothoraces should be drained, irrespective of size, by the method shown below. Tensioning is particularly likely to occur during the pressure changes of anaesthesia, ventilation, or air transfer.

Haemothorax

Haemothorax occurs with blunt and penetrating trauma. Slow or moderate bleeding usually arises from intercostal or internal mammary vessels, but massive bleeding is usually from aorta, subclavian, or pulmonary vessels. Clinical signs vary but there will be reduced breath sounds, dullness to percussion, and tachypnoea. In 85 per cent of cases, haemothorax can be treated by chest drain alone, using a large-size tube (40 Fr.) in the fifth or sixth intercostal space in the mid-axillary line (Table 17.14). If necessary, blood can be collected in a sterile container for autotransfusion using suitable apparatus. Careful note is taken of the volume of blood drained; over 1 litre leads to suspicion of major vessel injury but surgical intervention is not needed if the patient is stable, the bleeding ceases, and a post-drainage chest X-ray is satisfactory and shows:

- complete evacuation of all blood;
- full lung expansion;
- no signs of other injury such as mediastinal widening or 'apical cap' suggesting vascular injury.

Thoracotomy is required for patients with massive rapid blood loss (more than 1 litre and with continued bleeding) or with continued slower loss (100–200 ml/hour for 2–4 hours) or for those where blood cannot be fully evacuated by drainage. At thoracotomy, parenchymal bleeding is arrested by deep sutures or stapling (ensuring endobronchial bleeding is not continuing) or by resection of damaged lung.

Injuries to major airways

Tracheobronchial injury can occur with blunt or penetrating trauma. Respiratory embarrassment on arrival at hospital may be caused by damage to the upper respiratory tract. Injury to the larynx or trachea cause respiratory distress and surgical emphysema of the mediastinum and root of the neck Damage to a bronchus proximal to the pleural reflection causes a similar pattern of surgical emphysema. Diagnosis of upper airway injury requires experienced fibre-optic bronchoscopy with a team standing by to secure the airway. Mainstem bronchi are usually injured in deceleration accidents with shearing of the mobile lung and bronchi from the fixed trachea. The clinical signs include haemoptysis, subcutaneous emphysema, and persisting pneumothorax with a major air leak after chest drainage. Treatment is surgical, with early primary repair through a lateral thoracotomy.

Pulmonary contusion

Pulmonary contusion is a common cause of death after chest injury, particularly in patients with multiple injuries or who later develop pneumonia or ARDS. Pulmonary contusion is often progressive in its effects, with a relatively normal chest X-ray soon after injury but a deteriorating clinical course and hypoxaemia hours or days later. The effects of pulmonary contusion are compounded by rib fractures or a flail segment. Initially there is haemorrhage into alveoli and interstitium. Within hours, the alveolar wall becomes thickened and oedematous; by 48 hours, there is an inflammatory cell infiltrate and loss of surfactant, leading to reduced lung compliance. Overinfusion of crystalloid seems to aggravate the local oedema, and fluid balance must be maintained carefully. Management includes good analgesia, humidified oxygen, and physiotherapy. There is little evidence to support the use of methylprednisolone or mechanical ventilation with positive end expiratory pressure (PEEP) as prophylactic measures in pulmonary contusion.

Cardiac injuries

Penetrating cardiac injuries

Penetrating cardiac injuries are usually caused by knife or gunshot wounds but occasionally fragments of fractured ribs or sternum penetrate the heart. All injuries of this type are potentially life threatening from tamponade, haemorrhage, myocardial damage, or coronary artery disruption. The right ventricle is most commonly involved because of its anterior position in the chest. Left ventricular injuries are more often immediately fatal. Knife wounds may partially seal or produce tamponade but do not usually destroy much myocardium, in contrast to gunshot injuries.

Most patients with major cardiac injuries die before they reach hospital and those that arrive need treatment within minutes of arrival if lives are to be saved. As emergency services have improved, more of these patients are presenting for treatment. Every penetrating wound of the chest should be viewed as a potential cardiac injury, particularly if the entry wound is in the high-risk area between nipples or scapulae or the entry and exit wounds suggest that a bullet has passed across the mediastinum.

Blunt cardiac injuries

Blunt cardiac trauma is common after deceleration accidents. Life-threatening arrhythmias, cardiogenic shock, or cardiac arrest may occur suddenly and without warning symptoms or signs. If cardiac injury is suspected, echocardiography should be performed. A pericardial effusion strongly suggests a blunt cardiac injury.

Emergency department thoracotomy

Emergency thoracic surgery is best performed by an experienced cardiothoracic surgeon in a fully equipped cardiothoracic theatre, but cases periodically present that require more urgent treatment. Patients with penetrating thoracic injury who arrest

Table 17.15 Indications for immediate thoracotomy in thoracic injuries

Injury	Clinical picture	Treatment
Cardiac wounds	Penetrating parasternal wound in hypotensive patient Cardiac tamponade	Pericardiocentesis as immediate life-saving measure Median sternotomy (or left thoracotomy) for repair
Lung, heart, or great vessel injuries	Haemorrhage >1000 ml and continuing	Thoracotomy in fifth intercostal space on side of bleeding
Major tracheobronchial injury	Inadequate ventilation due to major air leak	Secure airway; thoracotomy on side of leak
Rarely, diaphragmatic rupture	Irreversible hypoxia	Reduction of herniated organs and diaphragmatic repair, usually via laparotomy

shortly before arrival or within the emergency department should undergo immediate thoracotomy, usually through a left anterior approach. Salvage is less likely following blunt thoracic injury and patients who arrive lifeless should not undergo operation. Immediate thoracotomy will be required for imminent exsanguination from thoracic injuries, cardiac tamponade with continuing haemorrhage, and, less commonly, for major tracheobronchial injury or diaphragmatic rupture with irreversible hypoxia (Table 17.15).

Management of cardiac injuries

Cardiac tamponade

Penetrating trauma to the heart can result in accumulation of blood in the space between the heart and the indistensible pericardium. As little as 50 ml can embarrass the cardiac action. Tamponade can be recognized clinically by the signs of Beck's triad, but the signs are subtle. This consists of *pulsus paradoxus* (a drop of 10 mmHg or more in systolic pressure during inspiration), muffled heart sounds, and distended neck veins, but these signs can be difficult to elucidate in the resuscitation room. In addition, there is usually a tachycardia in an attempt to maintain cardiac output. Chest X-ray may show an enlarged cardiac shadow and there are low-voltage complexes on ECG. Any patient with a parasternal wound and hypotension must be considered to have tamponade until it can be excluded.

Immediate management of cardiac tamponade

If there is major cardiac embarrassment, pericardiocentesis, although potentially hazardous, should be considered, both to confirm the diagnosis and to buy time while preparing for emergency thoracotomy. The technique is as follows: using a long cannula, non-clotting blood typical of tamponade can be drawn off, and aspiration of as little as 30 ml may produce a dramatic improvement. The cannula should be left in place while the patient is taken for urgent thoracotomy in the operating theatre.

Emergency thoracotomy for cardiac injury

If the patient remains *in extremis* after pericardiocentesis, an emergency room thoracotomy should be performed. Otherwise, it is better to move the patient to an operating theatre. In either case, the optimum approach is through a median sternotomy. This allows all areas of the heart and intrapericardial vessels to be explored and repaired and simplifies the procedure in the unlikely event of the patient requiring cardiopulmonary bypass. Thoracotomy via a fourth or fifth space anterolateral incision may be used by some surgeons if unfamiliar with median sternotomy, or if a sternal saw is not available.

Internal mammary artery damage is sought and dealt with by ligation and the pericardium opened longitudinally, taking care to avoid the phrenic nerve. Blood and clot is removed and the heart examined carefully to find the cardiac wound or wounds. The whole circumference of the heart must be inspected as wounds may transfix the heart; the heart needs to be elevated to see the posterior wall. A ventricular bleeding site can be controlled temporarily by finger pressure, and an atrial wound with a vascular clamp.

Myocardial wounds are repaired using non-absorbable polypropylene mattress sutures. Cardiac movement can be reduced temporarily by inflow occlusion. Special attention must be paid to knot tension to avoid the suture cutting out; sutures can be applied over Teflon pledgets if necessary. Damage to coronary vessels is avoided by applying horizontal mattress sutures beneath the vessel (Fig. 17.3). No attempt should be made to repair valvular or septal defects at the life-saving operation; these can be repaired electively later if necessary. Coronary vessel damage occurs in about 10 per cent of penetrating cardiac injuries. If a coronary artery has been divided, the ends can be ligated to control haemorrhage. The heart should then be observed for arrhythmias and if none develop within 10 min, the chest can be closed. If an arrhythmia develops, ligatures should be removed, haemorrhage controlled by pressure, and direct repair of the vessel considered using cardiopulmonary bypass. If the vessel is lacerated, repair is preferable to ligation. Unfortunately the results of coronary artery repair or bypass grafting in trauma cases are poor. Air embolism is common after penetrating cardiac wounds and air should be aspirated from the ventricles at operation.

Cardiac contusion

The incidence and importance of cardiac contusion is confused as there is no standard investigation of value. Measurements of enzymes, ECGs, and echocardiography have no predictive value and the patient should be managed according to manifestations of damage, particularly pump failure and arrhythmias. Signs of significant cardiac contusion are usually clearly evident and manifest early. Cardiac failure should be monitored by cardiac output measurement using a Swan–Ganz catheter, and is usually treated successfully with inotropes. Patients suspected of cardiac contusion should be monitored continuously for arrhythmias for 24 hours and antiarrhythmic treatment employed if necessary. After 24 hours, the risk is minimal.

The widened mediastinum

In blunt thoracic trauma, the aorta is the vessel most likely to be injured, particularly after high-velocity deceleration impact such as a motor vehicle accident or a fall. The usual site of rupture is just distal to the origin of the left subclavian artery. At this point, the ligamentum arteriosum fixes the aortic arch above a mobile descending thoracic aorta. Complete transsection causes death at the scene of the accident in 80 per cent of cases, but if there is a partial rupture with intact adventitia, the patient may survive for at least a few hours. However, about 50 per cent will die within 24 hours if untreated (about 2 per cent each hour). The patient is usually shocked and the earliest sign is a widened mediastinum on chest X-ray. Rarely, femoral pulses may be absent.

Most patients with a widened mediastinum do not have aortic injury but the consequences of missing an aortic rupture are so catastrophic that angiography should be used liberally. CT scanning is accurate in diagnosing mediastinal haemorrhage but is inferior to angiography for detecting aortic rupture. Arch angiography should be carried out in a hospital where cardiothoracic surgery is available.

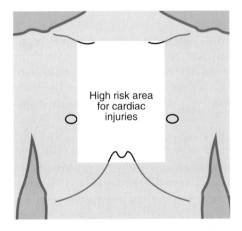

High risk area for cardiac injuries

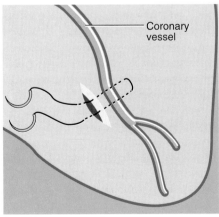

Coronary vessel

Horizontal cardiac mattress sutures

Figure 17.3 Surgical management of penetrating injuries to the heart.

These patients often have multiple injuries, and priorities need to be set concerning the order of treatment. If a patient with a widened mediastinum is obviously bleeding, it is unlikely to be from the aorta as this would rapidly cause death, and other sources of bleeding should be sought and treated (usually abdominal or pelvic). If the diagnosis of aortic rupture is confirmed, the patient can be transferred directly to the operating theatre for aortic repair or graft replacement of the torn arch under cardiopulmonary bypass.

Oesophageal injuries

Oesophageal injuries usually result from penetrating injuries to the neck or chest. The oesophagus lies close to the trachea and great vessels and penetrating oesophageal injuries may also damage these other structures. Conversely, if surgical exploration is performed for tracheal or great vessel injury in the chest, the mediastinal pleura should be opened and the oesophagus carefully inspected for injury.

Perforation or rupture should be suspected if a patient with a penetrating chest injury has haematemesis or bloody nasogastric aspirate, if subcutaneous emphysema is found in the root of the neck or pneumomediastinum, or if missile fragments are seen in the posterior mediastinum on chest X-ray. In a stable patient, the diagnosis needs to confirmed early using a contrast swallow. Repair should be carried out early. The cervical oesophagus can be repaired in two layers via a longitudinal incision anterior to the sternocleidomastoid muscle. The upper and mid-oesophagus can be approached through a right thoracotomy and the lower oesophagus through a left seventh interspace incision. Some surgeons buttress oesophageal repairs with a muscle flap of intercostals, rhomboids, or diaphragm. A chest drain is left in for at least 7 days until a satisfactory contrast swallow has been performed.

If the lesion is only discovered later, repair is unwise because of contamination, and conservative management should be instituted. The oesophagus should be 'defunctioned' using a nasogastric tube (unless there is a complete transsection), the chest drained and jejunal or parenteral feeding commenced.

2.4 Abdominal and pelvic injuries

Introduction

The abdominal viscera harbour an enormous potential for causing morbidity and mortality after injury through the mechanisms of haemorrhage or sepsis. Deaths resulting from abdominal and pelvic trauma often turn out to have been potentially preventable if appropriate action had only been taken. Treatment may be inadequate because peritoneal signs can be subtle or absent, particularly if there are other associated injuries, such as a head injury, or if the patient has been drinking alcohol. As many as one-third of the patients requiring laparotomy do not have worrying abdominal signs when first examined. Management therefore requires systematic initial evaluation and appropriate diagnostic procedures, but most importantly, when immediate surgery is not needed, the patient

must be reviewed continually until out of danger. In general, about 20 per cent of patients with blunt abdominal trauma require operation, 30 per cent of those with stab wounds but over 90 per cent of those with abdominal gunshot wounds.

Evaluation

Experienced surgeons find assessing the injured abdomen difficult, but several warnings are of value. The anatomical extent and compartmentalization of the abdomen should be recalled. Upper viscera are protected by the rib cage and extend as high as the nipple. Abdominal and thoracic injuries coexist sufficiently often to make the concept of *torso trauma* a valuable one. Penetrating injuries may affect both cavities, and the same is true of blunt injury. A patient with injuries to the right upper and lower limbs and the right-side ribs almost certainly has experienced right-sided abdominal trauma whether or not signs are apparent. Likewise, pelvic viscera are protected within a bony cage but extend low enough to be injured through the perineum or buttock. The retroperitoneal viscera are also protected, but are remote from the examining hand or lavage fluid, and may be injured by flank or back wounds.

Physical signs are unreliable predictors of injury; 30–50 per cent of patients with significantly injured abdomens will not exhibit signs, whereas some 25 per cent with apparently positive signs have no significant injury. The misleading findings may be due to abdominal wall injury, shivering, or anxiety. Positive signs must be acted upon within the context of the entire patient, either by a confirmatory investigation or operation. The drawback of performing a non-therapeutic laparotomy lies not so much in the small risk of its complications but more in the wastage of time valuable for the treatment of extra-abdominal injuries.

Given the incidence of false-negative examinations, all supportive clinical data must be borne in mind before declaring an abdomen uninjured. The principal mechanism is serial re-examination and observation, but specific investigations are often needed in addition to the history of injury and any identified associated injuries which may give pointers. The site of external contusion or bruising gives a clue as to a potential underlying injury, and the mark of a seat belt (London's sign) is noteworthy. Lower-right rib fractures may be associated with liver disruption, lower-left rib fractures with splenic disruption, and epigastric contusion may be associated with duodenal perforation or pancreatic fracture across the vertebral column. Fracture of lumbar transverse processes is associated with renal injuries, and pelvic fractures are associated with bladder rupture, urethral injuries, and iliac vessel damage.

Abdominal injuries associated with rapid deceleration tend to cause disruption of organs at the junctions of fixed and mobile parts of the intestine (e.g. jejunum near the ligament of Treitz, the terminal ileum, or at either end of the transverse colon). Blunt injuries tend to damage solid viscera or tethered lengths of gut. Penetrating injuries, on the other hand, typically occur along the track or trajectory of the instrument or missile that causes the injury and more often afflict small bowel and stomach. Caution is required with bullet injuries as the track is often tortuous. High-velocity weapons cause cavitation damage, to which the abdominal solid viscera are especially vulnerable. Commonly associated injuries should thus be sought during surgery. Thus if the liver is obviously injured, the diaphragm may be injured; if the portal vein is damaged, the common bile duct and hepatic artery may be damaged. Similarly, duodenal injuries are associated with pancreatic, vena caval, or common bile duct injuries, and the rectum is often damaged if bladder injuries are present.

Methods of clinical assessment

Immediate abdominal surgery is occasionally required to control haemorrhage, and failure to identify this need will inevitably be fatal. More commonly, major injuries to vascular structures and viscera bleed remarkably slowly and permit resuscitation to be accomplished or even mask the presence of continuing bleeding. Following a completed initial survey, the abdomen is examined fully during the systematic examination of the patient. This must include inspection of the back and flanks and rectal examination. The importance of acting on positive findings is worth reiterating. The presence of bowel sounds is no reassurance and the use of abdominal girth as an observation is mentioned only to be condemned. Girth may change insignificantly during the emptying of most of the circulating volume into the abdomen. Anal sphincter tone should be assessed as a reflection of anal or spinal injury and the rectal wall palpated for integrity and the presence of blood. A **high-riding prostate** suggests post-membranous disruption of the urethra. This or other signs of urethral injury (meatal blood, perineal bruising) necessitate retrograde urethrography before urinary catheterization is attempted. The testes should be examined for injury, and in a suspected pelvic fracture perineal or vaginal laceration must be excluded. Repeated springing of a fractured pelvis should be avoided lest further haemorrhage be precipitated. Open wounds should be inspected for obvious signs of peritoneal breaches and multiple or exit wounds sought. The presence of **haematuria** demands investigation by urography/cystography, and blood in the nasogastric aspirate requires a water-soluble contrast swallow. Plasma amylase level should be checked and, if raised, investigated by CT scanning, unless (as is often the case) concomitant findings require more urgent investigation and operation.

Table 17.16 Indications for laparotomy for abdominal injury

Hypotension and evidence of abdominal injury (bruising/wound/tenderness)

Peritonitis

Continuing intra-abdominal haemorrhage

Abdominal gunshot wound

Stab wound with peritonism, hypotension, or major evisceration

Positive diagnostic peritoneal lavage

Gastrointestinal perforation or bleeding

Specific visceral injuries not appropriate for conservative treatment

Following blunt injury, some 20 per cent of patients will require laparotomy. The main indications are shown in Table 17.16.

Abdominal stab wounds

About 20 per cent of stabbed patients have significant intra-abdominal injury and need laparotomy, but most do not. Clear indications for surgery should be acted on directly, but for many patients, the first step is to determine whether the peritoneum has been breached by exploring the wound under local anaesthesia. If it has, then peritoneal lavage can be employed. If negative, as in most cases, conservative management is appropriate. Conservative management is also appropriate for those who eviscerate only a small plug of omentum. However, approximately one-third of patients with significant intra-abdominal injury from a stab wound are free of signs at presentation and must be reassessed clinically at intervals. Many bowel perforations are sealed spontaneously by omentum without causing peritonitis.

Stab wounds of flank and back should be managed along similar lines. Although paravertebral muscles are thick, the loin muscles are easily penetrated, and damage to viscera such as the colon, pancreas, vena cava, and kidneys is likely to occur. In these cases, peritoneal lavage will not exclude visceral damage. In the stable patient, about whom doubt persists, contrast enhanced CT enema (CT after opacification of upper and lower gut and kidneys) is valuable in avoiding the overlooking of injuries (such as small wounds to the retroperitoneal colon).

Abdominal gunshot wounds

Abdominal gunshot wounds nearly always cause significant injury. Only about 10 per cent of cases have no intra-abdominal injury at laparotomy and these are usually attributable to a tangential missile track that fails to traverse the abdominal cavity. Seventy five per cent have more than one visceral or vascular injury and 50 per cent have small bowel injury. Urgent laparotomy is mandatory in all cases.

Recent studies have challenged the value of administering intravenous fluids to shocked patients with penetrating torso trauma before the operating room is reached. Earlier fluid administration to elevate blood pressure may simply stimulate further haemorrhage. However, the importance of rapid surgery has been established beyond doubt.

Diagnostic tests

Diagnostic procedures are needed when there is doubt about the presence of abdominal injury. Uncertainty can arise if the patient's responses are dulled by injury or intoxication, confused by adjacent thoracic, pelvic, or abdominal wall injury, or where the patient is inaccessible to further assessment on account of transfer to another unit or because prolonged investigation or treatment of non-abdominal injury is necessary. The principal contraindication to investigation is an established indication for laparotomy. These indications include those shown in Table 17.16, as well as obvious signs of specific visceral injury such as rectal bleeding with pelvic fracture, diaphragmatic rupture on chest X-ray, free air in the peritoneal cavity or retroperitoneal area, ruptured duodenum or intraperitoneal rupture of the bladder on a contrast study, or substantial injury to the renal artery or kidney on radiological investigation. In these circumstances, general investigations for intra-abdominal injury are not appropriate. In abdominal stab wounds, similar indications also apply, with the addition of significant evisceration. Haematemesis, rectal bleeding, or haematuria are strong indications for laparotomy after stab wounds.

Diagnostic peritoneal lavage

Diagnostic peritoneal lavage (DPL) for investigation of possible intra-abdominal injuries has proved to have a high sensitivity (99 per cent) and, depending on which criteria are applied, a false-positive rate as low as 1 per cent. The procedure is simple, rapid, accurate, and cheap.

Indications for DPL in suspected abdominal injury include:

- patients with diminished sensorium (head and spinal cord injury or alcohol or drug use);

- injury to structures adjacent to the abdominal cavity, such as ribs, lumbar vertebrae, and pelvis;

- where clinical examination of the abdomen leaves doubt;

- where re-assessment will not be possible for some time;

- when a source of significant haemorrhage is not found on initial assessment.

The principal limitation of the technique is its oversensitivity. Blunt trauma frequently causes minor injuries to the liver or spleen which bleed transiently but are of little threat. These often give rise to a (true) positive lavage and result in a laparotomy

Table 17.17 Mini-laparotomy technique for diagnostic peritoneal lavage (DPL)

1. Intubate and empty stomach and bladder
2. Aseptic technique, local anaesthesia if needed
3. 5 cm midline wound just below umbilicus, place retractors
4. Incise linea alba vertically
5. Open peritoneum between artery forceps, under direct vision
6. Egress of >20 ml free blood or intestinal contents requires laparotomy
7. Infuse 1000 ml warmed saline (adult) and tip patient to mix
8. Siphon out fluid (often only 300–500 ml) and analyse
9. The following criteria necessitate laparotomy:
   >100 000 RBCs/mm^3
   or >500 WBCs/mm^3
   or positive Gram stain or presence of food particles
10. Fluid appearing in chest drain or urinary catheter indicates laparotomy
11. In the presence of a pelvic fracture: enter above umbilicus to avoid haematoma and accept only free blood or intestinal content as positive

which is non-therapeutic because the bleeding has already stopped. This serves to emphasize the importance of adhering to accepted criteria of a positive lavage—deviation from these results in a less accurate assessment. Relative contraindications to DPL include multiple previous operations, pregnancy, and possibly obesity. In addition, the technique should be modified in the presence of a pelvic fracture. Used sensibly, complications are rare. The morbidity rate of DPL is about 1 per cent and includes perforation of small bowel, mesentery, bladder, and retroperitoneal vascular structures. These can be further reduced by employing a **mini-laparotomy technique** (Table 17.17). Egress of free blood on opening the peritoneum usually makes the need for surgery obvious. The quoted criterion for positivity of 100 000 RBCs/mm^3 of lavage fluid detects as little as 10 ml of blood diluted in 1 litre. It is important to be aware that DPL is often negative in isolated small perforations of hollow viscera or diaphragm, it fails to detect retroperitoneal injury, and is non-specific as regards the organ injured.

It is not acceptable to treat a patient conservatively in whom a positive lavage has been obtained. DPL can be performed rapidly in the resuscitation room in unstable patients. Its greatest use is perhaps in confirming intra-abdominal haemorrhage and thus determining management priorities in an unstable polytrauma victim.

Computed tomography

CT is an important technique in the early evaluation of abdominal and pelvic injuries but is only suitable for stable patients. Its limitations are based on the availability of equipment and experienced personnel, cooperation of the patient, and the need for oral or intravenous contrast agents. CT can image the retroperitoneum and identify specific injuries, but is not foolproof. Experience is still required to interpret scans, and significant volumes of blood, as well as intestinal and pancreatic injuries, can be missed, particularly during the first 12 hours after injury. CT is valuable for defining the extent and configuration of complex pelvic fractures. By identifying the source of haemorrhage, it can permit conservative management of certain carefully selected, stable, solid, visceral injuries.

Ultrasonography

The role of ultrasonography is expanding and it is regularly used in many parts of the world. Ultrasound is sensitive for demonstrating free intraperitoneal fluid as well as the location and extent of solid organ haematomas. It is particularly useful in the pregnant patient in avoiding radiation and use of contrast media. However, ultrasound is of little value in assessing hollow visceral perforation, it is intensely operator-dependent and, even in expert hands, misses very significant injuries in 10 per cent or so of cases. A negative scan provides no reassurance in the face of other findings suggesting intra-abdominal injury. Ultrasonography is valuable during conservative management of liver injuries, when sequential scans can monitor the volume of intra-abdominal blood after an initial CT scan (see below).

Laparoscopy

With increasing experience, diagnostic laparoscopy under local anaesthesia has been helpful in identifying diaphragmatic injuries. However, a major limitation is the difficulty of performing a comprehensive examination of the entire abdomen, pelvis, and retroperitoneum; the procedure has not replaced the investigations already described.

Plain X-rays

Plain or lateral decubitus abdominal X-rays can give valuable information: free or retroperitoneal gas may be seen and radiopaque missiles, such as bullets, shotgun pellets, and glass, may be revealed. Bony injuries with known association with specific visceral injuries may be seen.

Emergency laparotomy for intra-abdominal bleeding

It is very occasionally necessary to perform an emergency operation for catastrophic intra-abdominal bleeding. This may involve left thoracotomy to cross-clamp the descending aorta or laparotomy to compress the aorta or pack the abdominal cavity in the emergency room. However, the outcome from such procedures is poor, with average survival only 1–3 per cent, but on rare occasions they are life saving. In most cases it is better to transfer the patient quickly to the operating theatre.

Operative technique

In the operating theatre, the patient is placed supine on the operating table. If bleeding is rapid, simultaneous connection of the patient to monitoring equipment and anaesthetic preparation should be performed. An extremely unstable patient should be prepared and draped before induction of anaesthesia because the combined effects of anaesthetic agents inducing hypotension and releasing the abdominal wall tamponade may cause rapid loss of blood pressure. Additional large-bore intravenous lines and an arterial line for haemodynamic monitoring should be placed, but these procedures must not delay the start of surgery. Autotransfusion apparatus should be prepared if available and adequate quantities of blood for transfusion ordered. Intravenous antibiotics should be given to cover gut flora. Skin preparation should be from neck to knees (including flanks) so that extension into the chest for sternotomy, thoracotomy, or chest tube insertion, or access to the groins to harvest saphenous vein for vascular repair, can take place without further preparation.

A long mid-line incision should be made rapidly. If there is massive blood loss without bowel contamination, auto-transfusion can be performed. Some authors have even advocated its use if there is bowel contamination. If there is massive haemoperitoneum, inflow can be controlled by compressing the aorta at the oesophageal hiatus by hand or with a specially designed instrument to compress the aorta against the vertebral bodies. Blood and clot is then rapidly evacuated from the peritoneal cavity by scooping it out manually and by suction. The abdomen is then searched carefully, concentrating on the areas most likely to be the site of haemorrhage. In blunt trauma, solid organs are the most likely sites of haemorrhage, whereas in penetrating trauma, the path of the missile or blade needs to be followed to determine the source. All parts of the abdomen should be packed with large gauze packs, then these can be removed individually to seek sources of bleeding and control each in turn. Usually, haemorrhage is controlled by packing and this allows a pause to enable the anaesthetist to catch up with transfusion, and the theatre staff to obtain further equipment and assistance if necessary.

Adequate haemostasis must be achieved by **definitive surgery** or **damage control surgery**. Definitive surgery is the preferred treatment, but is likely to be achieved successfully only when injuries are limited in number and complexity. It is well established that prolonged and bloody operations performed on patients already shocked, hypothermic, and often endotoxic tend to result in coagulopathy and other features of multiple organ failure. The approach of 'damage control surgery' has therefore emerged, where complex injuries are temporarily treated as quickly as possible. This might include packing solid viscera, stapling closed (but not resecting) damaged bowel, and placing temporary vascular shunts. Closure is usually a simple running suture to skin as the patient will return to theatre for definitive surgery within 36 hours, after correction of hypothermia, acidosis, and coagulopathy.

Splenic haemorrhage

If the spleen is bleeding, it should be mobilized into the midline by freeing the lateral and superior peritoneal attachments and then mobilizing the spleen and the tail of the pancreas posteriorly. The spleen can then be thoroughly inspected to see whether repair is possible. Splenic repair techniques include pledgeted suture repair of parenchymal lacerations, ligation of specific bleeding vessels in the hilum, partial splenectomy, or the use of an absorbable mesh bag to compress the fragments of the spleen together and control haemorrhage. In adults there is a small but very real risk of overwhelming post-splenectomy infection (less than 0.7 per cent), which is often fatal. The risk is greater in children. If the bleeding cannot be controlled rapidly, or if there is continuing bleeding from other areas, splenectomy is the best solution.

Liver haemorrhage

Massive liver bleeding is very difficult to control and perihepatic packing and transfer to a specialized unit is the accepted method of management. If the liver is the only source of major bleeding within the abdomen, aortic compression can be released to allow reperfusion of the other abdominal organs and the inflow to the liver controlled using Pringle's manoeuvre. This involves cross-clamping the porta hepatis with either fingers or a vascular clamp via the opening of the lesser sac. If the Pringle manoeuvre does not control bleeding, injury to the hepatic veins or inferior vena cava (IVC) must be suspected. Most liver lacerations are minor and have stopped bleeding by the time of surgery, and these should be left alone. Actively bleeding lacerations are explored and bleeding vessels ligated. Liver lacerations may occasionally be re-approximated using sutures over pledgets, but large buttressing sutures can result in continuing intrahepatic ooze with subsequent necrosis and liver abscess. Extension of the laceration by finger fracture may be necessary to identify and ligate damaged vessels or biliary radicals. Partial hepatectomy is sometimes necessary to remove devitalized parts of the liver, but this is often counterproductive as it increases blood loss and coagulopathy. If hepatic veins or inferior vena caval damage is suspected, the liver should be mobilized fully. If control cannot be obtained, then insertion of a cavo-atrial shunt will occasionally permit a successful repair. With bursting or star-shaped injuries, the best method of controlling haemorrhage is to pack around the liver with large gauze swabs and close the abdomen to allow the patient to recover, rewarm, and restore coagulopathy. Absorbable mesh wraps have been used to reapproximate fragments of the liver to control haemorrhage. Packs are removed 36–48 hours later at a planned 'second-look' laparotomy.

Control of contamination

The entire bowel must be carefully examined from oesophageal hiatus to rectum. The stomach is inspected anteriorly and posteriorly, followed by the duodenum. The ligament of Treitz is located to follow the small bowel to the ileocaecal valve. The colon is then examined thoroughly. This may require opening the lesser sac, Kocherizing the duodenum, and mobilizing left and right colons for inspection. Areas of bowel injury may be controlled temporarily with clamps, staples, or sutures. Once all the sites of rupture have been located, definitive repair or resection is performed.

Inspection of the rest of the abdomen

The abdomen should be examined methodically. Both sides of the diaphragm must be palpated while re-examining the liver and spleen. The gallbladder and biliary system must be examined and the pancreas examined through the lesser sac. The right colon should be mobilized to examine fully the duodenum, and the duodenum itself mobilized by Kocher's manoeuvre (i.e. dividing the lateral peritoneum) to allow inspection of the head of the pancreas, the aorta, vena cava, and right kidney. If necessary, the left colon can be mobilized to examine the left kidney or great vessels. Pelvic organs in the female must also be inspected.

Retroperitoneal haematoma

Retroperitoneal haematomas discovered at laparotomy can be categorized into three zones:

(1) centrally over the great vessels and pancreas and duodenum;

(2) flank/perirenal area;

(3) pelvic retroperitoneal area.

Whether or not to explore a retroperitoneal haematoma depends on the mechanism of injury (i.e. blunt or penetrating), the location of the haematoma, and whether it is expanding. All penetrating retroperitoneal haematomas must be explored to control haemorrhage and confirm integrity of other retroperitoneal structures, such as ureters. Zone 1, or central retroperitoneal haematomas, following blunt trauma should be explored because of the risk of injury to the great vessels, duodenum, or pancreas. Exploration of zone 2 haematomas depends on whether preoperative information is available regarding function or injury to the kidneys, as well as findings at operation (see renal injury, below). If renal exploration is necessary, the blood supply to the kidney should be controlled at the pedicle, if possible, before entering the haematoma. This lessens blood loss and decreases the risk of nephrectomy when repair would have been possible. Pelvic haematomas mainly occur following pelvic fractures, and exploration should be avoided unless there is major injury to the common or external iliac vessels. Even then, repair of complex vascular injuries may be impossible and packing is the better option.

Thoracic bleeding

If abdominal haemorrhage is controlled and yet the patient remains hypotensive, the thorax is the most likely source of blood loss once bleeding into fractures has been allowed for. If an initial chest film did not show features of massive haemothorax, pericardial tamponade is possible. The pericardium can be approached from below the xiphisternum and, if blood is found, the chest can be opened via a median sternotomy to fully expose the pericardium.

Hypothermia

This is a serious problem in patients undergoing resuscitation and laparotomy for massive blood loss. Hypothermia disrupts normal physiological functions, particularly blood coagulation. Hypothermia can be minimized by warming intravenous fluids and blood and warming gases in the ventilator circuit, as well as by employing a limited initial operative procedure.

Enteral nutrition

Early enteral feeding after major multiple injury has been shown to reduce the rate of subsequent sepsis when compared with parenterally fed patients. There is much to be said for surgically placing a feeding jejunostomy during a laparotomy for major injury.

Management of specific abdominal injuries

Liver and spleen

Conservative treatment of injuries to the liver and spleen has been advocated, particularly in children, because it has been widely recognized that many injuries to these viscera stop bleeding spontaneously. Provided a patient is stable and remains so, and there are no other indications for surgery, non-operative treatment may be employed. Patients are usually investigated by CT scan and further investigated during the observation period by CT or ultrasound to monitor progress. Recurrent hypotension or continuing haemorrhage of lesser magnitude will require operation. This may occur unexpectedly, so it as an absolute prerequisite that these patients are managed in a high-dependency environment from which rapid 24-hour access to theatre is available. The risk of secondary haemorrhage persists for some time but the actual risks have not been clearly defined, so controversy persists about the duration of bed rest and hospitalization needed. Different reported series of conservative treatment of splenic injury have shown disparate results, with success recorded in 24–96 per cent of cases. Conservative treatment of liver injury is appropriate for simple lacerations or haematomas in which bleeding appears to have stopped and in which there is less than 250 ml blood in the peritoneum on CT assessment. With bed rest, a successful non-operative outcome can be achieved in 60–70 per cent of cases. Patients referred in stable condition with known hepatic injury need CT to delineate the injury pattern if this has not been done already. **Angiography** can be used to identify and embolize bleeding segmental arteries. A decision can then be made about removing any perihepatic packing previously placed once coagulopathy, acidosis, and hypothermia have been corrected.

Gastric injuries

Gastric injuries usually result from penetrating trauma. The principal pitfall is to miss a hidden exit wound or second site of injury through failing to examine the posterior wall adequately. Gastric instillation of methylene blue can help in this respect. Dead tissue, if any, should be resected and two-layer repair carried out. A nasogastric tube should be left in place.

Penetrating duodenal injuries

Penetrating duodenal injuries are seen but blunt rupture is more common in UK practice. This should be suspected in any patient with free gas in the abdominal cavity, retroperitoneal air, or bloody nasogastric aspirates. If laparotomy is not otherwise clearly necessary, an upper GI contrast study should be conducted, using water-soluble contrast. The common rupture is transverse, across the second part. Again, it can be missed at operation and full Kocherization should be employed during laparotomy to examine the area for trauma. Small defects may be repaired primarily. With larger defects or tissue loss, it may be necessary to close the defect by anastomosis to a Roux loop of jejunum or to bring a loop of jejunum up as a serosal patch for a larger primary repair. With more complex injuries it is probably wise to divert the food stream using a gastro-jejunostomy with pyloric closure. Alternatively, a **triple tube technique** can be employed. Here, a gastrostomy and proximal jejunostomy is used to drain the duodenum, while a slightly more distal jejunostomy initially drains the jejunum but can later be used for enteral feeding. These measures should be supplemented by gastric acid suppression medication. The principal complication is duodenal fistula and an external drain is advisable.

Pancreatic trauma

Pancreatic trauma is uncommon but serious and usually follows high-speed traffic accidents where the pancreas is impacted against the spinal column. Problems arise from haemorrhage (either from the vascular parenchyma or adjacent major vessels) or from leakage of pancreatic juice with subsequent necrosis and sepsis. Hyperamylasaemia is suggestive and should be sought in every patient with abdominal injury, but is neither pathognomonic nor present in every case. Even early CT has a significant false-negative rate and does not entirely exclude significant trauma. The principal question in assessing an injured pancreas is whether or not the duct has been damaged. For this, endoscopic retrograde pancreatography will occasionally be useful, provided the patient is stable and without an established indication for operation. When the ducts are intact, bleeding may be stopped by careful suture or omental plugging. Drainage is traditional. Ductal injuries should be managed by an experienced pancreatic surgeon, if necessary following transfer. Ductal rupture to the left of the portal vein is best managed by distal resection. In stable patients with injury at or just to the right of this, a distal pancreaticojejunostomy can preserve pancreatic tissue. Injuries to the head are difficult: resection carries a formidable mortality in non-expert hands and again anterior or distal Roux drainage may be the best option. Combined complex duodeno-pancreatic injuries may be managed by combined diversion procedures or by resection. The common complications are fistulas, delayed haemorrhage, and sepsis.

Small bowel injuries

Small bowel injuries are managed by repair or by resection when necessary. With mesenteric haematomas or lacerations, care should be taken to ensure that the associated small bowel is viable. Under adverse systemic circumstances, exteriorization as a stoma should be considered. Colonic injuries are more worrisome on account of the greater risk of sepsis. Any crushed or non-viable tissue must be resected. Clean lacerations may be repaired provided the patient is normotensive, the edges are viable, there has been minimal contamination and the injury is less than 6 hours old. Otherwise exteriorization is the safer option, particularly for the inexperienced trauma surgeon. Under favourable circumstances, right colonic resection with ileocolic anastomosis would be reasonable but colo-colic anastomosis would seldom be appropriate.

Rectal injuries

Similar considerations to the above apply to rectal injuries, where primary repair should be selective and always protected by a proximal stoma as well as presacral drainage. Injuries below the peritoneal reflection may be missed on cursory laparotomy and again require presacral drainage, colostomy, and rectal washout. Damage to the anal sphincters should not be repaired primarily but rather haemorrhage controlled, drainage instituted as necessary, and a stoma created. Early specialist opinion and repair should be arranged.

Pelvic fractures

Definitive care of pelvic fractures should be undertaken by an orthopaedic surgeon but the abdominal surgeon may become involved with the consequences in several ways. On presentation, it may not be clear whether hypovolaemia and lower abdominal signs are due to pelvic bony bleeding or to intraperitoneal injury or both. Obviously intraperitoneal injury must be diagnosed and dealt with, but there is much to be said for avoiding operation in patients with a haematoma related to a fracture, lest haemorrhage be worsened or infection introduced. Peritoneal lavage via the modified technique discussed earlier can help differentiate these possibilities, and pelvic radiographs are essential. Early external fixation can reduce bleeding from certain fractures, while in others, arteriography and embolization are of value. If laparotomy proves necessary, it is advisable to disturb the pelvic haematoma as little as possible. If pelvic haemorrhage continues, prolonged efforts to ligate vessels are inappropriate and packing should be employed at an early stage. Pelvic haemorrhage can be massive—either acutely or over a period of a few days—and expert multidisciplinary management may be needed to save the patient.

2.5 Urinary tract injuries

Renal trauma

Introduction

Most renal injuries occur in males between 20 and 40 years of age and result from blunt trauma. The majority occur in road traffic accidents, and sports injuries account for most of the rest. About 10 per cent of children with significant renal injury do not have haematuria. Penetrating injuries may be iatrogenic or result from knife wounds or missile injuries. Management of renal injury with haematuria remains controversial. In general, treatment in the UK is more conservative than in the USA. It is advisable to involve a urological surgeon early on.

Blunt injury

The kidney is relatively protected from blunt injury by its anatomical position and by its energy-absorbing layer of perinephric fat. However, the kidney remains vulnerable to direct impact over the lower posterior ribs and to thoraco-abdominal compression injuries which may cause renal crushing between the lower ribs and the spinal column.

The renal pedicle is the only fixed anchor point of the kidney and deceleration injuries may cause disruption of the renal vascular pedicle, with either complete avulsion or intimal damage leading to thrombosis. Congenitally abnormal kidneys and kidneys in abnormal positions are particularly prone to trauma in even minor accidents. Hydronephrotic and polycystic kidneys fall into the former category and pelvic and transplant kidneys into the latter. Haemophilia may first present as haematuria after minor trauma. If the patient is anuric, this may be due to clot obstruction, particularly if there is a solitary kidney.

The severity of renal injuries varies and the signs do not necessarily reflect the severity or potential for further problems. Minor injuries to the kidneys may pass unnoticed. For a renal injury to make its presence known, the capsule of the kidney must rupture (which causes a perirenal haematoma) or a calyx must be torn, leading to haematuria or, if there is full-thickness laceration of the kidney, urinary extravasation may occur into the surrounding tissues. Finally, in more severe injuries the main renal vessels may be damaged by avulsion, giving rise to a large retroperitoneal haematoma, often with hypotension.

Classification of blunt renal injuries

1. Minor injuries include contusion without disruption and minor fractures of only the outer cortex. These cause intrarenal bleeding without breach of the capsule and thus a subcapsular haematoma. Raised pressure within the kidney from a haematoma may cause ischaemia of adjacent renal tissue.

2. Major injuries may show a breach of the renal capsule or fracture of renal substance through the whole cortex extending into the collecting system. The renal pelvis may be ruptured, producing extravasation of urine, particularly if previously hydronephrotic. Substantial blood loss or leakage of urine or both, and the degree of each, depends on the depth of parenchymal fracture. Eighty per cent of these patients will have macroscopic haematuria, but the others have only microscopic haematuria or no haematuria. The integrity of Gerota's fascia is the most important determinant of blood loss. There may be separation of renal fragments and local devascularization, but the kidney remains substantially viable.

3. Catastrophic injuries include renal fragmentation or injuries of the renal vascular pedicle. In the fragmented kidney, one or more portions of renal substance becomes separated, leading to extensive haemorrhage and usually a leak of urine. The shattered kidney may have several major lines of disruption which destroy its structure. These kidneys are rarely salvageable.

4. Arterial injuries are of two types:

   (a) Total disruption with separation of the ends of the artery or of the artery from its aortic origin occurs. Total disruption leads to brisk initial blood loss before spasm arrests further haemorrhage but causes acute and complete ischaemia.

   (b) Intimal trauma may lead to arterial thrombosis. This often allows some blood flow to continue. If there is more than one renal artery supplying a kidney and only one is damaged, part of the kidney may remain viable. Injuries to the renal vein or inferior vena caval injuries are less likely to stop bleeding spontaneously and haemorrhage may be massive.

Penetrating renal injury

The most common cause of renal injury nowadays is iatrogenic trauma, inflicted inadvertently by instruments during percutaneous nephrolithotomy. Injuries are usually relatively minor and can be managed conservatively once the extent of injury is known. Similar injuries may be inflicted by knife wounds. Penetrating injuries may puncture the renal pelvis or upper ureter, leading to urinary leakage.

Presentation

A history of blunt trauma to the renal area, together with loin bruising, tenderness, and haematuria are the classical clinical features of renal trauma. If there is swelling in the renal area or fractures of lower posterior ribs or lumbar transverse processes, renal injury is extremely likely. Lesser renal injuries may produce renal tenderness and mild haematuria (often only detectable on testing). A loin mass usually signifies a substantial haematoma which later manifests as bruising in the loin. The presence and severity of haematuria, however, is not related to the extent of injury (see above). In frank haematuria, clot colic may occur. Major renal disruption is usually associated with hypovolaemic shock and a distended, tense abdomen. Urgent laparotomy may be unavoidable. Macroscopic haematuria is also suggestive of bladder injuries, 83 per cent of which are associated with fractures of the pelvis.

Investigation

In investigating the patient with possible renal injury, it is vital to establish that the injured kidney is not anatomically or functionally solitary by intravenous urography (IVU) or contrast enhanced CT scan. During investigation of haematuria, if the clinical picture suggests renal injury, begin with renal imaging. If lower-tract injury seems more likely, begin with urethro-cystography. If plain abdominal X-rays have been taken, they may show soft-tissue shadowing in the renal area or loss of psoas shadow caused by perinephric haematoma. Bony injuries to ribs or spine may also be seen.

Injudicious attempts at catheterizing an injured urethra may convert a simply treated partial tear into a complete one, which is difficult to treat. Therefore patients with signs of urethral damage, namely blood at the meatus, perineal bruising, or a high-riding prostate, should undergo gentle urethrography first. If needs dictate, a suprapubic catheter can be inserted as an immediate alternative. Cystography is easily performed to diagnose bladder rupture and involves instilling 300 ml contrast through a catheter under gravity.

If urgent laparotomy is required and renal injury likely, a single dose of intravenous contrast should be given so that a single-shot intravenous pyelogram (IVP) can be taken immediately or on the operating table. This is a valuable investigation even if it only establishes that there is a normal contralateral kidney. An 80 ml bolus of water-soluble contrast is given and 10 minutes later an abdominal film is taken. This will show the number of functioning kidneys present and give an indication of major damage—important information before laparotomy. The nephrectomy rate may be higher if urgent exploration is needed but this must be carried out in an unstable patient.

A little more time is usually available to allow investigation to proceed. The choice of primary investigation for suspected renal injury lies between intravenous urography (Table 17.18) with

Table 17.18 IVU findings following renal trauma

Pre-existing renal tract abnormalities may be revealed, including a solitary or misplaced kidney

Unilateral lack of renal function, suggesting interruption of blood supply (or a missing kidney)

Discrete areas of loss of function, suggesting fragmentation or vascular damage

Distortion of the calyceal pattern

Localized extravasation of urine, demonstrating penetration of the pelvicalyceal system

Divergence of the ureters suggests that there is a large retroperitoneal haematoma. This may contain as much as 4 litres of blood

tomography and contrast enhanced CT. Ultrasonography does not demonstrate renal function but can demonstrate intrarenal, perirenal, and retroperitoneal haematomas, parenchymal tears, and major disruption of the kidney. Ultrasound scanning is invaluable for following progress of a damaged kidney.

CT scanning employing intravenous contrast material gives reliable information about the severity of renal damage. CT can also define accurately the size and position of perirenal haematomas. This is likely to become the gold standard for renal trauma investigation in places where the investigation is available.

If a non-functioning kidney is found on IVU, or if there is clinical suspicion of a pedicle disruption, **arteriography** is required urgently. It is required less often following CT. In arterial separation, the injury is obvious on arteriography, whereas in intimal injury, some contrast may pass beyond the disruption. Injuries to arterial branches may be seen and there will be extravasation of contrast in fracture dislocations. If segmental vessels continue to bleed, therapeutic embolization may be used (e.g. after iatrogenic injury). Arteriography should also be considered if there is gross haematuria lasting longer than 10 days or clinical suspicion of an arteriovenous fistula. Radioisotopic scanning is of little value in acute injury but is useful later to demonstrate non-perfused segments after fracture dislocation.

Management of renal injuries

Substantial damage occurs in only about 15 per cent of renal injuries in the UK, and a much smaller proportion have devastating fragmentation or pedicle disruption. Mild injuries are treated with bed rest, fluids, and observation, with serial collection of urine samples to determine diminishing haematuria. Even after simple contusion, frank haematuria may persist and cause clot colic. If, however, there is no renal tenderness nor a palpable mass and only microscopic haematuria, early discharge from hospital is safe. Serial ultrasound examinations may be useful and blood pressure should be measured at follow-up. Further imaging may be indicated by clinical progress.

More substantial injuries should still be treated conservatively with rest, intravenous fluids, blood transfusion if necessary, and careful monitoring. Regular clinical examinations of the renal

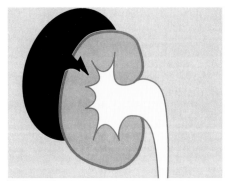

Perirenal haematoma

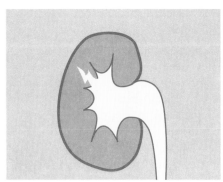

Torn calyx

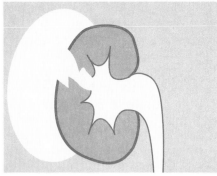

Complete rupture

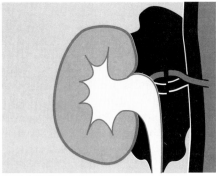

Avulsion of vessels

Figure 17.4 Potential indications for intervention after renal injury.

Table 17.19 The indications for intervention after renal injury

Penetrating wounds
Secondary haemorrhage
Infection of perirenal haematoma
Collection of extravasated urine
Early onset hypertension

mass should be performed by the same person. Paralytic ileus is common. In most, haematuria ceases and the haematoma gradually absorbs. In some cases, bleeding continues and the patient deteriorates. Depending on the severity, arteriography or laparotomy is needed. Potential indications for intervention after renal injury are shown in Table 17.19 and Fig. 17.4. Exploration should be through a midline incision and vascular control should be obtained before opening Gerota's fascia. This manoeuvre reduces the rate of nephrectomy and offers the opportunity of examining the intra-abdominal organs for an associated injury. When exposing and controlling the renal pedicle, it is wise to gain control of the renal vein before the renal artery. The haematoma can then be evacuated and the kidney examined carefully. If the kidney is repairable, this is carried out and the injured kidney can be wrapped in omentum, which is believed to decrease the postoperative complication rate. Remember that 25 per cent of patients have multiple renal arteries and partial nephrectomy may thus be an option. The bare area should be patched with omentum.

Some patients settle initially but develop recurrent pain and expansion of the loin mass 5–10 days after injury because of further blood loss or extravasation of urine. Many require nephrectomy but urological involvement or consultation will have been obtained.

Devastating injuries or pedicle injuries require urgent laparotomy. Usually there is multiple trauma with other abdominal injuries, including liver, spleen, bowel, or other major vessel disruptions. Nephrectomy is often the only option to arrest haemorrhage, but the surgeon must be sure that there is more than one functioning kidney. In isolated pedicle injury, arterial repair may be possible and usually requires an interposition saphenous vein graft. However, one rarely gets there in time and the overall outcome is disappointing. Even if the kidney survives, renal function (estimated isotopically) tends to be poor.

Some advocate early exploration of a ruptured kidney to confirm diagnosis, remove detached fragments of parenchyma, suture lacerations, and effect haemostasis. However, in inexperienced hands this leads to an unnecessarily high nephrectomy rate. After a major injury, prophylactic antibiotics and careful follow-up are needed, whichever approach is adopted.

Not all of these complications will require surgical exploration of the kidney as some can be managed with ultrasound-guided drainage methods; specialist radiological help should be obtained.

Management of penetrating renal trauma

Penetration of the kidney by a stab wound or trauma complicating percutaneous nephrolithotomy does not always require renal exploration. Non-operative management of minor degrees of renal injury carries a low morbidity. Unless there is a clinical indication of severe renal damage or continuing bleeding then surgery is not required. Concomitant injuries should be considered in the usual ways.

Management of injury to the renal pedicle

Injury to the renal pedicle is suspected when there is only partial or no visualization of the kidney on intravenous urography. The diagnosis should be confirmed with renal arteriography if possible. Success in managing the renal pedicle injury depends on minimizing the delay between injury and repair. This time interval is governed by the presence of other injuries, but if the kidney is to be saved, early surgical revascularization is the key. If the delay is longer than 18 hours, the kidney is likely to fail and nephrectomy may be the better option. The decision to perform vascular repair or nephrectomy depends on the general condition of the patient, the presence of pre-existing renal disease, and the condition of the involved and contralateral kidney.

Ureteric damage

Most ureteric injuries are iatrogenic and occur during gynae-cological, colorectal, or vascular surgical procedures. Penetrating abdominal injury is the most common cause of ureteric damage by an external route. Ureteric damage can occur as a result of blunt trauma, particularly in children, who may develop avulsion of the upper ureter following hyperextension of the trunk when struck from behind. When iatrogenic damage occurs during the course of surgery, it is often associated with severe pelvic disease that distorts the anatomical configuration of the tissues, for example tumour or endometriosis. On other occasions there is an unrecognized congenital abnormality, such as double ureter.

Late complications of renal injury

After arterial damage, the devascularized kidney atrophies and is likely to cause renal hypertension. Treatment may require partial nephrectomy or nephrectomy. Extravasation of urine into the perinephric tissues (**urinoma**) predisposes to infection and abscess formation. Extravasation is easily demonstrated with ultrasound. Many cases resolve with conservative treatment but others require external drainage using ultrasound guidance. Transient hydronephrosis caused by haematoma compressing the ureter usually recovers spontaneously.

An arteriovenous fistula may develop later and this may be particularly dangerous if there is a communication between the renal artery and vein. Arteriovenous fistula is rare and can follow percutaneous surgery. Minor vessel fistulas can be treated with immobilization but surgery is needed if the fistula is at the pedicle.

Management of the damaged ureter

Recognition at the time of damage during surgery

Urological help or opinion should be sought. The treatment depends on the site of damage and the extent of the injury.

Partial transsection of the ureter, if clean and involving less than half of the ureteric circumference, can be repaired by simple suture and drainage. Sutures should be absorbable. If the ureter is transsected completely, an end-to-end transverse spatulated anastomosis should be carried out. The repair should be supported by an indwelling stent which can be removed later by cystoscopy. If the ureter is injured distally, below the level of the iliac vessels, the ureter can be reimplanted into the bladder. The preferred technique is to use a **psoas hitch** after ligating the contralateral superior vesical artery. Alternatively, a Boari bladder flap may be used to replace the gap between the bladder and the ureteric end. Whichever method is used, the surgeon should ensure a tension–free anastomosis and should support the anastomosis with an indwelling stent. In cases where there is loss of ureteric length, a transuretero-ureterostomy can be performed. Here, the injured ureter is mobilized and swung across to the intact ureter and anastomosed end to side. Occasionally a simple cutaneous ureterostomy will be the best immediate option.

Late recognition of a damaged ureter

This is a more serious problem because the intervening delay leads to a localized urinary leak and infection and the possibility of ureteric obstruction. This requires operative management and may ultimately lead to a nephrectomy. Reconstruction is much safer if performed when the urine is sterile, so it is essential that a MSU for culture and sensitivity is obtained as soon as the injury is suspected. A high-dose intravenous urogram is performed to assess the level of the ureteric damage and this can be confirmed by a retrograde ureterogram. This complication must be managed by immediate operative drainage and definitive reconstruction when the acute phase is over. Percutaneous nephrostomy can be used to divert urine away from the point of leakage in preparation for the eventual surgical repair.

If a ureter is inadvertently ligated during a surgical procedure, it often passes unnoticed, as the contralateral kidney takes over its function of urine production. If the urine contained in the hydronephrotic kidney becomes infected, the patient presents with a **pyonephrosis**. This is confirmed by abdominal ultra-sonography which demonstrates the hydronephrotic ureter and renal calyces above the level of ligation. It can be treated initially by a tube nephrostomy and definitive reconstruction later if there is sufficient functioning renal tissue in the affected kidney.

Bladder injury

Traumatic rupture of the bladder may be **intraperitoneal** or **extraperitoneal**. Urine may cause little in the way of peritoneal signs, at least initially. Extraperitoneal rupture of bladder or urethra allows urine to track along the pelvic and perineal tissue planes and may lead to spreading cellulitis. When the diagnosis is suspected clinically, cystography will confirm it, or it may be discovered at a laparotomy for other injuries. Intraperitoneal rupture requires exploration and suture repair (using two layers of absorbable material). This approach is also advisable for most traumatic extraperitoneal ruptures. Postoperatively, catheter drainage of urine for 10 days should be employed.

Urethral injuries

Damage to the urethra anywhere along its length heals by scar formation, which narrows the lumen of the urethra, and a stricture inevitably follows. Scarring is worse if there is infection, extravasation, haematoma, or loss of urothelial lining. It follows, therefore, that the early management of any type of urethral injury must be directed towards preventing infection and extravasation of urine and avoiding further damage to the urethral lining.

Categories of urethral damage

Understanding the two broad categories of damage to the urethra requires a knowledge of the anatomical subdivisions of the urethra. The **posterior urethra** begins at the bladder neck and ends as it passes through the urogenital diaphragm. It is subdivided into the upper **prostatic urethra** and the lower **membranous urethra**. In adults, the prostate acts as a shock absorber for direct damage and hence the more common site of damage or rupture of the posterior urethra is in its lower, membranous part. This type of injury is commonly associated with **pelvic fractures.**

The anterior urethra is subdivided into the proximal bulbous, central pendulous urethra, and the distal glandular urethra. The bulbous urethra is the most common site of injury because it is curved and can be damaged by overvigorous catheterization or instrumentation. It is also the part of the urethra which is crushed against the under surface of the pubic symphysis as a result of a perineal blow. The anatomical spaces into which extravasation of urine is likely to occur following urethral damage need to be understood: if the damage lies above the urogenital diaphragm, then urinary extravasation occurs upwards into the retropubic space. If there is complete transsection of the urethra, the bladder and the prostate are dislocated from the pelvic floor. If the leak occurs below the urogenital diaphragm (i.e. in the bulbous urethra), extravasation occurs into the scrotum, penis, and lower abdominal wall, but the bladder and prostate retain their anatomical continuity with the pelvic diaphragm.

Recognition of possible urethral damage

Pelvic or perineal trauma with inability to pass urine and the presence of blood at the external urinary meatus suggest a **urethral rupture.** On rectal examination the prostate may be riding high and replaced by a boggy mass of haematoma and urine. This indicates a rupture of the membranous urethra. Urethral injury is excluded by taking a single X-ray film after syringe instillation of 20 ml of contrast into the urethra. If the contrast flows into the bladder without extravasation, a significant urethral injury can be excluded and a small indwelling urethral catheter can be passed safely. On the other hand, periurethral extravasation indicates urethral injury and urethral catheterization should not be attempted.

Management of urethral damage

Anterior urethral injury

These injuries vary from simple contusion to complete urethral rupture with extensive extravasation of urine into the scrotal tissues. The treatment depends on the type of injury. For simple contusion, no treatment is usually required; the haematuria will clear quickly and cause no long-term complications. If the urethral urothelium is lacerated, either partially or completely, the likelihood of stricture formation after healing is high. The safest way of dealing with this type of problem is to insert a suprapubic catheter to divert urine flow and limit the amount of extravasation. The injury is allowed to settle and is assessed later by further urethrography to assess the continuity and the amount of stricture formation as a result of healing. A stricture can be treated by regular dilatation or by surgical urethroplasty.

Posterior urethral injury

This commonly arises following pelvic fractures. The diagnosis is made by retrograde urethrography together with intravenous urography.

Classification of posterior urethral injuries

- Type 1 injury involves stretching of the urethra and compression of the bladder by pelvic haematoma. The ureter is not disrupted and treatment involves urethral catheterization until the haematoma settles. This type of patient often suffers sacral nerve plexus damage and may have difficulty in initiating micturition once the trauma has settled.

- Type 2 urethral injury involves partial or complete rupture of the urethra but without dislocation of the prostate. This is best treated by a suprapubic catheter followed by a voiding cystourethrogram performed after 2–3 weeks to assess the integrity of healing. If extravasation no longer persists and the urethra is of normal calibre, the suprapubic catheter can be removed. However, this injury will, more often than not, lead to a urethral stricture later.

- Type 3 injury is when the prostate is dislocated from the urogenital diaphragm. The bladder and prostate are elevated away from the lower urethral segment. The timing of surgical correction remains controversial. These patients will inevitably develop a severe urethral stricture in time and may become impotent and develop urinary incontinence because of injury to the lower part of the urethral sphincter. A suprapubic catheter is essential initially to divert urine away from the trauma site, but urologists debate the best method of bringing the prostatic urethra close to the upper part of the bulbar urethra. The time-honoured method of 'railroading' a Foley catheter through into the bladder and applying external traction is still advocated by some. However, the modern trend is to perform the Turner–Warwick isotonic operation, designed to leave the patient with a short, simple stricture that can be treated more easily at a later date.

2.6 Blast and gunshot injuries

The assessment and management of specific penetrating injuries has been discussed elsewhere, but a few general comments are appropriate.

Missile injuries

Missiles may be bullets or fragments from an explosive device. Missile injuries cause tissue damage along the wound track. If damage is confined to the track, this is classified as a **low-energy-transfer wound**. If there is damage outside the track, caused by the transfer of excess kinetic energy from the missile, the injury is known as a **high-energy-transfer wound**. However, every case does not fit neatly into this classification. The kinetic energy of a missile is proportional to the product of its mass and the square of its velocity. Rifles and machine guns have a high initial velocity, giving high kinetic energy to the missile. These cause high-energy-transfer wounds, whereas hand guns and most bomb fragments have subsonic velocity with lower kinetic energies. These cause low-energy-transfer wounds. The amount of energy transferred from a bullet also depends on its pattern of flight or **yaw angle**. The damage caused varies enormously according to the angle at which the bullet strikes the skin, and the same weapon may cause completely different injuries under different circumstances. A bullet travelling parallel to its long axis may 'drill' through a patient, causing relatively little damage. Conversely, a tumbling bullet is likely to cause extensive injuries.

High-energy missiles may cause a great deal of tissue damage around the missile track. A temporary cavity forms within the tissues. Some tissues (e.g. lung) recover from this stretching whereas others (liver, spleen, brain) are destroyed. Muscle occupies an intermediate position. If bone is struck, secondary fragments may cause even more extensive damage. There is also a large amount of wound contamination caused by the negative-pressure wave following the high-pressure wave, which sucks debris into both entry and exit wounds and disseminates it widely, causing gross wound contamination. Low-energy-transfer wounds are usually less contaminated because the missile drags in only small quantities of clothing or debris, which are confined to the track. However, any velocity of missile that penetrates the skin may kill the patients if vital organs are damaged. It is worth emphasizing that missiles may follow remarkably tortuous courses as they tumble and ricochet within the body. The literature is full of case reports describing unusual combinations of injuries and entry points, many of which proved survivable.

Management of missile injuries

Patients are often unaware of the extent of their injuries. Entry wounds may be surprisingly small but exit wounds are likely to be much larger, particularly in high-energy-transfer injuries. Initially the basic ABCDE assessment and resuscitation techniques are applied. If a chest injury is suspected, there may be a tension pneumothorax or haemothorax.

If there is an abdominal injury, antibiotics and tetanus prophylaxis should be administered as early as possible because of possible contamination with bowel contents. If hospital admission is delayed, systemic antibiotics should be administered en route.

Surgical management follows basic principles: dead tissue and foreign materials must be excised and wounds should not be closed until healing free from infection is likely. Delayed primary closure is usually performed around day 5 if practicable. It is difficult to determine the amount of tissue damage caused by any missile because, as stated earlier, this varies with velocity, yaw, fragmentation, contamination, delay, circumstance, and tissues involved. Experienced military surgeons stress that it is important to treat the wound and not the weapon. Within a civilian hospital environment, it is relatively straightforward to re-examine or re-explore wounds, if necessary with repeated débridements, until the surgeon is satisfied that all dead tissue has been excised. Doubtful tissue at initial operation will declare itself at planned re-exploration. In a military setting, where operative delay, gross contamination, and multiple casualties are likely, undue reliance on antibiotics without adequate early excision leads to horrific mortality from wound infection. These lessons constantly have to be relearnt, often the hard way. However, a balance sometimes has to be struck when it would be necessary to delve deep into dangerous territory for a bullet or missile fragment which is not causing active problems.

Explosives and blast injuries

Explosions result from war, terrorist incidents, or major accidents, and they often cause multiple casualties. Injuries may be caused by blast waves, missiles, or by casualties thrown through the air. In a conventional explosion, damage is caused by the very rapid expansion of hot gases which may propel missiles. The primary effects are caused by the **blast shock wave**, the release of radiant heat causing burns, and the **blast wind**, a rapidly moving column of gas and debris.

Primary blast shock wave

This is a wave of high pressure that spreads out from the centre of the explosion, travelling at just over the speed of sound. The power of this high-pressure wave is increased many times when it reflects from solid objects such as walls. Therefore the more serious injuries occur when people are hit in an enclosed space. The shock waves passes through the tissues, causing the greatest damage where there is a change in tissue density. Maximum damage occurs where there is a tissue–gas interface, such in the upper or lower respiratory tract and the gastrointestinal tract. Tympanic membrane rupture is very common and this is the most susceptible part of the body to blast damage. Perforations usually heal spontaneously but very high pressure waves may cause direct sensory neural damage to the cochlea, causing nerve deafness. Olfactory nerve damage results in anosmia.

Lung damage (blast lung)

This affects up to 5 per cent of patients involved in explosions. The primary disorder is alveolar rupture and haemorrhage, causing massive contusion leading to acute respiratory failure. Pneumothorax may occur and air may enter the pulmonary circulation, causing coronary occlusion, cardiac arrest, and cerebral neurological damage. Positive-pressure ventilation increases the risk of air embolism. In these cases air may be seen in the retinal vessels on fundoscopy.

Abdominal injury

Massive abdominal organ damage is rarely seen in survivors of blast injury. The most common injuries are multiple contusions of intestinal contents and secondary perforation caused by ischaemia, which may be delayed for up to 5 days.

Blast wind

This is a column of gas, and later air, that moves out from the centre of the explosion at very high speed. Blast winds are often channelled by surrounding obstructions and injuries are unpredictable. Close to the blast there may be total destruction of victims. Further away, traumatic amputations often occur, with nerves avulsed at a higher level than other structures.

Flash burns

Certain types of explosive cause a sudden release of energy, generating a wave of hot gas sufficient to cause flash burns and smoke-inhalation injuries. There may be superficial burns to the hands or face, and smoke inhalation may result in delayed symptoms. Staff must be alert to the development of oedematous airway obstruction, and prophylactic intubation must be considered. Patients exposed to flash burns should be admitted to hospital for rest and oxygen therapy if smoke inhalation is suspected. Delayed respiratory failure may occur as a result of blast lung, smoke inhalation, or systemic microemboli, and a period of close observation is essential.

Forensic responsibilities

Doctors have a duty to assist in the investigation of crimes and should collect information that may help. All material relating to the incident should be preserved and labelled, with its origin noted and recorded. This includes debris from wounds, clothing, fragments of missiles and explosives. Examination of the patient should be noted carefully and recorded, by photography if possible, including entry wounds and exit wounds.

2.7 Soft-tissue injuries

The most common causes of soft-tissue injuries are road traffic accidents and, to a lesser extent, accidents in the home, bites, injuries during sports, and assaults. It is important in all such injuries to keep very accurate clinical records, including Polaroid photographs to be stored in the clinical notes. This is particularly useful if medicolegal proceedings arise later. A classification of soft-tissue injuries is given in Table 17.20.

Principles of management

Management can be considered under three headings:

1. **Cleaning and irrigation.** The wound needs to be cleaned under local or general anaesthesia and irrigated with saline or

Table 17.20 Classification of soft-tissue injuries

1. Superficial abrasions. These cause partial-thickness skin loss, which usually epithelializes without surgical intervention
2. Superficial lacerations with a sharp margin. The shape of the wound may be irregular
3. Penetrating lacerations and puncture wounds. These are usually caused by broken glass, e.g. windscreen injuries. There are likely to be underlying foreign bodies
4. Human and animal bites, with or without tissue loss. These usually have an irregular edge and are invariably contaminated
5. Avulsion and degloving injuries, usually of limbs. These follow a shearing or crush injury. Injuries can range from elevation of a small skin flap to extensive loss of superficial tissues
6. Heavily contaminated injury with full-thickness skin loss. There is a high incidence of foreign material driven deeply into the wound

cetrimide to wash away loose foreign particles. With extensive grazes containing road dirt or multiple foreign bodies, it is necessary to remove these with a sterile scrubbing brush or by picking them out individually from the wound. If these foreign bodies are not adequately removed, the wound looks ugly and may have multiple tattoos from ingrained debris.

2. **Débridement of the wound.** All bleeding should be stopped before deciding about how much débridement is needed. Undercut margins are trimmed and small irregular wounds with possible ischaemic flaps are excised cleanly. The aim is to convert a ragged wound into a tidier wound with vertical margins, which would allow better primary closure, if appropriate. In the face, blood supply is so good that minimal trimming is performed before closure.

3. **Decisions about closure.** If the wound can be regarded as relatively clean, then it may be decided to close the wound primarily after adequate débridement. Systemic antibiotics should be given and the patient immunized against tetanus or receive a booster dose if indicated. If there is a high risk of infective contamination of the wound, it is best to leave the wound open and allow it to heal by secondary intention. In wounds where there is a risk of a retained foreign body, X-rays should be taken if it is likely to be radiopaque (e.g. glass). If non-radiopaque material, such as wood, is suspected, then careful exploration of the wound should be performed before closure.

Specific injuries

Animal bites

All bites are potentially infective and patients should be treated with prophylactic penicillin. It is customary to leave these wounds open because of the potential infective complications and then to close them secondarily once infection risk has passed. Healthy granulation tissue is very resistant to infection and granulating wounds can be closed if there are no residual pockets of infection or dead tissue. If there is soft-tissue loss as a result of the bite, specialist plastic surgical advice should be obtained.

Shearing and degloving injuries

Avulsion of the skin and subcutaneous tissue by a twisting mechanism ruptures the musculocutaneous and perforating vessels and devascularizes the outer soft-tissue cover. Assessing the extent of devitalized tissue in these injuries is difficult and plastic surgical help may be needed to decide on the extent of tissue removal. The wound will inevitably require good-quality skin cover. This is best provided by full-thickness flaps in most cases, but split-skin grafts can sometimes be used. If there is an associated skeletal injury, then a muscle flap may be required to cover exposed bone. Again, there is the need for expert plastic surgical advice.

Pretibial injuries

The partially avulsed V-shaped skin flap laceration following injury to the pretibial area is a common injury in elderly women and is difficult to treat effectively. The area has a poor blood supply and even a proximally based flap is likely to be poorly perfused and will not heal easily. If the flap is obviously ischaemic, all dead tissue needs to be excised and the defect covered with a split-skin graft.

Facial injuries

These commonly occur in association with faciomandibular fractures. Fracture reduction and stabilization should precede repair of any soft-tissue injuries. Lacerations of the mouth and full-thickness lip injuries are repaired primarily in three layers, reconstituting the mucosa, muscle, and skin. The cutaneous

Table 17.21 Types of vascular trauma

Type of trauma	Typical sites	Principles of management
Penetrating trauma		
Stab wounds	Root of neck Abdominal aorta Femoral artery or vein (often accidental in personnel involved in meat preparation)	1. Is patient exsanguinating from the wound or internally? If so, can external pressure control loss while preparing for operation? 2. Are there signs of ischaemia distal to the injury? If so, arteriography before surgery, perhaps on-table, may be essential 3. At operation, try to obtain control of arterial supply remote from site of injury before exploring wound. Access must be excellent 4. Repair all large vessels damaged, both arteries and veins, if possible with autogenous saphenous vein
Gunshot wounds	Abdomen Chest Popliteal fossa ('knee capping')	As for stab wounds. Damage is likely to be much greater, especially if high-velocity injury. All dead tissue must be excised, blood vessels reconstructed, and wounds left open for delayed primary closure. However, blood vessels must be covered (e.g. by muscle mobilization). Antibiotic prophylaxis essential
Glass	Radial artery, brachial artery	Injury usually superficial but plain X-rays reveal deep fragments of glass. Exploration if bleeding actively or if distal ischaemia. Arteriography if in doubt
Fractures and dislocations	Pelvis	Retroperitoneal haemorrhage may be severe. In unstable fractures with increased pelvic volume (see later), external fixation may be necessary. Continuing haemorrhage may require arteriographic embolization of internal iliac arteries. Direct exploration of pelvic vessels is not advisable
	Lower limb Hyperextension injury to knee	Vascular repair of popliteal vessels may be inappropriate if tibial nerves transsected and the limb is useless
	Femoral and tibial fractures	Rarely cause vascular injury but early arteriography if in doubt (and early surgical repair, perhaps with shunting, if appropriate)
	Upper limb—supracondylar fracture of humerus	Early reduction of fracture. Arteriography if perfusion in doubt
Crush injuries	Lower limb	Depends on extent of tissue damage and on duration since trauma. If tissue damage is severe and delay great, primary amputation prevents **crush syndrome** caused by release of myoglobin and other agents from crushed muscle
	Chest—aortic rupture	90% of aortic injuries in surviving patients occur at the aortic isthmus where it is tethered by the ligamentum arteriosum. On arteriography, a contained false aneurysm is the most common finding, but extravasation, an intimal flap, or partial occlusion may be seen. Surgical repair required
Iatrogenic injury	Iliac artery during lumbar disc surgery	Exploration by arterial surgeon as soon as injury is suspected. Delay and particularly transfer between hospitals can be fatal
	Femoral artery during inguinal hernia repair	Usually local pressure will arrest haemorrhage. Formal repair not usually required
	Femoral or brachial artery during cardiac catheter of after insertion of aortic balloon pump	Early exploration and repair by experienced surgeon. Controlled compression under ultrasound guidance used in some units. Arteriography if doubt about extent of damage or ischaemia

junction should be identified carefully and then accurately reconstituted to avoid an unsightly repair.

2.8 Vascular trauma

Introduction and principles of management

Blood-vessel trauma is as old as history, but, until recently, management has been limited to attempts at staunching haemorrhage by cautery or application of dressings. Ambroise Paré, the French military surgeon, rediscovered ligation of accessible vessels in the sixteenth century, but conditions were primitive and deaths from infection and secondary haemorrhage were common. Amputation was the only treatment available for ischaemia due to arterial injury. Even during the First and Second World Wars, arterial injuries were almost exclusively managed by ligation, largely because of the high risk of secondary haemorrhage from the vascular repair. This was due to infection resulting from wound contamination and the absence of antibiotics. The scientific management of vascular trauma had to wait for the advent of direct vessel suture and grafting techniques, which were first successfully applied during the Korean War in the 1950s (Hughes 1958).

Vascular trauma (Table 17.21) occurs in military and civilian settings and the principles of management are similar. High-velocity bullets cause devastating tissue damage in warfare and, less commonly, in civilian practice. Civilian trauma occurs chiefly with personal violence (stab and low-velocity gunshot wounds), road traffic accidents (blunt and penetrating trauma, often in association with other injuries), accidents with glass panels, sports injuries, and inadvertent trauma during medical and surgical procedures. In addition, arterial (and venous) injury may occur as a result of injectable drug abuse.

Managing vascular trauma may require, on the one hand, extremely urgent action to arrest exsanguinating haemorrhage, and, on the other hand, informed and skilled clinical assessment to recognize deficient blood supply or a potential delayed haemorrhage. In limb trauma, early recognition of ischaemia is crucial to the success of limb salvage. This will often require arteriography. Similarly, failure to recognize the significance of retroperitoneal haemorrhage after an abdominal stab wound, for example, may result in delayed concealed haemorrhage from an aortic puncture, which is potentially fatal. Vascular trauma unrecognized at the time of injury may present months or years later in the form of a false aneurysm or an arteriovenous fistula.

Vascular trauma occurs most often in young people, and the vessels injured are likely to be healthy and therefore more easily repaired than atherosclerotic and calcified vessels. But challenges remain—the ideal synthetic vascular graft is yet to appear, associated injuries to bone and nerve increase morbidity, and reconstructions may undergo thrombosis and become infected.

The role of arteriography

Arteriography is a vital tool in the management of arterial trauma. Good results require a surgeon with a low threshold for ordering an arteriogram and an experienced radiologist.

Arteriography can provide answers to many urgent questions. For example: Is the arterial circulation of the lower limb in continuity? If not, where are the abnormalities, or is there an aortic tear? Arteriography may also be used as a route for therapeutic embolization.

The femoral approach is most frequently used, provided femoral pulses are palpable, as it is the most familiar, the most versatile, and the safest route. Abnormal findings (in approximate order of frequency) include extraluminal contrast injection, abrupt arterial occlusion, arterial transsection, arteriovenous fistula, intimal flaps, intraluminal thrombus, luminal narrowing, arterial dilatation, venous extravasation, and an extravascular mass.

Arteriographic embolization may be appropriate to occlude certain bleeding vessels, using selective catheterization. The technique is important in managing massive retroperitoneal haemorrhage from pelvic fractures by embolizing internal iliac arteries. It has also been used successfully in controlling bleeding from liver, spleen, pancreas, and genitourinary tract, but general guidelines remain to be defined by experience. Embolic methods may also be employed in managing arteriovenous fistulas.

Problems associated with vascular trauma

Haemorrhage

The amount of bleeding from damaged blood vessels depends on:

◆ the diameter of the damaged vessels;

◆ whether veins or arteries are damaged;

◆ whether the trauma has produced a complete transsection or an opening in the side of a vessel in continuity;

◆ whether there is sufficient surrounding tissue pressure to restrain rapid haemorrhage;

◆ whether clotting and platelet mechanisms are intact.

In general, arteries are more forgiving of trauma than veins because their muscular, elastic walls contract to reduce the size of the defect. This is particularly effective if the vessel is completely transsected. A deep artery with a small wound may not exhibit signs of rapid haemorrhage, instead forming a false aneurysm with leakage of blood restrained by surrounding fibrous tissue. A false aneurysm, however, is a time bomb that may rupture catastrophically at any time. Thus, if the nature of the trauma or other signs suggests deep-vessel injury, meticulous arteriography should be performed if logistically possible.

The principles of surgical management of overt haemorrhage are given in Table 17.22. Overt or 'revealed' haemorrhage from a surface wound can usually be controlled temporarily by local pressure via a substantial gauze or gamgee dressing. This allows time to replace blood volume and induction of anaesthesia prior to exploratory surgery.

Arteries larger than 3 mm should be repaired unless there is evidence of good distal perfusion from collateral circulation.

Table 17.22 The principles of surgical management for overt haemorrhage

1. Arteriography if extent of injury is not obvious

2. Adequate exposure. The planned incision must allow proximal control prior to exploration, and provide full access to the injury, allowing for extension if unexpectedly extensive injuries are discovered. Detailed descriptions of blood-vessel exposure are given in specialized books such as (Bongard 1991)

3. Proximal control of arterial haemorrhage

4. Exploration of the wound to determine the injuries and to search for foreign bodies

5. Delineation of the extent of vascular injury (i.e. arterial, venous, or both), which vessels are involved, and the type of injuries

6. Application of clamps for local control

7. Local repair by direct suture or interposition grafting using autogenous vein

End-to-end repair by direct suture is preferred, provided the ends can be apposed without tension. If this is not possible, an interposition graft is needed. Autogenous saphenous vein is preferable to synthetic graft material because of the high risk of infection after trauma. For large vessels, long saphenous vein can be harvested, opened longitudinally, and a large vessel fashioned by spiralling the opened vein around a silicone tube drain and suturing the edges.

Large veins should be repaired by direct suture if possible, but ligation of veins is less likely to result in deficit than ligation of arteries. Small veins are thus usually ligated.

Where haemorrhage is concealed (i.e. within one of the body cavities), arteriography (and possibly venography) is usually regarded as mandatory. Thus, a patient suffering a crushing chest injury may have an aortic isthmus tear, and a patient with an abdominal stab wound may have injured the aorta or other great vessels. When the heart has been stabbed, arteriography is rarely useful and it is better to proceed immediately to surgical exploration.

In pelvic fractures, distinction should be made between lateral compression injury, anteroposterior compression injury, and vertical shear injury. Lateral compression fractures are often impacted and stable. The pelvis is infolded, reducing its volume and providing tamponade for injured vessels. The other types of injury tend to tear vascular structures as well as increasing pelvic volume, which allows unrestrained blood loss.

There is some disagreement about the best form of management of unstable pelvic fractures with continuing haemorrhage. Some surgeons advocate early application of an anterior frame external fixator to decrease pelvic volume, decrease blood loss from cancellous bone surfaces, minimize shear forces and consequent further vessel damage, and allow earlier patient mobilization.

Angiography and therapeutic embolization of pelvic arterial bleeding is indicated in patients who remain haemodynamically unstable as a result of pelvic retroperitoneal haemorrhage. Surgical exploration of these patients is often unsatisfactory because of the extent of venous injury. If arterial haemorrhage can be controlled by internal iliac embolization, venous haemorrhage will cease as a result of tamponade from thrombus, provided transfusion is adequate.

Ischaemia

Ischaemia caused by arterial injury is most likely to occur in the extremities. It occasionally occurs in a viscus, particularly a kidney, by avulsion of the pedicle after blunt abdominal trauma.

Limb ischaemia from a simple arterial injury (such as a femoral artery stab wound) is relatively easy to recognize by the usual signs of pallor, coldness, and loss of pulses. However, when a patient has suffered more extensive local injuries with crushing or fractures, particularly if shocked and hypotensive, the periphery may appear cold, oedematous, and pulseless, and yet be adequately perfused. In such cases, a 'wait and see' policy is inappropriate because of the danger of tissue damage if the limb is critically ischaemic and the likelihood of propagated thrombosis developing in underperfused arteries and veins distal to the injury.

In displaced fractures, the limb should be assessed before and after reduction as reduction may restore arterial circulation. If arterial injury is suspected, reduction must not be delayed beyond 2 hours of potential ischaemic time.

In limb injuries, pulses are examined and only passed as satisfactory if unequivocally palpable. If there is doubt, a Doppler ultrasound flow detector may be used, but the operator must have the experience to distinguish a normal pulse from a poor collateral pulse. It is better to err on the side of caution and perform urgent arteriography if any doubt remains, so that necessary treatment can be initiated early.

Arteriography will usually reveal the site and often the cause of peripheral ischaemia. This may be arterial transsection, crushing injury with fracture of the inner layers of the vessel or flap formation, or compression of the artery by a fragment of bone.

The principles of management of traumatic ischaemia are similar to those for haemorrhage, described above, with the following additional points:

- early exploration and revascularization is needed to prevent tissue damage;

- an indwelling shunt (e.g. Pruitt shunt) may be used to revascularize the periphery temporarily while repair is under way;

- if there is a ragged or stretch injury causing mural damage and thrombosis, repair is likely to need an interposition graft; arterial 'spasm' is overdiagnosed and the appearances are usually due to mural damage;

- fasciotomy (Table 17.23) should be performed if revascularization has been delayed by more than 2–4 hours (either outside or inside hospital). In doubtful cases, tissue compartment pressures can be measured and fasciotomy performed if pressure rises above about 30 mmHg.

If a limb injury is so extensive as to render the limb useless by virtue of either tissue loss or damage to blood vessels and nerves,

Table 17.23 Compartment syndrome and fasciotomy

This occurs if the pressure within a closed compartment of a limb rises to a level that compromises the circulation of the tissues within that space, causing ischaemia of muscles and nerves. If prolonged, tissue necrosis results, and this was originally described as Volkmann's ischaemic contracture. The cause of compartment syndrome is not wholly understood, but in the case of traumatic limb ischaemia, probably represents the injurious effects of reperfusion after severe ischaemia. The resulting cellular damage allows fluid to 'leak' from microscopic vessels into the interstitial space

Compartment syndromes occur most commonly in the four compartments of the leg. These comprise anterior, lateral, and deep and superficial posterior compartments

After delayed revascularization, all four compartments need to be decompressed by fasciotomy. The usual method is via a single parafibular incision, although partial fibulectomy is employed occasionally

or else has been the subject of prolonged crush entrapment, then a primary amputation is the best option. The standard sites of election apply, with every effort being made to preserve useful joints, even if a short stump results.

In the case of crush injury, amputation in the field at the site of injury may be advisable to prevent crush syndrome. In any case, all dead tissue must be excised to avoid the risk of gas gangrene.

Late effects of arterial trauma

False aneurysms may develop months or years after arterial injury. The original injury is constrained by surrounding tissue but blood continues to leak slowly outside the vessel, expanding the false sac. This is likely to rupture eventually and should be repaired surgically. Repair is usually a simple matter as the arterial defect is often small.

Arteriovenous fistulas may develop immediately or at any time after a vascular injury. The initial injury damages an artery and a vein lying in close proximity and allows blood to flow from artery to vein. This results in local dilatation of veins, which are often visible as a knot of vessels with a palpable thrill and an audible continuous machinery murmur. Arteriovenous fistulas may be amenable to treatment by arteriographic embolism or else the fistula can be divided surgically and the vessels repaired individually.

Venous problems

Damaged veins have little contractile ability after injury, either muscular or elastic, and consequently continue to bleed until tamponaded by surrounding tissues or the pressure of blood and clot. Many veins can be safely ligated, but where drainage is via a single main vein, such as the common femoral, the vein should be repaired when possible, usually before the arterial repair, or else signs of venous obstruction will ensue.

Bibliography

Bongard, F., Johs, S.M., Leighton, T.A., Klein, S.R. (1991). Peripheral arterial shotgun missile emboli: Diagnostic and therapeutic management—case reports. *Trauma-Injury Infection and Critical Care.* **31**, 1426–31.

Carrico, C.J., Thal, E.R., and Weigelt, J.A. (1998). *Operative trauma management.* Appleton and Lange, Connecticut.

Demetriades, D., Charalambides, D., Lakhoo, M. (1993). Physical examination and selective conservative management in patients with penetrating injuries of the neck. *Br. J. Surg.,* **80**, 1534–6.

Driscoll, P. and Skinner, D. (1998). *Trauma care beyond the resuscitation room.* BMJ Publishing, London.

Eaton, C.J. (1992). *Essentials of immediate medical care.* Churchill Livingstone, London.

Gentleman, D. and Jennett, B. (1981). Hazards of inter-hospital transfer of comatose head injured patients. *Lancet,* **2**, 853–5.

Hardy, D.G. (1989). The early management of head injuries. *Current Practice in Surgery,* **1**, 118–24.

Klein, J.S. and Weigelt, J.A. (1991). Disaster management, lessons learned. *Surgical clinics of North America,* **71**, (2), 257–66.

Pearn, J. (1985). The management of near drowning. *BMJ,* **291**, 1447–52.

Ridley, S.A., Wright, I.H., and Rogers, P.N. (1990). *Secondary transport of critically ill patients,* pp. 289–300.

Royal College of Surgeons of England Commission on the provision of surgical services (1988). *The management of patients with major injuries.* Royal College of Surgeons of England, London.

Skinner, D., Driscoll, P., and Earlam, R. (ed.) (1991). *ABC of major trauma.* BMJ Publishing, London.

West, J., Trunkey, D., and Lim, R. (1979). Systems of trauma care. *Arch. Surg.,* **114**, 455–60.

West, J., Cales, R., and Gazzaniga, A. (1983). The impact of regionalization: the Orange County Experience. *Arch. Surg.,* **118**, 740.

CHAPTER 18

Abdominal surgical emergencies

M. Whyman and Paul Thomas

1 Introduction

The 'acute abdomen' is still one of the most common surgical emergencies. The skill required to look after patients with acute intra-abdominal disease is acquired by first recognizing the common diseases likely to be present and then understanding the pathological changes occurring in the acute phases of these disorders. Some acute conditions, such as leaking aneurysm, require immediate surgical correction; others require urgent surgery after a period of active resuscitation (e.g. perforation or strangulated hernia). A proportion can be managed conservatively with the intention of converting an emergency into an elective condition (e.g. acute cholecystitis or diverticulitis). This concept of 'defusing' an emergency situation wherever possible and allowing the disease to settle before carrying out elective surgery is important. The management of the acute abdomen still presents a challenge to every surgeon, primarily because of these differing priorities. Developing the skills of 'timing' is an essential component of training in emergency abdominal surgical care.

It must also be borne in mind that certain acute abdomen patients should not be subjected to surgery at all. The elderly, demented patient with generalized peritonitis is one example. The situation is often complex and a decision to operate may require considerable care in collecting background information, assessing risks of operation, and discussion with relatives.

Most acute problems can be classified as inflammatory (secondary to either infection or ischaemia) and the remainder are mostly encompassed by haemorrhage and mechanical intestinal obstruction (Table 18.1).

2 Investigations and their interpretation

Evaluation of the history and examination usually suggests appropriate investigations. The predominant symptom is

Table 18.1 Causes of the acute abdomen

Inflammatory disorders	Appendicitis
	Diverticulitis
	Cholecystitis
	Pancreatitis
	Bowel perforation
	Ischaemic bowel
	Pyelonephritis
	Colitis
	Salpingitis and other gynaecological problems
Haemorrhage	Intraluminal
	Intraperitoneal
Mechanical obstruction	Extraluminal causes, e.g. hernia, adhesions
	Intramural causes, e.g. tumours
	Intraluminal causes, e.g. constipation, gallstones

usually pain. The nature of the pain, taken together with the presence and site of the signs of peritoneal irritation, should allow a narrow differential of likely diagnoses to be made. Some urgent investigations are useful to confirm a firm clinical diagnosis and others are helpful in assessing the overall physiological state of a patient systemically unwell as a result of the intra-abdominal pathology.

2.1 The blood picture

Full blood count (FBC)

The haemoglobin concentration is critical when dealing with haemorrhage, but in any situation where surgery is considered, the oxygen-carrying capacity of the blood is an anaesthetic consideration.

The white cell count is a useful adjunct when assessing the systemic effects and severity of local inflammation and can help in distinguishing between the presence of acute inflammation and an abscess and, indeed, between the presence or absence of disease at all. However, the test is not specific enough to be relied upon without supporting evidence.

C-reactive protein is now widely used as a non-specific but fairly sensitive inflammatory marker.

Electrolytes and urea

Intestinal secretions are often lost through vomiting or diarrhoea, or both, or become sequestrated in the intestinal lumen. Electrolyte and water loss results in dehydration and hypovolaemia, and the recognition and treatment of these abnormalities is a critical part of the resuscitation of the emergency surgical patient. The amounts of water and electrolyte lost are not always in the same proportion and the surgeon needs to recognize this when assessing the blood biochemical results. Haemoconcentration, as indicated by a raised haemoglobin and haematocrit, accompanied by normal concentrations of electrolytes, may reflect a reduction in total electrolyte content.

Table 18.2 Other causes of elevated plasma amylase

Perforated peptic ulcer
High small-bowel obstruction
Intestinal ischaemia
Biliary obstruction

Plasma amylase

In acute pancreatitis, the plasma amylase rises in the early phase of the disease and if the disease resolves within 2–3 days, the level falls accordingly. If the peak is missed, it is possible to measure the urinary concentration of amylase, which lags behind the plasma levels. Since the reference range for plasma amylase varies from lab to lab, the surgeon needs to know the levels that are considered diagnostic for pancreatitis in the local laboratory. However, the result must always be considered in relation to other clinical findings because other conditions also raise the plasma amylase and may need to be considered (Table 18.2).

2.2 Plain soft tissue X-rays

Presence of free gas beneath the diaphragm on an erect CXR is strong evidence of an intestinal perforation (Table 18.3). However, the absence of gas does not mean that a perforation is not present. If there is need for further investigation of this, a 'right side raised' lateral cubitus abdominal film (horizontal beam) after the patient has been lying on one side for 10 minutes can reveal as little as 1 ml of gas overlying the liver.

A supine abdominal X-ray is used to diagnose small-bowel obstruction when there is a central distribution of gas and fluid distension (Table 18.3). The bowel shows either a featureless pattern (ileum) or a 'pile of coins' appearance (jejunum). In addition, there may be a relative or absolute lack of colonic gas, depending on whether the obstruction is new or has been present for some time. Erect abdominal films were discouraged by radiologists for some years but are now enjoying a remission. Most surgeons find erect films easier to interpret in this respect.

2.3 Abdominal ultrasonography

This has become an increasingly important emergency investigation and there is now a case to be made to train surgeons to carry out the technique. However, since ultrasonography is still principally carried out by radiologists, there is a need for the surgical trainee to know when to call for an 'emergency' scan. It is rarely needed at night except in two possible instances: suspected rupture of abdominal aortic aneurysm (no investigation or a CT scan may be preferred) and septicaemia due to pyonephrosis, where very urgent drainage may be required.

2.4 Contrast radiology

Most cases of intestinal obstruction can be diagnosed clinically and confirmed if necessary by plain abdominal X-rays. Contrast

Table 18.3 What to look for on emergency chest and abdominal X-rays

Finding	Interpretation
Chest X-ray	
Free subdiaphragmatic gas	Abdominal visceral perforation[a]
Mediastinal widening	? Thoracic aortic aneurysm[b]
Lung mass	? Bronchogenic carcinoma or metastases[b]
Pulmonary oedema	Requires treatment before surgery
Plain abdominal X-ray (AXR)	
Air	
◆ Dilated bowel	Obstruction
◆ In biliary tree	Gallstone ileus
◆ In gallbladder	Emphysematous cholecystitis (very rare, usually very ill, cholecystectomy urgently needed)
On both sides of bowel wall	Abdominal visceral perforation
With fluid level (erect)	Abscess
Calcification	
Around pancreas	Pancreatitis (may be old)
In ureteric line	Ureteric calculus
Adjacent to vertebrae	? Aortic aneurysm
Right upper quadrant	Gallstones (10 per cent are visible on AXR)
Left upper quadrant	? Splenic artery aneurysm
Fluid	
Multiple levels in gut	Obstruction/ileus (beware in gastroenteritis)
Gastric fluid level	Gastric outlet obstruction
Air/fluid level elsewhere	Abscess

[a] Unless laparotomy, etc. has been carried out within past 2 or 3 weeks.

[b] Might affect decision-making in major emergency surgery (e.g. AAA).

radiology is rarely required except occasionally in postoperative obstruction when there is clinical uncertainty whether the dysfunction is due to ileus or an adhesive band, or for determining whether an obstructed colon is truly obstructed or has 'pseudo-obstruction'. It is essential that a water-soluble contrast medium is used (gastrografin) rather than barium sulphate, because of the tendency for the latter to solidify if left in a non-functioning segment of colon. In suspected renal colic, particularly in the elderly, an emergency IVU which confirms obstruction can be useful to rule out a leaking aortic aneurysm.

2.5 Abdominal paracentesis and peritoneal lavage

These techniques (Fig. 18.1) are standard methods of assessing whether there has been significant intraperitoneal haemorrhage. If a positive decision to perform a laparotomy has already been made (e.g. a perforating injury such as a knife or gunshot wound), then this test should not be performed. In cases of doubt (e.g. where a concealed blood loss is suspected), it is reasonable to perform a four-quadrant abdominal paracentesis. However, in recent years peritoneal lavage is preferred for suspected intra-abdominal haemorrhage in hypovolaemia, as it is more sensitive. Inexperienced surgeons are often anxious about performing this on a conscious patient, but in practice the method is most often required in a ventilated patient with multiple injuries.

2.6 Abdominal CT scan

This technique is not often used in the initial assessment of the acute abdomen. It can be helpful if there is doubt about the ultrasound findings in a possible leaking abdominal aneurysm, and it is used extensively in the later assessment of patients with severe attacks of acute pancreatitis and sometimes in the elderly with suspected colonic cancer or other intra-abdominal malignancy.

2.7 Emergency endoscopy

This is used in the assessment and treatment of gastrointestinal haemorrhage. The organization of a gastrointestinal endoscopy service varies in different hospitals, but it is vital that an upper gastrointestinal endoscopy be obtained early in the course of a bleeding episode. The result determines the further management of the patient. In many hospitals, general surgical trainees are required to be competent in upper gastrointestinal endoscopy. At least one of the special techniques used to control bleeding endoscopically should be learned. It is often argued that 'emergency' endoscopy is usually not necessary and that 'urgent' endoscopy within 24 hours is acceptable. However, it would pay the reader

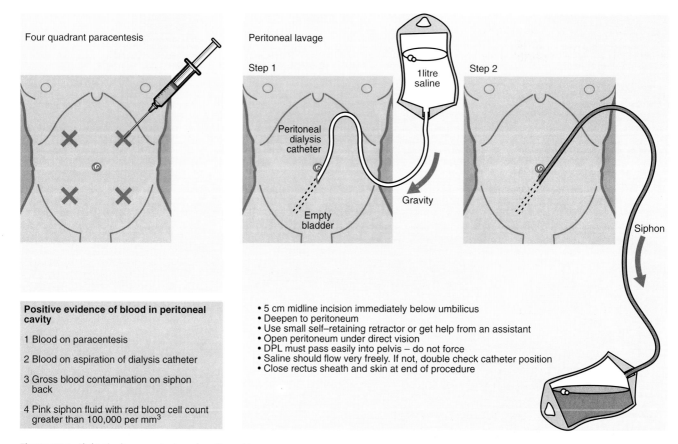

Four quadrant paracentesis

Peritoneal lavage

Step 1

Peritoneal dialysis catheter

1 litre saline

Gravity

Empty bladder

Step 2

Siphon

Positive evidence of blood in peritoneal cavity

1 Blood on paracentesis

2 Blood on aspiration of dialysis catheter

3 Gross blood contamination on siphon back

4 Pink siphon fluid with red blood cell count greater than 100,000 per mm³

- 5 cm midline incision immediately below umbilicus
- Deepen to peritoneum
- Use small self–retaining retractor or get help from an assistant
- Open peritoneum under direct vision
- DPL must pass easily into pelvis – do not force
- Saline should flow very freely. If not, double check catheter position
- Close rectus sheath and skin at end of procedure

Figure 18.1 Abdominal paracentesis and peritoneal lavage.

to bear in mind the possible advantages of endoscopy within a few hours of admission to hospital. The result might dictate:

(1) the intensity of medical and nursing observation required (i.e. ward, HDU, or ITU);

(2) the potential need for transfer to a specialist unit (e.g. for variceal bleeding);

(3) the need to inform senior surgical staff at an early stage if the patient is at high risk of rebleeding, rather than later when haemodynamically unstable.

2.8 Laparoscopy

This is particularly useful to distinguish appendicitis from gynaecological conditions, and in cases of uncertain peritonitis it can be used as a pre-laparotomy diagnostic test. Therapeutic emergency laparoscopic surgery can be used for appendicitis, perforated duodenal ulcer, and acute cholecystitis, although the results are still subject to scrutiny.

3 Understanding the signs of peritonitis

Apart from gastrointestinal haemorrhage, most abdominal emergencies are caused by inflammatory changes in the visceral

and parietal peritoneum—'peritonitis'. The signs and symptoms of peritonitis should be well understood because important clinical decisions depend on the interpretation of abdominal signs, particularly tenderness. In particular, being able to differentiate between simple tenderness, as might be found in acute duodenal ulcer, and signs of peritonitis, as occur with perforated ulcer, is important

3.1 The signs of peritoneal irritation

The inflamed peritoneum causes pain when disturbed and this gives rise to physical signs which allow a positive diagnosis of peritonitis to be made (Fig. 18.2).

- **Tenderness with rebound.** In this unkind test the tender area is slowly pressed and then quickly released. The patient is unaware of the intention to release and the rapid rebound of the anterior abdominal wall provokes severe pain. A more useful variant is simply to percuss over the area of greatest tenderness. When positive, this is extremely painful.

- A variant can be used when examining rectally for pelvic peritonitis by pressing gently on the recto-vesical pouch and then releasing the pressure rapidly. A modern variant of Murphy's test for an inflamed gallbladder involves asking the patient to inhale deeply while palpating the gallbladder area. The downward movement of the inflamed gallbladder hits the examining hand and the patient experiences pain.

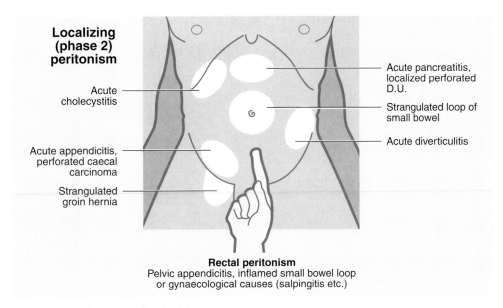

Figure 18.2 Likely diagnoses according to site of peritonitis

◆ **Guarding.** This may be involuntary or voluntary. The patient knows that pressure on the area where there is pain is likely to hurt. In anticipation of this, the anterior abdominal wall muscles are reflexly or, to some extent, voluntarily contracted to prevent movement of the peritoneum. It can be difficult on occasions to distinguish between voluntary and involuntary guarding. Under these circumstances it can be useful to ask the patient to bend the knees and hips a little, and, particularly in children, to keep the examining hand still while the patient is asked to take a deep breath (i.e. a sort of Murphy's sign used throughout the entire abdomen).

◆ **Rigidity.** This is an involuntary continuous contraction of the abdominal wall musculature and is associated with a generalized peritonitis. It is often combined with the absence of diaphragmatic breathing because, in severe cases, this is also painful.

3.2 Localizing the site of peritonitis

Irrespective of its position within the abdominal cavity, inflammation of the **visceral peritoneum** is poorly localized and is perceived centrally (phase 1: visceral pain). This is because the visceral peritoneum derives its sensory innervation from the sympathetic nervous system. For foregut structures, the pain is perceived in the upper abdomen, for midgut structures, in the periumbilical area and for hindgut structures, in the suprapubic area. When the inflammation spreads to the **parietal peritoneum**, the somatic nervous system provides the sensory input and localizes the pain accurately in the affected part of the abdominal cavity (phase 2: parietal pain). This shift in the site of pain, together with more precise localization is often an indicator of transmural inflammation, and its position an indicator of the likely diseased organ. Phase 1, however, may be absent,

particularly if the stimulus for inflammation does not originate within the wall of an affected organ, (for example, blood or gastrointestinal contents free within the peritoneum). The extent of peritonitis from the extent of tenderness (e.g. localized right iliac fossa peritonitis occurs in appendicitis and may become generalized with perforation and spreading infection). Conversely, a powerful response from the body may keep the peritonitis localized, as in an appendix mass, and the abdominal signs remain localized.

4 Scheme for management of the acute abdomen

1. Make a 'working' diagnosis from the history, examination and investigations. It is possible to make a fairly precise diagnosis early on in most cases of acute abdomen, but if doubt remains, it is sensible to observe the patient in hospital and use the changing clinical condition to indicate a changing clinical state. Increasing pain, a rising pulse rate and temperature indicate an increasing inflammatory response and a worsening clinical condition, which may be an indication for exploratory surgery.

2. Decide whether the patient needs immediate transfer to the operating room for life-saving surgery—CEPOD 'emergency

Table 18.4 Indications for emergency laparotomy

Peritonitis
Haemorrhage
Visceral perforation
Trauma from penetrating injuries

Table 18.5 Criteria for adequate resuscitation in massive haemorrhage

BP rises towards normal
CVP returns towards normal
Falling pulse rate
Urinary output >30 ml/hour

Table 18.6 CEPOD classification of surgical emergencies according to the urgency of operation required

Emergency	Immediate operation with simultaneous resuscitation, e.g. major haemorrhage
Urgent	Operation after rapid resuscitation e.g. intestinal obstruction
Planned	Operation after initial conservative management, designed to remove the cause of the problem, e.g. cholecystectomy
Scheduled	Operation on the next convenient operating list, usually during the same admission

surgery' category (Tables 18.4 and 18.6). General surgical conditions requiring the most urgent surgery include massive haemorrhage after trauma or a ruptured aneurysm. Rapid initial colloid resuscitation is required to improve the perfusion of the brain, kidneys, and coronary vessels, followed by crystalloid infusion to replace lost electrolyte and water. Universal donor blood may have to be given, but bank blood should be prepared rapidly and given early before shock supervenes. The criteria used to indicate adequate resuscitation are shown in Table 18.5.

3. Decide on a definite treatment policy. If the diagnosis is known, the treatment protocol will follow (see later for various conditions) and it usually becomes clear whether the immediate treatment is operative or non-operative (Table 18.6). In problem cases, observation for changes in clinical signs and response to treatment, and the appropriate use of investigations, guides the surgeon in managing the case.

4.1 The acute abdomen of uncertain aetiology

In about one-third of cases of acute abdomen, no definite immediate diagnosis can be made with confidence. Immediate surgery is not needed and the surgical policy is one of observation. This time-honoured method is based on one principle—namely that a patient's vital signs, together with local signs of tenderness, reflect the severity of the underlying problem. If the cause of the problem is uncertain, then a period of observation will usually demonstrate a change for the worse or for the better. If the condition worsens, an exploratory laparotomy may be needed without a specific diagnosis, although with increasing sophistication of non-invasive scanning procedures, and in some cases, diagnostic laparoscopy, such blind laparotomy is required less commonly now than before.

Table 18.7 Checklist before emergency laparotomy is undertaken

- Patient sufficiently investigated and fully resuscitated
- Adequate bank blood available (blood recycling equipment for major haemorrhage if available locally)
- Antibiotics given
- Thrombo-prophylaxis started
- Waterproof apron is on
- Abdomen has been examined under anaesthesia
- Sucker ready (two for trauma)
- Diathermy plate on and unit working
- Large packs open for trauma cases

4.2 Emergency exploration of the abdominal cavity

Whatever the cause, once a decision is made to carry out a laparotomy the surgeon needs to be decisive and well organized (Table 18.7). Morbidity and mortality are potentially much higher in emergency surgery and care and preparation should be shared between surgeon and anaesthetist.

Incision

Before opening the abdomen, it is worthwhile examining the abdomen carefully under anaesthesia, in case a mass is revealed which was not palpable with the patient awake.

In many cases, the diagnosis is suspected and the point of access is determined by the most likely diagnosis. However, the working diagnosis may be incorrect and the incision may need to be extended. For this reason, most surgeons favour a midline vertical incision, sited first in the middle abdomen if the source is uncertain (the 'incision of indecision') or in the upper or lower abdomen if, for example, a perforated peptic ulcer or diverticular abscess, respectively, is suspected.

Transverse incisions, while favoured by a few surgeons for elective surgery, give poor access to remote areas of the abdomen, particularly if a change of tack is required. If appendicitis is the likely diagnosis, most surgeons would commence with a grid-iron or Lanz incision and close it if the diagnosis is found to be remote. If possible, in patients who have undergone previous abdominal surgery, the incision should include an area of 'virgin' abdominal wall and the peritoneum opened at this point to minimize the risk of damaging adherent bowel.

Laparotomy for peritonitis

Staff should wear plastic aprons before scrubbing. Upon opening the peritoneum, fluid is found. This ranges between clear, non-odorous fluid through varying thicknesses of pus to frank faeces. The smell of the fluid may give some clue. Fluid from a perforated duodenal ulcer is usually odourless, whereas fluid contaminated with small bowel contents has a distinctive, slightly faeculent smell, which is particularly nauseating if there is infarcted bowel. Faecal perforation smells as you would expect.

The aim is to discover the source of the peritonitis, usually a perforation or infarcted segment of bowel. In the latter case, a diagnosis of obstruction with perforation will usually have been made before operation. Any fluid should be sucked out first without removing bowel from the abdomen, by gently displacing the bowel and employing a sump sucker to avoid damage to the bowel wall. Systematic suction from above downwards is best. Start with the subphrenic spaces above right and left lobes of liver, then both paracolic gutters, working down to the pelvis. Specimens of fluid should be sent for bacteriology and, if malignancy is suspected, for cytology for malignant cells.

A pointer to the site of perforation is usually given by the increasing serosal inflammation and fibrin deposition on the bowel wall as the source is approached. The most common are sigmoid diverticular perforations. Gastric and duodenal perforations are less common nowadays but are still found in the elderly, often those taking NSAIDs. Sigmoid perforations range from a pinhole or 'gaseous' perforation which excites minimal fluid response, through purulent perforations, to frank faeces lying free in the peritoneal cavity. In the last case, there is a grave risk of septicaemia.

The initial incision may need to be extended as the area of interest is approached. If the appendix is perforated, this often excites a purulent reaction. If the fluid is clear and there is patchy fat 'necrosis' (i.e. chalky areas of saponification on intra-abdominal fat), a preoperative diagnosis of acute pancreatitis has been missed. If all these areas are negative, the next step is to examine the small bowel in detail. It should all be withdrawn from the abdomen and examined carefully on both sides from one end to the other. If there are multiple adhesions from previous surgery, this can be complicated and require careful freeing of adhesions in order to inspect it.

It is unusual not to find an abnormality, although this does happen sometimes and it leaves the surgeon with uncertainty about possibly having missed a small abnormality. As long as a careful examination of all the abdominal contents and the retroperitoneum has been made, there is little further that can usefully be done at laparotomy.

5 Common intra-abdominal emergencies

5.1 Gastrointestinal haemorrhage

Patients with potentially serious bleeding from the gastrointestinal tract should receive the combined care of physicians and surgeons.

Table 18.8 Principles of management of a patient with gastrointestinal haemorrhage

Assess the amount of blood lost and replace it

Determine the site of the bleeding

Assess whether bleeding is continuing

Decide when active intervention is required to stop the bleeding

Unfortunately, they are often looked after by one and not the other and the timing of important decisions often suffers because of this. The particular problems of GI haemorrhage relate to:

◆ the 'hidden' nature of the haemorrhage;

◆ the difficulty of accurately measuring the volume of blood lost; and

◆ the difficulty in pinpointing the precise source of bleeding.

The principles of management involved are similar whether the bleeding is arising from the upper or lower gastrointestinal tract (Table 18.8).

Assessing blood loss

The volume of blood lost from a gastrointestinal bleed cannot be measured directly, except for that portion which is revealed by haematemesis or melaena (and hence quantifiable). An immeasurable amount of blood is contained within the GI tract and the loss can only be estimated from the pathophysiological responses to the blood loss (i.e. the changes in pulse, blood pressure, and central venous pressure). A nasogastric tube can be useful for detecting continuing blood loss from the upper GI tract.

Responses to blood loss vary from patient to patient. While haemorrhage is continuing, this makes it difficult to correlate changes in physiological variables with the need for specific volume replacement. When the bleeding has stopped, the total replacement volume required to return the variables to normal indicates the approximate amount lost by haemorrhage. The physiological response to bleeding depends on its rate. For rapid blood loss **in a previously fit patient** the approximate changes in variables are shown in Table 18.9.

If blood loss is judged to be substantial (i.e. with appropriate changes in pulse and blood pressure), then a urinary catheter should be used to monitor hourly urine output and a central venous sensor should be placed for pressure measurement. In a failing heart, it may be necessary to assess left heart function by

Table 18.9 Changes in physiological variables after rapid blood loss for a fit 70 kg man

	Blood loss			
	<750 ml	750–1500 ml	1500–2000 ml	>2000 ml
Pulse rate	<100	>100	>120	>140
Blood pressure	Normal	Normal	Low	Low
Respiratory rate (breaths/min)	14–20	20–30	30–40	>35
Urine output (ml/h)	>30	20–30	5–15	<5

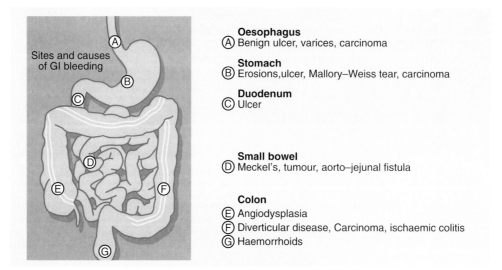

Figure 18.3 Potential sites of gastrointestinal bleeding.

inserting a pulmonary wedge pressure sensor (Swan–Ganz or flotation catheter).

Determining the site of bleeding

No surgeon likes to operate for exsanguinating gastrointestinal haemorrhage without knowing in advance where the bleeding is coming from. One of the surgeon's priorities is an early attempt to locate the bleeding (Fig. 18.3); this message needs to be got across to all who take care of patients with GI bleeding, medical and surgical. Most bleeding originates either in the foregut (oesophagus, stomach, and first two parts of the duodenum) or the colon and rectum. Active bleeding from the small intestine is fortunately rare and if it does occur, it is usually from a Meckel's diverticulum or angiodysplasias (often multiple). It is helpful, therefore, to localize the bleeding to the upper or lower GI tract.

The history may indicate the likely site, particularly if the patient has ingested non-steroidal anti-inflammatory drugs, including aspirin. Haematemesis always means that the bleeding is arising from the upper tract. Melaena can result from bleeding anywhere in the GI tract (although it is usually high up and the blood becomes altered during its passage through the GIT). The presence of bright-red blood in the stool usually indicates large bowel haemorrhage but, occasionally, rapid haemorrhage from a peptic ulcer can have the same effect. The 'hidden' nature of blood loss and the difficulty of localizing the bleeding point have stimulated the evolution of investigatory protocols (Figs 18.4 and 18.5).

Recognizing continuing or recurring haemorrhage

Gastrointestinal bleeding tends to be intermittent, particularly as there is a tendency for it to slow or stop as the blood pressure falls as a result of blood loss. Following resuscitation, the blood pressure returns towards normal and, unless the source of the bleed has occluded, there is a likelihood of recurring haemorrhage. There is no difficulty in recognizing massive continuing haemorrhage. This is likely to be accompanied by melaena,

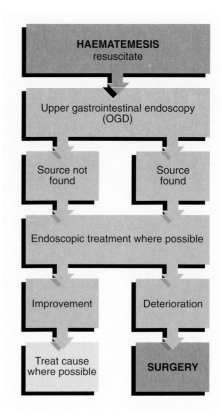

Figure 18.4 Management of haematemesis.

bleeding per rectum, or haematemesis. Where bleeding is slower, continuing, or recurring, haemorrhage is indicated by the following:

◆ a falling haemoglobin level or a low haemoglobin level despite blood replacement—a patient must never be discharged from hospital until the haemoglobin level has been shown not to be falling on successive days;

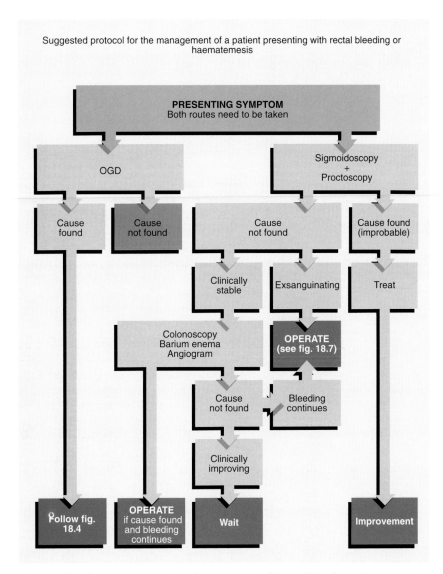

Suggested protocol for the management of a patient presenting with rectal bleeding or haematemesis

PRESENTING SYMPTOM
Both routes need to be taken

OGD

Sigmoidoscopy
+
Proctoscopy

Cause found

Cause not found

Cause not found

Cause found (improbable)

Clinically stable

Exsanguinating

Treat

Colonoscopy
Barium enema
Angiogram

OPERATE
(see fig. 18.7)

Cause not found

Bleeding continues

Clinically improving

Follow fig. 18.4

OPERATE
if cause found and bleeding continues

Wait

Improvement

Figure 18.5 Suggested protocol for the management of a patient presenting with rectal bleeding or haematemesis.

♦ a falling or continually low central venous pressure despite adequate fluid replacement; and

♦ further episodes of hypotension and tachycardia.

Need for active intervention—endoscopy or surgery?

The standard initial treatment for a significant gastrointestinal bleed includes:

1. Peripheral venous access for fluid replacement. The ideal replacement is fresh, compatible blood. In the initial stages, circulating volume is required and colloid in the form of gelatin solutions is commonly given. However, this does not replace oxygen-carrying capacity and should be used only until blood is available.

2. Urinary catheterization for hourly output monitoring.

3. Central venous pressure measurement to assess the response to fluid replacement and for early indications of rebleeding.

4. Correction or anticipation of clotting abnormalities likely to arise from massive blood loss and fluid replacement. This includes fresh, frozen plasma for clotting factors and platelet concentrate transfusion. As a rule, it is preferable not to operate on a patient with an INR greater than 3 or platelets less than 50 000 per mm^3.

5. The use of anti-ulcer therapy if there is a peptic ulcer, despite the fact that no single treatment has been shown beyond all doubt to reduce the rebleeding rate.

If the bleeding is likely to arise from the upper GI tract, upper GI endoscopy should be performed within 12 hours of admission, and more urgently if bleeding is rapid. This is for both diagnostic and therapeutic purposes. Most patients with an upper gastrointestinal bleed do not require more active intervention. The endoscopic findings which indicate that endoscopic treatment for bleeding is required are as follows:

Table 18.10 Non-surgical methods of arresting gastrointestinal bleeding

Nd/Yag laser coagulation of bleeding points

Direct bipolar coagulation

'Hot tip' heat probe which has a heating coil in its tip

Direct injection of alcohol, 1/10 000 adrenaline (epinephrine), or other sclerosants such as polidocanol

Table 18.11 Tips for the surgical endoscopist

Do emergency endoscopy in theatre wherever possible

Obtain consent for proceeding to surgery before sedation is given

Have adrenaline (epinephrine) for injection, etc. already drawn up. You may get only one chance

Use a large scope with steerable tip

Have an anaesthetist present, preferable giving the sedation and ready to proceed to general anaesthesia if surgery is necessary

♦ a single, visibly bleeding vessel;

♦ clot overlying a vessel (**Dieulafoy lesion**);

♦ a visible vessel in the base of an ulcer.

However, overzealous endoscopic treatment can precipitate further bleeding and treatment should be restricted to the lesions listed above. The types of endoscopic treatment available are listed in Table 18.10 and tips for the surgical endoscopist are given in Table 18.11.

Some clinicians are reluctant to intervene in elderly patients in the belief that surgery worsens the prognosis. This is not so: given the correct indications, early surgery (after failed non-surgical methods) gives the best chance of survival in elderly patients with continuing haemorrhage. Surgical intervention should be considered after transfusion of 7 units of blood, or if a patient over the age of 50 has a second bleed. Delay is likely to give rise to problems with consumption coagulopathy and cardiovascular failure. These are general guidelines, but close liaison between physician and surgeon will enable correct decisions to be made. Every hospital receiving such patients should have local written protocols for dealing with these patients. We would advise that they should include instructions that physicians should inform the duty surgeons about all upper GI haemorrhage patients. This avoids delay in treating the patient when surgery becomes necessary. It is also desirable for one surgical firm, once informed, to retain responsibility for that patient. This prevents procrastination as each subsequent surgical firm decides on 'a short period of observation'.

Surgical options for definitive lesions once surgery has become necessary

Upper gastrointestinal lesions

Bleeding duodenal ulcer

Access to the bleeding gastroduodenal artery is obtained by a longitudinal incision in the duodenum. The vessel is underrun both above and below the bleeding point using an 0 suture. Nowadays, the pylorus should be preserved if possible. A small biopsy of the ulcer edge or duodenal mucosa can be tested in theatre for *Helicobacter pylori* (e.g. Clotest). Medical treatment to suppress gastric acid secretion is usual (but of unproven benefit). If *H. pylori* positive, the patient should have elimination treatment when taking oral fluids. Nowadays, definitive gastroduodenal anti-ulcer surgery is very rarely indicated and could be considered mutilating except in carefully selected cases.

Bleeding gastric ulcer

The type of surgery depends on the position and type of the ulcer. Traditional surgical treatment involved a Billroth I partial gastrectomy, or oversewing of the duodenal stump and formation of a gastrojejunal anastomosis, a Polya gastrectomy. However, unless malignancy is likely, most surgeons nowadays would act as for duodenal bleeding above, but would take four-quadrant biopsies of the ulcer edge in case of malignancy.

Bleeding gastric erosions

This is one of the most difficult problems to deal with because of the widespread nature of the bleeding points and there is no definitive surgical therapy. A subtotal gastrectomy may be necessary if medical treatment has failed and life-threatening haemorrhage continues. However, by that time the prognosis is likely to be grave. In this situation all other factors (age, concomitant disease, coagulation state) have to be considered before embarking on such high-risk surgery.

Bleeding varices

It is first necessary to exclude a bleeding peptic ulcer, because this is the source of haemorrhage in 25 per cent of patients thought to be bleeding from varices. The optimal interventional treatment for bleeding varices is injection sclerotherapy via a flexible endoscope. However, varices can be difficult to detect and their injection should perhaps be left to those with particular expertise. If injection sclerotherapy fails, oesophageal transsection using a stapling device is one surgical option. An emergency portosystemic shunt is rarely a realistic option. The underlying hepatic cirrhosis means that these are high-risk patients whose long-term prognosis is poor. There is a high chance of rebleeding in the near future. Probably the most important thing a surgical trainee can do is to become familiar with the use of a Linton, Minnesota, or Sengstaken–Blakemore tube (see Fig. 18.6), so that time can be bought while the patient is transferred to a specialist unit.

Lower gastrointestinal lesions

Most bleeding from the lower GI tract stops spontaneously with conservative treatment. Causes include:

♦ **Diverticular disease**: common; bleeding is rarely heavy. There may be several episodes of painless bleeding, sometimes requiring transfusion but surgery is almost never required

♦ **Ischaemic colitis**: uncommon; usually occurs in elderly patients. Unlike diverticular bleeding, bleeding is usually

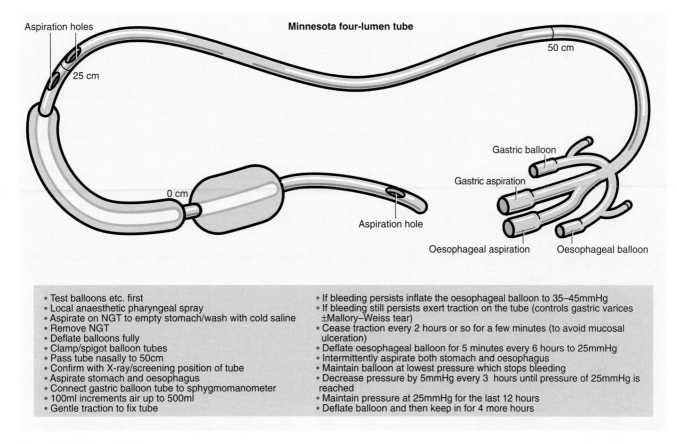

Minnesota four-lumen tube

Aspiration holes

25 cm

50 cm

Gastric balloon

Gastric aspiration

0 cm

Aspiration hole

Oesophageal aspiration

Oesophageal balloon

- Test balloons etc. first
- Local anaesthetic pharyngeal spray
- Aspirate on NGT to empty stomach/wash with cold saline
- Remove NGT
- Deflate balloons fully
- Clamp/spigot balloon tubes
- Pass tube nasally to 50cm
- Confirm with X-ray/screening position of tube
- Aspirate stomach and oesophagus
- Connect gastric balloon tube to sphygmomanometer
- 100ml increments air up to 500ml
- Gentle traction to fix tube

- If bleeding persists inflate the oesophageal balloon to 35–45mmHg
- If bleeding still persists exert traction on the tube (controls gastric varices ±Mallory–Weiss tear)
- Cease traction every 2 hours or so for a few minutes (to avoid mucosal ulceration)
- Deflate oesophageal balloon for 5 minutes every 6 hours to 25mmHg
- Intermittently aspirate both stomach and oesophagus
- Maintain balloon at lowest pressure which stops bleeding
- Decrease pressure by 5mmHg every 3 hours until pressure of 25mmHg is reached
- Maintain pressure at 25mmHg for the last 12 hours
- Deflate balloon and then keep in for 4 more hours

Figure 18.6 Minnesota tube.

preceded by abdominal pain. Bleeding here is also self-limiting

◆ **Malignancy**: common; never exsanguinating. Tends to be small quantities, passed persistently; mixed with stool if high up, fresh blood if low down, sometimes coating stool.

◆ **Angiodysplasia**: persistent, recurrent, sometimes severe. Diagnosis is suspected if bleeding continues. Diagnosis can only be made on colonoscopy, which is difficult in the acute phase. Treatment is usually with endoscopic diathermy.

◆ **Fulminating ulcerative colitis**: the bleeding is not usually the most significant symptom here. Need for urgent operation is usually determined by risk of perforation.

When bleeding continues, specialist investigation is required. If it appears to be coming from the rectum, flexible endoscopy may be useful. If a specific bleeding point is seen within the rectum or anal canal, then endoscopic underrunning or coagulation can be used to stop the haemorrhage. If the bleeding appears to arise higher up, highly selective arteriography may localize the bleeding area, provided the bleeding rate is greater than 1 ml/min. If the bleeding is at a lower rate but persistent, an isotope scan after reinjecting the patient's own radiolabelled red cells allows detection of the build-up of blood in part of the bowel and should define the site within an area.

Surgical options for massive GI haemorrhage from an unknown site

If all investigations have proved negative, or if the rate of bleeding requires immediate life-saving surgery, an emergency operation is likely to be required. There should be time to perform an upper gastrointestinal endoscopy before the abdomen is opened because it is such an important indicator of the source of the bleeding.

At laparotomy, examination of the entire bowel is performed, looking for evidence of pathology that might be the cause of the bleeding (Fig. 18.7). One would pay special attention to:

◆ dilated intraperitoneal or retroperitoneal veins, indicating a high portal venous pressure;

◆ scarring in the first or second part of the duodenum, indicating a chronic peptic ulcer;

◆ an obvious gastric lesion;

◆ a Meckel's diverticulum;

◆ a palpable colonic lesion, such as a cancer or diverticular disease.

Another feature often mentioned as an indicator is the level at which blood is found in the alimentary tract. If blood is aspirated from the nasogastric tube, then the bleeding point is in the foregut. Blood in the distal small bowel must not be assumed

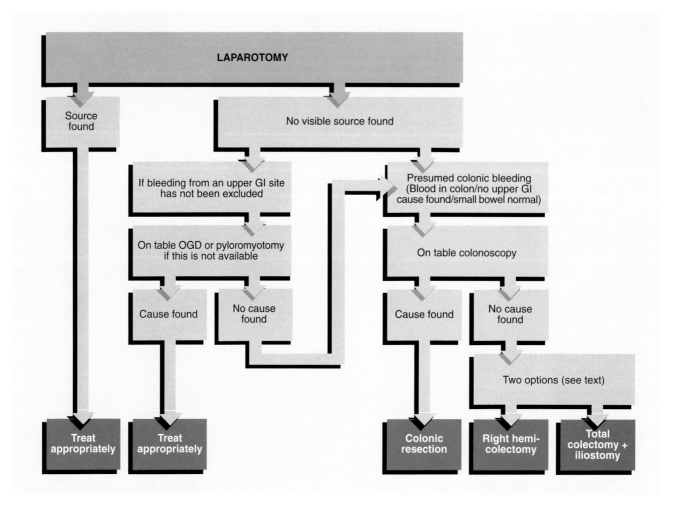

Figure 18.7 Operating for gastrointestinal bleeding from an unknown source.

to have arisen from the upper gastrointestinal tract because it can pass retrogradely from the colon. Similarly, blood confined to the colon does not exclude an upper GI bleeding point. Blood restricted to the left or right sides of the colon does not accurately locate the bleeding point. In short, the surgeon should not rely on the level of blood in the GIT unless it is found in the stomach or duodenum. If the source of bleeding is not apparent at laparotomy, then the options are to open the duodenum or stomach (if there is blood in the foregut) or carry out on-table endoscopy. This might include colonoscopy, if there is blood in the colon, or operative endoscopy of the entire small bowel via an enterostomy (see Fig. 18.7).

The most difficult decision arises when the bleeding is assumed to be colonic but the exact source cannot be located. As long as one can be sure that the bleeding is not coming from the rectum, the safest option is a total colectomy and ileostomy. This maximizes the chances of stopping the bleeding. In the worst case, and the patient continues to bleed, one would then be able to determine easily whether it was arising from the rectum or from the upper gastrointestinal tract. An alternative to a total colectomy is a right hemicolectomy, on the basis that a large proportion of these cases are bleeding from angiodysplasia of the right colon.

When this is successful, the patient is cured and left with a continuous gastrointestinal tract and the result is satisfactory. If the bleeding continues, however, the patient needs a second major operation. The decision on the extent of the first operation is not easy unless investigations have indicated a likely bleeding point; in this case there are no other current investigations to help the surgeon to make the correct decision.

5.2 Intra-abdominal inflammatory diseases

Acute appendicitis, acute cholecystitis, and acute diverticulitis

Although different in their aetiologies, these three conditions are linked by a common pathological process, and the general principles of assessment and treatment of each emergency are similar.

Basic pathology

The affected viscus becomes acutely inflamed and, eventually, transmural inflammation involves the overlying peritoneum (phase 1). If the pathological process continues to abscess formation (phase 2), there is then the risk that abscess rupture

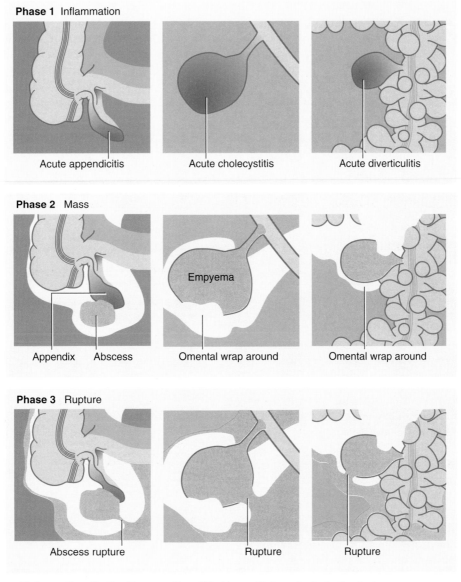

Figure 18.8 The phases of inflammation affecting the appendix, gallbladder, and inflamed colonic diverticula.

may follow (phase 3) and contaminate the peritoneal cavity (Fig. 18.8).

Phase 1

This represents the phase of 'acute inflammation'. Clinically there are local signs of peritonitis and systemic upset, indicated by a mild pyrexia, tachycardia, and a white cell count of less than 20 000 per mm³. The site of tenderness indicates the likely organ involved. It should not be forgotten that organs which are aberrant in position give rise to tenderness in unusual areas, for example, a high appendix can be confused with acute cholecystitis, and pelvic appendicitis is likely to have the maximal signs of peritonitis on rectal examination.

Phase 2

This represents the phase of 'abscess' formation. There is often a localized perforation which is limited by an omental barrier

between the inflamed organ and the peritoneal cavity. There is likely to be a palpable mass accompanied by more severe vital signs (e.g. swinging pyrexia, systemic toxicity, and a leucocytosis >20 000/mm³). The site of the mass indicates the nature of the underlying disease (e.g. appendix abscess, diverticular abscess, or empyema of the gallbladder). The omentum wraps itself around the diseased organ as a protective mechanism. If it contains an inflammatory phlegmon as distinct from pus, then it is regarded as a 'mass' rather than an 'abscess'. However, it is not always possible to distinguish between the two.

Phase 3

This is the phase where perforation of the diseased viscus occurs with resultant generalized peritonitis. This may occur if an abscess ruptures or if a perforation of the viscus occurs without omental wrapping. The systemic upset is marked and the abdominal physical signs do not localize the site of the primary pathology because the peritonitis is generalized.

Management

The essential steps in the successful management of these three conditions are:

(1) recognition of the specific condition, this is largely based on the site of the initial local tenderness;

(2) accurate placing of the condition into its correct 'phase';

(3) choosing the relevant treatment.

Specific treatments

Phase 1

- **The appendix**. The recommended treatment is appendicectomy.

- **The gallbladder**. Immediate cholecystectomy is not recommended but the initial management involves gastrointestinal rest with intravenous fluids, nasogastric aspiration, and antibiotics effective against *Escherichia coli*. Ultrasonography usually demonstrates gallstones and the case can be made for an early cholecystectomy. Often these cases can be put on the next convenient operating list.

- **The sigmoid colon**. Acute diverticulitis is managed non-operatively with systemic antibiotics effective against colonic bacteria (e.g. *E. coli* and *Bacteroides* spp.). Recovery is usual and the diverticular disease is demonstrated by contrast study after the inflammation has settled. One attack of diverticulitis is not an indication for subsequent colonic resection.

Phase 2

The finding of a palpable swelling indicates either an inflammatory mass or an abscess. The significance as regards treatment is that a mass is more likely to respond to antibiotic therapy, and therefore it is helpful to scan the palpable swelling ultrasonographically to determine whether there is a fluid centre indicating pus. If so, there may be an advantage in aspirating the pus under ultrasound control. Otherwise the presence of pus is an indication for active drainage and not for the use of antibiotics.

- **The appendix**. A 'mass' can be treated with antibiotics effective against large-bowel bacteria. Response to treatment is assessed by a reduction in the size of the mass, a return of the temperature to normal, and a fall in the white cell count. An 'abscess' requires drainage either at open surgery or by external needle drainage. At surgery, drainage may be accompanied by appendicectomy. Whether or not drainage is performed, it is advisable to perform an interval appendicectomy after 1–2 months to prevent recurrent appendicitis. However, there are no recent trials to indicate that this is essential.

- **The gallbladder**. A palpable gallbladder is usually because omentum has become wrapped around the inflamed gallbladder. However, it should be distinguished ultrasonographically from a mucocoele or an empyema. If adjudged to

be a 'mass', then treatment is the same as for acute cholecystitis. If thought to be an 'abscess', the gallbladder should be drained transcutaneously through the liver substance under ultrasound direction, or alternatively the gallbladder should be removed surgically. One reason for operating is the risk of gangrenous change scattered throughout the gallbladder, which would lead to perforation. Laparoscopic cholecystectomy is not contraindicated in empyema of the gallbladder but it is likely to be more difficult, with a higher rate of conversion to open surgery. If surgery is undertaken in a sick patient with empyema, it is still reasonable to simply carry out an open cholecystostomy.

- **The sigmoid colon**. The principles are exactly as for the gallbladder. A 'mass' is treated with antibiotics (**acute diverticulitis**). An abscess is drained, although it is usual to do this at open operation because of the risk of precipitating a faecal peritonitis if needle aspiration is used. Note that a diverticular abscess is usually associated with a localized perforation of a diverticulum. The operation of choice is sigmoid resection, with closure of the upper rectum and a proximal colostomy (i.e. Hartmann's procedure). Proximal drainage alone via a defunctioning colostomy has the disadvantage of allowing a continuing faecal leak because the colon between the colostomy and the perforation empties through the perforated diverticulum. This procedure cannot be recommended as safe. Immediate colonic resection with a primary anastomosis is a possible alternative treatment but can be hazardous because of local infection and the unprepared colon. The latter can be overcome by 'on-table' lavage and, in expert hands with minimal peritoneal soilage, it is a feasible 'one-stage' procedure.

Phase 3

This is characterized by generalized peritonitis and the immediate cause may not be obvious. The finding of free gas within the abdominal cavity usually indicates a perforation of a peptic ulcer or sigmoid colon. Very rarely, an appendiceal perforation produces free intraperitoneal gas.. The principles of care involve adequate resuscitation and then emergency surgery.

- **Perforated appendicitis**. Treatment involves appendicectomy and peritoneal lavage if there is extensive contamination, with saline warmed to 37 °C. Antibiotic cover is required both pre- and postoperatively.

- **Perforated cholecystitis**. This is usually due to 'speckled' gangrene of the gallbladder wall. The surgical option nearly always has to be cholecystectomy. Occasionally the gallbladder is so diseased and adherent to structures in the porta hepatis that only the distal part can be removed safely and a cholecystostomy performed. Biliary contamination of the peritoneal cavity requires lavage at the end of the definitive procedure.

- **Perforated diverticular disease**. The aim is to remove the source of the peritoneal contamination and remove any risk of further peritoneal contamination in the postoperative period. This is a condition with a high mortality and no unnecessary risks should be taken. Therefore an anastomosis should be avoided. The safest operation is a Hartmann's resection with a proximal colostomy and closure of the rectal stump. Peritoneal lavage and antibiotics are again important additional steps to limit infective complications.

Assessing progress in inflammatory conditions

Most patients who are treated conservatively improve, and this is reflected objectively by a return of the temperature, pulse, and white cell count towards normal. In the few who do not settle and remain static, or even deteriorate, it is important to recognize this early so that interventional treatment can be used. Close attention to the pattern of the temperature chart and the associated white cell count are accurate signals of what is happening.

Acute pancreatitis

Introduction

Acute pancreatitis is the result of pancreatic autodigestion secondary to activation of the normally inactive pancreatic digestive enzymes within the gland. The aetiological factors that predispose to this are well recognized, but the final pathway by which this happens is ill understood (Table 18.12).

Table 18.12 Aetiology of acute pancreatitis

- Biliary stones
- Alcohol
- Certain drugs: thiazide diuretics, steroids
- Viral disorders, e.g. mumps, polyarteritis nodosa
- Hyperparathyroidism
- Congenital pancreatic abnormalities, e.g. pancreas divisum
- Pancreatic trauma
- Periampullary carcinoma
- A group of patients in whom no cause is found

Acute pancreatitis causes both local and systemic effects (Fig. 18.9). The initial acute inflammatory reaction within the pancreas varies in severity and this is reflected in the clinical picture. Mild epigastric pain with localized signs of peritonitis are associated with a mild oedematous change within the gland This type is usually quick to resolve and does not threaten the patient.

However, if the insult is severe, the pancreas can be destroyed rapidly with progress to pancreatic necrosis. This group of patients is at risk of dying, both initially, from the metabolic changes secondary to the systemic release of pancreatic enzymes, and then later from the septic complications relating to the necrotic pancreas. It is important not to underestimate the severity of this disease. While most patients have a mild attack, the disease can suddenly alter its severity and proceed to major pancreatic damage. About 10 per cent of patients still die from an attack of acute pancreatitis, and no case of acute pancreatitis should be taken lightly.

Pathology

An understanding of the pathophysiological effects of acute pancreatitis can help in its clinical recognition and management. Damage to a metabolically active organ such as the pancreas produces systemic sequelae as well as local inflammatory responses. The systemic effects are predominant during the early phase. Later, progressive pancreatic destruction and necrosis means that the local effects of acute pancreatitis become more evident as time passes.

The early phase of acute pancreatitis

The essential point about this phase is the enormous metabolic insult the body receives as a result of destruction of the pancreatic acinar cell population. The comparison is sometimes made to a large internal 'burn' of the retroperitoneum. This accounts for the loss of tissue exudate into the locality of the pancreas but does not emphasize sufficiently the escalating systemic effects caused by leakage of pancreatic enzymes.

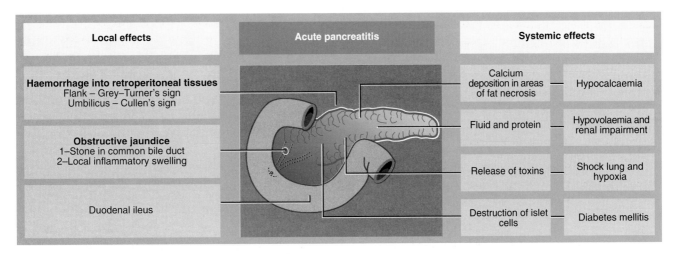

Figure 18.9 The local and systemic effects of acute pancreatitis.

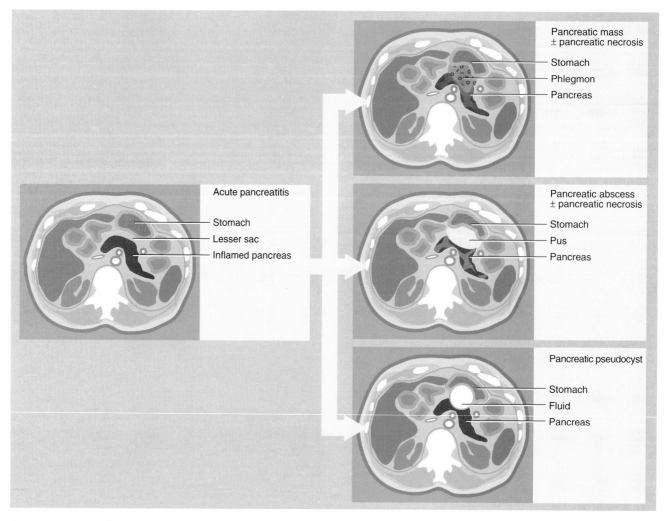

Figure 18.10 Intermediate and late pathological changes in acute pancreatitis.

Late pathological changes in the pancreas and peripancreatic tissues

The lesser sac of the peritoneum, because of its immediate anterior relationship to the pancreas, acts to localize the inflammatory changes following the initial damage (Fig. 18.10). It can fill with inflammatory tissue (pancreatic phlegmon), pus (pancreatic abscess), or later with fluid (pancreatic pseudocyst). If the inflammation is sufficiently severe, the pancreas is in danger of losing its blood supply (pancreatic necrosis). The later management of acute pancreatitis is directed towards the recognition of these conditions.

Diagnosis of the phases of acute pancreatitis

Decision making in surgery depends on understanding the underlying disease and its pathological stage. During the hospital stay of a patient with acute pancreatitis, the following four questions should be asked:

1. Is the diagnosis acute pancreatitis?

2. Is the attack mild or severe?

3. Is the pancreas viable ?

4. Does the lesser sac contain pathological material?

Is the diagnosis acute pancreatitis?

Patients usually present with severe epigastric pain accompanied by signs of peritonism in that area. The degree of systemic upset depends on the severity of the attack and can vary from no systemic change to catastrophic collapse. The only diagnoses likely to be considered are perforated peptic ulcer or acute chole-cystitis, although occasionally myocardial infarction can masquerade as pancreatitis. In the absence of free intraperitoneal gas and with a high plasma amylase, the diagnosis of acute pancreatitis is virtually certain. The pancreas can be scanned by ultrasound and evidence of swelling is consistent with acute inflammation. On very rare occasions, there may be real doubt about the diagnosis, particularly if the plasma amylase appears to be normal. This may be a false negative if the peak of amylasaemia has passed or if the serum is lipaemic. In the former case, urinary amylase persists longer, and, in the latter case, serial dilution of the serum may produce a positive result. If the clinical condition is deteriorating, it may be necessary to perform a laparotomy or laparoscopy.

Is the attack mild or severe?

The changing nature of this disease means that it is often difficult to predict precisely which group a patient belongs to. Patients may appear seriously threatened on admission and yet respond to resuscitation without subsequently developing the peripancreatic infection or necrotic changes that determine a poor prognosis. Unfortunately the reverse may apply, and from an innocent start the disease may progress rapidly to a fatal conclusion.

Prognosis in acute pancreatitis

There is no single criterion that can be used to predict the outcome from this disease. In particular, the level of plasma amylase is not an indicator of the severity of the attack. Two main prognostic systems using multiple clinical and biochemical variables have been developed (Table 18.13) but both are disadvantaged by the fact that each of the variables is given the same weight, irrespective of the severity of the abnormality.

An alternative method, which does make allowance for weighting and allows a patient's condition to be recalculated after initial treatment, is the APACHE II scoring system. This may be more sensitive in identifying the attacks that carry a poor prognosis, but it is not a clinical tool in widespread use for this purpose.

Is the pancreas viable?

In the most severe cases, the pancreas becomes ischaemic and the necrotic tissue acts as a reservoir of continuing sepsis. When compared with necrosis of other intra-abdominal organs, such as loops of bowel or gallbladder, the logical treatment for pancreatic necrosis would seem to be its surgical removal. The consensus view is that the presence of necrotic pancreas is not in itself an indication for pancreatic necrosectomy unless supportive intensive therapy is failing. In departments that support an aggressive surgical approach to pancreatic necrosis, it is essential to know whether the gland is necrotic. The best method for determining this is contrast enhanced CT scanning. Intravenous injection of contrast medium enhances a vascularized pancreas but there is no uptake in pancreatic necrosis.

Does the lesser sac contain pathological material?

In the initial stage of the disease, the swollen gland expands into the lesser sac because of the acute inflammation. In most cases this will resolve. If the disease progresses, a mass of inflammatory tissue may develop within the lesser sac and give rise to

Table 18.13 Prognosticating systems in acute pancreatitis

Ranson prognostic system	Imrie (1978) prognostic system
Each sign is given a score of 1	Each sign is given a score of 1
Severe disease is predicted with a score of over 3	Severe disease is predicted with a score of over 3
Mortality according to score:	
<3 0.9%	
3–4 18%	
5–6 50%	
>6 90%	
On admission	**During the first 24 hours**
Age > 55 years	Age >55 years
WBC > 16 000/mm^3	WBC >15 000/mm^3
Fasting blood glucose > 11.2 mmol/litre (200 mg%)	Blood glucose >10 mmol/litre
LDH>350 IU/litre	Blood urea >16 mmol/litre
AST (SGOT) > 250 sima-frankel units %	Pa_{O_2} < 8 kPa
	Plasma calcium < 2.00 mmol/litre
During the initial 48 hours	Plasma albumin < 32 g/litre
Haematocrit decrease greater than 10%	LDH > 600 U/litre
Rise in blood urea nitrogen over 1.8 mmol/litre (5 mg%)	AST or ALT > 100 U/litre
Serum calcium < 2.00 mmol/litre	
Central Pa_{O_2} < 8 kPa (60 mmHg)	
Base deficit > 4 mEq/litre	
Estimated fluid sequestration > 6 litres	

ALT, alanine transaminase; AST, aspartate transaminase; LDH, lactate dehydrogenase; WBC, white blood cells.

a palpable epigastric swelling. This is likely to be tender, with mild systemic toxicity indicated by a low-grade pyrexia and a moderate increase in the white cell count ($< 15\,000/mm^3$). This may fully resolve or it may deteriorate by liquefying with abscess formation. In this case, the patient becomes more toxic (high pyrexia/high white cell count) and it is more likely that the underlying pancreas is necrotic. All of these changes are likely to occur within the first 2 weeks of the attack, and regular ultrasound scanning during this period is a helpful means of assessment. At a much later stage (4–6 weeks) the lesser sac can be filled with non-infected fluid (pancreatic pseudocyst) and this may be asymptomatic.

Management of acute pancreatitis

Conservative management of acute pancreatitis is the mainstay of treatment. Attention to fine detail of maintaining physiological support is the chief determinant of a successful outcome in this disease if it is severe. There is no evidence that drugs such as aprotinin, glucagon, or anticholinergics add anything to the treatment described below.

Analgesia

Patients are in severe pain and opioid analgesia is required. Pethidine is theoretically preferable to morphine because it has a less contractile effect on the ampulla of Vater.

Metabolic resuscitation

Intravenous therapy

1. **Fluid replacement**. The degree of hypovolaemia is related to the severity of the attack. In more severe cases, there is fluid sequestration within the abdominal cavity and monitoring of fluid replacement by central venous pressure measurements is required. The type of fluid needed is initially a mixture of colloid and crystalloid, depending on the degree of shock.

2. **Blood transfusion**. Hypoxia in acute pancreatitis is likely to be due to ARDS. If there is anaemia, the oxygen-carrying capacity of the blood should be optimized by transfusion.

3. **Protein infusion**. Plasma protein infusion may be required because of loss, primarily from the retroperitoneal insult and then later in the course of the disease if sepsis leads to hypoproteinaemia.

4. **Intravenous nutrition**. This is seldom needed during an attack of acute pancreatitis but may be important if the patient goes on to develop septic complications. Nutritional support is an integral part of intensive therapy.

Pulmonary support

Arterial blood gases must be monitored regularly as occult respiratory failure is common and added inspired oxygen may be required. In more severe cases, oxygen therapy by mask may be insufficient and formal assisted ventilation with endotracheal intubation, often with PEEP (positive end expiratory pressure) may be needed.

Renal support

Acute renal impairment is a reflection of hypovolaemia; adequate fluid replacement ought to avoid renal complications. In severe cases there may be a need for dopamine support or even dialysis if acute tubular necrosis develops.

Plasma calcium

Calcium is sequestrated in the areas of fat necrosis and the ionized calcium levels fall. Correction with intravenous calcium is required to avoid the onset of paraesthesiae and tetany.

Plasma glucose

Destruction of a significant proportion of the pancreatic islet cell population can result in temporary diabetes mellitus which requires treatment with insulin.

Antibiotic therapy

Acute pancreatitis is not an infection and yet antibiotics are widely prescribed in its immediate treatment. In mild attacks there is no justification for them to be used. However, if there is judged to be a risk of pancreatic infection (e.g. the presence of a phlegmon or an occluded bile duct by a gallstone), then antibiotics should be used.

ERCP

The benefit of early ERCP and sphincterotomy to remove bile duct stones remains under scrutiny. It can be beneficial but should not be employed if the patient is improving.

Multiorgan dysfunction in acute pancreatitis

It is evident that successful conservative management of severe acute pancreatitis relies on multiorgan metabolic support. Failure to reverse any of these changes can be the precipitating factor in the cascade of multisystem failure and this is why the disease poses such a threat. Early recognition of failure to respond to conventional supportive therapy should allow judicious referral for intensive therapy. It is during this period of intensive therapy that the patient is likely to develop problems that relate directly to pancreatic infection secondary to pancreatic necrosis.

When intensivists find difficulty in reversing the organ failure, there may be a need to establish drainage of the lesser sac collection and perhaps remove some of the necrotic pancreas. Initially, peripancreatic fluid collections thought to be abscesses can be drained under ultrasound control. This provides a specimen for microbiology to allow a correct choice of antibiotic and, in some cases, achieves adequate drainage. If this fails, then open surgery should provide adequate drainage by a combination of peritoneal lavage and indwelling external drains. At this stage some units would advocate removal of necrotic pancreas but results are equivocal. In cases where there are multiloculated collections of pus, the abdominal cavity may be left unclosed as a laparostomy.

Pancreatic pseudocyst

A pseudocyst is a collection of fluid accumulating within the lesser sac, usually following acute pancreatitis. However, it can

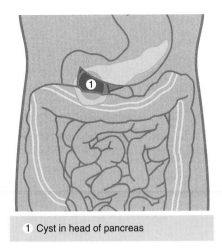
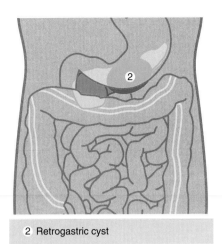
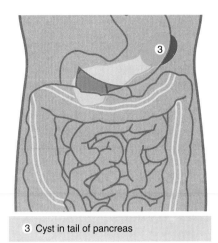

| 1 Cyst in head of pancreas | 2 Retrogastric cyst | 3 Cyst in tail of pancreas |

Figure 18.11 Sites of pancreatic pseudocyst.

arise in children after blunt abdominal trauma. The pseudocyst varies in size and can occupy different parts of the lesser sac because of local adhesions (Fig. 18.11). This may be important if surgical drainage is needed because the cyst may have to be drained into different parts of the alimentary tract.

A pseudocyst is a late complication of acute pancreatitis and does not occur within the first 2 weeks of an attack. However, a persistently raised plasma amylase may provide a clue that one is developing. It is recognized initially by ultrasound scan, but as it increases in size it is likely to become palpable. The decision to treat depends on the symptoms (many are totally asymptomatic) and concern about potential complications (Table 18.14).

Cysts can be drained externally by needle drainage under CT or ultrasound control. This is a less invasive method than internal surgical drainage and is a sensible first step in the management of a symptomatic cyst. The fluid aspirated should be analysed for amylase and cytology, although an underlying

Table 18.14 Indications for the active treatment of a pancreatic pseudocyst

- Pressure symptoms on stomach and duodenum
- Rupture into the peritoneal cavity
- Weight loss
- Pain
- Haemorrhage
- An infected cyst

malignancy would be unusual. Cysts drained in this way may recur rapidly if there is a connection with the main pancreatic duct. If so, surgical drainage needs to be considered (Fig. 18.12). All surgical drainage procedures require an anastomosis between the cyst wall and a neighbouring part of the alimentary tract. The cyst wall is by definition granulation tissue (pseudo-

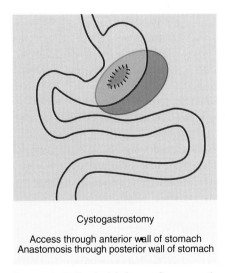
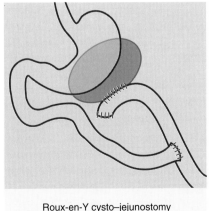
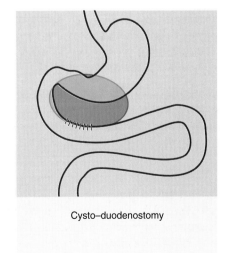

Cystogastrostomy

Access through anterior wall of stomach
Anastomosis through posterior wall of stomach

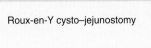

Roux-en-Y cysto–jejunostomy

Cysto–duodenostomy

Figure 18.12 Surgical drainage of a pancreatic pseudocyst.

cyst) and the thicker this is, the safer the procedure. Hence surgeons try to delay surgery long enough for the cyst wall to mature. The chosen method of drainage depends on the site of the cyst.

It is unusual these days for a patient to require open surgical drainage as it is an operation that can be carried out laparoscopically. The major complication associated with surgical drainage is secondary haemorrhage. This can be torrential as it originates from the splenic artery which lies in proximity to the pseudocyst.

The timing of intervention in acute pancreatitis

Cholecystectomy

A delay of 3 months between the attack of acute pancreatitis and cholecystectomy results in 40 per cent of patients having a further attack. Immediate laparoscopic cholecystectomy is not recommended, but surgery within the first month is sensible. Prior to surgery a prediction of likely stone in the common bile duct should be made. Some surgeons would recommend a diagnostic ERCP in all patients, others would select on the basis of abnormal liver function tests and a wide bile duct on ultrasound. Alternatively, laparoscopic operative cholangiography can be used in all cases, thereby avoiding ERCP. Each surgeon needs to develop his or her own approach, but with the common objective of leaving the patient safe and stone free.

ERCP

ERCP allows the extrahepatic biliary tree to be visualized, the presence of stones diagnosed, and their removal by duct sweepage and possible sphincterotomy. The technique carries a risk of complications, including precipitation of pancreatitis and possible duodenal perforation; the incidence of these problems is related to the experience of the endoscopist. The use of ERCP in all cases of gallstone pancreatitis does not stand critical assessment. The stones in acute pancreatitis are generally small and pass into the duodenum in 85–95 per cent of cases. In addition, the longer the time interval between the attack of pancreatitis and ERCP, the smaller the likelihood of there being stones in the ducts. The inference, therefore, is that as long as the patient is not getting clinically worse, ERCP can be held in reserve. However, if there is persistent obstructive jaundice or worsening pancreatitis, then early ERCP is essential.

Gallstone pancreatitis—its management in acute pancreatitis

Acute pancreatitis which arises directly as a result of biliary stones is a more complicated problem than pancreatitis secondary to other causes. In addition to the clinical changes directly attributable to the pancreatic inflammation/necrosis there are the potential problems that arise from the complications of the gallstones themselves. The most severe problems arise when there are stones within the common bile duct. It is believed that most attacks of gallstone acute pancreatitis are related to the passage of small stones through the extrahepatic biliary system. Patients classified as having 'idiopathic' pancreatitis may have

lithogenic bile containing stones too small to be demonstrated by ultrasonography.

Bile-duct stones may cause a persistent pancreatitis as well as obstructive jaundice. The latter may be exacerbated by ascending cholangitis or by pressure on the bile duct from the swollen pancreas. Occasionally there may be an associated acute cholecystitis and this needs to be managed as for acute cholecystitis occurring alone.

The role of emergency surgery in pancreatitis

The general view is that acute pancreatitis should not be treated surgically, although there are situations where surgery might be used:

1. If the original diagnosis is in doubt and a perforated or gangrenous intestine cannot be excluded.

2. If a patient with acute pancreatitis and obstructive jaundice fails to progress, and ERCP has been unsuccessful, then surgical drainage of the extrahepatic bile ducts (e.g. T-tube drainage) should be performed.

3. If sepsis complicates pancreatic necrosis or a pancreatic abscess, then pancreatic necrosectomy may be needed. This is most frequently used late in the course of the disease and hence is associated with a group of patients with a high mortality. Use of this procedure earlier in the course of the disease has not been shown to improve prognosis consistently.

4. If an associated acute cholecystitis fails to respond to conservative management, then emergency cholecystectomy is needed.

5.3 Intra-abdominal abscesses

Introduction

The anatomical configuration of the peritoneal cavity creates distinct spaces that allow localization of intraperitoneal infection. The omentum participates in the process by acting as a mobile blanket, the task of which is to localize purulent collections. The anatomical structure of the abdominal cavity means that there are well-recognized areas that are common sites for abscess formation (Fig. 18.13a), and the site involved will usually be determined by the underlying cause. As most intra-abdominal abscesses are related to specific inflammatory conditions, it is possible to relate an abscess in one site to its likely underlying cause (Table 18.15). If there has been generalized peritonitis, then the infection gravitates into the pelvic or subphrenic spaces (Fig. 18.13b). The transverse mesocolon divides the peritoneal cavity into the supracolic and infracolic compartments and the gravitational flow of infection from the upper abdomen towards the pelvis is directed along the paracolic gutters.

Causes of intra-abdominal abscesses

It is unusual for an abscess to arise *de novo* without peritoneal contamination from a diseased intra-abdominal organ or as a result of injury—either a penetrating wound or surgery.

Spontaneous infection is improbable without an underlying reason, and if no local reason can be found, then a state of general immunocompromise should be considered.

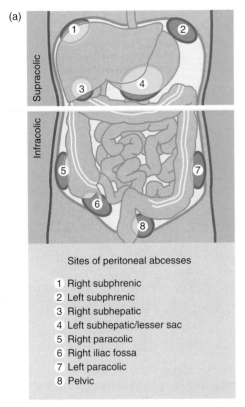

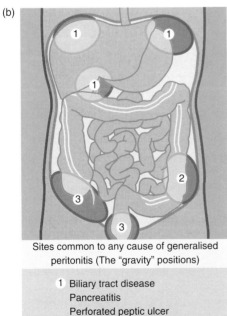

Sites of peritoneal abcesses

1 Right subphrenic
2 Left subphrenic
3 Right subhepatic
4 Left subhepatic/lesser sac
5 Right paracolic
6 Right iliac fossa
7 Left paracolic
8 Pelvic

Sites common to any cause of generalised peritonitis (The "gravity" positions)

1 Biliary tract disease
  Pancreatitis
  Perforated peptic ulcer
2 Diverticulitis
3 Appendicitis
  Salpingitis
  Perforated Ca caecum

Figure 18.13 Common sites for intraperitoneal abscesses.

Table 18.15 Common causes of abdominal abscess formation

Intra-abdominal disease	Trauma	Primary
Appendicitis	Penetrating, gun or knife	*Mycobacterium tuberculosis*
Cholecystitis	Blunt	Pneumococcus
Acute pancreatitis	Surgical, e.g. leaking anastomosis	Gonococcus
Acute diverticulitis	Iatrogenic: endoscopy, laparoscopy, biliary stents, etc.	Staphylococcus
Acute salpingitis		
Perforated peptic ulcer		

Diagnosis and localization of abscesses

In most patients with an intra-abdominal abscess, it will be evident that the site of the abscess is intra-abdominal. This is either because of previous surgery or because of pre-existing abdominal pathology. The patient is unwell, has a 'swinging' pyrexia, and the white cell count is high. A large abscess may be palpable on rectal examination or abdominally. Most collections can be recognized by ultrasonography although CT scan may be more sensitive and should be employed if no abnormality is seen on ultrasonography. A plain X-ray may occasionally show a fluid level in an abscess cavity. If these methods fail, there may be a need to resort to radionuclide scanning using either gallium-67, or indium-111 or technetium–labelled leucocytes.

Management
Abscess drainage

The first-line treatment is now needle aspiration using ultrasound or CT guidance, provided the cavity can be approached without endangering other nearby structures. Continuous drainage is established by inserting a 'pigtail' catheter. Access to the cavity offers the opportunity to perform sinogram contrast studies (useful if there is thought to be a connection with the alimentary tract) and cavity irrigation. If the cavity is multilocular, surgical drainage may be better and this would certainly be the case if the abscess was lying within coils of small intestine. Open drainage should be followed by drain insertion and the drain removed only when the clinical state indicates improvement and sinography shows obliteration of the cavity. Where possible, surgical drainage should avoid crossing the peritoneal cavity in order to restrict further contamination. Furthermore, the resultant track works better if it allows gravitational drainage. In cases of multiple or recurrent abscesses, the surgeon may choose to leave the abdomen open as a laparostomy.

Pelvic abscess

A pelvic abscess lies in the pelvis anterior to the rectum and posterior to the bladder and vagina. It is palpable on rectal examination as a mass pushing into the anterior wall of the rectum (Fig. 18.14). These abscesses eventually drain spontaneously into the rectum and this route can be used for elective drainage, although there is always a concern that blind drainage

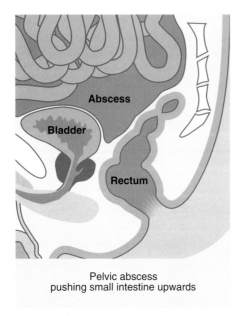

Pelvic abscess
pushing small intestine upwards

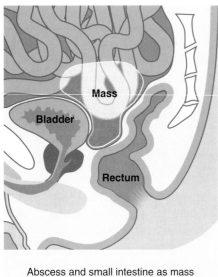

Abscess and small intestine as mass
in rectovesical pouch

Figure 18.14 Pelvic abcess.

Table 18.16 Antibiotic therapy and abscesses

Antibiotics are beneficial if the predominant pathological feature is acute inflammation but not if there is an abscess

Antibiotics can limit systemic effects during abscess drainage

Culture and sensitivity of aspirated pus is important in the investigation of an intra-abdominal abscess

Needle aspiration of pus combined with relevant antibiotic therapy may prove to be a better alternative to surgical drainage

may be followed by small intestinal contents as well as pus. If drainage via this route is chosen, ultrasound should be used to ensure that the abscess is elevating small bowel away from the pelvis rather than the abscess lying between loops of pelvic small bowel. Alternative ways of achieving drainage are by needle aspiration from above, using ultrasound guidance, or by open surgical drainage.

Antibiotic therapy

The treatment of an abscess is proper drainage and this need not be combined with systemic antibiotics (Table 18.16). Indeed, it is generally felt that antibiotics fail to reach the centre of an abscess and are likely to be ineffective. Patients have often been started on antibiotics before the appearance of an abscess and occasionally this masks the clinical features of a purulent collection. Their continued use can be justified if there are systemic signs of infection.

5.4 **Strangulated external hernias**

Strangulation occurs in a hernia when the blood supply of its contents becomes impaired (Table 18.17). Why hernias become strangulated is not understood, except that the smaller the size of the neck of the hernia, the more likely it is to strangulate. A small increase in the pressure at the neck can impair the venous return from the hernial contents and this results in swelling of

Table 18.17 The relative frequency of strangulated hernias

Common hernias strangulate most commonly; inguinal hernia is the most common strangulated hernia

As a proportion of each type of hernia, femoral and umbilical hernias strangulate most frequently

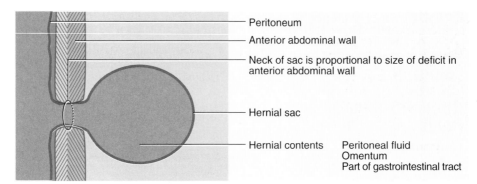

- Peritoneum
- Anterior abdominal wall
- Neck of sac is proportional to size of deficit in anterior abdominal wall
- Hernial sac
- Hernial contents — Peritoneal fluid
  Omentum
  Part of gastrointestinal tract

Figure 18.15 Anatomy of a hernia.

the hernial contents, which increases the venous pressure at the neck even more. Venous infarction may then follow. If this vicious circle continues, the pressure at the neck approaches arterial pressure and arterial infarction of the contents follows.

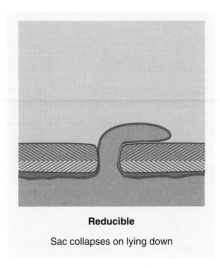

Reducible

Sac collapses on lying down

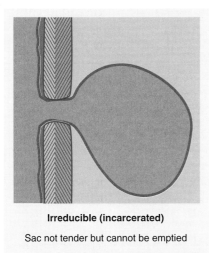

Irreducible (incarcerated)

Sac not tender but cannot be emptied

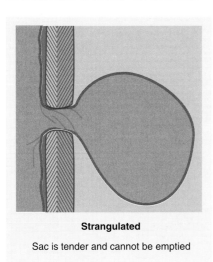

Strangulated

Sac is tender and cannot be emptied

Figure 18.16 Clinical types of hernia.

Components of hernias

The basic components of all external hernias are the same and differ only in the anatomical relationships of the hernial neck (Fig. 18.15). All hernial sacs are extensions of the peritoneal lining of the abdominal cavity and the size of the neck of the sac is determined by the defect in the anterior abdominal wall.

Clinically a hernia can be categorized in order of frequency into reducible, irreducible (incarcerated), and strangulated (Fig. 18.16), and this classification should be used to assess the timing of surgery. Strangulated hernias require immediate surgery whereas the others can be dealt with electively.

Clinical features of strangulation

The dominant clinical feature of a strangulated external hernia is the appearance of a painful swelling at the site of a hernial orifice. The remainder of the clinical picture depends on the content of the sac and, in particular, whether there is an associated intestinal obstruction caused by a loop of small bowel being caught in the sac. The general physical state of a patient with a strangulated hernia containing only omentum is much better than that of a patient who has the added fluid losses that accompany small bowel obstruction or entrapment. Pre-operative resuscitation becomes a major component of the care in the latter, and it is a fine balance between the time needed for this and the urgency of relieving the ischaemic loop of bowel. However, resuscitation must be performed before surgery is undertaken. NCEPOD demonstrated conclusively that most deaths from strangulated hernia are a result of inadequate resuscitation rather than delayed surgery.

Content of the sac

The sac usually contain a plug of omentum or a loop of small bowel. On occasions there may be any part of the circumference of the bowel wall included (**Richter's hernia**), a Meckel's diverticulum (**Littre's hernia**), or a double loop of small intestine where the loop on the inside is strangulated (**Maydl's hernia**) (Fig. 18.17).

Strangulated femoral hernia

As this is a common hernia to strangulate, it is described here in detail. The principles involved apply to all strangulated external hernias but the management of the strangulated femoral hernia often confuses the trainee. This is largely because of irrelevant discussions about the various surgical incisions employed to deal with the problem. It is important to understand the stepwise nature of the operation and the decisions that need to be taken at each step.

Aims of the surgery

There are three aims (Fig. 18.18):

1. To reveal the contents of the sac.

2. To remove the contents if there is irreversible damage, or to reposition them in the peritoneal cavity if the contents are viable.

3. To repair the hernia.

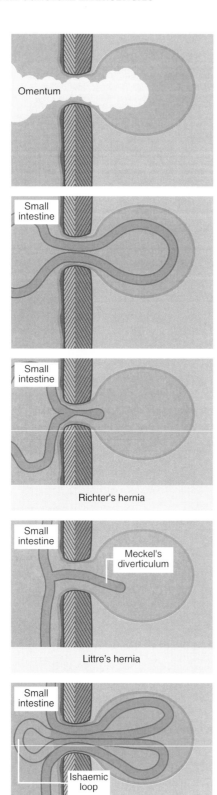

Figure 18.17 Hernia: content of the sac.

The first part of the operation involves an extraperitoneal approach to the hernial sac. The operation can be carried out using several different skin incisions (low/Lockwood, inguinal/Lothiesen, pararectal/McEvedy, midline/Henry), but any strong feelings about the 'correct' one indicate a personal preference rather than a definite advantage. It is essential that each surgeon becomes familiar with an approach that allows the different parts of the operation to be achieved with confidence and safety.

Phase 1: Revealing the contents of the sac

On opening the sac there may be dark fluid, which suggests ischaemic contents. This fluid may be infected and care should be taken to avoid unnecessary spillage. The contents need to be assessed and at this point a decision needs to be made whether to proceed to laparotomy. There are several possibilities:

1. Infarcted or viable omentum. This can be removed without the need to open the abdomen and is followed by excision of the sac and repair of the hernia.

2. If a viable loop of small intestine is found, it should be drawn downwards to ensure that there are no ischaemic areas at the neck of the hernia. If the whole loop is viable, an attempt should be made to reduce the loop into the abdomen. This may require widening of the neck of the hernia by stretching or division of the lacunar ligament. Failure to reduce the hernia is an indication for entering the abdomen.

3. A loop of infarcted bowel is found. This is an indication for entering the abdomen since a resection cannot usually be carried out without so doing.

4. A loop of bowel of doubtful viability is discovered. This also is an indication for a laparotomy so that the viability can be checked after the pressure at the hernial neck has been removed.

5. Dark fluid is found but there is a suggestion that the hernial content has slipped back into the abdomen. This may indicate a possible Richter's hernia and also occurs with a strangulated inguinal hernia where the constricting band is often found to be the external oblique aponeurosis. If dark fluid alone is found, it is safer to explore the abdomen.

Phase 2: The intra-abdominal procedure

The abdomen has been entered to:

◆ reduce the hernia;

◆ assess the viability of the hernial sac contents;

◆ carry out definitive bowel resection and anastomosis.

Reducing the hernia

The neck of the hernia is the usual constricting site and has to be widened to reduce the hernia. The anatomical boundaries of the neck determine whether this can be done easily and safely. The necks of inguinal, umbilical, and incisional hernias are formed by the anterior abdominal wall and there is little danger of

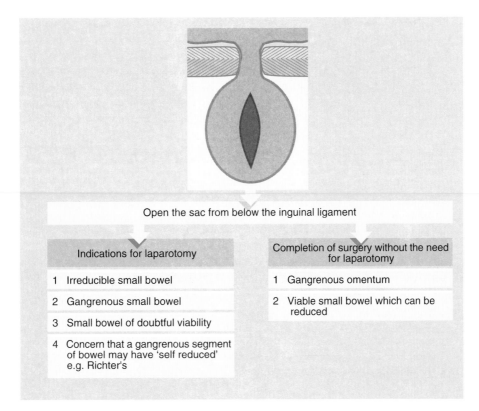

Open the sac from below the inguinal ligament

Indications for laparotomy	Completion of surgery without the need for laparotomy
1 Irreducible small bowel	1 Gangrenous omentum
2 Gangrenous small bowel	2 Viable small bowel which can be reduced
3 Small bowel of doubtful viability	
4 Concern that a gangrenous segment of bowel may have 'self reduced' e.g. Richter's	

Figure 18.18 Surgical options when operating on a femoral hernia.

damaging structures, apart from intra-abdominal organs that may be adherent to the deep surface of the neck. In femoral hernias, the neck is bordered laterally by the femoral vein and the only part of the neck that can be widened safely is the medially placed lacunar ligament (Fig. 18.19). This can be difficult to access when approaching from below, and occasionally there is an abnormally placed obturator artery which can be damaged if the ligament is divided blindly. It is therefore preferable to widen the neck under direct vision from inside the abdomen.

Assessing tissue viability

Hernial contents once reduced from the sac may be:

- Obviously gangrenous; needs to be removed.

- Pink and viable: the tissue is often bruised as a result of entrapment in the hernial sac and should not be confused with non-viability;

- Tissue of doubtful viability. If the tissue is easily removed (e.g. omentum), then it should be resected. An ischaemic loop of bowel should be wrapped in warm saline packs, the anaesthetist asked to give 100 per cent oxygen, and the surgical team needs to wait. An improving colour, visible peristalsis in the affected bowel, and mesenteric arterial pulsations all indicate viability, although if there is doubt, it is safer to resect the affected segment.

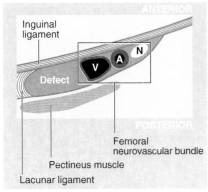
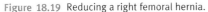
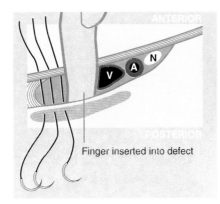
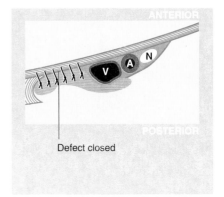

Figure 18.19 Reducing a right femoral hernia.

Resection of small intestine

The length of bowel resected in a strangulated femoral hernia is usually small because of the small size of the sac. The resection margins should be chosen well away from the ischaemic area, and after resection an end-to-end anastomosis in one (seromuscular) or two layers is fashioned.

Repair of the hernia

This is carried out in two stages:

1. **Herniotomy**: the sac is removed by transfixing it, dividing it at the neck, and then invaginating it into the peritoneal cavity (when operating from below).

2. **Herniorrhaphy**: the defect is closed by carefully placed sutures between the inguinal ligament anteriorly and the fascia over the pectineus muscle posteriorly, with care taken to avoid damaging or compressing the laterally lying femoral vein. One way to ensure the latter is to place the left index finger against the femoral vein laterally, while the sutures are placed medial to repair the defect.

5.5 Obstruction of the gastrointestinal tract

Introduction

The alimentary tract can obstruct anywhere along its length. The causes vary according to the site and relate to the prevalence of

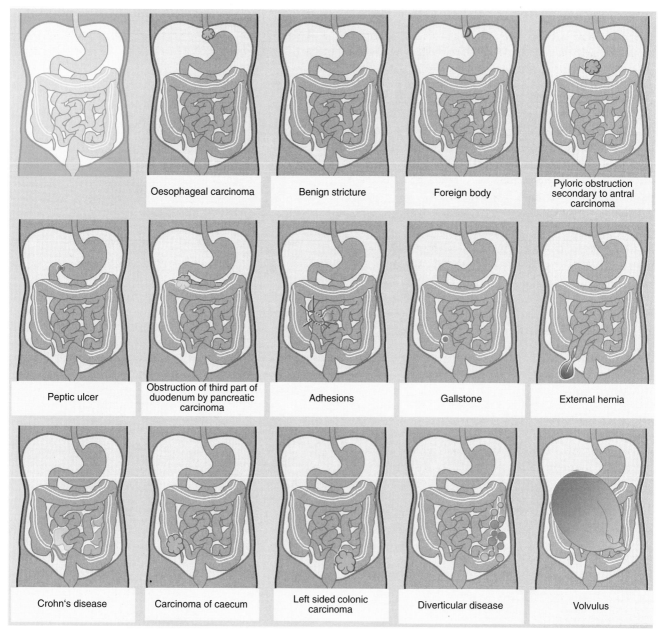

Oesophageal carcinoma	Benign stricture	Foreign body	Pyloric obstruction secondary to antral carcinoma
Peptic ulcer	Obstruction of third part of duodenum by pancreatic carcinoma	Adhesions	Gallstone	External hernia
Crohn's disease	Carcinoma of caecum	Left sided colonic carcinoma	Diverticular disease	Volvulus

Figure 18.20 Sites of gastrointestinal tract obstruction.

diseases at that site (Fig. 18.20); for example, malignancy is much more common in the upper and lower parts of the tract. It also relates to the mobility of intestinal loops; for example, small bowel is more likely to enter hernial sacs than either stomach or colon. Small-bowel obstruction is the most common form of obstruction and is most often caused by adhesions from either previous surgery or an external hernia.

The changes that occur secondary to obstruction are:

◆ Dilatation of proximal loops of bowel by intestinal contents and swallowed air.

◆ Increased proximal peristalsis. The initial contractions are responsible for the colicky pain that is a feature of small-bowel obstruction.

◆ The distal loops of bowel collapse as gas is absorbed, and are unable to function effectively.

◆ The gastrointestinal secretions proximal to the block continue to be formed and add to the dilatation of the bowel. This results in progressive dilatation of the alimentary tract and fluid will eventually be lost by vomiting. The onset of vomiting is early when the obstruction is high (e.g. pyloric stenosis). The fluid sequestered in the intestine is effectively 'lost' from physiological function because it lies outside the tissue fluid spaces. The volume lost varies with the length of dilated bowel. Hence, in a low small-bowel obstruction there is greater fluid sequestration. Dehydration and electrolyte abnormalities are common when this occurs.

Levels of obstruction of the GI tract

From the clinical viewpoint it is useful to consider obstruction at various levels in the gastrointestinal tract (Fig. 18.20):

◆ oesophagus;

◆ distal stomach;

◆ third part of the duodenum distal to the ampulla;

◆ small bowel distal to the duodeno-jejunal flexure;

◆ large bowel.

In each case of obstruction the clinician should attempt to position the likely level of blockage, using the history, clinical examination, and plain and contrast radiology. As this is often an emergency, sophisticated investigations may not be readily available and the diagnosis is made on clinical grounds.

The obstructed oesophagus

This is not usually an emergency presentation (Table 18.18) unless a foreign body or a solid food bolus has impacted on a

Table 18.18 Causes of oesophageal obstruction

Primary carcinoma of oesophagus
Secondary carcinoma of carinal nodes
Benign stricture secondary to reflux
Foreign body, particularly in children

Table 18.19 Causes of gastric outlet obstruction

Carcinoma of the stomach
Benign narrowing secondary to peptic ulceration
External pressure from a pancreatic carcinoma

narrowed oesophagus. There is a history of progressive dysphagia through dysphagia for solids, liquids, and then total obstruction even for saliva. Food intake is virtually nil and rapid weight loss is a constant feature of malignant oesophageal obstruction. A past history of oesophageal reflux ought to indicate a benign cause, but this needs to be confirmed by contrast studies and upper gastrointestinal endoscopy and biopsy.

Gastric outlet obstruction

The most common cause of gastric outlet obstruction (Table 18.19) is now carcinoma of the gastric antrum, although a generation ago most cases were caused by benign peptic ulceration. This is now less common because of two factors: the

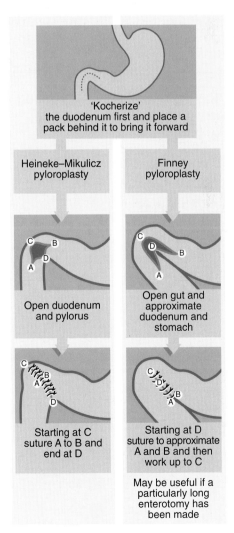

Figure 18.21 Common types of pyloroplasty.

spontaneous reduction in the incidence of the disease and the use of effective antacid drug therapy and antibiotic elimination of *H. pylori.*

Vomiting undigested food without bile is the predominant symptom and it occurs early in the course of the disease. It is possible to lose significant volumes of water and electrolytes if the vomiting is prolonged, although it is now unusual to see the metabolic alkalosis that often used to accompany obstruction due to benign disease. The stomach does not contract in response to the obstruction, so colicky pain is not a feature, although the presence of mucosal ulceration may give rise to epigastric pain and discomfort. Weight loss is a regular feature because little digested food is reaching the absorptive surface of the small intestine. Because of this there is constipation characterized by the occasional passage of low bulk 'rabbit pellet stools'. Most cases resolve on conservative treatment but, if this fails, a pyloroplasty may become necessary. The main types are shown in Fig. 18.21.

Duodenal obstruction distal to the ampulla of Vater

Duodenal obstruction distal to the ampulla of Vater (Table 18.20) is most commonly caused by a carcinoma in the head or uncinate process of the pancreas, and tends to be a late feature of the disease. It is often seen in a patient whose obstructive jaundice has been treated earlier by endoscopic stenting. Vomiting occurs early and the vomitus contains bile as well as duodenal and pancreatic juice, as long as the obstruction is distal to the ampulla of Vater. Electrolyte and metabolic disturbances are more likely to occur than with pyloric stenosis and need correction as a priority.

Table 18.20 Causes of duodenal obstruction distal to the ampulla of Vater

Carcinoma of the head of the pancreas
Duodenal carcinoma
Carcinoma of the hepatic flexure of the colon
Pressure from the superior mesenteric artery
Aganglionosis of the duodenal loop

Table 18.21 Causes of small-bowel obstruction

Adhesions
External hernias
Carcinoma of caecum
Intraluminal gallstone 'gallstone ileus'
Small-bowel tumours
Crohn's disease
Intra-abdominal abscesses

Obstruction of the jejunum and ileum: 'small-bowel obstruction'

Small-bowel obstruction (Table 18.21) is characterized by a combination of distension, vomiting, and abdominal colic. However, the precise combinations of these features depends on the level of the obstruction in the small bowel (Fig. 18.22).

This type of obstruction is particularly hazardous to the patient because of the metabolic changes, with fluid and electrolyte losses, and because of the risk of infarction in a 'closed-loop' obstruction.

Most small-bowel obstructions due to adhesions are caused by external compression by an adhesive band. The risk of ischaemia is less if there is not a closed loop. However, every case has to be assumed to have the potential to develop ischaemic changes and with a deteriorating situation—increasing pain, rising pulse and temperature, and signs of peritonitis—a laparotomy should be carried out without delay.

Obstruction of the colon and rectum: 'large-bowel obstruction'

The competence of the ileocaecal valve determines the clinical picture in large bowel obstruction. Obstruction is sometimes precipitated by a bolus of solid faecal material impacting on a stenosing carcinoma of the left colon. The proximal distension is a reflection of the raised intracolonic pressure. This is much higher if the ileocaecal valve is competent, producing a **closed loop obstruction** (Fig. 18.23). If the valve is incompetent, the distal force extends retrogradely and an apparent small-bowel

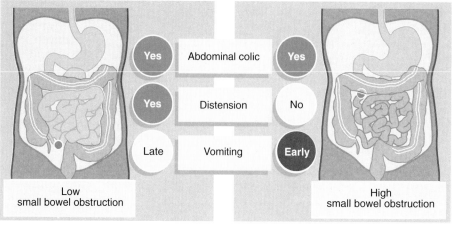

Figure 18.22 Level of the obstruction in the small bowel

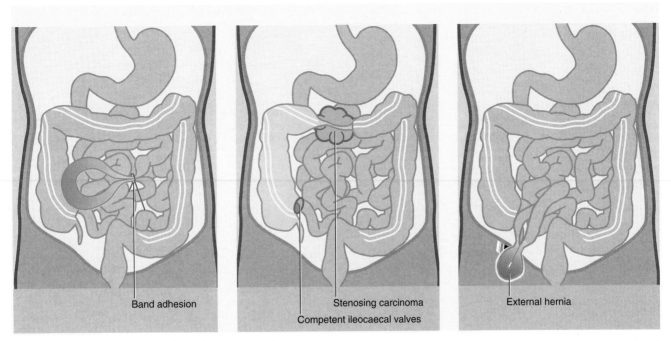

Figure 18.23 Types of closed loop obstruction.

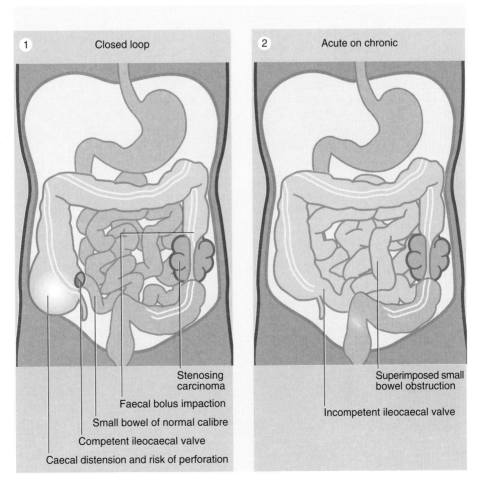

Figure 18.24 Large bowel obstruction.

Table 18.22 Causes of large-bowel obstruction

Carcinoma of the colon and rectum

Constipation

Diverticular disease

Volvulus

Pseudo-obstruction

obstruction is seen—so-called 'acute on chronic' intestinal obstruction (Fig. 18.24). The danger of a closed loop obstruction is caecal perforation, and one of the indications for urgent surgery is tenderness over the caecum or a dilated caecum on plain abdominal X-ray. The fluid and electrolyte losses are more significant with an 'acute on chronic' obstruction because of the extent of fluid sequestration in the small bowel.

In any case of large-bowel obstruction the possibility of 'pseudo-obstruction' needs to be considered. The clinical and radiological impression is of obstruction but there is no demonstrable physical block. This is seen as an emergency most frequently in the elderly, particularly if there has been a period of immobility (e.g. postoperative orthopaedic patients). There may be an associated electrolyte abnormality. The condition is characterized by dilatation of the colon and rectum around to the anal canal. The discovery of a dilated rectum full of soft faeces should alert the clinician to this possibility.

Confirmation of the level of obstruction

The clinical history and examination will probably give clues to the level of an obstruction and to the diagnosis. Confirmation is obtained by soft-tissue abdominal X-rays, which show proximal dilatation of bowel. The pattern and position of the distended bowel can be used to determine the point of obstruction. In a normal abdomen, abdominal X-rays demonstrate air–fluid interfaces (fluid levels) only in the gastric fundus and duodenum. In obstruction distal to these points, multiple 'fluid levels' should be visible on erect abdominal X-ray. Traditionally, both erect and supine films have been requested, but radiologists are often content with the supine film. Surgeons prefer to see fluid levels and favour the two-film approach.

Management of small and large intestinal obstruction

This is a surgical emergency where the surgeon has to use judgement to ensure that false decisions are not made. Not all patients with intestinal obstruction require surgery, and in those who do there is not always the need to carry this out immediately. Nevertheless, if a patient is developing a loop of ischaemic bowel, this needs to be recognized clinically. Early surgery, and the timing of surgery related to the amount of resuscitation required, should be planned, and this can be a demanding process.

Resuscitation

Patients admitted with intestinal obstruction have lost a variable amount of fluid and electrolytes, and the initial management is directed at estimating clinically how much has been lost. The process of resuscitation takes priority over every other aspect of treatment in the early phase (Table 18.24). Not all patients require central venous pressure measurements, but if there is clinical dehydration, this indicates a major fluid loss (at least 4 litres) and intensive care and monitoring should be considered.

One of the real difficulties in the emergency situation where a decision has been made to operate (e.g. a strangulating hernia or a closed-loop large-bowel obstruction) is the requirement to judge when resuscitation is sufficient to allow surgery to be carried out safely. This is an area where close liaison between the surgeon and anaesthetist is required, but the surgeon needs to have the knowledge necessary to be objective about the relative needs for resuscitation and surgery. There comes a time, in some cases, when resuscitation cannot improve the situation any

Table 18.24 Management of small and large intestinal obstruction

Establish intravenous access

Restore blood pressure and pulse to normal: colloid or blood for immediate life-threatening hypotension, sodium chloride and potassium for further electrolyte replacement, 5% dextrose for water replacement

Measure urinary output via catheter (maintain >30 ml/h)

Consider central venous pressure line (maintain CVP at 5–10 cmH$_2$O)

Table 18.23 Features of intestinal obstruction at various levels

Level	Pylorus	Third part of duodenum	Ileum	Large bowel: competent ileocaecal valve	Large bowel: incompetent ileocaecal valve
Pain	None	None	Colicky	Discomfort due to colonic distension	None
Vomitus	Gastric content, undigested food, no bile	Early, contains bile	Depends on the level and duration of obstruction	None	Copious vomiting
Metabolic changes	Loss of H$^+$, Na$^-$, K$^+$, Cl; loss of water	Loss of H$^+$, HCO$_3$, Na$^+$, K$^+$, Cl, H$_2$O. Alkalosis less likely because of HCO$_3$ loss	As for duodenal obstruction	Minor losses of fluid and electrolytes	Major loss of water and all electrolytes

further until definitive surgery has been carried out. It should not be forgotten that the process of resuscitation continues both per- and postoperatively.

Small-bowel obstruction

Obstruction due to hernia

All cases of obstruction caused by an external hernia require urgent surgery. It is unlikely that the obstruction will resolve without surgery and ischaemic changes in the loop of bowel entrapped within the sac are more likely to occur the longer the delay between the onset of symptoms and surgical relief. The only situation where surgery may not be needed immediately after resuscitation is where a large incisional hernia containing bowel is present, and it is judged that the obstruction is caused by the adhesions between loops of bowel rather than at the neck of the hernia.

Obstruction due to adhesions

Cases of adhesive obstruction are usually managed conservatively initially, with intravenous fluids, nasogastric suction, and alimentary rest. This allows the loop of bowel to untwist. This is recognized clinically by a reduction in abdominal distension and nasogastric aspirate volume, return of bowel sounds, increase in the urinary output, and eventually a bowel action. The risk of this treatment is the development of an ischaemic loop of entrapped intestine. The first symptom suggesting this is in the nature of the pain. In uncomplicated small-bowel obstruction, the bouts of colic are separated by pain-free periods.

Bowel ischaemia can be accompanied by a constant background pain which has bouts of colic superimposed. If this is the picture and there are signs of peritoneal irritation (either per abdomen or per rectum), then a laparotomy should be carried out. Some cases fail to settle and yet do not develop signs of developing intestinal ischaemia. There is no firm rule to decide how long a patient should be allowed to settle on conservative treatment before advising surgery, but 4 days should be the upper limit. During this period the resuscitative process must be completed so that the patient is as fit as possible if surgery becomes necessary. 'Never let the sun set twice on a case of non-resolving intestinal obstruction' is another rule of thumb which has its advocates and may be sensible if the attack is the first. In patients with recurrent bouts of obstruction secondary to adhesions, it may be too precipitate if there are no signs of impending ischaemia.

Other causes of small bowel obstruction

Even if the cause of the obstruction is not known, the principles outlined above for adhesive obstruction can be applied. The two indications for operating after an initial period of 'drip and suck' are a failure to resolve and the development of tenderness as a harbinger of peritonitis. If a patient does settle and there has been no history of previous abdominal surgery, then it is wise to investigate by contrast follow-through radiology to determine whether there is a stenosing small-bowel lesion.

Large-bowel obstruction

When faced with a case of large-bowel obstruction the surgeon should ask the following questions:

1 **Is this a mechanical or pseudo-obstruction?** The radiological finding of a dilated rectum and colon with gas present in the rectum suggests a pseudo-obstruction. The management of this is conservative and rarely should surgery be necessary for peritonitis suggesting the likelihood of ischaemia. Treating a large-bowel obstruction over several days by 'drip and suck' can be a worrying period if there is any uncertainty about the diagnosis. It is therefore sensible to organize a contrast enema to confirm the diagnosis. Then, in the certain knowledge of a non-obstructed colon, the conservative treatment can proceed. In fact, the routine use of a diagnostic emergency contrast study in virtually every case of large-bowel obstruction can be justified, particularly if stenting is available for obstructed left-sided carcinoma. In this way the correct treatment is always chosen.

2. **Is it possible to relieve the mechanical obstruction by enemas?** Constipation alone can cause large-bowel obstruction and therefore bowel clearance may relieve the block. There may be a stenosing colonic lesion which has become blocked off completely by a bolus of faeces. If this can be cleared, then the obstruction is relieved and confirmation of the underlying tumour can be obtained from urgent contrast study or colonoscopy. Any surgery can be carried out electively after suitable bowel preparation. Similarly, sigmoid volvulus can often be relieved in the short term by the passage of a flatus tube via a sigmoidoscope. Elective or semiurgent surgery may then be undertaken in a resuscitated and prepared patient.

3. **Does the patient require immediate surgery?** This would only take place after adequate resuscitation and the only indication for this is a closed-loop obstruction caused by a loop of sigmoid colon in a strangulated, sliding left, inguinal hernia; a strangulating sigmoid volvulus unrelieved by passage of a flatus tube; or in any instance where there is caecal tenderness or excess dilatation. Otherwise, surgery can be delayed and the patient placed on the next available daytime operating list.

Laparotomy for intestinal obstruction (excluding external hernias)

Introduction

The incision needs to allow complete access to the abdomen and pelvis, and therefore a midline approach is recommended. There may be a previous scar and, if this is used, the abdomen should be entered either just above or below the limit of the wound, so as to reduce the chances of injuring bowel attached to the underside of the wound. On entering the abdomen, note the colour and consistency of the 'free fluid' and also the presence of the unpleasant smell of gangrenous tissue. A swab for culture and sensitivity should be taken. The caecum should be inspected because it helps locate the site of obstruction—dilatation indicates a more distal bowel occlusion. A full examination of the abdominal contents should be performed.

Small-bowel obstruction

The site of obstruction can be found by following the intestine down from the duodeno-jejunal flexure to the point at which the dilated intestine collapses to its normal size. This marks the obstruction. If it is caused by a simple adhesion, the band is divided and the operation is complete. If the adhesions are more complex, they may need to be divided, and this can be difficult if there are loops of bowel adherent in the pelvis. This requires careful and time-consuming dissection, working on the principle of 'dealing with the easier parts of the operation first and this in due course makes the difficult parts easier'. It is at this point that the risk of inadvertent damage to the small bowel is at its highest. Any small defect can be repaired in two layers, but if more extensive damage occurs, it is wise to perform a resection. The major technical problem facing the surgeon is how two ends of unequal diameter should be anastomosed. In most cases, the end of the narrower bowel should be closed after resection and the wider end anastomosed end-to-side to the narrower end (Fig. 18.25). No matter how simple the surgical relief of obstruction, saline lavage of the peritoneal cavity should complete the procedure since bacteria are likely to have transgressed the obstructed bowel wall. Assessment of bowel viability is sometimes necessary, using the criteria discussed earlier in this chapter.

Large-bowel obstruction

The aims of treatment are:

- relief of the obstruction;

- removal of the source of the obstruction;

- consideration of restoration of intestinal continuity, depending on the fitness of the patient and the experience of the surgeon.

The first task is to determine the site of obstruction and its likely cause. The distended colon can be a difficult organ to examine fully, particularly in the region of the splenic flexure.

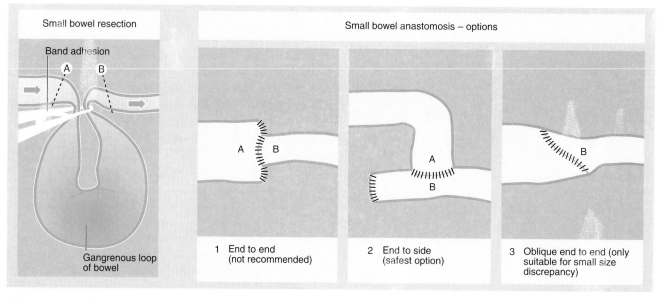

Figure 18.25 Small-bowel resection and anastomosis.

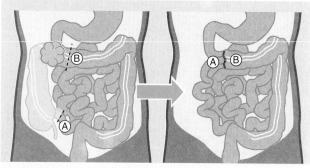

Right hemicolectomy

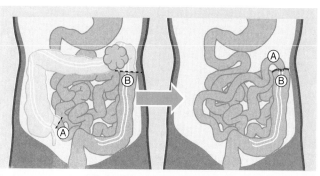

Extended right hemicolectomy

Figure 18.26 Hemicolectomy

Colonic obstruction between the caecum and the descending colon

Obstructing lesions in this zone can all be dealt with by a right (or an extended right) hemicolectomy (Fig. 18.26). This removes the obstruction and allows restoration of intestinal continuity. The proximal bowel is small intestine and its size approximates to the collapsed colon distal to the block. Also there is no necessity for an on-table colonic lavage because the small bowel contents are fluid. The rate of anastomotic dehiscence after right hemicolectomy approximates to that after left-side colonic resections. This may be due to the relative inexperience of the operating surgeon, but the fact underlines the importance of the principles behind all successful intestinal anastomoses, which are: good blood supply to the bowel ends, lack of tension in the anastomosis, absence of solid faeces in the proximal gut, absence of nearby infection or tumour, and good surgical technique. Side to end anastomosis is wise in most cases.

Obstruction in the sigmoid colon and upper rectum

There are numerous options here. The simplest is to defunction the distal obstruction with a colostomy (Fig. 18.27). In contrast to perforated diverticular disease, where a colostomy alone is inadequate and hazardous, in obstruction a colostomy does defuse the situation and allow further elective surgery when the patient is fitter. It is not the treatment of choice, but is a safe option and one that has to be used if the distal tumour is irremovable or inaccessible. Tumour excision is the preferred treatment. In most surgeons' experience, the safest option after excision is to close the distal bowel and form a single-lumen end colostomy (Hartmann's type procedure). In more ideal circumstances, it may be possible to perform a primary anastomosis after an on-table colonic lavage (Fig. 18.28). The colon is washed with water at 37 °C through a Foley catheter introduced after excising the appendix (an alternative route is through the side wall of the distal ileum). Effluent is collected in a closed system

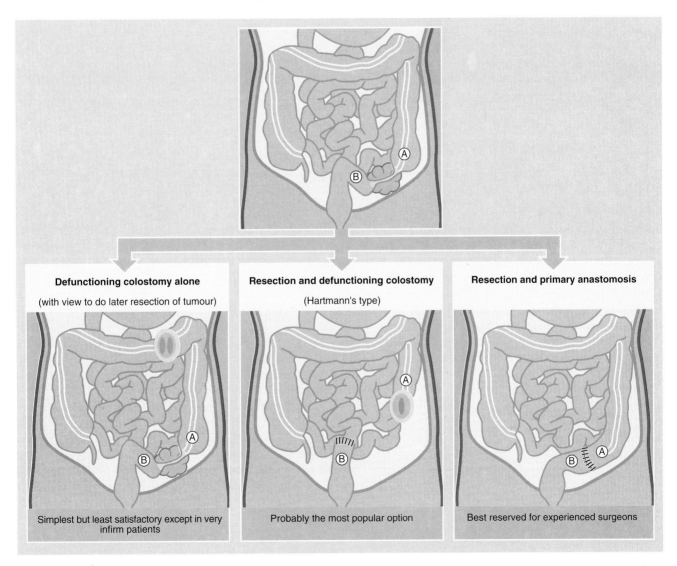

Defunctioning colostomy alone

(with view to do later resection of tumour)

Simplest but least satisfactory except in very infirm patients

Resection and defunctioning colostomy

(Hartmann's type)

Probably the most popular option

Resection and primary anastomosis

Best reserved for experienced surgeons

Figure 18.27 Colostomy.

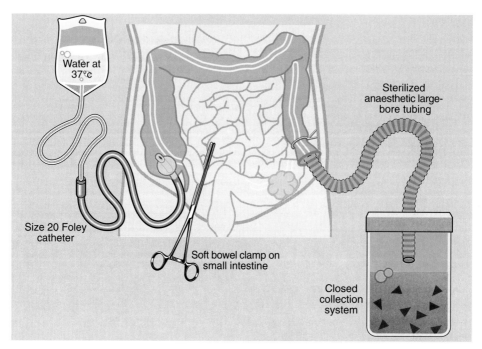

Figure 18.28 On-table lavage.

and preparation is complete when the effluent is clear. The proximal catheter is removed or it may be left *in situ* as a caecostomy.

5.6 A perforated viscus producing generalized peritonitis

Introduction

Localized perforations of intra-abdominal organs are more common than a perforation that gives rise to a generalized peritonitis. The localizing function of the omentum in severe inflammatory disease of the appendix, gallbladder, and sigmoid colon allows most of these conditions to be recognized before they burst into the general peritoneal cavity. The incidence of perforations has dropped dramatically in the past 20 years, mainly due to a reduction in the incidence of peptic ulcer disease. Perforating anterior duodenal ulcers in young and middle age were once common and most of the present data available on perforated ulcers relate to this type of perforation.

Table 18.25 Causes of visceral perforation

Acute diverticulitis in sigmoid colon

Acute appendicitis

Anterior duodenal ulcer/peptic ulcer

Carcinoma of caecum/colon

Stab wound

Gunshot injury

Endoscopic perforation

Small-bowel diverticulum/fish bone

Table 18.26 Factors determining outcome following a perforated viscus

- Age
- Nature of peritoneal contaminant
- Extent of peritoneal soiling
- Associated shock and dehydration
- Length of time between perforation and treatment

The other causes (Table 18.25) have remained constant, except for perforations due to stabbings, and the slow increase in perforations in the elderly caused by the use of non-steroidal anti-inflammatory drugs.

Determinants of outcome of a perforated viscus

The main factor that determines the outcome is age (Table 18.26). Patients over the age of 70 are less able to cope with the infection and fluid losses that form part of this disorder. In addition, there is a need to treat as soon after the perforation as possible, and the longer the time interval, the greater the risk of hypovolaemia, shock, and septic complications. The likelihood of these arising also depends on the nature and extent of the peritoneal soiling. Generalized peritonitis caused by faeces secondary to a diverticular perforation is more dangerous than an endoscopic colonic perforation occurring during colonoscopy in a patient who has had bowel preparation.

Diagnosis

Patients with generalized peritonitis are in severe pain and have board-like rigidity on abdominal examination. The associated systemic symptoms caused by sepsis and hypovolaemia are variable, but every patient needs some form of resuscitation. An erect chest X-ray is the simplest investigation to confirm free intraperitoneal gas, although a right-side-raised lateral decubitus film is more precise. This free gas may be apparent clinically if there is loss of liver dullness to percussion. The cause is usually apparent from the history (indigestion/peptic ulcer, NSAIDs/gastric or duodenal perforation, trauma, right iliac fossa pain in appendicitis), although surgery may be needed to determine the exact cause. A plasma amylase should always be measured, particularly if there is no free gas visible on X-ray, as acute pancreatitis can mimic a perforated peptic ulcer. Contrast radiology is almost never needed as the diagnosis is a clinical one, and barium should never be given if there is a possibility of it escaping into the peritoneal cavity.

Management

The initial treatment is similar to any other cause of 'acute abdomen' with the initial emphasis placed on assessing the need for resuscitation. No surgical treatment should be carried out until this phase is complete, unless there is associated bleeding, for example, in trauma patients. At that point the patient needs a laparotomy, except in a few sick, elderly patients who are thought to have a perforated peptic ulcer. This group can be treated conservatively if their general condition is poor, and particularly if the peritonitis is localized. The chance of survival with non-operative treatment may then be better.

Operative treatment

The principles of operative care in generalized peritonitis are:

- Perform a complete intra-abdominal examination at laparotomy to establish the cause.
- Deal with the perforation by either removal of the cause or repair.
- Perform peritoneal lavage and insert drains into the peritoneal spaces at risk of collecting infected material.

Perforated gastric ulcer

This is rare, but the underlying cause is usually a benign gastric ulcer. The standard treatment is a Billroth I gastrectomy, but this depends on the position of the ulcer (a proximal ulcer would not be removed by this operation) and the fitness of the patient to survive a longer procedure. An acceptable alternative is biopsy or removal of the ulcer and simple closure, although having resected the ulcer it can be difficult to close the defect well, leaving partial gastrectomy as the only option.

Perforated duodenal ulcer

A simple closure of the ulcer is the accepted standard procedure. This is carried out by open or laparoscopic surgery. At open operation, sutures are inserted transversely across the perforation and the repair can be patched with a piece of omentum.

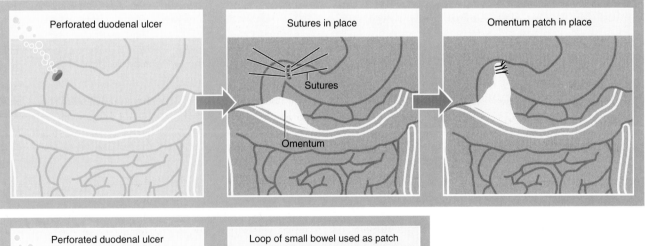

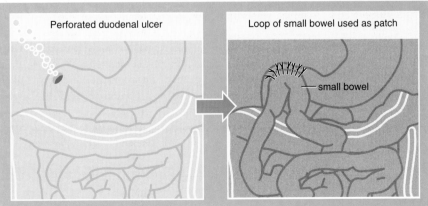

Figure 18.29 Repair of a perforated duodenal ulcer.

In difficult closures, the serosal surface of a loop of small bowel is a useful adjunct to closure (Fig. 18.29).

The aim of surgery is to close the defect and wash out the peritoneal cavity. This group of patients are at high risk and the mortality rises with increasing age. Prior to the introduction of specific H_2 receptor antagonists or proton-pump inhibitors (and latterly, *H. pylori* elimination therapy), the debate revolved around the need for a definitive antiulcer procedure and whether this should occur at the initial surgery or later when the patient had recovered from the emergency. This is no longer required as medical treatment is safer and as effective.

Perforated appendicitis

Remove the appendix and wash out the abdominal cavity if necessary.

Perforated diverticular disease

The treatment needed is the same as that for emergency surgery for a paracolic abscess, as discussed earlier. This condition carries a high mortality and no undue risk should be taken, particularly by performing primary anastomoses in less than ideal circumstances. A Hartmann's procedure is recommended. Treatment by colostomy alone is not recommended because the faecal leak will continue.

Perforation secondary to trauma

This is a result of:

◆ intraluminal trauma secondary to diagnostic, or more likely from therapeutic, endoscopy (e.g. colonoscopic polypectomy); or

◆ direct trauma from a penetrating abdominal wound.

The extent of local damage needs to be assessed at surgery. Wounds of the colon need to be closed, but the closure should, if possible, be protected by a proximal stoma because the bowel is full of faeces. Wounds in the upper and mid parts of the gastrointestinal tract can be repaired safely, or perhaps excised and a primary anastomosis performed.

Peritoneal lavage

Peritoneal soiling secondary to the perforation acts as a potential nidus for peritoneal infection and should be minimized by peritoneal lavage after definitive surgery. The likelihood of infective complications is highest when the appendix or the colon perforates, less when the gastroduodenal segment leaks, and smallest following perforation of the small intestine. When there is generalized contamination of the peritoneal cavity, the abdomen should be lavaged with normal saline (to maintain isotonicity), warmed to 37 °C, and in large volumes (at least 5 litres). The patient should be given systemic antibiotics effective against gut organisms, but, in addition, tetracycline (1 g/l) can be added to the normal saline.

Toxic dilatation of the colon

This is a rare surgical emergency but because of its high associated mortality every surgical trainee should understand

Table 18.27 Causes of toxic megacolon

Ulcerative colitis
Crohn's disease
Pseudomembranous colitis secondary to antibiotic therapy
Bacterial colitis (*Campylobacter*, *Salmonella*)
Parasitic colitis (amoebic dysentery)

the priorities of care of such a patient. Colonic dilatation predisposes to perforation and faecal peritonitis. The care of patients is usually shared between gastroenterological surgeons and physicians, and decisions need to be taken together. The important questions to be answered are as follows:

What is the cause of the megacolon?

The infective causes of a toxic megacolon (Table 18.27) can be treated successfully without surgery, but before considering surgery it is vital to exclude an infection. There is usually not a long history of inflammatory bowel disease because the megacolon occurs as the first indication of the disease. Stool cultures, rectal biopsy, and tissue culture and antibody testing for *Clostridium difficile* must be done before surgery is advised.

When should medical treatment stop and surgery be used?

The immediate management involves resuscitation with intravenous fluids and antibiotics. It is likely that the patient has been started on high doses of corticosteroids. These have the disadvantage of suppressing the inflammatory response, which makes assessment of the acute abdomen less reliable. Unless the colon perforates, surgery is not required immediately and time is needed to resuscitate and to ensure that the cause of the toxic dilatation is not infective.

The important investigation to assess the response to medical treatment is the plain abdominal X ray. Dilatation of the colon (usually the transverse), which either fails to resolve or increases, is an indication for surgery. No arbitrary time periods should be used to help decide whether surgery is indicated—in practice, once dilatation of the colon has occurred surgery is highly likely to follow.

What type of surgery should be carried out?

A life-saving procedure is required, with the aim of removing the diseased colon without perforating it during the procedure, and not risking a subsequent peritonitis from a leaking anastomosis. Therefore a subtotal colectomy with an end ileostomy is the treatment needed. This allows the patient to recover and does not compromise reconstructive 'pouch' surgery if indicated at a later date.

Bibliography

Balsano, N. and Cayten, CG. (1990). Surgical emergencies of the abdomen (in the elderly). *Emerg. Med. Clin. North Am.*, **8**, (2), 399–410. [Because of concomitant illness, these patients generally have a substantial operative risk. Further, the symptoms and signs in these patients are frequently milder and less specific than in younger adults with the same conditions.]

Gough, I.R. (1993). Computer assisted diagnosis of the acute abdomen. *Aust. N.Z.J. Surg.*, **63**, (9), 699–702.[Computer-assisted diagnosis (CAD) has been claimed to improve the accuracy of assessment of the acute abdomen but non-computerized structured clinical data collection with performance feedback results in improvements comparable to those of CAD.]

Jones, P.F. (1990). Practicalities in the management of the acute abdomen. *Br. J. Surg.*, **77**, (4), 365–7.

Jones, P.F., Krukowski, Z.H., and Youngson, G.G. (ed.) (1999). *Emergency Abdominal Surgery*, (3rd edn). Chapman & Hall Medical, London.

Madonna, M.B., Boswell, W.C., and Arensman, R.M. (1997). Acute abdomen—outcomes (in children). *Semin. Pediatr. Surg.*, **6**, (2), 105–11. [The outcome for children with an acute abdomen is discussed, including appendicitis, intussusception, malrotation, inflammatory bowel disease, intestinal obstructions, and non-organic pain.]

Munson, J.L. (1991). Management of intra-abdominal sepsis. *Surg. Clin. North Am.*, **71**, (6), 1175–85. [The management of intra-abdominal sepsis includes drainage of septic foci, débridement of devitalized tissue, and prevention of continuing peritoneal contamination. An algorithm is presented to aid the thought process.]

Paterson-Brown, S. (1993). Emergency laparoscopic surgery. *Br. J. Surg.*, **80**, (3), 279–83.

Saeian, K. and Reddy, K.R. (1999). Diagnostic laparoscopy: an update. *Endoscopy*, **31**, (1), 103–9.

Zinner, M.J., Schwartz, S.I., and Ellis, H. (1997). *Maingot's Abdominal Operations*, (10th edn). Appleton and Lange. Stanford CT.

The acute abdomen. *Surgical Clinics of North America*, **77**, (6), 1997 includes reviews of:

The acute abdomen in the critically ill patient.

Inflammatory bowel disease.

Antibiotics for the acute abdomen.

Gynecologic causes of the acute abdomen and the acute abdomen in pregnancy.

The role of minimal access surgery in the acute abdomen.

Advances in imaging of the acute abdomen.

The acute abdomen. An overview and algorithms.

CHAPTER 19

Elective upper gastrointestinal surgery

Abrie Botha, Frances Hughes, Dion Morton and Paul Thomas

1 Introduction

For a general surgeon, the foregut includes the embryological foregut and midgut, and the associated solid organs. This chapter deals sequentially with the common, and some not so common, disorders of the oesophagus, stomach, duodenum, liver, biliary tree, pancreas, and spleen.

2 Oesophagus

2.1 Anatomy (Fig. 19.1)

Structure

The oesophagus is a narrow, muscular tube, approximately 2.5 cm in diameter and 25 cm in length. The muscle coat is largely orientated longitudinally so that sutures placed longitudinally tend to cut out. It has a relatively thick mucosa, lined with squamous epithelium, lying upon a thick and strong submucosa, which provides the tensile strength for a sutured anastomosis. There is no serosal layer.

Relations

The oesophagus starts posteriorly in the neck at the level of the cricoid cartilage (15 cm from the incisor teeth), and courses virtually straight down in front of the vertebral column to the gastro-oesophageal junction at the level of T10. Approximately 5 cm of oesophagus is in the neck, 15 cm in the chest, and 5 cm in the abdomen. The proximal 12 cm is directly related posteriorly to the prevertebral fascia, but below the tracheal bifurcation, the oesophagus veers away from the vertebral bodies, and the descending aorta becomes a postero-lateral relationship. It is anteriorly directly related to the trachea; below the carina it is related to the pulmonary artery, the pericardium over the right atrium, the diaphragmatic hiatus, and left lobe of the liver. In the neck its lateral relations are the thyroid lobes, and in the chest, the parietal pleura. The azygos vein crosses the oesophagus laterally in the right chest cavity just above the tracheal bifurcation, whereas in the left chest cavity the oesophagus is crossed by the thoracic duct and arch of the aorta. The abdominal oesophagus has the gastrohepatic ligament on the right and the gastric fundus on the left as lateral relations.

Blood supply and lymphatic drainage of the oesophagus

There are no named oesophageal arteries other than the 2–3 small oesophageal arteries arising from the anterior surface of the descending thoracic aorta (Fig. 19.1). All the others are small branches from arteries named for their supply of other organs. The cervical oesophagus is supplied by branches of the inferior thyroid artery, the thoracic oesophagus by branches of the bronchial and oesophageal arteries, and the abdominal oesophagus by branches of the left gastric and splenic arteries. After penetrating the muscularis, these arteries form an extensive submucosal network of communicating arcades. The venous drainage of the oesophagus follows a similar pattern. The lymphatic drainage of the oesophagus is via numerous communicating longitudinal channels in the submucosa that give off branches at intervals to the surface channels (Fig. 19.1). These surface lymphatic channels drain into regional nodes in the neck, chest, and abdomen, respectively.

Innervation

The parasympathetic nerve supply of the oesophagus is from the vagus nerves, which form an oesophageal plexus below the tracheal bifurcation (Fig. 19.1). Near the diaphragm, these vagal fibres converge into anterior and posterior vagal trunks. The sympathetic supply is from the cervical and thoracic sympathetic chains. The autonomic nerves stimulate oesophageal contraction and peristalsis, and are both secretomotor and sensory.

2.2 Physiology

The oesophagus functions primarily as a conduit to deliver swallowed pharyngeal contents into the stomach. It occasionally transports gastric contents in the reverse direction. These functions are under delicate and complex central and local neuromuscular control. The oesophageal muscle fibres (striated in the upper third and smooth in the lower two-thirds) are arranged as an outer longitudinal and an inner circular layer. The upper oesophageal sphincter consists of a sling of cricopharyngeal muscle fibres which are contracted at rest. The lower oesophageal sphincter, consisting of a 5 cm length of considerably thickened circular muscle, is also contracted at rest. The two sphincters sequentially relax when a peristaltic wave passes down the oesophagus at the end of swallowing. The tone of the

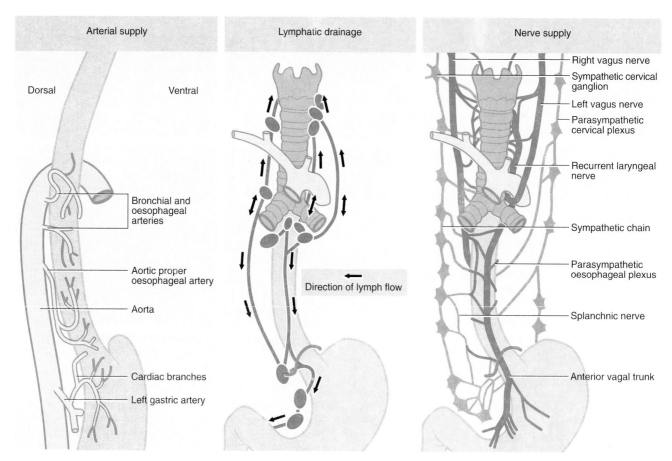

Figure 19.1 Anatomy of the oesophagus.

lower oesophageal sphincter is normally increased after a meal, to prevent reflux. If acid reflux is detected by the sensory nerves in the lower oesophagus, reflex peristalsis is set in motion to clear the oesophagus, and disruption of this function is an important factor in reflux oesophagitis. Venous engorgement in the submucosal plexus of the lower oesophagus also helps to protect against acid reflux.

2.3 Carcinoma of the oesophagus

Incidence

Oesophageal cancer is the ninth most common cancer worldwide. The age-adjusted incidence in the UK is 10 per 100 000 males and 2 per 100 000 females per year. This means that the average acute general hospital with a catchment population of 200 000 would expect about 10–12 new cases per year. In the West there has been a slow increase in oesophageal cancer over the past four decades, particularly adenocarcinoma of the lower oesophagus. Lower-third adenocarcinomas now comprise the majority of oesophageal cancers in the West.

Diagnosis

Oesophageal cancer presenting as **dysphagia** usually signifies advanced disease (i.e. the cancer is likely to have infiltrated the muscularis propria and metastasized to lymph nodes). Unfortunately, early cancer is usually diagnosed incidentally during the investigation of reflux symptoms when areas of oesophagitis or Barrett's mucosa have been biopsied at random. In such cases, adequate biopsies in both depth and volume need to be taken of at least six different sites of a suspicious lesion. Upper gastrointestinal endoscopy and barium meal can be complimentary investigations for dysphagia. Endoscopy gives an excellent view of the mucosa and can demonstrate mucosal lesions and strictures, but is less satisfactory for demonstrating functional abnormalities and the precise anatomical site of lesions to aid surgery. These investigations are usually performed sequentially, with endoscopy following the barium meal. Many units, however, have adopted endoscopy as the sole investigation for dysphagia.

Investigation and staging

The diagnosis of oesophageal carcinoma should first be confirmed histologically. After this, it is important to assess the presence and extent of local and metastatic spread in order to accurately stage the disease and plan the appropriate treatment. The TNM classification for staging oesophageal cancer according to the UICC system is presented in Tables 19.1 and 19.2.

Barium studies

A barium swallow (and meal for lower-third tumours) provides a good assessment of the longitudinal extent and an idea about the likely depth of penetration of oesophageal carcinoma. Of those tumours longer than 5 cm, 75 per cent are either unresectable or have metastasized.

Table 19.1 The TNM staging system

T factor	T_x	Primary tumour cannot be assessed
	T_0	No evidence of primary tumour
	T_{is}	Carcinoma in situ
	T_1	Tumour invades lamina propria or submucosa
	T_2	Tumour invades muscularis propria
	T_3	Tumour invades adventitia
	T_4	Tumour invades adjacent structures
N factor	N_x	Regional nodes cannot be assessed
	N_0	No regional node metastases
	N_1	Regional node metastases
M factor	M_x	Presence of distant metastases cannot be assessed
	M_0	No distant metastases
	M_1	Distant metastases

Table 19.2 TNM staging of oesophageal cancer

Stage	T	N	M
0	T_{is}	N_0	M_0
I	T_1	N_0	M_0
IIA	T_2, T_3	N_0	M_0
IIB	T_1, T_2	N_1	M_0
III	T_3, T_4	N_1	M_0
IV	Any T	Any N	M_1

Endoscopy

The precise site (distance from incisors and gastro-oesophageal junction), type (polypoid, ulcerating, infiltrating) and size (longitudinal and lateral) of tumour can be assessed and photographed. Endoscopic ultrasound has the potential to be more accurate than other methods for assessing the depth of tumour infiltration and involvement of peri-oesophageal lymph nodes; however, these advantages have not yet been proven conclusively.

CT scan

Spiral CT scanning of the chest and abdomen is used by some units as the sole preoperative staging investigation. Unfortunately CT is not precise in assessing depth of penetration (and therefore operability), nor lymph-node involvement or metastases that are smaller than 2 cm in diameter.

Abdominal ultrasound

Ultrasonography is of some value for assessing the abdomen, but up to 30 per cent of liver metastases may be missed, as well as peritoneal deposits and lymph-node involvement.

Laparoscopy

Diagnostic laparoscopy may enhance the accuracy of staging lower-third oesophageal tumours by diagnosing coeliac lymph-node involvement, small peritoneal and omental deposits, or liver metastases. In addition, peritoneal lavage can be performed for cytology as well as biopsy of suspicious lesions. **Laparoscopic ultrasound**, using a probe applied directly to the surface of the liver, has not so far added significantly to the accuracy of laparoscopic inspection.

Magnetic resonance imaging

MRI has not yet been shown to have any advantages over the above investigations in the staging of oesophageal cancer.

Selecting treatment options for oesophageal cancer

Treatment may be aimed at **relief of dysphagia** and **long-term survival**. For early and small cancers that have not metastasized (stages I and II), surgical resection is the treatment of choice. The hospital mortality after oesophagectomy is under 10 per cent in most units and the 5-year survival for all resectable tumours ranges from 5 to 20 per cent, reflecting the very poor outcome for advanced tumours despite aggressive surgery. Palliative oesophageal resection, where obvious tumour mass is left behind, is associated with high postoperative morbidity and survival measured only in months, and is not recommended. Such unresectability is best diagnosed during preoperative staging, but is occasionally determined only during surgery. Resection is best avoided in these patients and alternative palliative treatment should be employed to help the patient through his or her last few months.

In advanced squamous carcinoma, some survival benefit has been achieved by preoperative chemotherapy and radiotherapy. The same benefits have not been shown for adenocarcinoma, but several clinical trials are currently under way to assess the potential benefits of multimodality treatment for all stages of oesophageal cancer. Dysphagia is completely relieved by surgery, but due to the loss of lower oesophageal sphincter and stomach,

a change in the eating pattern can be expected. Chemoradiation results in substantial, but incomplete, relief of dysphagia.

Patient fitness is crucial in selecting treatment, as oesophageal surgery, as well as chemotherapy and radiotherapy, are substantial insults which are not in every patient's best interests. Patients all need careful assessment to match the individual with the best available and most appropriate treatment. Particular attention should be paid to cardiovascular, respiratory, psychological, and nutritional status. If a patient is deemed unfit for surgery or chemoradiation, minimally invasive therapies are usually employed for palliation of dysphagia.

Oesophagectomy (Fig. 19.2)

On current evidence, surgical resection is the only treatment that can be judged even potentially curative, even though 5-year survival rates of advanced disease are universally poor. The most commonly performed operation in the UK is a subtotal oesophagogastrectomy employing both a laparotomy (to mobilize the stomach) and a right thoracotomy (to resect the tumour), the so-called **Ivor Lewis operation** (Fig. 19.2).

Ivor Lewis oesophagogastrectomy

At laparotomy the stomach is mobilized by kocherizing the duodenum, dividing the greater and lesser omenta just lateral to the gastro-epiploic arcades, and ligating and dividing the short gastric, left gastric, and posterior gastric vessels. The right gastro-epiploic and gastric vessels are carefully preserved. The abdominal part of the oesophagus is then mobilized and the oesophageal hiatus enlarged. Lymph nodes along the hepatic, splenic, and left gastric arteries are dissected free *en bloc* with the proximal stomach ('one-field' lymph-node clearance). A feeding jejunostomy is frequently placed for postoperative nutrition. Some surgeons also perform a pyloroplasty before closing the abdomen.

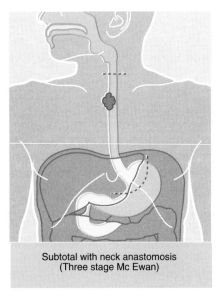

Subtotal with neck anastomosis
(Three stage Mc Ewan)

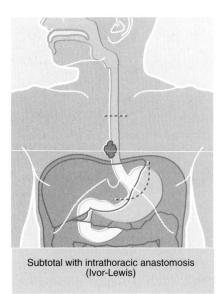

Subtotal with intrathoracic anastomosis
(Ivor-Lewis)

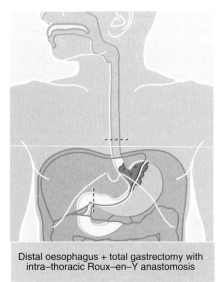

Distal oesophagus + total gastrectomy with
intra–thoracic Roux–en–Y anastomosis

Figure 19.2 Surgical resection of the oesophagus.

The patient is then placed in a left lateral position and a right postero-lateral fifth space thoracotomy is performed. The oesophagus is mobilized along its full length to the apex of the chest by dividing the inferior pulmonary ligament, azygos vein, and mediastinal pleura. Tracheo-oesophageal, subcarinal, right and left bronchial, para-aortic, supra-diaphragmatic, and para-oesophageal nodes are dissected free *en bloc* with the thoracic oesophagus ('two-field lymph-node clearance'). The stomach is then pulled into the chest, the oesophagus transsected near the apex of the chest, the stomach transsected longitudinally along the greater curve to create a 5 cm wide gastric tube, and the oesophagogastric anastomosis fashioned. The anastomosis is most commonly hand sewn using a single layer of full-thickness monofilament sutures, or alternatively can be stapled with a size 28, circular, end-to-end stapling device (Fig. 19.3).

One or two size 28F chest drains are placed prior to closure. Most patients require stabilization on an intensive care ward for 24 hours after operation. Postoperative analgesia, chest physiotherapy, fluid balance, thromboembolic prophylaxis, and nutritional support are of cardinal importance. The integrity of the anastomosis is checked with a gastrografin swallow on day 5, after which oral intake is commenced if the anastomosis is intact. The chest drains are removed after solid food has been consumed successfully, usually on the seventh postoperative day. Most patients can be discharged after a second week in hospital, by which time all other tubes and drains will have been removed.

Patients should be warned that their normal eating pattern will be permanently disturbed and that they will lose about 10 per cent of their preoperative weight before their eating pattern and weight will stabilize.

Total oesophagectomy

For proximal-third oesophageal cancers, which are usually squamous, a **total oesophagectomy** should be performed. The first two parts of this three-part operation are similar to the Ivor Lewis procedure, but a right or left cervical incision is then performed for mobilizing the cervical oesophagus, pulling the stomach into the neck and fashioning an oesophagogastric anastomosis in the neck. Removing the cervical lymph nodes completes a 'three-field' lymph-node clearance. The entire oesophagus may also be mobilized by other methods, including transhiatal blunt or sharp dissection, or by employing thoracoscopic instruments.

Distal oesophagectomy

For tumours confined to the gastric cardia, some surgeons prefer to perform a distal oesophagectomy via a left thoracotomy incision. The thoracotomy may be either an extension of an oblique or midline laparotomy or a second incision. This operation can also be performed through a single, curved thoraco-abdominal incision, with or without dividing the costal margin, and making a semicircular peripheral and postero-lateral incision in the diaphragm. The left-sided approach is also indicated for proximal gastric tumours that infiltrate the distal

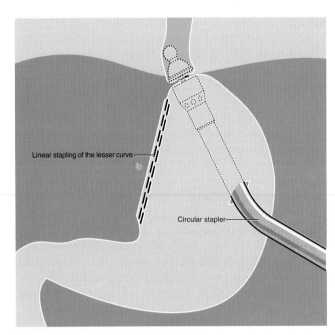

Linear stapling of the lesser curve

Circular stapler

Figure 19.3 Linear and circular stapling devices are commonly used in resection of lower third oesophageal tumours.

oesophagus, where a total gastrectomy and distal oesophagectomy is usually performed, followed by a Roux-en-Y oesophagojejunal reconstruction.

Chemotherapy for oesophageal cancer

Combination chemotherapy using two or three drugs can be effective in shrinking the tumour mass of both adenocarcinomas and squamous cancers. Drugs employed include cisplatin, vinblastine, bleomycin, 5-fluouracil, epirubicin, and mitomycin C. However, no randomized trial has yet shown any survival benefit in using chemotherapy either as sole treatment or as neo-adjuvant or adjuvant therapy pre- and postoperatively. Potentially curative regimens should therefore be used only in the setting of clinical trials and the empirical use of chemotherapy should be discouraged. Palliative chemotherapy has a small role, as does chemotherapy intended to 'downstage' large tumours when the aim is a subsequent curative resection.

Radiotherapy

Radiotherapy alone versus surgery for oesophageal cancer has not been tested in a randomized trial. Preoperative as well as postoperative radiotherapy versus surgery alone has been tested in several randomized trials, but no survival benefit has been shown. The rate of local recurrences seemed to be reduced, but these benefits were offset by increased radiation-related complications. Thus the empirical use of either pre- or postoperative radiotherapy outside clinical trials should be discouraged.

Chemoradiation

Chemoradiation has been shown to result in substantially improved survival versus radiotherapy alone in the treatment of oesophageal cancer. Chemoradiation alone has not been tested against surgery alone, but a few trials have compared neo-adjuvant chemoradiation versus surgery alone. No great overall survival advantage has yet been shown; however, the small subgroup of patients that had a complete pathological response after chemoradiation did survive longer.

Stenting

The simplest and most effective way of palliating malignant dysphagia is to place a stent across the tumour. Ideally, a single treatment session should palliate the patient to the end of his or her life. Stents need to have a lumen of at least 10 mm and the ends should both extend at least 5 cm beyond the tumour. **Plastic stents** (e.g. Atkinson, Cook, and Celestin) can be placed endoscopically by pulsion under X-ray control, after pre-dilatation of the tumour. About 25 per cent of patients can eat normally after intubation, but the rest remain dysphagic and some have to remain on a liquidized diet. Unfortunately, stent insertion is associated with a complication rate of up to 40 per cent and a mortality rate of 5–16 per cent (i.e. similar to surgery). The main complication is perforation of the oesophagus. This is usually treated conservatively with antibiotics, stopping oral intake, and placing a chest drain. Other complications include bleeding, aspiration pneumonia, chest pain, tube migration, tube obstruction by food or tumour ingrowth, and severe reflux symptoms.

Expandable metal stents (e.g. Wallstent, Ultraflex, and Gianturco) can be inserted radiologically without prior oesophageal dilatation. Insertion of metal stents is potentially associated with lower morbidity and mortality than that of plastic stents, but this still has to be proven. The stents are substantially more expensive than plastic stents.

Oesophageal recanalization

The neodymium yttrium aluminium (Nd:YAG) laser is the preferred method of tumour destruction for oesophageal recanalization in the treatment of malignant dysphagia. A sapphire tip is fitted to the end of a standard quartz laser fibre, and the laser energy heats it to extreme temperatures that destroy tissues in contact with the tip. Compared with the earlier technique of using a laser beam alone to destroy tissue, lower power settings (10–40 W) can be used and greater control is possible. For either technique, the laser fibres can be passed down the biopsy channel of a standard endoscope. The tip of the endoscope needs to be modified with a heat-protecting disc. After recanalization, swallowing is no better than with stenting and patients have to return monthly for up to six repeat procedures. Oesophageal perforation is a risk with laser therapy, but the overall morbidity and mortality is lower than with stenting. Oesophageal recanalization can also be achieved by other techniques, including absolute alcohol injection and electrocoagulation.

2.4 Gastro-oesophageal reflux disease

Incidence

Gastro-oesophageal reflux (GOR) is a physiological process and the normal lower oesophagus has effective mechanisms for counteracting and clearing the small amounts of acid refluxed during the day and at night. Although GOR is usually asymptomatic, up to 60 per cent of people experience symptomatic reflux at some time in their lives. Only when reflux symptoms become persistent or when complications of acid reflux such as oesophagitis, ulceration, stricture, or Barrett's oesophagus occur, does it become a disease, so-called gastro-oesophageal reflux disease (GORD).

Diagnosis

GORD can occur at any age. It has been associated with lifestyles that include high alcohol intake, smoking, stress, overeating of fatty and spicy food, and obesity. It appears to be a disease of the Western world and is rare in Asia. The most common symptoms are heartburn, epigastric and retrosternal pain, and reflux of acidic fluid into the back of the throat. When **oesophagitis** has set in, patients may also complain of dysphagia and painful swallowing (**odynophagia**). Atypical presentations include cardiac-like chest pain; respiratory symptoms such as sore throat, hoarse voice, and wheezing; erosion of teeth by acid; and atypical abdominal pain. Since these symptoms may also be associated with early oesophagogastric cancer, empirical treatment of patients over 40 years of age with antiacid drugs, without confirming a diagnosis, should be resisted.

Investigation

Unless there is endoscopic evidence of oesophagitis, the diagnosis of GORD relies heavily on the imprecise tools of oesophageal pH monitoring and manometric studies. Both of these tests are still being improved, and the quality and interpretation of data generated by the probes varies considerably between different laboratories.

Endoscopy

The purpose of endoscopy is to diagnose the presence and grade of oesophagitis (Table 19.3), to biopsy any suspicious lesion, and to assess whether there is evidence of Barrett's metaplasia or a hiatus hernia. With endoscopic proof of GORD, further investigations are not indicated unless surgery is planned.

Ambulatory pH monitoring

Ambulatory measurement of oesophageal pH over 24 hours can provide useful information to help determine whether a patient suffers from **pathological oesophageal reflux** and whether the symptoms may be ascribed to the episodes of reflux. Six data subsets that appear to provide the most useful clinical information have been described (Table 19.4).

Table 19.3 Endoscopic grading of oesophagitis (Savary)

Grade I	Single erosion or exudative lesion
Grade II	Multiple erosions or exudative lesions, involving more than one longitudinal fold
Grade III	Circular erosive or exudative lesions, or both
Grade IV	Ulcer(s), stricture(s), or short oesophagus, singly or in combination

Table 19.4 Normal values in ambulatory pH monitoring

% Time pH < 4, total	4.2
% Time pH < 4, upright	6.3
% Time pH < 4, supine	1.2
Reflux episodes, total (n)	50
Episodes > 5 minutes	3
Longest episode (minutes)	9.2

From these data, the following can be estimated:

◆ whether a patient's lower oesophageal pH is less than 4 for longer in a 24 hour period than in controls;

◆ whether the falls in pH occur during the day or night;

◆ whether the total number of reflux episodes is greater than expected;

◆ whether there is a delay in clearing the lower oesophagus of acid;

◆ what is the longest period that the lower oesophagus is exposed to acid.

It is important to know whether substantial falls in lower oesophageal pH are associated with symptoms. Some investigators feel that GORD should not be diagnosed when less than 50 per cent of reflux episodes are associated with symptoms (**50 per cent symptom index**).

Oesophageal manometry

Oesophageal manometry can be performed by pulling a measuring catheter through the lower and upper sphincters (**pull-through technique**) or by leaving a static measuring catheter in the oesophagus while the patient swallows water (**static manometry**). If necessary, static tubes can be left in for several days for ambulatory manometry. Newer catheters can measure both pH and pressure and are used for combined ambulatory 24-hour pH and manometry studies. With suspected reflux, the purpose of performing manometry is to exclude one of the three well-characterized primary oesophageal motility disorders (i.e. **achalasia**, and the spastic disorders, **diffuse oesophageal spasm** and **nutcracker** oesophagus). Unfortunately, most motility disorders detectable with current technology do not fit the above definitions neatly and have to be grouped together as **non-specific motility disorders** (NSMDs). Unfortunately, a diagnosis of NSMD is of little clinical significance. When a patient has GORD as well as a NSMD, treatment of the GORD, including surgery when necessary, should take preference. Some NSMDs may improve after the successful treatment of GORD.

Radiology

Swallowing barium liquid or barium-coated marshmallows may provide information about the function as well as the structure of the oesophagus, although it is not a sensitive test for oesophageal reflux. The same applies to scintigraphy using food labelled with radio-isotopes.

Acid perfusion and other provocation tests

Attempts to correlate a patient's symptoms with either acid in the oesophagus or oesophageal spasm have previously centred on infusing hydrochloric acid into the oesophagus or injecting parasympathomimetic substances, such as bethanechol, intravenously. Ambulatory pH and manometry have largely superseded these tests.

Treatment options

When a diagnosis of GORD is made based on symptoms and endoscopy, the treatment follows a stepwise progression from simple lifestyle adjustments plus antacids, via acid suppression therapy, and acid suppression plus pro-kinetic therapy, to antireflux surgery.

Lifestyle adjustment

Lifestyle adjustment centres on the following:

(1) changing the eating pattern (i.e. small meals, not lying down after meals, avoiding late night snacks);

(2) changing the diet (i.e. decreasing intake of fatty foods, alcohol, coffee, citrus food, chocolate, and tomato-based food);

(3) losing weight;

(4) stopping smoking;

(5) elevating the head end of the bed at night.

These adjustments can be combined with the use of over-the-counter antacids (aluminium and magnesium complexes, e.g. Maalox®), antacids combined with alginates (e.g. Gaviscon®), or mucosal protective agents such as sucralfate.

Acid suppression

Proton-pump inhibitors such as omeprazole and lansoprazole result in lower intragastric pH than the H_2 receptor antagonists such as ranitidine and cimetidine, and have been shown to be more effective in relieving symptomatic GORD and healing oesophagitis. A 6-week course of therapy usually achieves a response in 80 per cent of patients. More than 50 per cent of patients relapse after cessation of treatment and these patients may benefit from long-term acid suppression using a maintenance dose of a proton-pump inhibitor (e.g. 10 mg of omeprazole or 15 mg of lansoprazole per day). Non-healing oesophagitis and oesophageal ulcers should be biopsied to exclude dysplasia and cancer.

Pro-kinetic drugs

Cisapride, metoclopramide, and domperidone can be used to assist with oesophageal clearance of refluxed acid and to increase gastric emptying. Whereas cisapride on its own is as effective as the H_2 antagonists in curing GORD, the combination of cisapride with a proton-pump inhibitor does not seem to provide benefit over using either drug on its own.

Surgery

When contemplating antireflux surgery, both surgeon and patient must be aware of the potential benefits as well as the drawbacks. Whereas surgery is effective in abolishing acid reflux and thus reflux-associated symptoms and complications, it almost invariably results in new symptoms such as dysphagia, gas bloating, inability to belch, and flatulence. These symptoms may be as troublesome in the long run as the original reflux symptoms. It is therefore important for surgeons to monitor and audit patients' quality of life before and after the operation, and to compare their outcomes with patients treated with medical maintenance therapy alone.

Nissen's fundoplication (Fig. 19.4) is the most commonly performed antireflux procedure and can be performed either by laparotomy or laparoscopy. The principles of the operation are as follows: to approximate the diaphragmatic crura behind the oesophagus with two or three sutures, to wrap the gastric fundus around the back of the lower oesophagus, and to suture this 360° wrap loosely ('floppy wrap') together in front of the oesophagus by one or two sutures over a distance not more than 2 cm. Neither the lesser curve nor the fundus should be mobilized excessively. The mechanism of how this operation works is not fully understood and several surgeons have designed different operations, based on their own hypotheses of the mechanism of gastro-oesophageal reflux, in their quest to reduce postoperative side-effects. Partial posterior wraps were designed by Toupet and Lind, whereas a partial anterior wrap has been described by Watson.

For patients with a short oesophagus, preventing the gastro-oesophageal junction being reduced below the diaphragm, Collis designed a gastroplasty followed by a Nissen-type 360° posterior wrap. No surgeon has extensive experience with many different types of antireflux procedures, and most practise one type of repair based on individual preference rather than scientific evidence.

2.5 Barrett's oesophagus

Barrett's oesophagus is defined as replacement of at least the lower 3 cm of oesophageal mucosa by columnar cells, shown histologically as either gastric or intestinal metaplasia. When Barrett's metaplasia is present, reflux oesophagitis is associated with a higher incidence of benign ulceration, bleeding, and stricturing. There is also a risk of dysplasia in the Barrett's mucosa, leading to adenocarcinoma. Low-grade dysplasia is reversible with medical and surgical antireflux therapy, but high-grade dysplasia is thought to be irreversible and a direct precursor of carcinoma in situ. The true incidence of Barrett's mucosa in the general population and its association with the increasing incidence of oesophageal adenocarcinoma is not known, and owing to high cost and low yield, guidelines on the standard follow-up of newly diagnosed Barrett's metaplasia do not exist. There is also some controversy on the treatment of high-grade dysplasia found in an area of Barrett's mucosa. After confirmation of high-grade dysplasia by two or more histopathologists, some surgical units advise oesophagectomy, whereas other units place such patients on an endoscopic surveillance programme, usually 6–12 monthly.

2.6 Other motility disorders

Patients with motility disorders present with dysphagia, odynophagia, chest pain, and occasionally respiratory complications of aspiration. They usually present in a younger age group than cancer, and the history frequently spans months to years rather than weeks.

Achalasia

Achalasia is the best defined and therefore most easily recognized oesophageal motility disorder. The diagnosis is based on lack of relaxation of the lower oesophageal sphincter on swallowing and absence of peristalsis in the oesophageal body. The incidence is about 1 in 100 000 people per year. Medical therapy with smooth muscle relaxants such as nifedipine is of limited benefit, whereas injecting the lower oesophageal sphincter with

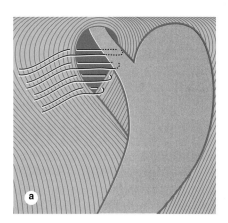 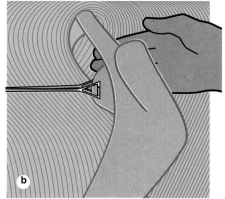 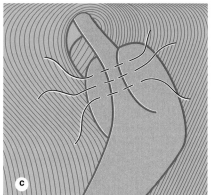

Figure 19.4 Technique of Nissen's fundoplication.

botulinum toxin provides somewhat longer relief. The mainstay of treatment is either balloon dilatation or surgical myotomy. The balloon used for dilatation is 2.5–3.5 cm in diameter and therefore substantially larger than the 1.5–2.0 cm balloon used for dilating peptic and malignant strictures. There is thus a higher risk of perforation. The risk of late gastro-oesophageal reflux is less with balloon dilatation than with surgical myotomy, but relief of dysphagia is better with surgery. A **Heller's cardiomyotomy** can be performed, either by thoracotomy, laparotomy, or laparoscopy. The myotomy should include the distal 5 cm of oesophagus and the proximal 1 cm of stomach, and extend through the full thickness of muscle. There is an incidence of postoperative reflux of up to 50 per cent and so it is advisable to perform a Nissen fundoplication at the same time. **Pseudo-achalasia** caused by a small submucosal cancer at the cardia has a shorter history. Endoluminal ultrasound and open biopsy are often required to confirm the diagnosis.

Diverticula

A **pharyngeal pouch** or hypopharyngeal diverticulum is thought to arise as a result of cricopharyngeal dysfunction, either a restrictive myopathy or achalasia. In addition to dysphagia and aspiration, patients may have a gurgling sensation and a bulge in the neck. The treatment is cricopharyngeal myotomy with or without a diverticulectomy. The usual technique is via a right or left neck incision and a posterior approach to the oesophagus, although some surgeons use an endoscopic approach, employing a rigid oesophagoscope and linear stapler. **Epiphrenic diverticula** present with dysphagia and are treated by diverticulectomy and myotomy through a left thoracotomy.

Hypermotility

The hypermotility or spastic disorders of the oesophagus are often diagnosed when other diagnoses have been excluded. The terms **diffuse oesophageal spasm** and **corkscrew oesophagus** are often used interchangeably, as demonstrating specific features in a range of oesophageal hypermotility. In contrast to achalasia, primary peristaltic waves are propagated along the oesophagus in these disorders. The treatment is largely medical, with the main emphasis on antireflux therapy.

Non-specific dysmotility

Non-specific oesophageal hypo- or hypermotility is frequently detected by manometric or barium investigation of chest pain and reflux symptoms. These findings have little clinical relevance and treatment should be focused on specific diagnoses such as gastro-oesophageal reflux.

2.7 Oesophageal rupture

Iatrogenic rupture

Most iatrogenic oesophageal injuries occur during diagnostic or therapeutic endoscopy. When the perforation is small and not causing systemic signs, conservative treatment using nasogastric tube drainage, stopping oral intake, and using intravenous antibiotics usually suffices. Large perforations in patients undergoing palliative treatment of oesophageal malignancy are also treated conservatively, but perforations causing systemic upset in patients with benign disease should be repaired surgically without delay.

Spontaneous and traumatic rupture

Spontaneous perforation after vomiting (**Boerhaave's syndrome**) or after blunt or penetrating trauma, should be repaired surgically. If surgery is delayed, primary repair may be unwise and oesophageal resection is then indicated. Primary reconstruction can frequently be performed, but in some cases it is best to perform a total oesophagectomy with a cervical oesophagostomy, treat the mediastinal and pleural infection, and reconstruct or replace the oesophagus after several weeks.

2.8 Hiatus hernia

Sliding

A sliding hiatus hernia results when widened diaphragmatic crura result in a bulging lower oesophagus and mediastinal prolapse of the gastro-oesophageal junction. It is very common, and is associated with gastro-oesophageal reflux. Surgical repair is only indicated as part of an antireflux operation (see Fig. 19.4).

Rolling (para-oesophageal)

A rolling or para-oesophageal hernia occurs when the lower oesophagus and cardia remain in their normal intra-abdominal position but the fundus and gastric body 'rolls' through a widened hiatus into the posterior mediastinum. This type of hernia is potentially more serious and occurs frequently in the elderly. Acute complications include acute gastric dilatation, gastric volvulus (Fig. 19.5), and bleeding or penetrating peptic ulcers that erode mediastinal structures. Chronic complications include intermittent cardiac and respiratory embarrassment. Although some surgeons argue that all rolling hernias should be repaired, most would agree that acute or chronic complications are definite indications for surgery. Via an abdominal approach, most rolling hernias can be reduced by simply pulling. The hernia is thereafter repaired and an anterior gastropexy performed. For acute cases, pulling may tear the stomach, with resultant mediastinal contamination. In these cases a left thoraco-abdominal approach is safer.

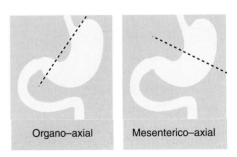

Organo–axial   Mesenterico–axial

Figure 19.5 Types of gastric volvulus.

3 Stomach

3.1 Anatomy

Structure

The stomach is a bag-like structure with a capacity of about 1 litre. Its wall consists of a thick mucosa, submucosa, muscle layer, and serosa, and it is completely invested in peritoneum apart from a small, bare area adjacent to the cardia. The **cardia** is the most fixed part and is at the level of T10, with a surface marking just left of the xiphisternum. The pylorus is very mobile, and is usually situated at the level of L1. The **fundus** is the part projecting above the cardia, the **body** is the curved vertical part, and the pyloric **antrum** the distal horizontal part leading to the **pylorus** or sphincter between the stomach and duodenum. The greater curve is much longer than the lesser curve and, when fully mobilized, the fundus can be stretched to the pharynx.

Relations

The stomach is an entirely intraperitoneal organ and is anteriorly related to the left lobe of the liver, the left hemi-diaphragm, the left costal margin, and abdominal wall muscles. Its posterior relation is the lesser sac (i.e. left diaphragm, spleen, left adrenal, pancreas, and left kidney). On the left, the greater curve is attached to the diaphragm, spleen, and greater omentum, and thereby to the transverse colon. On the right, the stomach is related to the lesser omentum and thereby the liver.

Blood supply and lymphatic drainage of the stomach

The stomach receives its blood supply from the three branches of the coeliac axis—the hepatic, splenic, and left gastric arteries—as well as some from the left inferior phrenic artery (Fig. 19.6). The hepatic artery gives rise to the right gastric artery (which runs in the mesenteric border of the lesser omentum) and, via the gastroduodenal artery, to the right gastro-epiploic artery (which runs in the mesenteric border of the greater omentum). The left gastric artery runs in the mesenteric border of the lesser omentum, whereas the splenic artery gives rise to the left gastro-epiploic artery, the short gastric arteries from the anterior aspect of the splenic hilum, and the posterior gastric arteries from the posterior aspect of the splenic hilum. Penetrating arteries from the mesenteric arteries form a rich submucosal network, which allows extensive devascularization of the stomach during resection and reconstruction. The accompanying veins drain into the portal system.

Lymphatic channels drain to nodes along the arteries within the mesenteric borders (within 2 cm of the stomach wall) and then to nodes along the branches of the coeliac axis and aorta (Fig. 19.6). Extensive communications exist between the lymphatic channels and nodes of the coeliac axis and para-aortic areas, which explains lymph node metastases distant from the primary tumour.

Innervation

The anterior abdominal vagus nerve gives off a hepatic branch, a pyloric branch, and a branch that forms the anterior gastric division. The posterior abdominal vagus gives off a coeliac branch and also forms a posterior gastric division. In the years prior to H_2 antagonists, proton-pump inhibitors, and *H. pylori* elimination, several operations, such as trunkal, selective, and highly selective vagotomies, were designed and performed as peptic ulcer therapy.

3.2 Physiology

The first function of the stomach, particularly the proximal stomach, is as a receptacle or store of an ingested meal, which on some occasions can be of substantial volume. The proximal stomach also secretes acid, pepsinogen, and intrinsic factor,

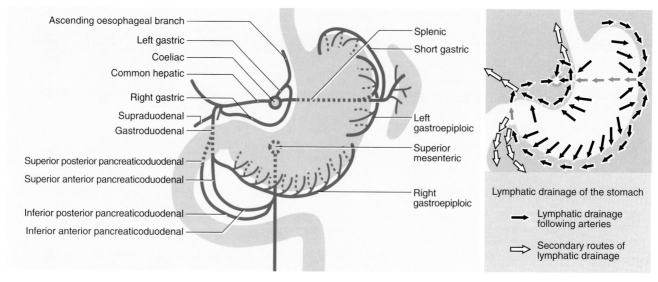

Ascending oesophageal branch
Left gastric
Coeliac
Common hepatic
Right gastric
Supraduodenal
Gastroduodenal
Superior posterior pancreaticoduodenal
Superior anterior pancreaticoduodenal
Inferior posterior pancreaticoduodenal
Inferior anterior pancreaticoduodenal

Splenic
Short gastric
Left gastroepiploic
Superior mesenteric
Right gastroepiploic

Lymphatic drainage of the stomach

→ Lymphatic drainage following arteries

⇒ Secondary routes of lymphatic drainage

Figure 19.6 Anatomy of the stomach.

which are important in sterilizing ingested food and contributing to digestion. Another major function of the stomach is to mix the ingested food, and this is predominantly in response to antral gastrin and parasympathetic nerve stimulation. Although the precise control of gastric emptying of chyme through the pylorus is poorly understood, we know that division of the vagus nerves interferes with the process. Gastric resection therefore invariably results in altered eating, digestion, upper gut flora, and absorption, with almost invariable weight loss, abdominal discomfort, and altered bowel habit postoperatively.

3.3 Cancer of the stomach

Incidence

World-wide, gastric cancer is the second most common cancer after lung cancer. In the UK the age-adjusted incidence is 27 per 100 000 males and 11 per 100 000 females per year. An average acute general hospital with a catchment population of 200 000 will therefore expect 30–40 new cases per year. There has been a slow decrease in the incidence of gastric cancers over the past few decades, particularly the incidence of distal cancers, although proximal gastric cancer is definitely on the increase.

Diagnosis

Advanced gastric cancer presents with dyspepsia (indigestion) or anaemia, whereas early cancers (disease confined to the mucosa and submucosa) are usually asymptomatic. The first line of investigation for someone over the age of 40 years with a new onset of dyspepsia should be endoscopy. A barium meal is sometimes used as a screening test, but is less accurate, particularly in early cancer. In Japan, the only country where gastric cancer is the most common malignant disease, annual screening is provided for everybody over the age of 40. This has resulted in an increase in the diagnosis of early cancer, which makes up 58 per cent of all gastric cancers diagnosed. In the Western world the opposite is true, with less than 5 per cent of gastric cancer diagnosed early, and over 50 per cent of patients having inoperable disease at the time of diagnosis.

Investigation and staging

Since the mainstay of treatment is surgical resection, investigations are geared towards assessing operability, and limiting the proportion of 'open-and-close' laparotomies. A useful approach to staging gastric cancer is endoscopy, followed by a chest X-ray, CT scan, or ultrasound of the liver, and a diagnostic laparoscopy. The TNM classification and staging of gastric cancer are presented in Tables 19.5 and 19.6.

Endoscopy

Endoscopy enables the macroscopic type, the site and the size of a gastric tumour to be identified, and can also be used for resecting small tumours confined to the mucosa. Endoscopic ultrasound can be used to assess the depth of penetration and lymph-node involvement. Poor prognostic features are macroscopic type 4 (diffusely infiltrating), proximal location (C), size

Table 19.5 TNM classification of gastric cancer

T factor	T_1	Tumour limited to mucosa and submucosa
	T_2	Tumour involves muscularis propria or serosa
	T_3	Tumour penetrates serosa
	T_4	Tumour infiltrates contiguous organ
N factor	N_0	No nodal metastases
	N_1	Involvement of perigastric node within 3 cm of primary tumour
	N_2	Involvement of perigastric node more than 3 cm from primary tumour, or nodes along the coeliac, hepatic, left gastric, and splenic arteries
		Involvement of any other abdominal nodes is classified as M_1
M factor	M_0	No evidence of distant metastases
	M_1	Evidence of distant metastases

Table 19.6 Staging of gastric cancer

Stage	
IA	$T_1 N_0 M_0$
IB	$T_1 N_1 M_0$ or $T_2 N_0 M_0$
II	$T_1 N_2 M_0$ or $T_2 N_1 M_0$ or $T_3 N_0 M_0$
IIIA	$T_2 N_2 M_0$ or $T_3 N_1 M_0$ or $T_4 N_0 M_0$
IIIB	$T_3 N_2 M_0$ or $T_4 N_1 M_0$ or $T_4 N_2 M_0$
IV	Any case with M_1

greater than 5 cm, and penetration of the tumour into the serosa or adjacent organs (T_3 and T_4).

Barium meal

A barium meal is sometimes booked as a first-line investigation, but is much less accurate than endoscopy for diagnosis. In skilled hands a barium meal can provide information on the site, size, and depth of penetration of the tumour.

CT scan

A CT scan is useful for assessing liver metastases, but is inaccurate for assessing intraperitoneal metastases. The presence of liver metastases signifies an incurable tumour.

Ultrasound

As with CT scanning, ultrasound is used mainly to search for liver metastases.

Laparoscopy

Laparoscopy is the most accurate technique of assessing the presence and extent of peritoneal and omental metastases. At laparoscopy, lavage for cytology is performed and any peritoneal deposits biopsied. A laparoscopic ultrasound probe improves the accuracy of detecting liver metastases and lymph-node deposits. Localized peritoneal metastases can be resected, but they signify a poor prognosis and resection alone can not be considered curative.

MRI

MRI scanning has not proved a useful staging investigation.

Selecting treatment options for gastric cancer

Surgical resection of the tumour and all involved lymph nodes is the only potentially curative treatment. Subtotal gastrectomy is the standard resection for middle and distal cancers ('M', 'A', and 'MA'), and total gastrectomy is the standard for proximal cancers ('C', 'CM','CMA') (Fig. 19.7a). Most surgeons add a D2 lymph-node clearance according to the definitions of the Japanese Research Society for Gastric Cancer. Achieving clear resection margins as well as lymph-node clearance is usually feasible for stage I and II tumours. However, tumours that penetrate to the serosa or into adjacent organs, or have extensive lymph-node metastases, are more difficult to clear (Fig. 19.7b). Incomplete or palliative surgical resection is associated with a higher morbidity and mortality than curative resection, and survival beyond 2 years is unusual. In these cases the minimum surgery to relieve symptoms such as bleeding, outflow obstruction, or dysphagia should be performed, and extensive resections avoided. For gastric outlet obstruction due to a distal gastric cancer, a palliative gastroenterostomy may be appropriate in sick patients, although a distal gastrectomy generally gives better palliation. Whereas a palliative distal gastrectomy may be quite feasible, palliation of proximal tumours, particularly those that infiltrate the lower oesophagus, is more difficult: a total gastrectomy and distal oesophagectomy can rarely be justified as a palliative procedure. The same principles of palliative surgery apply when peritoneal or liver metastases are present, although localized peritoneal metastases in the lesser sac can be excised *en bloc* with the tumour and lymph nodes.

Gastrectomy

The usual approach is via an upper midline incision that skirts the umbilicus and extends up the midline, then to the left of the xiphisternum. Good-quality self-retaining retractors are employed to provide strong 45° upward traction on the left costal margin, lateral retraction of the wound edges, and adjustable retraction of the liver. After placing a pack behind the spleen, the antral part of the greater omentum is dissected free of the transverse colon and the plane between the omentum and transverse mesocolon is developed down to the pancreas, thereby exposing the middle and right colic veins. The right gastro-epiploic vein is ligated and the omental bursa is dissected off the body of the pancreas working towards the right until the gastro-duodenal artery is encountered beneath the duodenum. The right gastro-epiploic artery is ligated at its origin and lymph node group 6 is lifted up with the stomach. The rest of the omentum is dissected off the colon up to the spleen, where the left gastro-epiploic artery is identified and ligated near its origin. The lesser omentum is divided close to the liver up to the hepatoduodenal ligament; here the right gastric artery is divided at its origin. The duodenum is divided and its end oversewn. By lifting the stomach forward, the coeliac artery as well as the hepatic, splenic, and left gastric arteries are displayed and are then

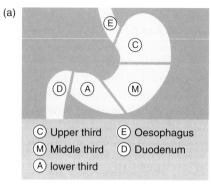

(a)

C Upper third   E Oesophagus
M Middle third   D Duodenum
A lower third

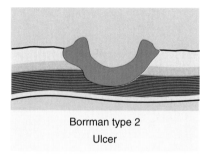

(b)

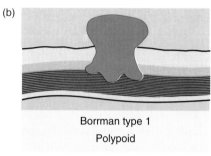

Borrman type 1
Polypoid

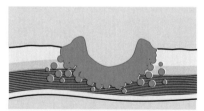

Borrman type 2
Ulcer

Borrman type 3
Ulcer in infiltrating cancer

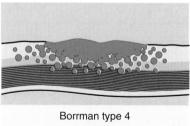

Borrman type 4
Diffusely infiltrating

Figure 19.7 Cancer of the stomach: (a) sites; (b) infiltration.

carefully cleared of lymph nodes. The left gastric artery is ligated and divided at its origin, its lymph nodes swept up with the stomach, and the lesser omentum is further divided up to the cardia. This completes the dissection for a **subtotal** gastrectomy.

Bare areas are then created on the lesser and greater curves and the stomach is stapled across from just below the cardia on the lesser curve to a variable distance below the spleen on the greater curve. The gastric remnant receives its blood supply from the splenic artery via the short gastrics and posterior gastric arteries. For a **total** gastrectomy with splenic preservation, the short gastric and posterior gastric vessels are divided, the abdominal oesophagus is mobilized, and the oesophagus transsected just below the hiatus. Tumours high on the greater curve are associated with a high incidence of metastases to the splenic hilar nodes and *en bloc* splenectomy is advisable in these cases. However, when a splenectomy and/or distal pancreatectomy are performed as part of a gastrectomy, the morbidity and mortality are significantly increased. Reconstruction after both subtotal and total gastrectomy is best achieved by a Roux-en-Y loop of jejunum passed through the transverse mesocolon and performing an end-to-side gastrojejunal or oesophagojejunal anastomosis.

Chemotherapy

Chemotherapy for gastric cancer should be used only in the setting of a clinical trial, and several trials of neo-adjuvant and adjuvant chemotherapy for gastric cancer are currently under way. Palliative chemotherapy can be considered for patients fit enough to withstand it.

Radiotherapy

Radiotherapy has only a small role in the treatment of gastric cancer.

Palliative treatment

Other palliative options such as stenting and endoscopic laser are rarely applicable in the stomach.

Other gastric tumours

Several different benign and malignant tumours are found in the stomach; all are rare. In addition to the relatively common **gastric fundal polyps** of middle-aged women, the two more likely rare tumours to be encountered are gastric lymphoma and leiomyoma.

Lymphoma

Primary gastric lymphomas present in the same age group and with the same symptoms as gastric adenocarcinoma. Owing to the submucosal location, preoperative biopsies are frequently negative. When diagnosed, staging of the lymphoma by CT scanning is indicated, although the diagnosis is often made on frozen section or postoperative histology. Surgery for gastric lymphoma should follow the same principles as for adenocarcinoma. Chemo- and radiotherapy should be planned in association with a haematologist.

Leiomyoma

Small leiomyomas are common in people aged over 50 years and are usually asymptomatic. The main presenting complaint of the larger tumours is bleeding. Because of the submucosal location, preoperative biopsies are usually negative, and the diagnosis is made on endoscopic or radiological appearance. The treatment is local excision with a cuff of normal surrounding stomach wall. Tumours larger than 6 cm may be leiomyosarcomas, but the histological differentiation from leiomyoma is difficult. Treatment of leiomyosarcoma is by surgical resection, and neither chemo- nor radiotherapy adds any additional benefit.

3.4 Gastritis/duodenitis and gastric/duodenal ulcer

Inflammatory conditions of the stomach and duodenum include a large variety of conditions that can broadly be grouped together.

Gastritis and duodenitis

Acute erosive gastritis is caused by mucosal ischaemia after major burns or shock (so-called stress ulcer), and by certain drugs, such as non-steroidal anti-inflammatory agents, corticosteroids, and alcohol. This form of gastritis can present with pain or upper gastrointestinal haemorrhage. Most cases of **duodenitis** and **acute infective gastritis** occur in the presence of *H. pylori* infection, and are thought to be precursors of ulceration. **Chronic gastritis** is invariably associated with mucosal atrophy and is frequently associated with *H. pylori* infection. It does not lead to erosions or bleeding. Chronic gastritis can involve predominantly the antrum (*H. pylori*-associated), body (associated with pernicious anaemia), or involve the whole stomach (associated with intestinal metaplasia, dysplasia, and cancer).

Gastric and duodenal ulcer

A **gastric** or **duodenal ulcer** is defined as a defect in the mucosa that penetrates to the muscularis propria. Duodenal ulcers are invariably benign, but for gastric ulcers, malignancy has to be excluded by biopsy. These ulcers are commonly associated with *H. pylori* infection, although it is not clear which comes first, the ulcer or the infection. Cure of these ulcers is by medical therapy, usually involving eradication of *H. pylori*. Short-term relief is provided by acid suppression using H_2 antagonists or proton pump inhibitors. Surgery is reserved for complications such as bleeding, perforation, and gastric outflow obstruction. Very rarely, acid-reducing surgery has to be undertaken for resistant or recurrent ulceration. The different types of vagotomy (i.e. trunkal vagotomy with a drainage procedure, selective and highly selective vagotomy), as well as partial gastrectomy (antrectomy) with either Billroth I or Polya-type reconstruction, is well described in specialist textbooks.

H. pylori

Helicobacter pylori is a spiral-shaped bacterium that colonizes the human stomach. Several serological subtypes exist. Its presence is strongly associated with gastric and duodenal ulcers. The diagnosis is by urea breath-testing, blood serology, or biopsy CLO testing. Direct causality has been established between *H. pylori* infection and ulcer development, and eradication of the infection results in permanent healing of the ulcers. *Helicobacter pylori* has also been incriminated in the aetiology of distal gastric cancers and gastric lymphomas, but probably plays no part in the increasingly more common proximal gastric cancers.

Bleeding and perforation

Emergency surgery for either bleeding or perforated peptic ulcers should be restricted to dealing with the emergency only. Bleeding gastric ulcers are best excised for histological examination, whereas bleeding duodenal ulcers should be underrun. Perforated ulcers should be closed and patched with a tongue of omentum.

Non-healing ulcers

Non-healing or recurrent ulcers may suggest an underlying gastrinoma causing **Zollinger–Ellison syndrome**. Management of these patients focuses on localizing and excising the gastrinoma from the pancreas.

4 Biliary stones

Gallstones are estimated to be prevalent in 10 per cent of the adult population of the UK, and about 80 per cent of people with stones are asymptomatic. Ultrasonography identifies a high proportion of incidental gallstones and the option to leave the stones untreated is being taken increasingly. Where treatment is carried out, the aims are to remove the stones with the gallbladder and to remove any stones that may have migrated or formed within the extrahepatic bile ducts. Removal of gallbladder stones without removing a diseased gallbladder is followed by a 50 per cent chance of gallstone recurrence within 3 years. In recent years, the upsurge of minimally invasive surgery has resulted in an increase in the number of cholecystectomies performed in both the USA and the UK.

4.1 Clinical management

Assessing the location of the stones

Gallbladder stones are most readily demonstrated by ultrasonography. The possible presence of associated bile-duct stones can be inferred from the following:

- a history of acute pancreatitis or recent jaundice;
- a dilated bile duct on ultrasound;
- an elevated plasma bilirubin or alkaline phosphatase.

Ultrasonography can sometimes demonstrate bile-duct stones, but they are best demonstrated preoperatively by endoscopic retrograde cholangiography (ERC). However, this is an invasive test with an attendant morbidity. For example, there is a high incidence of acute pancreatitis in young women undergoing the

Table 19.7 The complications of gallstones

Stones in the gallbladder	Biliary pain
	Acute cholecystitis
	Empyema of the gallbladder
	Gallbladder perforation and peritonitis
	Carcinoma of the gallbladder
Stones in the extrahepatic ducts	Acute pancreatitis
	Obstructive jaundice
	Ascending cholangitis
Stones in the gastrointestinal tract	Intestinal obstruction: 'gallstone ileus'

procedure. Magnetic resonance cholangiography is a noninvasive imaging technique which has successfully identified bile-duct stones. However, equipment is expensive and is not yet widely available. It is likely that in time MR cholangiography will largely replace ERCP for diagnostic bile-duct imaging.

Deciding whether treatment is necessary

About 20 per cent of patients with gallstones are likely to develop symptoms or complications (see Table 19.7) and these are generally regarded as the main indications for surgical treatment. The finding of asymptomatic gallstones was rare before the widespread use of ultrasound, but even now the majority of those with stones are likely to present with a gallstone complication as the first indication that they have the disease.

Asymptomatic gallstones

A strong case can be made for leaving these alone. There is a small risk of developing primary gallbladder cancer, although stones larger than 3 cm carry an increased risk. Prophylactic cholecystectomy has been suggested for immunosuppressed patients, young women of childbearing age, diabetics, and patients due to have organ transplants. It has been predicted that up to a quarter of patients with asymptomatic stones can be expected to develop symptoms over 10 years—an incidence too low to justify advising people with incidental stones to undergo elective cholecystectomy.

Symptomatic stones

Cholecystectomy should be advised if stones are symptomatic because of the likelihood of recurrent problems, provided the patient is fit enough to withstand treatment safely. Classical biliary colic is the symptom most likely to respond to cholecystectomy but where the diagnosis is equivocal, up to 1 in 5 patients' symptoms are not cured by cholecystectomy.

Acalculous cholecystitis

Acute acalculous cholecystitis is seen predominantly in very ill patients on the intensive care unit and is probably caused by splanchnic ischaemia. It is best treated conservatively with percutaneous or endoscopic drainage followed by interval cholecystectomy. Chronic acalculous cholecystitis is thought to be due to gallbladder dysmotility, but as there are no accurate diagnostic tests, it is a difficult diagnosis to prove. Other causes of upper gastrointestinal symptoms should be sought and treated appropriately prior to considering cholecystectomy in the absence of stones. Postoperative symptoms frequently persist. Positive predictors of successful treatment for acalculous cholecystitis are the presence of cholesterol crystals and confirmation of dysmotility on preoperative cholecystokinin scintigraphy.

4.2 Treatment options

Management of gallbladder stones

Cholecystectomy

If the preoperative assessment suggests that there are gallstones present only in the gallbladder and the symptoms or signs warrant treatment, then cholecystectomy is advocated. The range of methods employed includes conventional open cholecystectomy, mini-cholecystectomy, and laparoscopic cholecystectomy (Table 19.8). Mini-cholecystectomy seems to confer little advantage over conventional cholecystectomy except in terms of the size of the scar. It carries no convincing evidence of any reduction in analgesic requirements or recovery times, and there is the potential disadvantage of poor access if the operation proves difficult.

Principles of cholecystectomy

The detail of cholecystectomy is given in Chapter 14 and only the principles are covered here. The key stage in this operation is accurate identification of the structures around Calot's triangle (Fig. 19.8a). The gallbladder neck is put under traction to tent the peritoneum, which is incised. The underlying cystic artery and duct are exposed by blunt dissection. The junction of the cystic duct with the common hepatic duct is identified to prevent inadvertent division of the common duct. The cystic artery is identified and divided on the surface of the gallbladder to avoid damage to the right hepatic artery (Fig. 19.8b). Division of

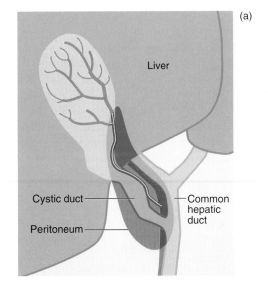

(a)

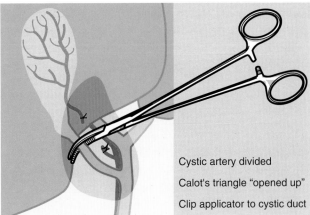

(b)

Cystic artery divided

Calot's triangle "opened up"

Clip applicator to cystic duct

Figure 19.8 Calot's triangle at open cholecystectomy.

Table 19.8 Advantages and disadvantages of open and laparoscopic cholecystectomy

	Advantages	Disadvantages
Laparoscopic cholecystectomy	Less invasive	Higher incidence of bile-duct injuries
	Less pain	Surgery often takes longer
	Faster recovery	Definite learning curve
	Improved pulmonary function	Some surgeons unable to learn the technique
	Possible reduced stress response	Tends to be expensive in equipment terms
Open cholecystectomy	Fewer anatomical complications (established technique)	Invasive
	Easier access to bile duct if required	More painful
	In competent hands, virtually never causes major bile-duct injuries	Longer recovery period
	Can deal with unexpected pathology	
	No unexpected open surgery—patient knows what to expect	
	All laparoscopic surgeons need to know how to perform an open cholecystectomy	

the cystic artery allows Calot's triangle to be opened up, aiding the accurate identification of the cystic and common hepatic ducts. The cystic duct can be cannulated before it is divided and an on-table cholangiogram performed. A 'fundus first' cholecystectomy should be considered, particularly if there is likely to be any difficulty in identifying the anatomy. Whether the gallbladder is mobilized before or after division of the cystic duct, care should be taken to stay on its surface, to avoid entering the liver substance or damaging the right hepatic duct in the region of the gallbladder neck. These principles remain the same whether an open or laparoscopic approach is used.

Laparoscopic cholecystectomy is the procedure of choice for the treatment of gallbladder stones. Concern about bile-duct injuries now seems to be decreasing and although the risk of damage is still higher than for open surgery, the dangers associated with the learning curve for innovative surgery have diminished for two reasons: the standard of equipment has improved and there are sufficient numbers of skilled trainers. It has been suggested that as experience in laparoscopic cholecystectomy increases, the need for open cholecystectomy may disappear. Conversion rates for laparoscopic to open cholecystectomy are 2–4 per cent, but higher in patients who have required preoperative ERC. It seems improbable that the need for open surgery will disappear altogether, and all patients who undergo laparoscopic surgery must be informed of the possibility of open conversion.

Non-operative treatment of gallbladder stones

A number of non-operative options are available for gallbladder stones for patients who are unfit for surgery. Medical dissolution therapy is suitable for solitary cholesterol stones less than 1 cm in diameter, in a functioning gallbladder. Chenodeoxycholic acid or ursodeoxycholic acid can be taken orally. Treatment takes at least 6 months, and 50 per cent of patients develop recurrent stones within 5 years. These factors markedly restrict the number of patients suitable for this treatment. **Extracorporeal shockwave lithotripsy** can be used in combination with medical dissolution therapy, but recurrent stone formation is likely to be similar to medical therapy alone. However, recurrent stones are usually cholesterol rich and amenable to medical therapy. **Methyl tertbutyl ether** can be instilled into the gallbladder following percutaneous, transhepatic, gallbladder puncture. This procedure does not require a functioning gallbladder, and could be applicable to patients not fit for surgery. However, it is not often used.

Management of common bile duct stones

Patients may present with both common bile duct and gallbladder stones or may present some time after cholecystectomy with bile-duct stones. It is generally assumed that the stones are residual in the latter case, although it is possible for them to arise *de novo* in the extrahepatic ducts. Primary intraduct stones alone are commonly seen only in the Far East and are associated with duct parasitic infestation by *Ascaris lumbricoides*. The natural history of common bile duct stones is not known, but

the grave complications of jaundice, ascending cholangitis, and acute pancreatitis, indicate that removal should be performed. Surgical exploration of the common bile duct (CBD) via the supraduodenal (common) or transduodenal routes in combination with an open cholecystectomy increases the morbidity and mortality of the procedure. The huge expansion of interventional ERC has considerably reduced the need for surgical exploration of the CBD, and standard endoscopic techniques and mechanical lithotripsy now successfully remove 95 per cent of common bile duct stones.

ERC in the management of bile-duct stones

ERC can both diagnose and remove stones from the common bile duct, making it the initial treatment of choice for bile-duct calculi. The principles of removal include identification of the ampulla of Vater with a side viewing endoscope, cannulation of the bile duct, radiological confirmation of stones, introduction of an electrocautery wire, sphincterotomy, passage of either a balloon or basket retriever, and removal of stones. Balloon dilatation of the ampulla is occasionally used in younger patients with small duct stones, because of uncertainty concerning the long-term complications of sphincterotomy.

If the common bile duct can be cannulated retrogradely, the limiting factor is the size of the stone. If stones exceed 1 cm in diameter, there may be difficulty in manipulating the extractor past the stone. If stones are embedded at the lower end of the bile duct, removal may be inhibited for the same reason. These problems may be surmountable by disintegrating the larger stone using extracorporeal shockwave lithotripsy under ultrasound control, or intracorporeal laser using cholangioscopy or fluoroscopic control, prior to a further endoscopic attempt at stone removal. However, these technologies are expensive and not widely available. In jaundiced patients where the stone cannot be removed at the initial ERC, a biliary stent may be placed across the obstruction to allow biliary drainage. Further attempts at stone removal can be made once the jaundice has settled.

The main dangers of ERC are duodenal perforation, bleeding following the sphincterotomy, acute pancreatitis, and ascending cholangitis. The morbidity and mortality from therapeutic ERCP is approximately 10 per cent and 1 per cent, respectively.

Surgical management of common bile duct stones

This has now become an uncommon operation in institutions with easy access to ERC. Nevertheless there is still a need for this type of surgery and the need often arises when less invasive treatments have failed. Under these circumstances, it is likely that that the operation will be difficult, particularly because of the decreasing experience surgeons have in this type of procedure.

The indications for surgical exploration are less defined than they used to be. Prior to the availability of ERC, the possible presence of bile-duct stones was inferred from the history of jaundice, deranged liver function tests, or a history of acute pancreatitis. The presence of stones was confirmed on peroperative cholangiography and exploration, and stone removal performed at the same open operation.

ERC and laparoscopic biliary surgery

When laparoscopic cholecystectomy was introduced, surgeons were careful to avoid operating without ensuring that the bile duct was clear of stones. Liver function tests (LFTs), ultrasound, intravenous cholangiography, and ERC were the main diagnostic tools. ERC was used frequently when there was a clinical suspicion or a biochemical suggestion there may be a stone in the duct. The need to clear the extrahepatic ducts is still imperative, but the approach has altered as experience has accumulated. ERC is now used less in its diagnostic role because of concerns about the small but significant risks associated with the investigation.

If patients can be shown to have bile-duct stones on pre-operative investigation with ultrasound or have abnormal LFTs, then a diagnostic ERC is indicated. An alternative is laparoscopic on-table cholangiography. If stones are found, an intra-operative decision needs to made on how they should be removed. The options are laparoscopic or open bile-duct exploration, or else to complete the cholecystectomy and arrange for an ERC postoperatively.

Indications for open surgical exploration of the common bile duct

There are three possible scenarios where common bile duct exploration is required:

(1) planned open common bile duct exploration;

(2) failed ERC;

(3) unexpected identification of common bile duct stones on a laparoscopically performed operative cholangiogram.

Planned open surgery

Although laparoscopic cholecystectomy is the preferred method for removing the gallbladder, world-wide, this may not be possible because of the expense. Thus, a large proportion of biliary surgery is still being performed in the traditional way. Access to ERC is similarly limited, and the sequence of open cholecystectomy, on-table cholangiography, and bile-duct exploration where indicated is still relevant. A further indication for open surgery is when endoscopic access to the ampulla is restricted because of previous gastric surgery (e.g. a Polya-type gastrectomy).

Access to the bile duct at surgery can be via a supraduodenal choledochotomy or transduodenally through the ampulla of Vater. Most stones can be removed supraduodenally and the duct can be examined peroperatively using a flexible or rigid choledochoscope to ensure stone clearance. The usual problem with this technique is ensuring that the lower end of the common bile duct has been completely cleared of stones. The presence of a stricture may prevent entry of the choledocho-scope into the duodenum. Hospital stay is prolonged by the need to decompress the extrahepatic ducts with a T-tube.

The morbidity of ERC as well as the improvement in laparoscopic instrumentation has encouraged surgeons to develop the skills required for laparoscopic on-table cholangiography and bile-duct exploration. On-table cholangiography is easily performed with custom-made kits or via a catheter inserted into the cystic duct through the subcostal port. The choledochoscope may be inserted via the subcostal port into the cystic duct for small stones, or choledochotomy performed for larger stones. Irrigation alone may dislodge some stones, but Dormia baskets or balloon sweepage may be required. Removal of the catheter and clipping the cystic duct, or closure of the choledochotomy around a T-tube completes the procedure.

Failed ERCP

When a patient is known to have a bile duct stone and it cannot be removed by ERC, laparoscopic duct exploration will also be difficult. Failure suggests a large stone, impaction, or an associated stricture. These stones are unlikely to dislodge with irrigation, Dormia baskets, or balloon trawling via laparoscopic ports, and conversion to open surgery is frequently required. Despite an increasing reported success rate from experienced laparoscopic surgeons, this situation would be regarded by most as an indication for open exploration of the duct.

Stones identified by laparoscopic on-table cholangiography

The management of duct stones discovered intraoperatively is controversial. Removal may necessitate conversion to open operation with conventional common bile duct exploration or laparoscopic duct exploration and stone removal. The decision is determined by the available expertise and an assessment of the likelihood of the stone being removable, based largely on its position and size. If the surgeon lacks the skills required for minimally invasive choledochotomy and wishes to avoid conversion to open duct exploration, then laparoscopic chole-cystectomy may be performed and postoperative ERC arranged for stone removal. This has the obvious disadvantage that if this fails, the patient requires a further general anaesthetic and open duct exploration. Cholecystectomy under these circumstances should never be done if the patient is jaundiced, as the duct system is likely to be distended and the cystic duct clips may slip postoperatively; this is always a risk when this approach is taken, even in the absence of jaundice.

Routine peroperative cholangiography, performed where ductal stones were not suspected, identifies stones in 10 per cent of cases. This contrasts with the 5 per cent of cases where the ducts are not imaged, who present with postcholecystectomy chole-docholithiasis, thus suggesting that a large number of ductal stones pass spontaneously or else do not give rise to symptoms.

Surgical exploration of the common bile duct

Supraduodenal exploration

Most surgeons choose to explore the bile duct in this way. Its chief advantage is the easy access to the duct without the need to open the duodenum. The chief disadvantage is the uncertainty about the state of the lower end of the duct and the fact that the surgeon can never be entirely sure that all stones have been removed.

The duct is opened in a longitudinal direction and a sample of bile taken for culture. Stones can be removed with a combination of Desjardins forceps, balloon sweepage, and duct irrigation, ensuring that the lower end is cleared by passing the instruments through the ampulla into the duodenum. This manoeuvre can be aided by kocherizing the duodenum and exploring from the left of the patient. A postexploratory duct check with a flexible endoscope can minimize the risk of leaving stones behind.

Insertion of a T-tube

In general, it is unwise to simply close the bile duct after exploration; the duct needs to be decompressed with a T-tube to avoid the major complication of a postprocedure biliary leak caused by a retained stone. Impaction at the lower end of the duct would increase the intraduct pressure and decompress through the sutured duct closure. The size of the T-tube depends on the diameter of the duct, but care must be taken to avoid the lower limb of the tube straddling the ampulla as this is a possible cause of postoperative pancreatitis. It is customary to close the duct around the tube by placing sutures above the tube. When the tube is removed, the direction of force required to do so is downwards and this should avoid 'unzipping' the duct closure. The T-tube is removed between 7 and 10 days later, once the patency of the duct has been confirmed by a T-tube cholangiogram. If this test shows a retained stone, the tube is left in place while plans are made to remove the stone either by ERC or basket clearance via the T-tube track.

Transduodenal exploration of the bile duct

If a stone is lodged at the lower end of the bile duct then a transduodenal exploration (Fig. 19.9) may be required. There is a significant increase in morbidity with this procedure and it should only be undertaken after failure of more conservative measures. It requires complete mobilization of the duodenum and palpation of the ampulla on the medial duodenal wall. The essential part of this operation is to cannulate the bile duct and not the pancreatic duct before performing the sphincterotomy. If the wrong duct is divided, then a fatal postoperative pancreatitis may follow. There is no need for T-tube drainage of the duct following sphincterotomy.

It is occasionally impossible to dislodge stones from the lower end of the common bile duct and a choledochoduodenostomy may be required.

Bile duct injuries after laparoscopic cholecystectomy

Large American meta-analyses show that injury of the common bile duct is more common after laparoscopic than open cholecystectomy. The England and Wales audit commissioned by the Royal College of Surgeons showed a fivefold reduction in bile duct injuries over 4 years as the learning curve progressed.

The incidence of major bile-duct injuries appears to be the same in open and laparoscopic cholecystectomy, but minor injuries are more common after laparoscopic procedures. Identified mechanisms of injury include tenting of the bile duct by traction on the neck of the gallbladder, diathermy injuries, and failure to convert to open surgery when the anatomy cannot be safely demonstrated. If recognized during surgery, immediate repair is advised and the type of surgery required depends on the extent of the injury. The techniques vary from simple suture to Roux-en-Y bile-duct reconstruction. Bile-duct injuries may present in the postoperative period with the onset of jaundice or with clinical evidence of a major bile leak. The investigation of choice is an immediate ERC, which will demonstrate an occluded duct or a free intraperitoneal leak.

Bile leaks

The incidence of bile leaks after cholecystectomy is small and many can be managed conservatively; however, early diagnosis is imperative. Major bile-duct injuries may present with jaundice, but biliary peritonitis causes very few symptoms in the immediate postoperative period, so a high index of suspicion is required. Excessive pain or distension following laparoscopic cholecystectomy requires ultrasound scanning and ERCP if doubt persists. Leaks result from cystic-duct clip disruption (due to insecure placement or the presence of common bile duct stones), unclipped ducts of Luschka, or a small tangential hole in the bile duct with otherwise intact anatomy. Treatment options include percutaneous drainage, ERCP and stone extraction, stenting, or surgery and reconstruction. After Roux-en-Y reconstruction, recurrent bile-duct strictures are common (15–18 per cent), so a long follow-up period is required.

5   Other biliary tract disorders

5.1   Biliary tract malignancies

Gallbladder neoplasms

These may be benign or malignant. Benign polypoid tumours include lipomas, fibromas, papillomas, and adenomas. Pseudopolyps may be formed by inflammation surrounding cholesterol crystals in the wall. They are usually identified as an incidental finding in the specimen following cholecystectomy. Occasionally gallbladder polyps are seen on ultrasound scans for epigastric pain. They are predominantly cholesterol polyps and are unlikely to be the cause of the pain. However, larger **adenomatous polyps** may have malignant potential, particularly when fewer than three are present and they are larger than 10 mm in diameter. If these are identified on ultrasound scan, then cholecystectomy is recommended.

Carcinoma of the gallbladder represents 3–4 per cent of gastrointestinal cancers. Gallstones are present in 80–90 per cent and an association has been demonstrated with 'porcelain gallbladder', chronic typhoid carriers, and sclerosing cholangitis. Patients tend to present with advanced disease or else the

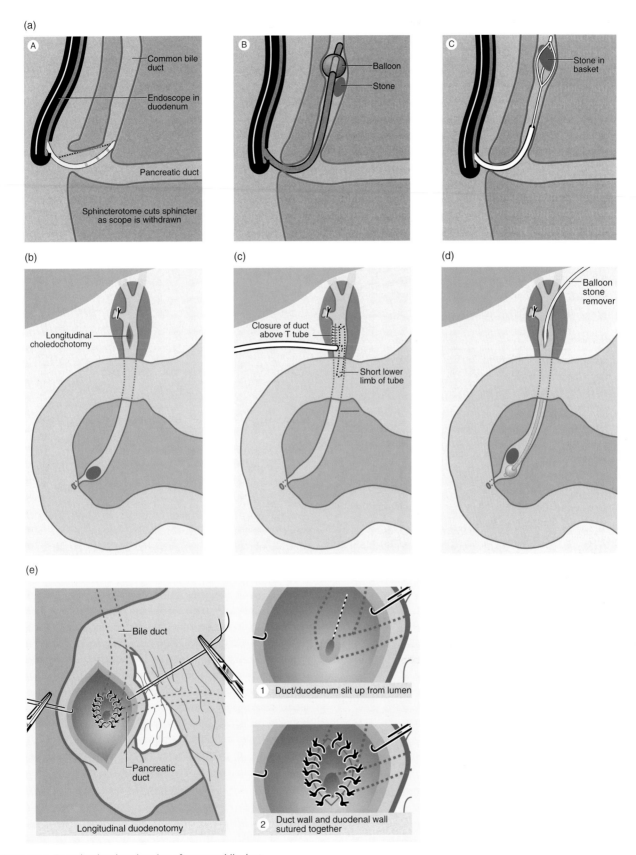

Figure 19.9 Transduodenal exploration of common bile duct.

diagnosis is made as an incidental finding after cholecystectomy for gallstones.

Staging of carcinoma of the gallbladder

Nevin's staging describes stage I carcinoma of the gallbladder as confined to the mucosa, stage II to the muscle layers, stage III penetrates the serosa, stage IV involves local lymph nodes, while stage V penetrates contiguous organs.

The treatment of gallbladder cancer is controversial. When serosal involvement has occurred, overall 3-year survival is only 7 per cent and this is not substantially improved by liver resection. This suggests that surgical resection may be inappropriate. For stage I and II disease identified incidentally in cholecystectomy specimens, further resection is recommended to ensure regional lymph-node clearance, together with a 2 cm margin of gallbladder bed and possibly resection of bile ducts. The 5-year survival for potentially curative resection is 52 per cent. A role for chemotherapy and radiotherapy has not been substantiated in gallbladder cancer.

Bile-duct neoplasms

Most bile-duct neoplasms are malignant, with papillomas and adenomas being very rare.

Cholangiocarcinoma

Cholangiocarcinoma represents 1 per cent of all gastrointestinal cancers. It is more common in the Far East where *Clonorchis sinensis* infestation is a major aetiological factor. Twenty to 50 per cent of cases of cholangiocarcinoma are associated with choledocholithiasis. Other associations include sclerosing cholangitis and choledochal cysts. The common aetiological factor seems to be biliary stasis. Cholangiocarcinomas are usually adenocarcinomas, and generally grow slowly, infiltrate locally, and metastasize late.

Presentation and investigation of cholangiocarcinoma

Ninety per cent of cases present with obstructive jaundice. The diagnosis is made with ultrasonography to demonstrate dilated ducts and ERC to demonstrate the anatomy, take biopsies, and cytological material. The tumours are classified according to position: **intrahepatic**, **proximal** (involving the right and left hepatic ducts), **middle**, and **distal**. For planned curative resection, preoperative investigation including ERCP, contrast enhanced CT scan, and angiography with portal venous phase imaging should ascertain resectability. Portal venous invasion, bilateral intrahepatic duct involvement, and extensive or bilateral involvement of the hepatic arterial or portal vein branches denotes inoperability.

Treatment of cholangiocarcinoma

Curative resection depends on the position of the tumour. Distal tumours are treated by excision of the biliary tree with pancreaticoduodenectomy; those which invade the unilateral intrahepatic biliary tree require hepatic resection; whereas the remainder require excision of the supraduodenal biliary tree and related lymph nodes. The treatment of tumours of the hepatic duct confluence remains controversial but resection with partial hepatectomy is possible.

Only 20 per cent of tumours are resectable; for the rest, surgical bypass provides the best palliation. If this is not possible, stents may be passed into the dilated biliary tree endoscopically or placed via the percutaneous transhepatic route. Most stents occlude at 4–6 months and will then require replacing. Expandable metallic stents have a slightly longer lifetime. No role of radiotherapy or chemotherapy has been established for cholangiocarcinoma. Following resection, the operative mortality is up to 5 per cent and the 5-year survival is 5–20 per cent.

5.2 Sclerosing cholangitis

This is a condition of unknown aetiology in which there is progressive fibrous obliteration of the biliary tract. It is an immune complex disorder with 70–80 per cent of cases associated with ulcerative colitis and, to a lesser extent, Crohn's disease. It is more common in males and the predominant age of onset is 40–50 years. It usually presents with cholestatic jaundice, although the diagnosis may be suggested by an incidental finding of raised alkaline phosphatase in patients with inflammatory bowel disease. The clinical course is variable, ranging from a protracted progression over many years to a rapid onset of liver failure and death in a few months. Sclerosing cholangitis is also associated with cholangiocarcinoma. In 80 per cent of cases there is diffuse involvement of the whole biliary tree. The diagnosis can be difficult, but is usually confirmed on cholangiography and staging investigations, as described earlier, if carcinoma is suspected.

Initial treatment is symptomatic, attempting to control pruritis and cholangitis. Indications for surgery are failure to control symptoms, progressive jaundice, and recurrent cholangitis and progressive cirrhosis.

The most effective form of treatment prior to the development of cirrhosis remains unclear. However, resection and long-term transhepatic stenting seems superior to endoscopic dilatation or percutaneous stenting in terms of reduction in bilirubin, 5-year survival, and time to requiring liver transplantation. Patients who develop cirrhosis should undergo liver transplantation, although recurrent sclerosing cholangitis can occur. After liver transplantation, published series suggest that where cholangiocarcinoma is an incidental finding in the pathological specimen, survival is unaffected. Patients with diagnosed cholangiocarcinoma rarely survived 6 months and transplantation cannot therefore be recommended in these cases.

5.3 Choledochal cysts

A choledochal cyst is a congenital dilatation of the extrahepatic bile ducts; this may include intrahepatic ducts. Any part of the system can dilate (Fig. 19.10); when there is intrahepatic dilatation, the condition is known as **Caroli's disease**. This is an autosomal recessive hereditary disorder with a poor prognosis

(a)

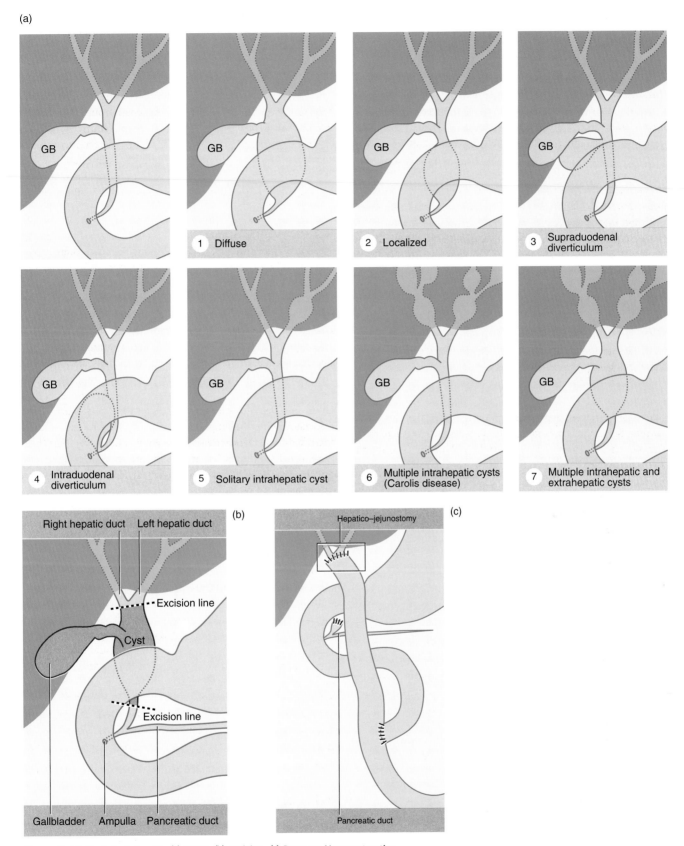

1 Diffuse

2 Localized

3 Supraduodenal diverticulum

4 Intraduodenal diverticulum

5 Solitary intrahepatic cyst

6 Multiple intrahepatic cysts (Carolis disease)

7 Multiple intrahepatic and extrahepatic cysts

(b)

Right hepatic duct   Left hepatic duct

Excision line

Cyst

Excision line

Gallbladder   Ampulla   Pancreatic duct

(c)

Hepatico–jejunostomy

Pancreatic duct

Figure 19.10 Choledochal cysts: (a) types; (b) excision; (c) Roux–en–Y reconstruction.

because of the development of intrahepatic stones, abscesses, ascending cholangitis, and ultimately cirrhosis.

Patients with a choledochal cyst present with jaundice, abdominal pain, and an abdominal mass. About one-third of cases present in childhood. The diagnosis is confirmed by ultrasound and ERCP. ERCP may demonstrate the anomalous junction of the pancreatic duct and the extrahepatic ducts; this leads to a very high amylase content in the extrahepatic bile. For resection of the cyst to be accomplished without damage to the main pancreatic duct, this junction has to be delineated carefully and this may best be achieved intraoperatively.

The most serious consequence of choledochal cyst is malignant change, with an overall risk of between 2.5 and 4 per cent. Because of this, excision is the recommended treatment rather than drainage via an internal anastomosis. An aetiological factor appears to be contact between the biliary epithelium and the pancreatic juice (with its high amylase content) via the anomalously sited pancreatic duct. Surgery therefore has to achieve two objectives: to separate the pancreatic juice from the biliary tract and to excise as much of the cyst wall as possible. The usual method is to excise the dilated part of the duct, close the distal bile duct proximal to the entry of the pancreatic duct, and effect biliary drainage by reconstruction with a hepatico-jejunostomy.

5.4   Extrahepatic obstructive jaundice

The clinical picture of icterus, pale stools (due to the absence of bile pigment), and dark urine (due to the urinary content of conjugated bilirubin) makes this diagnosis straightforward. The confirmation of a dilated extrahepatic biliary system by ultrasound avoids confusion with jaundice due to hepato-cellular dysfunction or, less commonly, liver replacement by metastatic cancer. The management is directed to the following considerations:

1. What is the cause of the jaundice? The history usually indicates that the jaundice is obstructive, but is not reliable in identifying the cause. Gallstones and pancreatic cancer are the most common causes and should feature high in the differential diagnosis (see Table 19.9).

2. Is the jaundice likely to resolve without intervention?

3. If intervention is required, what preparation is required before intervention in order to minimize complications?

4. How to treat the cause.

Table 19.9 Causes of obstructive jaundice

---
1. Gallstones
2. Carcinoma of the head of the pancreas
3. Periampullary cancer: bile duct, ampulla, duodenum
4. Obstruction of the porta hepatis by enlarged lymph nodes
5. Chronic pancreatitis
6. Benign stricture: iatrogenic, primary sclerosing cholangitis
---

Biliary imaging

Biliary ultrasonograpy

This is nearly always the first investigation. It can demonstrate extrahepatic duct dilatation and confirm the diagnosis of obstructive jaundice. It provides accurate imaging of stones in the gallbladder, a reasonable idea of the level of duct obstruction and shows the presence of liver metastases. It does not, however, provide reliable information on the distal third of the common bile duct, or of the presence of small masses (2 cm or less) in the head of the pancreas.

CT scanning with intravenous contrast

This technique is generally the investigation of choice for the pancreas. Spiral CT scanning has improved the speed of scanning in recent years and allows finer resolution of detail. CT can usually identify and differentiate between pancreatic carcinoma, chronic pancreatitis, acute pancreatitis, and pseudocyst formation, any of which may be obstructing the distal common bile duct. However, an important limitation is the ability to differentiate between a localized area of chronic pancreatitis and a small pancreatic carcinoma (which may even coexist). In addition, small cholangiocarcinomas are rarely visible. Both these diagnostic problems may be resolved by ERCP.

ERCP

This is most widely used therapeutically for extracting gallstones from the common bile duct, but is also an important diagnostic investigation for small pancreatic-head tumours, cholangiocarcinomas, and to identify the ductal changes of chronic pancreatitis.

Magnetic resonance cholangio-pancreatography

Magnetic resonance cholangio-pancreatography (MRCP) has recently been added to the biliary tract imaging armamentarium. It is non-invasive and avoids ionizing radiation. The images are acquired relatively rapidly but equipment and expertise not widely available. The technique has been shown to be 80 per cent sensitive in detecting common bile duct stones and 71 per cent sensitive in identifying normal biliary ducts compared with ERCP.

Is the jaundice likely to settle without intervention?

Most cases will not settle without intervention. The exception is when the jaundice follows an acute episode of biliary infection—either as a result of ascending cholangitis or when the inflammatory changes of acute cholecystitis involve the common hepatic duct (**Mirizzi syndrome**). Antibiotic treatment should always be used to treat the acute process, leaving the management of the gallstones for a later date. Complete duct occlusion, however, requires some immediate form of intervention.

Preparation of the jaundiced patient prior to timely intervention

The systemic disturbances brought about by the obstructive jaundice may lead to the following clinical problems:

(1) disruption in clotting factors owing to the failure of intestinal absorption of the fat-soluble vitamin K;

(2) susceptibility to acute renal failure, particularly in the presence of hypovolaemia and sepsis—**hepatorenal syndrome;**

(3) the potential to develop septicaemia as a result of a primary biliary infection.

Any procedure or operation performed on a jaundiced patient must take these factors into account and appropriate prophylactic measures must be taken to anticipate them. These include aggressive hydration, prophylactic broad-spectrum antibiotics, and daily injections of intramuscular vitamin K. If emergency intervention is required (surgical or endoscopic), fresh frozen plasma should be available.

Treating the cause of the obstruction

Gallstones are the most common cause of obstruction and their management has been covered earlier. The principle is to remove the duct stones endoscopically and then to prevent recurrence by performing cholecystectomy—in elderly or unfit patients this may be omitted. If the duct stones cannot be removed endoscopically, temporary drainage is achieved by placement of a bile-duct stent.

Curative resection is rarely possible for malignant obstruction of the extrahepatic duct system and most obstructive cases are palliated by endoscopic stenting.

6 Pancreas

6.1 Malignant tumours of the pancreas

Adenocarcinoma of the pancreas

The aetiology of adenocarcinoma of the pancreas is unknown but factors which have been implicated include cigarette smoking, alcohol, and diabetes mellitus. The prognosis is poor and the common adenocarcinoma has a 5-year survival of only 1–2 per cent. This is explained partly by the retroperitoneal

---

> **Box 19.1 Malignant tumours of the pancreas**
>
> 1. Adenocarcinoma of the pancreas usually presents late; 85 per cent of tumours are inoperable (i.e. incurable) at the time of presentation.
> 2. Curative surgery is possible for early tumours. Surgery should be undertaken by specialist surgeons to minimize morbidity.
> 3. Good palliation can be achieved by endoscopic stenting or surgical bypass.
> 4. Most of the rarer islet-cell tumours grow more slowly, and may benefit from debulking procedures.

location of the pancreas which allows tumours to enlarge to a size that makes them inoperable before producing symptoms. Experience dictates that adenocarcinoma of the pancreas must be regarded as incurable in nearly all cases. Management should focus on identifying the few cases that may be operable (up to 15 per cent) and endeavouring to avoid unnecessary surgery on the remaining 85 per cent of cases. Malignancies arising from other tissues within the pancreaticoduodenal segment (periampullary carcinomas) have a better prognosis, and surgery offers a greater chance of cure. Thus, the outlook for periampullary carcinomas is less bleak, with a 5-year survival as high as 40 per cent following resection. On the whole, these lesions justify a more aggressive approach.

Endocrine tumours of the pancreas

Pancreatic endocrine tumours are much less common than adenocarcinomas and have a variable malignant potential (Table 19.10). They are generally slow growing. They may present with symptoms caused by excessive hormone secretion (**insulinoma, gastrinoma**), or identified because of a mass effect (**non-functioning islet-cell tumour**). About 10 per cent of endocrine tumours are associated with multiple endocrine neoplasia type 1. This condition is inherited in an autosomal dominant fashion, and these patients should be screened for associated endocrine tumours, for the benefit of the patient and his or her relatives. The prognosis of different tumour types varies, but is often determined by the presence of multifocal

Table 19.10 Tumours of the pancreas

Tissue of origin	Histological type	Prognosis
Ductal	Adenocarcinoma (>80%)	Long-term survival rare
	Cystadenocarcinoma	50% 5-year survival
Acinar	Acinar cell carcinoma	Long-term survival rare
Islet	Insulinoma	10% are malignant
	VIPoma	50% are malignant
	Gastrinoma	60% are malignant
	Glucagonoma	60% are malignant
	Non-functioning	60% are malignant
Non-epithelial	Lymphoma (5%)	Responsive to chemotherapy

disease. It is important to emphasize that good relief of symptoms can often be achieved by palliative resection. Symptomatic metastases can be treated by therapeutic embolization at selective arteriography.

Clinical picture

Tumours occur most commonly in the **head** of the pancreas. Obstruction of the common bile duct means that they present with obstructive jaundice, often without pain. The absence of stones means that the bile is unlikely to be infected and cholangitis is an uncommon feature. In addition, the gallbladder is not fibrosed by inflammation and hence is able to dilate as a result of back pressure—**Courvoisier's sign**.

Tumours in the **body** and **tail** of the pancreas are more silent and present with insidious epigastric pain and weight loss. They invariably present at an advanced stage. Pain radiating through to the back indicates invasion of the coeliac plexus. Unexplained upper abdominal pain warrants abdominal CT scan to exclude pancreatic disease.

Investigation for a possible pancreatic cancer

1. A pancreatic mass can be detected by ultrasonography or CT scanning. Either of these investigations have a specificity of greater than 90 per cent, and a sensitivity of about 80 per cent. In cases where there is doubt, particularly for small tumours (<2 cm) such as periampullary carcinomas, diagnostic ERCP is required.

2. Once a mass has been demonstrated, the need for a tissue diagnosis must be addressed. This should be sought in all cases identified as being inoperable by CT scan (or by arterio-portography if performed). A tissue sample will occasionally diagnose a lymphoma which is likely to respond to chemotherapy. Concern about tract seeding and the significant false-negative biopsy rate make preoperative tissue diagnosis, in potentially resectable cases, unwarranted. Such lesions require excision in any case and this obviates the need for preoperative biopsy. Carrying out resection without biopsy inevitably means that the occasional case of focal pancreatitis is treated by radical surgery.

3. When required, a biopsy can be obtained preoperatively using fine-needle aspiration or Trucut core biopsy guided by ultrasound or CT scanning. In the rare case when a suspicious pancreatic lesion is first identified peroperatively, trans-duodenal Trucut biopsy (preferably after kocherizing the duodenum) minimizes the risk of a consequent pancreatic fistula.

4. Operability needs to be assessed systematically and progressively. If CT scanning raises doubt about local invasion or encasement of the portal vein, selective superior mesenteric artery arterioportography may help to clarify the picture, although spiral CT scanning with or without three-dimensional reconstruction of the vessels has reduced the need for arteriography. A chest X-ray, and CT scanning of the liver should be employed to exclude metastatic spread.

5. If the lesion appears operable, laparoscopy should be considered. This can identify small peritoneal deposits, which are not visible on scanning. Laparoscopic peritoneal lavage and cytology of the fluid has also been advocated to identify inoperable disease. Direct organ ultrasound scanning at laparoscopy and at ERCP is currently being evaluated. If any of these modalities suggests advanced disease, then attempted curative resection should not be undertaken. The purpose of these investigations is to minimize the number of laparotomies for inoperable disease. About 85 per cent of tumours are excluded from resection by these measures.

Selection of patients for attempted pancreatic resection

It is a commonly stated opinion that no patient should undergo resection for carcinoma of the pancreas because of the very poor prognosis. It is important to emphasize, however, that small lesions, completely resected, without nodal spread, have a 5-year survival of over 20 per cent. Patients to be considered for resection should fit the following criteria:

(1) fit for major surgery;

(2) have a primary tumour less than 3 cm in diameter;

(3) have no evidence of local invasion or distal spread.

It is interesting to note that 30 per cent of patients with pancreatic carcinoma have been diagnosed as suffering from maturity-onset diabetes within the preceding 2 years. It may be that this represents a suitable high-risk population for screening for early lesions.

In expert hands, resection should have a mortality of less than 5 per cent and a morbidity of less than 15 per cent. The patient must be aware of the risks of major surgery and the small chances of cure before such major surgery is undertaken.

Radical surgical excision for carcinoma of the pancreas

Whipple's operation (pancreaticoduodenectomy)

This is the most common operation performed because operable tumours nearly always lie in the pancreatic head. Tumours in the body and tail are rarely resectable. The same procedure is also used for resecting carcinomas of the ampulla, duodenum, or distal common bile duct. For lesions that are not in close proximity to the first part of the duodenum, a modified 'pylorus preserving' Whipple's operation is generally preferred, because of its reduced disturbance to digestion.

Postoperatively, patients may require pancreatic supplements to facilitate digestion of fats, and proton-pump inhibitors to minimize the potentially damaging effects of unopposed gastric acid secretion on the small bowel.

Pancreaticoduodenectomy comprises three stages:

(1) assessment of resectability (Fig. 19.11a);

(2) *en bloc* resection of the duodenum, distal common bile duct, head of pancreas, ± the gastric antrum (Fig. 19.11b);

(3) reconstruction (Fig. 19.11c).

(a)

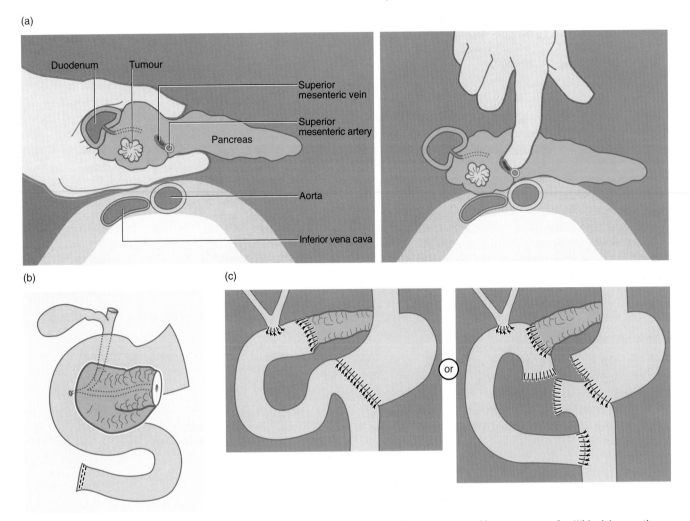

(b)

(c)

Figure 19.11 Whipple's operation: (a) assessing resectability; (b) the operative field after the resection; (c) anastomoses after Whipple's operation.

The principle of assessment is that no irreversible manoeuvre should be performed until the decision to proceed to resection has been taken. This requires a careful laparotomy, including assessment of lymph nodes in the free edge of the lesser omentum and porta hepatis. Suspicious nodes can be sent for frozen section. The inferior surface of the transverse mesocolon should be examined for local infiltration, particularly around the uncinate process. The retroperitoneum is assessed following full mobilization of the duodenum and head of pancreas from the vena cava. The lesser sac should then be opened to look for spread into the para-aortic and left gastric lymph-node chains. Finally, the plane between the neck of the pancreas and the superior mesenteric vein can be opened by blunt dissection to exclude involvement of the vein.

If all these sites are clear, resection can now proceed, usually by transsection of the common bile duct and stomach, with appropriate division of the lesser and greater omentum. The proximal jejunum is then divided, excluding the duodenal loop. The short segment of proximal small bowel mesentery is then divided close to the jejunal border for safety, along with the remaining attachment of the duodenum to the body of the

pancreas. This can produce troublesome bleeding behind the transverse mesocolon and the haemostatic clips are often best underrun with a fine suture. Prior to division of the neck of the pancreas over the superior mesenteric vein, two tied stay sutures should be passed through the superior and inferior borders of the pancreas to ligate the pancreaticoduodenal vessels. The pancreas can now be divided with a scalpel using a Kocher's dissector to protect the underlying vein. By gently reflecting the pancreatic head to the right, the final attachments of the pancreatic head to the portal vein can be divided. Again, underrunning the clips with a fine suture reduces the risk of bleeding from the short venous channels that run into the vein. Care must be taken to protect the superior mesenteric artery during this procedure, as it can be drawn to the right by traction on the duodenum.

Reconstruction requires three separate anastomoses. Usually the proximal divided end of jejunum can be advanced via a retrocolic route to anastomose to the remaining pancreas. The bile duct can be anastomosed end-to-side onto the anti-mesenteric border of the same loop. A separate, more distal loop of jejunum can be brought up to anastomose to the stomach.

Alternatively a Roux-en-Y loop can be fashioned to reduce subsequent bile reflux into the stomach.

The role of total pancreatectomy

More radical surgery has been advocated to reduce recurrence from multifocal disease and incomplete local tumour clearance. Operations include total or regional pancreatectomy, and total pancreatectomy with excision of the portal vein and superior mesenteric artery as they pass through the pancreas. Realistically, however, the number of cases which are suitable for the more radical approach is small and it is unlikely that justification could be provided by scientific analysis. Removal of all of the pancreas deals with the possible multifocal origin of pancreatic cancer and allows for a wider lymphatic clearance of the disease, but it cannot address the problem of microscopic residual disease in the retroperitoneum. The inevitable diabetes mellitus and loss of exocrine pancreatic function have to be balanced against the theoretical advantages of the wider excision.

Adjuvant therapy

Radiotherapy and monochemotherapy have not shown any survival advantage, either alone or as adjuvant therapy following surgical resection. However, multiagent adjuvant therapy has recently been shown to result in a survival advantage following 'curative' surgery. This is currently being evaluated in a European study.

Palliative treatment of pancreatic carcinoma

Insertion of a biliary stent to drain the bile duct

This is the preferred method of relieving jaundice, because of the low morbidity and reduced hospital stay. It has two drawbacks:

(1) the stents need to be changed periodically (50 per cent within 3 months);

(2) 15 per cent of patients go on to develop duodenal obstruction and may require surgery to relieve this late in the course of the disease.

Surgical relief of jaundice by a 'double bypass' technique (choledochojejunostomy and gastrojejunostomy)

Choledochojejunostomy and gastrojejunostomy are not the usual first-line therapy, but should be considered in younger patients with a longer life expectancy and also in patients with larger primaries who are more likely to develop gastric outlet symptoms. This treatment is otherwise held in reserve for situations where stenting alone fails. It is also used if, at laparotomy for attempted curative resection, the tumour is found to be inoperable, as this avoids a further laparotomy later for duodenal obstruction.

Cholecystojejunostomy can be used as an alternative to bile duct anastomosis if access to the duct is difficult. There is a risk, however, that a low cystic duct junction will become obstructed by the tumour.

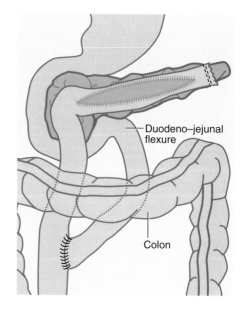

Figure 19.12 Longitudinal pancreaticojejunostomy.

Pain relief

Pain relief with narcotic drugs or coeliac axis block, or both, is a particularly important aspect of the management of the late stages of this disease.

Radiotherapy and chemotherapy

External-beam radiation, combined with 5FU as a radiosensitizer, results in marginally improved survival.

6.2 Chronic pancreatitis

This is summarized in Table 19.11. The range of procedures for chronic pancreatitis include:

(1) pancreatic duct decompression by pancreaticojejunostomy;

(2) pseudocyst drainage;

(3) interruption of pain pathways by coeliac plexus block; however, this is not effective in the long term;

(4) pancreatic resection.

Pancreatography demonstrates the sites of pancreatic duct strictures and dictates which of these procedures is logical.

Chronic pancreatitis most commonly affects men in their late middle age, with a history of long-standing excessive alcohol

Table 19.11 Chronic pancreatitis

Rare, but with marked geographic variation

Alcohol abuse is the most common aetiology

The main elements of treatment are abstinence from alcohol, oral pancreatic supplements, control of diabetes and provision of good analgesia

Operations are only indicated in the small group of patients who fail to respond to pain-relieving measures consumption. It is also less commonly seen following recurrent acute pancreatitis. However, in a substantial proportion of cases the cause in unknown. Chronic pancreatitis is generally a progressive condition that is characterized by periods of severe exacerbation and spontaneous remission.

The main aspects of treatment are pain control, often requiring opiate analgesia during exacerbations, dietary supplements to improve malabsorption, control of diabetes, and abstinence from alcohol. In most cases, the disease burns itself out over a period of years, but in a small group of patients surgery is required to control florid disease or deal with its complications.

The diagnosis is based primarily on the history, together with supportive evidence of chronic pancreatic damage. The pivotal investigations are CT scanning showing deformity, cystic degeneration, and calcification, and ERCP with demonstration of ductal abnormalities. Corroborative evidence may have been provided by the finding of calcification on a plain abdominal X–ray, hyperglycaemia, and steatorrhoea. Formal assessments of exocrine functions are only rarely required and in equivocal cases. In general, they lack the necessary sensitivity in early disease for which they would be most clinically useful, and are most effective in diagnosing gross insufficiency, which is usually clinically obvious. Careful assessment of the extent of disease by CT scanning and ERCP are essential for planning surgery.

The clinical importance of chronic pancreatitis is as a cause of chronic abdominal pain and as an important differential diagnosis in pancreatic cancer. The correct diagnosis may sometimes be reached only following resection (see Table 19.12).

Selecting cases suitable for surgery

Patients with chronic pancreatitis are usually debilitated from poor nutrition, immunocompromised from chronic alcohol abuse, and suffering from chronic respiratory disease from smoking. As a result, patients are high risk of early postoperative complications and late mortality (>30 per cent at 5 years) from intercurrent disease. Surgery should therefore be offered only to those who are most likely to receive long-term relief of symptoms (70 per cent of cases in published series). Abstinence from alcohol should be a requirement as continued drinking is likely to cause disease progression and early recurrence of symptoms. Cases with localized disease or duct dilatation are most likely to benefit from surgery.

Surgical options in chronic pancreatitis

Marked duct dilatation (>7 mm) is amenable to drainage. This is usually best achieved by laying open the duct and anastomosing it side-to-side, usually to a Roux loop of jejunum (longitudinal pancreaticojejunostomy, Fig. 19.12). This is especially appropriate for chronic pancreatitis because the duct commonly contains several short strictures, and the procedure achieves drainage of the whole duct and minimizes the chances of later

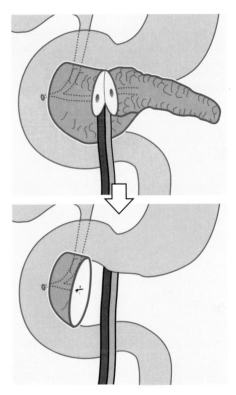

Figure 19.13 Distal pancreatectomy.

Table 19.12 Differentiation between chronic pancreatitis and carcinoma of the head of the pancreas

Common features	Chronic pancreatitis	Pancreatic cancer
Obstructive jaundice	May fluctuate	Usually progressive
Calcification (CT)	Common; may be florid	Rare; usually localized
Cysts (US or CT)	Common and multiple	Rare, seen in cystadenocarcinoma
CBD obstruction (ERC)	Smooth, tapered stenosis	Abrupt cut-off
Pancreatic duct	Multiple strictures	Sharp cut-off
Obstruction (ERP)	'Chain of lakes'	Distal dilatation
Vascular occlusion (CT)	Rare	Stricture of SMV/portal vein
Selective (arteriography)	Splenic vein thrombosis common	

CT, computed tomography; ERC, endoscopic retrograde cholangiography; ERP, ; SMV, ; US, ultrasound.

stricturing at the anastomosis. Localized disease in the head or tail of the pancreas may be amenable to resection.

Distal pancreatectomy (Fig. 19.13) was at one time combined with drainage into a Roux loop, but it has been shown that the duct will inevitably undergo stricture formation. Thus the procedure is only performed in the presence of proximal obstruction. As this is a benign disease, an attempt should be made to preserve the spleen, but local inflammation can make this a risky undertaking.

Subtotal pancreatectomy can be performed without resection of the duodenum (**duodenal-preserving proximal pancreatectomy**). In this procedure, a rim of pancreatic tissue is left in order to preserve the blood supply to the duodenal loop, and the head of the pancreas is resected, leaving the common bile duct intact and draining via the ampulla. The morbidity from such major surgery and the associated loss of endocrine and exocrine function means that this procedure is rarely employed.

Surgery for the complications of chronic pancreatitis

Pancreatic cysts

After pain, this is the most common reason for surgery in this condition. Pancreatic pseudocysts may complicate acute and chronic pancreatitis, and their management is similar. Large cysts (5 cm or greater) that have been present for longer than 6 weeks are unlikely to resolve spontaneously. They may give rise to symptoms because of compression of other structures such as the common bile duct or the duodenum. This may result from infection, especially after repeated bouts of external drainage, or because of bleeding, usually due to erosion of adjacent vessels. In chronic pancreatitis, it can be difficult to know if pain is primarily due to the cyst, or if the cyst is merely a manifestation of underlying parenchymal disease and duct occlusion. In these cases a preoperative ERCP to assess the state of the duct may be helpful, but often the dilemma can only be resolved by cyst drainage.

Internal drainage is the procedure of choice. This can be achieved via a cysto-gastrostomy or a cysto-duodenostomy, but is preferentially performed by Roux–en–y cysto-jejunostomy (Fig. 19.14). This excludes the cyst contents from food and bile and should prevent activation of the pancreatic secretions until they are within the jejunum. The optimal point of drainage can be inferred from the CT scan, where the cyst wall is thin (and extrapancreatic). This may be via the lesser sac through the stomach, anterior or posterior to the second part of the duodenum, or through the transverse mesocolon. Careful assessment of these areas should be made at operation. It is worth emphasizing that safe anastomosis is best achieved by suture to the fibrous wall of the cyst, and that the friable, surrounding inflammatory tissue should be removed from the area of fenestration and anastomosis.

Biliary obstruction

This can be due to occlusion by a pseudocyst, but is more commonly due to fibrosis around the common bile duct as it passes through the pancreas. As chronic pancreatitis is a progressive condition, definitive bypass (choledocho-jejunostomy) or resection of the head of the pancreas is required.

Haemorrhage

This is a rare complication, usually occurring in the presence of a pseudocyst. If cyst drainage has been performed, haemorrhage manifests as bleeding into the GI tract. If not, the pseudocyst may form part of the wall of a false aneurysm. For this reason it is always best to aspirate the cyst, prior to fenestration. If there is doubt preoperatively, then selective angiography should be performed. The treatment of choice for a false aneurysm is selective arterial embolization. The most commonly involved major vessel is the splenic artery.

Infection

This is a serious complication, for which preventative measures should be taken. Although it may occur spontaneously, it most commonly follows instrumentation. Percutaneous drainage of

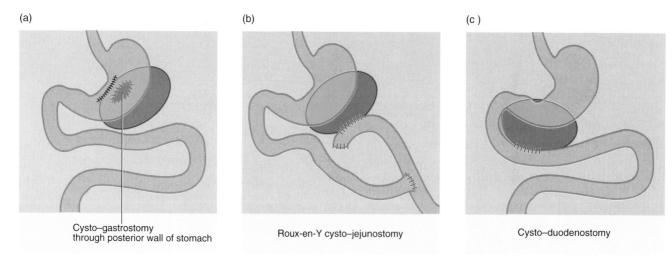

(a)   (b)   (c)

Cysto–gastrostomy through posterior wall of stomach

Roux-en-Y cysto–jejunostomy

Cysto–duodenostomy

Figure 19.14 Surgical drainage of a pancreatic pseudocyst (a) Cysto-gastrostomy; (b) Roux-en-Y cysto-jejunostomy; (c)cysto-duodenostomy.

established pseudocysts it unlikely to be beneficial and should therefore be resisted. Infection may also follow ERCP. Percutaneous drainage should always be covered by antibiotics, especially if a cyst is suspected. ERCP should only be performed in the presence of a pseudocyst if it is likely to influence management (e.g. if resection of the pancreatic head is being considered as the primary procedure).

7 Liver surgery

7.1 Liver anatomy

Performing surgery on the liver requires familiarity with its internal architecture (Fig. 19.15) in order to plan resections, minimize blood loss, and maintain the blood supply and biliary drainage of the remaining tissue. The capacity of normal liver parenchymal cells to hypertrophy and undergo hyperplasia allows resection of up to 75 per cent of the organ to be undertaken safely. However, it should be noted that this regenerative capacity is impaired in the cirrhotic liver. Early recovery of function is also impaired by obstructive jaundice.

Liver resections are most commonly performed for treatment of primary and secondary malignancies. Anatomical resection is preferable to enucleation so that satisfactory resection margins of 1 cm or more can be achieved. Local resection is sometimes employed in cirrhotic livers with small primary tumours in order to preserve sufficient functional parenchyma. In adults, the most common primary tumours are **hepatocellular carcinoma** and **cholangiocarcinoma**. The most common secondary tumours considered for resection are metastases from colorectal primaries (see below). Operability is determined by:

- the general health of the patient;
- the number and distribution of metastases within the liver;
- the presence of extrahepatic disease;
- the site of the tumour in the liver;
- the function of the uninvolved liver tissue.

Unfortunately, most primary malignancies are inoperable at the time of presentation. With hepatocellular carcinomas, at least two-thirds of cancers develop in a cirrhotic liver and the remaining liver cells have insufficient residual function to compensate for a major anatomical resection. Intrahepatic cholangiocarcinoma most commonly presents with obstructive jaundice as a result of a tumour at the confluence of the right and left hepatic ducts. Surgery would involve an extended resection which greatly increases the risk of postoperative hepatic decompensation.

7.2 Investigation of a hepatic mass

Hepatic masses may be solid or cystic and these can be readily differentiated by ultrasound scanning. The increased use of abdominal scanning for a wide range of conditions is bringing to light increasing numbers of incidental asymptomatic lesions.

Liver lesions detectable on ultrasound:

1. **Simple cysts** were historically believed to be rare, but are now known to be present in 1 per cent of the population. Cysts are multiple in 50 per cent of cases. Nearly all are asymptomatic, although large cysts may produce pressure symptoms. Cysts are smooth-walled, rounded lesions. It is important to differentiate a simple cyst from a hydatid cyst. The latter usually

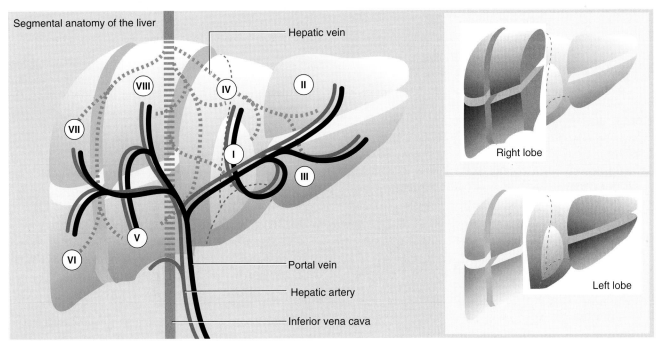

Figure 19.15 Anatomy of the liver.

contains daughter cysts, but if there is doubt serological tests should be performed. The diagnosis of a simple cyst is confirmed by aspirating clear fluid.

2. A **pyogenic liver abscess** can present in a subacute fashion, with night sweats, anorexia, and weight loss, making the clinician suspicious of an underlying neoplasm. However, an ultrasound scan readily differentiates an abscess from a solid tumour. The plasma liver enzymes, particularly alkaline phosphatase, are often elevated. Lesions of this type should be aspirated for culture and Gram staining. With the availability of accurate localization techniques, the initial treatment should be by percutaneous drainage (often multiple) and appropriate antibiotic therapy. Transpleural drainage should be avoided because of the risk of causing an empyema. Abscesses that fail to resolve with conservative measures require surgical drainage.

3. **Hydatid cyst of the liver** may present as an asymptomatic mass. These cysts have a typical appearance on ultrasound scan, when the encased daughter cysts can be clearly seen. The presence of thick calcification in the wall indicates the main cyst is dead, although some small daughter cysts may still contain live brood capsules. The lesions should not be biopsied as this may result in peritoneal contamination. The diagnosis should be confirmed by a specific complement fixation test. Treatment usually involves primary medical therapy with flubendazole and secondary surgery. Old calcified cysts can be left if they are asymptomatic, and cysts deep in the liver parenchyma may be better treated medically and expectantly.

4. Solid hepatic tumours are often identified incidentally by abdominal ultrasound scanning, performed for investigation of unrelated problems. Asymptomatic lesions are more likely to be benign (Table 19.13). Rapidly growing malignant lesions become painful because of stretching of the capsule.

Basic investigations for all solid lesions should include plasma liver enzymes to look for evidence of underlying liver pathology, plasma tumour markers (CEA, AFP, CA19–9), and a contrast-enhanced CT scan. In the presence of normal results from the blood tests, and no specific features of malignancy on CT scanning, asymptomatic lesions can often be safely treated expectantly and the patient reassured. If the lesion(s) are suspected of being adenomas or focal nodular hyperplasia, any corticosteroid treatment should be withdrawn. Symptomatic lesions may require definitive histological diagnosis unless a

Table 19.13 Benign liver tumours

Cholangioadenoma	Very common, incidental finding at laparotomy
Haemangioma	Usually asymptomatic; can be treated expectantly
Hepatic adenoma (focal nodular hyperplasia)	Promoted by steroids, the oral contraceptive pill; may progress during pregnancy
Cystadenoma	Rare, not neoplastic

haemangioma is the likely diagnosis. Ultrasound or CT-guided percutaneous biopsy is usual, although the results can be misleading for some benign lesions. Biopsy should not be carried out if there is any suggestion of malignancy as resultant seeding along the needle track would make the tumour inoperable.

Markedly elevated AFP should be considered diagnostic of hepatoma and the patient investigated as to resectability. Metastatic disease is usually suspected because of a previous primary tumour resection. Again, elevated tumour markers can be considered diagnostic, particularly if the lesion was not present on a previous scan. Diagnostic difficulties in asymptomatic lesions can occasionally be aided by MRI scanning. In particular, T_2-weighted images can confirm a haemangioma.

Assessing the resectability of liver tumours

The prognosis for primary hepatic malignancy is poor, with an overall 5-year survival of less than 10 per cent. The role of surgical resection is limited because of multifocal disease, late presentation, and underlying cirrhosis. Despite this, surgery offers good palliation in selected cases and occasional long-term cure. In appropriate cases, liver resection now carries a low morbidity and mortality when carried out by trained liver surgeons. As with all major upper abdominal surgery, underlying respiratory disease adds to the morbidity and slows postoperative recovery.

Resection is regarded as appropriate if the following criteria are met:

1. There is sufficient residual liver to compensate for the reduced liver function.

2. There is no invasion of the common bile duct, portal vein, vena cava, or spread beyond the liver. Assessment may require selective angiography in addition to contrast-enhanced CT scanning and chest X-ray. Angiography also provides anatomical information on the presence of accessory or anomalous arteries supplying the liver.

3. There is no spread beyond the liver capsule. This may be best assessed at laparoscopy. This is also the most sensitive method for identifying small peritoneal deposits. It can also be used to acquire a liver biopsy, and perform intraoperative ultrasound scanning.

7.3 Liver resection (right hepatectomy)

Right hepatectomy (Fig. 19.16) can be considered in four stages:

Access

This is best achieved via a 'rooftop' upper abdominal incision, with a midline extension upwards. The liver should then be fully mobilized from its peritoneal attachments.

Control of major blood vessels

Having assessed the tumour, with or without intraoperative ultrasound, and excluded macroscopic spread, it is necessary to achieve control over the blood supply and venous drainage. This

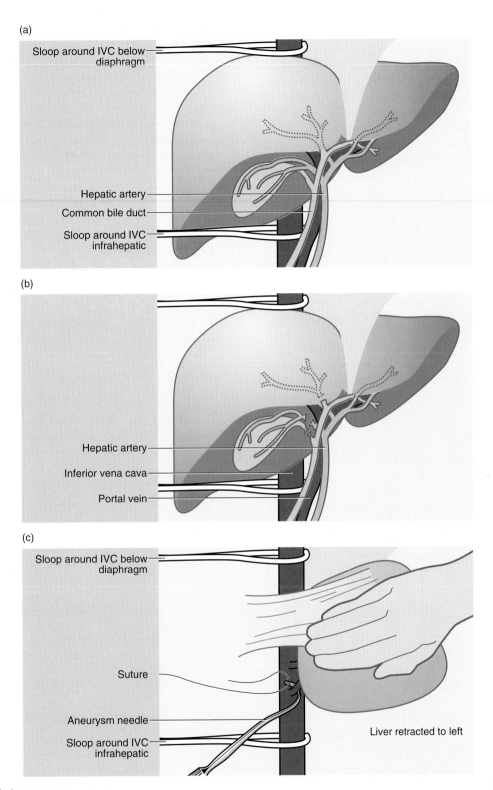

(a)

Sloop around IVC below diaphragm

Hepatic artery

Common bile duct

Sloop around IVC infrahepatic

(b)

Hepatic artery

Inferior vena cava

Portal vein

(c)

Sloop around IVC below diaphragm

Suture

Aneurysm needle

Sloop around IVC infrahepatic

Liver retracted to left

Figure 19.16 Right hepatectomy.

requires placing a silicone sling around the suprahepatic vena cava below the diaphragm and the infrahepatic cava, above the renal veins. For a right hemi-hepatectomy (also known as right hepatectomy), the right superior adrenal vein can be ligated at this stage. The vein is identified by dividing the peritoneum over the right side of the vena cava.

Dissection of the porta hepatis

A 'fundus first' cholecystectomy allows identification of the lateral border of common hepatic bile duct and the portal vein behind it. The fascial coverings can be laid open by extending the incision into the portal hepatis, exposing the left and right ducts. Access may be improved at this stage by dividing the tissue bridge across the umbilical fissure. The right duct is then divided between artery forceps, and the proximal limb is oversewn. The distal end of the duct can be ligated. The right hepatic artery is now identified and divided to expose the right portal vein. This is also divided between artery forceps, taking care not to tear the short branch to the caudate lobe that often branches off posteriorly. All the portal structures are best oversewn as ligatures tend to slip off during manipulation of the liver. A line of demarcation will now become apparent on the liver, identifying the principal vascular plane.

Resection

Prior to resection, the right hepatic vein should be identified as it enters the cava. It usually has an extrahepatic course sufficient to allow it to be divided prior to liver resection. Access can be improved by early ligation of the short hepatic veins entering the posterior surface of the liver. These can be approached from the right side by dislocating the right hepatic lobe anteriorly, and divided between fine ties. Great care must be exercised as any tear in the vena cava or right hepatic artery at this stage results in major blood loss and possibly air embolism. Once sufficient length of right hepatic vein has been exposed, it should be divided between vascular clamps and the cut ends oversewn with a vascular suture.

The line of resection should pass from the left side of the hepatic vein into the gallbladder bed. The liver capsule can be divided with diathermy and the liver substance fractured by blunt finger dissection or with an ultrasound dissector. The purpose of either manoeuvre is to identify the small intrahepatic vessels or ducts which are then individually ligated with fine sutures. Very small vessels can be divided by diathermy. As the dissection proceeds it is helpful to gradually open the fracture site by lifting the liver forward. Major haemorrhage can be controlled by clamping the cava, and if necessary, temporarily clamping the free edge of the lesser omentum (**Pringle's manoeuvre**). As the dissection deepens, the larger branches of the portal structures are identified and ligated. Deep to these, the major hepatic vein tributaries are encountered. Once the posterior liver surface is reached, any remaining short hepatic vein branches into the cava must be identified and individually ligated. Major haemorrhage is usually from these vessels or from branches of the middle hepatic vein. After resection, one or two wide-bore tube drains are placed in the hepatic bed. Good haemostasis is essential as a degree of coagulopathy is likely to follow surgery. Oozing from the liver surface may be controlled with haemostatic gauze or a proprietary collagen spray.

Complications of liver resections

Haemorrhage

This can be minimized by careful surgical technique. Post-operative bleeding should prompt aggressive replacement of clotting factors with fresh frozen plasma, cryoprecipitate, and platelets, as required. Any bleeding leads to impaired liver function and exacerbates any underlying coagulopathy.

Infection

Pneumonia and pulmonary collapse commonly complicate liver resection and the risk needs to be minimized by pre- and post-operative physiotherapy. Collections of blood and bile in the liver bed should be actively sought by ultrasound scanning, and drained percutaneously if identified.

Acute liver failure

This is a rare complication in the absence of jaundice or cirrhosis. However, once it has developed, successful conservative management is unlikely.

7.4 Non-surgical therapy of liver tumours

Liver tumours are not generally responsive to radiotherapy and high doses of radiotherapy result in damage to the liver parenchyma. Systemic chemotherapy may help reduce symptoms of pain but cannot be offered in the presence of jaundice. Locoregional chemotherapy is currently under trial for irresectable hepatomas: an antitumour agent, SMANCS, can be given via a hepatic artery cannula, in the form of a preparation suspended in ethiodol which is selectively taken up by hepatoma cells. Preliminary findings have indicated a very high response rate. This may provide a therapeutic alternative for the treatment of unresectable liver cell tumours. Percutaneous ethanol injection has been used to palliate hepatoma. Injection into the parenchyma at the periphery of the tumour produces coagulative necrosis followed by granuloma formation, fibrosis, and local vessel thrombosis. In small tumours, it has produced results similar to resection.

Transplantation has been used for tumours limited to the liver, and has the theoretical advantage of removing multifocal disease. The short-term survival is good, but unfortunately, recurrence is early and aggressive, presumably due to the necessary immunosuppressive therapy. For this reason it is not currently considered to be a satisfactory therapeutic option.

7.5 Hepatic colorectal metastases

The liver is the most common site of metastatic disease in colorectal cancer. Liver metastases develop in over two-thirds of all cases of colorectal cancer and have been identified as a major determinant of survival. Survival is dependent on the extent to which the liver is replaced by tumour, ranging from a mean of 3 months for a heavy tumour load to 25 months for a solitary metastasis.

Liver resection is now considered an important therapeutic option in selected cases of metastatic colorectal cancer. Large series have shown 5-year survival in excess of 25 per cent for selected cases, compared with less than 1 per cent for untreated solitary metastases. However, no prospective randomized trial has been performed.

Good prognostic factors include:

◆ three or fewer lesions;

◆ metastases confined to one lobe;

◆ no lesion larger than 5 cm;

◆ no macroscopic metastases at the time of primary resection.

The timing of liver resection for operable metastases found at primary surgery is controversial. It is generally felt that those discovered unexpectedly should be assessed in the light of the primary tumour pathology before considering resection, although some surgeons do perform planned synchronous resection. Following liver resection, 15–40 per cent of patients subsequently develop further hepatic metastases. One-third of these are suitable for further liver resection.

Recent studies have also been performed to assess locoregional therapy in the treatment of unresectable hepatic metastases. Therapeutic options include cryotherapy and alcohol injection. Cryotherapy is administered at open operation using liquid nitrogen circulated through insulated probes placed in the tumour under ultrasound guidance. Disease-free survival of 25 per cent at a median follow up of 2–3 years has been reported.

The only treatment that has been assessed in a prospective fashion is locoregional chemotherapy, via an hepatic artery catheter. Phase II pilot studies have indicated a response rate of 60 per cent and an overall survival advantage. A multicentre trial of systemic versus locoregional chemotherapy is currently under way. Hepatic artery perfusion is preferred over portal venous perfusion because hepatic tumours derive their blood supply preferentially from the hepatic artery (unlike the liver parenchyma).

The optimal management of hepatic metastases from colorectal carcinoma is not yet established. However, patients with disease limited to one lobe should be considered for resection. Patients with unresectable metastases can be offered locoregional chemotherapy. For the present this therapeutic option ought to be restricted to patients entered into prospective randomized trials.

8 Portal hypertension

Raised pressure within the portal venous system is most commonly due to cirrhosis and in Western society this is usually secondary to alcohol. Extrahepatic causes are less common and include **prehepatic** (portal vein thrombosis) or **posthepatic** (Budd–Chiari syndrome) causes. Raised portal venous pressure results in diversion of venous flow via collaterals into the systemic venous system, bypassing the liver. Clinically, the most important collaterals are the submucosal veins in the distal oesophagus, which become congested, forming oesophageal varices. These varices are at risk of spontaneous rupture and potentially life-threatening haemorrhage. Gastric and rectal varices are seen less commonly, but are similarly predisposed to haemorrhage. Portal hypertension may also be complicated by

Table 19.14 Management of bleeding oesophageal varices

- Acute management requires resuscitation, replacement of clotting factors and pharmacological lowering of portal hypertension
- Emergency endoscopy and sclerotherapy is the treatment of choice. Banding of varices may be performed when acute bleeding settles
- Balloon tamponade may be required for sustained or massive haemorrhage
- Follow-up sclerotherapy is required in all cases
- Transjugular intrahepatic portosystemic shunting if bleeding fails to respond
- Emergency surgery carries a prohibitively high operative mortality and should probably be restricted to oesophageal transsection
- Elective portosystemic shunting should be restricted to young, fit patients with good liver function. This is a small group, often with portal hypertension caused by a thrombosed portal vein

ascites or encephalopathy. Portal hypertension only requires treatment for its complications—the most important and life-threatening being bleeding oesophageal varices.

8.1 Management of oesophageal varices

Up to 60 per cent of acute variceal haemorrhage ceases spontaneously. Acute management is medical, requiring aggressive supportive therapy and pharmacological therapy to reduce portal venous pressure (Table 19.14). This usually includes a vasopressin infusion and sublingual nitroglycerine. Vasopressin alone causes systemic vasoconstriction so nitrate is added to counteract this. Somatostatin and its analogues has been shown to reduce splanchnic blood flow selectively but it is not yet widely used. Emergency endoscopy is required to confirm the source of bleeding and, where possible, treatment with emergency sclerotherapy. In patients with persistent major haemorrhage, sclerotherapy may not be possible. After initial control of bleeding with sclerotherapy, endoscopic variceal banding may be more effective in reducing further haemorrhage.

Persistent or massive haemorrhage may be controlled by balloon tamponade using a modified Sengstaken (Minnesota) tube (Fig. 19.17). Others prefer the intragastric Linton balloon, which allows sclerotherapy while compressing varices at the oesophagogastric junction. The Minnesota tube has four lumens, two connected to balloons for the stomach and the lower oesophagus, one for aspiration of the stomach, and one for aspiration of the upper oesophagus. The tube is passed via the mouth. Once the stomach is reached, the gastric balloon is inflated first, and the tube pulled up to provide tamponade of the gastro-oesophageal junction. The oesophageal balloon can then be inflated to 40 mmHg. The balloons should be decompressed within 12 hours to minimize the risk of ulceration. Endoscopic sclerotherapy should be re-attempted within 12 hours. The tube should not be replaced after sclerotherapy, because of the increased risk of ulceration.

The early mortality from an acute variceal haemorrhage approaches 50 per cent. Survival is closely related to the severity of underlying liver disease. This is related to the increased risk of

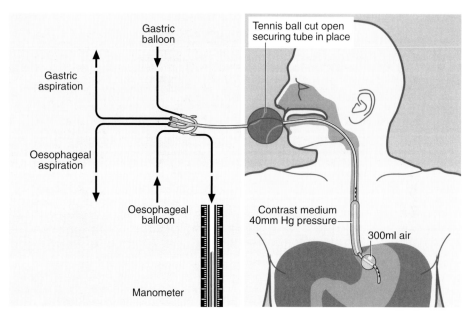

Figure 19.17 Sengstaken (Minnesota) tube.

rebleeding and concomitant hepatic failure. Following an acute variceal bleed, the patient has a 70 per cent risk of a further haemorrhage unless further treatment is instigated. This risk is greatest in the 2 months after a bleed. Follow-up sclerotherapy has been shown to control rebleeding in up to 90 per cent of cases. For cases that rebleed despite these measures, consideration should be given to surgery, but unfortunately many have insufficient reserve of liver function to undergo a portosystemic shunt.

Transjugular intrahepatic portosystemic shunt (TIPSS) is a recently introduced therapeutic option (Fig. 19.18). It can be used to control portal hypertension, even in the acute situation. The right hepatic vein is cannulated via a transjugular approach and a stylet passed into the portal vein under radiological control. The tract is dilated and held open using an expandable metallic stent. This procedure can result in immediate control of the portal hypertension and may replace surgery for the acute setting. Unlike surgically constructed portosystemic shunts, TIPSS does not disrupt the extrahepatic vasculature. This may be important if transplantation is indicated. Thirty to 50 per cent of TIPS shunts thrombose within a year and require revision.

8.2 Surgery for portal hypertension

Stapled transsection of the oesophagus

This is principally indicated in acute variceal bleeding resistant to sclerotherapy. Having mobilized the abdominal oesophagus, an endoluminal circular stapler is inserted via an anterior gastrotomy. The gun is advanced just beyond the gastro-oesophageal junction. A strong tie is placed between the anvil and cartridge. The gun is then fired, resecting a short segment of oesophagus, and effecting re-anastomosis. This procedure is

complicated if there are large collateral vessels around the oesophageal hiatus. These are best divided between ligatures early on to avoid bleeding. Scarring around the hiatus is also encountered if repeated sclerotherapy has been employed. Early rebleeding following transection is uncommon, but new varices form in time and should be treated by injection sclerotherapy.

Oesophagogastric devascularization is also advocated in the acute situation, and can be used in combination with oesophageal transection. It is a more lengthy procedure in the presence of portal hypertension and is less widely used in these unstable patients.

Division of the short gastric vessels can be employed as an adjunctive procedure if gastric fundal varices have been identified at endoscopy.

Portosystemic shunts

Introduction

Experience has determined that these procedures (Fig. 19.19) do not alter the prognosis of bleeding oesophageal varices. Shunting reduces portal venous pressure but the accompanying encephalopathy is exacerbated by the decreased function of the cirrhotic liver, and this means that the patient does not benefit overall. As a consequence, surgical shunts are usually restricted to a small group of young patients with satisfactory liver function.

Techniques of surgical portosystemic shunting

1. **End-to-side or side-to-side portocaval shunting** is achieved by dividing the portal vein in the free edge of the lesser omentum, and anastomosis of the proximal limb to the underlying inferior vena cava. This procedure is the 'gold standard' for achieving the surgical objective of a sustained fall in the portal venous pressure and long-term patency.

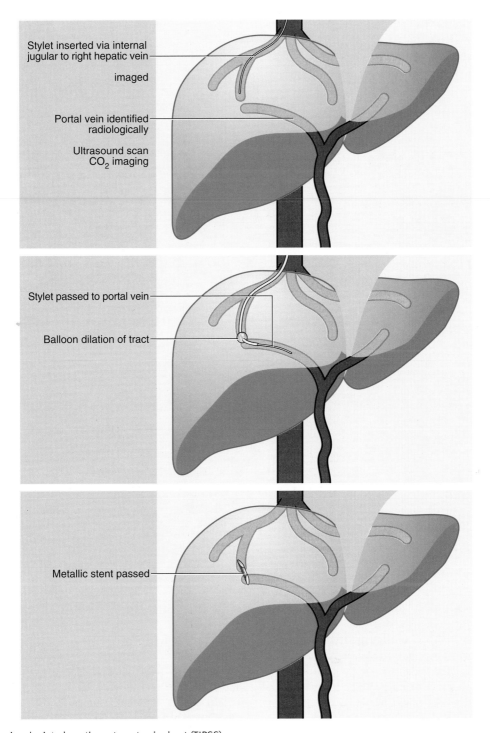

Stylet inserted via internal jugular to right hepatic vein

imaged

Portal vein identified radiologically

Ultrasound scan CO₂ imaging

Stylet passed to portal vein

Balloon dilation of tract

Metallic stent passed

Figure 19.18 Transjugular intrahepatic portosystemic shunt (TIPSS).

Concern about the procedure centres on the complete loss of portal blood flow to the liver, potentially increasing the risk of encephalopathy.

2. The conventional **lienorenal shunt** requires a splenectomy and anastomosis of the portal end of the splenic vein to the left renal vein. The narrower calibre of these vessels necessarily results in a lower long-term patency rate for the shunt.

The reported reduced incidence of encephalopathy may reflect thrombosis of the shunt and probably results in an increased recurrent bleed rate.

3. The **mesocaval shunt** involves the formation of a side-to-side shunt between the infracolic superior mesenteric vein and the inferior vena cava, usually using an autologous vein graft such as the internal jugular vein. No reduction in the incidence of

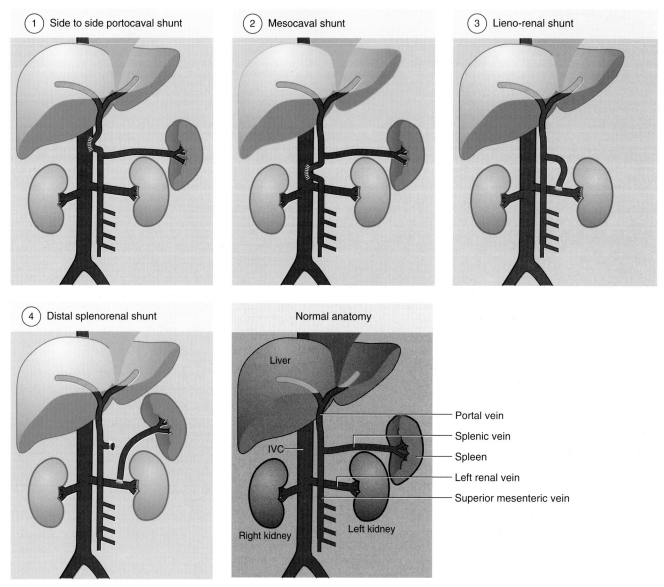

Figure 19.19 Portosystemic shunts.

encephalopathy has been demonstrated but the procedure may be applicable when liver enlargement, as in Budd–Chiari syndrome, limits access to the portal vein. All of these procedures have a high incidence of postoperative encephalopathy (variably reported between 10 and 50 per cent) that may be refractory to treatment.

In an attempt to reduce the incidence of postoperative encephalopathy, selective portocaval shunts have been advocated. These attempt to decompress the oesophageal varices, leaving the main portal circulation undisturbed. The procedures are more technically demanding, and although the incidence of early encephalopathy is probably reduced, the long-term benefits remain unproven. The distal splenorenal shunt involves anastomosis of the distal splenic vein end-to-side to the left renal vein. In addition, the gastric collaterals are selectively divided, preserving only the short gastric vessels.

9 The spleen

The spleen is a friable and vascular organ, protected in the upper abdomen by the overlying rib cage. It has a number of important, but not essential, functions relating to immunity and destruction of mature red blood cells and platelets. The most common indication for splenic surgery is its removal following (blunt) trauma (Table 19.15). This often follows injury to the overlying rib cage. Staging laparotomy has been used widely for Hodgkin's lymphoma; however, improved imaging and changes in therapeutic regimens have rendered this procedure largely obsolete. The most common reason for elective splenectomy is now for hypersplenism.

Hypersplenism may result in pancytopenia or thrombocytopenia alone. This is caused by a combination of increased platelet destruction and sequestration in the spleen, and is invariably associated with splenomegaly at the time of surgery.

Table 19.15 Indications for splenectomy

Indication	Notes
Trauma	Major disruption requires excision but attempts at preservation may be indicated for minor trauma
Spontaneous rupture	
Hypersplenism	Primary or secondary
As part of cancer surgery	Gastrectomy (to obtain lymph-node clearance)
	Distal pancreatectomy (proximity)
	Lymphoma staging

The most common causes in the West are primary haematological disorders (e.g. idiopathic thrombocytopenia), but infection is more common in developing countries. These patients usually have an associated reduction in platelet count and often impaired platelet function, and the operation is likely to require a covering platelet transfusion, best given at the time of clamping the splenic artery. Broad-spectrum antibiotics are required for patients with an impaired immune state. Splenectomy should also be accompanied by a careful laparotomy, looking for splenunculi (present in 10–30 per cent of the population).

9.1 Spleen preservation

Increased awareness of the long-term complications of splenectomy have precipitated a move towards spleen preservation, particularly in children. Non-operative treatment of splenic injuries is possible in haemodynamically stable patients, but requires close observation. Hospitalization for 10–14 days is recommended. A blood transfusion requirement of greater than 2–4 units suggests that surgery is indicated. Following trauma, minor lacerations can be repaired with Teflon buttresses, cyanoacrylate adhesives, or microfibrillar collagen. In addition, surrounding the spleen with a proprietary Vicryl bag is sometimes employed. Partial resection for localized trauma and marsupialization of splenic cysts are all advocated where possible. Retroperitoneal reimplantation of splenic tissue has been shown to maintain some function, although its effect on immunity is uncertain.

Splenectomy results in thrombocytosis. Although this is desirable in hypersplenism, it predisposes to thrombosis and pulmonary embolism in later life. Altered immunity predisposes to overwhelming infection, particularly from capsulated organisms such as *Pneumococcus*. This occurs in approximately 4 per cent of patients but has a mortality of 50–75 per cent. In order to minimize these side-effects, pneumococcal vaccine is given, preferably at least 2 weeks before surgery. In addition *Haemophilus influenzae* type *b* vaccine and meningococcal vaccine are recommended. Re-immunization should been performed every 5 years. Long-term, low-dose antibiotic prophylaxis is also advocated, particularly in children and young adults. In patients with thrombocytosis, low-dose aspirin should be prescribed.

9.2 Splenectomy

This is usually performed via an upper midline or a left subcostal incision. However, for massive splenomegaly, a left thoraco-abdominal incision may be required.

The aim is careful mobilization of the spleen from its peritoneal attachments so that it can be delivered into the wound, before division of the splenic artery and vein. It is convenient to start by drawing the spleen caudally and dividing the diaphragmatic attachments first (Fig. 19.20). The spleen can then be drawn medially and the lateral peritoneum divided. By gently drawing the spleen forward, the lienorenal ligament can be felt and divided. The inferior pole is then freed by division of the omental attachments, if necessary, between clips. Further mobilization can now be performed by blunt finger dissection. Care should be taken to divide the vessels close to the hilum to avoid damage to the tail of the pancreas.

If difficulty is encountered in delivery of the spleen, prior ligation of the splenic artery should be considered. The splenic artery can be identified by exposing the superior border of the pancreas in the lesser sac. The artery can be ligated safely at any point along the body of the pancreas on the left side of the abdomen.

Laparoscopic splenectomy has been performed, but has not been successful in reducing hospital stay and recovery time, as these are usually prolonged by the underlying medical condition. Mobilization is performed as for open splenectomy, and the pedicle divided with a vascular stapler. The spleen is then placed in a large endobag. The spleen is fragmented with either a liquidizing instrument or macerated with the surgeon's finger. The procedure is very time consuming, owing to the difficulty of removing a large organ through a porthole. This requires piecemeal removal, thus destroying the organ structure and hindering histological examination. Laparoscopic splenectomy is contraindicated in trauma, massive splenomegaly, where multiple perisplenic adhesions are present, and malignancy.

Bibliography

Jamieson, G.C. (1996). Recent developments in upper gastrointestinal surgery. *Aust. N.Z.J. Surg.*, **66**, (1), 46–9.

(1992) *Guidelines for good practice in and audit of the management of upper gastrointestinal haemorrhage.* Report of a Joint Working Group of the British Society of Gastroenterology, the Research Unit of the Royal College of Physicians of London and the Audit Unit of the Royal College of Surgeons of England. *J. Roy. Coll. Phys. Lon.*, **26**, 281–9. [This clearly sets out a set of standard guidelines for managing upper GI haemorrhage for both physicians and surgeons. Stratification of risk and indications for endoscopy are covered clearly and explicitly. A scheme for auditing the results of treatment is also set out lucidly. These recommendations or similar ones should form the ground rules for any hospital department managing upper GI haemorrhage]

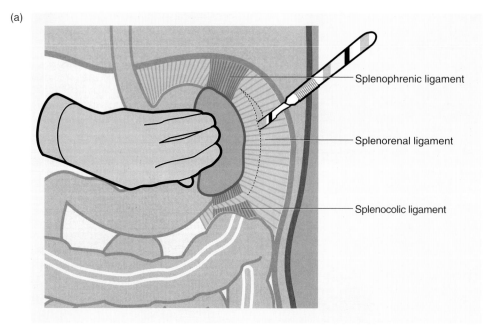

(a)

Splenophrenic ligament

Splenorenal ligament

Splenocolic ligament

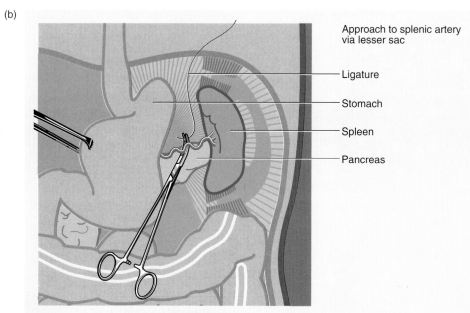

(b)

Approach to splenic artery via lesser sac

Ligature

Stomach

Spleen

Pancreas

Figure 19.20 Splenectomy.

Cancer of the pancreas

Huguier, M. and Mason, N.P. (1999). Treatment of cancer of the exocrine pancreas. *Am. J. Surg.*, **177**, (3), 257–65. [The outcome of cancer of the exocrine pancreas remains poor and opinions are divided over the optimal management. The indications, contraindications, and techniques for resection, palliation, chemotherapy, radiotherapy, and other treatments are discussed. Irrespective of tumour size or spread, resection gives the best survival rates, but careful patient selection is required. The place of adjuvant therapies remains controversial and further controlled trials are required to demonstrate their efficacy.]

Yeo, C.J. (1999). The Whipple procedure in the 1990s. *Adv. Surg.*, **32**, 271–303.

Yeo, C.J., and Cameron, J.L. (1999). Pancreatic cancer. *Curr. Probl. Surg.*, **36**, (2), 59–152.

Oesophageal and gastric cancer

Byrne, J.P. and Attwood, S.E. (1999). Duodenogastric reflux and cancer. *Hepato-Gastroenterology*, **46**, (25), 74–85.

Cuschieri, A. (1999). Surgical treatment of patients with invasive gastric cancer: dogma, debate and data. *Europ. J. Surg. Oncol.*, **25**, (2), 205–8.

Ellis, F.H., Jr (1999). Standard resection for cancer of the esophagus and cardia. *Surg. Oncol. Clin. North Am.*, **8**, (2), 279–94. [A review of 505 operations for cancer of the oesophagus found 90 per cent resectability, 3.3 per cent hospital mortality, 34 per cent postoperative complication rate, and 24.7 per cent adjusted actuarial 5-year survival rate. Neoadjuvant therapy or extended resection did not improve the results.]

Falk, G.W. (1999). Endoscopic surveillance of Barrett's esophagus: risk stratification and cancer risk. *Gastrointest. Endoscopy*, **49**, (3, Pt 2), S29–34.

Karpeh, M.S., Jr and Brennan, M.F. (1998) Gastric carcinoma. *Ann. Surg. Oncol.*, **5**, (7), 650–6.

Kuipers, E.J. (1999). Review article: exploring the link between *Helicobacter pylori* and gastric cancer. *Alimen. Pharmacol. Therap.*, **13**, (Suppl. 1), 3–11. [Cancer of the distal stomach, both the intestinal and diffuse type, is strongly associated with *Helicobacter pylori* colonization, which causes chronic active inflammation and eventually leads to loss of gastric glands, and atrophic gastritis, associated with intestinal metaplasia and dysplasia. Forty to 50 per cent of infected subjects develop these conditions, but they are rare in non-infected subjects. Infection with *H. pylori* plays an important role in the aetiology of atrophic gastritis and gastric cancer, particularly the intestinal type. Studies suggest an eightfold increased risk for both conditions. The age at which infection occurred and the presence of cagA as a marker for more pathogenetic *H. pylori* strains are important factors.]

Dyspepsia and peptic ulceration

Anand, B.S. and Graham, D.Y. (1999). Ulcer and gastritis. *Endoscopy*, **31**, (2), 215–25.

Moayyedi, P. (1998). What is the optimum strategy for managing dyspepsia? *J. Gastroenterol.*, **33**, (Suppl. 10), 44–7.

Hepatobiliary disorders

Edye, M. (1997). Current laparoscopic approaches to pancreatico-biliary disease. *Europ. J. Gastroenterol. Hepatol.*, **9**, (8), 744–9. [In pancreatic malignancy, staging by laparoscopy is valuable, with some operators able to perform definitive laparoscopic palliative bypass at the same sitting. Intraoperative laparoscopic sonography has potential in the evaluation of choledocholithiasis, hepatic metastases, and the staging of pancreatic cancer. Innovative options to deal with bile duct calculi include antegrade sphincterotomy and intraoperative stent placement.]

Gibbons, J.C. and Williams, S.J. (1998). Progress in the endoscopic management of benign biliary strictures. *J. Gastroenterol. Hepatol.*, **13**, (2), 116–24.

Tait, N. and Little, J.M. (1995). The treatment of gall stones. *BMJ*, **311**, (6997), 99–105.

Pancreatitis

Beger, H.G., Rau, B., Isenmann, R., and Mayer, J. (1998). Surgical treatment of acute pancreatitis. *Ann. Chirurg. Gynaecol.*, **87**, (3), 183–9.

Frey, C.F. (1999). The surgical management of chronic pancreatitis: the Frey procedure. *Adv. Surg.*, **32**, 41–85.

Gupta, R., Toh, S.K., and Johnson, C.D. (1999). Early ERCP is an essential part of the management of all cases of acute pancreatitis. *Ann. R. Coll. Surg. Engl.*, **81**, (1), 46–50.

Kemppainen, E., Puolakkainen, P. *et al.* (1998). Diagnosis of acute pancreatitis. *Ann. Chirurg. Gynaecol.*, **87**, (3), 191–4.

Lillemoe, K.D. and Yeo, C.J. (1998) Management of complications of pancreatitis. *Curr. Probl. Surg.*, **35**, (1), 1–98.

Neoptolemos, J.P., Raraty, M., Finch, M., and Sutton, R. (1998). Acute pancreatitis: the substantial human and financial costs. *Gut*, **42**, (6), 886–91.

Salim, A.S. (1997). Perspectives in pancreatic pain. *HPB Surg.*, **10**, (5), 269–77. [This review describes mechanisms important in the causation of pain in chronic pancreatitis. Medical and surgical techniques for treating the pain are described.]

Gastro-oesophageal reflux disease

Chekan, E.G. and Pappas, T.N. (1999). The laparoscopic management of gastroesophageal reflux disease. *Adv. Surg.*, **32**, 305–30.

Corvera, C.U. and Kirkwood, K.S. (1997). Recent advances. General surgery. *BMJ*, **315**, (7108), 586–9. [See comments.]

DeMeester, T.R., Peters, J.H., Bremner, C.G., and Chandrasoma, P. (1999). Biology of gastroesophageal reflux disease: pathophysiology relating to medical and surgical treatment. *Annu. Rev. Med.*, **50**, 469–506.

Galmiche, J.P., Letessier, E., and Scarpignato, C. (1998). Treatment of gastro-oesophageal reflux disease in adults. *BMJ*, **316**, (7146), 1720–3.

Horgan, S. and Pellegrini, C.A. (1997). Surgical treatment of gastroesophageal reflux disease. *Surg. Clin. North Am.*, **77**, (5), 1063–82.

Peters, J.H. (1997). The surgical management of Barrett's esophagus. *Clin. North Am.*, **26**, (3), 647–68.

Watson, D.I. and Jamieson, G.G. (1998). Antireflux surgery in the laparoscopic era. *Br. J. Surg.*, **85**, (9), 1173–84. [The development of laparoscopic techniques has led to reports

of large clinical series. This approach reduces the early
morbidity of surgery but complications such as
para-oesophageal herniation, pneumothorax, and
oesophageal perforation may be more common. A short,
loose laparoscopic Nissen fundoplication is appropriate for
gastro-oesophageal reflux disease. However, long-term
outcomes will not be available for some years.]

CHAPTER 20

Colorectal surgery

*Mike Saunders, John Abercrombie and
Paul Thomas
with W.G. Everett and John McGregor*

1 Introduction

The surgical principles employed in most colorectal procedures have been steadily evolving over the past 120 years. Standard methods for resection of all parts of the colon have now been formalized and technical advances have been made with stapling devices which sometimes obviate the need for a permanent stoma in patients with low rectal carcinoma. The ability to anastomose bowel low in the pelvis at the level of the anorectal ring is the key advance, which allows low anterior resections and ileal pouch procedures to be undertaken. However, it is still necessary to pay close attention to the details of patient preparation if morbidity and mortality are to be kept at a minimum.

Relatively little is known about colonic physiology; in part, because access to study the colon is difficult. However, the anorectal region is better understood. In specialized units anorectal physiology forms an integral part of the work-up for functional colorectal disorders. Its application to clinical problems is limited but it is a valuable research tool in studying the pathophysiology of incontinence and other pelvic-floor disorders.

A thorough history and general examination should be conducted in conjunction with a more specific anorectal assessment. A brief review of the range of tests is included here.

2 Investigations and their interpretation

2.1 Endoscopic assessment

Proctoscopy and sigmoidoscopy

These complimentary investigations are the most commonly used to examine the rectum and lower sigmoid colon but not before a digital rectal examination has been performed. These examinations are easiest with the patient lying in the left lateral position, and the legs flexed at the hips and knees. The buttocks overlap the near edge of the couch and the feet the far edge. A knee–elbow position can be adopted for this examination, but it is awkward and undignified for the patient. The rectum can be visualized in all cases, except when it is coated with soft faeces, and the rectosigmoid junction lies about 15 cm from the anal margin. Inspection beyond this level may prove difficult because of angulation, or rigidity caused by sigmoid diverticular disease. Nevertheless, it is possible to diagnose inflammatory bowel disease, polyps, and cancers by recognizing their macroscopic appearances and taking appropriate biopsies. A large-diameter 'operating' sigmoidoscope can be employed to enable complete polyp removal in an anaesthetized patient.

A flexible sigmoidoscope is easier to pass into the sigmoid colon than a rigid instrument and causes less discomfort. The examination may be continued up into the descending colon without the need for specific bowel preparation or sedation. This provides further access to polyp and cancer sites but is no substitute for total colonoscopy.

Colonoscopy

Colonoscopy is a more difficult procedure because of the length and tortuosity of the colon. A clean and empty (prepared) colon is essential for this examination and this is achieved by a combination of diet restriction and purgation. The two most commonly reported complications of colonoscopy are perforation of the colon and haemorrhage from polypectomy sites (approximate incidence 0.5 per cent). A variety of unusual complications have been recorded, including intracolonic explosion during diathermy. Complications are rare for an experienced colonoscopist. The procedure may be unpleasant and uncomfortable, and patients often require intravenous analgesia and sedation. Monitoring of the patient's vital signs during the procedure and in the recovery phase is mandatory. The colonoscopy provides far superior information about the colonic mucosa than contrast radiology. Lesions can be assessed, biopsied, and in the case of polyps, snared and removed. Contrast radiology is still widely requested as a first-line investigation, but colonoscopy is now the investigation of choice for many colorectal disorders and provides a useful second-line investigation after barium enema.

2.2 Radiological investigations

Plain abdominal X-ray

Faecal loading of the colon and rectum is indicated by a speckled opaque appearance and is indicative of constipation. Lucent areas on the radiograph may reflect the distribution of gas within the colon and rectum. Intestinal transit can be assessed by plain abdominal X-ray taken 5 days after the ingestion of a known number of radiopaque, polyethylene shapes. A normal transit rate is recorded when 80 per cent or more of the shapes have gone.

Contrast (enema) studies

Barium sulphate or a water-soluble contrast (e.g. gastrografin), given as an enema, is used to outline the colonic wall. When combined with air insufflation in a 'double-contrast' technique, fine detail of the mucosa can be obtained. Preparation for an elective contrast enema necessitates purgation with laxatives. A well-prepared bowel is essential since the presence of retained faecal residue may be mistaken for colonic filling defects. In large bowel obstruction, colonic patency should be assessed by a water-soluble contrast study to exclude pseudo-obstruction.

Ultrasonography

Transabdominal ultrasound is the investigation of choice for small amounts of ascites and is very accurate in distinguishing between cystic and solid masses. It is extremely effective in imaging the liver and identifying the presence of subphrenic collections. Biopsies, aspirations, and drainage procedures can be undertaken accurately with ultrasound guidance. Overlying bowel gas may impair the image, restricting its more widespread use in the abdomen. The recent development of a rotating ultrasound probe has allowed endoluminal applications, particularly in the rectum. This seems to provide high-quality information for staging rectal cancers as well as detecting early recurrences. However, difficulties exist in identifying pathological lymph nodes reliably and distinguishing recurrent cancer at an anastomosis, particularly when it is stenosed.

Computed tomography and magnetic resonance image scanning

Computed tomography (CT) scanning is used extensively in the evaluation of the primary and metastatic colonic and rectal carcinomas. The diagnostic yield is further improved if contrast is given, either orally, as enemas or intravenously. CT provides accurate localization for biopsy and drainage techniques. Magnetic resonant imaging (MRI) has further expanded diagnostic imaging by providing excellent anatomic delineation using multiplanar images. Moreover, it does not require ionizing radiation or contrast media. However, lengthy image acquisition may allow bowel movement to degrade the images. MRI is very valuable in assessing anal fistula disease and has been shown to be as accurate as the opinion of an experienced fistula surgeon examining a patient under anaesthesia.

Nuclear medicine imaging and angiography

Successful management of profuse lower gastrointestinal haemorrhage depends upon accurate localization of the source. Selective mesenteric artery angiography and radiolabelled red cell scans both have a place. Other radioisotopic techniques sometimes encountered are radiolabelled white cell scans, used to look for occult infection or the extent of inflammatory bowel disease. Novel tumour localization techniques for the diagnosis of recurrent colorectal cancer using radiolabelled antibodies to tumour antigens are currently being assessed.

Defecating proctography

A videoproctogram records the evacuation of a barium suspension, simulating defecation. The anorectal angle can be measured, a rectocoele or rectal prolapse identified, and functional assessments of colonic or ileoanal reservoirs made. This approach has improved the understanding of a wide variety of anorectal motility problems and is described in detail later in this chapter.

3 Principles of safe elective colorectal surgery

Certain procedures are necessary in preparing patients for colorectal surgery under general anaesthesia. Most important is a careful history and physical examination, with particular attention to the cardiovascular and respiratory systems. Baseline investigations include urine analysis, haemoglobin estimation, and renal function tests. An electrocardiograph is required if an abnormality is suspected. In overt or suspected malignant disease, a chest X-ray is taken to determine the presence of pulmonary metastases. Serum is saved for cross-matching if a blood transfusion is likely to be required; for example, when pelvic dissection is anticipated at least 3 units of blood should be available.

Infection is the major cause of morbidity and hospital mortality in colorectal surgery. Any procedure involving transsection of the colon has this high potential for infective complications. Contamination is minimized by ensuring that the colon is empty at the time of surgery. The problem of systemic absorption of colonic bacteria is covered by using prophylactic antibiotic therapy and the likelihood of an anastomotic leak is reduced by meticulous dissection and anastomotic technique.

3.1 Bowel preparation

The colon may be emptied by whole-gut irrigation (e.g. polyethylene glycol electrolyte solution: Golytely®) or a combination of oral aperients (e.g. sodium picosulphate: Picolax®) and distal enemas (e.g. sodium acid phosphate 10 per cent: phosphate enema) prior to elective surgery. The process takes at least 24 hours and although patients are usually in hospital, admission is not always necessary. Patients should take only a liquid diet during this period of preparation. If preoperative bowel preparation is inadequate or is contraindicated by an obstructing lesion, on-table lavage may be employed.

3.2 Antibiotic therapy

The bowel may be 'sterilized' with oral antibiotics preoperatively. However, this is not now generally recommended because it disrupts the complex bowel ecosystem and may allow unwanted organisms to predominate, resulting in antibiotic-associated colitis, including pseudomembranous enterocolitis. The aim of antibiotic prophylaxis in colorectal surgery is to achieve systemic bactericidal levels during the period of resection and anastomosis. Most prophylactic antibiotic regimens combine an antianaerobic agent (metronidazole) with a broad-spectrum aerobic antibiotic to target Gram-negative bacilli (cephalosporin: cefuroxime). Optimal tissue levels can be achieved by intravenous administration prior to induction of anaesthesia.

3.3 Surgical technique

Position and exposure

Patients must be positioned safely in a way that gives easy access to the surgical field. The patient lies supine for most right-sided colonic resections. A head-down tilt improves access in the lower abdomen, whereas a head-up and lateral tilt exposes the splenic flexure more easily. Where access to the pelvis in left-sided colonic and rectal lesions is required, a lithotomy–Trendelenburg (Lloyd-Davies) position is used (see Chapter 5). A midline incision provides good exposure and can easily be extended to give access to the whole abdomen. It interferes least with the abdominal wall, leaving both iliac fossae clear for stomas.

Anatomical considerations

Many elective colorectal operations are for cancer. For these, excisional surgery requires circumferential and longitudinal clearance together with removal of as much lymphatic field as practicable. The blood supply to the colon and rectum deter-

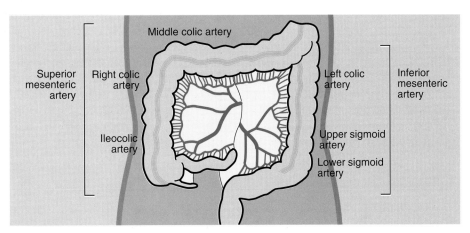

Figure 20.1 The blood supply to the colon—the route map for segmental resections.

mines the extent of removal of lymph-node fields (Fig. 20.1). For cancers of the caecum and right colon, the ileocolic and right colic pedicles are ligated near their origins, whereas transverse colonic cancers require ligation of the middle colic vessels. For left-sided cancers, the inferior mesenteric artery can be taken at its origin and the inferior mesenteric vein ligated together with the left colic artery. There is no evidence that high ligation of the inferior mesenteric artery *above* the origin of the left colic artery improves the recurrence rate of cancer compared with ligation below it. Problems may also arise with resection of the splenic flexure because it is at the junction of two vascular fields. When ligation of both middle colic and inferior mesenteric arteries are thought to be necessary, it is probably best to fashion an anastomosis between the terminal ileum and the descending colon. For poor-risk patients, an alternative would be to ligate the left colic artery alone and perform only a limited segmental resection. For inflammatory bowel disease and other benign conditions, it is unnecessary to remove the vascular pedicles so completely. However, the same principles of preserving the blood supply remain.

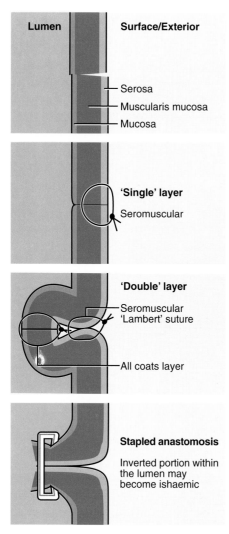

Figure 20.2 Techniques of anastomosis in the large bowel.

Bowel anastomosis

A sound anastomosis depends upon good surgical technique (Fig. 20.2) and preserving adequate perfusion of the bowel ends to be anastomosed. The colon needs to be mobilized sufficiently to allow apposition without tension. Direct anatomical apposition of the bowel ends gives the most rapid gain in tensile strength. There has been much debate on the best method for anastomoses but there are sound theoretical reasons for a single layer of interrupted sutures for most anastomoses. This method employs the least amount of suture material with minimal interference to the blood supply, and is technically straightforward and reliable.

Use of drains and covering colostomies

There are few indications for using drains in elective colorectal surgery. Most anastomoses become rapidly surrounded by omentum and small bowel, which help seal potential defects. In contrast, the anastomosis of a low anterior resection of the rectum lies within the avascular sacral hollow in which there is a tendency for blood and serum to pool. Drainage will keep this space free of haematoma and allow the surrounding tissues to support the anastomosis.

Technical difficulties are occasionally encountered, more often with low pelvic anastomoses. Established infection increases the risk of anastomotic failure and a temporary proximal defunctioning stoma can be used in these situations. Interestingly, drains themselves may increase the likelihood of anastomotic leakage by preventing surrounding tissue from adhering to the external surface of the anastomosis.

4　Stoma care

W.G. Everett and John McGregor

4.1　Siting a stoma

Accurate siting of a stoma is of great importance. If a stoma is badly positioned, the patient's ability to lead a full and active life is compromised and no amount of skilled nursing care can compensate for it. Before siting the stoma, a detailed explanation of the anticipated surgery should be given, along with the reasons behind the need for a stoma. Ideally, the patient should be fully assessed before surgery (although this is rarely possible in emergency surgery), taking the following into consideration:

◆ occupation

◆ hobbies

◆ sport and leisure

◆ general lifestyle

◆ type and style of clothes worn

◆ physical disabilities (e.g. impaired vision, arthritis)

◆ physical abilities and manual dexterity

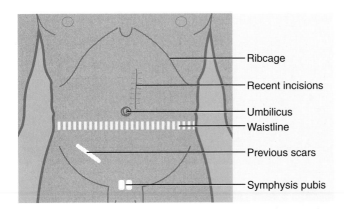

Figure 20.3 Sites to avoid when siting a stoma.

- deportment
- culture and religious beliefs
- obesity and abdominal sag (especially when sitting).

The patient's abdomen then needs to be appraised in order to avoid adverse features in siting the stoma (Fig. 20.3).

4.2 Standard sites for different types of stoma

Stomas are usually placed one-third to halfway between the umbilicus and the anterior superior iliac spine (Fig. 20.4) unless there are specific contraindications. Once the position has been determined, a mark is made on the skin with a permanent marking pen. The patient should be able to see this mark. For some patients, wearing an appliance prior to surgery is helpful to test the suitability of a chosen site before the stoma is created surgically. In emergency cases, a detailed stoma assessment cannot usually be undertaken, but if a stoma is anticipated, the site should at least be marked beforehand by the surgeon.

4.3 Problems of a badly sited stoma

The aim of stoma design and placement is for the patient with a stoma to be able to return to a virtually normal life; this will not be possible if the stoma is badly sited:

1. The patient must be able to see the stoma site, otherwise independent care is impossible.

2. If adhesion of the appliance to the skin is impaired by irregularities in the skin or nearby structures or wounds, this will cause leakage, odour, and skin excoriation. This seriously interferes with normal daily activities, exacerbates psychological problems, and delays rehabilitation.

3. Pain and discomfort around the stoma is likely to prevent the wearing of normal clothing.

4. Work activities may dislodge the appliance or cause discomfort, resulting in delayed return to work.

5. Sports and hobbies may have to be curtailed unless the appliance is attached robustly. Sometimes special arrangements need to be made for particular sports (e.g. swimming).

4.4 Complications with stomas which generally do not require surgery

Skin problems

Causes:

- inappropriate appliance
- incorrect size or fit
- poor seal
- too frequent or unnecessary changing of appliance
- sweating
- allergy

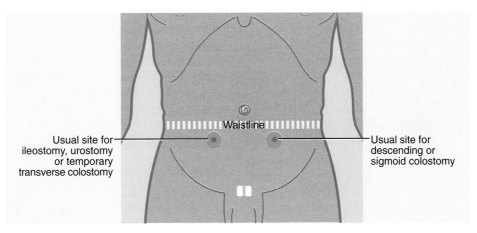

Figure 20.4 Standard sites for different types of stoma.

- psoriasis or eczema

- poor hygiene

- radiotherapy

- poor general health and malnutrition

- drug interactions.

Most skin problems can usually be alleviated by attention to the underlying problem, assisted by various skin protective materials, including barrier creams and hydrocolloid wafers.

Stoma retraction

Stoma retraction usually occurs as a result of insufficient mobilization of the bowel or too much tension on the stoma when sutured to the skin. Provided the stoma remains viable and does not detach from the surrounding skin, retraction can usually be managed using appliances with inbuilt concavity, or devices that create concavity.

Constipation

Constipation usually responds to dietary advice and education about what is a balanced diet and the importance of fibre and adequate fluid intake. If that fails, bulking agents such as Fybogel® should be tried before other types of aperients.

Diarrhoea

The consistency of the bowel effluent depends on which portion of the bowel has been exteriorized. The more proximal the stoma, the more fluid the effluent. The effluent tends to become thicker with time as the patient's body adapts to the stoma, but various oral drugs can be given to help. These include Imodium® and Lomotil® for small-bowel stoma and codeine phosphate for colonic stomas. Diarrhoea may be due to other factors, listed below. In this case, management is of the underlying condition.

Some causes of diarrhoea:

- previous bowel resections and short bowel;

- residual diseased bowel (e.g. Crohn's disease);

- radiotherapy;

- intestinal infection;

- dietary effects (e.g. curries and spices; tomato pips and skins);

- drugs;

- emotional stress and worry.

4.5 Complications which may require surgery

Ischaemia

The bowel may be ischaemic from the outset because of impaired blood supply to the bowel end, tension on the mesentery, or constriction as it passes through the abdominal wall. Such ischaemia may be **partial**, where the mucosa sloughs but the muscular wall survives, or **complete**, when the bowel end sloughs entirely, detaches from the abdominal wall, and drops back into the abdomen, causing peritonitis. Occasionally, ischaemia occurs later due to an inappropriately fitting appliance constricting the stoma.

An ischaemic stoma is dusky or purplish from the outset and fails to 'pink up' over the first few hours. However, necrosis and sloughing usually take a few days to develop fully. The questions for the surgeon are whether to refashion the stoma and, if so, when. If the stoma is clearly not viable or falls back into the abdomen, revision is necessary and this may be urgent. If necrosis is confined to the mucosa, this will eventually slough and can be lifted out, revealing a healthy, pink stoma.

Stenosis

Stenosis is usually caused by lesser degrees of ischaemia, or separation and infection where the stoma is sutured to the skin. Granulation tissue is first formed, leading to fibrosis and stenosis. Stenosis may also occur as a result of active Crohn's disease. If the stenosis is mild, regular dilatation and stool softeners are all that are required. Severe stenosis will require revision.

Parastomal herniation

Parastomal herniation is frequently seen with end colostomies and less commonly with ileostomies and urostomies. Most hernias do not present a major problem to the patient, other than causing an unsightly bulge. However, intestinal obstruction occasionally occurs. Surgical repair is often unsuccessful, with a high recurrence rate. If surgery is needed, a better approach is to perform a full laparotomy and resite the stoma.

Prolapse

A length of inverted bowel may protrude through the stoma. It is most common in transverse loop colostomies. The distal end of the bowel usually prolapses, but sometimes both distal and proximal portions prolapse. This is a distressing and alarming condition for the patient, but with careful explanation, fitting of a larger appliance, and continued support, many patients cope well until the colostomy can either be closed or refashioned.

Recurrent carcinoma

Locally recurrent cancer at the stoma is usually associated with recurrent disease elsewhere in the abdomen. In such cases, further surgery is seldom indicated unless it is causing obstruction, when resection or revision of the stoma may be needed.

Crohn's disease

Recurrent or residual Crohn's disease may present as stenosis, fistulation, or a parastomal abscess. The bowel proximal to the stoma is usually involved and resection is often necessary via a laparotomy.

4.6 Stoma appliances

Over the past 25 years, a wide range of appliances has become available, driven by the needs of professional stoma therapists and enabled by the development of new materials. Most modern appliances are equipped with hypoallergenic barriers to protect the skin, and are constructed of odour-resistant plastics. The soft and flexible materials used for appliances provide the security and comfort needed to recover quality of life.

A wide variety of different appliances is available and the choice depends on the needs of the individual. Most patients need guidance and advice from a stoma-care nurse, who has the necessary training and expertise. Many manufacturing companies provide samples of their products so the patient can try out a range until a final choice is made.

Stoma appliances are available on prescription and those with permanent stomas are exempt from prescription charges in the UK.

Types of appliance

There are two basic types of appliance: the **one-piece appliance** consists of a collecting bag with an adhesive seal attached. After use, the complete appliance is removed and discarded, and replaced with a new one. The **two-piece appliance** consists of an adhesive base-plate (flange) that is fixed around the stoma and a collecting bag which is clipped on to it. The base plate remains *in situ* for several days but the bag is removed and discarded when necessary.

Drainable bags have an open end distally for evacuation of the contents. Patients with ileostomies need drainable bags because of the fluid nature of the effluent. Some colostomy patients with loose faeces do better with this type of appliance, particularly in the postoperative period.

Closed, non-drainable bags need to be discarded after each bowel action. Most patients with an end colostomy use this type of appliance.

Urostomy appliances are more complex. They are fitted with a drainage tap and an antireflux valve which prevents reflux of urine over the stoma when the patient is lying down or is very active. These features reduce the risk of leakage and the incidence of ascending renal tract infection.

Most appliances are available in clear or opaque plastic. A new concept is an appliance that can be flushed away, as it is made of a biodegradable material. At present, it is available only as a closed bag for colostomies but others are likely to follow.

For patients with an end colostomy, there are two alternatives to wearing a bag:

- **Irrigation**. With this method, the colon is washed out with water via the colostomy daily or on alternate days, producing a total evacuation of the colon. The wash procedure takes about 45 minutes. The patient then only needs to wear a small stoma cap. Not all patients are suitable for this and the appropriateness of the technique for an individual needs to be agreed between the patient, surgeon, and stoma nurse. If suitable, the procedure can be taught by the stoma-care nurse.

- **Plug**. This device, like irrigation, can restore continence and control for the patient but is only suitable for end colostomies. The plug is made of soft foam which, after being inserted into the stoma, expands to block the escape of faeces and flatus. Some patients can only wear the device for 2 hours, whereas others can use it for up to 24 hours.

5 Special instrumentation and innovative surgery

5.1 Staplers

Stapling devices have been developed as an alternative to manual techniques of suturing. In practice, they are generally reliable and safe. They produce a uniform anastomotic line and are undeniably rapid. However, their real advantage is in the restoration of bowel continuity, deep within the pelvis, where access may be limited. This has consolidated the place of sphincter-saving operations in the treatment of ulcerative colitis, familial adenomatous polyposis (e.g. ileo-anal pouch formation) and middle- or lower-third rectal carcinomas (e.g. low anterior resection and colo-anal anastomosis). It is rightfully argued that, despite the initial capital outlay, a real cost benefit is gained by preserving sphincter function and avoiding a stoma.

Double- and single-staple techniques

Three types of stapling device are commonly used in colorectal surgery: linear staplers, linear cutter, and circular stapling instruments. These instruments are frequently used to complement one another. For example, after the rectal stump has been closed with a linear stapler, a circular stapler can be used to restore bowel continuity. This is known as the double-staple technique. The linear cutter has the additional benefit of cutting between the inserted staple lines, thus minimizing spillage of bowel contents.

To achieve an end-to-end colorectal anastomosis on to a low-lying short rectal stump, the circular stapler is introduced from below through the anus (Fig. 20.5). The bowel ends are drawn together and compressed between a cartridge (containing stainless-steel staples as well as a circular cutting knife) and an anvil already secured within the proximal colon by a purse-string suture. By squeezing the instrument handles together, a double row of staples is pushed through the tissue ends, held between cartridge and anvil, and configured into a B-shape to join the ends. Simultaneously the circular knife creates a patent anastomosis on the luminal side of the staple line by excising the redundant tissue as two complete doughnuts. This technique can be modified as a single-staple technique for reversal of Hartmann's procedure.

Benefits and risks

It is claimed that the tissue damage is relatively less with the stapling process than with hand-sewn methods. Simultaneous

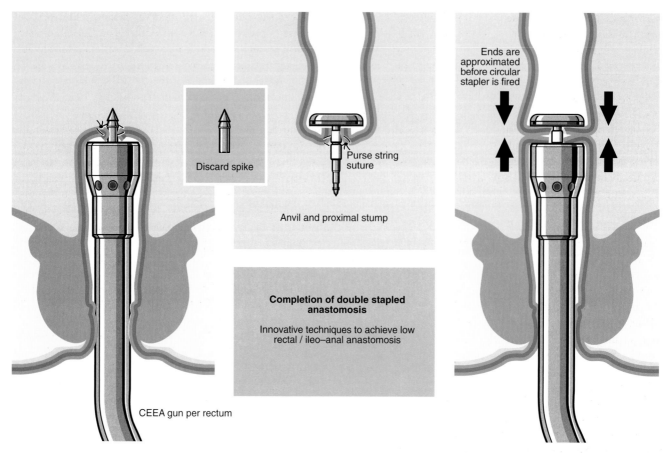

Figure 20.5 Technique of using a circular stapler for end-to-end anastomosis to a short rectal stump.

penetration, uniformity, and the B-shape configuration of the staples reduce handling trauma, oedema, and potential ischaemia. Furthermore, tumour cell adherence to staples is minimal. Unfortunately, a poorly constructed or, indeed, failed low colorectal staple line is catastrophic. It creates a dilemma for the surgeon inexperienced in restorative colorectal procedures and may lead to unnecessary sphincter sacrifice.

5.2 Minimal access (laparoscopic-assisted) surgery

Progress in laparoscopic colorectal surgery has been hindered by the need for high competence levels in minimal access surgery, by the limitations of instruments, and by concerns about the completeness of resection and potential for seeding malignant cells during laparoscopic-assisted resections for cancer. In general, the principles of surgical resection are similar to those applied in conventional open surgery; however, modifications are necessary and techniques must be adapted when access is limited.

Patient position, port position, and instrumentation

The patient needs to be placed in a well-secured and modified Lloyd-Davies position, with hips flexed less than usual. This allows a greater range of movement of instruments while maintaining transanal access. Furthermore, it allows for the adoption of the steep Trendelenburg position, which is often necessary for small-bowel repositioning. Port placement varies with operative site, patient's habitus, and the surgeon's preference. A common arrangement is one subumbilical port and one port in each of the four quadrants of the abdomen. This allows the surgeon a two-handed dissection technique with good retraction and optimum vision.

Accurate preoperative localization of the lesion is vital as some masses may not be readily visible with the laparoscope and direct palpation is no longer possible. Intraoperative laparoscopic ultrasound probes are available to assist localization, and facilities for on-table colonoscopy may be necessary, though these may add considerably to an already lengthy procedure.

Retrieval of the specimen

An intact specimen is required for accurate histological staging, and this poses a dilemma for the surgeon. It is often impractical to deliver a bulky lesion transanally. Furthermore, this manoeuvre exposes the rectum to the theoretical risk of seeding malignant cells. For this reason, a small laparotomy may be performed.

Extracorporeal versus intracorporeal anastomoses

Patients who need a laparotomy to facilitate specimen retrieval already have an access route through which to perform the anastomosis. Via the appropriately positioned incision, an extra-corporeal anastomosis may be performed by hand sewing or stapling. Alternatively, restoration of bowel continuity can be achieved by intracorporeal anastomosis. For left-sided resections, an end-to-end anastomosis is achieved using both linear (laparoscopic linear stapler) and circular stapling instruments. Procedures best suited to this technique include reversal of a Hartmann's operation and anastomosis after transanal removal of resected sigmoid diverticular disease, rectal prolapse, or polyps. Right-sided resections can be anastomosed intra-corporeally in a similar way to a stapled side-to-side technique at open surgery.

Pitfalls, cancer issues, and costs

Clear identification of vital structures (ureter, duodenum, major vascular pedicles) during laparoscopic colonic surgery may prove difficult, especially if the patient is obese. Furthermore, diathermy injury to these structures is a potential hazard. Nevertheless, reported morbidity is low, implying that laparoscopic colonic surgery can be performed safely. Aside from this, the safety of the laparoscopic approach to malignant disease is of greatest concern and dispute. It remains uncertain whether the same quality of dissection can be achieved using laparoscopy and whether this new technique is associated with a greater risk of malignant cell dissemination and subsequent implantation. Certainly, a small but important number of port-site recurrences have been reported after laparoscopic surgery for malignant disease. The time between laparoscopic surgery and presentation of wound metastasis ranges widely, from less than 1 week to almost a year. The most likely mechanism is direct implantation of viable exfoliated tumour cells.

Operative costs for laparoscopic colonic surgery, as compared to conventional open methods, are high and are not, in reality, offset by the shortened postoperative hospital stay. However, the longer operating time and current high prices for instruments and equipment will diminish with greater operative experience and more frequent use. Furthermore, economic justification must also be balanced against the improved cosmesis, reduced pain scores, and the accelerated return to normal activity reported after laparoscopic colonic surgery.

Outcome

Experience is very limited, with little more than 50 publications reporting the outcomes of almost 500 attempted laparoscopic colonic procedures. The concerns about long operating times, conversion rates, and postoperative stays have predominated. However, the prime aims of cancer surgery, namely long-term cure and reduced local recurrence rates, need to be addressed. No randomized controlled trial has yet been published, but prospective studies are currently being undertaken.

5.3 Intestinal pouch construction

Where patients lose the whole of the colon and rectum, as in ulcerative colitis and familial adenomatous polyposis, attempts to restore the reservoir function of the rectum and avoid a permanent stoma are often made by constructing a capacity pouch of ileum. Similarly, a low anterior resection or colo-anal anastomosis can be augmented by construction of a colonic pouch. The presence of a reservoir (**neorectum**) aims to reduce the high frequency, urgency, and nocturnal disturbance associated with a direct ileo-anal or colo-anal anastomosis.

Ileo-anal pouch

A range of pouch designs has been proposed (Fig. 20.6). The optimal volume of the reservoir approaches 300 ml and this is achieved using ileal loops of between 12 and 20 cm in length. The J-pouch is the most easily constructed and has found widest application. However, the three-limb S-pouch has a longer reach, making it particularly useful in patients with short, thickened mesentery and a long, narrow pelvis. Alternatively, the four-limb W-pouch with its greater capacity, it is claimed, is

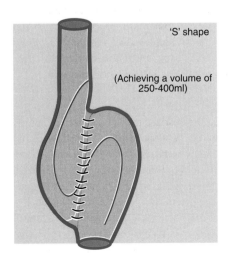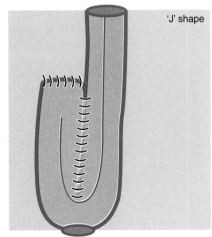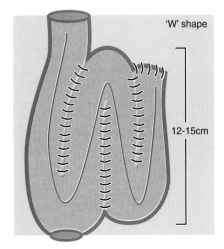

Figure 20.6 Types of ileal pouch.

associated with a lower frequency of defecation. Larger-capacity pouches are often troubled by erratic emptying and may need to be intubated. In all of these, the efferent limb of the pouch is anastomosed to the anal canal with retention of the anal sphincters (**restorative proctocolectomy**).

Colonic pouch

Functional outcome after sphincter-saving surgery for low rectal cancers has become a major consideration. Disappointingly, stool frequency and urgency are high and appear to be related to the length of the rectal stump. The colonic J-pouch is designed to improve this by creating a neorectal reservoir. A 6 cm limb for the pouch provides optimal function while minimizing evacuation difficulties. Data suggest that the initial advantage of a pouch over an end-to-end anastomosis is transitory and that after a year there is very little functional difference between the two procedures. It must be cautioned that pouches constructed from the colon are, at the very least, as susceptible to synchronous and metachronous tumours as the remaining colon and require equivalent surveillance.

6 Colonic diverticular disease

Diverticular disease of the colon occurs predominantly in the elderly and is a disease of Western communities. In developed countries, it is estimated that diverticular disease affects 70 per cent of the population by 85 years of age. The sigmoid colon is invariably involved with colonic diverticular disease. Pathophysiology links anatomical and neuromuscular defects with raised intraluminal pressure resulting in pulsion diverticula. Epidemiological evidence links the condition with a low-residue diet, particularly lacking in cereal fibre. Consequently, where high-fibre diets are customary a low incidence is recorded.

6.1 Clinical features of diverticular disease

The symptoms relating to diverticular disease are wide ranging and the signs vary according to the disease process. Some patients may exhibit extensive diverticular formation on contrast radiology (barium enema and CT scan) or colonoscopy, and yet have no symptoms. However, infection, fistula formation, bleeding, obstruction, and painful bowel dysfunction may be a consequence of diverticular disease (Fig. 20.7). Fortunately the majority of patients suffer no serious consequences of their diverticular disease, but complications can be severe and life-threatening. Mortality amongst patients requiring emergency surgery for complications of the disease is five times greater than among those undergoing elective procedures.

6.2 Surgery for diverticular disease

The emergency management of patients who present with acute diverticulitis and diverticular haemorrhage has been discussed in Chapter 18.

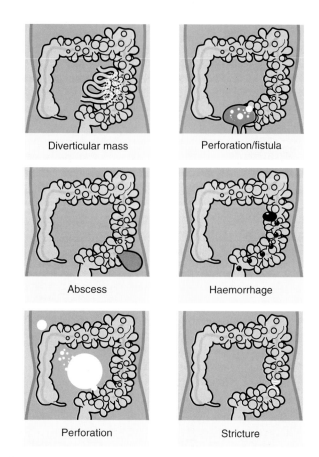

Figure 20.7 The consequences of colonic diverticular disease.

Principles of surgical resection of diverticular disease

Surgical resection for diverticular disease can be technically demanding and good judgement is required. The bowel is frequently foreshortened, thickened, and accompanied by a dense inflammatory process. A fixed sigmoid loop, deep within the pelvis, may be firmly adherent to adjacent structures (vagina, uterus, ureter, bladder, or pelvic side wall), perhaps obscuring an abscess or fistulous tract. Furthermore, there may be the unresolved issue of possible malignancy and it will be necessary to decide whether to separate the inflamed colon from the contiguous structures or to resect in a fashion consistent with cancer surgery.

Diverticula are most numerous in the sigmoid colon but are absent distal to the rectosigmoid junction. The number of diverticula more proximally will vary. The distal resection point must always include the upper rectum and the extent of resection should normally include all of the diverticula. The left colon must be mobilized sufficiently to allow an anastomosis between a disease-free segment of proximal colon and the rectum, under no tension and with a good blood supply. This may occasionally require removal of all of the left colon and anastomosing the transverse colon to the rectum. It is seldom necessary to use a defunctioning colostomy.

Operating for painful diverticular disease

Patients who recover from an attack of acute diverticulitis and who are subsequently shown on contrast studies to have diverticular disease should not be recommended to undergo colonic resection, but several attacks may alter this advice. The more difficult decision is when patients present with left-sided abdominal pain and diverticular disease but no objective signs of complications. It is impossible to assess the pain threshold in such patients—and resectional surgery cannot guarantee that the pain will be cured. The mechanism of pain is presumably colonic contractions and these may continue even after resection. Where possible, patients should be advised to avoid surgery if pain is the only problem—medical therapy is the main treatment for such cases.

Operating for fistulous complications

A colo-vaginal fistula is socially unacceptable. A colo-vesical fistula, producing pneumaturia and faeces in the urine, is not only socially unacceptable but also results in urinary tract infections and possible deterioration in renal function. Colo-intestinal fistulae with loops of small intestine, although rare, may produce short-circuiting of small-bowel contents and diarrhoea. For any of these conditions, corrective surgery is indicated. Where possible, the segment of involved colon should be excised. A diverting defunctioning proximal colostomy alone may help in cases of colo-vesical and colo-vaginal fistulae, but will not influence the problem where the small bowel is involved and should be employed only where more major surgery is regarded as unsafe. Preoperative attempts to demonstrate the fistula using barium enema, cystoscopy, or vaginal specular examination are often unsuccessful. Where there is clinical evidence of a fistula, a failure to image the fistula should not concern the surgeon—surgery is still needed.

The surgical principles are the same as for an uncomplicated resection. Additional considerations include:

1. Is the fistula into the vagina or bladder formally closed? Where there is a narrow track, it is often impossible to find it. In this case, it is best left alone.

2. The primary colonic anastomosis should be separated from the bladder or vagina by a plug of omentum. The omentum can be mobilized from the right side of the transverse colon and anchored to lie between the anastomosis and the presumed fistular site (**omentoplasty**).

3. The use of a defunctioning stoma. A fistula is the principal condition where a defunctioning stoma (ileostomy or colostomy) needs to be considered. Front-line colorectal surgeons have an aversion to using defunctioning stomas, particularly for a 'high' resection such as this. Nevertheless, anastomoses do leak, and it is demoralizing for patient to be left with the same symptoms from the fistula after correctional surgery. Surgeons at all levels of experience should not be ashamed to use a defunctioning stoma in this type of case. Each case should be judged on its merits but a stoma should never be used to protect a poor anastomosis. It is better to redo the anastomosis.

Operating for a sigmoid stricture

A proportion of cases will present with large-bowel obstruction and their management is discussed in Chapter 18. Elective surgery for a sigmoid stricture is a common event and the aetiology of the narrowing is often uncertain despite pre-operative colonoscopy. Diverticular disease and carcinoma do coincide and, if malignancy is a possibility, then the resectional principles should follow the guidelines for the management of colorectal cancer.

Outcome

Overall, high mortality (5 per cent) and morbidity (30 per cent) rates are recorded amongst patients requiring surgery for colonic diverticular disease. Much of this relates to emergency surgery and the resultant serious septic complications. Ideally, patients who are at high risk of developing complications should be identified for elective resection, but, unfortunately 50 per cent of those who require emergency operations for complications of diverticular disease have had symptoms for less than 30 days at the time of the presenting illness.

Long-term results of colon resection for complicated diverticular disease are good. Most patients are relieved of their complaint and all the infective sequelae, although they tend to more frequent stools as compared with preoperative status. Recurrent diverticulitis is rare following adequate resection and affects less than 5 per cent overall. However, in patients who have incomplete staged operative treatment and are left with a colostomy and defunctioned diverticular sigmoid, the disease and its complications may continue in the defunctioned section. This ought to be a rarity now, as resectional surgery is the norm even in the emergency situation.

7 Inflammatory bowel disease

Ulcerative colitis and Crohn's disease are the most common types of chronic inflammatory bowel disease and their highest prevalence is in northern Europe and the USA. The incidence and prevalence of ulcerative colitis has changed little over the years, but the rate of diagnosis of Crohn's disease has increased substantially. The peak age of onset for both diseases is 20–35 years and both have similar distributions with respect to geography, age, gender, race, occupation, and social class. Smoking appears to protect against the risk of ulcerative colitis but increases the risk of developing Crohn's disease.

The pathogenesis of ulcerative colitis and Crohn's disease is, at least in part, due to a complex interaction between genetic predisposing factors and (largely unknown) exogenous and endogenous mediators. This results in immune-mediated tissue injury that presents clinically as relapsing and remitting inflammatory processes. Although the gastrointestinal tract is principally affected, almost 30 per cent of patients with ulcerative colitis and Crohn's disease suffer additional extra-intestinal manifestations (Table 20.1).

Table 20.1 Extra-alimentary manifestations of inflammatory bowel disease

Sacroiliitis

Pyoderma gangrenosum

Uveitis

Aphthous ulceration

Sclerosing cholangitis

Erythema nodosum

7.1 Pathology

Ulcerative colitis

This condition is colon-specific and is characterized by extensive epithelial cell damage, crypt abscess formation, and an acute inflammatory cell infiltration. Typically, the process begins in the rectum and extends proximally to involve a variable length of the colon. However, in 20 per cent of patients, the disease involves the whole of the colon from the outset. The main symptoms are rectal bleeding, diarrhoea, and passage of mucus per rectum. Abdominal pain is seldom a prominent symptom in mild or moderate disease. Patients with a severely inflamed rectum suffer urgency of stools and tenesmus.

Crohn's disease

By contrast with ulcerative colitis, Crohn's disease may affect any portion of the gastrointestinal tract. Histologically, it is typified by patchy, chronic transmural inflammation containing non-caseating granulomas. More than 50 per cent of patients with Crohn's disease have ileocaecal involvement and 25 per cent have disease limited to the colon. Diarrhoea, whether due to mucosal inflammation, interruption of bile-salt reabsorption, or bacterial overgrowth secondary to stasis, is frequently a presenting symptom. Abdominal pain and systemic symptoms (malaise, anorexia, fever, weight loss) are more common than in ulcerative colitis. Additionally, symptoms may arise due to complications of the transmural inflammatory process. These include stricturing, perforation, and fistulation.

7.2 Risks of cancer and dysplasia in inflammatory bowel diseases

Patients with extensive chronic colitis since childhood, carry a risk for colorectal cancer between 15 and 20 times greater than for a comparable normal population. Somewhat surprisingly, when like is compared with like, the relative risks and the absolute 20-year cumulative incidence of large-bowel cancer are similar in cohorts of ulcerative and Crohn's colitis patients. In practice, however, many Crohn's patients are eliminated from risk by early colectomy for refractory symptomatic disease.

The value of surveillance for bowel cancer in these patients has been questioned, particularly in view of the high costs and dubious benefits. Furthermore, the significance of dysplasia as a marker of malignant potential remains controversial. However, patients with colitis for more than 10 years have a clinically important cancer risk. Currently, colonoscopy is usually undertaken at intervals of 2 years or less, with multiple biopsies to detect dysplasia or early colorectal cancer. It is important to emphasize that patients entering a surveillance programme must accept that a colectomy will need to be performed if high-grade dysplasia or a dysplasia-associated lesion or mass is found.

7.3 Medical care of inflammatory bowel disease

Ulcerative colitis and Crohn's disease alike, are prone to relapse and remission. Medical treatment is directed at achieving and maintaining remission of both clinical symptoms and mucosal inflammation. The cyclical nature of inflammatory bowel disease, particularly when diagnosed in young patients, will considerably disrupt patients' attempts to lead a normal life and thus counselling and support groups form an important part of management.

7.4 Surgical management

Ulcerative colitis

In some cases, surgical intervention is required as a matter of urgency; in others it can be planned after careful counselling (Table 20.2). The most common indication for surgery is failure of medical treatment to control symptoms adequately. Chronicity, or recurring moderate to severe relapses, often require repeated hospital admissions and interfere seriously with the patient's work and normal life. Elective surgery is mandatory for carcinoma complicating ulcerative colitis, and should also be performed in patients with high-grade dysplasia detected during surveillance Proctocolectomy is the only operation that totally eradicates this disease. Nevertheless, total disease eradication is not the only objective. If the objective is to remove the risk of malignancy, then a proctocolectomy is the operation of choice (there may be a case to spare the anorectal junction when a restorative ileal pouch is being constructed). Where the risk of malignancy is adjudged to be small and surgery is advised to control symptoms when medical treatment has failed, the rectum can be defunctioned and left in place, and symptoms controlled by a total colectomy and ileostomy.

Table 20.2 Indications for surgery in ulcerative colitis

Emergency
Toxic dilatation
Bleeding(rare)
Elective
Failed medical treatment
Malignant change
Severe dysplasia
Carcinoma

Total colectomy with ileostomy and mucous fistula

This is the safest procedure for patients undergoing emergency or urgent resection. By reducing both surgical trauma and operating time, which is often crucial in debilitated patients, a low mortality rate (< 3 per cent) can be achieved. However, retention of the rectum to limit the stress of surgery may lead to problems of local infection, continuing toxicity, and extra-intestinal problems. Furthermore, there may be poor acceptance of the ileostomy. Nevertheless, the procedure gains time for pathological confirmation of the diagnosis, patient counselling, and the option of definitive surgery.

Panproctocolectomy and permanent ileostomy

This is a safe elective procedure that removes all of the diseased colon and rectum but has the disadvantages of a permanent stoma and a perineal wound which may be a source of morbidity. None the less, the procedure is indicated for patients either unsuitable for restorative surgery (i.e. those with poor anal sphincter function or low rectal carcinoma) or those who have had major complications from pouch surgery and require excision of the pouch.

Koch pouch or continent ileostomy

Modification of the ileostomy into a flush stoma and continent reservoir can be achieved by retrograde intussusception of the ileum into a capacity reservoir. It is a complex procedure with a local complication rate approaching 30 per cent. The nipple valve is prone to slippage and the flush stoma to retract and stenose. This operation is now largely redundant, having been replaced by restorative proctocolectomy and ileo-anal pouch formation.

Total colectomy and ileorectal anastomosis

Controversy has prevented widespread acceptance of this operation: it is now rarely performed. A satisfactory functional outcome requires minimal disease activity in a distensible rectum together with good sphincter activity. Unfortunately, despite apparent careful selection, patients frequently complain of multiple bowel actions, nocturnal incontinence, and the need to rely on antidiarrhoeal medication. However, these symptoms often improve with time. Further concerns surround any additional morbidity and mortality from operative complications and the residual risk of later malignancy in the retained rectum. Detecting potential or early malignancy is a crucial issue in the follow-up of these patients. Long-term results of over 1000 cases of ileorectal anastomosis show an incidence of carcinoma of 3.4 per cent. Despite the disadvantages, ileorectal anastomosis may still have a role in restoring intestinal continuity following emergency surgery in elderly or unfit patients who have good sphincter function.

Restorative proctocolectomy with ileo-anal pouch formation

In suitable patients, this is currently the operation of choice for ulcerative colitis. It should never be advised if there is the slightest suggestion that the colon is affected by Crohn's disease. Restorative proctocolectomy is usually performed as a staged procedure which follows either emergency colectomy or is carried out electively for chronic symptoms of ulcerative colitis or complicating carcinoma. Patients must be well motivated to avoid an ileostomy in this way and should be advised of the possible complications and the range of functional outcomes. The common goal is to create a compliant reservoir allowing the patient an acceptable stool frequency and the ability to defer defecation and maintain continence. Most would accept 4–6 bowel actions per 24 hours with a night-time range of 0–3, depending upon the time of the last evening meal. Control of urgency and maintenance of continence are probably a reflection of the preoperative state of the anal sphincter function. A normally functioning anal sphincter is essential to success of the operation. Furthermore, great care must be taken to avoid excessive anal manipulation and dilatation during surgery.

Until recently, mucosal proctectomy with a pull-through anal anastomosis of the ileal pouch was the method of choice. However, this has been superseded by rectal transection at the pelvic floor and a stapled anastomosis to the upper end of the anal canal. Concerns about the potential risks of persistent inflammation or malignant change are to date unfounded. The functional advantages of retaining this anorectal zone seem considerable. However, regular surveillance and biopsy of this region is recommended.

Crohn's disease

In general, surgery for Crohn's disease aims to relieve the patient of the symptomatic complications rather than achieve a cure. Crohn's patients are frequently poorly nourished and may be receiving immunosuppressive treatment. Minimizing operative risk requires careful consideration about the timing and nature of the surgery as intervention should be as safe, conservative, and appropriately timed as possible.

Surgical treatment of small-bowel Crohn's disease, with particular reference to stricture and fistula management, is considered in Chapter 19. Perianal disease is discussed in Chapter 21. Crohn's disease of the colon and rectum may be focal or diffuse. As many as 25 per cent of patients with colonic disease have an apparently normal rectum. There is thus a strong incentive to perform an ileorectal anastomosis rather than commit the patient to a permanent ileostomy. However, if surgical resection is required, its nature is influenced by the extent and severity of the disease.

Severe (fulminating) Crohn's colitis

This is managed the same way as severe ulcerative colitis. Indeed, the diseases may be indistinguishable. If surgery is required, the procedure of choice is total colectomy with preservation of the rectum, ideally exteriorized as a mucous fistula. A temporary ileostomy is fashioned. Intestinal continuity is restored by ileorectal anastomosis once the patient has fully recovered and provided there is relative sparing of disease in the rectum.

Diffuse colitis with rectal sparing

This is managed with colectomy and ileorectal anastomosis. In principle, the longest length of rectum is retained to gain maximum fluid-absorbing capacity and prevent disabling diarrhoea.

Diffuse colitis with rectal involvement

When associated with significant perianal disease, this condition may require panproctocolectomy. The perineal dissection is performed in the intersphincteric plane, thereby leaving a relatively small empty space that may be left to heal by secondary intention.

Localized Crohn's colitis

Localized parts of the colon affected by Crohn's disease may be treated by segmental resection and primary anastomosis.

7.5 Counselling, support groups, and stoma care

Inflammatory bowel disease is frequently diagnosed in young patients and may interfere considerably with their ambitions and ability to lead a normal life. Careful and considerate counselling is valuable in this respect. Support groups for sufferers of ulcerative colitis and Crohn's disease can provide practical help, support, and further information. When patients require a stoma, a stoma therapist provides a key role in assessing the optimal stoma site, providing patient counselling, teaching stoma care, and dealing with stoma-related complications.

8 Colorectal neoplasia

8.1 Polyps

A polyp is the term used to describe any lesion that protrudes from an epithelial surface, in this instance into the bowel lumen. If it has a stalk, the polyp displays a **pedunculated** appearance. Alternatively, it may have a **sessile** form, presenting as a slightly raised nodule. Within the colon, polyps are usually derived from an overgrowth of epithelium, although occasionally they arise from the underlying connective tissue. Colorectal polyps may be classified is several ways, but a commonly used classification is shown in Table 20.3.

Juvenile polyps

Juvenile polyps occur most often in children, usually below the age of 10 years and they may be familial. Although present throughout the large bowel, these histologically distinct polyps are most common in the rectum. A low rectal polyp may pro-

Table 20.3 Classification of polyps

Non-neoplastic	Metaplastic
	Inflammatory
	Hamartomatous
Neoplastic	Adenomatous
	Tubular
	Tubulo-villous
	Villous
	Carcinoma

lapse through the anus, or it may present with rectal bleeding. Occasionally, a juvenile polyp may be found in the baby's nappy after spontaneous autoamputation. Juvenile polyps are not premalignant and may be removed endoscopically.

Peutz–Jeghers polyps

These polyps occur as part of a rare familial disorder, Peutz–Jeghers syndrome, and are associated with pigmentation around the lips. In addition to polyps in the colon, polyps may be found in the small bowel and stomach. Histologically, they are characterized by a branch-like excrescence of the muscularis mucosae. These polyps first present in childhood with bleeding or may cause obstructive symptoms due to intussusception. The polyps have a malignant potential, but treatment is limited because of their widespread nature. Surgery is usually restricted to complications as they arise.

Inflammatory polyps

These are composed of residual epithelial pseudopolyps which protrude above the surrounding ulceration and granulation tissue. The polyps are not premalignant. Inflammatory polyps are typically associated with inflammatory bowel disease, amoebiasis, and schistosomiasis. They are occasionally found at the site of previous colonic anastomoses and can be confused with local anastomotic recurrence.

Lipomas, leiomyomas, and haemangiomas

Lipomas and leiomyomas are commonly found but rarely give rise to symptoms. Typically, they are sessile, smooth, and covered by normal-looking mucosa. In general they need no treatment. Occasionally, large polyps may ulcerate and bleed. Haemangiomas can present with intermittent and sometimes severe colonic bleeding. Localization and distinction from angiodysplasia often proves difficult. Although benign, large haemangiomas are best treated by segmental resection.

Adenomatous polyps

Adenomatous polyps are composed of dysplastic epithelium, either lining the glands (**tubular adenomas**) or raised into a villous pattern (**villous adenomas**). The degree of dysplasia varies within and between adenomatous polyps. They are **premalignant** lesions and the risk of malignancy increases with the size of the adenoma and the severity of dysplasia. Malignancy is more likely in those with a villous configuration. Adenomas are frequently multiple and may coexist with carcinoma.

Most adenomatous polyps are asymptomatic and are discovered incidentally, for example by palpation during rectal examination or visualized on sigmoidoscopy. However, colonoscopy remains the best method of detecting them. Some adenomatous polyps cause bleeding, prolapse, or intussusception. If there are multiple adenomatous polyps in the rectum, diarrhoea or mucus discharge may result. Rarely, a large villous adenoma of the rectum presents with symptoms of hypokalaemia.

Complete removal of adenomatous polyp(s) should be performed, followed by accurate histological assessment. There

Table 20.4 Surveillance after removal of colonic polyps

1. Remove all polyps.

2. If polyps are adenomatous, further colonoscopy in 1 year.

3. If colon is clear, no further colonoscopy for 4 years unless symptoms return.

are several methods available for removal, including transanal excision under direct vision or using transanal endoscopic microsurgery (TEM), or by colonoscopic snare. It is acceptable to destroy small, sessile lesions using 'hot' biopsy forceps. However, surgical excision is the safest option for moderately sized sessile or large (> 5 cm) polypoid adenomatous polyps. If carcinoma is discovered within the polyp, it need not mandate further surgical treatment provided the lesion is well or moderately differentiated and the resection margin exceeds 2 mm (see Table 20.5). However, surveillance of the biopsy site will be needed. Once the colon is 'clean' of polyps, the patient should be offered repeat colonoscopy after 3 years, because of the risk of further adenomatous polyps developing. This may be extended to 5 years if the patient remains polyp free (Table 20.4).

Adenoma–carcinoma sequence

Evidence for the importance of the adenoma as a precursor of colonic cancer is largely derived from a series of observations on the prevalence and behaviour of adenomatous polyps in colorectal cancer and familial adenomatous polyposis. The significant features are:

Table 20.5 Management of colonic polyps according to histology (Note: numbering likely to change)

Histology of excised polyp	Futher immediate management	Colonoscopic surveillance policy
Invasive carcinoma (i) • Through muscularis mucosa or into stalk • Poorly differentiated • Incomplete removal	Consider bowel resection	Endoscope 3–5 yearly
Invasive carcinoma (ii) • Through muscularis muscosa or into stalk • Not poorly differentiated • Completely excised	Endoscopic surveillance	Endoscope at 6 months —if colon clear, repeat at 1 year. If clear at 1 year, repeat 3–5 yearly
Adenomatous or tubulovillous polyp with no evidence of malignancy	Remove any residual polyps colonoscopically	Surveillance 3–5 yearly

(1) the distribution of adenomatous polyps and carcinoma in the colon and rectum is identical;

(2) adenomatous polyps occur at a mean 5 years earlier than the mean age of patients developing colorectal cancer;

(3) one or more coincidental adenomatous polyps are found in 30 per cent of resected colon cancer specimens; in these patients, metachronous cancer occurs twice as commonly as in those without polyps;

(4) more than 70 per cent of patients with synchronous cancers have coexisting adenomas;

(5) adenomatous tissue and carcinoma frequently coexist in a polyp.

Familial adenomatous polyposis

Familial adenomatous polyposis (FAP) is inherited through an autosomal dominant gene with incomplete penetrance. The incidence is around 1 : 10 000 live births. It is characterized at the genetic level by a deletion on the p-arm (p21) on chromosome 5. It follows that within families of known patients, individuals can be identified by careful DNA screening. Furthermore, congenital hypertrophy of the retinal pigmented epithelium (CHRPE) is highly specific for FAP and can be detected on ophthalmological examination, often before polyps develop. It should be noted that 25 per cent of cases are due to new mutations and give no family history.

Sigmoidoscopic examination of the rectal mucosa can be used to confirm established disease. The affected colon and rectum are covered with hundreds of polyps. The disease develops in early adult life and within 10 years or a few more, invariably undergoes malignant transformation. FAP patients frequently have other abnormalities, including multiple osteomas, epidermoid cysts, desmoid (stromal) tumours, and periampullary tumours of the duodenum.

Early surgical intervention is advocated, before malignant transformation occurs. Total colectomy with ileorectal anastomosis, followed by outpatient surveillance of the remaining rectum with endoscopic treatment of polyps, as necessary, is frequently undertaken. However, this has the disadvantage that rectal cancer will develop later in some cases. This can be avoided by panproctocolectomy, although the patient requires a permanent ileostomy. A **restorative proctocolectomy** with an ileal pouch–anal anastomosis combats both these disadvantages and is now considered to be the treatment of choice.

Metaplastic and hyperplastic polyps

The terms metaplastic and hyperplastic are used synonymously for these common polyps. They are often multiple and are rarely larger than 5 mm in diameter and are slightly raised above the surrounding mucosa. They have a pale, uniform appearance and are most frequently seen in the rectum and sigmoid colon. Histological appearances are distinctive, yet their aetiology remains unknown. Metaplastic polyps have no malignant potential. Unless large numbers are seen on sigmoidoscopy, there is no indication to perform colonoscopy.

8.2 Colorectal cancer

This is the second most common malignancy in the Western world. Approximately 25 000 new cases are reported annually in the United Kingdom. The peak incidence is in patients aged 70–80 years. Half of all cases present when the disease is already beyond a surgical cure; disappointingly, the annual UK mortality of 19 000 has not changed significantly over the past 40 years. Although the aetiology of colorectal cancer has not yet been fully worked out, a combination of environmental and genetic factors appears to play an important part in the pathogenesis. Specific disorders that increase the likelihood of developing a colonic malignancy include inflammatory bowel disease (ulcerative colitis and Crohn's disease), familial adenomatous polyposis, and schistosomiasis. It is probable that mucosal malignant change is induced by contact with faecal chemicals (e.g. altered bile acids), but the detail of this is unclear.

Pathology

Adenocarcinoma arises from the epithelial lining of the colon and rectum. It may present as a polypoid, ulcerating, or stenosing lesion. Histologically, the cancer may range from a well-differentiated lesion with recognizable glandular structures to a poorly differentiated tumour. Local spread is by direct invasion through the muscle wall, into local structures. Distant metastasis commonly follows lymphatic channels to draining lymph nodes and may migrate further into the portal venous system. Alternatively, malignant cells may disperse within the abdominal cavity by transcoelomic spread and take root there.

Clinicopathological staging of colorectal cancer

Staging represents the anatomical extent of tumour spread estimated after operation, and should have a clinically meaningful correlation with prognosis. However, staging alone does not take into account many other factors (such as tumour grade) which affect prognosis and as such, should not be regarded as a *prognostic index*. Validation of any staging system requires scrutiny of large series of patients treated in standardized ways and with accurate and long-term data collection.

Dukes (1932) described a system of purely pathological staging rectal cancer which depended on the histological extent of tumour spread within the resected specimen. It correlated well with prognosis but, among other weaknesses, ignored evident distant metastases or bowel end involvement. In 1939, the Mayo Clinic demonstrated that the Dukes staging system applied equally well to colonic cancer. The definitive paper on Dukes staging by Dukes and Bussey (1958) was based on 2447 carefully documented patients treated at St Mark's Hospital, London and followed up over 24 years. Dukes later subdivided his C category into C1 and C2 according to whether the highest or apical node was involved or not. Turnbull *et al.* from the Cleveland Clinic in 1967 added a D stage if at operation there were distant metastases or tumour invading the abdominal wall or other organs, but this did not necessarily imply incurability.

The American Joint Committee for Cancer (AJCC) published recommendations for the staging of colonic and rectal cancer which followed the TNM principles laid down by the Union Internationale Contre Le Cancer (UICC) of 1968. This was based on a retrospective study of 1826 cases and used multiple regression analysis. It was later modified according to results of prospective analyses (AJCC 1992). The system recognized five stages depending upon the extent direct tumour spread (T), the

Table 20.6 Modified Dukes' classification for staging colorectal cancer

Stage A	Growth limited to the bowel wall
Stage B	Extension into the perirectal or colic fat, but no lymph-node metastases
Stage C1	Lymph-node metastases in the vascular pedicle, but the most apical node clear
Stage C2	Lymph-node metastases in the vascular pedicle, but the most apical node involved
Stage D (Turnbull)	Distant metastases or irremovable tumour because of parietal invasion or adjacent organ invasion

presence of lymph node metastases (N) at the presence of distant metastases at the time of operation. As it was based on post-surgical staging, it was labelled pTNM staging. The later version included an 'R' category for cases where residual tumour has been left but remains optional. Although the system correlated better with survival than modified Dukes staging especially in cases with a very good or very poor prognosis, however it remains complex and time consuming to implement. For the time being, the modified Dukes staging system seems the most useful. However, an initiative from the 1990 World Congress of Gastroenterology examined the six most commonly used staging systems and found all of them flawed. It recommended a standard international documentation system (IDS) be adopted for colorectal cancer with an standard comprehensive anatomical terminology. IDS consists of a minimal list of clinical and pathological features for documentation in prospective studies. The ultimate aim is to develop a standard staging system of greater efficacy. In the end, whether or not residual tumour has been left is likely to become the gold standard for prognostication and this is likely to eventually become achievable.

Dukes' classification (Table 20.6) addresses the stage of spread of the carcinoma and gives information about the general prognosis, including the probability of occult hepatic metastasis, which is a major factor affecting long-term survival. It is important to be clear which Dukes' classification or which modification of it is being discussed as many variants have been proposed and adopted in different places. Alternatively, more refined staging methods have been proposed, although none has been so widely adopted.

It is of considerable interest and importance that about 7 per cent of patients have synchronous bowel cancers (i.e. present at the same time as the principle cancer), and that within 10 years of a curative resection, almost 5 per cent of all patients will have developed a further (**metachronous**) malignancy in the remaining bowel.

Clinical features

The clinical presentation of colorectal cancer is largely determined by the part of the bowel involved (Table 20.7). Distribution is uneven around the colon and rectum, with almost 70 per cent distal to the splenic flexure. Moreover, 45 per

Table 20.7 Clinical presentations of colorectal cancer

Right-sided lesions	Occult blood loss
	Anaemia
	Obstruction
Left-sided lesions	Visible blood in stool
	Altered bowel habit
	Obstruction

cent of colorectal cancers are at, or below, the rectosigmoid junction. Left-sided lesions clearly predominate, but carcinoma of the caecum is becoming more common.

Preoperative assessment

A careful history together with a general abdominal, rectal, and sigmoidoscopic examination form an essential part of the assessment of the patient. Biopsy specimens are taken if a rectal cancer is identified for histological confirmation. Where sigmoidoscopy is normal, colonoscopy or barium enema examination should be performed to seek a more proximal lesion. This has the added purpose of excluding a synchronous tumour and is recommended before virtually all planned resections, once a cancer is found. If a satisfactory colonoscopy is impossible before resection, one should be carried out within the first postoperative year to exclude other polyps.

In rectal cancers, digital examination provides valuable information about the degree of invasion of the tumour into surrounding tissues. This can also be assessed by endoluminal ultrasonography or computed tomography of the pelvis. Abdominal ultrasonography or computed tomography will also assist in preoperative staging. However, the discovery of hepatic metastasis rarely precludes surgery as resection provides good palliation.

Hereditary non-polyposis colorectal cancer

The non-polyposis syndromes are inherited in an autosomal dominant fashion and patients can be identified as carrying a specific chromosomal abnormality. Patients fall into two categories:

1. **Lynch syndrome I**—hereditary site-specific colon cancer. This predisposes only to colorectal cancer.

2. **Lynch syndrome II**—with a predisposition to colorectal, endometrial, ovarian, and gastric cancer.

HNPCC families account for between 5 and 10 per cent of all colorectal cancers. The tumours are predominantly right sided, occur in the early 40s, and there is a higher incidence than normal of synchronous and metachronous lesions. Families may be identified by applying the Amsterdam criteria (Table 20.8) and if a family seems to fall into this category, decisions can be made as to whether referral for genetic screening is justified.

The significance of family history

It is uncertain whether medical concern about the family history of colorectal cancer patients has led to an overall improvement in the management of the disease. On the one hand, if what represented a 'significant' family history could be defined, then

Table 20.8 The Amsterdam criteria for suspecting HNPCC

Three or more relatives with colorectal cancer

At least one first-degree relative affected by the disease

At least two generations affected by the disease

One family member with colorectal disease should be under the age of 50

Table 20.9 Steps in managing a family member anxious about inherited colorectal cancer

1. Take an accurate family history

2. Is the family history significant?
   ◆ Several first-degree relatives with the disease
   ◆ Age of onset less than 40

3. What type of screening is advisable?
   ◆ A one-off colonoscopy
   ◆ Regular colonoscopies
   ◆ Refer for genetic counselling and screening

4. Discuss possible involvement of other family members in the screening process

individuals in such families could be targeted for screening with the expectation of a higher yield of preventable disease and perhaps cure. However, in the absence of such a definition, many people informed by the media that a family history is important, have reason for worry and seek reassurance. Most however, have little cause for serious concern.

A positive family history of colorectal cancer does not necessarily mean that other family members are likely to develop the disease (Table 20.9). Even when the evidence is strong for a genetic basis (young age of onset, several first-degree relatives having the disease) a genetic abnormality may not be identified, and even if it is, cancer development is not inevitable (Table 20.10). As with other forms of screening for genetic abnormalities, the decision to screen a family should not be taken lightly. The consequence of a person being shown to carry a gene but without there being a definitive preventative treatment can damage a life psychologically. Furthermore, the fact that a definitive genetic abnormality is not found does not allow total reassurance. Thus, experienced genetic counsellors should become involved before genetic screening is undertaken.

In practice, enquiries arise either from anxious family members without symptoms or parents concerned that their children may develop the disease. The recommended approach is similar for all groups and is considered here. The criteria for referral for genetic counselling need to be strict. Family sizes vary, and in

Table 20.10 Lifetime risk of colorectal cancer in first-degree relatives

Population risk	1 in 50
One relative affected	1 in 17
One first- and one second-degree relative	1 in 12
One relative under 45	1 in 10
Two first-degree relatives	1 in 6
Dominant pedigree	1 in 2

Table 20.11 Glossary of terms about colorectal cancer

1. Colon cancer versus rectal cancer	Colon and rectal cancers are often discussed separately when adjuvant therapy is considered
	Excision of lower sigmoid and rectosigmoid cancers involves excision of the upper rectum—so which group?
	Tumours within 15 cm of the anus should be regarded as rectal and the term 'rectosigmoid' should be abandoned
2. Surgical resection	• Aim to resect all local disease in the bowel wall and draining lymphatics
	• Local invasion of lateral pelvic wall, bladder, uterus, etc. makes wider resection desirable
	• Extensive lymph-node dissection does not improve survival or the incidence of local recurrence. Flush ligation of the lymphovascular pedicle at the aorta is not beneficial
	• Lymph-node metastasis is a sign of aggressive disease and an indication to consider adjuvant treatment. Benefits are uncertain and are under review in several clinical trials
	• After an operation the surgeon can classify it as potentially curative or palliative (if there is residual disease or evidence of metastases)
	• For fixed tumours, resection may not be possible and only a palliative defunctioning stoma (for pelvic tumours) or a bypass (for more proximal tumours) can be performed
3. Recurrent disease	
(a) Anastomotic recurrence	This is prone to occur with low colorectal anastomoses. Distal clearance is limited by proximity to the anal canal: the minimum recommended clearance is 2 cm
	Measures which may reduce the incidence of anastomotic recurrence are:
	• peroperative washout of the distal rectum with a cytocide;
	• when a double-stapled anastomosis is used, the cross staple line should be in an area of rectum already irrigated with cytocide
(b) Local recurrence	Most commonly occurs with rectal cancer and is likely to be related to the effectiveness of excisional surgery. Recurrent disease in the soft tissues of the pelvis or lateral pelvic nodes represents treatment failure but it is uncertain whether the cause is inadequate surgery or the biological behaviour of the disease
	Total excision of the rectal mesentery (TME, see later) reduces the incidence of local recurrence but it is not the only determinant—pelvic recurrence often occurs in tandem with distant metastases, suggesting that the systemic response has failed
(c) Metastatic disease	Nodal disease is an indicator of disease aggression with regard to the use of adjuvant therapy
	Liver metastases are often multiple and make the disease incurable, except in a small number of cases where liver resection is practicable and proves beneficial

small families few are at risk and few family members are likely to have had the disease. However, if a particularly young family member develops colorectal cancer, this must be regarded as significant. Patients or relatives must understand the uncertainties, discussed earlier, which may result from counselling and genetic analysis, and many families decide against referral at this point. Where the family history is weak, there is no need for genetic screening but clinical screening is wise. The choices are discussed below.

Prevention (screening)

Population screening may be beneficial in prevention and in early detection of colonic and rectal cancer. The method employed must be proven to be efficacious, furthermore it must safe, simple, acceptable, reliable, and cheap. Perhaps not surprisingly, no single method matches these stringent requirements. The current favourite relies upon detecting unseen blood in the stool (Haemoccult®, Faecotest®). Patients who are positive for faecal occult blood proceed to flexible sigmoidoscopy or colonoscopy. Disappointingly, audit of the final outcome of population screening for colorectal cancer with faecal occult blood testing

reveals not only that the test is a poor predictor of underlying neoplasia, but that the apparent improved survival achieved by detecting early lesions can be explained by lead-time bias. Screening of high-risk groups may improve the yield. For example, people from families with a history of cancer, polyposis, and inflammatory bowel disease are at increased risk. Likewise, patients who have had adenomatous polyps or colorectal cancers treated merit close surveillance.

Planning treatment for colorectal cancer

As with other common malignancies, the care of patients with this colorectal cancer often involves doctors in other disciplines, particularly medical gastroenterology. Surgeons often conduct the initial management and thus tend to determine the general direction of therapy. Surgical resection is the principal form of treatment and the morbidity and mortality of surgery has improved steadily in recent years. However, the same cannot be said of the disease outcome. Thus other advances are needed to improve the outcome, including earlier diagnosis and perhaps adjuvant treatment. This can be a confusing field because of the number of current clinical trials taking place. Part of the difficulty stems from confusion about terminology and it may be helpful to draw up a series of definitions (Table 20.11).

Pre- and postoperative adjuvant treatments

Whenever additional therapy is considered, its purpose must be clear: is it intended for palliative or salvage reasons or is it intended to increase the chances of cure i.e. true 'adjuvant' therapy? This distinction is not always possible, but to compare the effectiveness of different treatments, attempts must be made.

The objectives of adjuvant therapy in colorectal cancer are to reduce the incidence of local recurrence and metastatic disease. Radiotherapy and chemotherapy are the two most commonly used treatments. In rectal cancer, the primary aim of radiotherapy is to reduce the local recurrence rate, whereas chemotherapy for both rectal and colonic cancer is intended to reduce the incidence of metastases. Relatively few patients die from local recurrence unless associated with metastases, so irradiation should not be expected to alter survival. Nevertheless a recent Swedish study on the use of preoperative radiotherapy for patients with rectal cancer rather surprisingly demonstrated a survival advantage as well as a reduction in the incidence of local recurrence.

Preoperative adjuvant therapy—potentially curable cases

Colon cancer

There is no evidence to support the use of either radiotherapy or chemotherapy prior to surgery in colonic cancer.

Rectal cancer

The value of preoperative chemoirradiation in operable rectal cancer is a matter of intense debate. Swedish studies suggest that preoperative irradiation not only reduces the incidence of local pelvic recurrence but also provides a survival benefit. Surgery should take place within a week of finishing irradiation to avoid operating when the fibrotic process has become established.

Postoperative adjuvant therapy

Adjuvant chemotherapy during the immediate postoperative period is attractive because it follows surgical debulking of the tumour mass when the quantity of residual tumour is either small or absent. Provided the tumour cells are sensitive to the cytocidal action of the agents used, the therapy ought to improve survival, but herein lies the problem. The main agent used in the treatment of colorectal cancer is 5–fluorouracil (5FU). This has a variable effect on colorectal tumour cells. Its potency can be enhanced by combining it with folinic acid. This modulates the action of 5FU by enhancing its enzyme poisoning effects on cell metabolism. An alternative approach is to use immunotherapeutic agents such as interferon, interleukin, and small-molecular-weight immunomodulators such as levamisole or cimetidine.

Colonic cancer

There is no evidence to support the use of postoperative irradiation in colon cancer. The case for adjuvant chemotherapy is undergoing various trials at present. In the QUASAR trial, the chemotherapy regimens being tested are intravenous 5FU coupled with either high- or low-dose folinic acid. In addition, a comparison is being made between oral levamisole, an immunostimulant, and placebo capsules among the chemotherapy group of patients. The study is designed to look specifically at the possible value of chemotherapy in Dukes' B and C patients.

Rectal cancer

Chemotherapy

Several Scandinavian studies have studied prospectively agents such as 5FU, leucovorin, and levamisole in postoperative rectal cancer (Dukes' B and C) and have not shown a survival advantage.

Radiotherapy

There is no evidence that routine postoperative irradiation reduces the incidence of local recurrence in patients who are thought to have had a curative surgical resection. What is less clear is whether irradiation helps in patients thought likely to have a increased risk of developing local recurrence. These include those where the surgeon considered removal to have been incomplete or where there is pathological evidence of tumour at the resection margin. This question may be answered by the proposed CRO7 trial (Table 20.12) which compares preoperative radiotherapy with selective postoperative chemoradiotherapy in rectal cancer.

Salvage and palliative treatment

Patients found to have tethered or fixed rectal tumours are sometimes referred for preoperative irradiation in an attempt to reduce the size of the tumour and make surgery possible ('downstaging'). This must be regarded as a salvage procedure. Similarly, any treatment directed at metastatic disease has to be regarded as palliative. This situation needs to be handled with sensitivity and a humane, open approach. After discussion, some patients will choose not to have treatment and this view should be respected. If chemotherapy is chosen, there are two trials in place in the UK into which patients may be entered (CRO5 and CRO6, see Table 20.12).

The plethora of trials currently available should answer the important questions about the effectiveness of adjuvant and palliative treatment. However, it must be remembered that any improvements in survival from these treatments are at best small and that the most effective curative treatment for colorectal cancer is effective surgery if the stage allows it.

Cancer of the right colon

Right-sided colonic cancer, with or without obstruction, is treated by right hemicolectomy and primary anastomosis. This procedure removes a small length of distal ileum, the caecum, ascending colon, and the proximal third of the transverse colon. The blood supply to this segment is chiefly via the ileocolic artery and the integrity of the anastomosis (given good surgical

Table 20.12 Clinical trials in progress testing the effectiveness of adjuvant and palliative treatment of colorectal cancer

Metastatic colorectal cancer

CRO5: a randomized trial of intravenous versus intrahepatic arterial 5FU and leucovorin for colorectal liver metastases

CRO6: a randomized trial comparing two durations and three systemic regimens in the palliative treatment of advanced colorectal cancer

Clinically operable adenocarcinoma of the rectum

CRO7 – Randomize into:

| A | Preoperative radiotherapy (25 Gy) Surgery and pathology assessment | B | Selective postoperative chemoradiotherapy Surgery and pathology assessment Patients at risk of local recurrence receive chemoradiotherapy (45 Gy and 5FU) |

Selecting patients with colorectal cancer for trials of additional treatment

Potentially operable cancer of the rectum	*Metastatic colorectal cancer*	
CRO7 trial	Liver metastases only	Metastases at any site
	Operable	Inoperable
	Surgery	CRO5 trial

technique) depends on the vascular supply from the distal ileal arterial branches and the middle colic artery. For cancers of the distal transverse colon, **extended right hemicolectomy** is the appropriate treatment. This procedure removes the ascending and transverse colon together with the middle colic artery. The blood supply of the remaining colon then relies on the proximal branches of the inferior mesenteric artery contributing to the marginal artery. This **watershed** area, between the superior and inferior mesenteric arterial blood supplies, located around the splenic flexure, is likely to be relatively ischaemic when compared with other parts of the colon, and the blood supply to the cut ends of the colon should be carefully assessed prior to anastomosis.

Cancer of the left colon

Left-sided colonic cancer may be treated by wide excision including the splenic flexure, descending and sigmoid colon (left hemicolectomy), and primary anastomosis. The arterial integrity of the proximal and distal ends then depends upon the middle colic artery (from the superior mesenteric artery) and the middle rectal arteries (Fig. 20.8). Alternatively, a non-obstructing cancer within the sigmoid loop may be excised by a sigmoid colectomy and primary anastomosis. The sigmoid loop usually lies free in the abdominal cavity but can be fixed to local structures by the disease process. Greater mobility is obtained by freeing the lateral peritoneal adhesion; this opens up the retroperitoneum to reveal the left ureter. The junction between the sigmoid colon and rectum is marked by the transition in the longitudinal musculature from three taenia coli to the complete smooth-muscle layer of the rectum.

The presence of intestinal obstruction has traditionally influenced attitudes away from performing a primary anastomosis. In the past, left-sided colonic obstruction was treated by a three-stage procedure. This involved a proximal defunctioning colostomy, followed later by resection of the cancer with anastomosis and later by closure of the colostomy. In most

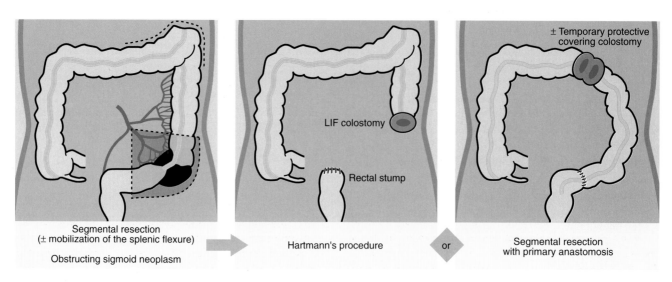

Segmental resection
(± mobilization of the splenic flexure)

Obstructing sigmoid neoplasm

LIF colostomy

Rectal stump

Hartmann's procedure

or

± Temporary protective covering colostomy

Segmental resection with primary anastomosis

Figure 20.8 Anatomy of resections for left-sided colonic cancer.

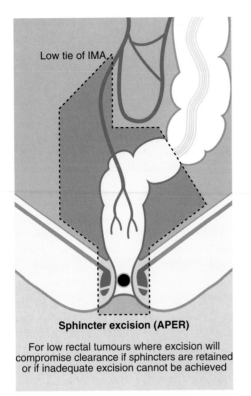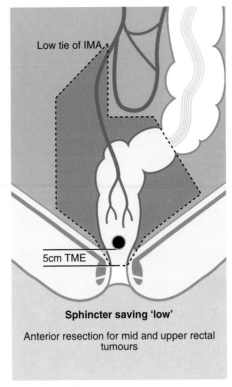

Figure 20.9 Anterior resection (sphincter-saving resection) and abdomino-perineal resection of the rectum for rectal cancer.

centres in recent years, this has been reduced to two stages (Hartmann's operation) with resection and colostomy as the primary procedure. The proximal colon is exteriorized as an end colostomy and the distal end may be brought to the abdominal surface as a mucous fistula, or closed off. Restoration of bowel continuity entails the second stage. Contemporary surgical management of obstructing left colonic lesions goes a step further, aiming to achieve resection and primary anastomosis in a single stage. This can be achieved either by on-table lavage, which clears upstream faecal material and reduces the disproportion in lumen size between proximal and distal cut ends, or, alternatively, by subtotal colectomy and anastomosis of ileum to distal colon or rectum.

Cancer of the rectum

The two procedures commonly used for surgical treatment of rectal cancer are anterior resection (sphincter-saving resection) and abdomino-perineal resection of the rectum, which leaves a permanent colostomy (Fig. 20.9). The main determinant of which procedure is performed is the distance of the cancer from the anal margin. There is a fine balance between the necessity to achieve a clear distal margin in excess of 2 cm in order to minimize local recurrence, and consideration of the functional outcome. An anastomosis involving the anorectal transition zone not only reduces the rectal reservoir but may also impair internal anal sphincter tone and so compromise anal control and continence. An intact external anal sphincter is rarely sufficient to maintain complete continence, particularly if the

stool is loose. However, a greater residual rectal reservoir can be achieved by fashioning a colonic pouch, as described earlier. Apart from the tumour site, other important factors include the stage and degree of differentiation of the cancer. Extension through the bowel wall, particularly invasion of the mesorectum, requires wide lateral clearance. In addition, poorly differentiated adenocarcinomas often infiltrate the mucosa widely and necessitate greater longitudinal clearance margins, perhaps as much as 5 cm.

Anterior resection

Anterior resection is considered the standard approach for cancers of the upper and mid-rectum. It may also be undertaken for selected distal rectal cancers where adequate, safe clearance can be achieved without disturbance of the anal sphincter complex. The operative details are available in standard operative texts but it is worth stressing that effective surgery must pay special attention to three areas in particular:

◆ The need for 2 cm of distal luminal clearance.

◆ The lymph nodes which drain the rectum lie in the rectal mesentery and total excision of the mesentery (**total mesorectal excision**; TME) is regarded as essential if all nodes are to be removed and thereby reduce the incidence of local recurrence. This means that the mesorectum has to be removed down to the level of the pelvic floor in all cases. With high rectal cancers it is often feasible to achieve a distal luminal clearance of 2 cm without carrying the dissection of the mesorectum down to the pelvic floor—a good reason why the mesorectum is often only partly excised.

- The lateral pelvic wall is often a site of tumour invasion and, wherever possible, clearance should be achieved in this direction.

The aim of surgery is to try to achieve clearance as defined above and then to allow the pathologist to assess whether there are clear **circumferential resection margins** (CRMs).

Abdomino-perineal resection

An abdomino-perineal excision of the rectum (**synchronous combined excision of the rectum**) may be necessary for very low rectal cancers encroaching on the anorectal transition zone. The upper rectum is mobilized in exactly the same way as for an anterior resection and it is carried down into the pelvis as far as technically feasible. The perineal operator then dissects upwards around the anal sphincteric ring and through the levator ani pelvic sling to meet the abdominal operator. The perineal cavity is closed around drains, the pelvic peritoneal floor is reconstituted by the abdominal surgeon and a left iliac fossa permanent colostomy is brought onto the abdominal wall.

Alternative procedures for rectal cancer may be considered. For example, Hartmann's operation involves resection of the rectum without an anastomosis and the proximal colon exteriorized as an end colostomy. Frequently, this operation is designed to give palliative control, although it is sometimes used as the initial procedure for acute cases, particular where the operator is not a colorectal specialist. Local excision can be effective, using **trans-anal endoscopic microsurgery** on a selected group of small, well-differentiated tumours of the rectum. However, early experience gives cause for concern because of the high incidence of local recurrence. Other approaches include endoscopic resection, electrocoagulation (diathermy) or laser destruction, photodynamic therapy, or radiotherapy, used alone or in combination. These methods, too, are prone to local recurrence because of inadequate clearance or tumour implantation. None the less, symptom and tumour control can be achieved, particularly in very frail and elderly patients unsuitable for major surgery. Endoscopic resection frequently achieves good control and may be repeated whenever necessary.

Mortality and morbidity

In general, the operative mortality for cancer surgery of the colon and rectum should be less than 5 per cent. Indeed, some centres claim a rate less than 2 per cent. However, outcome is inevitably influenced by case mix. Concurrent cardiorespiratory problems, particularly in the elderly, are principal causes of death after surgery. Furthermore, operative mortality is higher if the surgery is undertaken for colonic obstruction or perforation.

The surgeon and surgical technique are important determinants of anastomotic leak rate. In any patient, an anastomotic dehiscence is likely to be life threatening. Although there is a small risk of leakage from any colonic anastomosis, the risk is greater in low colorectal anastomosis.

Less serious complications include wound infection and genitourinary dysfunction. Perioperative prophylactic antibiotic therapy minimizes the incidence and severity of wound infection. Avoidance of damage to the autonomic nerves within the pelvis can greatly reduce postoperative urinary retention and later impotence.

Follow-up

Clinical review after resection of a colonic or rectal cancer is aimed at detecting recurrent or metastatic disease. This assumes that treatment will be better if these complications are found early. This may be a forlorn hope, however, as potentially treatable recurrent disease is rarely detected. Furthermore, reliable detection requires more than clinical examination. Patients at greatest risk should be targeted, with analysis of serum markers, regular colonoscopy, and hepatic ultrasound. Moreover, rectal endosonography can detect local extrarectal recurrence after anterior resection

9 Functional bowel disorders

9.1 Rectal prolapse

This condition affects children and adults. It may be surprisingly well tolerated, although it frequently causes discomfort and distress, forcing some adult sufferers into self-inflicted social exclusion. Rectal prolapse can be partial (incomplete) or complete. A partial prolapse is limited to the mucosal layers of the rectum, whereas complete rectal prolapse involves the two layers of rectum and the intervening peritoneal sac, with or without contained small bowel. Mucosal prolapse is most common in children. In contrast, 85 per cent of adults with full-thickness rectal prolapse are women and invariably of advanced age.

Aetiology

The precise aetiology of rectal prolapse remains unknown. In children, the causal factors include diarrhoea, constipation, or poor defecatory habits. Mucosal prolapse in adults may be associated with large haemorrhoids. In elderly patients there is invariably a history of constipation and prolonged straining at stool, with consequent attenuation of the pelvic floor musculature and anal sphincter mechanism. Rectal prolapse is not thought to be causally associated with childbirth or parity. Theoretically, a complete rectal prolapse may result from a concealed intussusception of the proximal rectum, which in turn is predisposed to by poor rectal fixity or an excessively deep rectovaginal or rectovesical pouch.

Clinical features

Children

A rectal prolapse is usually first noticed by a parent after the child has defecated. There is sometimes discomfort and a small amount of mucus discharge or blood. The child is otherwise well. The prolapse is usually easily reduced. Rectal prolapse must be distinguished from a prolapsed rectal polyp or colonic intussusception. Careful palpation between finger and thumb invariably reveals that the prolapse consists only of the mucosal layer.

Adults

Symptoms in rectal prolapse are frequently compounded by concomitant poor sphincter function. Defecation invariably produces prolapsing rectal tissue and may require manual reduction; rarely is it irreducible. Discomfort, discharge, and rectal bleeding are frequent complaints. In some patients, coughing, sneezing, and, indeed, merely standing may precipitate prolapse. Not surprisingly, three-quarters of these patients have faecal incontinence. On examination the anus is patulous and the anal sphincter weak. The patient may be able to 'strain down' the prolapse, or indeed it may well be evident. Close inspection of the mucosa may reveal granularity and ulceration (**solitary rectal ulcer**).

After reducing the prolapse, it is important to perform a sigmoidoscopy. A large prolapsing polypoid tumour of the rectum or sigmoid colon can be indistinguishable at first sight.

Surgical correction

Partial (incomplete) prolapse

Minimal rectal prolapse can be managed by a haemorrhoidectomy-type procedure, where the lower rectal mucosa is removed. Particular care must be taken to avoid circumferential excision of anal-canal skin as this will lead to an anal stenosis. Where the anal sphincter is very lax, a postanal repair operation may be necessary in addition.

Complete rectal prolapse

Many surgical techniques have been described and they may be broadly divided into perineal and abdominal procedures.

Encircling sutures (Thiersch technique)

Through two small incisions at the anal margin, wire, nylon, or silastic is threaded around the anal sphincter to support the prolapse and induce fibrosis of the anal canal. Difficulties arise when the tension is incorrect or the sling migrates and cuts through the skin.

Delorme's operation (partial excision of the rectum through the anus)

With the rectum fully prolapsed, a circumferential incision is made through the mucosa 1 cm above the dentate line. The mucosa is then stripped from the underlying muscle coat as far as is possible, in a sleeve-like fashion. The muscle wall is plicated with sutures and the mucosal edges approximated prior to gentle reduction.

Abdominal rectopexy

This procedure (Fig. 20.10) aims to prevent rectal intussusception by fixing the rectum to the presacral fascia using sutures after mobilizing the rectum as for an anterior resection. The operation can be performed open or laparoscopically. Earlier operation placed foreign material in the retro-rectal space and wrapped it to a greater or lesser extent around the rectum. Materials included polyvinyl alcohol (Ivalon) sponge (**Well's operation**) and polypropylene or polyester mesh (**Ripstein's operation**). The fibrous reaction then held the rectum in place. Operations involving implants are rarely employed nowadays because the suture operation is simpler and has fewer potential complications. Some surgeons seek to identify the defect in the pelvic floor and narrow it by placing sutures across the two limbs of puborectalis muscle in front of or behind the rectum.

Continence after abdominal rectopexy is improved in almost half the patients. Paradoxically, the main complication is the high incidence (60 per cent) of constipation. This is most likely to be related to impaired rectal immobility, combined with a large, redundant sigmoid loop.

9.2 Constipation

Constipation describes infrequent or irregular and sometimes painful defecation of hard stools. Its assessment is based on considering the possible underlying causes (Table 20.13) and with a careful history and detailed examination, including sigmoido-

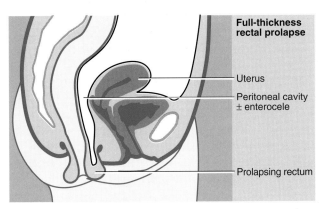

Full-thickness rectal prolapse

Uterus

Peritoneal cavity ± enterocele

Prolapsing rectum

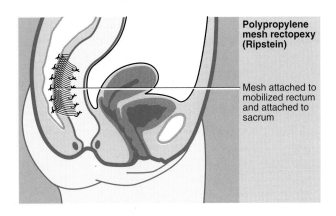

Polypropylene mesh rectopexy (Ripstein)

Mesh attached to mobilized rectum and attached to sacrum

Figure 20.10 Abdominal rectopexy.

Table 20.13 Causes of constipation

Functional
  Aganglionic megacolon
    Hirschsprung's disease
    Chagas disease
  Idiopathic megacolon
  Irritable bowel syndrome
  Slow transit
  Dietary
  Depression
  Drugs, e.g. iron, antidepressants

Medical diseases
  e.g. Myxoedema

Colorectal lesions
  Carcinoma
  Diverticular disease
  Crohn's disease
  Colonic strictures

scopy. In older patients presenting with constipation, and in any patient with constipation of sudden onset, a double-contrast barium enema is indicated. Surgery has a very limited role in the treatment of primary constipation, although patients with this complaint are commonly referred to surgeons.

In a few patients, constipation proves to be refractory to dietary measures and supplementary laxatives. Careful re-evaluation is necessary, together with specialized investigations of anal and colonic function. It is vital to distinguish between slow colonic transit and anorectal dysfunction, thereby identifying conditions such as Hirschsprung's disease, or severe idiopathic constipation with its associated megacolon and megarectum. The treatment of Hirschsprung's disease is surgical. Idiopathic constipation may be improved by combination therapy (enemas, suppositories, and osmotic laxatives). Moreover, behavioural management and psychotherapy may help. Failing this, surgery is indicated, although the best procedure for intractable constipation is far from evident. A Duhamel procedure or resection with colo-anal anastomosis are suggested for megarectum, whereas a colectomy and ileorectal anastomosis may relieve a functional colonic condition. Alternatively, a defunctioning loop ileostomy can provide enormous relief. In short, surgery is best avoided in this condition.

9.3 Faecal incontinence

Introduction

Faecal incontinence may be defined simply as the involuntary passage of faeces though the anal canal. Estimates of its prevalence suggest that a surprisingly large number (1 : 1000) of people are affected. Incontinence, however, is merely the symptom and often reflects a much more complex underlying physiological problem than the name implies. These patients frequently have abnormalities of sensation, evacuation, and sphincter function. Unravelling the precise pathogenesis of the symptom is complicated by the fact that the finer complexities of anorectal physiology are still relatively poorly understood. Abnormalities in either the external or internal sphincter, anal sensation, rectal sensitivity, or lowered rectal compliance all appear to be able to cause the symptom.

Aetiology of faecal incontinence

The causes of faecal incontinence can be considered under two categories: disorders in which the anorectal continence mechanism is abnormal, and disorders where incontinence occurs despite normal anorectal physiological function. The latter group is easily forgotten but highly important. Constipation with overflow, ulcerative colitis, villous adenoma, and carcinoma of the rectum are good examples of causes of this kind of 'pseudoincontinence'. In the former group the abnormality lies within the continence mechanism. Since the external anal sphincter is under conscious control, the abnormality may lie anywhere between the brain and the bottom.

Most incontinence in the UK is caused by pudendal neuropathy, obstetric injury to the anal sphincters, and iatrogenic injury to the anal sphincters. All three factors are sometimes encountered in a single patient.

Assessment of faecal incontinence

The most important part of the assessment of an incontinent patient is the history. This gives clues to the aetiology of the problem (i.e. obstetric injury or long, forceps-assisted labour). Careful assessment and documentation of the incontinence is vital, with particular reference to the social effects on the lifestyle of the patients. It is easy to get carried away in the decision-making process by seductive apparent abnormalities seen on investigation. This may lead to excessive treatment for minor symptoms, a combination seldom rewarded by good results from surgery.

Care must be taken fully to explore the nature of the incontinence. Are patients able to perceive rectal filling? Are they able to discriminate flatus from faeces? Are they able to defer defecation or does the incontinence occur in the absence of any warning? Do they have symptoms suggestive of urgency? Are there associated symptoms such as urinary incontinence? Assessment of their ability to evacuate the rectum is important. Often patients with what appears to be clear-cut faecal incontinence also have major evacuatory difficulty. They may have to resort to excessive straining or even digital evacuation.

Investigation of the incontinent patient

Care must be exercised to exclude a serious organic pathology, such as a carcinoma or inflammatory bowel disease. There should be a low threshold for investigation of the colon by colonoscopy or barium enema. There are then a bewildering variety of evaluations which may be made on anorectal function. Physiological assessment of anorectal function provides useful information, adding to the history and examination.

Anorectal manometry

Anorectal manometry is the measurement of anal canal pressures, traditionally using a station pull-through technique, with the patient at rest and squeezing their anal sphincters. This yields the resting and squeeze anal canal pressures and the functional anal canal length (length of the anal canal high-pressure zone). Anal canal pressures may be measured by a variety of techniques, including water- or air-filled microballoons, and solid-state intra-anal transducers. Recently the advent of integrated computer software has allowed highly sophisticated measurements, using multilumen, water-perfused tubes, to become available. There is a reasonable body of evidence showing most of these techniques to be reliable and reproducible. Manometry documents the starting point prior to any intervention, providing a useful baseline. Manometry is extremely useful in the diagnosis of Hirschsprung's disease where the recto-sphincteric relaxation reflex can be shown to be absent.

Balloon rectal distension test

Rectal sensory function is assessed by the **balloon rectal distension test**. A balloon is passed into the rectum and then distended at a constant rate with either air or water at 37 °C. Patients are asked to report when they first become aware of any rectal sensation ('threshold volume'), when they feel the desire to defecate ('defecatory desire volume'), and when they can tolerate no further filling of the rectal balloon ('maximum tolerated volume'). The balloon distension test gives a reasonable impression of rectal sensitivity, although it is not without its limitations. Repeatability studies have shown the technique to be reproducible and reliable, although it is well known that variations in the rate of distension of the balloon will result in different values being obtained. When a highly compliant rectal balloon is used, a pressure transducer may be placed inside the balloon and thus a calculation of rectal compliance can be made. The clinical significance of rectal compliance is unclear at present and it is probably a measurement best left to research for the moment. Ambulatory rectal manometry may also play a place in patients with a history of marked urgency of defecation. Rarely, extremely high pressure waves may be seen, implying a primary rectal motor dysfunction.

The anal canal is a highly sensate area. Diverse techniques have been described, including mucosal electro- and thermo-sensitivity. Both are validated methods but mucosal electrosensitivity is probably more widely used. Abnormalities of anal sensation have been identified in incontinent and diabetic patients, but the significance of these observations is unclear.

Neurophysiological assessment

Neurophysiological assessment may include pudendal nerve terminal motor latencies (PNTML) and single-fibre electromyography (SFEMG). To measure PNTML a customized finger stall (PICTURE) is placed in the rectum. The pudendal nerve is then stimulated at the sciatic notch on each side. The time taken from the application of the stimulus to the beginning of the wave of depolarization in the external anal sphincter is measured. This is often prolonged in incontinence associated with protracted labour, when there may be a traction pudendal neuropathy. SFEMG is a much more sensitive test of neuromuscular damage and may be used to assess the degree of denervation and reinnervation that has occurred in the external sphincter. However, SFEMG requires several perineal needle punctures in each patient and is understandably unpopular.

Proctography

Proctography has a relatively minor place in the investigation of incontinence. The patient's rectum is filled with a radiopaque paste to mimic stool. The subject is then placed on a radiolucent lavatory and invited to pass the paste while being screened radiologically. A variety of abnormalities may be seen, including rectocoeles and intrarectal prolapse. An important feature on proctography is the identification of an occult evacuatory disorder in a patient whose primary complaint is of incontinence.

The anatomy of the sphincter complex

The anatomy of the sphincter complex may be imaged in a variety of ways. Intra-anal ultrasound has become the most widely used modality. Detailed images of both internal and external anal sphincter anatomy may be obtained with a high-frequency, 360° rotating head device. This has now replaced the more painful technique of EMG sphincter mapping which had been previously, and painfully, employed. Recent advances in imaging software have allowed three-dimensional reconstructions to be created from intra-anal ultrasound.

Treatment of faecal incontinence

Surgical treatment for incontinence is a last resort. Results from all the different procedures tend to be unpredictable and benefits are often relatively poorly sustained in the long term, even after an initially encouraging response.

Non-surgical treatment

There are no hard and fast rules concerning the dietary and drug treatment of faecal incontinence. Careful counselling of the patients and, sometimes long, slow experimentation with a combination of agents may be needed before resorting to an operation. Bulking agents and increased dietary fibre may be helpful. Many patients, especially those with an habitually low fluid intake, find these measures quite constipating. Loperamide is used widely, appearing to have diverse pharmacological actions, including reduction of stool weight, frequency, urgency, and slowing of intestinal transit. Anticholinergic agents are well known to slow intestinal transit, but these agents tend to be unsuitable for prolonged use because of the high incidence of side-effects, such as dry eyes and mouth. More traditional remedies such as kaolin may also be worth trying. It is now accepted that many patients have a concomitant disorder of rectal evacuation. A combination of a constipating agent along with a stimulant to aid evacuation (i.e. bisacodyl) can be effective.

Several studies have been published showing that biofeedback may be effective, at least in the short term. In principle, biofeedback involves providing the patient with a visible or audible indicator of external anal sphincter contraction. They can then be taught an exercise regime designed to maximize muscle function. However, this approach does nothing to counter the pathogenesis of the incontinence. Most authors have found that the benefits from biofeedback are not sustained well in the longer term.

Surgery for incontinence

The results from the myriad surgical options are best treated as unpredictable. It is vital when counselling patients to be crystal clear about any potential benefits and disadvantages before surgical treatment is begun. The risks of surgery, including the potential need for a stoma in the event of complications, must be included in the discussion. The surgical options fall into three groups:

- repair of a damaged sphincter;
- pelvic-floor repair;
- sphincter augmentation.

Sphincter repair

External anal sphincter repair would appear to be the operation that has the most likelihood of long-term success, provided there is no pudendal neuropathy. This procedure is usually carried out after sphincter trauma, obstetric or iatrogenic injury. The anatomical abnormality is usually relatively straightforward to repair.

At operation, the external sphincter is dissected anteriorly and the intersphincteric plane developed. There is usually a bridge of fibrous connective tissue between the divided ends of the sphincter. The anterior segment of sphincter is fully mobilized back to healthy muscle laterally. The fibrous scar is then divided at its midpoint and an overlapping repair is fashioned, usually using two rows of interrupted, non-absorbable sutures.

Meticulous bowel preparation is thought to be important in minimizing the risk of postoperative infection. Infection can destroy the repair, and great care must be taken to avoid it. Most authors now avoid the use of a temporary stoma to cover the procedure. However, it is important to remain vigilant, since severe postoperative sepsis may require temporary faecal diversion.

The published results from external anal sphincter repair are excellent, with reports of at least 65 per cent of patients gaining full continence. However, more recently there have been some worrying observations that these results may not be maintained in the longer term.

Some authors have reported reparative procedures for internal anal sphincter defects, including direct repair and plication. The results from such operations are not clear and few coloproctologists use them regularly.

Pelvic-floor repair

Procedures to repair the pelvic floor are generally carried out for patients with extensive sphincter damage or pudendal neuro-pathy. The concept behind these operations is that little can be done to improve the muscular function of the sphincter apparatus and the pelvic floor is reconfigured to lengthen the anal canal or to increase the angulation at the anorectal junction.

Results from these procedures is unpredictable. Some patients are undoubtedly improved, but a minority, as many as a third, may be worsened. Long-term follow-up suggests that improvements in continence are not well maintained. A small number of patients may find that they exchange a problem with continence for difficulty in evacuation. Physiological assessment of the effects of pelvic-floor repair has been carried out by several authors. These reports have shown increased functional sphincter length, increased angulation, and even increased sphincter pressures. However, these reports are hard to interpret, consistency of surgical technique and physiological assessment is not evident.

The two most commonly practised operations are postanal repair and anterior pelvic-floor repair.

Postanal repair

First described by Parks, this procedure has been practised widely. Recently it seems to be used less, although it probably still has a place in the elderly. The procedure is carried out through a curved transverse incision, approximately 3 cm behind the anus. The external sphincter is exposed and then the intersphincteric plane is developed. Retracting the rectum forwards and the sling of the external sphincter backwards, Waldeyer's fascia is exposed and divided transversely. Mass sutures are placed between the opposing halves of the pubo-rectalis sling after gently freeing the rectum from its attachments to the pelvic floor. These are then tied, completing the repair.

Anterior pelvic-floor repair

Anterior pelvic-floor repair is similar in principle. A curved anterior perineal incision is employed. The external sphincter is exposed and dissected free in the intersphincteric plane posteriorly. The rectovaginal plane is entered anteriorly and above. The rectovaginal plane is then developed until the pillars of puborectalis can be visualized on either side above the external sphincter. The sides of puborectalis are then approximated and the external anal sphincter is plicated.

Sphincter augmentation procedures

When a sphincter is destroyed, either by injury, infection, or neuropathy, conventional surgical procedures hold little hope of success. A wide variety of muscle transposition procedures have been developed to attempt to augment the native sphincters. The electrically stimulated neoanal sphincter is a novel approach, taking the gracilis muscle from the thigh, wrapping it around the anal canal and employing electrical stimulation to convert it from its fast twitch to a slow twitch phenotype. The muscle can then be left in a tonic contraction, behaving as a sphincter. Patients are able to control the function of their neosphincter using a hand-held telemetry device acting on their implanted neural stimulator. This procedure is a formidable undertaking and has an appreciable morbidity and failure rate. No patient should be considered for it unless they understand that they may end up with a stoma if it is not a success.

There has been a recent resurgence in interest in the artificial bowel sphincter. This is an adaptation of the AMS 800 artificial urinary sphincter. Early reports from across Europe suggest that it is a feasible option, although not without its attendant problems.

Bibliography

Books

Keighley, M.R.B. and Williams, N.S. (1999). *Surgery of the Anus, Rectum and Colon* (second edition) Saunders Press

Williams, N.S. (Ed) (1996). *Colorectal cancer.* Clinical Surgery International series no. 20. Churchill Livingstone, Edinburgh.

Colorectal cancer

Bonaiti-Pellie, C. (1999). Genetic risk factors in colorectal cancer. *Eur. J. Cancer. Prev.*, **9**, Suppl 1:S27–32.

Cady, B. (2000). The changing role of the surgical oncologist. *Surg. Clin. North. Am.*, **80**, 459–69.

Dorrance, H.R., Docherty, G.M., O'Dwyer, P.J. (2000). Effect of surgeon specialty interest on patient outcome after potentially curative colorectal cancer surgery. *Dis. Colon. Rectum.*, **43**, 492–8.

Gee, I.R., Mayberry, J.F. (2000). A study of colo-rectal carcinoma in the Asian and European populations in the city of Leicester from 1981 to 1991. *Public Health*, **114**(1): 53–5.

Greelish, J.P., Friedberg, J.S. (2000). Secondary pulmonary malignancy. *Surg. Clin. North Am.*, **80**, 633–57.

Hill, M.J. (1999). Mechanisms of diet and colon carcinogenesis. *Eur. J. Cancer Prev.* **9**, Suppl 1: S95–8.

Jonker, D.J., Maroun, J.A., Kocha, W. (2000). Survival benefit of chemotherapy in metastatic colorectal cancer: a meta-analysis of randomized controlled trials. *Br. J. Cancer*, **82**, 1789–94.

Kronborg, O., Fenger, C. (1999). Clinical evidence for the adenoma-carcinoma sequence. *Eur. J. Cancer Prev.*, **9** Suppl 1: S73–86.

Lavery, I.C., Lopez-Kostner, F., Pelley, R.J., Fine, R.M. (2000). Treatment of colon and rectal cancer (review). *Surg. Clin. North Am.*, **80**, 535–69.

Lev-Chelouche, D., Margel, D., Goldman, G., Rabau, M.J. (2000). Transanal endoscopic microsurgery: experience with 75 rectal neoplasms. *Dis. Colon Rectum.*, **43**, 662–8.

Longo, W.E., Virgo, K.S., Johnson, F.E., Oprian, C.A., Vernava, A.M., Wade, T.P. *et al.* (2000). Risk factors for morbidity and mortality after colectomy for colon cancer. *Dis. Colon. Rectum.*, **43**, 83–91.

Lynch, H.T., Lynch, J.F. (2000). Hereditary nonpolyposis colorectal cancer. *Semin. Surg. Oncol.*, **18**, 305–13.

Sharma, S., Saltz, L.B. Oral chemotherapeutic agents for colorectal cancer. (2000). *Oncologist*, **5**, 99–107.

Parc, Y., Frileux, P., Schmitt, G., Dehni, N., Ollivier, J.M., Parc, R. (2000). Management of postoperative peritonitis after anterior resection: experience from a referral intensive care unit. *Dis. Colon. Rectum.*, **43**, 579–89.

Gillams, A.R., Lees, W.R. (2000). Survival after percutaneous, image-guided, thermal ablation of hepatic metastases from colorectal cancer. *Dis. Colon. Rectum.*, **43**, 656–61.

Swedish Rectal Cancer Trial (1997). Improved survival with pre-operative radiotherapy in respectable rectal cancer. *N. Engl. J. Med.*, **336**, 980–7.

Winawer, S.J., Stewart, E.T., Zauber, A.G., Bond, J.H., Ansel, H., Waye, J.D. *et al.* for the National Polyp Study Work Group (2000). A comparison of colonoscopy and double-contrast barium enema for surveillance after polypectomy. *N. Engl. J. Med.*, **342**, 1766–72.

Windham, T.C., Pearson, A.S., Skibber, J.M., Mansfield, P.F., Lee, J.E., Pisters, P.W., Evans, D.B. (2000). Significance and management of local recurrences and limited metastatic disease in the abdomen. *Surg. Clin. North Am.*, **80**, 761–74.

Crohn's colitis

Geoghegan, J.G., Carton, E., O'Shea, A.M., Astbury, K., Sheahan, K., O'Donoghue, D.P. *et al.* (1998). Crohn's colitis: The fate of the rectum. *Int. J. Colorect. Dis.*, **13**, 256–9.

Murray, J.J. (1998). Controversies in Crohn's disease. *Bailliere's Clinical Gastroenterology.* **12**, 133–55.

Prabhakar, L.P., Laramee, C., Nelson, H., Dozois, R.R. (1997). Role for segmental or abdominal colectomy in Crohn's colitis. *Dis. Colon Rectum.*, **40**, 71–8.

Rubio, C.A., Befrits, R. (1997). Colorectal adenocarcinoma in Crohn's disease: A retrospective histologic study. *Dis. Colon. Rectum.*, **40**, 1072–8.

Familial adenomatous polyposis

Bjork, J., Akerbrant, H., Iselius, L., Alm, T., Hultcrantz, R. (1999). Epidemiology of familial adenomatous polyposis in Sweden: Changes over time and differences in phenotype between males and females. *Scand. J. Gastroent,* **34**, 1230–5.

Clark, S.K., Neale, K.F., Landgrebe, J.C., Phillips, R.K.S. (1999). Desmoid tumours complicating familial adenomatous polyposis. *Brit. J. Surg.*, **86**, 1185–9.

Navaratnam, R.M., Chowaniec, J., Winslet, M.C. (1999). The molecular biology of colorectal cancer development and the associated genetic events. *Annals. Roy. Coll. Surg. Engl.*, **81**, 312–19.

Petersen, G.M., Brensinger, J.D., Johnson, K.A., Giardiello, F.M. (1999). Genetic testing and counseling for hereditary forms of colorectal cancer. *Cancer.* **86** (11 Suppl.), 2540–50.

Sondergaard Galle, T., Juel, K., Bulow, S. (1999). Causes of death in familial adenomatous polyposis. *Scand. J. Gastroent.*, **34**, 808–12.

Stucchi, A.F., Becker, J.M. (1999). Pathogenesis of pouchitis. *Problems Gen. Surg.*, **16**, 139–50.

Tiret, A., Parc, C. (1999). Fundus lesions of adenomatous polyposis. *Current Opinion in Ophthalmology.* **10**, 168–72.

Young, C.J., Solomon, M.J., Eyers, A.A., West, R.H., Martin, H.C., Glenn, D.C., Morgan, B.P., Roberts, R. (1999). Evolution of the pelvic pouch procedure at one institution: The first 100 cases. *Aus. & N.Z. J. Surg.*, **69**, 438–42.

Diverticular disease

Isbister, W.H., Prasad, J. (1997). Emergency large bowel surgery: A 15 year audit. *Int. J. Colorect. Dis.*, **12**, 285–90.

Kohler, L., Sauerland, S., Neugebauer, E. (1999). Diagnosis and treatment of diverticular disease: Results of a consensus development conference. *Surg. End.*, **13**, 430–6.

Makela, J., Vuolio, S., Kiviniemi, H., Laitinen, S. (1998). Natural history of diverticular disease: When to operate? *Dis. Colon Rect.*, **41**, 1523–8.

Merad, F., Hay, J-M., Fingerhut, A., Yahchouchi, E., Laborde, Y., Pelissier, E., *et al.* (1999). Is prophylactic pelvic drainage useful after elective rectal or anal anastomosis? A multicenter controlled randomized trial. *Surgery.*, **125**, 529–35.

Stevenson, A.R.L., Stitz, R.W., Lumlay, J.W., Fielding, G.A. (1998). Laparoscopically assisted anterior resection for diverticular disease: Follow-up of 100 consecutive patients. *Annals. Surg.*, **227**, 335–42.

Stollman, N.H., Raskin, J.B. (1999). Diverticular disease of the colon. *J. Clin. Gastroent.*, **29**, 241–52.

CHAPTER 21

Perianal surgery

Peter Lunniss

1 Introduction

Patients, and indeed many non-surgical clinicians, tend to describe most anal conditions under the umbrella terms 'haemorrhoids' (pertaining to bleeding) or 'piles' (pertaining to prolapse). Rectal bleeding is one of the most common symptoms referred to surgical outpatient clinics and most causes relate to problems within the anal canal. However, patients with anal problems also present with anal pain, discharge, and soiling, and it is important to be able to evaluate the symptoms in relation to the likely diagnosis. This depends primarily on taking an adequate history. Managing the problem hinges upon a thorough understanding of the relevant anatomy and physiology. Whereas most cases present as elective problems, the inflammatory complications associated with pathology in this area also present as surgical emergencies and the trainee needs to be able to recognize them.

Examination of the conscious patient, whether in the clinic or in the accident department, must include a full examination of the anorectum with the patient in the left lateral position. It includes inspection, careful palpation both within and without the anal canal with an adequately lubricated digit, rigid (and sometimes flexible) sigmoidoscopy, and proctoscopy. If pain or other factors prevent a full examination in the awake patient and there is doubt about the diagnosis, arrangements must be made for the patient to undergo an examination under anaesthesia (EUA).

2 Surgical anatomy

2.1 The pelvic floor

The pelvic floor is formed by the levator ani group of muscles, the components of which are named according to their attachments. The most important muscular component of anorectal anatomy is the puborectalis. Through this muscular diaphragm pass the rectum and anal canal posteriorly and the

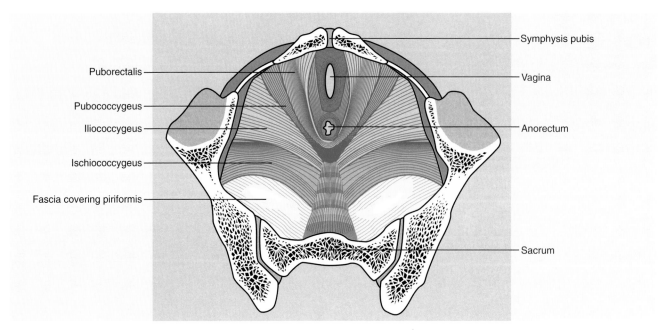

Figure 21.1 Muscles of the pelvic floor viewed from above.

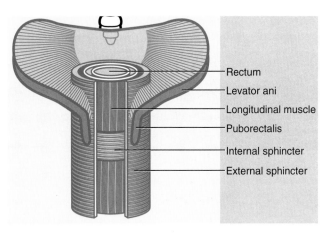

Figure 21.2 The 'pelvic funnel'.

urethra and vagina anteriorly (Fig. 21.1). It is important, especially in the assessment of anorectal infection, to realize that the pelvic floor is not a flat sheet but a funnel (Fig. 21.2). The puborectalis envelops the lower rectum on three sides but not anteriorly, and continues inferiorly as the external sphincter of the anal canal. This sphincter is physiologically and histochemically indistinguishable from the puborectalis. The puborectalis muscle is responsible for the forward angulation of the anorectal junction, and is easily felt in the conscious patient as a posterior ridge (Fig. 21.3), but is less easy to palpate under anaesthesia. The length of anal canal surrounded by striated muscle is shorter anteriorly than posteriorly because of the arrangement of the puborectalis sling, a fact which can be important in managing anterior fistulas in women.

2.2 The external anal sphincter

The external sphincter is made up of type 1 fibres and is supplied from sacral roots 2, 3, and 4 via the pudendal nerve.

The sphincter has only minimal activity at rest, but is brought into play when the desire to pass rectal contents needs to be overcome, usually for reasons of social nicety. Neurogenic or mechanical disorders of the external sphincter lead to a sense of urgency and an inability to withhold defecation, with urge incontinence for flatus, liquid, or formed stool. The classical description of the external sphincter as three distinct bundles—subcutaneous, superficial, and deep—is somewhat arbitrary. However, the subcutaneous portion may be regarded as anatomically separate from the remainder. This is because the terminal ramifications of the conjoined longitudinal muscle which enclose it insert into the perianal skin (Fig. 21.4).

2.3 The internal anal sphincter

The internal anal sphincter is a direct continuation of the circular smooth muscle coat of the rectum, which has developed specialized properties. The internal sphincter is in a state of tonic contraction at rest and contributes about 75 per cent of the resting anal tone. Disruption of the internal sphincter may therefore lead to soiling and passive incontinence of rectal contents. Under general anaesthesia and with an anal retractor opened in the anal canal, the lower edge of the internal sphincter may be felt easily as a firm band, where it forms the upper border of the **anal intermuscular groove**. The internal sphincter is crossed by fibroconnective tissue fibres derived from the medial aspect of the conjoined longitudinal muscle as this runs down the intersphincteric space. These fibres cross in an inferomedial direction at the upper end of the anal canal and superomedially below the dentate line (Fig. 21.4). In axial or longitudinal section, these fibres can be seen to endow the so-called circular muscle with a spiral arrangement, with the axis of rotation opposite at each end of the anal canal. Contraction of the internal sphincter therefore appears to both shorten the

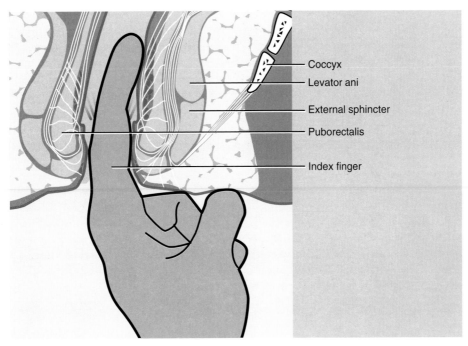

Figure 21.3 Palpating the anorectal junction.

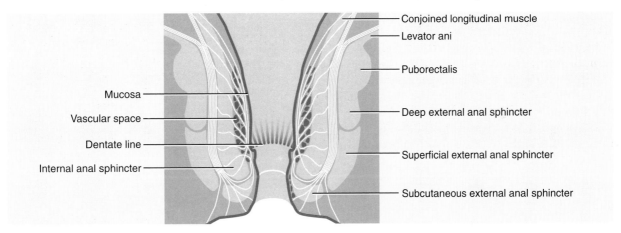

Figure 21.4 Anorectal anatomy in the coronal plane.

anal canal and to reduce its luminal diameter. The fibres that cross the internal sphincter intermingle with those of the subepithelial space and support the overlying anoderm and mucosa.

There is a condensation of these supporting fibres at the level of the dentate line, which Sir Alan Parks named the **mucosal suspensory ligament**. This description is important, since this ligament separates the vessels of the superior haemorrhoidal plexus (related to internal haemorrhoids) from those of the inferior haemorrhoidal plexus (related to thrombosed external piles), as well as separating the marginal space from the submucous space (see below).

2.4 The intersphincteric space

Between the internal and external sphincters lies the **intersphincteric space**. On its medial aspect runs the conjoined muscle of the anal canal, formed as a continuation of the longitudinal smooth muscle coat of the rectum, augmented by fibres from the puborectalis. In the fetus, this structure is easily seen, but with age it is gradually replaced by fibrous and connective tissue. There is conjecture as to the possible roles of the conjoined longitudinal muscle, but it would appear to act as a supporting mechanism for the other components of the sphincter complex by virtue of the ramifications which pass from it—medially across the internal sphincter, laterally across the external sphincter, and inferiorly to the skin of the anal margin. The other reason the intersphincteric space is clinically important is because the anal glands lie within it, thought to be responsible for the majority of 'idiopathic' anal fistulas. The function of the anal glands is unknown. They have been shown to secrete mucus but the mucus has a different composition from that of the rectal mucosa. By comparative anatomical studies, they have been shown not to be vestigial remnants of the sexual scent glands. Infection of the anal glands, however, is probably responsible for the majority of cases of acute anorectal infection, with bacteria passing retrogradely up the anal ducts from the crypts at the dentate line to form an abscess in the gland in the intersphincteric space. This cannot then discharge spontaneously back into the anal lumen because of the tone of the internal sphincter. Anal glands may also be found superficial to the internal sphincter, but these are not important clinically, since infection in such glands should be able to drain spontaneously and resolve.

2.5 The lining of the anorectum

An appreciation of the lining of the anorectum is important. The skin of the perineum is hairy, stratified, squamous, keratinized epithelium. The distal end of the anal canal is lined by stratified, squamous, non-keratinized epithelium up to the level of the dentate line. The dentate line may be regarded as the site of fusion of the embryological proctodeal ectoderm and the hindgut. In practical terms, it is the site of the **anal crypts**, where the ducts of the anal glands open into the anal lumen. It is also the site of the majority of internal openings of cryptoglandular or idiopathic anal fistulas. The dentate line has its name by virtue of its likeness to a row of teeth, with the sides of the teeth passing cephalad as the **rectal columns of Morgagni**. It is also

known as the **pectinate line** because of its likeness to a comb. The dentate line is a watershed for lymphatic drainage: lymphatic drainage (which accompanies the arteries) above the dentate line passes superiorly to the inferior mesenteric nodes, but below the dentate line passes inferiorly to the inguinal nodes. In the region of the dentate line there is also the highest concentration of sensory nerve endings. The sensory component of the anal canal is important for the conscious discrimination of intestinal contents passing over it, and also in the unconscious reflex by which the internal sphincter relaxes to allow 'sampling' of the rectal contents. Continence may be regarded as the coordinated activity of the muscular components of the sphincter complex, orchestrated by intact sensation.

Above the dentate line is the so-called **transitional zone** of the anal canal, not to be confused with the transitional epithelium of the urinary tract. This area represents a gradual change from flattened squamous-type cells to the true columnar epithelium of the rectum. Above the dentate line the epithelium is relatively insensitive, although an appreciation of stretch can be elicited.

2.6 The anatomical spaces of the anal sphincter complex

The arrangement of the muscular and supporting tissues of the anal sphincter complex means that there are several well-defined anatomical spaces in relation to them (Fig. 21.5). These spaces are important in the spread of infection, and accurate identification of the site of infection is fundamental to correct management. It is for this reason, amongst others, that surgeons should be able to describe their findings in a way that is easily understood by others; the simplest and most objective method of description is by drawing, and the St Mark's Hospital fistula operation sheet is an excellent example of how this may be done (Fig. 21.6).

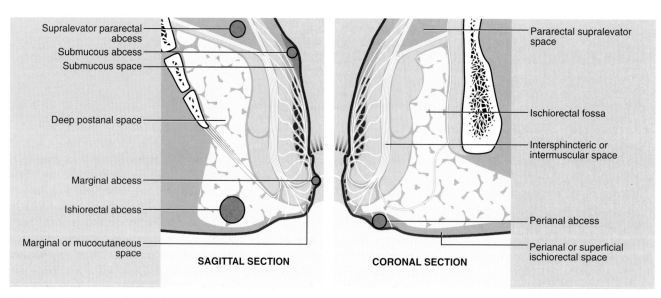

Figure 21.5 Pararectal and perineal spaces.

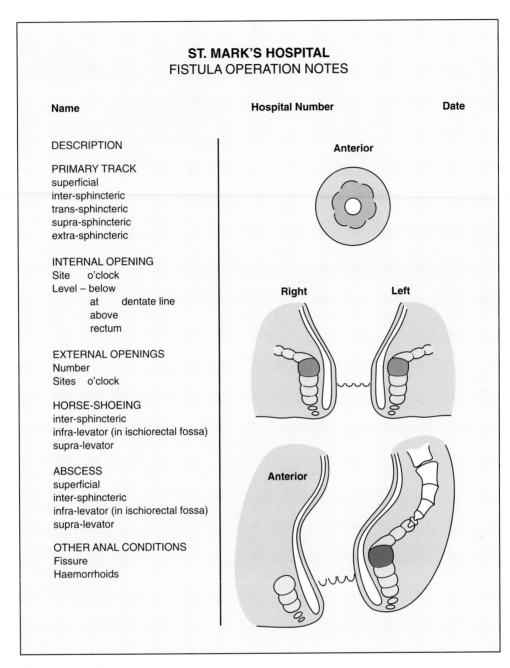

ST. MARK'S HOSPITAL
FISTULA OPERATION NOTES

Name   **Hospital Number**   **Date**

DESCRIPTION   **Anterior**

PRIMARY TRACK
superficial
inter-sphincteric
trans-sphincteric
supra-sphincteric
extra-sphincteric

INTERNAL OPENING   **Right**   **Left**
Site   o'clock
Level – below
         at   dentate line
         above
         rectum

EXTERNAL OPENINGS
Number
Sites   o'clock

HORSE-SHOEING
inter-sphincteric
infra-levator (in ischiorectal fossa)
supra-levator

ABSCESS   **Anterior**
superficial
inter-sphincteric
infra-levator (in ischiorectal fossa)
supra-levator

OTHER ANAL CONDITIONS
Fissure
Haemorrhoids

Figure 21.6 St Mark's Hospital fistula operation sheet.

3 The principles of perianal surgery

3.1 Preparation for surgery

The incidence of postoperative surgical infection following perianal surgery is remarkably low considering the fact that the wounds are continually bathed by bacteria-loaded faeces. The blood supply of the perineum is excellent, rather similar to that of the scalp and face, and it is probably this that allows effective healing to occur in the presence of obvious infected material. It is not necessary to empty the colon completely prior to local perianal surgery unless complex surgical procedures such as postanal or sphincter repair are planned. It is sufficient to simply empty the rectum by the use of suppositories or an enema. This only needs to be done if it can be carried out without the patient's obvious discomfort, and is therefore contraindicated in painful conditions such as anal fissure and prolapsed haemorrhoids. It is usual to shave the perineal area preoperatively, although this is more effectively performed under anaesthesia using a large scalpel blade over well-lubricated skin. Prophylactic antibiotics are not generally used unless there are specific indications (e.g. evidence of systemic infection from acute anorectal infection or major reconstructive surgery).

3.2 Types of anaesthesia

Most operations are performed under general anaesthesia which allows adequate exposure and dilatation of the anal canal not possible in a conscious patient. A similar level of anaesthesia can be obtained with a spinal anaesthetic, and minor excisions and drainage of perianal haematomas can be performed under infiltrative local anaesthesia.

3.3 Position on the operating table

1. The left lateral (Fig. 21.7) is the customary position for the standard sigmoidoscopy/colonoscopy/proctoscopy, but is not commonly used when patients are anaesthetized.

2. The lithotomy position (Fig. 21.8) is used for all examinations under anaesthesia and for minor and intermediate perianal operations. In principle, the buttocks project beyond the end of the table and the hips are flexed beyond the right angle with legs in stirrups outside the poles.

3. The Lloyd-Davies position (Fig. 21.9) is used for operations that require pelvic dissection as well as perineal dissection,

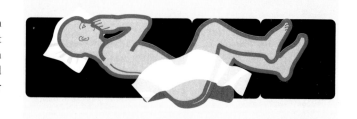

Figure 21.7 Left lateral position on the operating table

and is not used for perineal surgery alone. The legs are not flexed to a right angle as they would get in the way of the abdominal operator; the coccyx lies beyond the end of the table, and the sacrum is lifted off the table by a sacral rest.

4. The prone jackknife position (Fig. 21.10) is sometimes used for operations involving the anterior aspect of the anal sphincters, and operations requiring greater exposure of the buttocks (pilonidal disease, hidradenitis suppurativa). This position is used more commonly in the USA, where much

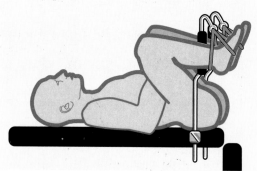
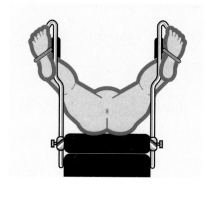

Figure 21.8 The lithotomy position on the operating table.

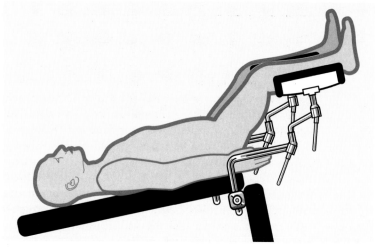
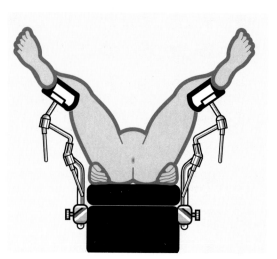

Figure 21.9 The Lloyd-Davies position on the operating table.

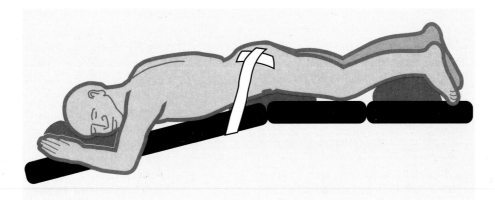

Figure 21.10 The prone jackknife position on the operating table.

perianal surgery is performed under local or epidural anaesthesia. It affords easier surgical access, but some anaesthetists are reluctant to employ this position because it may compromise thoracic excursion if the torso is incorrectly placed.

4 Special care and problems in the postoperative period

4.1 Wound care

Most anal wounds are allowed to heal by secondary intention. Primary closure is probably associated with an increased risk of breakdown caused by infection from faecal contamination. The fibrosis that follows healing by secondary intention can result in a narrowing of the anal canal. Attention to maintaining skin bridges when operating on the anal canal is an important means of preventing this complication. The standard form of dressing is the wound pack. This maintains an open wound and allows it to granulate, but should be sufficiently light as not to delay healing. Daily digital examination of the wound before cleaning and redressing prevents premature bridging at the wound apex. Inevitable regular contamination of the wound by faeces means that the perineum should be bathed regularly and certainly after each bowel action.

4.2 Secondary haemorrhage

The cause of secondary haemorrhage is infection at the operative site. A sizeable vessel must be eroded for significant haemorrhage to occur. In practice, haemorrhoidectomy is the only procedure when this is likely to occur. It happens about 7–10 days after surgery and, if local pressure cannot control the bleeding, it will require reoperation. The usual finding is an arterial bleeding point in relation to the transfixion ligation of the haemorrhoidal pedicle.

4.3 Anal stenosis and fibrosis

Reference has been made to the potential problem of anal stenosis, which could follow excision of an excess of the anal skin circumference. The process of healing by fibrosis, however, can also be used to the patient's advantage when operating on fistulas. In operations where portions of sphincter muscle are divided, the resulting gap becomes filled with fibrous tissue and this contracts to brings together the remaining sphincter muscles. The process also allows operations to be performed in stages, with the strength of the fibrous tissue used to maintain sphincter competence. However, sufficient time must be allowed for the fibrosis to mature before more muscle is divided.

4.4 Recurrent perianal problems

The usual cause of this is inadequate treatment of the primary disease process. This can vary from the simple continuance of constipation to recurrent fistulas.

5 Particular perianal problems

5.1 Pruritis ani

Pruritis ani is a common and embarrassing condition, in the majority of cases of which, unfortunately, no specific cause is found. Classically of an intermittent nature and aggravated by stress, the symptoms may drive the anxious individual into a state where his or her life is dominated by an overwhelming need to scratch the perineum, which, of course, exacerbates the condition. Pruritis is a difficult condition to manage, and a confident approach by the clinician is paramount, especially if no specific cause can be identified and treated. Common predisposing conditions include primary skin disorders affecting the perineum; fungal, viral, and parasitic infections; and, not uncommonly, hypersensitivity reactions to washing agents, lavatory paper, and even topical agents applied in the hope of relieving the condition. Itching may occur as a result of anal seepage, which may occur with haemorrhoids, fissure, fistula, proctitis, prolapse, or malignancy. It may also result from minor incontinence secondary to anal surgery and from liquid stool from any cause.

Clues to the cause in an individual are provided by a detailed history and both a methodical examination of the local area and a general dermatological examination. Skin scrapings for fungi should be taken before the perianal skin is lubricated. A useful part of the examination is the 'cotton-wool test', in which minor anal seepage can be detected by placing a cotton-wool ball at the anal orifice and then inspecting it for stains.

Treatment depends upon finding any predisposing cause and treating that, but the majority of sufferers do have an obvious cause. For them, strict advice about anal hygiene is recommended, given in a confident manner. This includes bathing the perineum with water (and not soap) after defecation, instead of cleaning with tissue, avoiding rubbing to dry the area, wearing cotton underwear, and, if necessary, positioning a cotton-wool plug (one-third of the size of a proprietary cotton-wool ball) at the anal margin to prevent anal seepage.

5.2 Haemorrhoidal disease

Not only is the prevalence of haemorrhoids unknown, but much conjecture and controversy exists as to the aetiology, pathogenesis, and treatment of the condition (Loder *et al.* 1994). 'Haemorrhoids' should only be identified as such when they are symptomatic, and should not be treated unless they produce symptoms (or there is doubt as to their nature). The proctoscopic diagnosis of haemorrhoids far exceeds the prevalence of symptoms. The proportion of people presenting with symptoms to their family doctor, and thence possibly to the surgical clinics, is highly dependent upon cultural and psychosocial factors. Haemorrhoids may be regarded as pathological anal cushions. Anal cushions are normal and important structures which distend to effect a complete seal at the anal canal to prevent leakage of gas, liquid, or solid. This is a function that cannot be achieved by an intact sphincter mechanism alone. This distensibility is afforded by the vascular plexuses contained within them, which in turn are supported by a scaffold of subepithelial smooth muscle and fibroconnective tissue. This fibroconnective tissue is connected to the intersphincteric space structures (see earlier). The nature of this supporting framework and its connections across the sphincter complex allow a state of relative relaxation and vascular filling, with anal cushion distension at rest. During defecation, however, the subepithelial tissues may be pulled upwards and outwards to allow atraumatic descent of stool. Certainly, the differing pharmacological properties of the constituent muscle components of the complex *in vitro* would support this attractive concept. Unfortunately, with age, and probably in an accelerated manner in those people who develop symptomatic haemorrhoids, there is a gradual caudal displacement of the anal cushions, a process that may be augmented by the high anal pressures found in afflicted patients. Although constipation has been regarded historically as an important aetiological factor, this has not been substantiated by the (few) prospective studies performed, although straining at stool, or even just sitting on the lavatory with a relaxed perineum would allow such displacement of the cushions.

Miles' (1919) description of the three terminal branches of the superior rectal artery supplying the three anal cushions is one of those 'facts' that have been accepted more than challenged. More recent work suggests that there are, on average,

five terminal branches; and only a proportion of the population has their anal cushions in the classical 3, 7, and 11 o'clock positions. The terminal branches supply the vascular dilatations within the anal cushions which, in turn, drain freely into the superior, middle, and inferior rectal veins. The bleeding from haemorrhoids is bright red, not because it is arterial, but rather venous with a high oxygen tension.

Patients with haemorrhoids may complain of a variety of symptoms. The nature of the bleeding is characteristic—separate from the motion and either seen on the paper after wiping or as a fresh splash into the pan. Pain is not commonly associated with the bleeding and a history of pain should alert the clinician to the possibility of another diagnosis. Pain may be present, however, and is probably due to congestion of the masses below the hypertonic internal sphincter. Fresh bleeding in the absence of other gastrointestinal symptoms is not associated with an increased probability of colorectal malignancy compared to the rest of the population, but this does not mean that investigations to exclude a more proximal cause should be denied, especially in patients over the age of 40 years. Haemorrhoids and cancer may coexist, and it is therefore imperative in patients who fall into an age group where colon carcinoma is common that the colon should be examined thoroughly before the bleeding is attributed to piles. Indeed, some patients do not seek local treatment for their haemorrhoids on being assured that their bleeding is not from a suspicious cause.

Another common symptom is perianal itching. This may be due to the secretions of the rectal mucosa overlying the displaced cushions low down or even outside the anal canal, or due to loss of the complete seal afforded by the cushions, with flecks of stool escaping along the gutters between the pathologically enlarged cushions. The two forms may be differentiated by placing a cotton-wool ball at the anal margin and noting the colour of the stain.

Patients may also complain of true 'piles' (Fig. 21.11)—lumps that appear at the anal orifice during defecation and which return spontaneously into the anal canal (second degree), have to be replaced manually or which lie permanently outside the anus (third degree). It is apparent on examination that many so-called fourth-degree piles cannot be reduced because it is the external skin component which is irreducible. These tags presumably arise through intermittent congestion and oedema when the internal components prolapse. There is indeed a subgroup of patients in whom the main complaint is one of difficulty in cleaning after evacuation and in whom the internal component has abated; in these patients a simple 'anal tidy up' with tag excision is all that may be required to bring symptomatic relief. True strangulated haemorrhoids usually present via the Accident and Emergency department and are associated with severe, constant, unremitting pain, with large pile masses protruding from the anal orifice with gross oedema and later ulceration.

Management of symptomatic haemorrhoidal disease

Exclusion of other causes of rectal bleeding is the first priority; but it is reasonable for treatment of symptomatic piles to be

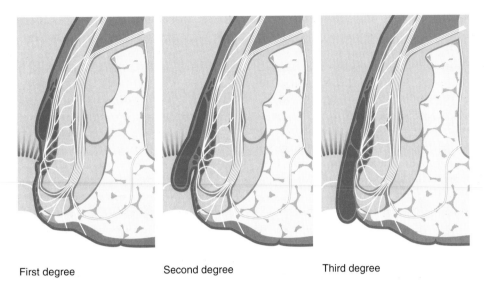

First degree   Second degree   Third degree

Figure 21.11 Grading of haemorrhoids.

initiated during the first consultation, while investigations of the proximal large bowel are awaited. In an ideal world, colonoscopy would be the investigation of choice, as this procedure is diagnostic, allows biopsies to be taken of mucosal abnormalities, and can also be therapeutic. In practice, barium enema is used most frequently because of the patient numbers involved.

The variety of treatments available, as in many other pathologies of the anorectum, implies that there is no single 'all healing' method. Time should be spent assessing the defecatory habits of the patient; the bowel frequency and stool consistency, the time spent in the act of defecation, and the time spent cleaning the perianal area. Although hard stools are often blamed, as many people are afflicted with symptoms after bouts of frequent loose stool. It would appear to make sense, therefore, to try and educate the patient into passing soft, bulky stools (akin to a fresh cow pat) without undue straining or sitting on the lavatory pondering other matters. Advice about dietary manipulation carries little compliance, and it is generally easier and more acceptable to advise supplementary dietary fibre (of a palatable variety) and to ensure an adequate fluid intake. Avoidance of foodstuffs that exacerbate symptoms would also be sensible. Although a minority of patients are happy and are helped by these simple means, most seek further local treatment.

In the case of small but vascular first- or second-degree haemorrhoids, submucosal injection of 5 per cent phenol in arachis or almond oil is useful. There are no rules about the optimal volumes to inject, some favour about 2 ml per pile body and others up to 20 ml injected circumferentially. The aim of the injections is simply to cause fibrosis, which both obliterates the vascular channels and hitches up the anorectal mucosa to prevent prolapse. Our preference is to use 5 ml injected under direct vision submucosally into the apex of the pile pedicle. This must be a pain-free procedure, any pain meaning that the injection is in the wrong place and should be stopped immediately. Phenol injections are not without risk and it is the surgeon's responsibility to check every ampoule of phenol.

Injections that are too superficial are visible as the mucosa rises rapidly and turns white; this leads to superficial mucosal sloughing but rarely to septic complications, as the circular muscle provides an effective barrier to the spread of infection. However, injections placed too deeply can have disastrous consequences, such as chronic prostatitis, pelvic infection, and rectovaginal fistula. It is usual to see the patient again after 8 weeks, to assess response and, if necessary, re-inject. No more than three sets of injections should be given: a need for more means that this treatment is not working and the fibrosis caused by repeated injections makes subsequent haemorrhoidectomy more difficult, with an increased risk of internal sphincter disruption.

For more bulky piles, banding is a logical treatment. The Barron's bander is a commonly available device (Fig. 21.12). Application must be performed under direct vision. It is easier if the patient holds the proctoscope in his or her right hand once the desired position has been achieved; the patient's hand never

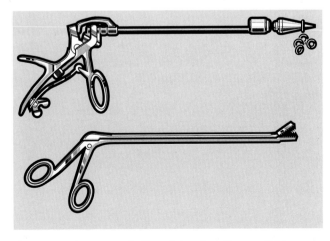

Figure 21.12 Instruments for Barron's banding of haemorrhoids.

moves and it allows the operator two free hands, one to grasp the mucosa at the pile base with the grasping forceps and the other to place the bander over the forceps and release the bands. Again this must be a pain-free procedure. There is no good evidence against banding three piles at a single session, and we advocate loading the bander with two rather than just one rubber band. Because banding works through ischaemic necrosis and secondary scarring, the patient must be warned of bleeding after about 10 days. Pain felt immediately after banding means that the bands have been placed too low on to the sensitive anoderm and should be removed carefully with a narrow scalpel blade. Any bleeding should cease with direct pressure from a cotton-wool ball, or one soaked in dilute adrenaline (epinephrine). Some patients feel rather faint after banding, and they must be allowed time to lie down and recover before leaving the clinic. It is imperative that a full explanation of the rationale and side-effects is explained before any treatment is given.

Other local outpatient remedies exist, such as cryotherapy and photocoagulation, but these are generally less available and there is no good evidence that any one method carries any significant advantages over the others.

Indications for surgery in haemorrhoidal disease

If there is any doubt about the diagnosis of haemorrhoids when the patient is seen in the clinic, arrangements should be made for admission and EUA and biopsy. The other strong indication for surgery is bleeding sufficient to cause anaemia (other causes having been excluded). Beyond these, indications for surgical intervention are more relative than absolute. Failure to control symptoms from first- or second-degree piles by more conservative approaches is an appropriate indication; and attempts at conservative management of symptomatic third-degree piles are nearly always unsuccessful, and there seems little point in banding or injecting piles that are 'beyond the point of no return'.

Haemorrhoidectomy using a modification of the technique described by Milligan and Morgan in 1937 is the most commonly performed in UK. However, it carries an unfavourable reputation with the public, because of horror stories about postoperative pain, especially after defecation. Psychosocial factors and personality traits are probably important determinants of outcome, but a lot can be done through careful explanation of the reasons for advising the procedure. The presence of an intra-anal dressing is in fact the strongest independent factor associated with postoperative pain, and if careful surgical technique is employed, then patients are usually very satisfied with the outcome. The benefits of surgery must be balanced against the risks, and these must be explained, specifically loss of the finer aspects of continence, the risk of anal stenosis, and the possibility of recurrence.

Contraindications to surgical excision include general frailty and high anaesthetic risk. Local contraindications include patients with a patulous anus associated with pudendal neuropathy, and perhaps with mechanical sphincter disruption. These patients may be only just continent before haemorrhoidectomy, but the removal of the anorectal lining may tip them into frank incontinence for all rectal contents. For those in whom doubt exists about sphincter strength, it is prudent to perform anorectal physiological assessment before embarking on surgery.

Operative technique

The technique is performed under general anaesthesia, with the patient in the lithotomy position. It is our preference to infiltrate the anoderm between the pile masses and subcutaneously with adrenaline (epinephrine)1 : 250 000 to reduce bleeding and to help preservation of skin bridges. Forceps are applied to the skin-covered external components of the haemorrhoids, and retraction of these exposes the internal components, which are grasped in turn with another pair of artery forceps (Fig. 21.13). After incision of the skin in a V shape, dissection of the haemorrhoid from the underlying internal sphincter may be performed with scissors or with coagulating diathermy. Traction on the buttock by an assistant, combined with the operator's index finger within the anal canal, helps delineate the internal sphincter, which should be visible throughout the dissection. The dissection proceeds well up the anal canal towards the anorectal junction, the sides of the mucosal dissection converg-

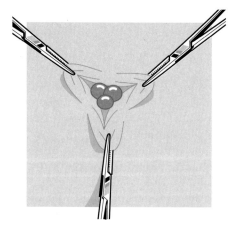
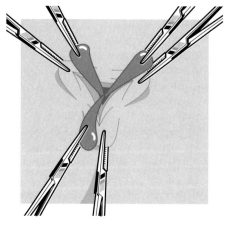

Figure 21.13 Technique of haemorrhoidectomy.

ing towards the apex of the pile pedicle to ensure preservation of mucocutaneous continuity. The pile pedicle is transfixed with an absorbable suture, the pile excised with scissors, and, after inspection to ensure haemostasis, the suture cut long. The three pile masses are excised in turn, with care to leave mucocutaneous bridges—it is far safer to leave haemorrhoidal tissue behind than risk anal stenosis. If there are prominent secondary haemorrhoids beneath these bridges, these can be filleted out by scissor dissection. Haemostasis must be absolute at the end of the procedure, before a soft absorbable 'Spongistan' anal dressing is inserted. Laxatives are prescribed (Milpar®, 10–15 ml twice daily, and Fybogel®, one sachet twice daily) and the patient asked to bathe daily and after each bowel action. Patients are allowed home after a satisfactory bowel movement, usually on the third or fourth postoperative day, and are seen in the clinic after a few weeks to ensure that there is no stenosis. If stenosis occurs, the use of an anal dilator is advised (inserted for 10 minutes twice daily after lubrication of the anus and dilator with 2 per cent lignocaine (lidocaine) gel). Patients must be warned of the possibility of bleeding at around the tenth postoperative day, and should keep taking their laxatives until reviewed in the clinic.

Emergency haemorrhoidal problems

Prolapsed strangulated haemorrhoids

In this emergency condition, severe third-degree piles prolapse through the sphincter ring and swell as a result of increased venous pressure. The increase in size of the pile prevents spontaneous retraction. The piles are often of long standing but may develop rapidly in the late stages of pregnancy. The emergency is often precipitated by straining at stool. Failure of pile retraction is then followed by oedema of the surrounding external component and a concentric ring of strangulated piles is seen on inspection of the anal canal. The inner ring forms the strangulated (and often gangrenous) internal component and the outer ring is formed by the external oedematous component.

Most strangulated prolapsed haemorrhoids are managed conservatively. The essence of treatment is to allow the internal component to reduce in size to a level where it reduces spontaneously. Treatment includes relief of local discomfort combined with methods of speeding up the resolution of local oedema. Ice packs may help shrinkage but patients need to be told that it will be several days before the symptoms begin to improve.

Non-operative management is usually advocated because emergency haemorrhoidectomy is thought to be associated with an excess risk of portal pyaemia, secondary haemorrhage, anal stenosis, and incontinence. In experienced hands, however, the emergency procedure has been shown to be as safe as the elective, and also saves the patient a possible readmission for elective haemorrhoidectomy. Occasionally, an EUA combined with an anal stretch is used in an attempt to reduce the haemorrhoids. In general, this does not work, and is quickly followed by a recurrence of the piles, and also carries the well-documented risks of traumatic disruption of internal and

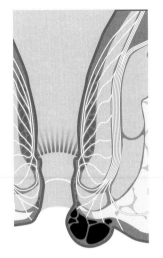
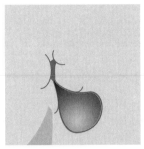

Figure 21.14 Thrombosed external pile (perianal haematoma).

external sphincters. Lateral anal sphincterotomy, similarly, has lost credibility in this situation. One advantage of conservative regimens is that the fibrosis associated with recovery from strangulation can sometimes produce a spontaneous resolution of haemorrhoids when everything has settled.

Thrombosed external haemorrhoids

This represents spontaneous thrombosis in external haemorrhoidal vessels and presents as a very painful, blue, firm, olive-like swelling in the perianal skin (Fig. 21.14). It is distinct from the usual haemorrhoidal problem and is not always associated with internal haemorrhoids. The immediate aim of treatment is to relieve the perianal pain, which can be done by opening the thrombus under local anaesthesia through a radial incision and evacuating the contained clot. This produces an immediate improvement in symptoms and nothing further needs to be done. If the patient presents after 48 hours of onset of symptoms, then it is likely that the clot is undergoing organization and evacuation is not easy. In these circumstances, it is advisable to pursue the conservative line, and if the residual skin tag causes problems, it can be dealt with accordingly.

5.3 Acute anorectal infection

Acute anorectal infection is common, with about 4000 emergency surgical admissions a year in England and Wales. An understanding of the aetiology and anatomy is fundamental to correct management. It is perhaps unfortunate that, in the UK, treatment is often left to a junior member of the on-call team, in the early hours of the morning after the more 'glamorous' emergencies have been operated upon. Patients with acute anal infection present with a story of increasing pain in the region, usually a lump, and occasionally a purulent or bloody discharge, and fever. The condition of high intermuscular abscess is uncommon, but must be considered in the differential diagnosis in a patient with fever, vague deep anorectal pain, perhaps difficulty in passing urine, but in whom no abscess is visible but where digital examination of the anorectum is extremely

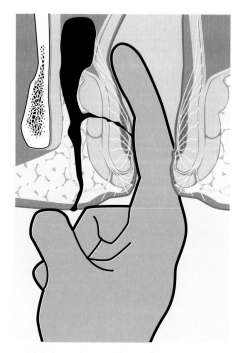

Figure 21.15 Digital examination of a patient with an anal fistula.

painful. The anatomy of the tissue spaces has been shown earlier (Fig. 21.5). For the most part, anorectal infection may be divided into non-specific (i.e. not peculiar to the anorectum), including boils, pilonidal abscess, and hidradenitis suppurativa, and specific (i.e. intimately related to the anorectum).

Pilonidal disease and hidradenitis are usually easy to recognize. Cutaneous boils can present as both perianal and ischiorectal abscesses. The key to distinguishing them from anal problems may be found in the microbiology of the pus. Grace and his co-workers demonstrated in 1982 that abscesses from which skin organisms are cultured have nothing to do with fistulas, whereas culture of intestinal organisms and intestine-specific anaerobes points to an underlying fistula or abscess which will recur if not dealt with appropriately. The incidence of anorectal infection from skin organisms is divided equally between the sexes, whereas infection due to gut organisms is more common in men, reflecting the similar (unexplained) male predominance of the chronic condition, the anal fistula.

A history of previous infection at the same site is also indicative, but not diagnostic, of a communication with the anorectal lumen. Although microbiology is extremely sensitive, it is not 100 per cent specific, in that cutaneous boils in the perianal area may be infected with gut organisms; also the results of culture are, of course, not available at the time of the first operation. A more specific indicator of an underlying fistula may be found in the surgical anatomy (Lunniss and Phillips 1994), that is, the presence or absence of infection within the intersphincteric space. However, this requires a knowledge of surgical anatomy and a level of surgical skill not expected in junior trainees, and where the potential for serious iatrogenic injury is considerable.

Most cases arise spontaneously and are not associated with underlying diseases, but occasionally they are a presentation of established inflammatory bowel disease and can be associated with underlying diabetes and other immunosuppressed states. If present, these should lead to a more diligent and speedy approach to management than might otherwise occur.

Urgent treatment

The patient should be examined under anaesthesia in the lithotomy position. After skin preparation, the skin is carefully shaved—this allows more comfortable dressing changes, and also helps to prevent delay of healing by ingrowth of hair into the granulating wound. Inspection shows whether the abscess is perianal or ischiorectal. The area should then be palpated with a well-lubricated finger to determine the relation of the abscess to the anal sphincter complex, and whether there is supralevator infection, either high intermuscular within the rectal wall, or outside the rectal wall in the pararectal space. After sigmoidoscopic assessment of the rectal mucosa, and conventional proctoscopy, the anal canal can be opened with an Eisenhammer anal retractor and gentle pressure over the site of the abscess may reveal a discharge of pus through the internal opening. If no internal opening is revealed, then the question of whether the infection is cryptoglandular or simply cutaneous remains. Subsequent management depends upon the experience of the surgeon.

The safest management is simply to drain the abscess, through a cruciate incision over the most fluctuant part of the abscess cavity. The cavity should be broken down gently with the index finger, care being taken not to enter the rectal ampulla by deep extension through the abscess cavity. Instruments should never be passed deep into the abscess cavity and any form of manipulation should be accompanied by the opposite index finger placed inside the rectum to allow assessment of the position of the anorectal musculature (Fig. 21.15). An iatrogenic communication caused at this stage of the operation results in an extrasphincteric fistula, which is an iatrogenic disaster. Pus should be sent for microbiological culture, which need not include a detailed search for anaerobes but simply whether the organisms are skin or gut type. Samples of the abscess wall should also be sent for histological appraisal, and it is also prudent to send separate specimens of both pus and tissue to look for tuberculosis. The cavity should then be lightly packed with gauze soaked in saline or an antiseptic, with instructions that the dressings be changed daily after a bath, and laxatives prescribed. Further management depends on the results of microbiology. Should skin organisms alone be cultured, then the patient can be reassured that the wound will heal uneventfully and with minimal risk of recurrence. If gut organisms are cultured, then an underlying fistula is likely. Some surgeons adopt a wait and see policy, since some cases will be cured by simple drainage even if the infection is cryptoglandular in origin. Others advocate a careful search for a fistula and treatment of it under elective conditions once the acute inflammatory changes have settled. Certainly those patients who present with recurrent infection at the same site should undergo an EUA.

Experienced surgeons may prefer to take a more aggressive approach at the time of acute infection. This is certainly associated with much lower rates of recurrence and fistula formation, but also carries the potential for iatrogenic damage to the sphincters, which may ultimately prove more troublesome than the presenting complaint. Our own preference is to counsel the patient fully preoperatively about the potential findings and the operative strategies available according to the surgical findings, and to arrive at a mutually agreed plan. Certainly, if primary fistulotomy is contemplated, the patient must be warned of the possibility of loss of the finer aspects of continence, balanced against the risks of protracted treatment. If an internal opening is evident, then it is safe to assume a fistula exists. If no internal opening can be detected, then the presence of a covert fistula may be determined by exploration of the intersphincteric space.

The abscess is opened via a radial incision with diathermy (which results in a relatively bloodless field) and the incision extended medially, if necessary, to the anal verge, to allow dissection of the intersphincteric space. If there is pus in the space, irrespective of the site of the presenting abscess, then there will be a fistula. If the abscess is perianal or in the superficial ischiorectal space, then the internal sphincter is laid open to the level of the dentate line to eradicate the intersphincteric infection (the precursor of the fistula). If the abscess is in the ischiorectal fossa and there is associated intersphincteric infection, then treatment depends upon the level at which the infection crosses the external sphincter. If the surgeon is sure that that the fistula is low and a good length of intact sphincter is preserved, then primary fistulotomy is reasonable. If there is any doubt about the level, or if it is felt that primary fistulotomy would result in excessive sphincter sacrifice, then the internal sphincter is laid open to the level of the dentate line (to drain the intersphincteric space) and a loose seton passed along the path of the fistula across the external sphincter. Of course, if no intersphincteric infection is found, then there should be no fistula, and the abscess is simply drained with no sphincter division whatever. If the sphincter is divided, then this necessitates an intra-anal dressing—the most comfortable and easily changed is the so-called 'Concorde' dressing, comprising a gauze square soaked in antiseptic over which is laid a Surgicell square, and this folded so as to resemble the wings of the aeroplane, and passed up to the apex of the wound with the index finger. If a loose seton is used, this can then be left for 3 months. About half the patients will suffer no further problems after removal at that time, and the others are treated in the same way as those with an established chronic fistula.

Management of high infection

Fortunately, infection high in the anorectal complex occurs relatively rarely as an acute problem, and perhaps it would be less common if the underlying fistula were dealt with adequately at the time of initial presentation rather than allowing subdued spread after incomplete primary drainage. The surgeon must be able to distinguish infection within the rectal wall (Fig. 21.16) from that outside the wall (Fig. 21.15). The former can be managed safely by draining it into the rectum by dividing the

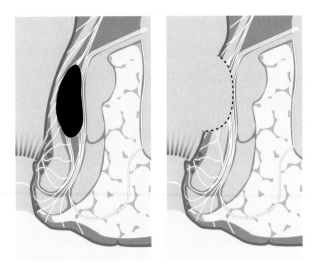

Figure 21.16 Intermuscular abscess and its treatment.

circular muscle, whereas the latter, if drained in the same way, might result in an extrasphincteric fistula. Careful palpation can differentiate the two: intermuscular infection is felt as a soft bulge in the rectal wall, whereas pararectal or high ischiorectal infection feels like bony, hard induration (in comparison with the contralateral side).

If the infection is outside the rectal wall, then management depends upon its origin and is outside the realms of the surgical trainee. The origin of supralevator pararectal infection may be truly pelvic, by for example appendicular, diverticular, or gynaecological inflammation, or indeed from malignancy. The correct operative approach in these cases is via the abdomen. Rarely, an acutely infected postrectal dermoid cyst may present as discharge at the posterior perineum, and this is usually approached through an intersphincteric route. Infection at this site may also arise through the cephalad extension of a transsphincteric fistula through the levators, as depicted in Fig. 21.17, or from a suprasphincteric fistula; these should be dealt with via the perineum. If there is any doubt, then surgical treatment should be delayed until the source has been identified.

5.4 Anal fistula

In Western Europe the incidence of anal fistulas is approximately 10 : 100 000, and is much more common in men than in women. Although relatively uncommon, fistulas may cause much misery to patient and surgeon. From the outset, it is important for the patient to understand that treatment is essentially a balance between eradicating the pathology and avoiding incontinence, and that a satisfactory outcome requires the patience of both parties. Most fistulas thought to be caused by persisting infection of the anal glands in the intersphincteric space (the cryptoglandular hypothesis; Parks 1961), but anal fistulas are also seen in association with other specific conditions, such as inflammatory bowel disease, tuberculosis, malignancy, actinomycosis, lymphogranuloma venereum, trauma, and foreign bodies. Anal fistulas communicate between the anal canal and the perianal skin and may be considered the chronic sequel of

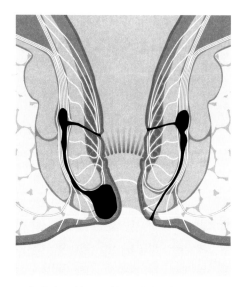

Figure 21.17 Varieties of intersphincteric fistula.

the parent condition, acute anorectal infection, despite the fact that many years may elapse between the two clinical conditions.

Patients with anal fistulas complain of intermittent anal pain and discharge, either purulent or mixed with blood, the two symptoms often inversely related, with the pain increasing until it eases off when the pus drains through the external opening. There is often a history of acute anal infection, which might have been treated surgically or have settled after spontaneous discharge of pus. Sometimes, it will have settled insidiously, leaving a fistulous opening on the perianal skin. Patients with intersphincteric fistulas are more likely to have sought surgical intervention at the acute perianal abscess stage than those with trans-sphincteric fistulas at the equivalent ischiorectal abscess stage. This is presumably because of the differences in tension (and therefore pain) that develop within the confines of the terminal ramifications of the conjoined longitudinal muscle and within the loosely areolar-filled tissue of the ischiorectal fossae.

Surgical management of anal fistulas depends upon accurate knowledge of both anorectal sphincter anatomy and the course of the fistula through it. The classification most commonly used in UK is that devised by Sir Alan Parks at St Mark's Hospital, based upon a study of 400 fistulas treated there (Parks *et al.* 1976). The cryptoglandular hypothesis is central to this classification, which holds, first, that the majority of fistulas arise from a primary abscess in the intersphincteric space, and, secondly, that the relation of the primary track to the external anal sphincter is paramount in surgical management. This classification has stood the test of time, although does not include those low intersphincteric fistulas that result from an anal fissure, and subcutaneous tracks arising from superficial infection. These two types are relatively minor, but are seen much more commonly in district hospitals than in tertiary referral centres.

According to Parks classification, there are four main fistula types—intersphincteric, trans-sphincteric, suprasphincteric, and extrasphincteric—each of which may be further subdivided according to the presence and course of any secondary tracks.

1. The **intersphincteric fistula** (Fig. 21.17) passes from the anal canal across the internal sphincter, downwards between the internal and external sphincter, and opens onto the perineal skin. Such fistulas are most commonly simple, but others end with a high blind track, or have an internal opening into the rectum, or no perineal opening, or even have a pelvic extension, or arise through pelvic disease.

2. The primary track of the **trans-sphincteric fistula** (Fig. 21.18) passes through the external sphincter at varying levels into the ischiorectal fossa. Such fistulas may be uncomplicated (a), consisting only of the primary track opening onto the skin of the buttock; or can have a high blind secondary track which ends either below (b) or above the levator ani muscles (c).

3. **Suprasphincteric fistulas** (Fig. 21.19) run up in the intersphincteric plane to loop over the top of the puborectalis

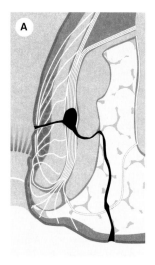
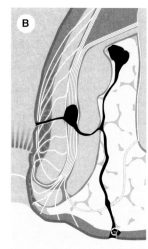
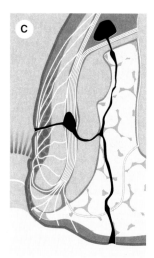

Figure 21.18 Varieties of trans-sphincteric fistula.

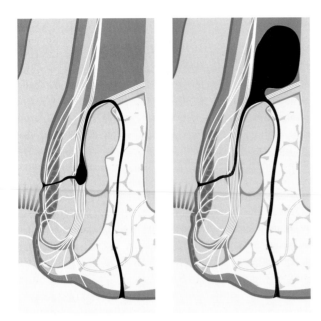

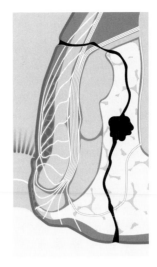

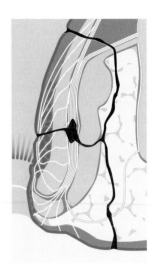

Figure 21.20 Extrasphincteric fistula.

Figure 21.19 Suprasphincteric fistula.

muscle and thence to pass down through the levator ani and ischiorectal fossa to reach the skin of the perineum. They are often associated with a supralevator abscess

4. **Extrasphincteric fistulas** (Fig. 21.20) run without relation to the sphincters and are classified according to aetiology. Some are undoubtedly iatrogenic in origin, arising from over-zealous probing of the ischiorectal fossa in a patient who presents with an ischiorectal abscess. The underlying fistula here is usually trans-sphincteric.

It is important to understand the basic primary tracks of the four recognized types of anal fistula. Superimposed on these primary tracks are extensions or secondary tracks which may be blind or which may open onto other parts of the perineal skin,

or indeed back into the anorectal lumen (most usually because of injudicious probing). Besides vertical and horizontal spread, infection may also spread circumferentially along any of the three tissue planes: intersphincteric (or intermuscular, which implies no restriction to below the anorectal ring), ischiorectal, or pararectal (Fig. 21.21).

The differentiation of fistulas into 'high' and 'low' is often a point of confusion, not least because it has been used to mean different things by different coloproctologists. A sensible and useful way of implementing this terminology is to describe as 'high' all fistulas that would cause significant functional morbidity if laid open at a single-stage fistulotomy. The remainder, where it would not cause major incontinence, would be called 'low'. This does not imply that laying open a 'low' fistula is not associated with functional morbidity, but rather that the incidence and severity of symptoms is less. Milligan and Morgan in 1934 emphasized the importance of the anorectal ring (anatomically the puborectalis) in maintaining continence.

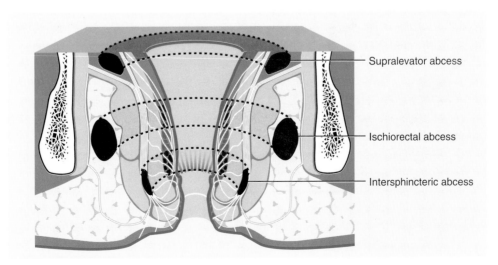

Figure 21.21 Extension of anorectal abscesses.

Certainly dividing this muscle during fistula surgery leads to unacceptable incontinence to all rectal contents in nearly all patients. Thompson's (1962) division into simple (95 per cent) and complex types was based on whether the internal opening was below (simple) or above the anorectal ring (complex), and also, whatever the level of the internal opening, whether laying it open would divide less than 75 per cent of the length of the sphincter musculature (simple) or more than 75 per cent (complex).

Assessment of anal fistulas

In the clinic

Clinical assessment of anal fistulas involves five essential points, enumerated by Goodsall and Miles at the turn of the century:

◆ the location of the external opening;

◆ the location of the internal opening;

◆ the course of the primary track;

◆ the course of any secondary tracks ('lateral burrowings');

◆ the presence of other diseases complicating the fistula.

Of these, perhaps the more important are the relative positions of the internal and external openings (which indicates the likely course of the primary track) and the presence of a high secondary track, especially supralevator, suggested by palpable induration. The distance between the external opening and the anal verge may assist differentiation between an intersphincteric and a trans-sphincteric fistula. The greater the distance, the higher the likelihood of a complicated upward extension. The position of the external opening also gives a clue to the likely site of the internal opening (Fig. 21.22). Goodsall's rule states that for openings anterior to the transverse anal line, the fistula usually runs radially into the anal canal; for openings posterior to this imaginary line, the track is usually curvilinear and opens into the anal lumen in the midline posteriorly. The exceptions to this rule include anterior openings more than 3 cm from the anal margin, which may represent anterior extensions of

posterior horseshoe fistulas, fistulas associated with Crohn's disease, or fistulas arising from carcinoma of the anal glands.

The internal opening may be felt digitally as an indurated nodule or pit, or seen at proctoscopy (especially with the Graeme Anderson proctoscope), aided if necessary by gentle downward retraction of the dentate line. This may expose openings concealed by prominent anal valves. Outpatient assessment must include sigmoidoscopy, but beyond this, more information can only be obtained safely and comfortably from EUA or special investigations. Probing fistulas in the clinic is both painful and dangerous, and rarely yields useful information. Special investigations are generally reserved for 'difficult' fistulas, difficult because of recurrence despite expert treatment, or difficult because of uncertainty during assessment under anaesthesia.

Examination under anaesthesia

EUA in the lithotomy position allows a more detailed assessment of the geography of fistulas which would be too uncomfortable in the awake state, but carries the disadvantage of the sphincters being in a relaxed state. This can occasionally make accurate judgement of the level of the fistula difficult. Examination, as in the clinic, begins with inspection, within and without the anal canal. Several manoeuvres have been proposed to aid in finding the internal opening. These include digital massage of the track and watching for a bead of pus to appear in the lumen, gentle passage of a probe through the external opening (if the track is low and straight); injection of dilute hydrogen peroxide down the track which will demonstrate the internal opening by the site of frothing, and the injection of various dyes (e.g. methylene blue). However, if the initial appearance of the dye is missed, the whole anorectal lining becomes stained. Furthermore, if a track is transsected, the surrounding tissues become stained, making further dissection difficult.

The primary track can usually be inferred by identifying the internal and external openings and feeling between these two points with a well-lubricated finger. Careful probing can help delineate primary and secondary tracks; if both openings are

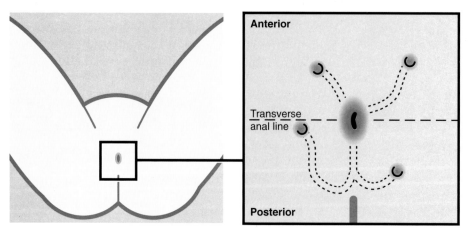

Figure 21.22 Goodsall's rule.

seen but a probe cannot easily be passed from one to the other, it is possible that a high extension exists; a probe passed via each orifice may then delineate the primary track. High induration should alert the surgeon to the possibility of supralevator infection, and the persistence of granulation tissue after curettage also indicates a secondary track.

Special investigations

Most anal fistulas are relatively simple, both in their course and ease of satisfactory surgical treatment. All surgeons with experience in this area know of patients in whom clinical assessment proved incorrect, or they could not be sure of what exactly was going on, or they were afraid of aggressive surgery because of the risk of incontinence. In any of these instances, extra information would be useful but most special investigations have been relatively unhelpful. **Fistulography** is relatively insensitive and non-specific, in that it may fail to demonstrate (usually secondary) tracks, and, more worryingly, may indicate the presence of tracks and openings which do not exist. Endoanal ultrasound was shown in initial studies to yield no more information than could be obtained by expert examination, failing to demonstrate pathology beyond the focal range of the probe (i.e. above and lateral to the sphincters, areas that often provide the most difficulties in management). Probes of different frequency would image more distal pathology but at the expense of imaging intrasphincteric pathology. **Intraoperative endosonography** shows promise when used in conjunction with hydrogen peroxide, but there have been no published prospective studies to date. **Computed tomography** of the perineum is technically difficult in all but the axial plane, sphincter resolution is poor, and important information such as the relation of the tracks to the levators can only be inferred since these muscles are not well identified. Like conventional fistulography, CT also involves ionizing radiation and the need for contrast media.

The advent of **MRI** has allowed a significant advance in anal fistula assessment, and has been shown in prospective studies to be at least as accurate as experienced coloproctological examination, demonstrating tracks that may be missed at surgery and which are the cause of fistula persistence (Lunniss and Phillips 1994). However, the investigation is expensive and there are some economic arguments for reserving it for the difficult, complex, or recurrent fistula.

Anorectal physiological studies in patients undergoing fistula surgery have shown that although the external sphincter is important in maintaining continence, perhaps less consideration has been given in the past than merited to the sensitive anoderm and internal sphincter. For the majority of low fistulas, any deficit in continence is more likely to be due to surgical division of these two structures rather than the voluntary muscle, and although such postoperative symptoms are relatively minor, they are common (up to 50 per cent incidence of soiling and/or occasional flatus incontinence). There is therefore a strong argument to try and preserve as much sphincter as possible. The problem is that no operation for

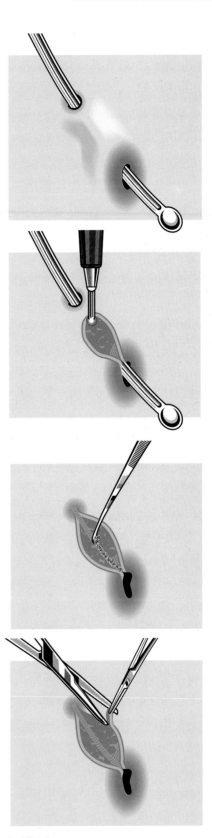

Figure 21.23 Anal fistulotomy.

fistula is as good as traditional laying open at actually getting rid of the fistula, something the surgeon must discuss with the patient before embarking on one of the more complex procedures available. Preoperative physiological tests are not really predictive of functional outcome, but when faced with what is likely to be a difficult problem, it is prudent to obtain baseline studies.

Surgical management of anal fistulas

Fortunately, 90 per cent of all anal fistulas are easy to treat. These are intersphincteric or low trans-sphincteric types which can be managed safely by laying open of the fistula tract. A probe is passed along the primary track between internal and external openings, an assessment made of the amount of sphincter above the level of the probe, and if appropriate, the track laid open by scalpel blade or cautery (Fig. 21.23). The laid-open track is curretted and granulation tissue sent for histological appraisal. Careful examination of the laid-open track will reveal if there are any secondary tracks. These should be thoroughly curretted or laid open, according to their position.

Intersphincteric extensions are best treated by extending the internal sphincterotomy to allow drainage into the anorectal lumen. Infection in the ischiorectal fossa can be safely laid open without fear of sphincter damage, and although the wounds so created may appear at first sight alarmingly large and disfiguring, they will heal uneventfully with remarkably little deformity as long as the pathology has been eradicated. In the USA, drainage catheters are sometimes preferred in order to reduce wound size but this carries the risk of inadequate drainage and later recurrence. In order to allow good healing, it is wise to freshen the edges and perform a 'back-cut of Salmon', and in

order to reduce the size of the wound, to suture the fibrous edge of the track to the divided skin (**marsupialization**).

In the case of a posterior horseshoe fistula, the limbs of the horseshoe often need to be laid open before easy access and assessment of the level of the primary track is possible (Fig. 21.24). In such circumstances, the probe should be passed via the external opening(s) along the track towards the coccyx in the posterior midline and this part of the track laid open. Division of the fibres connecting the sphincter to the coccyx can safely be performed, and this allows good access to the retrosphincteric space where the primary track across the sphincters is not infrequently found.

The wound should be dressed with light packs into the apices of the wound and a laid-on, non-adherent dressing placed along the primary track, similar to that described after primary fistulotomy. Postoperatively the patient should be asked to bathe daily and after each bowel action, and the wounds explored digitally and irrigated to prevent bridging. For simple fistulas, if the wound is healing well, the patient may be discharged with appropriate instructions to patient, spouse, and district nurse, and the patient followed up at regular intervals in the outpatient clinic. In the case of difficult fistulas, or those in which the wound is not granulating well, a second EUA should be performed to ensure that no secondary tracks have been missed.

The complex fistula

Fistulas may be complex because either there are multiple secondary tracks or the primary track crosses the sphincters at a level where fistulotomy would be expected to result in significant functional morbidity. In the first case, the key is to deal with the secondary tracks, often through multiple stages, until one is left with just the primary track crossing the sphincters. This may turn out to be low enough to lay open with confidence. If not, then the fistula becomes complex for the second reason. The most important aspect of the management of a patient with a high primary track is to recognize this possibility at the first examination and to avoid damaging the sphincter through failure to appreciate the level of the track. Indicators of difficulty include the presence of induration between the rectal wall and puborectalis, and whether a probe passed through the external opening travels in a path parallel to the axis of the anal canal. In either of these circumstances, it is best to accept the possibility of a high fistula-in-ano or even an extrasphincteric fistula arising from pelvic disease and refer the patient to a specialist fistula surgeon.

Sphincter-conserving techniques

The range of differing techniques advocated for treating high fistulas is a reflection of the fact that none has excellent results. This arises mainly because the high fistula is extremely difficult to manage, with a balance between cure and continence having to be achieved. Unfortunately, different techniques cannot be compared objectively because there are no randomized trials. This is because fistula classification is not uniform (and one surgeon's high fistula may be another surgeon's low fistula), and

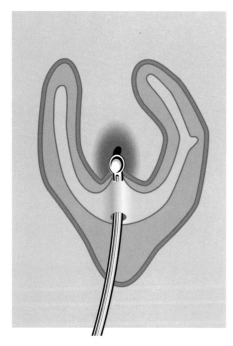

Figure 21.24 Horseshoe fistula.

because surgeons are likely to use only those methods that they have found useful themselves. These methods include **setons** (which may be loose (Thomson and Ross 1989), tight (Held *et al.* 1986) or 'chemical' (Shukla *et al.* 1991), fistulotomy and immediate reconstruction of the divided sphincters (Parkash *et al.* 1985), core-out fistulectomy (Lewis 1986), advancement flaps (Jones *et al.* 1987), intersphincteric approaches (Matos *et al.* 1993), rerouting of the track (Mann and Clifton 1985), and even laser vapourization of the track (Slutki *et al.* 1981) or sealing off the track with fibrin glue (Abel *et al.* 1993). Each method has its group of protagonists who claim results which may or may not be reproducible by others; the clever surgeon is one who has all these methods in his or her armamentarium so as to employ the most appropriate method for any particular circumstance. The clever surgical trainee, on the other hand, is one that recognizes a fistula to be difficult and does not try and deal with it alone!

5.5 Anal fissure

An anal fissure is a tear in the ectodermal portion of the anal canal and it is usually found in either the 12 o'clock or the 6 o'clock position around the anal circumference. It commonly occurs after a bout of constipation and is a very painful condition which can interfere with normal bowel function. Patients find themselves in a vicious circle where they appreciate that the next bout of defecation will be painful and hence they avoid passing a stool and become progressively more constipated. When the bowels are eventually opened, the tear is made worse.

A diagnostic feature of an anal fissure is anal pain after defecation. In chronic cases, the skin at the lower part of the fissure becomes swollen and can be used as a marker of an anal fissure—the so called 'sentinel pile'. This may be the only sign of a chronic anal fissure as it is often too painful to examine the patient proctoscopically. Under these circumstances it is best that the examination in outpatients is abandoned and the patient is admitted for an EUA to determine the exact problem. This can be done as a day case and is combined with a full sigmoidoscopic examination to exclude associated inflammatory bowel disease. Most cases of anal fissure have no underlying aetiology other than a bout of constipation. It is commonly seen in mothers in the postpartum period, where their anal pain has been mistakenly attributed to the presence of piles, commonly seen during pregnancy.

It is important to assess whether a fissure is acute (short history, shallow fissure) or chronic, (long history, deep fissure, and sentinel pile), as conservative management is less likely to be of help in the chronic situation. In acute fissures, a combination of a bulk laxative, locally applied local anaesthetic gel, and possibly the use of an anal dilator form the basis of conservative management. An average of 50 per cent of acute fissures respond to non-operative measures, and acute fissures affecting the anterior part of the anal canal are more likely to respond. Laboratory studies have suggested that high maximal resting anal pressures and reduced perfusion at the fissure base are the causes of spontaneous healing of the established chronic fissure, but whether these observations are primary factors or epiphenomena is uncertain. Reduction in anal pressure with topical

nitrates has been shown to alleviate symptoms in the majority of patients, but compliance may be limited due to the associated headaches reported in 30 per cent of patients, and persistence of symptoms associated with a chronic fissure despite conservative measures usually implies the need for operative treatment.

Two operative treatments are used for treating non-responsive anal fissures. These are forcible dilatation of the anal sphincter muscles and lateral internal anal sphincterotomy. Pain relief following anal dilatation is usually rapid, but the main objection is the unacceptable level of incontinence for flatus and for faeces which follows as a result of the variable disruption of internal and external sphincters. It is for this reason that the operation should not be performed. Lateral anal sphincterotomy, on the other hand, is less likely to result in serious continence problems and is the treatment of choice in patients with an established chronic fissure. However, defects in continence do occur after anal sphincterotomy—up to 30 per cent of patients may experience some incontinence, particularly for flatus, irrespective of the type of sphincterotomy. All patients must therefore be adequately counselled preoperatively.

Operative details of lateral anal sphincterotomy

The procedure (Fig. 21.25) is usually carried out under general anaesthesia but can be performed under local anaesthesia in outpatients. The patient is placed in the lithotomy position on the operating table and full examination, including sigmoidoscopy, is carried out to rule out rectal disease. An anal retractor is introduced and gently stretched to reveal the inferior edge of the internal sphincter laterally, which is palpable. Dilute adrenaline (epinephrine) solution (1 : 250 000) may be infiltrated on either side of the internal sphincter at either the 3 or 9 o'clock positions, to open up the tissue planes and reduce bleeding. A small circumferential incision over the taut lower border of the internal sphincter is made and the intersphincteric plane between the internal and external sphincters is developed up to the level of the dentate line. The internal sphincter is also separated from the anal skin and mucosa and then divided up to the dentate line. The overlying skin incision is then closed with absorbable sutures.

There is a subgroup of patients with chronic anal fissure in whom the aetiology is manifestly not one of anal canal hypertonicity, and in whom sphincter division for fissure would carry an unacceptable risk of incontinence. These include patients who have had previous fistula surgery or suffered obstetric injury. For these patients, the principle of introducing a vascularized skin flap into the bare area from which the fissure has been excised is attractive, and can give good symptom relief, at least in the short term, with no deterioration in anal sensation or resting pressure. When this technique is employed for patients with hypertonicity of the anal canal with fissures, the results of island advancement flaps are probably not as good.

5.6 Perianal Crohn's disease

The characteristic and diverse perianal manifestations of Crohn's disease can pose major challenges to both physician and surgeon (Lunniss and Phillips 1994). There is little information about its prevalence in the Crohn's population. This is because there is no standard definition of perianal Crohn's disease (PACD) and because most published data come from specialist centres. Recognition is further complicated because:

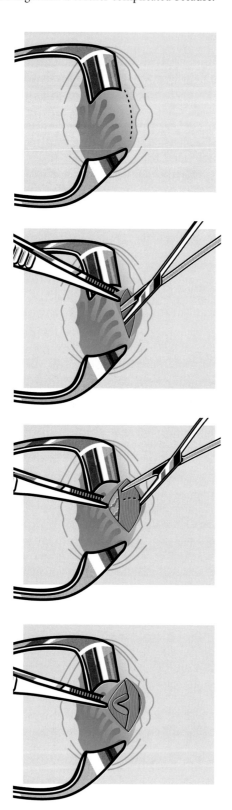

Figure 21.25 Lateral anal sphincterotomy.

- asymptomatic pathology may not come to the attention of the clinician;

- patients with Crohn's disease may have perianal pathology of a non-inflammatory origin;

- anorectal Crohn's disease may be the first manifestation of the systemic disorder, occurring years before other gastro-intestinal manifestations become evident.

PACD may be found in up to 75 per cent of patients with Crohn's disease, the incidence varying with the site of gastro-intestinal pathology, with higher rates the more distal the disease. The spectrum of PACD has been divided by Hughes (1978) into:

(1) those primary conditions with activity reflecting that of the intestinal disease (i.e. fissures, ulcerated piles, and cavitating ulcers); and

(2) secondary lesions, either mechanical (skin tags, strictures, epithelialized fistulas) or infective (abscesses and fistulas), for which local treatment should be determined by the local severity.

The observation that lesions in PACD can improve symptomatically and even heal spontaneously, combined with the significant potential for iatrogenic problems caused by aggressive surgery, has led surgeons to adopt a highly conservative approach. Certainly, complete resection of proximal disease and maintained remission does have an ameliorating effect on PACD, and intense medical management similarly has been shown beneficial for perianal conditions. The reported effects of faecal diversion away from the perineum are more diverse.

Just as with the gastrointestinal disease, the severity of symptoms and interference with lifestyle incurred by PACD are highly diverse, and patients probably self-select towards surgical management and eventually proctectomy in the worst cases, rather than because optimum medical treatment is unavailable. The combination of severe drug-resistant proctocolitis and PACD usually heralds the eventual need for proctectomy, and in selected cases it may be prudent to consider this surgical option at an early stage.

In principle, asymptomatic manifestations of PACD should be left well alone. Medical treatment of intestinal disease may be expected to result in sustained healing of fissures in patients with Crohn's disease in whom the fissure is the only manifestation of PACD. Low symptomatic fistulas may be approached in a way similar to their idiopathic equivalents, whereas management of more complex tracks should be directed more towards effective drainage to prevent recurrent septic painful exacerbations. Selected patients with little in the way of proctocolitis and with symptomatic ano-recto-vaginal fistulas may benefit from attempts at local repair, for which the procedure employed depends upon the level of the fistula. Very low anovaginal tracks can be cured by laying them open, with little risk of functional disturbance; high fistulas communicating with the vaginal vault have to be approached via the abdomen; whereas those in between may be treated with vaginal or rectal advancement flap techniques.

Patients with PACD may become incontinent for several reasons: the liquid nature of the stool together with macro- or microcolitis causing increased frequency of defecation; reduced rectal compliance; loss of gastrointestinal length by resection of involved segments (especially if the ileocaecal valve has been resected); and mechanical trauma to the sphincters. Sphincter disruption might result from infection, from surgery employed to treat infection, and women, from obstetric trauma. Patients with major incontinence due solely to sphincter disruption (and in the absence of rectal disease) are likely to benefit from sphincter repair.

5.7 Faecal incontinence

Continence to rectal contents depends upon a multitude of factors, some of which need to be closely co-ordinated. These include: stool consistency, rectal volume and compliance, anorectal sensation, voluntary and involuntary anal sphincter function, and a distensible anal mucosa. Most cases of incontinence seen in coloproctological practice result from trauma to the sphincters, mainly obstetric, but also iatrogenic (e.g. after surgery for fistula-in-ano), or pudendal neuropathy. Congenital anomalies and other neurological disorders are rare. Most patients are multiparous women in whom both anatomical disruption of the sphincters and neuropathy are likely to contribute to the problem. Sphincter trauma may arise also through repeated sphincter dilatation (either social or surgical) or as part of major trauma (civilian and war).

Pudendal neuropathy leading to neurogenic faecal incontinence may follow years of straining at stool, through traction damage to the pudendal nerves or by direct trauma to the sacral nerves during prolonged labour. Conduction defects have been shown to lead to denervation/reinnervation changes in the puborectalis/external anal sphincter complex, and also lead to impaired internal sphincter function and reduced anal sensation. In the anorectal physiology laboratory, this can be assessed by the measurement of pudendal nerve terminal motor latency or by the more painful single-fibre electromyographic assessment of muscle fibre density in the external anal sphincter.

Obstetric causes of mechanical sphincter disruption are increasingly being recognized and acknowledged as such in the UK, possibly because women feel more able to point out and seek help for their symptoms. Another reason is the advent of, and now widespread availability of, endoanal ultrasound, a relatively non-invasive method which currently has no equal in the assessment of internal and external sphincter integrity. Sphincter disruption is seen fairly commonly after forceps deliveries, but the patient may not present until middle age. At this point, the added effects of pudendal neuropathy swing the balance from a controllable nuisance to a situation which is seriously socially embarrassing.

Thorough assessment of sphincter function is required in order to plan appropriate treatment. A careful history must be taken, including a detailed obstetric history and previous anal surgery, and the precise type and degree of incontinence should be assessed. Clinical examination is complemented by anorectal

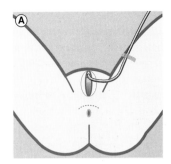
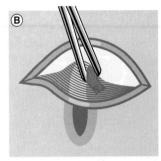
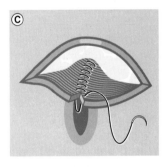
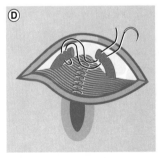
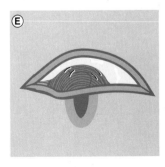

Figure 21.26 Anal sphincter repair.

physiological tests and endoanal ultrasound. Many patients with borderline incontinence derive great benefit from a reduction in the intake of dietary fibre, together with the use of stool hardeners, such as codeine phosphate and loperamide (the latter also augments internal sphincter tone). However, surgery remains the mainstay of treatment in those in whom sphincter disruption or neuropathy can be demonstrated.

For patients with sphincter disruption as the cause, the aim of surgery is to resect all scar tissue and to achieve an overlapping plication of the muscle ends to create a complete ring of functional muscle around the anal canal (Fig. 21.26). This procedure aims primarily to restore external sphincter function; whether it augments internal sphincter function is unclear.

About 90 per cent achieve an excellent short-term functional result after repair for obstetric injury while up to 70 per cent with other causes of sphincter damage derive some improvement. This is probably because of the lesser degree of disruption and scarring in obstetric cases. Thus attempts at repair are usually worthwhile if continued incontinence or a permanent stoma are the only alternatives.

In cases of incontinence associated with pudendal neuropathy but with intact sphincters, the operation of **postanal repair** may give good results in a proportion of patients in the short term, but a much smaller percentage would appear to derive long-term benefit. The aim of the operation (Fig. 21.27) is to narrow the anorectal angle by moving the anorectal junction anteriorly and cranially (this helps provide a mechanical barrier to the passive descent of stool into the anal canal), and to lengthen and tighten the anal canal. This increases resting anal tone and sometimes incidentally improves anal sensation. A good functional outcome appears to depend most upon changing the postoperative resting sphincter pressures.

In patients with sphincter disruption and pudendal neuropathy, there is argument for combining the above two procedures in a single 'total pelvic repair'.

More recently more complex procedures have been used to try to restore continence in patients in whom sphincter surgery alone is not indicated. These include implanting an artificial bowel sphincter or creating an electrically stimulated neosphincter using the gracilis muscle. The development of these techniques has led to the realization that patients often have coexistent incontinence and disorders of rectal evacuation, which limits the success of these procedures and for which, in some patients, some form of procedure to enable antegrade irrigation of the colon (e.g. the colonic conduit), is required.

5.8 Perianal warts

The incidence of perianal warts, or **condylomata accuminata**, is increasing in the population. The condition is caused by the human papillomavirus. The condition is almost invariably sexually transmitted, with the highest rates seen in homosexual males, although heterosexuals are not immune. There is often a history of other sexually transmitted diseases. As a consequence, and because of the increased 'availability' of sexual health clinics, only a minority of patients with this condition are referred to colorectal clinics, usually with warts resistant to the remedies of the specialist in sexual medicine. Apparent resistance to treatment is, however, more often to do with reinfection than failure of treatment.

Patients with perianal warts usually complain of itching, bleeding, and perianal lumps. There may also be symptoms from warts elsewhere on the genitalia. The presentation of the

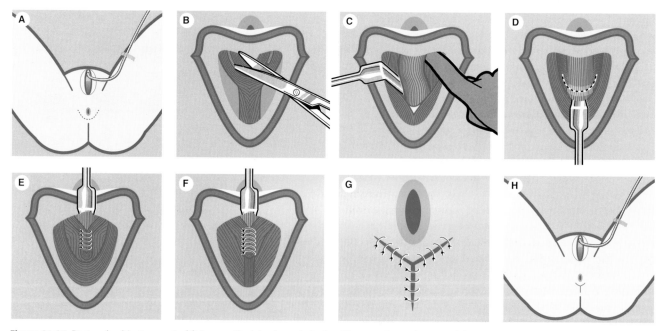

Figure 21.27 Postanal sphincter repair. (A) A curved incision is made in the skin posterior to the anus; (B) The anterior skin flap is retracted anteriorly and the sphincters exposed; (C) The intersphincteric plane is developed to display Waldeyer's fascia; (D) Waldeyer's fascia is divided; (F) Interrupted 2/0 polydioxanone sutures are placed to approximate the two sides of the puborectalis sling; (G) The skin is closed with 3/0 Vicryl Rapide® (note: this covers two drawings).

warts is variable, ranging from one or two discrete excrescences (within and without the anal canal) to massive cauliflower-like lesions obscuring the anal orifice. Warts may be apparent elsewhere on the genitalia, and rarely may resemble frank malignancy.

Surgical treatment is usually by scissor or diathermy excision under general anaesthesia. Individual warts are excised, leaving normal skin between. An EUA allows a thorough assessment, especially of warts within the anal canal, as well as those elsewhere on the genitalia. Before excision, the lesions are raised from the skin contour on a subcutaneous bleb of dilute adrenaline (epinephrine) (1 : 250 000). If there is concern about the degree of scarring following excision of large areas of skin, then removal may occur over several stages. Surgical excision requires fewer sessions than podophyllin application and has a lower recurrence rate. All specimens must be sent for histological assessment to ensure that there are no *in situ* or invasive malignant changes. Patients who turn out to have locally advanced invasive malignancy should be referred for combined chemotherapy and radiotherapy.

5.9 Pilonidal disease

A pilonidal sinus is a chronic inflammatory disorder comprising a midline epithelialized pit between the buttocks. This extends as a single or a series of granulation-tissue-lined tracks for a variable distance craniocaudally and laterally. These tracks almost invariably contain hair and end as a blind cul-de-sac or at another sinus opening. The condition is not seen before puberty and rarely over the age of 45—indeed its self-limiting nature combined with the relative lack of success of surgical treatment makes the doctrine of conservative treatment attractive. However, in some patients, recurrent acute or chronic infection make attempts at eradication worthwhile. The aetiology of the condition is uncertain, but it is likely to be a foreign-body reaction to shed hair which 'drills' into congenital midline pits. Hair is barbed and, when reversed, will penetrate further and further into the skin. Congenital pits are common incidental findings on examination but most are never associated with pilonidal disease. The highest incidence is in people who sit all day, particularly on hard seats, such as tractor drivers.

Abscesses form within the sinus, but discharge is prevented through the midline by fibrous septa between skin and sacral fascia, and secondary lateral tracks develop. These may pass caudally and create an appearance which resembles hidradenitis suppurativa or fistula-in-ano (both of which may coexist with pilonidal disease).

Patients usually present with an acute abscess or with a chronic discharging sinus. The acute abscess usually lies to one side the midline, although a midline pit is always visible. These abscesses are best treated by simple deroofing which effects drainage, and curettage of the cavity. They are then lightly packed with saline-soaked gauze. In up to 50 per cent of cases, this is sufficient and allows healing. So-called definitive pilonidal surgery at this stage is not justified.

The variety of treatments proposed for the chronic condition demonstrates the lack of reliability of any one, despite the quoted claims of their respective advocates. In addition, the morbidity of radical surgical treatments has encouraged some surgeons to adopt a much more conservative approach. The success of simple laying open of the tracks with curettage and packing probably relies upon the removal of hair from the wound, which heals by secondary intention. Weekly shaving of the area is wise in the convalescent period. Radical surgery includes excision rather than laying open of the sinuses, with the resulting defect being allowed to heal by secondary intention (our preferred method), or the edges closed primarily, or closed by rotation flap. Selection of patients for these more radical approaches must be performed carefully. Many patients with this condition are young and are poor attenders at follow-up clinics. In a few, there may be the possibility of self-induced harm preventing healing.

5.10 Hidradenitis suppurativa

Hidradenitis is a chronic recurring suppurative disease of skin bearing apocrine glands. Although more common in women, those cases involving the perineum (the apocrine circumanal glands of Gay) are more often seen in men. Like pilonidal disease, hidradenitis is not seen before puberty, and most patients present in the age range of 16–40 years. The aetiology is unknown, although obesity, acne, poor hygiene, and excessive sweating have been suggested as predisposing factors. It may be seen in a variety of endocrine disorders, suggesting that a relative androgen excess or increased target organ androgen sensitivity may be implicated.

Occlusion of the apocrine gland ducts leads to bacterial proliferation within the glands, rupture, and spread of infection to adjacent glands. Secondary infection causes further local extension, skin damage, and fibrosis, eventually leading to multiple communicating subcutaneous fistulas. In the primary stages, hidradenitis suppurativa presents with multiple tender, raised, red lesions in the perianal region; in its chronic form multiple sinuses are seen, with secondary infection leading to gross fibrosis and scarring. It may rarely extend into the anal canal, but never above the dentate line.

When the disease is seen in its early stages, antibiotics are the mainstay of treatment; these should be continued until complete resolution has been achieved. Acute abscesses may need to be treated by incision and drainage; but extensive sinus formation (as more commonly seen in hospital practice) necessitates surgical excision. The surgical alternatives are similar to the more radical treatments employed in managing pilonidal disease: excision with packing; excision with marsupialization; excision with primary closure; or excision with skin grafting or flap. Although the healing time associated with excision and healing by secondary intention is prolonged, it seems to give good results with low recurrence rates. Only very rarely is a defunctioning colostomy necessary when there are multiple lesions close to the anus.

5.11 Perianal disease in the HIV-positive patient

The rise in prevalence of AIDS sufferers and the anorectal lesions associated with the syndrome mean that more of these patients are attending the general surgical or colorectal outpatient clinic. Initial data on the surgical management of anal conditions associated with HIV positivity were dominated by a high surgical morbidity and mortality. However, advances in medical treatment which improve the general health of patients, especially in the earlier stages (CDC I and II), has improved healing rates of ulcerative conditions.

HIV patients suffer from the same sexually transmitted diseases (STDs) as the rest of the population, but particularly those associated with anoreceptive intercourse; up to 80 per cent of AIDS patients with anorectal disease have a history of previous STDs, including gonorrhoea, syphilis, and chlamydia. In addition, HIV patients suffer almost uniquely from various anal viral infections and benign and malignant tumours, such as squamous cell and cloacogenic carcinomata, lymphoma, and Kaposi's sarcoma.

Anorectal pathology in the HIV-positive or AIDS patient includes ordinary anal conditions as well as a range of conditions rarely found outside this group. These include: herpes simplex (HSV), cytomegalovirus (CMV), *Mycobacterium avium intracellulare* (MAI), *Candida albicans*, *Condylomata accuminata*, and non-specific primary HIV-induced anal ulcer.

Most HIV patients seen in the surgical clinic will already be under the care of an immunologist. A thorough history should include evaluation of the anorectal symptoms, age, HIV status, CDC classification, previous and current STDs, previous anorectal conditions and treatments, and current medication. Examination should be carried out with all precautions taken, and specific pathology, such as warts, vesicles, ulcers, fissures, fistulas, and abscesses, looked for. Proctoscopy and sigmoidoscopy should be performed and intra-anal or rectal ulcers biopsied. Biopsies should be sent for microscopy, viral cultures (including HIV, HSV, and CMV), acid-fast stain (for MAI), and Indian ink stain (for cryptococcus).

Anal condylomata of various viral types are probably the most frequent pathology, and there may be a higher incidence of dysplasia and *in situ* neoplasia than in HIV-negative homosexuals with warts. Such condylomata can be treated by surgical excision (or fulguration if more extensive) if local chemotherapy fails to control them, but the recurrence rate once initial control is established is as high as 50 per cent.

Herpetic ulcers are treated with topical and oral aciclovir; the isolation of CMV in ulcer biopsies indicates the need for intravenous ganciclovir. Ulcers in which no specific virus is isolated may respond to intralesional steroid injections.

Fissures and haemorrhoids should be treated conservatively —even injection or banding of piles appears ill-advised. Selected patients with true fissures (rather than ulcers) who have ceased anoreceptive intercourse may benefit from sphincterotomy but the risks of wound breakdown, infection, and incontinence are high, so dietary advice and the use of local anaesthetics are preferable. Painful abscesses should be drained, and if an underlying fistula is found (usually at the base of a cavitating ulcer), a loose, long-term seton inserted. A diverting colostomy may be indicated in a few patients with severe erosive ulceration of the perineum to control diarrhoea and to alleviate pain.

Treatment protocols for anorectal conditions in AIDS patients are still evolving, but a logical approach is one based on accurate diagnosis of the pathology and aetiology (largely dependent upon good biopsy analysis), together with surgical conservatism.

Bibliography

Abel, M.E., Chiu, Y.S.Y., Russell, T.R., and Volpe, P.A. (1993). Autologous fibrin glue in the treatment of rectovaginal and complex fistulas. *Dis. Colon Rectum,* **36**, 447–9.

Ambrose, N.S., Morris, D., Alexander-Williams, J., and Keighley, M.R.B. (1983). A randomized trial of photocoagulation or injection sclerotherapy for the treatment of first and second-degree haemorrhoids. *Dis. Colon Rectum,* **28**, 238–40.

Belliveau, P., Thomson, J.P.S., and Parks, A.G. (1983). Fistula-in-ano. A manometric study. *Dis. Colon Rectum,* **26**, 152–4.

Buchmann, P., Keighley, M.R.B., Allan, R.N., Thompson, H., and Alexander-Williams, J. (1980). Natural history of perianal Crohn's disease. Ten year follow up: a plea for conservatism. *Am. J. Surg.,* **140**, 642–4.

Choen, S., Burnett, S., Bartram, C.L., and Nicholls, R.J. (1991). Comparison between anal endosonography and digital examination in the evaluation of anal fistulae. *Br. J. Surg.,* **78**, 445–7.

Eisenhammer, S. (1978). The final evaluation and classification of the surgical treatment of the primary anorectal, cryptoglandular intermuscular (intersphincteric) fistulous abscess and fistula. *Dis. Colon Rectum,* **21**, 237–54.

Eu, K.-W., Seow-Choen, F., and Goh, H.S. (1994). Comparison of emergency and elective haemorrhoidectomy. *Br. J. Surg.,* **81**, 308–10.

Grace, R.H., Harper, I.A., and Thompson, R.G. (1982). Anorectal sepsis: microbiology in relation to fistula-inano. *Br. J. Surg.,* **69**, 401–3.

Haas, P.A. and Fox, T.A. (1980). A-,e-related changes and scar formations of perianal connective tissue. *Dis. Colon Rectum,* **23**, 160–9.

Held, D., Khubchandani, I., Sheets, J., Stasik, J., Rosen, L., and Reither, R. (1986). Management of anorectal horseshoe abscess and fistula. *Dis. Colon Rectum,* **29**, 793–7.

Hughes, L.E. (1978). Surgical pathology and management of anorectal Crohn's disease. *J. Roy. Soc. Med.*, **71**, 644–51.

Jones, I.T., Fazio, V.W., and Jagelman, D.G. (1987). The use of transanal rectal advancement flaps in the management of fistulas involving the anorectum. *Dis. Colon Rectum*, **30**, 919–23.

Keighley, M.R.B., Buchmann, P., Minervium, S., Arabi, Y., and Alexander-Williams, J. (1979). Prospective trials of minor surgical procedures and high fibre diet for haemorrhoids. *BMJ*, **2**, 967–9.

Khubchandani, I.T. and Read, J.F. (1989). Sequelae of internal sphincterotomy for chronic fissure in ano. *Br. J. Surg.*, **76**, 431–4.

Kuijpers, H.C. and Schulpen, T. (1985). Fistulography for fistula-in-ano. *Dis. Colon Rectum*, **28**, 103–4.

Lewis, A. (1986). Excision of fistula in ano. *Int. J. Colorect. Dis.*, **1**, 265–7.

Loder, P.B., Kamm, M.A., Nicholls, R.J., and Phillips, R.K.S. (1994). Haemorrhoids: pathology, pathophysiology and aetiology. *Br. J. Surg.*, **81**, 946–54.

Lunniss, P.J., Sultan, A.H., Sheffield, J.P., Talbot, I.C., and Phillips, R.K.S. (1994). The anal intersphincteric space. *Clin. Anat.*, **7**, 164.

Lunniss, P.J. and Phillips, R.K.S. (1992). Anatomy and function of the anal longitudinal muscle. *Br. J. Surg.*, **79**, 882–4.

Lunniss, P.J. and Phillips, R.K.S. (1994). Surgical assessment of acute anorectal sepsis is a better predictor of fistula than microbiological analysis. *Br. J. Surg.*, **81**, 368–9.

Lunniss, P.J., Barker, P.G., Sultan, A.H., Armstrong, P., Reznek, R.H., Bartram, C.I., Cottam, K., and Phillips, R.K.S. (1994). Magnetic resonance imaging of fistula-in-ano. *Dis. Colon Rectum*, **37**, 708–18.

Lunniss, P.J., Kamm, M.A., and Phillips, R.K.S. (1994). Factors affecting continence after surgery for anal fistula. *Br. J. Surg.*, **81**, 1382–5.

Lunniss, P.J. and Phillips, R.K.S. (1994). Extra-intestinal fistulae and perianal disease in Crohn's disease. *Europ. J. Gastroenterol. Hepatol.*, **6**, 100–7.

Mann, C.V. and Clifton, M.A. (1985). Re-routing of the track for the treatment of high anal and anorectal fistulae. *Br. J. Surg.*, **72**, 134–7.

Matos, D., Lunniss, P.J., and Phillips, R.K.S. (1993). Total sphincter conservation in fistula surgery: results of a new approach. *Br. J. Surg.*, **80**, 802–4.

McColl, I. (1967). The comparative anatomy and pathology of anal glands. *Ann. R. Coll. Surg.*, **40**, 3647.

McElwain, J.W., Maclean, D., Alexander, R.M., Hoexter, B., and Guthrie, J.F. (1975). Anorectal problems: experience with primary fistulectomy for anorectal abscess. A report of 1000 cases. *Dis. Colon Rectum*, **18**, 646–9.

Miles, W.E. (1919). Observations upon internal piles. *Surg. Gynecol. Obstet.*, **29**, 497–506.

Miller, R., Bartolo, D.C.C., Cervero, F., and Mortensen, N.J.M.C.C. (1988). Anorectal sampling: a comparison of normal and incontinent patients. *Br. J. Surg.*, **75**, 44–7.

Milligan, E.T.C. and Morgan, C.N. (1934). Surgical anatomy of the anal canal with special reference to anorectal fistulae. *Lancet*, **ii**, (1), 150–6, 1213–17.

Milligan, E.T.C., Morgan, C., Naunton Jones, L.F., and Officer, R. (1937). Surgical anatomy of the anal canal and the operative treatment of haemorrhoids. *Lancet*, **ii**, (II), 19–24.

Nyam, D.C.N.K., Wilson, R.G., Stewart, K.S., Farouk, R., and Bartolo, D.C.C. (1995). Island advancement flaps in the management of anal fissures. *Br. J. Surg.*, **82**, 326–8.

Parkash, S., Lakshmiratan, V., and Gajendran, V. (1985). Fistula-in-ano: treatment by fistulectomy, primary closure and reconstitution. *Aust. N.Z.J. Surg.*, **55**, 23–7.

Parks, A.G. (1954). A note on the anatomy of the anal canal. *Proc. R. Soc. Med.*, **47**, 997–8.

Parks, A.G. (1961). The pathogenesis and treatment of fistula-in-ano. *BMJ*, **i**, 463–9.

Parks, A.G., Gordon, P.H., and Hardcastle, J.D. (1976). A classification of fistula-in-ano. *Br. J. Surg.*, **63**, 1–12.

Phillips, R.K.S. (1989). Management of fistula-in-ano. *Curr. Med. Lit. Gastroenterol.*, **8**, 71–5.

Pinho, M. and Keighley, M.R.B. (1990). Results of surgery for idiopathic faecal incontinence. *Ann. Med.*, **22**, 426–47.

Schmitt, S.L. and Wexner, S.D. (1994). Treatment of anorectal manifestations of AIDS: past and present. *Int. J. STD & AIDS*, **5**, 8–10.

Scott, A., Hawley, P.R., and Phillips, R.K.S. (1989). Results of external sphincter repair in Crohn's disease. *Br. J. Surg.*, **76**, 959–60.

Shukla, N.K., Narg, R., Nair, N.G., Radhakrishna, S., and Satyavati, G.V. (1991). Multicentric randomized controlled clinical trial of Kshaarasootra (Ayurvedic medicated thread) in the management of fistula-in-ano. *Indian J. Med. Res.*, **94**, 177–85.

Slutki, S., Abramsohn, R., and Bogokovsky, H. (1981). Carbon dioxide laser in the treatment of high anal fistula. *Am. J. Surg.*, **141**, 395–6.

Sweeney, J.L., Ritchie, J.K., and Nicholls, R.J. (1988). Anal fissure in Crohn's disease. *Br. J. Surg.*, **75**, 56–7.

Thompson, H. (1962). The orthodox conception of fistula-in-ano and its treatment. *Proc. R. Soc. Med.*, **55**, 754–6.

Thomson, W.H.F. (1975). The nature of haemorrhoids. *Br. J. Surg.*, **62**, 542–52.

CHAPTER 22

Venous and lymphatic disorders

S. Sarin

1 Introduction

1.1 Historical

Ulcerating wounds of the lower limbs must have been treated by innumerable men of medicine in the past, but the association between ulcers and varicose veins is attributed to Hippocrates of Cos (460–377 BC), who was also the first to recommend incision of the varices and compression, to squeeze out the 'humours'. The rise of the Roman Empire saw Aulus Cornelius Celsus (AD 30) deal with the treatment of ulcers by bandaging with linen, and Galen (AD 130–200) is said to have popularized avulsion techniques of varicose veins. However, Galen's erroneous views of anatomy and physiology, based on comparative anatomical dissections (he had little access to human post-mortem specimens) and the dogmatic views of the Church, marked an enduring stagnation in the development of surgery in Europe throughout the Middle Ages.

Henri de Mondeville (1320) described compression of the whole limb to 'drive back the evil humours infiltrated in the leg and ulcer'. This was the first challenge to the writings of Galen, and marked the resurgence of European medicine with a return to the humoral school. Marianus Sanctus of Barletta (1555) was the first to associate varicosities with child bearing, and Ambroise Paré (1510–90) advocated mid-thigh ligation of varices and theorized that 'heaping up' of suppressed menstruation during pregnancy was the cause of varicosities in women. The relaxation of the Church's ban on human dissection paved the way for the anatomists, with Leonardo da Vinci (AD 1452–1519) producing over 770 anatomical drawings, many of which illustrated the venous system. The celebrated anatomist Vesalius (AD 1514–64) described the venous system in great detail, and both Fabricius (AD 1537–1619) and Alberti (AD 1585) publicly demonstrated venous valves.

The concept of blood circulation, using simple, fundamental observations, is attributed to William Harvey (1578–1657) and stimulated a range of mechanical theories. Wiseman (1676) rediscovered the association of varicose veins and ulceration. He also coined the term 'varicose ulcer' and developed a laced compression stocking. Home (1756–1832) later noted the importance of collateral vessels as a cause of recurrence after varicose vein ligation. An important mechanism was discovered in 1824 by Briquet, who suggested in his thesis that the calf muscle acted as a pump, but he wrongly believed that it normally caused blood to flow from the deep to the superficial systems via the communicating veins. Brodie (1846) described his clinical test for reflux down the long saphenous vein, involving application of digital pressure over the sapheno-femoral junction.

Gay (1866) and Spender (1868), writing independently, suggested that ulceration was not a direct consequence of varicosities but was caused by some other condition of the venous system, of which varicosities were another complication. They postulated that this 'other' condition was obstruction of the deep veins. They noted that ulceration could occur in the absence of varicose veins, providing there had been previous post-thrombotic damage to the deep veins.

Treatment of venous disease in the pre-twentieth century era was usually directed at the superficial varicosities. The close connection of deep venous pathology with superficial venous disease was suspected but not proven. In the twentieth century there has been a rapid expansion in technology which has facilitated investigation of every aspect of venous physiology, resulting in a greater understanding of the aetiology, pathophysiology, and treatment of venous disease.

1.2 Anatomy

The venous system of the lower limb can be divided into two main systems: the **superficial veins**, which drain the skin and superficial fascia, and the **deep veins**, which drain muscle and bone. Connecting the deep and superficial systems are the **communicating veins**. In addition, there are the capacious sinusoidal veins within the gastrocnemius and soleus muscles, which act as reservoirs for blood within the muscle pump. Both superficial and deep veins possess valves, which have the vital function of directing the venous return towards the heart. All the calf veins except the sinusoidal veins are densely valved, but the populations of valves falls off in a proximal direction, with the popliteal vein usually having two, the femoral vein between one and two, and the iliac veins one or none.

The superficial venous system

This consists principally of the long and short saphenous veins, together with a complex network of smaller interconnecting veins. The long saphenous vein is formed by union of the veins of the medial aspect of the foot. It then passes anterior to the medial malleolus, coursing behind the knee and passing anteriorly in the thigh, eventually traversing the cribriform fascia to join the femoral vein at the sapheno-femoral junction. There are numerous tributaries which join the long saphenous vein in the calf and thigh, and the anatomical distribution of these is extremely variable. The short saphenous vein drains the lateral part of the foot, running upwards, along the posterior aspect of the calf, to join the popliteal vein in the popliteal fossa. The precise anatomical location of the sapheno-popliteal junction is also variable (usually lying between 10 cm above and 10 cm below the knee crease in the posterior midline), and there are several connections with the long saphenous system around the knee.

The deep venous system

The medial and lateral **plantar veins of the foot** unite to feed the posterior tibial veins. The large, valveless sinusoids of the gastrocnemius and soleal muscle connect with the axial tibial veins or directly with the popliteal vein. The tibial veins unite at a variable level to form the popliteal vein, which then ascends in Hunter's canal as the **superficial femoral vein**. In the upper part of the thigh, the superficial femoral vein is joined by the **profunda femoris vein** to form the **femoral vein** which becomes the **common femoral vein** after union with the long saphenous vein at the sapheno-femoral junction.

The communicating veins

The deep and superficial veins of the lower limb are separated by fascia and joined by communicating veins, also known as **perforators**. Two types of perforator are described: the direct ones, connecting the superficial to the deep veins, and the indirect, connecting the superficial to the deep system via the muscle sinusoids. The larger and more consistent perforators are named (e.g. Cockett's group of communicating veins along the lower medial aspect of the calf, Boyd's perforator at the upper medial aspect of the calf, and Dodd's perforators along the medial aspect of the thigh; see Fig. 22.1).

1.3 Physiology

When a patient stands up, the pressure within the dorsal foot veins is equal to that exerted by the hydrostatic pressure of the column of blood between the heart and the foot. As a result of the arrangement of the valves within the deep veins, the calf muscle, on contraction, ejects blood proximally towards the heart. The arrangement of valves within the communicating veins appears to be designed to prevent blood from entering the superficial venous system. On relaxing the calf muscles, blood fills the sinusoids of the gastrocnemius and soleus from both the foot veins and the superficial venous system, thereby reducing the pressure within the superficial veins. In normal people, this pressure during ambulation is usually less than 50 per cent of the resting pressure on standing. Failure of the calf pump mechanism results in persistent **venous hypertension**, which is an important cause of the chronic skin changes associated with both varicose veins and the post-thrombotic limb.

1.4 Epidemiology of venous disease

Relatively little information has been available until recently detailing the extent of venous disease in the West. The Tecumseh Community Health Study, a longitudinal study of a population in Michigan USA, extrapolated their data to the whole USA

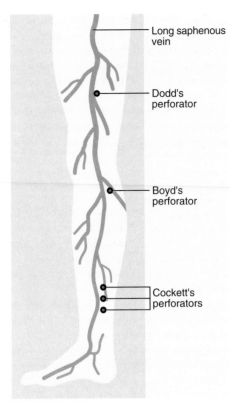

Figure 22.1 Perforating veins of the lower limb.

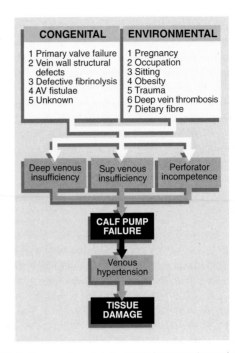

Figure 22.2 Factors predisposing to venous hypertension and deep venous thrombosis.

using 1970 census figures. They estimated that 24 million people have significant varicose veins (prevalence 12.9 per cent), while 6 to 7 million people have stasis changes in the skin of the legs (prevalence 3 per cent), and that between 400 000 and 500 000 have or have had a varicose ulcer (prevalence 0.1 per cent). Differences between populations in the prevalence of varicose veins have also become apparent. The range varies from 1 per cent (women in lowland New Guinea) to 53 per cent (women in South Wales) and appears to be higher in industrialized societies. Varicose veins are usually bilateral and are more common in the left lower limb.

In summary, these studies suggest that approximately 10 per cent of the Western population have significant varicose veins and 0.1 per cent have venous ulceration. Many surgeons estimate that over half of their operating time is devoted to treating venous problems, and most surgical trainees 'cut their teeth' on varicose veins.

1.5 Aetiology of venous disease

Ambulatory venous hypertension is undisputed as the consistent abnormality associated with venous disease. It is also generally agreed that venous hypertension is the initiating factor in the pathophysiology of the skin changes associated with venous ulceration.

Development of venous hypertension

The two main causes of varicose veins are hereditary factors and the effects of pregnancy.

Hereditary factors

Hereditary factors are likely to be important in the pathogenesis of venous hypertension. Males with venous abnormalities frequently have a family history on their male side, but varicose veins are so common in females (a positive family history can be obtained in up to 80 per cent of patients with primary varicose veins), it is difficult to differentiate the effect of environmental influences. Potential hereditary defects include: primary valvular defects, structural changes in the vein walls, arteriovenous fistulas, and defective coagulation predisposing to deep vein thrombosis (Fig. 22.2).

Primary valvular defects

Primary proximal valvular deficiency has been suggested as the cause of varicosities in the superficial veins. Some cadaveric studies have shown that there is often an absent common femoral valve in normal limbs but a more recent study failed to show a relationship between the absence of this valve and long saphenous vein varicosities. Another study showed that the number of valves in a varicose long saphenous vein were less than the number found in a normal long saphenous vein, but this was thought to be the result of venous dilatation rather than the cause. An American study compared the rate of incompetence of the iliofemoral valve in children of patients with varicose veins with normal adults; they found a higher rate of incompetence in the children—a classic example of a poorly designed study! Primary deep vein valve prolapse has also been described, but the experience of the St Thomas's group is that most patients with deep venous insufficiency have had previous deep vein thrombosis and that primary valve disease is relatively infrequent.

Structural changes in vessel wall

The development of varicose veins can be explained by postulating that initial dilatation of the vein wall results in valvular incompetence. The collagen content in the wall of varicose veins has been found to be lower when compared with normals and, more importantly, when compared with normal veins of patients with varicose veins of the contralateral limb. Certain clinical observations, for example that *in situ* vein bypass grafts rarely become varicose and even unsupported coronary bypass grafts (usually harvested from the long saphenous vein) never become varicose, support the concept that varicose veins may be associated with a primary defect in the veins which become varicose. The St Mary's group, using strain-gauge plethysmography and dorsal foot-vein pressure measurements, found some support for this concept by showing a reduced elasticity in the limbs of patients with varicose veins and 'high-risk' patients when compared with patients with normal veins.

Acquired factors

Pregnancy

Varicose veins frequently develop for the first time during pregnancy, particularly the second or third pregnancy. Although they frequently resolve to a greater or lesser extent a few months after delivery, many patients date the first appearance of their symptomatic veins to a pregnancy. Several factors are probably involved. The hormonal environment during pregnancy, predominantly high levels of progestogens, promotes relaxation of collagen. This is likely to affect the walls of susceptible veins to cause dilatation and valvular incompetence. Once overstretched, veins may not recover their competence and increased distal venous pressure may, as a result, lead to successive valve failure downstream and spreading varicosities. Other factors in pregnancy include increased blood volume, a hyperdynamic circulation, and pressure on pelvic veins by the enlarging uterus.

Arteriovenous shunting

In limbs with varicose veins, past thrombosis, or ulceration, the oxygen content of blood leaving the limb is higher than that found in the antecubital veins, raising the possibility of arteriovenous shunting in the lower limb. Further studies using radioactively labelled macroaggregates have, however, failed to demonstrate substantial shunting in patients with varicose veins.

Deep vein thrombosis

A patient who has suffered a thrombosis that extends into or above the popliteal vein has been shown to have a 40 per cent chance of developing a severe post-thrombotic syndrome within 6 years, and 75 per cent of these patients will become symptomatic. There is some evidence that early and effective treatment of the thrombosis may be beneficial in reducing the development of the condition.

Other factors associated with an raised prevalence of varicose veins include:

- being female;
- lack of dietary fibre;
- obesity;
- occupations involving long periods of standing.

Development of microcirculatory changes

The changes in the microcirculation with chronic venous insufficiency are well documented. There is enlargement of the local dermal capillary bed, but a *decreased* number of capillaries, which themselves are dilated and tortuous. There is also destruction of part of the microlymphatics, with increased permeability and backflow. The result of these changes is described by the pathological term 'lipodermatosclerosis': induration, inflammation, oedema, and erythema, classically on the skin of the gaiter area of the affected limb.

The cause of these changes has been much debated. The **venous stasis hypothesis**, described by Homans in the earlier part of this century, has been disproved. In fact, the blood flow through the microcirculation in lipodermatosclerotic skin is faster than in normal skin and the term 'stasis ulcer' should be abandoned. The St Thomas's group subsequently proposed the **fibrin cuff hypothesis**. This postulates a diffusion block to oxygen caused by polymerization of leaking fibrinogen to form fibrin 'cuffs' around the capillaries. There are theoretical arguments against such a postulate and later experimental work has demonstrated no diffusion block. While the presence of pericapillary fibrin cuffs in areas of lipodermatosclerosis is undisputed, it is likely that they are a manifestation of the damage inflicted upon the microcirculation rather than the cause. More recently, the Middlesex Hospital group have suggested that there is white blood cell trapping in the capillaries of limbs with persistent venous hypertension. The subsequent white blood cell and endothelial cell interaction results in activation of the granulocytes. The damage produced sets up a chronic inflammatory response which eventually results in the typical skin changes associated with venous hypertension.

2 Specialist investigations and their interpretation

2.1 Doppler ultrasound

The basis of Doppler flow detection is the principle that the frequency of a wave reflected from a moving object is changed in proportion to the velocity of the reflecting object. Hand-held ultrasound Doppler probes have been in widespread use for many years. Venous reflux testing may be performed with the patient standing using a modification of the Trendelenburg test. The femoral vein and saphenofemoral junction can be examined by insonating with the Doppler probe and locating the femoral vein lying medial to the femoral artery. Calf compression is applied by hand to produce forward flow, which may be detected in the groin. On relaxation of calf compression, a search is made for venous reflux. This is easily seen as an upward deflection of the trace when using a bi-directional Doppler system in connection with a chart recorder, or its characteristic sound can be sought without such complexity. The popliteal fossa can be examined similarly, searching for popliteal or short saphenous vein reflux. Narrow cuffs or tourniquets can be used to compress the superficial veins and assist in the differentiation of superficial from deep venous reflux. This method has the inherent difficulty that it is qualitative, and more importantly, it is difficult to determine which vein is being examined, particularly in the popliteal fossa. Thus the investigation is useful in experienced hands but is easily misinterpreted by less experienced users.

2.2 Duplex Doppler scanning

The combination of Doppler ultrasound with real-time B-mode (brightness mode) imaging has provided a means of localizing the Doppler sampled volume on the ultrasound image. Using a pulsed Doppler mode means that a precisely defined volume of blood can be studied to determine its velocity and direction of flow. The presence of flow in major vessels can be established and the location of venous reflux determined beyond doubt. The lower-limb veins may be identified in turn, either with the patient standing or lying with the feet dependent. Forward flow can be produced in the calf by manual calf compression and the presence of forward flow and reflux assessed in each vein of the lower limb in turn. Virtually all veins below the inguinal ligament can be imaged by this technique and the competence of individual valves determined. It has been shown to have a good correlation with venography in the assessment of venous reflux and thrombosis. This technique is even more demanding of training and experience than simple Doppler flow detection. It is also time consuming but reliable when properly performed.

Colour flow mapping of the Doppler signal provides additional sophistication. The Doppler shift of each pixel of the ultrasound image is electronically converted to a colour, according to direction of flow and different saturation depending on the velocity of flow. In effect, real-time images with colours representing flow of blood (e.g. blue for blood flowing away from the probe and red for blood flowing towards the probe) are obtained. This considerably simplifies the assessment of venous reflux. Other advantages of duplex scanning are that it is entirely non-invasive and can be repeated easily with minimum discomfort to the subject. The main disadvantage of duplex scanning in the assessment of venous disorders is that it is operator dependent. If the test is undertaken by a technician inexperienced in the surgical management of venous disease, interpretation of the results can be difficult. Secondly, the accuracy of the test is less for calf veins (either for reflux or thrombosis). Keeping these two points in mind, this test has proved extremely useful in preoperative assessment of primary varicose veins, recurrent varicose veins, preoperative marking of the sapheno-popliteal junction, venous assessment of lower-limb ulcers and diagnosis of acute deep-vein thrombosis.

2.3 Venography (phlebography)

Venography was the first means of investigating the venous system and is still in wide use today. Use of this modality enables direct assessment of the superficial and deep venous systems and an evaluation of venous valvular function. In experienced hands, images of lower-limb veins can be obtained, and the technique is still regarded by many as a reference standard in the investigation of deep vein thrombosis. Modifications that permit the assessment of valve competence in the deep and superficial systems have been described. These include retrograde (ascending) and descending venography. In clinical practice, ascending venography is used to detect evidence of venous thrombosis and descending venography evidence of venous reflux. However, it does require expensive equipment (the use of real-time screening is highly desirable), it is uncomfortable for patients and exposes them to ionizing radiation. Repeated radiological studies to assess the progression of venous disease are clearly undesirable. With the advent of duplex scanning the author has found venography of little value in general clinical practice, although it is still useful in assessing patients prior to deep venous reconstructive procedures.

2.4 Plethysmography

Sophisticated plethysmographic tests designed to assess venous function are usually used in a research setting but can be used to assess the outcome of surgical procedures. Some vascular laboratories provide plethysmographic data routinely. Of the plethysmographic tests, photoplethysmography (PPG) is widely available and easily performed. PPG uses variation in light absorption in the skin to estimate changes in venous volume indirectly. The principal chromophore in the skin is haemoglobin and so light absorption is largely dependent on the volume of blood in the superficial dermal venous plexuses. When these are full, the haemoglobin in the red blood cells absorbs light, and as venous pressure falls the plexuses become emptier and light absorption decreases. The method uses an infrared (805 nm) light-emitting diode within a probe fixed to the skin by double-sided adhesive tape, and a photoelectric cell arranged within the probe so that it measures light reflected from the skin. Following a standard procedure to empty the veins (e.g. repeated dorsiflexion of the ankle in a sitting patient), a graph reflecting the changes in light backscatter, is obtained. This represents the emptying of the limb during muscle contraction followed by gradual refilling during relaxation. It reflects both the action of the muscle pump in emptying the dermal venous plexus, and the presence of reflux within the superficial or deep venous systems allowing rapid venous refilling. From the trace, various indices can be measured, including the venous emptying and refilling times. The total refilling time, 95 per cent refilling time (as the upward slope may level off slightly or overshoot before returning to the baseline), 50 per cent refilling time (t_{Ω}), or the gradient of the slope have been suggested as standard measurements (Fig. 22.3). A 95 per cent refilling time is used by most laboratories and a value of less than 20 seconds has been regarded as evidence of venous reflux, although individual laboratories need to calculate their own values. The test is of little value in the primary diagnosis of venous disease. The author reserves it to assess the contribution of coexistent superficial venous disease to overall venous function in the presence of deep venous insufficiency.

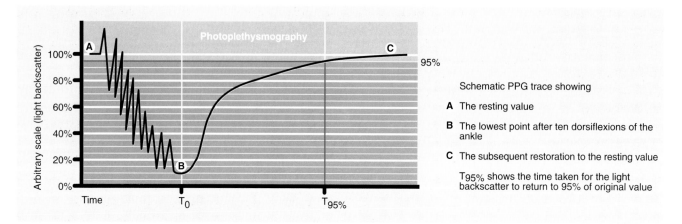

Figure 22.3 Photoplethysmography in the diagnosis of venous reflux.

3 Principles of therapeutic techniques

The cause of symptoms in patients with venous disease of the lower limbs is failure of the calf pump mechanism with persistent venous hypertension and subsequent microcirculatory changes. However, in many cases, the patient presents before venous symptoms have developed, with the main complaint of unsightly varicose veins. Treatment is directed towards improving venous function, limiting damage to the microcirculation and the cosmetic appearance of the limb.

3.1 Injection sclerotherapy

With the limb dependent, each of the offending veins is cannulated with a fine needle attached to a syringe. After raising the leg and emptying each vein in turn of blood, it is injected with 0.5 ml of **sodium tetradecyl sulphate** (STD Pharmaceutical) and then compressed with a dental roll or foam pad. The limb is then bandaged for between 2 and 6 weeks. Up to 20 varicosities can be dealt with at one session and the sessions can be repeated. This modification of an earlier technique was popularized by Professor Fegan of Dublin in the 1960s and 1970s and he claimed very good results if the injections were carried out properly. However, there are disadvantages: first, the technique is difficult to perform, and if incorrectly performed results in superficial thrombophlebitis, pigmentation of the skin, and sometimes necrosis of the overlying skin, any of which may result in litigation. Secondly, although injection sclerotherapy is effective in obliterating varicosities, it does nothing to deal with the source of venous hypertension. Studies looking at the results of sclerotherapy alone have found a recurrence rate approaching 70 per cent after 6 years. For these reasons the author tends to reserve this technique for dealing with small cosmetic veins below the knee, or residual varicosities after the source of reflux has been dealt with surgically.

3.2 Surgery

The main principle of surgery is the correction or obliteration of the source of venous hypertension. Reflux of blood down a vein is usually due to an incompetent valve, and particular attention is given to those sites where the superficial veins join the deep venous system.

Sapheno-femoral junction ligation

Ligation of the sapheno-femoral junction is usually performed under general anaesthesia, with the patient supine, the leg abducted and laterally rotated, and the knee slightly flexed. This operation is commonly referred to as the Trendelenburg procedure, although the operation actually described by Trendelenburg was excision of a portion of the long saphenous vein in the upper part of the thigh. An incision in the groin crease, just medial to the femoral artery and 2.5 cm below and slightly lateral to the pubic tubercle, gives good exposure of the sapheno-femoral junction and a good cosmetic result. The superficial fascia is divided in the line of the incision, the long saphenous vein is dissected out, and the sapheno-femoral junction identified and cleared. All tributaries joining either the femoral vein or long saphenous vein are ligated and divided using an absorbable ligature. Finally, the long saphenous vein is ligated flush with the femoral vein and divided distally. It is essential to ensure that the common femoral vein is adequately visualized and protected. In thin patients, even experienced surgeons have mistakenly ligated and divided the common femoral vein believing it to be the long saphenous. Such indefensible errors are less likely to occur if the anatomy is clearly defined. Many surgeons nowadays prefer to close the saphenous opening (foramen ovale) to completely dissociate the deep from the superficial system and reduce the possibility of neovascularization reconnecting the systems. Closure of the wound is achieved using interrupted absorbable sutures to the superficial fascia and a subcuticular suture to skin. Recurrent sapheno-femoral reflux is dealt with in a slightly different manner. The old scar is re-opened and the common femoral artery is identified first. Then the common femoral vein distal to the site of previous ligation is identified. The dissection continues (in 'fresh' tissue), working up towards the site of previous ligation where any recurrent connections can then be ligated and divided with confidence.

Stripping the long saphenous vein

Considerable controversy exists over the need to strip the long saphenous vein. Proponents argue that stripping produces a better immediate result and also a lower long-term recurrence rate. However, this must be weighed against the greater morbidity associated with stripping the vein, due to bleeding, pain, and wound infection, any of which may result in a prolonged hospital stay. More importantly, there is an increased incidence of injury to the saphenous nerve which runs adjacent to the vein in the distal calf. Finally, stripping the long saphenous vein results in the loss of a possible conduit suitable for later arterial or venous reconstruction. However, most of these objections do not apply if the long saphenous vein is stripped only from the groin to the upper calf. Certainly, saphenous nerve injury does not occur with this technique and the main benefit of stripping the long saphenous vein (i.e. a lower recurrence rate) is secured, as demonstrated in a recent randomized study.

Two techniques are in common use: extraluminal stripping and inversion stripping. In either case, the stripper is introduced via the cut end or an incision in the side of the long saphenous vein in the groin. The stripper is then passed distally, rotating it to ensure passage down the vein. The end of the stripper is identified at a convenient point below the knee and it is delivered through a small (< 1 cm) longitudinal incision over its end and the vein is ligated over the shaft of the stripper in the groin. If extraluminal stripping is to be undertaken, then a medium head is attached to the groin end of the stripper and the stripper pulled through subcutaneously. If inversion stripping is to be undertaken, one end of a ligature is tied to the proximal shaft of the stripper which is then pulled a few centimetres into the vein. The other end is then tied firmly to the vein and the stripper pulled through distally. The claimed advantage of inversion stripping is less bleeding (because the vein is stripped within its fascia) although this has not yet been adequately demonstrated.

Sapheno-popliteal junction ligation

As referred to earlier, the anatomical location of the sapheno-popliteal junction is extremely variable, with less than half located at the 'classical' site—2 cm above and lateral to the popliteal skin crease. For this reason, preoperative localization is essential and, in the author's practice, is achieved by duplex scanning. Under general anaesthesia, with a cuffed endotracheal tube, the patient is placed prone and a transverse incision is made over the site of the previously marked sapheno-popliteal junction. The popliteal fascia is exposed and incised vertically, taking care to avoid the popliteal nerve. The fat is retracted and the short saphenous followed to its junction with the popliteal

vein, where it is ligated and divided. The popliteal fascia must be closed securely with an absorbable suture to avoid painful herniation of popliteal fossa contents, and the incision is then sutured with a subcuticular suture.

Ligation of calf perforators

Although a popular undertaking in the recent past, these operations have finally fallen out of favour. The theoretical basis for undertaking such procedures is flawed and, despite numerous studies, no one has been able convincingly to prove their benefits. The traditional operations (e.g. Linton's subfascial ligation or Cockett's extrafascial ligation of medial calf-perforating veins) required long incisions and extensive disruption of tissues beneath the deep fascia. Not surprisingly, these operations were associated with many complications, particularly difficulties with wound healing, and should now rarely be used. A modern alternative is subfascial endoscopic perforator surgery (SEPS). If a medial calf perforator needs to be ligated, it should be marked preoperatively using duplex scanning or venography, and the perforator should be ligated beneath the deep fascia via a 1–2 cm incision. The fascial defect should then be closed with an absorbable suture material.

Multiple avulsions

Using a number 11 or 15 blade, a 2–3 mm incision is made over the previously marked varicosity and a fine-toothed clip or a vein hook is used to draw the underlying vessel wall out of the incision. The vein wall is then clamped with a heavier artery forceps and the vessel gently teased out. The operator should avoid excessive 'digging around' in the subcutaneous tissues as this will result in a poor scar and increases the risk of injuring adjacent cutaneous nerves. Stab incisions placed 3–4 cm apart will ensure that all the varicosities are removed. The incisions do not require suturing, although some surgeons prefer to appose the edges with Steri-strips® or staples.

Surgery to the deep veins

Surgical treatment of deep venous disease has been reported in only a few centres and the results are difficult to interpret for several reasons: incomplete follow-up, imperfect end points, and the performance of additional procedures at the same time as surgery to the deep veins (e.g. treatment of superficial venous disease). However, there is good evidence that correction of reflux in the venous systems of the lower limb in patients with venous insufficiency will lead to healing of venous ulcers and improvement in calf muscle pump function and this provides an incentive for continued investigation of these techniques. **Primary valve failure** within the deep venous system is the valvular abnormality most amenable to surgery, and is caused either by cusp prolapse, as described by Kistner, or dilatation of the valve ring. Techniques of valvuloplasty are employed: direct valvuloplasty involves 'reefing' of the incompetent valve cusps by fine sutures to restore competence. Indirect valvuloplasty has been performed by wrapping a Dacron cuff around the valve to reduce sinus dilatation and so restore competence. More commonly, deep valvular reflux is secondary to **post-thrombotic damage** which responds poorly to surgical intervention. In carefully selected cases, valve replacement techniques have been employed. This involves transplantation of superficial brachial vein valves to the site of deep venous reflux. Despite initial optimistic reports, objective, direct examination of valve function has shown a relatively low rate of competence and a high rate of thrombosis.

In summary, although interest in deep venous reconstruction has increased, surgical techniques to correct deep venous reflux remain experimental and without application for most patients.

The small group of patients who present with chronic venous insufficiency and symptoms of venous claudication secondary to isolated iliac vein or superficial femoral vein thrombosis are amenable to surgical treatment employing various bypass procedures. An essential prerequisite is a demonstration of raised deep vein pressures on exercising the limb. Techniques include femoro-femoral bypass using the contralateral long saphenous vein as the conduit (**Palma operation**) for occlusion of the iliac vein. This has been shown to have a 5-year patency of 75 per cent with satisfactory resolution of 'obstructive' symptoms. However, even in specialized centres, the experience with this type of procedure is small, emphasizing the small number of patients amenable to surgical treatment of deep venous disease.

3.3 Compression therapy

External compression therapy has been used since the times of Hippocrates in the treatment of venous disease. The main developments in this form of therapy have been in the materials used to achieve compression of the limb. The modern graduated compression stockings have resulted from evolution of elastic fibre and then of synthetic twisted fibre with 'memory'. Standards were established in the UK when the British Standard BS 6612:1985 was researched and published by the Textile and Clothing Standards Committee. This Standard grades compression into three classes, according to the maximum compression at the ankle. All compression classes fall to a similar level at the thigh. The classes are: class I, light (14–17 mmHg); class II, medium (18–24 mm Hg); and class III, strong (25–35 mmHg). The standard specifies the stiffness and durability of garments and requires them to be labelled by size, compression value, washing instructions, manufacturer, and BS number. Stockings must be fitted individually to achieve maximum benefit, ideally by a skilled surgical fitter. A wide range of off-the-shelf stockings is available and it is rare for custom-made stockings to be required.

The mechanism of action of compression therapy remains elusive but several clues exist. Reduction of oedema remains an important hypothesis and stockings may also alter microvascular dynamics favourably. There appears to be a beneficial action on the haemodynamics of the venous system, with suggestions including diversion of blood from the superficial to the deep systems, prevention of high-amplitude swings in pressure in the superficial veins during systole, 'support' of the superficial veins, and restoration of competence and enhancement of emptying of deep veins. By allowing the dilated vein walls to be more closely approximated, it is postulated that the valve cusps may regain function, allowing the muscle pump to work more efficiently.

Graduated or uniform compression?

Theoretical considerations suggest that graduated external compression (higher at the ankle) is more appropriate than uniform compression. Compression of the limb at any point should overcome the increase in venous pressure at that point. Therefore, the higher venous pressure at the ankle requires a greater external compression pressure than the lower venous pressure at the knee. Some studies have assessed venous function and found a greater improvement with the use of graduated rather than uniform compression. The amount of compression achievable is dictated by arterial pressure and inflow; thus a maximum external pressure at the ankle of 30–40 mmHg would appear to be satisfactory providing there is no evidence of arterial disease.

Stockings or bandages?

Graduated compression of the limb can be achieved by employing either commercially available elastic stockings or by application of bandages. The advantages of bandages are that they are cheap and relatively disposable. However, they require a considerable degree of skill to apply correctly and invariably lose compression soon after application, usually because of slipping and sometimes because of intrinsic factors in the material. Furthermore, simple bandages need to be reapplied several times a day to prevent ridges forming in oedematous limbs. Stockings, on the other hand, provide a standard degree of compression (though this may not be the same as that claimed by the manufacturer) and retain elasticity over many months. However, they are expensive and difficult to put on, the latter because of the infirmity of the majority of patients who require them and, particularly, in the presence of ulcers.

Our own preference is to use bandages in the presence of ulcers. The Charing Cross technique of four-layer bandaging is widely employed but requires training and skill in application. The use of several layers spreads the compression and absorbs exudate so that bandages need renewal once or twice a week (or more regularly if there is a large amount of exudate) until the ulcer heals. Once the ulcer has healed, or in post-thrombotic limbs without ulcers, we use commercially available class III graduated compression stockings (e.g. Venosan 2000®, Credenhill; or Sigvaris 503®, Ganzoni) which apply a ankle pressure of 30 mmHg and are suitable in most situations. The stockings are available in a variety of sizes designed to fit most leg shapes. It is important to realize that the stocking may need to be refitted once the initial oedema has reduced. The patient may also require help in putting on the stocking, and every encouragement should be given to ensure patient compliance.

Pneumatic compression

These techniques were originally developed for prevention of postoperative deep vein thrombosis, but it was noted that they increased venous return and also enhanced fibrinolytic activity in the blood. A controlled study evaluating a sequential compression device (Kendall Company, Mansfield, Mass., USA) reported an increased rate of ulcer healing and more healed ulcers after 13 weeks in the treatment group when used for two 3-hour sessions a day in the patients' home. The increased healing rate was achieved despite using graduated compression stockings in both groups. However, this machine is expensive and most institutions could not overcome the logistics of providing similar devices for home use.

Indications for compression therapy

Compression therapy is mainly used for limbs with deep venous disease or with a combination of deep and superficial venous disease which are unsuitable for surgery. Simple varicose veins can also be controlled effectively by stockings or tights, with compression values as low as 6 mmHg. Hosiery providing 5–10 mmHg compression and conforming to British Standards can be purchased (but not prescribed on NHS prescriptions). Deep venous thrombosis prevention in hospital patients requires medium compression stockings around 18 mmHg. In post-thrombotic syndrome, strong compression is required. The last should only be used if the doctor can be satisfied that the patient does not also have arterial insufficiency. Although stockings bring about substantial improvement in calf muscle pump function, symptoms, and oedema, it is not clearly established whether compression therapy can prevent complications such as lipodermatosclerosis or ulceration. However, circumstantial evidence is strong, as graduated compression has been shown to reduce the visible area of venous skin changes. Once an ulcer has developed, effective compression greatly enhances the healing of venous ulcers, ensuring that the patient can remain mobile while being treated on an outpatient basis. In recent years, prolonged periods of bed rest with elevation were employed for healing venous ulcers, but hospital admission is now reserved for treating complications such as cellulitis or for skin grafting of large ulcers. We reserve sequential pneumatic compression for those ulcers that show no improvement despite conventional compression therapy.

Once the ulcer has healed, the patient is advised to wear graduated compression stockings during the day as it is our experience that the ulcer commonly recurs once stockings have been discarded.

3.4 Drugs

Although the mainstay of treatment of venous disease remains surgery and compression therapy, a greater understanding of the microcirculatory pathophysiology has enabled rational pharmacotherapeutic approaches to be investigated. Several different groups of drugs have been tested but few have definite indications.

Diuretics

Oedema is a prominent feature in limbs with chronic venous insufficiency. The oedema is due to an increased capillary permeability and is protein rich, making it unsuitable for treatment with diuretics. Treatment of this type of oedema is more appropriately undertaken using leg elevation and compression therapy.

Antibiotics

The use of systemic antibiotics in the treatment of chronic venous disease or its complications cannot be justified. In particular, patients with superficial thrombophlebitis should not be prescribed antibiotics because the superficial areas of erythema and tenderness are invariably due to a sterile inflammation rather than infection. The only exception to this simple rule is the presence of cellulitis or systemic signs of infection.

Zinc

In 1970 a study suggested that serum zinc levels were lower than normal in patients with venous ulceration and that treatment with oral zinc supplementation promoted healing. Three subsequent double-blind, randomized studies could not reproduce the earlier claims and one must conclude that zinc supplementation is of no benefit in healing venous ulcers.

Hydroxy-rutosides

These drugs are flavanoid compounds derived from plant glycosides. There has been a revival of interest in these drugs with the demonstration that they can both reduce the capillary filtration rate in patients with chronic venous insufficiency and produce a corresponding reduction in clinical oedema. A number of studies have suggested that many of the symptoms of chronic venous insufficiency are also ameliorated by these drugs, although there is no evidence of a beneficial effect on the healing of venous ulcers. The current indication for this class of drug may be patients with chronic venous insufficiency with severe aching or pain, where an initial course has been shown to relieve symptoms.

Stanozolol

The concept of a diffusion barrier caused by pericapillary fibrin cuffs in chronic venous disease led to attempts to reverse their effects by enhancing fibrinolysis. Only one drug, stanozolol, a profibrinolytic anabolic steroid, has been extensively evaluated. Preliminary studies undertaken by the St Thomas's group were encouraging. However, a further study looking at healing of venous ulcers in 75 patients found no difference between the healing in the stanozolol or placebo groups. On the basis of the evidence to date, one can only conclude that stanozolol is of no value in the treatment of chronic venous insufficiency.

Pentoxifylline

The hypothesis that white blood cell trapping may, in part, be responsible for the damage to the microcirculation has allowed new avenues of drug treatment to be explored. Pentoxifylline has a multitude of actions on white cells, including reduction of neutrophil–endothelium adhesion, increased white cell deformability, and reduction of the production of free radicals by these cells. Additionally, it also promotes fibrinolysis and reduces whole blood viscosity by increasing red cell deformability. A rigorous multicentre, double-blind, placebo-controlled trial, set in Ireland, found that 23 of 38 ulcers healed in the treatment arm while 12 of 42 had healed in the placebo group. These differences occurred despite the use of conventional compression therapy in all. Certainly, this trial strongly suggests that venous ulcer healing can be enhanced by treatment with pentoxifylline. Whether continued treatment reduces the incidence of recurrence is uncertain.

Prostaglandin E₁

Reduction of white cell activation, inhibition of platelet aggregation and small vessel vasodilatation are some of the effects of prostaglandin E_1 (PGE_1) on the microcirculation. One randomized study investigated the effect of a daily 3-hour infusion for a period of 6 weeks. Although the number of ulcers healed was greater in the treatment group, this form of intensive, expensive treatment is unlikely to be widely accepted.

Local dressings

Many local treatments are available and are widely used in the treatment of skin complications of chronic venous disease. The huge variety of dressings and débriding agents available testifies to the fact that none is likely to be predominantly effective in promoting the healing of ulcers. The area affected by lipodermatosclerosis and eczema can be reduced by judicious local application of steroids; excessive or continuous use will cause thinning, and atrophy and should be avoided. When ulceration is present, the author's preference is to use daily changes of gauze soaked in normal saline while the ulcer is sloughy, to be replaced by calcium alginate when the base of the ulcer is well granulated.

4 Common emergency and elective conditions

4.1 Varicose veins

A vein is said to be varicose only when it is dilated and tortuous. For most patients, the main complaint is of unsightliness. Here, true varicose veins need to be distinguished from 'thread veins' or venous flares when planning treatment. Requests for consultation reveal other anxieties: a common (and often unstated) reason for referral is a worry that the patient's legs will deteriorate and 'end up like mother's'. Frequently this can be laid to rest by simple advice and reassurance. Tiredness and aching limbs are extremely common and should not be necessarily be attributed to varicose veins. In making a diagnosis, it is important that the history is appropriate and in proportion to the severity of varicose veins. Other causes of aching should be sought but may prove elusive. Aching caused by varicose veins is perceived throughout the leg, particularly towards the end of the day or after long periods of standing. Night cramps are often attributed to varicose veins and sometimes respond to treatment. Other presentations include ankle oedema, superficial thrombophlebitis, or acute haemorrhage from a varicosity. A 'bursting sensation' during exercise (venous claudication) is more consistent with venous outflow obstruction than primary varicose veins.

Having established the presence of varicosities, the initial purpose of examining the affected limb is to determine whether the superficial venous system alone is involved or whether there is coexistent deep venous disease. As detailed earlier, superficial venous incompetence is highly amenable to surgical treatment, whereas deep venous incompetence is not. Occasionally the varicosities are part of a venous malformation (e.g. Klippel–Trenaunay syndrome) or arteriovenous fistulas (congenital or acquired). The majority of patients presenting with simple varicose veins (i.e. without lipodermatosclerosis or ulceration) have only superficial venous disease. The examination is next directed at determining sources of reflux from deep to superficial venous systems. Within the outpatient setting, the standard tourniquet test is normally used, although the author has found a hand-held Doppler to be a useful adjunct and more accurate and reliable in many instances. In cases where the clinical examination does not provide a satisfactory answer, where there is suspected deep venous damage, and in all cases where the patient presents with recurrent varicose veins, a duplex Doppler scan examination of the lower limb veins should be performed.

Having diagnosed reflux in the superficial venous system and located the sources of reflux, the treatment options can be considered. Surgery should be recommended for cases where superficial venous insufficiency is associated with venous ulceration or eczema. Thereafter the decision to intervene can be influenced by a number of factors, including the patient's symptoms, the likely benefit of treatment, the patient's desire for treatment, and the resources available. Little is known about the natural history of primary varicose veins but it is safe to assume that progression varies with aetiology. Most 'hormonal' veins (i.e. following pregnancy) progress slowly—over a period of 10 years or more—whereas male-pattern inherited varicosities progress much more slowly. Where varicosities appear during teenage years, progression is likely to be more rapid.

The effect of long-term compression on progression is also unknown. Almost all retail outlets now stock aesthetically acceptable support hosiery and for some patients, with minor varicosities, this option, combined with reassurance, may be appropriate. Most patients, however, prefer to opt for surgical treatment and this can be undertaken as a day surgery procedure.

The precise operation performed depends on the clinical findings and the special investigations. Most operations are performed under general or spinal/epidural anaesthesia but publications have shown that many patients can be treated under femoral nerve block. In patients with primary varicose veins, the most common site of incompetence is the saphenofemoral junction (SFJ) with reflux into the long saphenous vein. In this case the operation consists of ligating the SFJ, multiple distal avulsions, and usually stripping of the long saphenous vein. The patient is consented appropriately and warned of the possible complications, in particular, that a permanent cure cannot be guaranteed and recurrence (i.e. new varicosities) are likely after about 10 years. In addition, the limb may have small patches of paraesthesia postoperatively but that these usually resolve with time. The site of reflux is marked, as are the individual varices, using a permanent marker. If the sapheno-popliteal junction is to be ligated, preoperative marking of the junction indicated by duplex scanning should be undertaken and the anaesthetist warned as a the patient will have to be turned prone in theatre. This entails an endotracheal tube whereas all other procedures can be undertaken with a laryngeal mask.

At the end of the procedure, the limb is bandaged using standard crepe or other light-elastic bandages, which can be removed 24 hours later and replaced with class II (or sometimes class III) compression stockings. Crepe bandages rapidly lose their elasticity and become lax soon after application and are unsuitable for maintaining compression. Some surgeons employ crepe bandages with a class II stocking over the top, both of which remain *in situ*. The duration of compression required is uncertain, although each surgeon has his or her own opinion. The purpose of postoperative compression is to reduce haematoma formation, bruising, and oedema and to maintain apposition of the walls of residual varicosities, allowing them to thrombose with minimal inflammation. To this end, this author's preference is to keep stockings on continuously for 2 weeks and during the day only for another 4 weeks. Others use 1 week and 1 week. On review in the outpatient department, any residual varicosities can be dealt with by injection sclerotherapy, although if the operation has been undertaken with care, this is rarely necessary.

4.2 Venous ulceration

Venous ulcers are classically described as shallow, irregularly shaped ulcers with a sloping edge and a granulating base, situated on the gaiter area of the lower limb. There is usually a history of varicose veins and/or previous 'thrombosis' of the lower limb, or a period of hospitalization for a fracture or back injury when a deep vein thrombosis (DVT) can be surmised. In a hospital setting, it is unusual to come across a previously untreated ulcer. None the less, all lower-limb ulcers should be assessed thoroughly. The main aim of examination and subsequent investigations are to establish whether the ulcer is truly of venous origin and, if so, to find the cause of the venous hypertension. Initial investigation should be directed at both the

arterial and venous systems. Doppler ankle pressures or ankle/brachial indices should be measured to exclude arterial disease and to confirm whether compression therapy can be applied safely. Duplex scanning is now the mainstay of assessing the venous system and may be used to give evidence of previous deep venous thrombosis with deep venous reflux. It is estimated that nowadays 90 per cent of newly referred lower-limb ulcers are venous in origin and of these 40–50 per cent are due to superficial venous insufficiency alone (Table 22.1). This is a considerable change from as recently as 20 years ago, when the majority were post-thrombotic. The decline has coincided with more rapid mobilization after parturition and after major surgery, together with prophylactic measures against DVT.

Surgical treatment of superficial venous disease will result in the ulcer healing and more importantly, remaining healed. In the presence of deep venous insufficiency, compression therapy (as described earlier) is used, provided it does not embarrass the arterial circulation. Additional simple measures, such as keeping the limb elevated when sitting, ankle exercises, and elevation of the foot of the bed are invaluable. The principle that all venous ulcers will heal with bed rest is still true and occasionally this can only be achieved with inpatient care. With large venous ulcers, healing can be speeded up by the use split-skin grafts, although if venous hypertension persists, the graft will inevitably fail. Although it is possible to persuade most venous ulcers to heal, the main problem is preventing recurrence. To this end, continued compression therapy has been shown to decrease recurrence rates, although compliance remains a problem.

Because of the significant healthcare costs associated with venous ulcers, recent studies have concentrated on accurately documenting the magnitude of this problem, both in terms of financial implications for the community and morbidity to the patient. A postal survey conducted in Scotland suggests that in the UK there are approximately 100 000 patients with active leg ulceration at any one time within a population of 400 000 with a history of leg ulceration. From these and other studies it seems that the majority of patients with ulceration are over 60 years of age, that most of the ulcers have been present for more than a year, almost half of the ulcers are 'recurrent', that few patients are ever seen by a specialist, and that most patients are not being treated with compression bandages (the only known effective treatment).

4.3 Axillary/subclavian vein thrombosis

Axillary vein thrombosis is most commonly encountered in men in their third or fourth decade, usually in the side with the dominant hand. There is usually a history of an episode of excessive use of the arm, with discomfort and swelling developing within 24 hours. The arm is cool to touch, slightly blue with oedematous hand and fingers. In extreme cases there may be venous gangrene of the fingers. Over the next few weeks, the collateral circulation develops with distended veins visible in the upper arm and shoulder girdle. The thrombosed axillary vein may be palpable as a thickened tender cord along the lateral aspect of the axilla. The main differential diagnosis is of acute

Table 22.1 Types of lower-limb ulcers

Ulcer type	Percentage occurrence
Venous	80–90%
Arterial	5–10%
Rheumatoid arteritic	<5%
Trauma	<5%
Neuropathic	<5%
Neoplastic	<1%
Others	<1%

ischaemia of the arm but this is usually excluded easily by palpation of the pulses. The aetiology of axillary vein thrombosis is multifactorial and most commonly termed 'idiopathic'—possibly because of a congenitally narrow space between first rib and clavicle. Recognized causes, including thoracic outlet obstruction (due to a cervical rib or band), external compression by malignant lymph nodes or a Pancoast tumour, should be excluded by thoracic outlet X-rays and a chest X-ray. Diagnosis is confirmed non-invasively by duplex ultrasonography or, if this modality is unavailable, ascending brachial venography.

Most patients present a few days after the onset of symptoms, where the only active management should be anticoagulation for 3 months after excluding haematological malignancies and thrombophilias. Pulmonary embolization occurs in less than 5 per cent of cases, although fatal cases are extremely rare. If the patient presents early (within 3 days) consideration should be given to chemical thrombolysis. In most patients the collateral circulation develops well enough for them to be symptom free within a few months.

4.4 Thrombo-embolic disease

A thrombosis is defined as a semisolid mass, formed of the constituents of blood occurring in a blood-containing vessel (Table 22.2). When a thrombosis occurs within a subfascial vein of the lower limb it is referred to as a deep vein thrombosis. Spontaneous coagulation is prevented by inhibition of the coagulation system by a complex physiological 'braking system' in which each component of the coagulation cascade is inhibited specifically. **Antithrombin III** is a protein that specifically neutralizes the activated serine proteases, the **protein C system** inactivates the cofactors, and the platelets are inhibited by **endothelial-derived prostacyclin** and the natural anticoagulant properties of the endothelial surface. Any fibrin formed within the vasculature can be removed by **plasmin**, a protein that degrades fibrinogen and fibrin molecules. Plasmin is generated on the surface of fibrin clots from the circulating precursor molecule plasminogen; thus fibrinolytic activity is relatively confined to the clot and there is no degradation of fibrinogen within the circulation. The most important physiological activator of plasminogen is **endothelial-derived tissue plasminogen activator** (tPA). Although the integrity of these systems is contributory to the prevention of peri- and postoperative venous thromboembolic disease, laboratory evaluation of these systems is not used to influence venous thromboembolic prophylactic regimens and is not routinely warranted.

The clinical diagnosis of DVT can be difficult because many patients have no symptoms or signs. It is far better to take all precautions to prevent DVT where possible. The most common

Table 22.2 Virchow's triad

Damage to the vessel wall
Changes in the constituents of the blood
Changes in the flow of blood

symptoms are those of pain and swelling of the calf. The more proximal and the more complete the DVT, the more severe the symptoms and signs. A mild pyrexia, tenderness in the calf, oedema of the ankle, warmth and distended superficial veins of the limb are sometimes observed. A white leg (**phlegmasia alba dolens**) may sometimes be seen and represents extreme venous outflow obstruction with oedema secondary to iliofemoral thrombosis. A blue leg (**phlegmasia caerulea dolens**) suggests venous gangrene. Homan's sign (pain or resistance on dorsiflexion of the foot) is inaccurate and should no longer be used. Signs of pulmonary embolism (i.e. pleuritic chest pain, haemoptysis, shortness of breath and, in extreme cases, collapse of patient) may, unfortunately, be the first signs of a DVT.

At the present time diagnosis of a DVT is made by ascending venography or by duplex scanning. Both tests have a sensitivity and specificity of over 90 per cent. Duplex scanning is slightly less accurate than venography at picking up deep calf vein thrombosis, whereas venography is less accurate than duplex scanning at detecting iliofemoral thrombus. The choice of test is usually determined by locally available facilities. Iodine-labelled fibrinogen and other isotope uptake tests are used only in the research setting and have little regular clinical application. If the patient presents with symptoms of pulmonary embolism, providing he or she is stable, a ventilation–perfusion scan can be performed to confirm or refute the diagnosis and is undertaken within 24 hours. Supportive evidence for a pulmonary embolism are the classical ECG changes (a S wave in lead 1, a Q wave in lead 3, and a inverted T wave in lead 3), a wedge-shaped area of consolidation on chest X-ray, and hypoxia combined with hypocarbia. In extreme cases, clinical signs may suggest severe pulmonary artery obstruction with continuing shock. Where thrombolysis or thrombectomy is contemplated, pulmonary angiography can be used to confirm the diagnosis.

As soon as a diagnosis of DVT is established, and sometimes if the clinical suspicion of a DVT or pulmonary embolism is high (prior to confirmatory tests being undertaken), the patient should be heparinized. An initial intravenous bolus of 5000 units of heparin should be followed by an intravenous infusion of 30 000 units over 24 hours. The rate of infusion should be adjusted to maintain the **activated partial thromboplastin time** at about twice the control level. Alternatively, 10 000 units subcutaneously twice daily will also achieve the desired anticoagulation, although it will be appreciated that accurate control may be more difficult to achieve. Low-molecular-weight heparins can give a smoother and perhaps more reliable anticoagulation by the subcutaneous route. The main purpose of anticoagulation is to prevent propagation of the thrombus. However, there is some evidence that heparin also causes a minor increase in fibrinolysis. Heparinization does not prevent embolism of the thrombus, although it is likely that the incidence of pulmonary embolism is reduced by anticoagulation.

The main clinical objectives in the treatment of DVT are to prevent fatal pulmonary embolism, reduce the severity of the presenting symptoms. and to reduce the severity of the post thrombotic syndrome.

Preventing pulmonary embolism can be undertaken by removing the thrombus by thrombolysis or thrombectomy. There is no evidence that thrombolysis prevents recurrent pulmonary emboli, it may in fact cause embolism by breaking up the thrombus. Surgical thrombectomy does not prevent recurrent embolism and should be undertaken only if it is thought to be the only way to save the limb. Placement of a inferior vena caval filter should be considered in patients at high risk of recurrent embolism. Direct operations to partially occlude the inferior vena cava (IVC) are no longer indicated. The first generation of vena caval filters (e.g. Mobin–Uddin umbrella, Greenfield filter) suffered particularly from 'migration' problems and have largely been replaced by newer designs (e.g. bird's nest filter). These are placed percutaneously under local anaesthesia via the right internal jugular or the femoral vein to lie within the IVC just distal to the renal veins. X-ray control is important. If the femoral route is used, the operator needs to ensure, preoperatively, that there is no thrombus present within the femoral or iliac veins.

Although they are effective at containing thrombi and having a low incidence of migration, the longer-term outcome of these filters is unknown. The principal indications for the use of an IVC filter are:

- the patient with recurrent pulmonary emboli despite adequate anticoagulation;

- the patient in whom anticoagulation is considered unsafe (e.g. recent haemorrhagic stroke);

- the patient who develops complications of anticoagulation therapy.

However, as the technique of insertion is now safe and the filters more reliable, indications for their use may include those patients with deep vein thromboses thought to be at high risk of embolization. Thrombi within the femoral and iliac veins, particularly those which are 'free floating', are thought to be responsible for most clinically significant episodes of pulmonary embolism.

Once the patient is stable, oral anticoagulation is commenced. The half-life of warfarin is 35 hours and it may take 3–4 days for full anticoagulation to take place. Heparin must be continued until the patient is adequately warfarinized. The effect of warfarin is assessed by measuring the prothrombin time and is expressed as the international normalized ratio (INR), the ratio between the patient's prothrombin time and the control time of a standardized animal-derived thromboplastin. An INR of between 2.5 and 3.5 is desirable. Oral anticoagulation is continued for 3–6 months, although the duration is probably more traditional than rational. Any benefit of the use of elastic stocking in reducing the incidence of deep venous insufficiency following a DVT is unproved, although the circumstantial evidence is highly indicative. It is our policy to provide the patient with compression stockings for at least 6 months as this reduces limb swelling and may reduce the incidence of the 'post-thrombotic syndrome'.

4.5 Prevention of deep vein thrombosis and pulmonary embolism

The incidence of clinical DVT in the population is estimated at 0.1 per cent per year, although it is likely that twice as many people have asymptomatic DVTs. Reviews of the literature in the early 1980s suggested that without prophylaxis as many as 30 per cent of patients after a general surgical procedure suffered a DVT and that the figure was even higher for patients undergoing pelvic and hip operations (Table 22.3). Without prophylaxis the incidence of fatal pulmonary embolism has been estimated as between 0.4 and 1.6 per cent. All patients within a hospital are at risk, including patients who have suffered myocardial infarction or a stroke. In these patients, the incidence of DVT is between 20 and 60 per cent.

Reduction of the incidence of DVT has been shown to reduce the number of pulmonary emboli but it is commonly argued that reducing the incidence of DVT has never been proved to reduce the number of fatal pulmonary embolic events. Although the large International Multicentre Trial published in 1975 (using subcutaneous heparin) did show a statistically significant reduction in fatal pulmonary embolism, the study is thought by many to be methodologically unsound, particularly as many (30–40 per cent) of patients who died did not undergo an autopsy. However, some evidence is present and the theoretical arguments for the use of DVT prophylaxis, sound. An overview of the subject, reviewing over 70 randomized trials in 16 000 patients, confirmed that the use of perioperative subcutaneous heparin reduced the incidence of DVT and also demonstrated a reduction in fatal and non-fatal pulmonary emboli.

Methods of prevention fall into two broad categories: mechanical and pharmacological. Graduated compression stockings, intermittent pneumatic compression, and electrical calf stimulation have all been shown to reduce the incidence of DVT. Of these, graduated compression stockings are the most used as they are cheap, easily obtained, and acceptable to the patient. Early mobilization plays an equally important role and may, in part, explain the apparent reduction in the incidence of pulmonary embolism over the past few decades. Of the pharmacological methods, subcutaneous heparin is probably the most popular; 5000 units of heparin are administered subcutaneously,

Table 22.3 Patients at particular risk for DVT

Fractures, particularly if multiple
Previous history of DVT
Major surgery, particularly in the pelvis
Coexisting malignancy
Immobility
Age (>40 years)
Obesity
Pregnancy
Obstructive jaundice
Pre-existing cardiac failure and other major cardiorespiratory co-morbidity

twice a day and this has been shown to reduce the incidence of both DVTs and pulmonary emboli. The main disadvantage is of a slightly increased risk of intraoperative bleeding. Low-molecular-weight heparins are now available and are marketed on the strength of a claimed lower incidence of intraoperative bleeding and a once-daily dosage regimen. Full anticoagulation is known to be the most effective way of reducing pulmonary embolism, although this benefit may be offset by an increased risk of postoperative bleeding. Intra- and postoperative infusion of Dextran 70 is thought to reduce the incidence of pulmonary emboli, particularly in hip operations, but has never been tested in a trial. It is also inconvenient as it requires an intravenous infusion to be maintained for the duration of treatment.

All methods of prophylaxis are more effective when started preoperatively and there is some evidence that a combination of methods produces a synergistic effect in the reduction of DVTs. Hospital audits have shown that if DVT prophylaxis is used on a selective basis for high-risk patients then the majority of patients do not receive any form of prophylaxis. It is therefore, this author's practice to provide every patient with graduated compression stockings and to administer low-dose subcutaneous heparin unless the patient is thought to be at a low risk of DVT. We reserve low-molecular-weight heparin for those patients where the operation is anticipated to be difficult (e.g. previous adhesions, previous local radiotherapy) and for those undergoing pelvic dissections. Some anaesthetists are reluctant to site epidural or spinal cannulae in the presence of low-dose heparin because of a perceived increased risk of bleeding and complications, although there is little evidence to support this reservation. If postoperative epidural analgesia is contemplated, then low-dose subcutaneous heparin should be administered on induction of anaesthetic, after the epidural has been sited rather than earlier.

Prophylactic measures should be continued at least until the patient is fully mobile, and in most cases until discharge from hospital. A recent study suggested that patients remain at risk of developing pulmonary embolism even after discharge from hospital, and in some surgical units the patient is advised to continue wearing the compression stockings for a few weeks after discharge.

4.6 Lymphoedema

The lymphatic system returns plasma proteins to the circulation. These proteins accumulate in the interstitial fluid and a normally functioning lymphatic system returns between 50 and 80 per cent of the total volume of intravascular protein to the bloodstream every day via the thoracic duct. Within a limb, the valveless terminal lymphatics drain into the valved lymphatic trunks, which in turn drain into the regional lymph nodes. Lymph flow depends on the intrinsic contractility of the lymph vessels, although extrinsic factors such as adjacent muscular activity are also important. Within a limb, the superficial and deep lymphatics (i.e. beneath the deep fascia) drain independently until their convergence at the regional lymph nodes. Accumulation of the protein-rich lymph in the interstitial

tissues is known as **lymphoedema** and is classified into primary and secondary lymphoedema.

Secondary lymphoedema

In the developed world, secondary lymphoedema is due mainly to either radiotherapy or surgical excision of the regional lymph nodes. Commonly, the most severe cases of lymphoedema occur in patients who have had a combination of the two treatments, particularly for breast cancer. Chronic infections with filaria (*Wuchereria bancrofti*) or chronic granulomatous disease (lymphogranuloma venereum, tuberculosis, sarcoidosis) produce a fibrotic reaction within lymph nodes and cause lymphatic obstruction.

Primary lymphoedema

Primary lymphoedema is associated with abnormalities of the lymphatics. Lymphatic hypoplasia is said to be the most common abnormality, although ectatic, hyperplastic, and mega-lymphatics have all been described. Lymphatic aplasia is relatively uncommon. The traditional classification of primary lymphoedema into congenital, praecox, and tarda is not helpful and does not aid management.

The clinical onset of primary lymphoedema is commonly delayed until the second or third decade. Although a small proportion of patients give a family history of swollen legs, true Milroy's disease (congenital familial lymphoedema) is relatively rare. The oedema is initially soft but with time becomes brawny because of subcutaneous fibrosis. Characteristically the oedema does not pit with finger pressure. The main presenting complaint is usually cosmetic deformity (i.e. swelling of the lower limb ascending from the ankle), although, in severe cases, recurrent skin infections occur with cellulitis, and impaired mobility may be significant problems.

Investigation of suspected lymphoedema

If the diagnosis of lymphoedema itself is in doubt (Table 22.4), a radionuclide-labelled albumin clearance study (injected subcutaneously) is indicated. Rapid clearance indicates venous oedema, whereas delayed clearance indicates lymphoedema. Lymphangiography is a well-established investigation in patients

Table 22.4 Causes of lower-limb swelling

Local
Deep venous thrombosis
Post-thrombotic syndrome
Disuse/dependent oedema (particularly in paralysed limbs or severe ischaemia)
Lymphoedema
Lipodystrophy
Klippel—Trenaunay syndrome

General
Cardiac failure
Renal failure
Hepatic failure
Hypoproteinaemia
Angio-oedema (acute)

suspected of having primary lymphoedema, although this investigation is only indicated if surgical intervention is contemplated. A subcutaneous lymphatic is identified and cannulated on the dorsum of the foot following a subcutaneous injection of patent blue dye. A slow injection of radiopaque contrast (Lipiodol®) outlines the lymphatic channels and eventually the pelvic lymphatics.

Treatment of lymphoedema

Treatment is directed at reducing the swelling of the limb, taking care of the skin, and urgently treating any infection. Most patients with lymphoedema respond to conservative measures, and surgery is only indicated if there is failure to control progressive lymphoedema or to improve functional disability of the limb. Simple measures of elevation of the foot of the bed and graduated compression hosiery are usually enough to control the oedema, although in unresponsive cases intermittent sequential pneumatic compression may be helpful (e.g. Flowtron pump). Daily care of the skin with the use of an emollient may prevent some of the skin changes, and any infection should be treated immediately.

Surgical procedures are only indicated when limb swelling becomes gross. It is directed at either debulking the limb or improving the lymphatic drainage. If the overlying skin is normal, then a Homan's procedure may be useful. In this procedure, skin flaps are raised and the underlying subcutaneous tissue removed down to the deep fascia and the skin flaps sutured, so that they lie directly on the deep fascia. If the skin is abnormal, then a Charles' procedure may be more appropriate. The skin and the subcutaneous tissues are removed, followed by split-skin grafting placed on the deep fascia. However, the grafted skin heals poorly and there is high postoperative morbidity. Various modifications of these two procedures are used and are sometimes successful at debulking the limb.

However, the cosmetic result is poor and these procedures should not be used where cosmesis is the main complaint.

Results of procedures aimed at improving lymph flow are not easy to assess but the overall impression is that they are not very successful. The buried dermal flap, as described by Thompson, has largely been abandoned, as have operations designed to join the superficial and deep lymphatic systems by excising strips of fascia. More promising are the so-called 'bridging' operations, where an omental or denuded small-bowel flap is placed on the cut surface of the groin lymph nodes. These procedures are only useful where the distal lymphatics are relatively normal but there is proximal (pelvic) lymphatic obstruction. The results of these procedures are difficult to assess and are only undertaken in surgical units with a particular interest in lymphatic disease.

Bibliography

Browse, N.L., Burnand, K.G., and Lea Thomas, M. (1988). *Diseases of the veins. Pathology, diagnosis and treatment.* Edward Arnold, London.

Coleridge Smith, P.D. (ed.) (1994). *Microangiopathy in venous disease.* R.G. Landes Company.

Collins, R., Scrimgeour, A., Yusuf, S., and Peto, R. (1988). Reduction in fatal pulmonary embolism and venous thrombosis by perioperative administration of subcutaneous heparin. Overview of results of randomized trials in general orthopaedic and urologic surgery. *NEJM*, **318**, 1162–73.

Tibbs, D.J. (1998). *Varicose veins and related disorders*, second edn. Butterworth Heinemann, Oxford.

Wells, P.S., Hurse, J., Anderson, D.R. *et al.* (1996). Accuracy of clinical assessment of deep venous thrombosis. *Lancet*, **348**, 983–7.

CHAPTER 23

Arterial surgery and lower-limb amputations

Clive R. Quick and Alun Davies

1 Introduction

Arterial surgery is largely about treating ischaemia and actual or potential rupture of vessels. The main underlying problems are degenerative arterial diseases, obliterative arterial disease (usually atherosclerotic), and aneurysmal disease. In addition, acute arterial trauma may demand the skills of a vascular surgeon.

Management of the majority of obliterative arterial disease depends on the severity of ischaemia in the lower limbs and the risk of stroke in extracranial arterial disease. Many patients can be managed conservatively, with interventional techniques reserved for those with the most severe symptoms or most at risk from complications. Similarly with aneurysms, surgery is reserved for those with warning symptoms suggesting imminent rupture, or those of a size or type known to be at risk of rupture.

Other than those with vascular trauma or one of the rare conditions affecting arteries in younger people, patients with arterial diseases are usually elderly and afflicted by widespread (and often occult) atherosclerosis and other disorders of the elderly. These are likely to reduce longevity and substantially increase the risks of surgery. Three-quarters of patients with obliterative arterial disease are, or have been, substantial cigarette smokers. This is a primary risk factor (i.e. predisposing to atherosclerosis) as well as a secondary risk factor (i.e. giving up reduces the rate of progress of atherosclerosis and reduces the risk of impairing long-term patency of any reconstruction). Thus, giving up the addiction of smoking is an important priority for the sufferer.

Co-morbid diseases include atherosclerosis of coronary arteries, carotid, and renal arteries, predisposing to myocardial infarction, stroke, and renal failure, respectively. It should be noted that patients with obliterative arterial disease are at much higher risk in this respect than patients with aneurysms.

Twenty five per cent of patients with obliterative peripheral arterial disease have diabetes, usually of maturity onset (type II) and many will suffer other degenerative diseases associated with ageing. These include chronic chest problems and benign prostatic enlargement. Thus, the general state of the patient and associated risk factors must be taken into account when planning treatment.

2 Clinical examination and investigations and their interpretation

2.1 Introduction

Investigating patients with arterial disease consists of three main components:

1. Can arterial disease explain the symptoms and signs and, if so, what is its severity? For example, in intermittent claudication, Doppler ankle pressure measurement before and after tread-mill exercise provides objective evidence of disease severity as well as degree of handicap. This phase helps characterize the disorder and will help to decide what is appropriate treatment

2. If the clinical findings and preliminary investigations suggest that an intervention is indicated, more information may be needed to decide whether an operation is technically feasible and to plan the type and level of the operation. For example, arteriography is often used as a 'road map' before recon-structive surgery to the lower limb.

3. If an operation is to proceed, clinical examination and inves-tigation of cardiac and renal function may be necessary (see Table 23.6). The extent of investigation depends on the inter-pretation of the symptoms and signs.

2.2 Clinical assessment of risk in patients undergoing arterial surgery

History: potential problem areas

1. Consider the role of any predisposing disorders: diabetes, smoking, high plasma fibrinogen, prothrombotic disorders.

2. Cardiac disease:

   - ischaemic heart disease, angina, previous myocardial infarction (particularly if within a year);

   - hypertension—generalized arteriopathy produces non-compliant arterial circulation, resulting in potentially hazardous swings of blood pressure during operation;

   - cardiac failure is particularly dangerous in major surgery;

   - arrhythmias, particularly atrial fibrillation and bifascicular block;

   - valvular heart disease, particularly mitral and aortic stenosis.

3. Pulmonary diseases:

   - respiratory failure;

   - chronic airways obstruction;

   - acute pneumonia.

4. Chronic renal failure from whatever cause is likely to be aggravated by aortic surgery.

5. Carotid artery disease and the risk of stroke. If history of TIAs or previous stroke, investigate in the same way as for an asymptomatic bruit, below.

6. Drugs: antihypertensives, particularly beta blockers (may impair peripheral circulation and may block physiological tachycardic response to blood loss), aspirin (increases surgical bleeding), and anticoagulants (ensure properly controlled in the low range of the prothrombin ratio).

7. Bleeding tendency.

In younger patients with aortic occlusion, particularly females, consider hypothyroidism as a cause, perhaps via its role in promoting homocysteinaemia.

2.3 General examination of the cardiovascular system

- Observe whether the patient can lie flat during examination and can walk up stairs.

- Inspect skin and mucous membranes for signs of polycy-thaemia, anaemia, or cyanosis.

- Examine for signs of cardiac failure—jugular venous pressure and lung bases.

- Auscultate for cardiac murmurs.

- Auscultate for arterial bruits in carotids, subclavians (in supraclavicular fossa), renals (posteriorly in loins), mesenterics (in epigastrium), and femoral arteries. If an asymptomatic carotid bruit is found, investigate with duplex Doppler to assess carotid artery stenosis. If stenosis is greater than 70 per cent, consider carotid endarterectomy as a first stage.

- Measure blood pressure in both arms (variation may indicate subclavian artery disease).

- Palpate the abdomen for aortic aneurysm.

Examination of lower limbs

- Inspect skin of legs and feet for ischaemic trophic changes and signs of arterial embolism.

- Inspect for local infection of lower limb, e.g. gangrene or an infected penetrating ulcer.

- Infection may cause systemic toxaemia as well as increasing the risk of infecting artificial graft material.

- Risk of clostridial gas gangrene after amputation.

- May be evidence of reduced resistance to infection in diabetes.

2.4 Ultrasound assessment

Simple ultrasound scanning for abdominal aortic aneurysm

Ultrasound scanning is a simple, quick, cheap, and reliable screening test for abdominal aortic aneurysm. There is a growing interest in population screening for asymptomatic

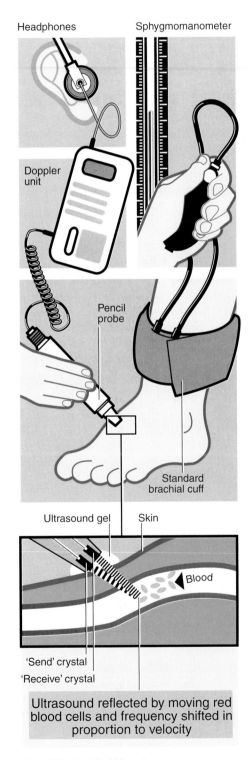

Figure 23.1 Use of the hand-held Doppler.

aneurysm which can be detected reliably in 98 per cent of those screened. Ultrasound can also demonstrate rapidly whether a patient presenting as an emergency with abdominal or back pain and collapse has an abdominal aortic aneurysm (although not whether it is leaking); the test should be performed as soon as the diagnostic possibility is considered.

Although ultrasound can show reliably the diameter of aortic, femoral, and popliteal aneurysms, it cannot show reliably the relationship of the aneurysm to the renal arteries, nor the complexities of tortuosity and secondary aneurysms of the iliac arteries.

Doppler ultrasound ankle pressure measurement and exercise tests

The hand-held Doppler (Fig. 23.1) is the basic instrument used in both clinic and vascular laboratory for evaluating patients with peripheral arterial disease, particularly to measure the ankle systolic pressure at rest and after exercise. This inexpensive, hand-held electronic instrument, introduced by Strandness and his colleagues in 1966, is invaluable in the day-to-day practice of vascular surgery. It consists of a small battery-powered electronic box which generates signals in the 5 megaHerz range, which activate a piezo-electric crystal at the tip of a pencil probe. This projects a continuous wave of ultrasound from the probe tip, via ultrasound connecting gel, through the skin into underlying blood vessels. The ultrasound beam is reflected back from moving red corpuscles and the reflected signal is received by a second piezo-electric crystal, also on the end of the pencil probe. The sender and reflected signal are mixed electronically to produce a beat frequency which falls in the audible range.

The portable Doppler is suitable only for arteries near the skin surface and is most frequently used for detecting peripheral pulses at the ankle. The main use of the hand-held Doppler is as a sensitive stethoscope for measuring limb systolic blood pressure. However, as the audible pitch is governed by the velocity of blood flow, a simple Doppler also gives some qualitative information about blood flow to an experienced user. A normal peripheral pulse has a biphasic or triphasic signal of high pitch (equivalent to high blood velocity); the second and third signals represent reverse flow. In contrast, in a diseased vessel the peak velocity is slow in being reached, the velocity is low, and the signal is described as 'damped'. This is caused by proximal arterial stenosis or occlusion so that the blood reaches the periphery via long, slender collateral pathways.

Ankle pressure measurement

In general, the ankle systolic pressure is at least as high as the brachial systolic, and in many cases is higher due to distal systolic amplification. Thus the systolic pressure is normally elevated at the ankle and the diastolic pressure reduced compared with the brachial, owing to the high resistance of the distal arterial system. In peripheral arterial disease, the resting ankle systolic pressure is lower than normal and its level corresponds roughly with the severity of arterial obstruction. In broad terms, if the ankle/brachial ratio is 0.8 or less, this indicates peripheral arterial obstructive disease.

In patients with critical ischaemia, Doppler measurement of resting ankle pressures alone is useful; these patients can rarely walk far enough to test exercise tolerance. The resting ankle systolic pressure in these patients is rarely above 60 mmHg; a pressure below 40 mmHg indicates impending gangrene or critical ischaemia. However, in the patient unable to use a treadmill, a supine exercise device such as a Stresster™ or a 2-minute hyperaemic test is of value. The latter involves arterial occlusion and measuring the ankle pressures immediately after release of the occlusion cuff. In patients with lower-limb trauma, where foot pulses are impalpable, Doppler detection of pulses and distal pressure measurement is useful in experienced hands to characterize a compromised arterial supply.

The ankle pressure is often expressed as a ratio with the brachial pressure, known as the ankle–brachial index (ankle systolic/brachial systolic), although this is less useful if the ankle systolic pressure is low.

Other Doppler assessment

If a pulse cannot be identified with a simple Doppler flow meter, two methods can be used to help identify a patent vessel. One is to place the limb in a dependent position to gain 'gravity assist'. The other is to use a device and technique called pulse-generated runoff (PGR). In this, a cuff is automatically inflated intermittently around the calf to a pressure of 250 mmHg while the distal vessel is insonated with the Doppler to see if a signal is heard from the vessel.

Box 23.1 Problems with ankle pressure measurement in patients with diabetes mellitus

Diabetic patients with impalpable ankle pulses sometimes have spuriously high ankle pressures when measured by Doppler, often in excess of 200 mmHg. This is due to arterial wall calcification which is incompressible. In these cases, pressure may be estimated by elevating the limb (as in Buerger's test) while listening to the ankle pulse. The height at which the pulse disappears gives an estimate of systolic pressure. Toe systolic pressure may also be measured by plethysmography and is more reliable than ankle pressure in diabetics because calcification of digital arteries is uncommon. In critical ischaemia, the toe pressure is usually below 30 mmHg. However, the apparatus required to perform this test is expensive.

Exercise testing

To assess the walking ability of patients with claudication, walking exercise under measurable and controlled conditions is required. Most conveniently, the patient walks on a motorized treadmill, and ankle pressures are measured before and afterwards. The fall in pressure and the rate of recovery is related to the severity of ischaemia and the ability of the patient's own collaterals to compensate. Exercise capability on a treadmill is not directly related to daily walking ability but can be reproducible and gives an idea of claudication distance and may reveal other causes of poor walking, such as breathlessness.

Indications for ankle pressure exercise testing

1. Confirming that symptoms are caused by arterial insufficiency rather than musculoskeletal causes.

2. Objective assessment of severity of arterial insufficiency. This is useful in the preliminary assessment of a patient, particularly if a diagnosis of critical ischaemia is in doubt. Objective assessment is also useful in observing the results of treatments such as reconstructive arterial surgery (or stopping smoking).

3. Early postoperative observation for patency of reconstructions where palpable pulses have not reappeared. Where available, colour duplex scanning is more precise.

4. During long-term follow-up for assessing improvement or deterioration. Unfortunately, early suggestions that pressure testing could anticipate graft occlusion have not proved reliable.

Duplex Doppler scanning

Introduction

This is a technological development which has become an indispensable part of the vascular surgeon's armamentarium. It enables accurate and reliable direct examination of arteries and veins deep within the body. The instrument incorporates a combination of B-mode (brightness mode) ultrasound scanning to image vessels, and frequency spectral analysis of blood flow using pulsed Doppler ultrasound to measure the velocity profile. It should be emphasized that the reliability of Duplex scanning is highly operator-dependent. Examination can be time consuming, but if a very specific question is to be answered, the test can usually be performed rapidly.

The B-mode scan

The B-mode scan produces an image of the vessel under study in longitudinal or transverse section. It reveals irregularities within the lumen and mature (but not recent) thrombus, as well as abnormalities of the vessel wall. The path and orientation of the Doppler element of the scan is indicated by a white line on the screen image.

Velocity profile

The instrument can be set to 'sample' blood flow at any point in the vessel, indicated by a steerable dot on the real-time image. The angle of incidence of the Doppler beam can be adjusted to enable flow velocity to be accurately calculated electronically.

A further development of duplex Doppler is colour-encoded flow imaging. With this instrument, false colour is added to the display to reveal the direction of blood flow (red one way, blue the other) and the velocity (intensity of colour). Whenever blood flow is encountered during scanning, the colour image 'lights up' on the grey scale display, making it easy to identify vessels and follow their course. A further advantage is that the colour display reveals flow in the whole lumen of the vessel rather than a small, sampled section, making it more practical to examine pelvic and abdominal vessels. The instrument is also helpful in examining deep veins of the lower limb in suspected thrombosis. The price of colour Duplex machines is falling every year, and in terms of capital cost and disposables, the average price of a duplex scan is one-sixth that of an arteriogram.

Applications of duplex Doppler

Extracranial cerebral vascular disease

Duplex scanning enables direct examination of the extracranial carotid and vertebral arteries to demonstrate blood flow velocity and luminal morphology. Duplex scanning is highly accurate in skilled hands and in many units has become the primary investigation for investigating extracranial vascular disease. Paradoxically, it is the frequency pattern (i.e. velocity profile) rather than the observed morphology which gives the most reliable information about stenoses. Duplex is now the investigation of choice for evaluating an asymptomatic bruit and for follow-up for restenosis after carotid endarterectomy.

A classification of scan characteristics found in different grades and types of stenosis has been recommended by the Seattle group and has found favour elsewhere. However, it is more usual to grade stenoses by percentage of stenosis. If plaque is identified on B-mode scanning, it can be rated as smooth or irregular. The latter is regarded as ulcerated and thus more likely to accumulate platelet thrombi, leading to embolism.

In patients with typical hemispheric symptoms, duplex scanning is used to confirm the diagnosis of extracranial arterial disease and also provides a baseline for follow-up. In patients unsuitable for arteriography because of allergy or renal failure, it can be used as the sole diagnostic test. Indeed, many surgeons have gone further and abandoned arteriography in unequivocal cases. This is because of the 1–2 per cent risk of cerebral arteriography precipitating a stroke.

Bypass grafts

Duplex is useful for marking out the saphenous vein before femoro-distal bypass surgery. It provides information about its diameter and branching, which indicate its suitability for grafting. After operation, duplex is invaluable for **graft surveillance**. Up to 25 per cent of vein grafts develop stenoses during the first year, which may need corrective surgery or angioplasty; stenoses can readily be detected by duplex.

Duplex is also valuable for direct examination of other arterial interposition grafts for patency (e.g. aorta–superior mesenteric, carotid–subclavian). This often avoids the need for arteriography.

Aorto-iliac occlusive disease

Duplex Doppler can be used to estimate the severity of aorto-iliac stenoses. This information is subject to unpredictable errors at present and as such remains supplementary to arteriography.

Mesenteric ischaemia

Coeliac and superior mesenteric arteries can be examined for patency and blood flow characteristics, both at rest and after a meal, thus enabling a positive diagnosis to be made or refuted in patients with suspected chronic mesenteric ischaemia.

Renovascular hypertension

Renal artery stenoses greater than 60 per cent can be detected by comparing peak flow velocity in renal arteries with the peak velocity in the adjacent aorta.

Varicose veins

In short saphenous varicosities, the level at which the short saphenous enters the popliteal can easily be demonstrated and marked before operation. In 'recurrent' long saphenous varicose veins after surgery, duplex can demonstrate whether communication persists between superficial and deep veins, for example at the sapheno-femoral junction.

Deep venous thrombosis and post-thrombotic limbs

Most of the deep veins of the leg can be visualized directly by duplex Doppler. The common and superficial femoral veins, the popliteal vein, and the three paired crural veins can be examined for the following features:

- compressibility by the probe (reduced if thrombus is present);

- the presence of echogenic thrombus within the lumen;

- changes in venous flow velocity in response to respiration and the Valsalva manoeuvre, and for changes in calibre of the vein during these manoeuvres.

- in post-thrombotic limbs, occluded veins and irregularity, and internal reflux demonstrating valvular insufficiency can be reliably demonstrated.

It should be noted that the profunda vein and the calf veins may not be adequately seen, and that clot formed within the previous 24 hours is not echogenic.

2.5 Radiology

Arteriography

Introduction

Arteriography is often wrongly used for assessment of chronic arterial insufficiency. It does not measure the rate of blood flow to the tissues, nor dynamic circulatory responses to exercise. Arteriography does provide a two-dimensional map of the arterial system, and demonstrates the site and severity of vessel stenoses and occlusions. Arteriography should therefore be reserved for those patients in whom reconstructive surgery or balloon angioplasty is intended and should not be ordered simply because a patient has intermittent claudication.

Indications for arteriography

The main indications for arteriography are:

- The patient with disabling claudication who is regarded as likely to benefit from surgery or endoluminal treatment.

- The patient with critical ischaemia where an attempt at limb salvage is to be made. This includes the diabetic with predominantly atherosclerotic problems.

- The acutely ischaemic lower limb. Wherever possible, pre-operative arteriography should be performed because of the notorious unreliability of distinguishing clinically between thrombosis and embolism. 'On-table' arteriography can be used (Box 23.2), especially if operation does not reveal embolism, and peroperative thrombolysis performed if appropriate.

◆ Although colour duplex is the investigation of choice for graft surveillance, arteriography is often used to confirm and further delineate any problems detected prior to intervention. Most departments prefer to use digital subtraction angiography (see below) for this purpose as the contrast dose is lower.

◆ Trauma affecting limb circulation. In fractures (open or closed), dislocations, and lacerations where peripheral pulses are absent and the periphery of a limb is cool and under-perfused, a strong normal Doppler signal usually means the arterial circulation is intact. If there is any doubt, however, an arteriogram should be obtained early to prevent ischaemic damage that is likely to result from delay.

◆ Abdominal aortic aneurysm. Some surgeons like to have pre-operative arteriography for aortic aneurysm replacement. This shows the relationship of the aneurysm to the renal arteries and also shows any other synchronous aneurysms (e.g. iliac, femoral, popliteal) and the patency of internal iliac arteries and the inferior mesenteric artery, as well as occlusive disease in arteries supplying the lower limb. All of these factors can have a bearing on how the operation is carried out. However, improvements in other modes of imaging (e.g. spiral CT and three-dimensional reconstructions) have rendered arteriography unnecessary except in coincident occlusive disease.

◆ Carotid artery disease. Many surgeons no longer demand arteriography for most cases and are satisfied with the information available from duplex Doppler assessment alone (see above).

Box 23.2 Technique of on-table arteriography

If an image intensifier is available, contrast material can be injected into the femoral artery and its passage followed down the limb with the C-arm. If not, a large X-ray-film case is wrapped in a sterile towel and placed beneath the limb; 20 ml of contrast material is injected into the femoral artery with a clamp proximal to it. A single exposure is taken on completion of the injection.

Digital subtraction angiography

A relatively recent development in angiography, this is a method of recording the X-ray images electronically in digital form, as opposed to the analogue form of conventional radiographic film. These digital images can be processed electronically to optimize the available information; this includes subtracting background detail (thus removing bony images) and enhancing the arteri-ographic profile. Background subtraction in real time can produce satisfactory vascular images with much lower concen-trations of contrast. The technique is known as digital sub-traction angiography (DSA) or digital vascular imaging (DVI).

DSA lacks some of the resolution of conventional arterio-graphy but has several advantages, including better imaging of distal vessels in the presence of proximal occlusions by the use of digital subtraction of the bony image, and the fact that lower volumes and concentrations of contrast material are used, making it safer than conventional arteriography. Most radio-logists prefer intra-arterial injection but satisfactory images for some purposes can be produced by central venous injection. DSA may also be used for screening of doubtful cases where conventional arteriography might not be justified. It can be used repeatedly for follow-up of disease or reconstructions.

CT scanning

CT scanning provides a more complete examination of aneurysms than ultrasonography. It is not more reliable for demonstrating diameter, but is better at showing the relation-ship to the renal arteries, and for showing pelvic aneurysms, especially if spiral CT scanning is available. CT can also demonstrate aortic wall thickness, which some surgeons believe is a better predictor of imminent rupture than diameter. The most useful application of CT in aneurysms is to reveal retro-peritoneal fibrosis associated with an inflammatory aneurysm. This condition is of unknown aetiology, which presents particular difficulties for surgical access and control. CT scanning will also demonstrate the presence of a horseshoe kidney, the isthmus of which overlies the lower end of the aorta and common iliac arteries, making operation much more difficult. Inflammatory aneurysms and horseshoe kidneys are both rare, but are best anticipated before surgery.

CT scanning occasionally shows retroperitoneal leakage of blood but cannot be relied upon to diagnose leakage where clinical evidence is equivocal. Leaking or ruptured aneurysm is essentially a clinical diagnosis and there is no reliable test for it, although spiral CT is improving in its diagnostic accuracy. However, it is better to be wrong on the operating table than in the post-mortem room.

Magnetic resonance angiography

MRI provides an alternative, non-invasive approach to angio-graphy. With this investigation, there is natural contrast between flowing blood in vessels and stationary soft tissues and this can demonstrate the vessel morphology without intravascular contrast medium. This phenomenon allows the production of MR angiograms. Multiple contiguous slices of tissue need to be imaged by a process known as volume acquisition. In the early days of MR, data acquisition times were long, and the technique was restricted to relatively immobile areas such as the cartotid arteries and the intracranial circulation. This limitation has largely been overcome by faster scanners and by techniques of enhancing the difference between blood and stationary tissue with intravenous contrast. Successful angiography can now be performed in all regions of the body with scan times of less than 30 seconds. With ECG triggered scanning, even the coronary arteries can be imaged, but not yet at a clinically useful resolution.

MR angiography is a rapid outpatient procedure that requires no more preparation than an intravenous injection. It carries none of the risks of ionizing radiation and is ideally suited to repeated or follow up examinations. If vascular surveillance cannot be performed by ultrasound, MRA is a satisfactory (though more expensive) alternative. Over the next few years, contrast enhanced MRA is likely to replace diagnostic angiography in centres with ready access to the equipment. Patients requiring open surgery can expect to have this planned entirely on non-invasive MR imaging. Traditional angiography will only be required for patients needing percutaneous intervention, e.g. angioplasty or stenting.

2.6 Angioscopy

Advances in the design of flexible endoscopes have allowed the production of small-diameter scopes (0.8–3 mm) which are beginning to be used for examining the luminal surface of vein grafts, arteries, and arterial reconstructions.

An angioscope can also be used to prepare a long saphenous vein for *in situ* bypass grafting. The vein is exposed only proximally and distally and the scope is passed along the vein from above to inspect the work of the valvulotome passed up from below. This ensures that all valves are effectively destroyed. Furthermore, the level of each tributary can be seen and can then be ligated through small separate incisions rather than the more usual full-length incision. Thus, a more thorough destruction of valves and a less traumatic incision should result. In experienced hands, a realistic maximum of 500 ml of irrigating fluid is required.

After angioplasty or atherectomy (removal of atheroma using rotating atherectomy catheters, for example), the luminal surface can be examined for loose flaps or debris and steps taken to correct defects.

The place of angioscopy has not yet become established in daily practice in most hospitals, largely because of the high capital cost, the extra time required, and the lack of definite proof of benefit. Perhaps its most useful application is as a completion procedure after carotid endarterectomy.

3 Instrumentation and principles of therapeutic techniques in arterial surgery

3.1 Introduction

Arterial surgery is one of the most unforgiving branches of surgery with little margin for error. The specialty is highly operator dependent and technical details are of crucial importance. Less than perfect operative technique, or failure to adhere to the important principles described here, will usually result in failure of the reconstruction. This will often leave the patient

Table 23.1 Desirable qualities of arterial clamps

Atraumatic so that the vessel wall is not damaged by crushing or fracture of plaques
Retain a firm grip on the vessel and do not slip while the arteriotomy is open
Easy to place, particularly in remote areas, and require minimal dissection for placement
Must not get in the way of the operator when in position

worse off than before operation and will risk limb loss or even loss of life.

In most cases, secondary failure of revascularization is due to incorrect or inappropriate technique. Problems include choosing a vessel at donor or recipient end of the reconstruction which cannot sustain sufficient blood flow to ensure patency, thrombosis of native arteries or grafts during clamping, or twisting or kinking of grafts during placement causing thrombosis.

Special instrument sets are always used for arterial surgery as general sets do not contain suitable instruments for displaying and handling arteries and clamping them without causing damage (Fig. 23.2).

Arterial clamps

In any reconstructive arterial surgery, vessels need to be opened. In order to do this without loss of blood and without obscuring the field of view, the main vessels proximal and distal to the arteriotomy need to be temporarily occluded, as well as all other branches feeding into the closed segment. (Table 23.1)

Special retractors

The standard 'basic set' retractors are used in abdominal arterial surgery. In addition, specially designed, fixed, self-retaining retractors are of benefit when operating on the abdominal aorta, for example the Omnitract. In this, a vertical bar is locked to the operating table and other bars locked to it, to which a variety of different shaped retractors may be firmly attached. The instrument enables firm, steady, and precise retraction in several directions at once. This reduces the number of assistants needed for aortic reconstruction and allows the assistants to concentrate on the particular needs of the operator. For these reasons it is sometimes known as the 'metal houseman'.

For the popliteal fossa there are other self-retaining retractors, similar to a Travers retractor, with one long blade and one short (e.g. the Browse retractor). More complex retractors have a small circumferential frame to which angled retractors can be attached.

Suckers

The standard metal sump sucker is useful for delicate dissection around arteries, particularly the iliac arteries. The outer cover is removed and the inner section employed to gently tease the tissues apart around the artery. Gentle, low-volume suction keeps the area clear of blood.

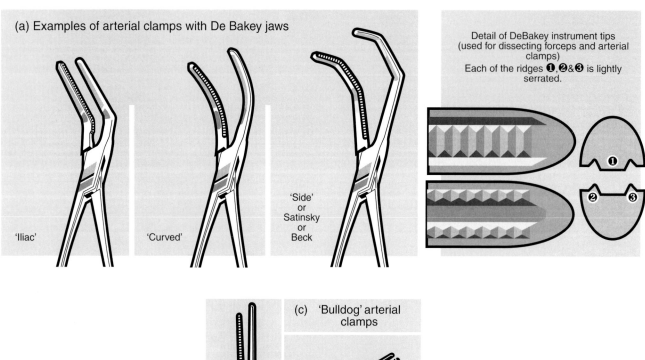

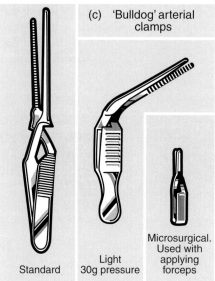

Figure 23.2 Instruments used in arterial surgery.

Tunnelling devices

Some arterial grafts need to be placed deeply, often over a long distance. A tunnelling device is a metal tube which may be curved, with a removable rounded end. It allows a small-diameter tunnel to be formed through the tissues with minimal trauma and provides a smooth conduit for the graft to pass through. The pathway is between muscles, as in a femoro-popliteal bypass graft, or through fat, as in extra-anatomic grafts such as a femoro-femoral crossover graft or axillo-femoral graft.

Magnifying loupes

Many vascular surgeons use magnification when operating on small blood vessels. This is most easily achieved by using loupes, which are magnifying lenses cemented or otherwise attached to

spectacles. They are usually constructed for one individual so that the lenses can be placed precisely. Quite small degrees of magnification, in the order of 2 to 3 times, give a remarkable increase in discriminatory ability, enabling potential defects in an anastomosis to be seen more clearly. These include:

- Splitting of the arterial wall layers can be seen.

- The inner layers of the vessel wall can always be confirmed visually to have been included in the suture line.

- Fine flakes of calcification can be circumvented.

- Sutures in tiny vessels can be placed precisely to avoid stenosis. This is most likely to occur at the toe of an end-to-side anastomosis (e.g. an *in situ* vein graft to an anterior tibial artery).

(b)

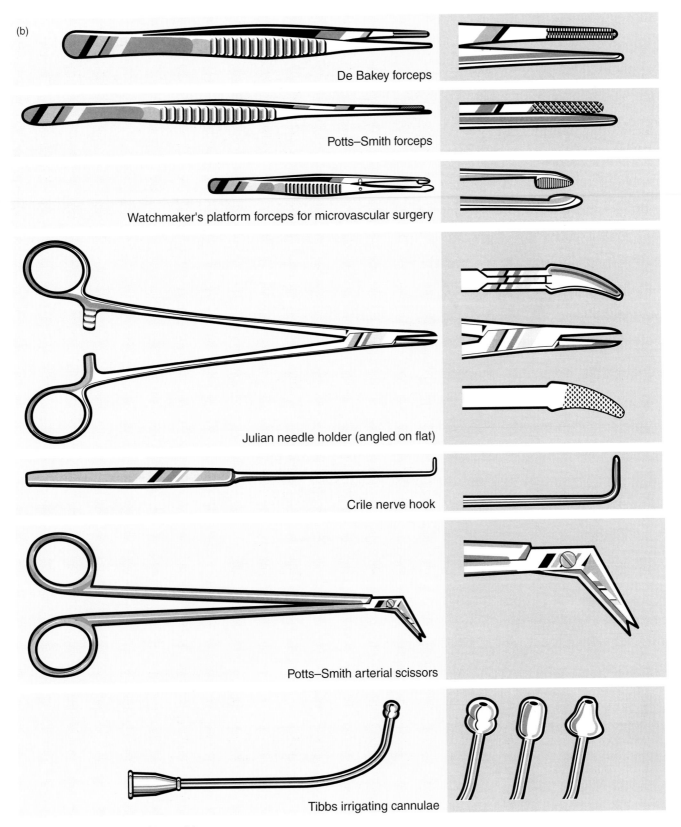

De Bakey forceps

Potts–Smith forceps

Watchmaker's platform forceps for microvascular surgery

Julian needle holder (angled on flat)

Crile nerve hook

Potts–Smith arterial scissors

Tibbs irrigating cannulae

Figure 23.2 Instruments used in arterial surgery.

(a) Arteriotomy closure

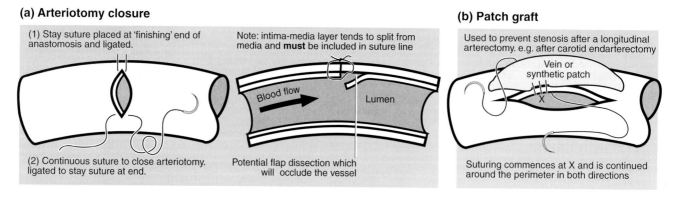

(1) Stay suture placed at 'finishing' end of anastomosis and ligated.

(2) Continuous suture to close arteriotomy. ligated to stay suture at end.

Note: intima-media layer tends to split from media and **must** be included in suture line

Blood flow

Lumen

Potential flap dissection which will occlude the vessel

(b) Patch graft

Used to prevent stenosis after a longitudinal arterectomy. e.g. after carotid endarterectomy

Vein or synthetic patch

X

Suturing commences at X and is continued around the perimeter in both directions

(c) End-to-end anastomosis

e.g. distal end of aorto-iliac bifurcation graft for aneurysm

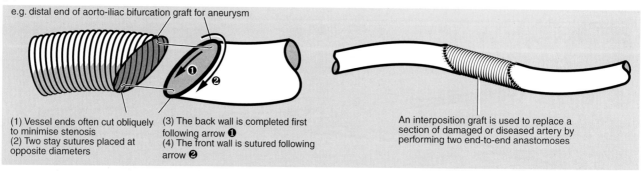

(1) Vessel ends often cut obliquely to minimise stenosis
(2) Two stay sutures placed at opposite diameters

(3) The back wall is completed first following arrow ❶
(4) The front wall is sutured following arrow ❷

An interposition graft is used to replace a section of damaged or diseased artery by performing two end-to-end anastomoses

(d) End-to-side anastomosis

e.g distal end of aorto-bifemoral graft for aorto-iliac occlusive disease or both ends of a femoro-popliteal bypass graft

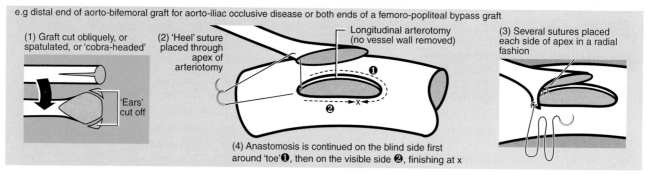

(1) Graft cut obliquely, or spatulated, or 'cobra-headed'

'Ears' cut off

(2) 'Heel' suture placed through apex of arteriotomy

Longitudinal arterotomy (no vessel wall removed)

(3) Several sutures placed each side of apex in a radial fashion

(4) Anastomosis is continued on the blind side first around 'toe'❶, then on the visible side ❷, finishing at x

(e) Inlay graft

e.g for abdominal aortic aneurysm

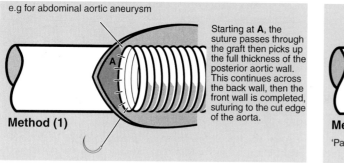

Method (1)

Starting at **A**, the suture passes through the graft then picks up the full thickness of the posterior aortic wall. This continues across the back wall, then the front wall is completed, suturing to the cut edge of the aorta.

Method (2)
'Parachute technique'

In this method, most of the posterior layer sutures are placed as shown before the graft is fully tightened down. This gives accurate visualization to place sutures when the aortic wall is in poor condition. The anastomosis is completed as in method (1)

Figure 23.3 Techniques of arterial suture.

♦ Inadvertent picking up the posterior wall of the vessel while placing sutures.

♦ Some arterial surgeons use magnification for anastomoses on larger vessels such as the femoral arteries. Particularly where the arteries are of poor quality, it enables precise placement of sutures and a more accurate anastomosis, reducing the chance of an intimal flap or other irregularity on the luminal surface.

3.2 Principles of vascular suturing

Suture materials

Non-absorbable materials are the rule in arterial surgery. These are always used for artificial grafts because the continued integrity of the anastomoses depends on the suture line remaining permanently intact.

In the early days of arterial surgery, grafts were sutured with silk. However, silk is a biological material and gradually degrades over the years; it is now believed that this was responsible for the large number of false (anastomotic) aneurysms that developed in the early reconstructions. In the early 1960s, braided poly-ester sutures appeared (trade names Tevdek and Ticron). This material was stronger than silk and, like polyester (Dacron) grafts, scarcely degraded with time. However, like silk, polyester has the inherent disadvantage of all braided materials, namely surface roughness. Each loop of a continuous suture line has to be individually tightened as it is placed, and a graft cannot be 'parachuted' into position after placing a number of loose sutures (Fig. 23.3). Furthermore, sutures tend to saw through the vessel wall, so sutures can cut out, particularly when vessel walls are of poor quality.

In the 1970s polypropylene (Prolene™) sutures first appeared and produced a revolution in arterial and cardiac surgery. This is a monofilament material with great strength, secure knotting properties and, most importantly, the capability of sliding easily through the tissues. This allows the operator to keep both edges of an arteriotomy or anastomosis separated and clearly in view while placing each suture, finally tensioning several sutures to bring the edges together. It also facilitates the '**parachute technique**' used to perform the posterior layer of the proximal anastomosis of an inlay graft for aortic aneurysm.

Gauge of suture

The gauge of suture used is to some extent a matter of personal preference, but in general, stronger sutures are used on larger vessels, and finer sutures on small, thin-walled vessels. Heavier gauges of suture have larger and thicker needles and this may influence the choice (Table 23.2)

Table 23.2 Gauge of sutures used in arterial surgery

Aorta	Iliacs	Femoral	Popliteal/tibial
2/0 or 3/0	3/0 or 4/0	4/0, 5/0, or 6/0	6/0 or 7/0

Needles

Vascular sutures are 'double-armed' (i.e. they have a needle at each end). This facilitates suturing in both directions around an anastomosis.

Vascular needles are nearly all half round in shape, and the majority are round bodied with a smooth, non-cutting tip. However, special needles are made for more resistant vessels. For example,

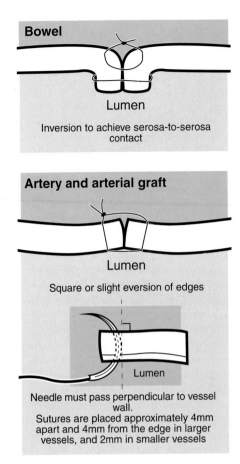

Figure 23.4 Techniques of arterial anastomosis.

the 'armour piercing' SX needle from Ethicon, is designed with a rigid square-section body and a short cutting point. This type of needle is of great benefit when tackling heavily calcified arteries, particularly abdominal aortic aneurysms. The Ethicon CC needle has a short trocar point and is useful for thick-walled small arteries.

Arterial suturing techniques

Arterial suturing is intended to achieve a smooth, non-thrombogenic internal surface to the reconstruction, ensuring that the inner layers of the vessel are secured without risk of leaving a 'flap' as a potential origin for a dissection, and without causing vessel stenosis. Where possible, the needle should be passed through from the inside to the outside of the artery to minimize separation of the layers.

The edges of an arterial anastomosis should be apposed either squarely or with slight eversion to minimize encroachment on the lumen (Fig. 23.4); this is in direct contrast to the inversion usually used on bowel.

Continuous suturing is preferred except for microvascular anastomoses. For anastomoses to a single calf vessel a continuous suture around the heel of the graft is often used, then at the toe of the graft six interrupted sutures can be used, thus preventing narrowing of the distal end of the anastomosis.

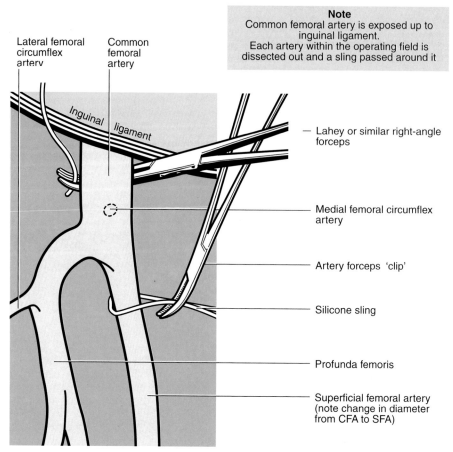

Note
Common femoral artery is exposed up to inguinal ligament.
Each artery within the operating field is dissected out and a sling passed around it

Lateral femoral circumflex artery

Common femoral artery

Inguinal ligament

— Lahey or similar right-angle forceps

— Medial femoral circumflex artery

— Artery forceps 'clip'

— Silicone sling

— Profunda femoris

— Superficial femoral artery (note change in diameter from CFA to SFA)

Figure 23.5 Exposure of femoral arteries.

3.3 Principles and techniques of arterial reconstruction

General principles of arterial reconstruction

Stages in arterial reconstruction include exposure of the arteries and control of all branches in the area to be operated upon, assessment of local conditions in relation to the treatment plan, anticoagulation, clamping, arteriotomy, the procedure proper (i.e. anastomosis, endarterectomy, embolectomy, or angioplasty), flushing, haemostasis and, finally, evaluation of the result.

Exposure of arteries and control of branches

It is important to expose sufficient length of the artery to allow it to be clamped securely both proximally and distally, leaving sufficient access to perform the bypass or endarterectomy safely and in a bloodless field. Detailed anatomy will not be covered here but the operator must understand the anatomy and technique of access for a range of standard exposures, such as the femoral artery, subclavian artery, brachial artery, the infrarenal aorta, the popliteal artery above and below the knee, and various approaches to the crural or tibial arteries more distally in the leg or foot.

For a bypass graft, the principle is to expose a proximal artery which has good inflow and a distal artery with potentially good outflow and low resistance.

A plane of dissection is developed close to the wall of the artery to expose all of its branches in the operative field. Silicone-rubber slings are looped around branches to identify each one and to assist with later clamping (Fig. 23.5). In general, arteries are sturdy and do not tear easily. In contrast, veins adjoining arteries can be damaged easily and may be difficult to repair. Examples are iliac veins lying behind iliac arteries, tributaries of the left renal vein as it crosses the aortic neck, and the profunda vein crossing the profunda femoris artery.

Assessment of local conditions in relation to the treatment plan

However carefully the patient has been assessed clinically and radiologically before operation, the vessels need to be checked for patency and for their suitability for reconstruction once exposed. This includes operative assessment of inflow (from the proximal vessel) by demonstrating a satisfactory 'squirt' of blood through the arteriotomy when the proximal clamp is briefly removed, and good back flow from the periphery when the distal clamp is removed. If a poor inflow is identified at surgery then intraoperative pressure measurements can be performed using a transducer, comparing the reading to brachial systolic (or radial artery) pressure. If no obvious discrepancy exists, then a stress test should be performed by the injection of papaverine, or other powerful vasodilator, into the exposed (unclamped) artery. This markedly reduces the peripheral resistance; if the arterial pressure falls by more than 20 mmHg this suggests there is a significant proximal stenosis, impeding the rise in flow required by the lowered peripheral resistance.

If there is no backflow, the vessel either has a long-standing occlusion or is occluded acutely by fresh thrombus or embolus. An operative or on-table arteriogram may be needed to resolve doubts. Many surgeons use operative angiography routinely for crural (below-knee) bypasses.

The arterial wall is visually checked for suitability for grafting by palpation (i.e. for flexibility, wall thickness, and calcification). If arteries are found to be unfavourable, the original treatment plan will have to be modified in the light of the new evidence. Having to extend a graft more proximally or more distally than was intended is not unusual in these patients who have widespread atherosclerosis.

Anticoagulation

Once the arteries are all exposed and branches controlled, the patient is usually anticoagulated systemically with intravenous heparin. The dose varies between surgeons. Many use a standard dose of 5000–7500 units, while others vary the dose according to body weight. In either case, small top-up doses may be required later if clots begin to form or after a given time interval (e.g. 1000 units per hour). Some surgeons simply flush the distal arterial tree with heparinized saline. It is rarely necessary to reverse the heparin with protamine at the end of the operation.

Clamping

Next, vascular clamps are applied, taking care to clamp the whole diameter of both proximal and distal arteries and to avoid areas of heavy calcification which may fracture. Small branches are controlled either by double loops of silicone sling held in artery forceps or bulldog clamps. Where possible, only those vessels involved in the current procedure are clamped so that arterial perfusion of distal structures can continue.

The procedure

The chosen arterial reconstructive procedure is then carried out as described below (e.g. anastomosis of a bypass graft, endarterectomy, or embolectomy).

Flushing and completion of the suture line

When nearing completion of a suture line, first proximal and then distal clamps should be released temporarily to ensure that forward and back bleeding is satisfactory and clotting has not occurred. This also flushes out any accumulated debris and reduces the amount of air passing into the distal arterial tree once the clamps are finally removed. Clamps are reapplied, the suture line completed and the clamps removed.

Haemostasis

Most suture lines bleed a small amount on declamping. Simple pressure with a swab for a timed 5 minutes is usually all that is needed for platelets to plug small leaks. Sometimes one or more fine interrupted sutures need to be placed if bleeding is substantial; arteries should be reclamped before this is carried out. If bleeding persists despite these measures, particularly if it has been a difficult and bloody operation, continued attempts at suturing usually aggravate the problem. In these circumstances, it is often useful to place a matrix of an absorbable haemostatic material around the anastomosis to assist the clotting process; examples are oxidized cellulose (e.g. Surgicel®) and alginate derivatives (e.g. Caltostat®). Transfusion of blood products may be needed to restore clotting factors.

Evaluation of the result

The most useful means of assessing reperfusion after reconstruction is to look for 'pinking up' of the extremity. This will usually occur within a few minutes of declamping. The blue or white foot will first demonstrate venous filling, then gradual return of pinkness. If this does not happen, a technical fault must be assumed and measures taken to overcome it. For example, thrombosis of the graft or distal arterial tree may have occurred, or the graft may be occluded by an intimal flap at an anastomosis.

It should be noted that the presence of pulsation in a graft does not necessarily mean that satisfactory flow is taking place. However, unequivocal return of ankle pulses does confirm successful revascularization.

Completion studies for quality control should always be performed. They can be simple Doppler assessment, flow measurements, angioscopy, or arteriography. Simple Doppler evaluation and arteriography should be available in any hospital where arterial surgery is performed.

Table 23.3 summarizes the problems associated with interventional treatment in arterial surgery.

3.4 Reconstructive techniques

Endarterectomy

Endarterectomy is now used mainly for carotid artery disease. The technique is also sometimes known as **thromboendarterectomy** or **disobliteration**.

For lower-limb arterial disease, endarterectomy has largely been superseded by bypass grafting, which has been shown to have more durable long-term results. Furthermore, bypass grafting is substantially quicker, less technically demanding, and results in less blood loss. Endarterectomy is occasionally employed to treat localized arterial occlusions (e.g. common femoral artery) or for local preparation of a diseased artery to accept a bypass graft.

The principle of endarterectomy is that occluded or stenosed arteries have a strong and nearly normal outer layer composed of the adventitia and the outer layer of media. There is usually a plane of cleavage between this and the inner layers consisting of

Table 23.3 Problems of interventional treatment in arterial surgery

Nature of problem	Cause of problem	Prevention and management
Peroperative haemorrhage	Most often a problem in aortic surgery, particularly ruptured AAA. With rupture, the body's attempts to arrest haemorrhage by thrombosis exhausts clotting factors and platelets, resulting in consumption coagulopathy; aggravated by further blood loss during surgery	(1) Take care to avoid damaging nearby veins during dissection (2) Obtain good exposure of arteries to allow clamping well away from the arteriotomy (3) In ruptured aortic aneurysm, make sure minimal time is lost between the patient's first symptoms of aortic rupture and applying a clamp to the aorta. Once good venous access has been established, the patient should be anaesthetized without delay. Further monitoring can be added once the aorta is controlled (4) In ruptured aortic aneurysm, appropriate blood products should be given in advance and during and after surgery (e.g. platelet concentrates and fresh, frozen plasma). Tests of clotting under these circumstances are often misleading
Swings in blood pressure liable to affect organ perfusion	Atherosclerotic patients have generally reduced arterial compliance and are more sensitive to changes in cardiac output and to blood losses	Careful intraoperative monitoring of blood loss, arterial blood pressure, and central venous pressure, and in patients with cardiac failure, left atrial pressure with a Swan–Ganz catheter
Problems of graft material availability and compatibility	In supra-inguinal areas, synthetic grafts are the rule and are well tolerated. In infra- inguinal areas, saphenous vein grafts are preferred but the patient's veins may be inadequate	Saphenous vein can be harvested from the opposite limb, or a composite graft can be made up of part saphenous vein and part cephalic vein from the arm. Wholly synthetic grafts of expanded PTFE give reasonably good results above the knee but are less suitable for femoro-tibial grafts. However, improved results have been found using a vein cuff or patch on the distal end (see later). Other possibilities are modified human umbilical vein graft and modified animal arteries, but these have generally proved unsatisfactory in the long term
Problems of access, especially to the perirenal aorta	The lower thoracic and the abdominal aorta lie deeply posteriorly and access requires displacement of lung or peritoneal contents. The perirenal aorta lies high in an abdominal incision requiring strong retraction. There is a rich venous plexus lying anterior to the aorta, including the left renal vein, which hinders access	Thorough mobilization of surrounding structures should be performed before attempting clamping. Renal arteries should be identified in high dissections and, if necessary, the left renal vein divided towards the right side to allow good access. Most surgeons prefer to re-anastomose the vein at the end of the operation
Problems of particular vessels: renals, iliacs, inferior mesenteric	(1) Renal arteries are difficult to access and are fragile and easily damaged (2) Iliac arteries tend to be bonded firmly to iliac veins lying deeply. These veins are easily torn and produce torrential haemorrhage	(1) Thorough dissection and careful handling are required (2) Iliac arteries can often be clamped without posterior dissection. Never pass sharp instruments blindly behind iliac arteries—dissect under direct vision with blunt instruments
Problems of iatrogenic embolism—'trash foot'	This is a particular problem with aortic aneurysm surgery. If the aneurysm sac is handled before the iliacs are clamped, thrombi may be released into the distal circulation and lodge as distal emboli in the legs and feet	Clamp the iliacs before handling the aortic sac and prior to proximal clamping (except in ruptured aneurysms)
Primary problems with revascularization	Failure to revascularize a limb may be due to: • Inadequate inflow or runoff (selection of unsuitable vessels) • Technical defects of suturing of anastomoses or placement of grafts • Graft thrombosis or embolism	 • Good preoperative arteriography and Doppler ultrasound plus peroperative clinical assessment of inflow and outflow, if necessary with operative angiography or pressure measurement • Training and supervision and taking care to be technically meticulous • Suitable anticoagulation during clamping, correct placement of grafts without twist or undue tension, and avoiding dislodging clot to form emboli
Secondary problems with revascularization—late graft failure	• Progression of atherosclerosis • Vein graft stenosis and occlusion	• Persuade patient to stop smoking; control hypertension; treat elevated cholesterol • Perform graft surveillance for first year and take remedial action if necessary

Table 23.3 *continued*

Nature of problem	Cause of problem	Prevention and management
	• Fibromuscular hyperplasia at anastomosis between PTFE graft and popliteal artery	• Use venous patch or cuff at distal anastomoses between* PTFE graft and below-knee popliteal artery
Iatrogenic mesenteric ischaemia	Uncommon. Affects the colon (left side) after division of the inferior mesenteric artery. Presents with abdominal pain and bloody diarrhoea 2–4 days after operation	Check perfusion of colon at operation before closure. Colonoscopy and biopsy if in doubt. If the condition is suspected later, early laparotomy, colonic resection, and colostomy are required. Graft infection is a serious risk
	The inferior mesenteric may be the sole source of blood supply to the sigmoid colon. After transverse colectomy and division of the marginal artery it may supply the whole of the left side of the colon	If the inferior mesenteric is divided during aneurysm replacement, always check the sigmoid colon for viability. If in doubt, reimplant the vessel into the graft
Problems of interventional radiology: thrombolysis, vessel damage, arteriovenous fistula, embolism, false aneurysms	Trauma at arterial puncture: includes tearing of the vessel wall, causing haemorrhage; dissection of the vessel wall (usually harmless but may cause an occluding flap); false aneurysms; and iatrogenic arteriovenous fistula. Thrombosis of arteries at the site of puncture or more distally, usually caused by problems with hypertonic contrast material or by embolism from displaced thrombus	Meticulous puncture technique using cannulae as small as practicable. Employing an access sheath means that catheters and balloon catheters can be replaced without further trauma. A period of effective pressure on the puncture site after the procedure is essential. Non-ionic contrast materials prevent intimal damage and reduce the risk of chemically induced thrombosis. Provisional injections of contrast during the procedure detects trauma early, allowing abandonment of unsatisfactory procedures
Iatrogenic trauma to spleen, bowel, nerves	• Heavy retraction during aortic surgery, particularly with table-fixed retractors, can damage solid organs • Veins lying closely bound to arteries can be torn during dissection • Nerves can be traumatized during dissection, e.g. femoral nerve in groin, lumbar nerves in posterior abdominal wall	• Avoid by careful placement of retractors with swabs beneath • Never pass sharp, pointed instruments blindly behind arteries that lie close to veins • Careful dissection
Aortic graft infection	Almost invariably occurs after the bowel has been opened during aortic surgery	If the bowel is opened during an elective aortic operation, consider abandoning the operation until 2–4 weeks later. Alternatively, soaking the graft in suitable antibiotics (e.g. rifampicin) may help to prevent infection. During the first year after grafting, use prophylactic antibiotics for procedures known to cause bacteraemia
Wound healing	Amputation wounds in ischaemic limbs may fail to heal because of inadequate blood supply	There is no predictive test of any value to determine amputation stump healing. If wound breakdown occurs, often a secondary 'trimming' procedure will allow healing. If this is unsuitable or fails, amputation at a higher level should not be delayed

* PTFE = polytetrafluoroethylene.

the rest of the media, the atheromatous plaque, and any occluding thrombus. This plane can be developed with endarterectomy instruments to allow removal of a core of occluding material, restoring full patency to the artery.

The technique has several drawbacks. It is difficult to 'finish' the endarterectomy distally without leaving a flap as a potential source of dissection. Some arteries are notoriously difficult to endarterectomize (e.g. external iliac), and repairing the artery after the procedure may cause stenosis. The roughened interior of the endarterectomized vessel, with exposed collagen, makes it highly thrombogenic. These problems account for the higher rate of failure of endarterectomy when compared with bypass procedures (where these are practicable).

Endarterectomy technique

After exposure, anticoagulation and clamping of the arteries, an arteriotomy is made and the plane of cleavage found. The inner

strata are mobilised around the full circumference with a Watson–Cheyne dissector (Fig. 23.6). In the carotid area, the core tapers at each end and the entire core can be removed without leaving a flap or shelf. If a flap is apparent, it should be tacked down with sutures. Where a longer endarterectomy is necessary, for example in the iliofemoral system, the core is divided transversely and a ring stripper passed over it and gently manipulated distally, freeing the core of tissue from the outer layers of the arterial wall. This plane is sometimes easy to develop, but the layers are often adherent (particularly in the external iliac) and the process can be tedious and prolonged. It may require further arteriotomies which will later need to be closed with patch grafts.

The distal limit of the endarterectomy must be scrutinized from within the artery via a further arteriotomy and the distal ledge of 'intima' carefully sutured to the arterial wall to obviate a flap dissection which could occlude the distal vessel.

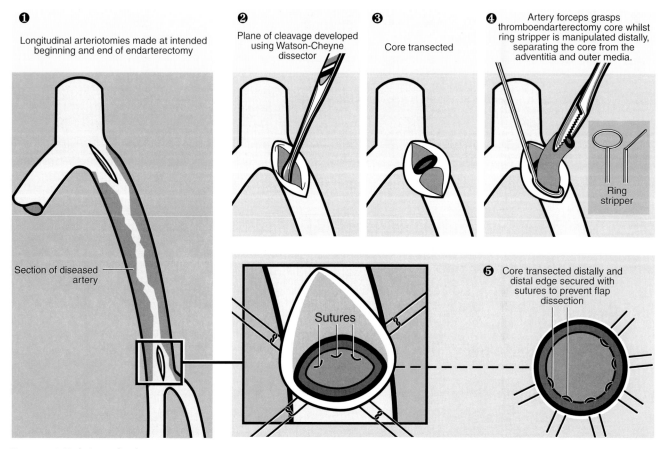

❶ Longitudinal arteriotomies made at intended beginning and end of endarterectomy

❷ Plane of cleavage developed using Watson-Cheyne dissector

❸ Core transected

❹ Artery forceps grasps thromboendarterectomy core whilst ring stripper is manipulated distally, separating the core from the adventitia and outer media.

Ring stripper

Section of diseased artery

Sutures

❺ Core transected distally and distal edge secured with sutures to prevent flap dissection

Figure 23.6 Technique of endarterectomy.

Indications for shunts

A temporary shunt is often used during carotid endarterectomy to allow flow into the distal internal carotid during the procedure. Some surgeons use a shunt in every case, while others only use one in patients they regard as having inadequate distal perfusion when the carotid artery is clamped. One indicator commonly employed is if there is a low 'stump pressure' (< 50 mmHg) in the distal artery. Others include changes developing in EEG monitoring or transcranial Doppler monitoring (TCD) of middle cerebral artery velocity.

Bypass grafting: anatomic and extra-anatomic

Introduction

Bypass grafting is the most common reconstructive technique used in arterial surgery. It has largely superseded thrombo-endarterectomy for treating stenosed or occluded arteries except in the carotid system. This is because grafting has been demonstrated to be less traumatic, quicker, and to give better long-term patency.

In general, synthetic materials are highly satisfactory for large proximal arterial grafts but are a poor second to autogenous saphenous vein where the graft originates below the inguinal ligament. Most grafts are termed **anatomic** because they run along a route similar to that of the vessel they replace (e.g. aorto-

bifemoral graft (Fig. 23.7), femoro-popliteal graft). In certain circumstances, an **extra-anatomic graft** is preferred which follows a novel course (Fig. 23.7). Examples include crossover femoro-femoral grafts and axillo-femoral grafts. These are used for one of the following reasons:

◆ a desire to reconstruct the aorto-iliac system without the extra trauma of opening the peritoneal cavity in an elderly or unfit patient;

◆ reconstruction after an anatomic reconstruction has failed;

◆ avoiding placing a graft in an infected field.

Grafts for the aorto-iliac segment

In the early days of modern arterial surgery in the 1950s, cadaveric homograft vessels were used as arterial replacements. However, the long-term survival of these grafts proved unsatisfactory as they tended to become aneurysmal after a few years.

Since there are no suitable alternative natural materials from which to construct grafts for the aorto-iliac segment, synthetic materials were used as soon as they became available. Early materials included nylon and Teflon, but polyester (Dacron) has gradually become the popular choice for synthetic aortic grafts. The earliest grafts were woven and impermeable, but suffered from rigidity, difficulty in passing needles, and fraying of the cut ends. Modern woven grafts are thinner walled and still

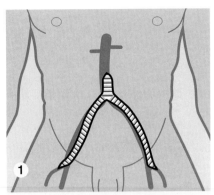

Retroperitoneal aorto-bifemoral or 'trouser' graft.
End to side or end to end of abdominal aorta.
End to side of common femoral and profunda.
This is an 'anatomic' graft.

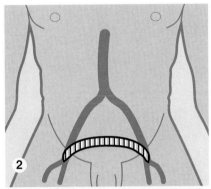

Femoro-femoral crossover graft for unilateral
disease.
Ends anastomosed to common femoral arteries.
Graft placed either deep to abdominal wall or in
subcutaneous fat.

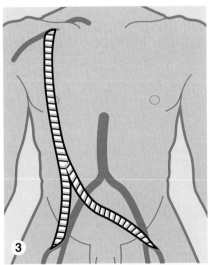

Axillo-bifemoral graft.
Proximal end anastomosed to axillary artery
below clavicle. Access by splitting pectoralis
major.
This and (2) are 'extra-anatomic' grafts.

Figure 23.7 Aorto-iliac grafting techniques.

impermeable, and although they suffer from the same disadvantages to a lesser extent, they are still preferred by some surgeons. Woven grafts cannot be made with a velour surface to encourage firm attachment of the neo-intima and perigraft tissues, and a potential space therefore persists around the graft where infection can lurk. Neo-intima may also become detached, creating a dissection and occlusion.

Knitted Dacron grafts are now more popular than woven grafts because they are easier to handle and to suture, they do not fray, and the inner, outer, or both surfaces of the graft can be made with a velour surface. Knitted Dacron has the disadvantage of high porosity and must either be preclotted with blood (usually the three-stage Sauvage technique), or else sealed with gelatin or collagen during manufacture. There is an increasing trend towards the use of these sealed and impermeable grafts, despite their greater cost.

All Dacron grafts are constructed with transverse corrugations that allow longitudinal elasticity and do not seriously interfere with blood flow. Grafts are made in either straight or bifurcated ('Y' or 'trouser') format or special formats (e.g. for axillo-femoral grafts). Diameters range between about 6 mm and 45 mm.

Aorto-iliac grafting techniques are illustrated in Fig. 23.7

Grafts for the femoro-popliteal segment

Where grafts originate below the inguinal ligament, the almost universal preference of graft material is autogenous saphenous vein. This has excellent handling properties and elasticity. It gives consistently better long-term results than any synthetic graft. However, a suitable saphenous vein is not available in up to 25 per cent of cases, either because it has been removed or is too narrow or varicose. Then a synthetic graft will usually provide a suitable substitute. The majority of synthetic grafts used in this segment are made of expanded PTFE (Teflon), constructed so as to be impermeable to blood yet porous enough to allow tissue ingrowth. Teflon is non-water-wettable; it is almost inelastic and demands a precise anastomotic technique. It goes under the trade names of Goretex, Impra and others, and is made in different diameters and lengths, and even in a tapered variety. Where the graft has to cross the knee joint, a variant with rigid external plastic reinforcing spirals may be preferred.

Femoro-popliteal bypass using a synthetic graft can be completed more quickly because time is not spent preparing a saphenous vein graft (Fig. 23.8). However, synthetic grafts need to become cheaper and better in terms of compliance and the ability to support an endothelial lining before they are likely to gain ascendancy over autogenous saphenous vein. More durable results have been obtained by using a vein cuff or patch at the distal anastomosis, particularly when the distal anastomosis in below the knee.

Saphenous vein grafts are also the first choice to replace arteries damaged by trauma (because of the risk of infection) and for other arterial bypass grafts where a small-diameter conduit is required. Examples include renal artery reconstruction and aorto-mesenteric bypass for superior mesenteric artery occlusion.

Percutaneous transluminal angioplasty

Introduction

Percutaneous transluminal angioplasty (PTA) using balloons has become an important technique in the treatment of arterial occlusive disease. It is extensively used in coronary artery disease and makes up as much as 50 per cent of arterial interventions for peripheral ischaemia.

The technique was first described by Grüntzig in 1974 and has rapidly spread since its introduction. As with most new techniques, the indications have only gradually become clear as a result of trial and error. Some of the early extremely promising results have relapsed with later re-stenosis or reocclusion, although repeat procedures are often possible.

Indications for angioplasty

Angioplasty succeeds best where there is a localized stenosis in a relatively large artery with good distal runoff. Thus, most consistent results have been obtained in iliac artery stenoses, followed by isolated and short superficial femoral artery stenoses.

Experienced operators obtain a greater success rate than beginners and will often succeed with unlikely material. An attempt at angioplasty is often justified if reconstructive surgery or amputation is the only alternative, and the patient is unfit. If angioplasty fails, it is unusual for the patient to be worse off as a result, and an alternative plan can be substituted. Angioplasty equipment and experience have developed rapidly and some operators have success even with long occlusions.

In general, the success rate is lower under the following circumstances:

◆ if an occlusion rather than a stenosis is treated;

◆ if a lesion is longer than 10 cm;

◆ if multiple lesions are treated in series;

◆ if the native vessel is of small diameter (e.g. anterior tibial artery);

◆ if the runoff is poor.

Angioplasty is sometimes used in conjunction with reconstructive surgery, either before, after, or during the operation. An example might be angioplasty of an iliac artery stenosis prior to performing a femoro-popliteal bypass graft to avoid the need for a two-level operation.

Technique of angioplasty

Equipment

Angioplasty catheters (Fig. 23.9) are made with balloons of various diameters and lengths and have two channels—one to inflate the balloon and the other to allow distal injections of contrast material or heparinised saline as well as pressure measurements across an arterial stenosis before and after treatment. The balloons are constructed of indistensible polyethylene, which allows inflation only to the predetermined diameter even under extreme pressure (up to 15 atmospheres or

more). Pressure is usually applied using specially designed screw syringes, with or without an attached pressure gauge.

Steps in angioplasty

1. Cannulation of artery. The ipsilateral femoral artery is usually the preferred choice of entry for infra-inguinal stenoses and often for supra-inguinal disease. However, a contralateral approach is required if suitable access is not possible

2. Angiography to define the lesion and select an angioplasty catheter with a balloon of appropriate length and diameter.

3. Passing a guidewire across the stenosis or occlusion.

4. Passing the balloon catheter over the guidewire under X-ray control, so that the radiopaque markers at each end of the deflated balloon lie at each end of the stenosis. This stage may include measurements of arterial pressure above and below the stenosis.

5. Inflation of balloon to a predetermined pressure. This varies with the arterial diameter and the nature of the lesion.

6. Repeat arteriography (and often pressure measurements) to confirm success.

These steps are illustrated in Fig. 23.9.

3.5 Techniques of treating acute ischaemia

Embolectomy

The invention of the Fogarty balloon embolectomy catheter, first described in 1963, transformed and expanded the practice of embolectomy. The Fogarty catheter enables distal thrombo-embolic material to be retrieved remotely via a small arteriotomy. Thus, thrombus could at last be retrieved from as far as the ankle via a femoral arteriotomy. Previously, embolic material and propagated thrombus could only be retrieved by direct arterial exploration and this rarely produced a satisfactory result. Fogarty catheters come in a variety of diameters from 2 to 8 Fr., with progressive increases in the size of balloon. Detailed use of these instruments is shown on page 516.

Thrombolysis

Introduction

Thrombolysis began in the early 1970s (Chesterman 1971; Dotter 1972) with the introduction of streptokinase, an enzyme derived from streptococci. Initially, the drug was used as a systemic agent, administered intravenously, to treat pulmonary embolism. This was soon abandoned because it was found to be ineffective for life-threatening embolism and at the same time produced a high rate of haemorrhagic complications. Complications were mainly caused by the high dosage needed for systemic effect with its unguided and generalized effects, particularly harmful at recent operation sites. However, systemic thrombolysis has recently found its place as a highly effective single-dose emergency therapy for acute myocardial infarction.

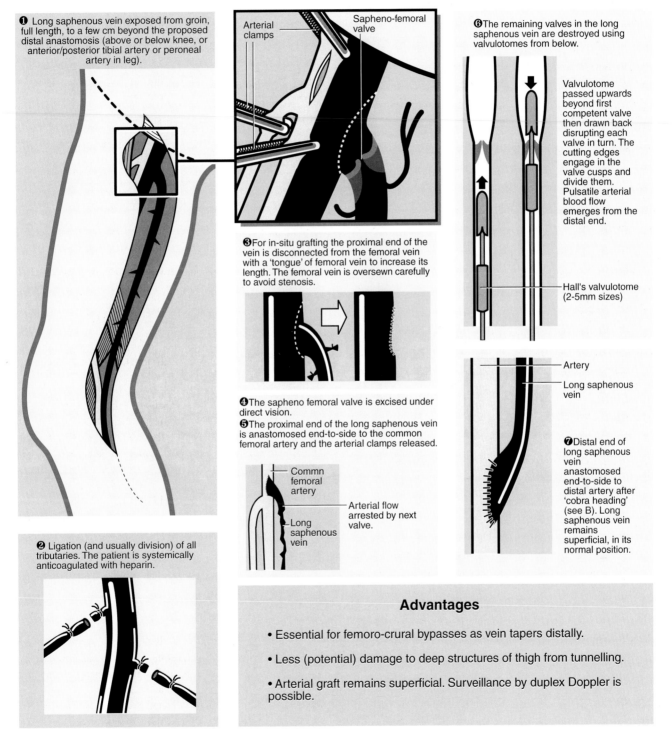

A **Preparation of long saphenous vein for in-situ grafting**

❶ Long saphenous vein exposed from groin, full length, to a few cm beyond the proposed distal anastomosis (above or below knee, or anterior/posterior tibial artery or peroneal artery in leg).

❷ Ligation (and usually division) of all tributaries. The patient is systemically anticoagulated with heparin.

Arterial clamps

Sapheno-femoral valve

❸ For in-situ grafting the proximal end of the vein is disconnected from the femoral vein with a 'tongue' of femoral vein to increase its length. The femoral vein is oversewn carefully to avoid stenosis.

❹ The sapheno femoral valve is excised under direct vision.
❺ The proximal end of the long saphenous vein is anastomosed end-to-side to the common femoral artery and the arterial clamps released.

Commn femoral artery

Arterial flow arrested by next valve.

Long saphenous vein

❻ The remaining valves in the long saphenous vein are destroyed using valvulotomes from below.

Valvulotome passed upwards beyond first competent valve then drawn back disrupting each valve in turn. The cutting edges engage in the valve cusps and divide them. Pulsatile arterial blood flow emerges from the distal end.

Hall's valvulotome (2-5mm sizes)

Artery

Long saphenous vein

❼ Distal end of long saphenous vein anastomosed end-to-side to distal artery after 'cobra heading' (see B). Long saphenous vein remains superficial, in its normal position.

Advantages

- Essential for femoro-crural bypasses as vein tapers distally.

- Less (potential) damage to deep structures of thigh from tunnelling.

- Arterial graft remains superficial. Surveillance by duplex Doppler is possible.

Figure 23.8 Techniques of femoro-popliteal bypass grafting.

B **Preparation of long saphenous vein for reversed saphenous vein fem-pop bypass Steps ❶ and ❷ as in A**

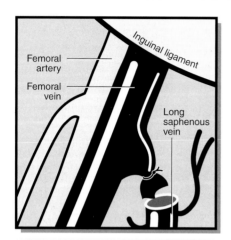

Femoral artery
Femoral vein
Inguinal ligament
Long saphenous vein

❸The long saphenous vein is removed ligating the proximal and distal ends in the patient.

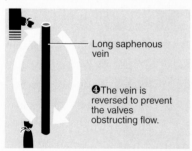

Long saphenous vein

❹The vein is reversed to prevent the valves obstructing flow.

❺Proximal and distal ends are shaped ('cobra headed').

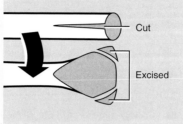

Cut

Excised

❻Long saphenous vein is placed superficially in thigh or deeply alongside superficial femoral artery using a tunnelling device.

❼Proximal ends anastomosed end-to-side to femoral and distal arteries

Synthetic and HUV grafts

For synthetic femoro-popliteal grafting, or human umbilical vein (HUV) graft , proximal and distal arteries are dissected as for vein grafts.

HUV grafts and Dacron grafts are usually anastomosed end-to-side as for long saphenous vein grafting.

PTFE (Goretex®, Impra®) grafts have improved long-term patency if a vein collar or patch is included in the distal anastomosis. This probably provides a 'shock absorber' for the pulse wave transmitted along a rigid graft and reduces the neointimal hyperplasia which develops after a few years in the native artery.

Without vein cuff

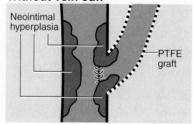

Neointimal hyperplasia

PTFE graft

With vein cuff

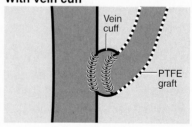

Vein cuff

PTFE graft

Advantages

• No problems with valves.

• Patency no worse than in-situ for fem-pop grafts.

• May be quicker.

• Easier than in-situ to bring proximal end to common femoral artery.

Disadvantages

• Unsuitable for anastomosis to distal arteries (eg tibials).

• If placed deeply - out of reach of duplex Doppler surveillance.

• Taper may make proximal anastomosis unsatisfactory.

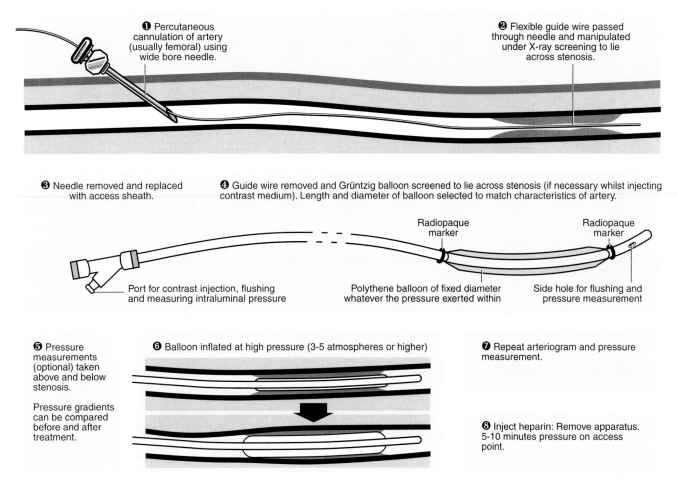

Figure 23.9 Technique of percutaneous transluminal angioplasty (PTA).

Attempts at systemic thrombolysis had never been effective in peripheral arterial occlusion, but in 1974, Dotter introduced a more refined technique of instilling a high local concentration of a thrombolytic agent directly into an occluding thrombus via a catheter. This technique ensures that small volumes of the lytic agent can be placed precisely into the occluding thrombus in the required concentration, yet the overall dose is small and systemic side-effects are minimized. The technique has become widely popular as the methodology, catheter equipment, and lytic agents have gradually improved. Like most new techniques, the most appropriate applications and contraindications have emerged by a process of trial and error.

Thrombolysis has become a valuable tool to treat arterial thrombosis and certain cases of arterial embolism, but must be used judiciously alongside traditional techniques of balloon embolectomy, emergency arterial reconstruction, and percutaneous angioplasty. It is not a panacea for all cases of acute ischaemia, but when used appropriately, may rescue limbs unsalvageable by any other technique. Thrombolysis is largely a percutaneous or minimally invasive technique and is most often performed by radiologists. However, the management of the patient must be an integrated venture between surgeon and radiologist. The surgeon must ensure that the limb is viable and

that it is safe to withhold operation for at least 12 hours. He must also stand by to carry out an urgent operation if thrombolysis runs into trouble of if a lesion requiring surgical correction becomes evident.

Applications of thrombolysis

Arterial thrombolysis is used chiefly for acute arterial occlusion, with the general proviso that the limb must be capable of surviving long enough for the procedure to be completed. In acute ischaemia, the chief applications of thrombolysis are:

- *in situ* thrombosis of an atherosclerotic artery (i.e. acute-on-chronic thrombosis);

- acute thrombosis of a popliteal aneurysm;

- acute occlusion of a PTFE bypass graft.

Until recently, it was thought that there was no point in attempting to declot a saphenous vein bypass graft because it would inevitably be irretrievably damaged by the process of thrombosis; however, there is emerging evidence that, provided intervention with thrombolysis is early, results comparable with PTFE can be obtained with vein grafts.

Obvious acute embolism is most effectively and quickly treated by balloon embolectomy because of the volume of occluding thromboembolic material and often because the severity of ischaemia precludes delay.

Thrombolysis has the unique advantage of being able to lyse thrombus in arteries beyond the reach of an embolectomy catheter. This may enable salvage of a limb where thrombosis or embolism has spread distally (e.g. popliteal aneurysm occlusion). Thrombolysis may be employed intraoperatively after proximal embolectomy if distal clearing is inadequate.

Thrombolysis is most effective with recent thrombus, although satisfactory results have been reported at 3 weeks or more after occlusion, provided the limb has remained viable in the interim.

In about one-third of cases treated successfully with thrombolysis, this is all that is necessary to restore and maintain perfusion. In the other two-thirds, perfusion is temporarily restored but the underlying cause of the occlusion is revealed. These underlying disorders must be treated before the patient is discharged, to prevent early re-thrombosis. The cause may be atherosclerotic stenosis (which is often amenable to angioplasty or may require reconstructive surgery) or anastomotic stenosis in a PTFE bypass graft due to fibromuscular hyperplasia.

Advantages and disadvantages of thrombolysis in treating acute ischaemia

Advantages

◆ May save a limb which is otherwise unsalvageable.

◆ Reveals the cause of occlusion, which is usually treatable by angioplasty or surgery.

◆ Reliably diagnoses untreatable disease in a limb.

◆ May reduce reperfusion injury because of slower revascularization.

Disadvantages

◆ Contraindicated in advanced or severe limb ischaemia (paralysed, numb limbs) because of inevitable delay in revascularization.

◆ Demanding of medical and nursing time—often takes 8 hours or more.

◆ Expensive equipment and lytic agents, particularly tPa.

◆ Only appropriate for about 50 per cent of cases of acute ischaemia.

Table 23.4 Factors in the choice of agent for thrombolytic therapy

Streptokinase	Recombinant tissue plasminogen activator (R-tPa)
Cheap	Expensive
High allergic potential, especially on reuse	Low allergic potential
Cannot be repeated (allergy)	Can be repeated
Works slowly (8–36 hours)	Works quickly (1–8 hours)

◆ Fails in about one-third of highly selected cases.

◆ High risk of complications, including haemorrhage.

Thrombolysis in practice

Choice of thrombolytic agent

The principal choice of agent is between streptokinase and recombinant tissue plasminogen activator (R-tPa), although a few centres are using urokinase and other agents. The lytic ability of the two main agents is probably similar, and their other relative merits are shown in Table 23.4. Both main agents have their adherents, but as the price of tPa falls, it is likely to become the agent of choice.

Techniques of treatment

Introduction

The plan of treatment should be agreed in advance between the radiologist and surgeon, and the surgeon must be available during treatment in case urgent surgery is needed. Negotiations include deciding at what point to abandon the procedure and proceed to surgery and on the management of underlying problems revealed by lysis. The patient needs to be observed in a high dependency area during treatment so that complications can be recognized early.

Where possible, the arterial system is catheterized from the opposite femoral artery (the contralateral approach), although a brachial approach may sometimes be used if femoral arteries are occluded. It is rarely advisable to enter the ipsilateral femoral artery because backwash of the lytic agent risks serious haemorrhage.

The main variables in treatment are in the choice of lytic agent and whether treatment is by bolus or infusion. Choosing between streptokinase and tPa should be governed by local experience of clinical effectiveness, but the large difference in cost may have a bearing on choice. As regards bolus or infusion, most clinicians no longer use single bolus injections, preferring either regular bolus injections, often at 15 minute intervals, or a continuous infusion. The choice is largely personal as results do not show a clear benefit for either method.

Technique

A standard technique is as follows:

1. Introduction of a valved operating sheath into the opposite femoral artery. Under local infiltration anaesthesia, the femoral artery is cannulated using a metal needle. A flexible guidewire is passed through the needle to lie within the femoral artery and the needle is removed and replaced with a plastic sheath. This provides a conduit for passing instruments and catheters into the artery without further wall trauma and without leakage of blood.

2. Diagnostic angiography. This is performed via a pigtail catheter passed over a guidewire across the aortic bifurcation. This demonstrates the site and extent of occlusion and may show any patent runoff vessels.

3. Physical break-up of the clot using a guidewire. Using fluoroscopic screening, the guidewire is passed distally into the occluding thrombus and across it several times to disrupt it.

4. Introduction of a thrombolysis catheter over the guidewire, which is then removed. The thrombolysis catheter is passed at least 2 cm into the thrombus (some prefer to pass it two-thirds of the way through the thrombus). Newer catheters have multiple slit-like side holes in the distal part for 'lacing' the thrombus with lytic agent.

5. Intermittent bolus injection or infusion of lytic agent.

6. If tPa is used, check lysis on repeat angiogram at 2 hours; if streptokinase is used, check at 6–12 hours.

7. Continue infusion/injection and intermittent angiography as above, advancing the catheter as the thrombus lyses and continuing until distal vessels are seen to be clear. If clearance is unsatisfactory after 24 hours, the procedure will usually be abandoned.

8. If a stenosis is found to underlie the acute thrombosis, consider immediate angioplasty or early reconstructive surgery.

Most radiologists employ heparin infusion near the end of the procedure to prevent rebound re-thrombosis.

If the limb deteriorates during treatment, this may be due to shifting of thrombus or debris distally.

Results of thrombolysis

In most series, only about 50 per cent of acutely ischaemic lower limbs have been regarded as suitable for thrombolysis. In addition, most units believe that acute upper-limb ischaemia should not be treated by lysis.

Using streptokinase in appropriate patients, effective lysis occurs in about two-thirds of patients in an average of 24 hours.

In a few late failures, arterial clearance occurs but venous obstruction prevents adequate revascularization. Using tPa, similar rates of clearance have been obtained but clearance is quicker, taking an average of 8 hours.

In general, one-third of successful cases need no further treatment, one-third require additional angioplasty, and one-third additional reconstructive surgery.

Complications of thrombolysis

Complications include haemorrhage (substantial bleeding in about 5 per cent), allergy to streptokinase in 5 per cent, distal embolism in 3 per cent, and transient stroke (presumed haemorrhagic) in 3 per cent. In one series, there was a 20 per cent amputation rate and a 7 per cent death rate following thrombolysis. This compares favourably with results from surgically treated patients with acute ischaemia. Table 23.5 summarizes the means by which complications of thrombolysis may be avoided.

3.6 Sympathectomy

Lumbar sympathectomy

Introduction

Open surgical sympathectomy for lower-limb occlusive disease is rarely employed nowadays and has been largely replaced by percutaneous chemical sympathectomy. Some surgeons perform the technique themselves but it is often carried out by anaesthetists.

Indications

Sympathectomy is a minimally invasive procedure designed to improve skin blood flow in the foot by blocking sympathetic vasomotor tone. It has no effect on muscle blood flow or overall limb perfusion and therefore has no place in treating inter-

Table 23.5 Avoiding complications of thrombolysis

Point of technique	Complication
Use contralateral femoral artery or brachial to enter arterial system	Minimizes risk of haemorrhage from entry point because of backwash of lytic agent
Special care if there is a recent operation site	Local haemorrhage
Special care with thrombosed Dacron grafts	Bleeding may occur through the wall even years after implantation
Avoid traumatic arterial puncture	Trauma may cause haemorrhage, elevation of an occluding flap, or arteriovenous fistula
Take care when applying prolonged pressure at puncture site after withdrawal of sheath	Pressure sufficient to occlude the femoral artery may allow thrombosis to develop distally
Ensure that the patient is heparinized immediately after the procedure	Re-thrombosis may occur in newly cleared vessels
Avoid delay in dilating strictures or surgically removing debris	Re-thrombosis may occur in newly cleared vessels
Do not prolong thrombolysis if progress is inadequate	Failure to revascularize by lysis may result in irreversible ischaemic changes if definitive surgery is delayed as a consequence. Complications related to catheter and lytic agent are more likely to occur with prolonged thrombolysis
Look for occult bleeding by careful observation of the patient in a high dependency area	Major concealed haemorrhage may occur during treatment (e.g. retroperitoneal)

mittent claudication. For the same reasons, the procedure has insufficient beneficial effect in patients with gangrene, particularly if infected. Its prime indication is in an attempt to 'tip the balance' in patients with early rest pain or ischaemic ulceration. There are no reliable tests to predict the likely success of sympathectomy, but using clinical criteria, about 50 per cent of patients undergoing the procedure are likely to benefit.

Technique

The procedure is performed under local infiltration anaesthesia. Most practitioners use an operating table and an image intensifier to localize the injections. The patient lies in a curled lateral position with the side to be treated uppermost. A 20-gauge spinal needle is passed from lateral to the erector spinae to touch the lateral side of the lumbar vertebral body at L3. It is then withdrawn slightly and passed beyond into the longitudinal space around the lumbar sympathetic chain.

Correct positioning is confirmed by injecting a small amount of contrast material which is seen to flow within a confined longitudinal space. Two more needles are similarly placed at L4 and L5 levels and then 5 ml of 6 per cent aqueous phenol (NOT liquefied phenol or phenol in oil) is injected into each needle.

Any beneficial effect will be recognized within 2–4 hours by the foot becoming warmer. This can be checked using a skin thermometer before and after the procedure and comparing the differential between left and right feet. Patients are usually able to return home the same or the following day. Complications are uncommon.

Even if the foot warms, ultimate success can usually only be confirmed by a favourable response observed over several days or weeks, with remission of rest pain and healing of ulcers.

3.7 Venous access for dialysis

Circulatory access in acute renal failure

Dialysis for renal failure requires intermittent access to part of the circulation with a high blood flow. In acute renal failure, a Scribner shunt used to be the most widely used form of temporary access. This was also used on a semipermanent basis in the early days of dialysis before subcutaneous arteriovenous fistulas were introduced.

A Scribner shunt was usually performed at the wrist and involves inserting a small cannula into both the radial artery and the cephalic vein. A silicone-rubber tube was connected to each cannula beneath the skin and formed a loop above the skin which could be opened to connect to the dialyser. Nowadays, acute renal failure is more often treated initially by haemofiltration, with circulatory access via indwelling catheters in a large artery and vein, often the femoral.

Circulatory access in chronic renal failure

For chronic dialysis, a more permanent solution to the problem of circulatory access is provided by the Cimino–Brescia fistula (Fig. 23.10). In this procedure, an artificial subcutaneous arteriovenous fistula is created by anastomosing the radial artery to the cephalic vein at the wrist. This causes gradual dilatation of the forearm veins over 2–3 months which can then easily be cannulated to remove and return blood for dialysis.

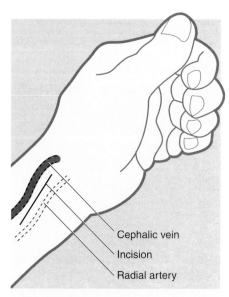

Usually performed under local anaesthesia in the non-dominant wrist using magnification (loupe or microscope)

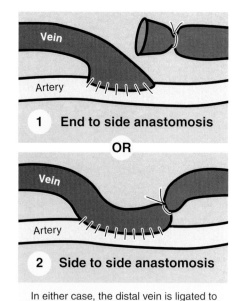

In either case, the distal vein is ligated to prevent dilatation of the hand veins.
The vessels are rarely more than 2mm in diameter, so success is dependent on meticulous technique.
This includes no handling of intima, avoidance of inverting adventitial edge and avoidance of picking up posterior wall of artery with needle.

Figure 23.10 Technique of Cimino–Brescia fistula for renal dialysis.

4 Principles of anaesthesia for arterial surgery

4.1 Introduction

Anaesthesia for aortic and carotid surgery are two of the most demanding tasks for an anaesthetist. The potential of arteriopathic patients to compensate for the stresses of surgery is invariably impaired by widespread vascular disease—atherosclerosis and arteriolar hypertrophy and constriction—both of which impair arterial compliance.

In particular, these patients are usually hypertensive, with evident or occult ischaemic heart disease and often have an impaired renal or cerebral blood supply, or both. They are often smokers with consequent lung disease.

4.2 Aortic surgery

During aortic surgery, there are rapid haemodynamic changes which can cause extreme swings in intravascular pressure. The causes include:

- the autonomic response to surgery (high levels of circulating catecholamines);

- haemorrhage (which may be sudden and catastrophic);

- the effects of clamping the aorta (rapid rise in cardiac afterload which may precipitate severe hypertension or left ventricular failure);

- unclamping the aorta (equivalent to haemorrhage of more than 1 litre of blood);

- the rapid inflow of metabolic products of ischaemia to the circulation (mainly hydrogen ions in the form of lactic acid).

4.3 Carotid surgery

During carotid artery clamping, it is vital to ensure that the brain remains perfused. After operation, the patient may be subject to unpredictable swings in blood pressure owing to the surgical trauma to carotid baroreceptor nerves. Thus peroperative and postoperative monitoring of cerebral function and blood pressure is vital and appropriate interventions should be taken early.

Table 23.6 Special tests for cardiovascular assessment

Exercise ECG—now recognized to be of little benefit over static ECG
Echocardiography, to assess areas of abnormal ventricular wall movement, ejection fraction, and valvular function
Isotope scans to assess regional myocardial perfusion and its reversibility with drugs
Coronary angiography if other tests indicate a high risk

4.4 Preoperative assessment of the patient for major arterial surgery

Introduction

Passing a patient as fit for surgery is an imprecise science and is based on a balance of probabilities. Given the presenting complaint (i.e. an aneurysm in danger of rupture or a state of lower-limb ischaemia), is the risk benefit to the patient in favour of surgery?

As regards cardiovascular assessment, hypertension, arrhythmias, and cardiac failure must be under good control. Cardiovascular function can be assessed at rest and under mild exercise stress. However, standard exercise routines cannot test the circulation to the levels of stress experienced in an aortic operation and are thus never completely satisfactory.

If there is a history of ischaemic heart disease or clinical cardiac examination, chest X-ray, or ECG at rest is abnormal, this warns of troubles ahead. However, if these test results are normal, this does not mean that this patient's cardiovascular system will withstand the stresses of operation. In cardiac cases, special tests of cardiovascular function should be employed (Table 23.6).

4.5 Preoperative preparation

An intensive care bed or equivalent must be available for postoperative care. A proportion of patients will not require this, but it is not possible to reliably predict operative or anaesthetic problems which will demand continuous postoperative care. For this reason, it would be negligent to perform elective aortic surgery without confirming that an ITU bed is available. In emergency aortic surgery, the demand for an ITU bed is even more pressing, but surgery must not be delayed because of the lack of an ITU bed.

It should be noted that an intensive care unit is an alien place in which to awaken after operation and patients benefit from a preoperative visit to the unit or at least a chance to meet the nurses who will be looking after them.

Prescribed cardiovascular drugs should be continued up to the stage of premedication and any anticoagulants modified according to a predetermined plan.

No special drugs are required for premedication. The choice depends on the condition of the patient, the anaesthetic technique to be used, and the anaesthetist's personal preference. It must, however, be sufficient to quell all fear which might provoke dangerous tachycardia and hypertension at induction.

4.6 The anaesthetic

Haemodynamic monitoring

Continuous haemodynamic monitoring is required because changes can be so rapid that they are likely to be missed by intermittent measurement. The minimum monitoring is direct measurement of arterial pressure (usually via a radial artery cannula, but note that blood pressure may be unequal in the two arms), and of cardiac filling pressure. The latter is usually achieved via a central venous cannula placed into the internal jugular vein.

There is still discussion about which patients need monitoring of pulmonary artery wedge pressure. The current consensus is in favour of selective use of a Swan–Ganz catheter in patients at particular risk of differential pressure between left and right atria, predominantly those with a left ventricular ejection fraction of less than 0.5. In addition, patients treated for left ventricular failure and patients with severe angina should be monitored in this way. There are drawbacks to the use of these catheters. They are technically more difficult to place than CVP lines and they are subject to inaccurate readings unless great care is taken in their use.

Blood loss during operation is continually monitored, both by suction volume and by swab weighing, so that blood replacement can be anticipated. Urine output is measured at regular intervals (usually hourly) via a urinary catheter draining into a burette. This gives reassurance that renal perfusion pressure and volume is maintained and provides an indirect measure of adequacy of fluid replacement.

Other monitoring

Standard anaesthetic monitoring is used, including continuous ECG trace, arterial oxygen saturation, and end-tidal CO_2.

Special points of anaesthetic technique in major arterial surgery

◆ The adrenergic response to surgery needs to be firmly suppressed.

◆ Sharp rises and falls of arterial pressure must be prevented during the stress moments of induction and intubation, clamping and unclamping the aorta, and episodes of rapid haemorrhage.

◆ Hypocapnia must be avoided.

◆ Ventilatory control is used to eliminate the carbon dioxide resulting from the lactic acidosis after aortic unclamping. Bicarbonate rarely needs to be given.

◆ Renal support is standard, using low-dose dopamine.

Analgesia

Standard intravenous opiate agents are used but long-acting local anaesthetics given via a low-thoracic or high-lumbar epidural catheter give excellent analgesia during operation and afterwards.

4.7 Fluid balance

This vital process involves titrating the fluid requirements against the measured loss of blood, the urine output, and the changes in intravascular pressure. Given the rigid, inelastic arterial circulation, with its limited ability to compensate for changes in fluid volume, fluid management works best if the anaesthetist is able to anticipate changes at different stages of the operation; for example, giving nitroprusside to dilate the rest of the circulation prior to aortic clamping and transfusing blood prior to aortic unclamping.

Fluid must be capable of being given rapidly. This requires at least one 12- or 14-gauge cannula and the availability of blood-warming apparatus and pressure infusers. Whole blood is undoubtedly the best replacement for blood loss. As bank blood is increasingly offered as packed cells with clotting factors removed, there is a trend towards methods of conserving the patient's own blood. These include:

◆ Predonation of two or more units of the patient's blood, collected over several weeks prior to elective surgery.

◆ Normovolaemic haemodilution (i.e. collecting blood from the patient immediately prior to surgery and replacing it with colloid) has several potential advantages over transfusion of bank blood: oxygen delivery is increased in patients by moderate acute normovolaemic anaemia; the blood is fresh and contains viable platelets if kept at room temperature. It also contains significant levels of labile clotting factors. Up to 2000 ml of blood can be removed safely from adults without cardiac disease immediately before an operation and replaced with an equal volume of colloid. When about 300 ml of (low haematocrit) blood have been lost at operation, autologous blood with a normal haematocrit is transfused. If blood loss is less than 2 litres, additional bank blood is rarely needed. The procedure is inexpensive, convenient for the patient, and flexible as regards operation scheduling.

◆ Spilled blood can be collected and autotransfused using either a 'cell saver' system, which washes the red cells and resuspends them in saline before transfusion, or the simpler Solcotrans system which anticoagulates the collected blood, which is filtered before return to the circulation.

4.8 Recovery

Recovery after arterial surgery depends on the magnitude of the operation and on the age and general fitness of the patient. Any operation that opens the abdomen has a longer recovery period than a peripheral arterial operation such as femoro-popliteal bypass graft, which requires a lighter anaesthetic and less analgesia. An aortic replacement for aneurysm causes considerable physiological trauma. This includes heavy blood loss and its

Table 23.7 Indications for elective ventilation for 12 hours or more after aortic reconstructive surgery

Large peroperative blood loss
Marked peroperative cardiovascular instability
Respiratory insufficiency
Likely need for emergency reoperation
Pre-existing episodes of left ventricular failure
Marked angina of effort

replacement, disruption of pulmonary and other vital functions which may require elective mechanical ventilation while physiological processes return towards normal, and a need for powerful postoperative analgesia. These patients are best assumed to require intensive care after operation and it is unwise to proceed to an elective operation unless a bed is available. In many units, patients can be admitted to ITU before operation and baseline measurements made and monitoring established before operation.

Intensive care management includes:

1. **Ventilation.** Opinions vary as to whether to ventilate patients for an elective period after operation. Some anaesthetists like to ventilate patients for an hour or two while setting up monitoring, and ensuring that the patient is stable in ITU before extubation because awakening may be associated with increased sympathetic activity, vasoconstriction, hypertension, and tachycardia. Table 23.7 shows some generally accepted indications for elective ventilation after major vascular surgery.

2. **Fluid management.** Continued blood loss and compartmental shifts demand continued haemodynamic and urine output monitoring, fluid replacement, and, if necessary, replacement of clotting factors and platelets. Excessive blood loss may need a return to theatre.

3. **Lower-limb circulation.** This needs to be assessed to ensure it is not impaired by embolism or thrombosis. If the feet are pink and warm with palpable pulses, circulatory integrity is assured. In contrast, a blue, cold foot is ischaemic and likely to need surgical attention to the arterial circulation. In doubtful cases, thermocouples attached to each big toe give an indication of reperfusion. Once the temperature rises above 27 °C, the omens are good. Doppler ultrasound can be used to measure ankle blood pressure. A level greater than 100 mmHg is generally satisfactory.

In most cases, 24 hours in the intensive care unit is sufficient to ensure that the patient is stable, self-ventilating, and with no continuing blood loss. At this point the patient may be returned to the general ward.

5 Common emergency and elective conditions

5.1 Peripheral arterial insufficiency

Introduction

In a patient with progressive atherosclerosis, there is a gradual patchy occlusion of large arteries of distribution and, at the same time, compensatory dilatation of collateral arteries circumventing the occlusion. This results in a battle to preserve function as well as survival of the organ or tissue supplied. In chronic arterial insufficiency, the balance becomes tipped against preservation if the narrowed arteries then undergo acute thrombosis.

For the peripheral arterial surgeon, chronic arterial insufficiency most often manifests as intermittent claudication. This represents a state of relative ischaemia of the lower limb, worst at the periphery, which is revealed by exercise. The limb is not in imminent danger of necrosis, and at rest, the volume of blood circulating through the limb is little different from normal. In more severe ischaemia, the blood flow volume at rest is impaired and 'rest pain' and other stigmata of critical ischaemia are likely to appear. The limb is now under threat and may be critically ischaemic.

Potential benefits of reconstructive arterial surgery

In general, the surgical treatment of atherosclerosis must be regarded as palliative since the underlying cause is unaffected and the disease is likely to progress unabated. Nevertheless, reconstructive surgery may have the obvious benefit of returning the patient to enjoy a productive life and, in many cases, maintain an independent existence. Reconstructive arterial surgery can thereby have profound economic and social benefits. A secondary effect may be to restore motivation, encourage abandoning harmful habits such as cigarette smoking, and enable the patient to exercise, all of which may prolong life.

Special risks in patients with ischaemic tissues

Patients with chronically ischaemic tissues are at particular risk as follows:

◆ Without revascularization, healing is impaired—amputation of a necrotic toe in an ischaemic leg will not heal; infection is liable to enter and become entrenched in the vulnerable tissue. This causes spreading tissue death and systemic sepsis.

◆ Heels and other bony prominences are susceptible to pressure sores and therefore particular care must be taken of these areas before, during, and after surgery. Loss of tissue over pressure points is often the result of neglecting this principle. It may result in extended hospitalization and often further operations for amputation or skin grafting.

Evaluation of chronic lower-limb ischaemia

When evaluating an ischaemic limb, it is important to grasp that there is a continuum of severity which ranges from mild claudication, brought on only by extreme exercise, to established necrosis. Management of both extremes is usually unambiguous but management of the middle range is more problematic. Furthermore, the rate of development and progression of ischaemia profoundly influences the management.

Chronic severe ischaemia develops gradually over days or weeks and can usually be investigated on an outpatient basis, whereas ischaemia of rapid or sudden onset is often more complete, requiring urgent hospital admission. This may fall within the definition of acute ischaemia (see below).

When deciding whether to investigate and when to treat patients with ischaemic symptoms, the important factors are:

Table 23.8 Less common causes of chronic lower-limb ischaemia

Underlying cause	Description
Occluded popliteal aneurysm	Popliteal aneurysms may thrombose, resulting in chronic ischaemia. Sudden thrombosis or embolism of thrombus accumulated within the aneurysm may cause acute ischaemia
Congenital popliteal artery entrapment	This is due to an abnormal insertion of the medial head of gastrocnemius. (This should be considered if a younger patient presents with claudication or an acutely ischaemic limb)
Cystic adventitial degeneration of the popliteal artery	This condition of unknown aetiology produces marked thickening of the popliteal artery wall. It should be considered in younger patients with ischaemia of the lower limb
Blood disorders producing hypercoagulability	In a small proportion of patients with an ischaemic lower limb, a blood disorder is the primary pathology. The blood disorder may only become apparent years later. Disorders include: polycythaemia rubra vera, essential thrombocythaemia, and blood neoplasias
Buerger's disease	Buerger's disease and similar disorders such as Takayasu's disease are much more common in Japan and the Far East. The aetiology is unknown but may be associated with variations in smoking material
Other forms of arteritis	These are very rare and usually associated with collagen disorders such as ankylosing spondylitis

◆ What is the functional defect or handicap? (Is any treatment necessary?)

◆ How severe is the ischaemia? (Does it need treatment and if so how radical?)

◆ Is ischaemia progressive and if so how rapidly? (How quickly is intervention needed?)

◆ Is there spreading infection? (Is amputation required?)

Most of these questions can be answered by clinical evaluation aided by simple ankle pressure tests. Arteriography is not a measure of physiological function and should be performed only when the decision to operate has been taken.

Critical ischaemia

Aetiology of severe and critical ischaemia

In Western countries, the usual cause of severe lower-limb ischaemia is atherosclerotic occlusion of large vessels of distribution. This can occur anywhere between the abdominal aorta and the tibial and peroneal arteries, often at multiple levels.

Diabetics have a higher incidence of atherosclerosis, which often manifests at an earlier age but follows a similar pattern to that of non-diabetics. Diabetic patients also suffer with neuropathic foot complications which are not predominantly ischaemic (see below). A third cause of foot problems in diabetics is probably 'small vessel disease' affecting digital arteries and resulting in isolated toe necrosis in an otherwise well-perfused foot.

In some Eastern countries, notably Japan, Buerger's disease is a more frequent cause of chronic, severe limb ischaemia. This is an occlusive disorder of younger people, affecting small distal arteries (and probably veins) which results in a centripetal pattern of necrosis and, often, stepwise amputations. It also affects the upper limb and is always associated with smoking. It is extremely rare in the West.

There are several other causes of severe lower-limb ischaemia which are much less common than atherosclerosis (Table 23.8).

Pathophysiology of critical ischaemia

In severe chronic ischaemia, the blood flow volume at rest is impaired and rest pain is likely to occur. This term should be reserved for a symptom complex in which the patient suffers severe pain in the skin of the foot which usually comes on at night (cardiac output falls during sleep, gravity assistance to flow to the foot is lost, skin vessels dilate with warmth). On waking, an hour or two after going to bed, the patient typically hangs the affected foot out of bed or walks around with some relief.

In more severe and protracted cases, the patient sleeps in a chair, often with the foot drawn up towards the chest, and develops dependency oedema and eventually, fixed flexion contractures of the knee. Ischaemic ulceration may occur (usually caused by slight trauma with non-healing due to ischaemia), and necrosis or gangrene may supervene. If toe necrosis is present, the toe alone may be involved or, more seriously, the web space or the deep layers of the foot.

Apart from the lack of blood supply, a further pathological process aggravates the condition. The normal microvascular defence system becomes inappropriately activated and vicious circles develop between activated platelets, activated leucocytes,

---

Box 23.3 Definition of critical ischaemia

It is important to define critical limb ischaemia precisely, so that clinicians agree that they are talking about the same condition when comparing the results of treatment. In 1992, the Second European Working Group on Critical Limb Ischaemia produced a consensus document which defined critical limb ischaemia as follows:

Critical limb ischaemia exists when there is:

1. persistently recurring rest pain requiring regular analgesia for more than 2 weeks, or ulceration or gangrene at the foot; plus

2. an ankle systolic pressure less than 50 mm Hg. In diabetics, this pressure criterion is replaced with absence of palpable ankle pulses because of the unreliability of pressure measurement due to arterial calcification.

and damaged endothelium, which, in association with local ischaemia, lead to irreversible tissue damage.

A patient who presents with typical signs and symptoms of severe ischaemia will almost certainly require some form of intervention. If the limb is critically ischaemic (see definition Box 23.3), the limb or even the patient's life may be lost if there is no intervention.

Intervention in severe ischaemia is needed for two main reasons. First, rest pain is intolerable because it is difficult or impossible to control with analgesia. Secondly, there is an appreciable risk of progression to gangrene and inevitable limb loss, particularly if there is skin breakdown and infection. Thus, even in patients in poor general health, active measures should be pursued with the intention of improving the perfusion of the lower limb, or amputation if this is impracticable.

In the UK, the incidence of critical ischaemia is 500–1000 per million population per year. About one in four will need a major amputation within a year of presentation.

Treatment of severe and critical lower-limb ischaemia

Introduction

Treatment for limb salvage is aimed at substantially increasing lower-limb arterial blood supply. The most effective methods of relieving arterial obstruction are by balloon angioplasty or reconstructive arterial surgery. In acute ischaemia, discussed later, thrombolysis is often appropriate as a first stage.

Medical treatments with prostanoids (e.g. prostacyclin) reverse many of the damaging effects of the activated microvascular defence mechanisms but, for the moment, should be seen as adjuncts to mechanical methods or as topics for research.

Sympathectomy is ineffective when survival of a limb is threatened by ischaemia, as it merely redistributes some of the available blood to the skin. It may, however, be effective in the early stages of rest pain or mild skin ulceration.

Factors to be considered in planning therapy

1. How urgently is treatment required? Wet gangrene or other evidence of spreading infection demands immediate hospital admission and treatment with intravenous antibiotics while investigating the pathological anatomy of the arterial tree or proceeding directly to amputation. Severe rest pain should similarly be given a high degree of urgency. If, however, the pain is manageable with analgesics and the condition is not deteriorating rapidly, investigation may proceed on an outpatient basis.

2. How severe is the threat to the viability of the limb and is the patient's life threatened by sepsis?

3. Are there any visible breaks in the skin caused by ischaemia where infection could enter (e.g. ulcers, fissures, tissue breakdown at the junction with necrotic tissue)?

4. Is infection spreading through the tissues of the limb (cellulitis)? This represents a real risk of systemic infection or septicaemia and declining renal function as a con-sequence.

5. What is the severity of ischaemia? This is assessed by clinical means (history of rest pain, presence of shiny, atrophic skin, ulceration, gangrene) and by Doppler ultrasound to determine ankle systolic pressure. Oxygen saturation probes, isotope clearance studies or plethysmography to measure blood flow and laser Doppler are presently research tools without clear application to daily surgical practice.

6. What is the extent of irreversible tissue loss? Will amputation be necessary even if revascularization is successful?. Without revascularization, major amputation above or below knee is inevitable if there is tissue necrosis, but with successful revascularization, the extent of tissue loss may be minimized. For example, minor digit amputations may be performed at the same time as reconstruction with a good prospect of healing. Often a **provisional amputation** to remove infected material is useful at the time of revascularization, with later fashioning of a formal stump.

7. Are there factors in the patient's general health which make reconstructive surgery inadvisable? Fixed flexion deformities of the knee or, more rarely the hip, may prevent a revascularized limb being useful. If the patient is bedbound or wholly wheelchair dependent, primary amputation may be the best choice. Continued cigarette smoking by the patient is likely to jeopardize arterial reconstruction in the long term and attempts should be made to persuade the patient to abstain.

Principles of surgical treatment of critical ischaemia

Reconstructive arterial surgery or, less commonly, angioplasty is used to restore peripheral perfusion. After clinical assessment, the next stage is usually to perform an arteriogram to demonstrate the extent and distribution of arterial stenoses and occlusions. Care should be taken to demonstrate any patent and potentially graftable arteries down to the foot, and if possible, show the integrity of the pedal arch.

In a patient with multiple stenoses or occlusions, is sometimes a matter of clinical judgement as to which is primarily responsible for the ischaemia and which, if corrected, would be likely to salvage the limb. However, in principle:

◆ Proximal occlusions should be treated first, even if the superficial femoral artery is occluded. If satisfactory inflow to the profunda femoris can be achieved, the operation is likely to succeed if there is reasonable runoff.

◆ An occluded popliteal artery should be bypassed unless collaterals are excellent. The popliteal is the single common pathway between the two arteries supplying the thigh and the three vessels supplying the calf.

◆ Long femoro-crural vein bypass grafts are often required in distal disease. The best of the three tibial vessels is chosen as the recipient of the graft. The choice is based on Doppler flow detection (if necessary assisted by pulse-generated runoff (PGR) which temporarily generates an artificial pulse using a calf compression device), duplex Doppler scanning, and arteriography (preoperative or on-table). Doppler-based investigations can detect up to 30 per cent more patent vessels at the calf than preoperative angiography; an audible flow signal in a tibial vessel often means that it will be a suitable recipient for a graft, and a lack of patent vessels on arteriography should not necessarily be equated with the need for amputation. A patent pedal arch on arteriography is a good prognostic sign in difficult cases with undetectable pulses.

Intermittent claudication

Introduction

The onset of claudication symptoms is probably precipitated by thrombotic occlusion of a stenotic artery. There is a span of severity ranging between mild claudication, which barely limits activity, and severe claudication with rest pain, bordering on critical ischaemia.

Superficially similar symptoms may be caused by spinal claudication in which the cauda equina is compressed by special stenosis or central disc protrusion. However, symptoms are very variable and walking is often easier uphill. CT scanning demonstrates the spinal compression.

Intermittent claudication is a relatively benign condition, with the unusual characteristic of tending to improve spontaneously with time in a least 50 per cent of cases. The risk of eventual amputation is low, even in untreated cases (less than 10 per cent). Indeed, most amputations for ischaemia occur in patients presenting first with critical ischaemia. With these facts in mind, the surgeon can predict a degree of spontaneous improvement, particularly if there are favourable changes in the patient's lifestyle.

This is often a more prudent course than proceeding rapidly to reconstructive surgery, with its appreciable risk of failure and amputation. Occasionally, a patient may demand a reconstructive operation, and although his wishes must be weighed in the balance, intervention should not be undertaken for claudication alone unless the following criteria can largely be met:

◆ giving up cigarette smoking;

◆ fairly good general health with a reasonable life expectancy;

◆ unless handicap is extreme, a period of 6 months, and possibly a year, after onset of symptoms should be allowed to pass for collaterals to develop;

◆ demonstration of reconstructable vessels with a realistic chance of operative success.

Making the diagnosis

The clinician's first task is to make an aetiological diagnosis. In most cases this will be atherosclerosis, but other conditions causing similar symptoms need to be excluded (see Table 23.8). An assessment is then made of how severe the ischaemia is in terms of potential tissue damage and how the arterial insufficiency affects exercise capacity.

Severity of ischaemia is assessed by clinical examination for palpable pulses and signs of trophic or nutritional changes in the feet and legs, by Buerger's test, and by ankle systolic blood pressures measured by Doppler ultrasound. In some units, colour duplex is the next investigation of choice. Arteriography is not a physiological study of function and should only be used in patients in whom interventional manoeuvres have been decided upon.

Next, the site or sites of obliterative arterial disease should be evaluated. These may be multifocal and may be bilateral. The pattern of arterial occlusion has a considerable bearing on the type of intervention that might be offered and, indeed, whether any intervention might be offered at all. For example a man in his fifties with aorto-iliac disease, who is unable to work because of severe claudication, is likely to have good distal vessels and therefore a relatively straightforward proximal reconstruction has a high chance of success. In contrast, an elderly man with good proximal vessels and severe disease below the knees on both sides would require complex, high-risk femoro-distal bypasses on each side, with a relatively high chance of failure as well as considerable physiological upset in undergoing two major operations. The operating time and hospital time must also be taken into account. Most surgeons would not consider complex distal bypasses in patients with symptoms of intermittent claudication alone because of the high price of failure.

In recent years, with the increasing popularity of balloon angioplasty, more patients who might not be considered for open reconstructive arterial surgery are nevertheless offered arteriography in the hope that angioplasty will be possible. As a result, more patients are being treated more successfully for arterial disease than was formerly the case.

Clearly the advisability of investigation and reconstructive surgery depends to a certain extent on the likelihood of spontaneous improvement of the symptoms. In most patients, any major degree of spontaneous improvement will have occurred within 6–12 months after the onset of symptoms, but stopping smoking will probably accelerate the rate of improvement. Other factors to be considered in deciding on operation or otherwise depend on a general physical examination and tests, as indicated below.

Factors in deciding which claudication patients should have further investigation with a view to intervention

◆ Age—younger patients generally demand greater mobility.

◆ Severity of handicap in relation to work and leisure activities.

◆ Willingness to give up smoking.

◆ Poor chance of adequate spontaneous improvement: long history, severe symptoms.

◆ Perceived danger of progression.

◆ Symptoms suggesting rest pain, and clinical examination showing trophic changes.

Table 23.9 Problems of femoro-popliteal bypass grafting operations

Finding	Action
At operation	
Occluded common femoral artery (CFA)	Endarterectomy of CFA, or interposition graft of Dacron or expanded PTFE before anastomosing proximal end of vein graft
Occluded or tightly stenosed popliteal artery	Explore popliteal artery more distally, if necessary, below knee
Saphenous vein largely unsuitable for grafting	Use Dacron or expanded PTFE graft or, if part of vein suitable, construct composite of part leg vein and part arm vein. PTFE grafts should have a distal vein collar or patch if anastomosed below the knee
Saphenous vein partly varicose	Excise varices and repair vein. Note: signs of old thrombosis should lead to rejecting the vein
Poor flow through graft	Assuming good inflow, check vein for mechanical defects—anastomotic narrowing, intimal flaps at anastomoses, residual valves in *in situ* grafts, twist of reversed vein grafts
Foot fails to 'pink up' on release of clamps	Mechanical defects in graft or thrombosis of proximal or distal artery or graft. Reopen graft and clear with a Fogarty catheter. If this fails, on-table arteriography to reveal defect
Early postoperative problems	
Haemorrhage	Re-explore site of haemorrhage
Foot loses perfusion	Re-explore graft and proceed as when foot fails to pink up (see above). Often technical error—twisting of graft, intimal flap, or retained valve cusp
Wound-edge necrosis	Await healing by secondary intention. Excise if necessary
Lymphatic leakage or lymphocoele in groin	Await spontaneous resolution, which may take 6–8 weeks, or inject patent blue dye into thigh and underrun site of leakage. Aspiration of lymphocoele is not helpful
Wound infection	Vein grafts are fairly resistant to infection. Treat with antibiotics. Synthetic grafts usually need to be removed, particularly if Gram-negative infection, and alternative means of revascularization found
Intermediate (30 days to 12 months)	
Arteriovenous fistula	Results from residual patent tributaries. Causes patches of skin necrosis. Treat by ligation
Vein graft occlusion after 30 days and less than 1 year	Anticipate by graft surveillance after 3 months. Most early graft failures are due to strictures, which develop in 25 per cent of cases during the early postoperative weeks. Surveillance may be by arteriography or duplex Doppler
Late	
Graft occlusion after 1 year	Usually due to disease progression. Manage according to symptoms, signs, and arteriography

◆ Favourable vascular anatomy and ease of surgical or endovascular treatment.

◆ Favourable cardiorespiratory risk assessment—blood pressure, cardiac failure, aortic stenosis and other valvular disorders, low cardiac output, chronic chest disease.

◆ Extracranial arterial disease with potential for stroke.

◆ Drug therapy: beta-blockers should be stopped.

◆ Blood disorders predisposing to thrombosis: polycythaemia, thrombocythaemia, prothrombotic states (previous spontaneous intravascular thrombosis).

◆ Level of ankle pressures before and after exercise.

Operations for claudication

As for critical ischaemia, the type of operation depends on which stenoses or occlusions are regarded as significant.

In general, if femoral pulses are impalpable, supra-inguinal reconstruction is likely to be needed. This may be aorto-iliac angioplasty, aorto-bifemoral grafting, or extra-anatomic grafting such as crossover femoro-femoral grafting.

If femoral pulses are good, distal reconstruction is likely to be needed. This is most often femoro-popliteal bypass grafting or occasionally profundoplasty or common femoral endarterectomy. Femoro-distal grafting is rarely undertaken for claudication alone.

If arteriography reveals aorto-iliac occlusion and superficial femoral artery occlusion but a good profunda and good distal vessels, supra-inguinal reconstruction alone is likely to succeed.

Potential problems of femoro-popliteal bypass grafting are summarized in Table 23.9.

5.2 Acute lower-limb ischaemia

Introduction

Acute lower-limb ischaemia is usually caused by arterial thrombosis, peripheral embolism, or by arterial trauma. In general, early operative or radiological intervention is required if a functional limb is to be preserved. In one well-documented series, 75 per cent of acutely ischaemic lower limbs were caused by embolism, and, with careful management, limb salvage rate was 90 per cent. However, early mortality was very high (40 per cent) and 5-year survival was only 40 per cent. More recently, the balance has swung very firmly in favour of acute-on-chronic thrombosis rather than embolism as the main cause of acute limb ischaemia in the West.

Distinguishing between thrombosis and embolism is crucial in determining the appropriate management and the chances of a successful outcome:

◆ Thrombotic acute ischaemia is most often an acute event on a background of chronic obliterative arterial disease, although the latter may have been previously asymptomatic. It may also occur with occlusion of an existing arterial reconstruction. Thrombotic acute ischaemia is becoming more frequent as people are living longer and obliterative disease increases proportionately. More unusual causes include thrombosis of a popliteal aneurysm or of a congenital popliteal artery entrapment. In certain blood disorders, notably polycythae-mia rubra vera, spontaneous thrombosis of normal arteries may lead to acute ischaemia. Managing any of these acute thromboses requires all the skills of an experienced arterial surgeon.

◆ Arterial embolism is becoming a less frequent cause of acute ischaemia. This probably relates to the declining incidence of rheumatic mitral valve disease and its associated left atrial dilatation containing thrombus, as well as better treatment of mitral stenosis and atrial fibrillation. The incidence of the other common cause, emboli originating on damaged endocardium after myocardial infarction, remains static.

◆ Arterial trauma secondary to fractures or penetrating wounds also falls in the province of the arterial surgeon. The pos-sibility of closed (or penetrating) arterial injury must be considered whenever limbs are injured. Many more limbs are lost as a result of failure to recognize, or delay in recognizing, post-traumatic ischaemia than by technical problems in reconstruction (see Chapter 17, Section 2.8).

Diagnosis of acute ischaemia

Recognizing ischaemia

The clinical signs of acute ischaemia are well known and include Pain, Pallor, Pulselessness, Paraesthesia, Paralysis, Perishing cold, fixed Pigmentation, and blistering. However, there are important subtleties in the diagnosis which depend on the severity and distribution of ischaemia, the state of the collateral circulation, and the stage in the natural history at which the patient presents.

Thus, an elderly patient with cerebral failure may present in an advanced stage with an obviously dead leg displaying all the above signs, whereas at the other extreme, a patient may present with a sudden onset of severe claudication and a leg which is clearly viable, if a little cool. All stages between these two extremes are seen. In general, pain, pallor, and pulselessness are early and reversible features, anaesthesia and paralysis are late signs in which ischaemic damage has occurred but the limb may be salvaged, whereas fixed pigmentation and blistering denote irreversible tissue death.

Pathophysiology of acute ischaemia

Acute occlusion of the main artery of supply

Arterial inflow ceases but venous drainage continues and the limb becomes pale. The severity of ischaemia depends on the volume of blood available through collateral vessels and determines both the severity of ischaemia and the rate at which a limb becomes irreversibly damaged. Patients with chronic arterial insufficiency are more likely to withstand acute occlusion of the main vessel because of collaterals already developed.

Fall in temperature of the limb

Once it loses the flow of warm blood, the limb cools and gradually assumes the ambient temperature. This has the benefit of slowing the metabolic rate in the ischaemic tissues. Artificial warming should be avoided as it increases the rate of autolysis in the ischaemic areas of the limb.

Loss of function in specialized tissues

Nerve ischaemia causes first pain, then a progressive loss of sensation and motor function. If sensation is diminished but not absent, full recovery is likely if blood flow is restored. When paralysis occurs, this is a more ominous sign and is caused by a combination of nerve ischaemia and muscle necrosis. Complete loss of motor function is usually irreversible. Attempts to revas-cularize the limb at this stage must be cautious and may be abandoned if muscle necrosis is found. Late revascularization usually requires the addition of fasciotomy to relieve the swelling that occurs with reperfusion, which is likely to compromise the blood supply.

Table 23.10 Clinical pointers to distinguishing thrombosis from embolism

Thrombosis	Embolism
Older patient	Younger patient
History of claudication or arterial reconstruction	Mitral stenosis, atrial fibrillation, or recent myocardial infarction
Known popliteal aneurysm or popliteal aneurysm in opposite limb—may have thrombosed	Known popliteal aneurysm or popliteal aneurysm in opposite limb—may have embolized
	Previous embolic event
	Acute bilateral ischaemia (saddle embolus), but beware aortic dissection
Absent pulses in opposite limb	Opposite limb pulses excellent and no history of claudication
	Known AAA
	Acute ischaemia of the upper limb

Table 23.11 Questions to be answered in assessing an apparently ischaemic lower limb

1. Is this acute ischaemia?	The diagnosis of ischaemia depends on applying the pathophysiological principles described in the text. Evidence of absent blood flow, based on the appearance of the limb, low skin temperature, and absent pulses, should enable the diagnosis to be made with confidence. Absent flow on Doppler ultrasonography is confirmatory
2. Is the ischaemia embolic or thrombotic?	Clinical diagnosis is notoriously unreliable (Table 23.10). Firm diagnosis usually requires urgent arteriography before intervention or on-table angiography
3. How reversible is the degree of ischaemia?	It is often believed that irreversible changes occur 6 hours after arterial occlusion. This may be true if all blood supply is cut off, but misleading where there is significant collateral circulation. Thus, the clinical signs should be assessed and a decision taken as to whether a primary amputation or an attempt at revascularization should be made
4. Should thrombolysis and possibly angioplasty be attempted?	If the limb is likely to remain viable for 8–12 hours, technical expertise is available, and angiography is favourable, thrombolysis has several advantages
5. Should embolectomy or reconstructive surgery be attempted?	This is the reverse side of the coin from thrombolysis and depends on clear clinical or arteriographic evidence of embolism (for embolectomy) or arteriographic findings and a decision not to perform thrombolysis
6. If amputation is required, at what level should it be performed?	The level of amputation depends on the findings at operation. All necrotic tissue must be removed and if a clear decision cannot be made, a provisional guillotine amputation is carried out and reamputation or delayed primary closure performed later

Necrosis of less-specialized tissues

Ischaemic muscle groups undergo autolysis and swelling. This is recognized clinically by muscle tenderness and pain with movement. Biochemical changes include release of intracellular potassium, accumulation of lactic acid, and breakdown products of muscle infarction such as myoglobin. Revascularization at this stage can release these toxic products into the general circulation and result in multiple organ failure with results similar to that found in the crush syndrome.

Established tissue death

The end point of untreated acute severe ischaemia is irreversible peripheral necrosis or gangrene. It is recognized by fixed blue or black pigmentation (i.e. which does not blanch with pressure) and blistering. The level of ischaemia is usually substantially more proximal than the skin necrosis would suggest, and revascularization may still be required to preserve the knee joint after performing provisional amputation of necrotic tissue.

Differential diagnosis

Causes of lower-limb pain such as deep vein thrombosis, sprains, and bruises, which may bear a superficial resemblance to acute ischaemia, lack the features of diminished perfusion associated with ischaemia. Acute ischaemia can confidently be diagnosed or excluded on clinical grounds, if necessary aided by Doppler ankle pressure measurement.

Differentiating between thrombosis and embolism on clinical grounds is unreliable even in expert hands. If there is doubt, an arteriogram should be performed before definitive treatment is commenced. Table 23.10 gives clinical pointers to the diagnosis.

Ischaemia due to trauma occurs only in an obviously traumatized limb (see below). If a popliteal aneurysm is palpable in the opposite limb, a complication affecting a similar aneurysm in the ischaemic limb is likely to be the cause. This may be due to thrombosis of the aneurysm or distal embolism from clot within the aneurysm. The diagnosis can be confirmed by arteriography, and if the limb is viable and expertise available, thrombolytic therapy can be instituted (Table 23.11). Popliteal artery occlusion caused by thrombosis in polycythaemia rubra vera may be suspected from the blood picture but confirmed only by arteriography. Again, thrombolytic therapy may be most appropriate.

Aortic dissection occasionally presents with acute lower-limb ischaemia. In this case, the dissection usually occludes the aortic bifurcation with the elevated flap. There is often a history of chest pain or acute cardiac failure due to aortic regurgitation, and the level of ischaemia is unusually high, often involving the buttocks and flank. Diagnosis can usually be confirmed on arteriography and treatment directed at fenestrating the abdominal aorta and resuspending the aortic valve if necessary.

Management of acute ischaemia

Introduction

Surgery of acute ischaemia (other than after trauma) has traditionally been delegated to junior surgeons, on the assumption that the cause is embolism and an embolectomy is within his or her capabilities to perform. However, recent studies, have revealed the appalling consequences of this policy in terms of limb loss (40 per cent failure of revascularization) and often loss of life (in excess of 25 per cent mortality). This can often be traced to a failure to recognize a diagnosis of acute thrombosis. It has been demonstrated that even in apparently clear-cut cases, it is often impossible to determine the cause of acute ischaemia on clinical grounds preoperatively without an arteriogram.

The scene is set for disaster if an inexperienced surgeon tackles an acutely ischaemic leg, assuming it to be due to an embolism, without a firm preoperative diagnosis. An embolectomy is often attempted out of hours, under local anaesthesia, without preparing the sequel if thrombosis of diseased arteries proves to be the cause. By the time this has been recognized (by the failure of embolectomy) and steps taken to set up a competent approach to the problem, several additional hours of ischaemia will have passed and the moment may be lost.

Thus, the early stages of diagnosis and management may be critical to saving the patient's limb and life.

Surgery for the acutely ischaemic lower limb

Immediate management

Anticoagulate the patient systemically immediately, to limit propagation of thrombus (5000–10 000 units heparin IV stat.).

The ideal next step is for all cases to be assessed by a competent arterial surgeon and to arrange urgent arteriography for all but the most obvious cases of embolism. This gives the opportunity for thrombolytic therapy if circumstances warrant it. If surgery is required, preparation can be made for adequate theatre time, an experienced arterial surgeon and anaesthetist, and on-table arteriography. If a firm diagnosis cannot be made, these facilities should be available to follow on if an attempt at embolectomy fails.

If arteriography shows embolism and the limb is viable, thrombolysis may be undertaken if technical constraints of access permit. If viability is in danger, embolectomy should be undertaken as a matter of urgency (see below).

If thrombosis appears to be the cause, thrombolysis should be undertaken if the limb is likely to remain viable for 6–8 hours, the expertise is available, and it is technically feasible (see above). Thrombolysis has the particular merit of being able to clear small distal vessels which are not accessible to embolectomy catheters. It is also possible to clear the system in patients who present late and in whom adherent thrombus would be difficult to clear mechanically.

Once the arterial system is cleared, the underlying stenosis is likely to become apparent and may be amenable to balloon angioplasty.

If thrombolysis is not the treatment of choice, a preoperative angiogram may have revealed sufficient run-in and runoff to plan a reconstructive bypass operation along the lines discussed earlier. Some surgeons prefer to carry out on-table angiography as this reduces delay in getting to theatre and may give better distal definition. However, this assumes minimally invasive techniques will not be employed instead.

Embolectomy for lower-limb embolism

Decision to intervene

This is based on a firm diagnosis of acute ischaemia due to embolism with physical signs which suggest that the condition is reversible.

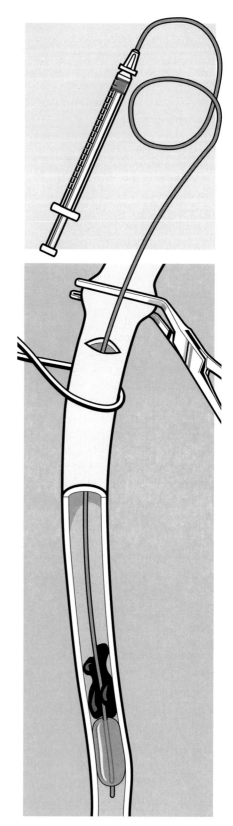

Figure 23.11 Embolectomy technique.

Preoperative preparation and anaesthesia

The choice of anaesthesia depends on the fitness of the patient and the choice of the surgeon and anaesthetist, but may be general, regional, or local. General or regional anaesthesia is preferable unless the patient has suffered a recent myocardial infarction, in which case local anaesthesia is safer. Systemic heparin should have been administered as described above.

Exposure

Access to the contralateral femoral artery is occasionally required, for example to remove embolism passing down the contralateral limb or to perform a femoro-femoral crossover graft. Both groins should be skin prepared and draped. Explore the femoral artery, exposing and controlling common femoral, superficial femoral, profunda femoris, and other small branches with slings. Clamp all vessels.

Procedure

◆ Make an arteriotomy just above the femoral bifurcation. A transverse arteriotomy is thought to cause less narrowing than a longitudinal arteriotomy after closure; however, a longitudinal arteriotomy allows easier anastomosis if a graft is required, and in the case of potential narrowing can be closed over using a vein patch.

◆ Examine the state of the arterial wall. If normal, this favours a diagnosis of embolism.

◆ Pass a size 4 Fogarty balloon catheter (without stylet) 10 cm down the superficial femoral, inflate balloon and draw back to retrieve embolus (Fig. 23.11). Balloon pressure is varied to keep it snugly in contact with the arterial wall. Pass the Fogarty to 20 cm and repeat the above at 10 cm intervals until all thrombus is retrieved and back bleeding occurs. Repeat for the profunda femoris (maximum 25 cm). If the catheter cannot be passed along the full length of the limb, the diagnosis of embolism is incorrect and thrombosis is the cause. This cannot be treated by Fogarty catheterization.

◆ Inject 20 ml heparin/saline (5000 units in 500 ml) into each artery.

◆ Check forward bleeding (from above) and then pass the Fogarty proximally up to the aortic bifurcation (about 20 cm).

◆ A completion arteriogram should be performed to confirm successful embolectomy.

◆ Close the arteriotomy and drain the wound with a suction drain.

◆ If the Fogarty catheter passes easily only as far as the knee and quantities of embolic material are retrieved, two techniques are available. Intraoperative thrombolysis may be tried. A solution of 100 000 units of streptokinase in 50 ml of normal saline is placed in a syringe in a syringe driver set at 2 ml/min. This is attached to a catheter which is passed down the distal artery and infused over 30 minutes. Further embolectomy

catheters are then passed and previously hard or adherent thrombus may then be retrievable. Alternatively, or if intra-operative thrombolysis fails, the popliteal artery should be opened below the knee and the trifurcation cleared of thrombus. In order to clear more than one vessel, a 'double balloon ' technique can be used, using one Fogarty catheter into each vessel via the same arteriotomy.

◆ If embolectomy fails, proceed immediately to arterial reconstruction, as described below.

Confirming success

The surgeon needs to be honestly objective in assessing reperfusion. Misplaced optimism at the end of an 'embolectomy' procedure often leads to limb loss or even eventually to death of the patient.

If embolic material is retrieved in substantial amounts and backbleeding occurs, the diagnosis of embolism is sustained. The foot should 'pink up' immediately on declamping and warm up within an hour. If under local anaesthesia, the patient will shortly be aware of sensation returning. Pulses will become palpable in most cases.

If these signs of success do not occur, then embolectomy has failed. Immediate steps should be taken to revascularize the limb, because the chance of success of deferred attempts diminishes rapidly. If all attempts at revascularization are unsuccessful, then amputation is likely to be needed later. It is not usually necessary for this to be done until a day or two later, after the patient has come to terms with the need for it.

In the long term after successful embolectomy, controversy remains about the benefits of anticoagulation versus the drawbacks. Anticoagulating patients with atrial fibrillation is recommended by most authorities these days to minimize the risk of embolism anywhere. There is probably little advantage in anticoagulating patients who embolize after myocardial infarction.

Arterial reconstruction for acute ischaemia following inadequate embolectomy

If there is inadequate forward flow when the proximal clamp is released and a Fogarty catheter fails to pass proximally, some form of supra-inguinal vascular reconstruction will be required. This may be aorto-bifemoral bypass, unilateral ilio-femoral bypass, or crossover femoro-femoral by pass, depending on suitability of proximal vessels for graft takeoff and operator choice.

If the Fogarty catheter passes only a short distance into the superficial femoral artery, the inference is that the vessel is occluded by atheroma and the acute ischaemia has been caused by acute-on-chronic thrombosis. On-table arteriography should be performed to assess the arterial anatomy, showing sites of occlusion and patent distal vessels.

Successful vascular reconstruction by femoro-popliteal bypass depends on the usual criteria of an adequate inflow and a low-resistance distal circulation—'a good runoff'. Inflow can

Table 23.12 Causes of diabetic foot complications

Factor	Pathophysiology	Consequence	Result
Neuropathic sensory loss	Loss of pain sensation. Unawareness of injury	Loss of protective reaction to injurious agents	Infection enters unnoticed sites of trauma. Patient does not seek treatment because the foot is not painful
Neuropathic motor loss	Denervation of small muscles of foot. Unopposed action of long extensors and flexors	'Clawing' of foot with increased vertical dimension. Loss of normal pressure distribution pattern on sole	Trauma from rubbing on footwear. Disordered pressure pattern of foot causing pressure necrosis and ulcers
Neuropathic autonomic loss	Diminished sweating. Loss of temperature control with opening of subcutaneous arteriovenous fistulas	Loss of lubrication and flexibility of skin. Diversion of nutrient blood supply away from skin surface	Cracking and fissuring of skin. Possible cutaneous ischaemia
Tendency to early and extensive atherosclerosis, often with a distal distribution	Arterial stenoses and occlusions	Ischaemic skin lesions. Poor healing	Critical ischaemia with rest pain and ulceration and gangrene
'Small-vessel disease' affecting digital arteries	Hypertrophic narrowing of digital arteries	Necrosis of individual toes, often with good pulses	Need for amputation. Note that this problem also occurs in poorly perfused limbs, which require revascularization before amputation

be crudely tested by releasing the proximal clamp and demonstrating a good 'spurt'. Intraoperative pressure measurement can be easily performed to check this. Runoff is not easily measured, but can be assessed by exploring the popliteal artery for patency and back bleeding, or by on-table arteriography.

5.3 The diabetic foot

Introduction

The diabetic foot is the greatest single cause of hospitalization amongst diabetics and yet it is largely preventable. The main underlying problem is neuropathy which, if neglected, can give rise to the 'pure' diabetic foot. Diabetes may also be associated with accelerated atherosclerosis causing peripheral arterial insufficiency and many diabetic foot problems are caused predominantly by atherosclerosis. A third, and least common, cause is probably diabetic small-vessel disease affecting the blood supply of digits. Here, a foot with strongly palpable pulses undergoes necrosis of an individual toe. This may occur in the absence of neuropathy and atherosclerosis. Table 23.12 summarizes these causes of diabetic foot.

Most diabetic foot problems can be identified as being primarily neuropathic or primarily atherosclerotic, but some patients have elements of both and these comprise the most difficult group to manage successfully. Typically, the neuropathic foot is red and warm with strong pulses, whereas the atherosclerotic foot is pale, cold, and pulseless.

Diabetics are also predisposed to infection and have greater difficulty overcoming established infection. This is probably due to a degree of immunocompromise coupled with disordered local tissue metabolism.

The neuropathic foot

Diabetic neuropathy is probably caused by microangiopathy affecting sensory, motor, and autonomic nerves:

◆ Sensory neuropathy causes loss of protective pain responses.

◆ Motor neuropathy denervates the small muscles of foot, allowing unmodified contraction of long extensors and flexors. This leads to distortion and uneven loading of the sole of the foot and an increased vertical dimension of the forefoot. Both of these make the insensitive foot more liable to trauma from footwear.

◆ Autonomic neuropathy abolishes sweating (dryness and splitting of skin) and causes loss of local vascular control. Arteriovenous communications open beneath the skin, diverting nutrient flow away from it. Damaged tissue thus heals poorly and is vulnerable to infection.

Pathology of the neuropathic diabetic foot

Microangiopathy causes thickening of arteriolar walls and impairs nutrition of nerves. Loss of sensation means the patient is unaware of abrasions caused by tight footwear, shoe nails, and foreign bodies. The lack of pain sensation abolishes the normal feedback which warns of a potentially serious condition occurring in the foot, originating with minor trauma, and the patient is not prompted to seek treatment.

Infection enters through a break in the skin and spreads without hindrance. This is because impaired tissue energy metabolism and the glucose-rich tissue environment favour bacterial growth. Necrosis of deep tissues follows and pyogenic infection spreads rapidly along tendon sheaths. By the time the patient is aware of the problem, irreversible tissue damage may have taken place.

If, in addition, the arterial supply is already compromised by atherosclerosis, the scene is set for gangrene and limb loss.

Presentation of the neuropathic diabetic foot

Patients most at risk of foot complications are elderly, poorly controlled, maturity-onset diabetics and younger, often neglectful, patients with long-standing type I diabetes. Patients with diabetic microangiopathic complications in the kidney or retina appear to have an increased risk of foot problems.

Diabetic ulcers always occur on the foot, either as perforating ulcers on the sole beneath the first metatarsal head or at other bony prominences such as the toes or the malleoli. The ulcers tend to penetrate deeply into the foot and there is often underlying necrotic and infected tissue. Ulcers on the sole have a characteristic appearance: the edge of the ulcer is often hyperkeratotic and the ulcer is a punched out necrotic crater with abrupt transition from healthy-looking skin. Surrounding tissues are usually well perfused (pink and warm). There is generalized sensory impairment but joint position sense and vibration sense is lost preferentially and can be estimated clinically. Peripheral pulses are usually palpable. The ulcer is often recent, usually over a bony prominence and is often preceded by minor trauma such as chiropody to toenails or footwear abrasion. Infection may spread rapidly causing extensive limb-threatening necrosis and potentially fatal septicaemia.

Maturity-onset diabetes may develop insidiously, so if a patient with a foot ulcer is not known to be diabetic, the urine and blood sugar should be tested. A diagnosis of diabetes may not mean that this alone is the cause of the ulceration and the possibility of atherosclerotic ulcers should be borne in mind.

Box 23.4 Foot complications of diabetes

- Painless, deeply penetrating ulcers. The infecting organism is usually *Staphylococcus aureus*. The necrosis spreads through the web space and along the tendon sheaths. Spreading infection causes venous thrombosis, which appears to be an important factor in tissue destruction.

- Painless necrosis of individual toes. These first turn blue then later become black and mummified. This may be caused by atherosclerotic arterial insufficiency, but, in some cases, occurs as a result of diabetic small-vessel disease affecting digital arteries. In non-diabetics, toe necrosis also occurs with arterial insufficiency, but the condition is painful.

- Extensive spreading skin necrosis associated with superficial or deep infection. This develops very rapidly and spreads proximally, threatening both limb and life.

- Chronic ulceration of pressure points and sites of minor injury without spreading infection.

Management of the neuropathic diabetic foot

Control of infection

Control of infection is the first priority in the management of diabetic foot problems. Minor foot lesions in the diabetic must be taken seriously and treated early with oral antibiotics and elevation.

If there is any sign of spreading infection or systemic involvement (i.e. fever, tachycardia, or loss of diabetic control), the patient should be admitted to hospital for intensive treatment with parenteral antibiotics and management of blood glucose control. The latter often requires temporary treatment with insulin.

Removal of necrotic tissue

If there is an abscess in the foot or evident necrosis, early surgery is required. This may involve desloughing of an ulcer, minor amputation, or even major amputation. The key to success is to remove all dead tissue and to leave the wound open. If performed correctly, these surgical procedures will eventually result in complete healing. Plaster casts may be used after surgery to allow patients to become ambulant while supporting the foot and distributing pressure evenly over the sole. A window can be cut to allow dressings to be applied to areas of skin loss.

Prevention

Clinicians dealing with diabetics need to recognize the high priority that should be given to prevention. There are now many well-established diabetic departments which aim to screen all diabetics for potential problems such as neuropathic feet, renal changes, and retinal problems. A neuropathic foot is an 'at-risk' foot and detailed advice on self-care should be given and professional chiropody services provided. Patients should be advised to take great care with footwear to ensure it fits well, to check the shoes periodically for foreign bodies and nails. There are several ranges of off-the-shelf special shoes available for patients unable to wear standard shoes, and individually designed and fitted insoles can be provided to distribute pressure over the sole.

Atherosclerosis in diabetics

Diabetics have a marked predisposition to atherosclerosis and are at greater risk of arterial insufficiency. Thus, whereas 1–2 per cent of the general population is diabetic, 25 per cent of patients presenting with peripheral ischaemia are diabetic. Atherosclerotic disease follows the usual pattern but tends to develop at an earlier age.

Management of atherosclerotic ischaemia is similar in diabetics and non-diabetics. For mixed disease, the contribution of arterial insufficiency needs to be established by the methods described earlier and, if severe, must be treated by revascularization procedures if there is to be any hope of healing. Given the frequently distal pattern of disease, with preserved superficial femoral and popliteal arteries, shorter distal bypasses between the popliteal and ankle or pedal vessels may be necessary. In contrast, the neuropathic diabetic foot can be treated by intensive antibiotics and local surgery.

5.4 Carotid artery disease

Introduction

Carotid endarterectomy enjoyed an enormous vogue in the 1970s and 1980s for treating transient ischaemic attacks, completed stroke, and asymptomatic carotid stenosis, particularly in USA. Later, papers demonstrating better results from medical management of carotid artery stenoses (antiplatelet medication) resulted in a swing away from surgery, but, recently, further comparative studies have been published in Europe and the USA showing that provided the carotid stenosis was greater than 70 per cent, surgery reduced the annual stroke rate from about 6 per cent (for the medically treated group) to about 1.5 per cent. Surgery, however, did not reduce the long-term mortality from carotid artery stenosis, which is comparable in the two groups at about 5 per cent per annum over 5 years, taking operative mortality of 2–3 per cent into account.

Currently about 2000 carotid endarterectomies are performed annually in UK, but this is set to rise now that favourable results for surgical treatment of severe stenoses have been demonstrated. At present, seven males are treated for carotid artery stenosis for every three females.

Investigation of carotid artery disease

After pursuing a number of unsatisfactory methods, the choice of initial investigation for suspected carotid artery stenosis is now duplex Doppler. Some units follow this with angiography if tight or equivocal stenosis is demonstrated. However, there is an appreciable risk of stroke from angiography and, latterly, many units perform angiography only if duplex studies suggest near occlusion or bilateral disease.

Indications for surgery

Full clinical trials of medical versus surgical treatment are continuing in Europe and the USA, but preliminary results have shown clear benefit for surgery in reducing the stroke rate if stenosis is between 70 and 99 per cent. Surgery demonstrated a reduced rate of ipsilateral stroke (out of 595 patients, 24 medically treated and seven surgically treated had suffered strokes within 3 months of treatment). This benefit continued to increase as time passed up to 30 months (US NASCET study). No benefit has yet been demonstrated in patients with 30–70 per cent stenosis. However, mortality is unaffected by endarterectomy, at 5 per cent per annum in both groups. Evidence is emerging from the ACAS trial that surgery should be offered to patients who are asymptomatic but have a greater than 60 per cent stenosis, confirmatory data is awaited from the European ACST.

The main clinical presentations found in most series of patients having carotid endarterectomy are transient ischaemic attacks and amaurosis fugax (70–85 per cent), after recovery from stroke (10–25 per cent), and less than 5 per cent each for progressing stroke/crescendo TIA, asymptomatic stenosis (prior to cardiac surgery or progression under observation), and global hemispheric symptoms.

Operative technique and intraoperative monitoring

The technique of carotid endarterectomy has been described earlier (Section 3.4). All patients should be kept on low-dose aspirin as an antiplatelet agent. Prior to surgery, patency of the internal carotid artery (ICA) to be operated on should be confirmed by duplex, ideally within 24 hours of the proposed procedure. Most operations are performed under general anaesthesia (although local anesthesia is becoming more popular) and the majority employ the routine use of a shunt, a Javed shunt being the most common type employed. Some teams prefer selective use of a shunt in patients with:

(1) low pressure in the distal internal carotid after clamping (low stump pressure);

(2) contralateral occlusion of the ICA;

(3) a fall of 50 per cent in the middle cerebral artery velocity on transcranial Doppler (TCD) monitoring;

(4) development of cerebral symptoms, such as falling consciousness, if the operation is performed under local anaesthesia.

The British joint vascular research group has published in favour of patching the carotid arteriotomy after the endarterectomy as this appears to reduce the postoperative occlusion rate. Overall, however, patches may only be appropriate for small arteries and consequently are more often required in females.

Results of carotid endarterectomy

The basis of comparing different series of patients

When comparing the overall benefits of medical versus surgical treatment, the following factors should be taken into account:

- perioperative and long-term mortality rate;

- perioperative and long-term stroke rate;

- early and late occlusion rate after surgery, and ipsilateral stroke rate resulting from this;

- long-term mortality and stroke rate of matched medically treated patients.

It is also important that nationally and internationally agreed definitions of cerebral complications are used. The following are widely accepted:

- A transient ischaemic attack results in a deficit which lasts up to 24 hours.

- A transient deficit lasts up to 3 weeks.

- An established stroke has occurred if a deficit is present after 3 weeks.

Early results of surgery

After carotid endarterectomy in units with a high throughput, the 30-day operative mortality is about 3 per cent, all from circulatory problems, predominantly myocardial infarction and stroke.

In addition, the perioperative non-fatal stroke rate is about 3 per cent, with about half having long-term major disability. The risk of perioperative stroke varies with the indication for surgery. Thus, there is a 2 per cent risk of stroke when treating TIAs and a 12 per cent risk where surgery is urgent for progressive symptoms. No particular risk factors for operative neurological deficit can be identified, even in retrospect.

About 5 per cent of patients suffer transient postoperative neurological deficit and 5 per cent suffer temporary cranial nerve damage. Two per cent of patients require early reoperation, usually for thrombosis of the reconstruction causing hemiplegia. In one series, about 5 per cent underwent silent occlusion of the operated carotid within 6 weeks of surgery, half of whom suffered a stroke.

Long-term results of surgery

After 5 years' surgical follow-up, the total mortality rate (including the operative mortality) is about 25 per cent (5 per cent per annum), which is virtually identical to several reports of medically treated patients. However, in a group of 150 patients with asymptomatic bruits not requiring surgery, the 5-year mortality rate was only 7 per cent (1.4 per cent per annum).

The total ipsilateral and contralateral stroke rate after 5 years' surgical follow-up (including the perioperative stroke rate) is about 7 per cent (1.4 per cent per annum). This compares favourably with a 6 per cent annual stroke rate in several large medically treated series and is virtually the same as the 5-year stroke rate in patients with asymptomatic bruits (i.e. 5.7 per cent or 1.1 per cent per annum).

About 4 per cent of patients develop late re-stenosis or occlusion of the reconstruction and about half of these are associated with stroke. The place of re-intervention is not yet established (Ellis 1987).

5.5 Abdominal aortic and lower-limb aneurysms

Introduction

Peripheral arterial aneurysms are found in later life, with the exception of so-called 'mycotic' (infective) aneurysms. The prevalence of aneurysms increases with age; it is rare to find aneurysms below the age of 60 years and almost unknown before the age of 50. This appears to represent a change in epidemiology from the nineteenth century, where the literature abounds with accounts of patients in their 30s or 40s with abdominal aortic aneurysms and popliteal aneurysms.

Abdominal aortic aneurysms are the most common aneurysms and, for reasons unknown, 95 per cent or more affect only the infrarenal aorta. Thoraco-abdominal aneurysms present a much greater surgical challenge, with a higher mortality, and are best treated in specialized units.

In about 25 per cent of cases, abdominal aneurysms are associated with aneurysms elsewhere. Popliteal aneurysms are the next most common. These are often found by chance but if they present with symptoms, the limb is often in danger from ischaemia. A popliteal aneurysm may cause peripheral ischaemia by several different means: thrombotic occlusion, embolism of accumulated thrombus, or, rarely, by rupture. There are two schools of thought about managing asymptomatic popliteal aneurysms—the interventionist (which advocates

prophylactic bypass grafting with saphenous vein) and the optimistic (which treats the aneurysm only when it becomes symptomatic). Both views can be supported by results of published series; however, with improved results from surgery there is increasing evidence to support intervention in asymptomatic popliteal aneurysms of greater than 2.5 cm diameter.

The aetiology of most aneurysms is undoubtedly degenerative, and atherosclerosis is found in many of them. However, it is likely that this relationship is fortuitous—elderly patients suffer from both conditions and they will inevitably sometimes occur together. The true aetiology probably involves changes in collagen or collagenase, elastin or elastase, yet to be characterized.

Certain groups of people have an increased risk of developing an aortic aneurysm. Incidence increases steadily with age, so older patients are more likely to have one. A first-degree relative (parent, child, sibling) of a patient with an aneurysm has a 20 per cent chance of having an aneurysm, and patients with hypertension (15 per cent) and peripheral arterial insufficiency (20 per cent) are also at increased risk.

Elective surgery for AAA

Mortality for elective abdominal aortic aneurysm has progressively fallen over the years, owing to improved preparation of the patient, more modern anaesthesia and intensive care, as well as better surgical technique. Mortality risk for all comers is still between 5 and 10 per cent in most centres but can be as low as between 1 and 5 per cent, and this would make screening a realistic proposition. Details of elective aneurysm surgery are not given here, but the technique is similar to that employed for ruptured aneurysm, described below.

Ruptured abdominal aortic aneurysm

Mortality from ruptured AAA

Ruptured abdominal aortic aneurysm is a common cause of collapse and sudden death in elderly males. Published figures for incidence undoubtedly underestimate the problem. Many patients who die suddenly in the community are wrongly labelled, as having myocardial infarction for example. Where careful post-mortem examinations of these patients have been performed, it has been shown that fewer than 50 per cent of patients with this diagnosis reach hospital and, of those that do, fewer than 50 per cent survive. Thus, the true average mortality for ruptured aneurysm is at least 80 per cent. In unselected post-mortem studies and anatomical dissecting rooms, as many as one-third of patients are found to have an abdominal aortic aneurysm and up to one-third of these have died of rupture. The most effective way of reducing the death rate from ruptured aneurysm may be population screening by ultrasound (see Chapter 1).

Many patients die without reaching hospital because the rupture is intraperitoneal. More often, the rupture is posterolateral and the retroperitoneal haemorrhage is contained for a variable period by the tamponade effect of retroperitoneal tissues.

Diagnosing rupture

The diagnosis must be considered if a male over 55 years or a female over 65 years presents with unexplained back or abdominal pain, particularly if accompanied by transient or continuing circulatory collapse. If an abdominal aneurysm is also palpable, the diagnosis of ruptured aortic aneurysm can be assumed. A high index of suspicion and appropriate rapid action will prevent a patient dying undiagnosed in the accident and emergency department or radiography department.

A history of collapse is highly significant in any patient with abdominal or back pain that fits the age criteria. It may have lasted only a few minutes, with the patient appearing to recover but often the pain appearing later. Half the patients with rupture will not have a palpable aneurysm because of obesity, guarding, or hypotension. If the blood pressure is low, ruptured aneurysm is even more likely. If the diagnosis is suspected but not definite, an emergency ultrasound (or CT scan), perhaps with portable equipment, will readily confirm the presence of an abdominal aortic aneurysm and will make the diagnosis more reliable.

The urgency of operation

There is a variable period in which operation has a chance of success between the initial leak and inevitable death from catastrophic haemorrhage. Medical treatment alone is of no value. Unfortunately, there is no way of predicting how long this 'window of opportunity' may last, so every case must be treated without delay. The diagnosis, once seriously considered, should be used to activate all necessary services to reduce the interval before clamping the aorta. This means alerting a senior surgeon, anaesthetist, operating theatre, intensive care unit, and blood bank for immediate operation. An ECG and chest X-ray should be taken to look for MI, chest problems, and possible thoracic aneurysm.

The nightmare scenario

In a typical case, an elderly patient collapses and a diagnosis of ruptured aneurysm is made. The urgency of operation means little history is available so the premorbid state is not known, and the preparation has to be rushed. The emergency will often be at night when the usual efficient daytime facilities and experience are not readily available.

The patient is brought to theatre with a low blood pressure, probably no urine output, and continues to lose blood. The anaesthetist wants to take time to put venous and arterial lines in, but the surgeon wants to get a clamp on the aorta as a matter of extreme urgency. An inexperienced theatre nurse has to prepare the instruments rapidly. The patient is conscious but anxious and sweaty with adrenaline output, making arrhythmias likely. Immediate induction of anaesthetic relaxes the abdominal wall and removes the tamponade effect, causing the blood pressure to plummet before the surgeon is prepared.

It is clear that in such a case, the outlook is grim. Improved speed of diagnosis and preparation for operation (i.e. ordering fresh frozen plasma and platelet concentrates, involving experienced anaesthetists early in resuscitation) can mean the difference between the patient surviving and dying.

Emergency surgery for abdominal aortic aneurysm

The decision to intervene

Emergency aneurysm surgery is demanding of hospital staff, it imposes great stress on the patient, and is extremely expensive. Mortality for this type of surgery is more than 50 per cent, although 70 per cent or more will survive the operation, the rest dying days or weeks later from complications such as multisystem failure. Thus the decision to operate should be taken only if the chance of a successful outcome is judged to be reasonable. Rapid diagnosis and immediate surgery greatly improves the chances of a successful outcome.

Factors to be considered in the decision to intervene include:

- The state of the patient on arrival at hospital—if the patient is unconscious, recovery is almost unknown. Similarly, if the patient has been critically hypotensive for a prolonged period (more than 1 or 2 hours) and hypotension fails to respond to intravenous infusion and there is no urine in the bladder, operation will be in vain.

- The patient's general state of health—a history of serious co-morbid conditions, particularly those likely to be aggravated by the stress of operation, may govern a decision not to operate. For example, refractory cardiac failure, chronic renal failure, or carcinomatosis. Dementia, especially if associated with extreme age, may be a contraindication to operate. In some cases, no sensible medical history can be obtained in the brief interval before operation; here, the patient should be usually be given the benefit of the doubt.

- Advanced age alone should not be a contraindication to surgery. Indeed, one series obtained a better survival rate in the over 80s.

- Previous refusal of elective repair should not necessarily be interpreted as a contraindication to emergency repair. The risk-benefit of repairing a small aneurysm in an elderly patient may have been judged too hazardous, yet operation may be indicated if the alternative is inevitable death.

Once the decision to operate is taken, it is vital to minimize the time between presentation and aortic clamping. This should never take more than 1 hour.

Perioperative preparation and anaesthesia

Adequate blood for transfusion (10–12 units) is required urgently and a central venous line and, if possible, a large-bore 12- or 20-gauge peripheral line is inserted immediately. The patient is taken directly into the operating room, bypassing the anaesthetic room, so that further preparation and induction of anaesthesia can occur with the surgeon ready to proceed immediately. Once muscle relaxation is induced, tamponade is lost and rapid exsanguination can occur. Rapid control of haemorrhage is usually required, but not at the expense of damaging other structures (e.g. mesenteric veins, left renal vein) in undue haste. Prior to induction, a urinary catheter is placed to monitor renal function via urine output and the abdominal and groin skin prepared (in case access to the femoral arteries is

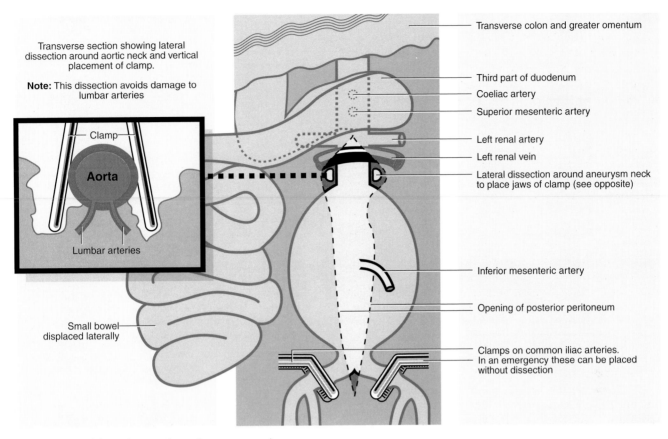

Figure 23.12 Applying a clamp to the aortic aneurysm neck.

required) and drapes put in place. Prolonged delay during anaesthetic preparation must be avoided because once the phase of rapid exsanguination occurs, clotting factors become rapidly exhausted and the chance of success is undermined. An arterial line can be placed once the aorta has been clamped.

Obtaining proximal control of the aneurysm

Access is obtained via a long midline incision. The method used depends on the rate of blood loss. If there is a large retroperitoneal haematoma without exsanguination, it is possible to identify the neck of the aneurysm in the usual way. The greater omentum is thrown upwards and the small bowel brought out of the right side of the wound. A longitudinal incision is made in the posterior peritoneum high up on the curve of the aneurysm and deepened to reach the aortic wall. This plane is followed upwards with blunt dissection until the pale neck of the aneurysm is reached. No attempt should be made to go round the back of the neck but the dissection is deepened each side of the neck so a large, almost straight, clamp can be placed vertically on the neck (Fig. 23.12). Initial proximal suprarenal clamping just below the diaphragm is preferred by some surgeons (see below).

Great care is taken to avoid damaging large retroperitoneal vessels, particularly the inferior mesenteric and left renal veins. These may not bleed at the time but bleed massively (and perhaps fatally) once volume is restored. The duodenum is separated from the aneurysm and the neck identified below the left renal vein. Finding the neck can be easier than in the elective case because the haematoma opens up the plane between aorta and posterior peritoneum (Fig. 23.13).

A particularly difficult situation occurs when a free intraperitoneal rupture is found on opening the abdomen. Iatrogenic free rupture can also be produced while attempting dissection around the neck of the aneurysm. In order to occlude the aorta while proper control is obtained, some surgeons use an **aortic compressor** to press the infra-diaphragmatic aorta posteriorly on to the lumbar spine. This is not always effective and may damage the pancreas. A better way is to open the aneurysm with a scalpel and immediately insert the left thumb into the aortic lumen to control flow. A size 20 Foley catheter, preloaded onto a catheter introducer, is then passed into the aorta and inflated. This temporarily occludes flow to the kidneys, but does allow an orderly dissection of the aneurysm neck. The aorta can then be cross-clamped in the usual way after dissection and the Foley catheter removed as the clamp is applied.

An alternative approach favoured by some surgeons is to obtain temporary control of the suprarenal aorta with a cross-clamp at the level of the diaphragm in all ruptured aneurysms, before attempting to approach the neck. This is a difficult technique to employ quickly, but is effective in experienced hands. The method involves: dividing the left triangular ligament of the liver, reflecting the left lobe of the liver to the patient's right side,

Non-leaking aortic aneurysm

Posterior peritoneum applied to neck of aortic aneurysm

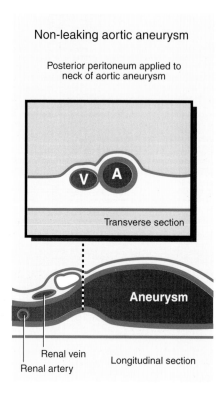

Transverse section

Aneurysm

Renal vein
Renal artery   Longitudinal section

Leaking aortic aneurysm

Retroperitoneal blood clot overlying neck of aortic aneurysm

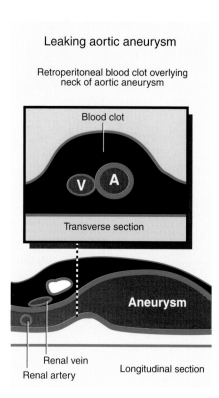

Blood clot

Transverse section

Aneurysm

Renal vein
Renal artery   Longitudinal section

Figure 23.13 Thrombus separating the posterior peritoneum from the neck of a ruptured aneurysm.

Box 23.5   Points of technique in ruptured aortic aneurysm surgery

1. Open the abdomen through a long midline incision.
2. Obtain proximal control of aorta and apply clamps to the iliac arteries.
3. Prevent clotting in distal vessels using systemic heparin (some surgeons prefer not to do this) or inject heparin/saline into iliac arteries.
4. Place retractors and explore the abdomen for complicating factors such as other aneurysms, GI cancer, shrunken kidneys. All involved can now relax and further anaesthetic lines can be placed.
5. Open the aneurysm, remove clot, suture backbleeding lumbar arteries, and ligate the inferior mesenteric artery.
6. Suture the proximal end of the inlay graft into the aneurysm using a continuous 2/0 or 3/0 Prolene suture (the graft should be non-porous, i.e. woven, or knitted Dacron impregnated with gelatin or fibrin). Use a tube graft if possible, a bifurcation only if there are definite iliac aneurysms: the prime purpose of the operation is to save life. Test the proximal anastomosis by clamping the graft and a trial release of the aortic clamp.
7. Perform the lower anastomosis in a similar fashion, look for backbleeding, taking care to flush debris and clot out of the vessels before completing the anastomosis.
8. Check carefully for haemorrhage.
9. Check lower limbs are perfused (colour and palpable pulses).
10. Check perfusion of sigmoid colon (because of ligation of inferior mesenteric).
11. Close aortic sac over graft.
12. Close posterior peritoneum and abdominal wall.
13. Send patient to intensive care unit.

---

dividing the peritoneum transversely over the lower oesophagus, splitting the right crus of the diaphragm along its fibres, and mobilizing enough of the aorta to apply a cross-clamp. The neck of the aneurysm is then approached and clamped as above and the clamp at diaphragmatic level removed.

Surgical management of ruptured abdominal aortic aneurysm

The actual aortic grafting (repair) is the same as that used in elective operations (Box 23.5). The potential hazards of this surgery are listed in Table 23.13.

5.6 Amputations

History of amputations

Early history

Amputation of limbs has a long history. In the early days, the need for amputation was probably small and most were probably carried out for trauma with infection. Hippocrates in 400 BC described amputation through necrotic tissue, but it was not until AD 50 that Celsus in Rome described the first flap

Table 23.13 Potential intraoperative hazards of ruptured aortic aneurysm surgery

1. Problems on opening the abdomen

Suprarenal aneurysm	If aneurysm extends above renal arteries, find site of rupture after gaining proximal control (usually at infradiaphragmatic level, above the stomach, by splitting the right crus of the diaphragm). If rupture is above renals, chances of success are very low and most would abandon the procedure. If aneurysm extends above renals but rupture is infrarenal, it is often possible to replace only the infrarenal portion of aorta to save patient's life
Inflammatory aneurysm	Thick, firm, inflammatory material lying across the anterior of aneurysm makes access to the neck difficult. Often bonds the duodenum to the aorta. Obtain temporary (suprarenal) control as above. Carefully dissect neck and reposition clamp
Horseshoe kidney	Kidneys joined in midline with the isthmus 'dragged' caudally by the inferior mesenteric artery, lying across the aneurysm. The isthmus cannot easily be divided. Therefore obtain proximal control as usual, occlude one renal artery temporarily, and divide the isthmus at line of demarcation. Oversew cut ends. Sometimes one half of the kidney must be sacrificed. Occasionally, the left side of the kidney can be mobilized and swung medially, allowing adequate access without sacrificing it

2. Damage to other structures during access

Inadvertent opening of bowel	The third part of the duodenum may be opened during separation from the aorta, or other gut may be damaged if adhesions are present. This represents a major problem with a great risk of graft infection. An elective operation should be abandoned, but for ruptured aneurysm, operation must proceed and rely on antibiotic cover and perhaps an antibiotic-impregnated graft (e.g. rifampicin-soaked gelatin-sealed graft) or an extra-anatomic bypass performed
Damage to veins	At risk when approaching aortic neck are the inferior mesenteric vein in the mesentery, the left renal vein and its tributaries across the aortic neck, the inferior vena cava if bonded to the aneurysm. Iliac veins are at risk when dissecting iliac arteries

3. Problems when inserting the graft

Access to aortic neck	Restricted access to aortic neck, or aneurysm very close to renals, makes proximal control difficult to obtain • If the aortic wall is of poor quality, there is a risk of traumatic perforation or splitting • Renal arteries can be damaged or embolized from clot in aneurysm • Suturing can be difficult and upper anastomosis is likely to leak
Arresting haemorrhage	Anastomotic bleeding: may be a technical fault requiring further suturing, but depletion of clotting factors ('red inking') is a common cause. Anticipate if bleeding is heavy by beginning fresh frozen plasma and platelet transfusions early. Wrap anastomoses with thrombogenic matrix (e.g. Surgicel®)
Failure to perfuse iliac arteries	After clamps removed, check distal perfusion by palpating femoral pulses and inspecting feet for 'pinking up'. Failure to revascularize may be due to a technical fault at lower anastomosis or a distal occlusion caused by thrombosis *in situ* or embolism. Do not wait to see if perfusion improves 'later'. Check distal anastomosis for patency; revise if necessary or consider femoro-femoral crossover graft. If okay, explore femoral artery in groin and pass Fogarty catheters proximal and distal to remove thrombus

4. Late complications An apparently successful operation may be followed by mortality because of late complications

Postoperative haemorrhage	Postoperative intra-abdominal blood loss which continues once clotting has been corrected prompts return to theatre. The source of haemorrhage is usually apparent and can be corrected by a suture or two
Acute renal failure	Often results from reperfusion injury following hypotension. Usually requires dialysis/haemofiltration. Recovery depends on extent of renal injury. Renal failure may be due to exacerbation of pre-existing renal failure or damage to renal arteries by aortic dissection or clamping or embolization
Myocardial infarction or cardiac failure	Profound swings in blood pressure may damage the myocardium, particularly if there is pre-existing coronary artery disease. Reperfusion injury also plays a part
Changes in fluid balance	Under- and over-transfusion may interfere with cellular metabolism and precipitate organ failure
Intestinal ischaemia	If mesenteric vessels are diseased, perfusion may depend on the inferior mesenteric. Ligation may cause intestinal ischaemia, most marked in the sigmoid colon. More extensive ischaemia is caused by hypotension and reperfusion injury
Sepsis syndrome	Probably caused by bacterial translocation (i.e. transfer of endogenous intestinal bacteria or endotoxins following intestinal ischaemia/reperfusion). May follow bacterial contamination after inadvertent opening of bowel, causing graft infection or other intra-abdominal infection. This is usually fatal

amputation in a text known as *De Medicus*. This was a scientific approach to surgery with amputation performed through healthy tissue proximal to the necrosis. Celsus also described the use of catgut ligatures and arterial forceps for the first time.

In the Dark Ages, these skills were forgotten and amputation surgery regressed to little better than butchery. After crudely severing the limb, hot iron cautery or molten tar was applied to the stump for haemostasis.

Military amputations

If a victim of conventional warfare survives injury, the limbs are the most commonly damaged part of the body. With the spread of gunpowder and the cannon ball in the fourteenth century, there was a massive increase in battlefield trauma. The battle of Crecy in 1346 was the first time firearms were used in a large-scale battle and resulted in great loss of life and limb. Treatment, however, remained primitive until the 1550s when Ambroise Paré, a French military surgeon, rediscovered the writings of Celsus, put them into practice and improved on the techniques.

Military amputation in the early days had a very high mortality. For example, Malgalene in 1842 reported a mortality of 62 per cent after above-knee amputation. This was probably largely due to gas gangrene implanted into wounds from soil contaminated with horse manure containing clostridial spores.

Carrey, another French surgeon working in Napoleonic times (early 1800s), discovered delayed primary closure for amputation wounds and was able to reduce mortality for battle amputations to 10 per cent. Delayed primary closure has remained a core of military surgery to this day, but has periodically been forgotten, with disastrous results.

Flap amputations

After Celsus's work had been forgotten, most amputations were performed by the circular or guillotine method, where all tissues are cut at the same level. Flap amputations were rediscovered in the Edinburgh school early in the nineteenth century, where Liston, Syme, and Ferguson used equal flaps of skin to close stumps. It was not until myoplastic flaps were introduced in the 1950s that a more physiological approach was adopted towards function after amputation.

Successful below-knee amputations using a myoplastic technique was first described by Kendrick in 1956. He was able to preserve many knee joints and obtained a remarkable ratio of six below-knee to one above knee-amputations. A similar technique was popularized by Burgess (1968) and the standard below-knee amputation is often known at the **Burgess flap**. In 1982, Robinson described a modification to the skin flaps, known as the **skew flap**, which has some advantages for early limb fitting as the stump is conical from the outset. Early hopes that healing would be better have unfortunately not been fulfilled in randomized trials.

Amputation prostheses

Crude peg legs have been in use as functional prostheses for centuries. These were made by carpenters and consisted of a platform upon which the patient kneeled with a short below-knee amputation, and a simple chair leg below. James Potts introduced the first articulated lower-limb prosthesis, the 'Anglesey leg', in 1800 for above-knee amputations, but prosthetic technology had to wait for modern materials to provide lightness, comfort, ease of use, and satisfactory simulation of joint function, which are the continuing goals of limb prosthetics. In developing countries, the simple, locally maid **Jaipur limb** is effective. This employs a hand-beaten sheet-metal socket (which can be shaped to accommodate later stump changes) and a simple rubber foot.

Incidence and types of amputations

There are about 6000 new amputees in England and Wales per annum and a total of 65 000 amputees were known to the Department of Health in 1986. This is undoubtedly an under-

Table 23.14 Indications for limb amputations in developed countries

Underlying pathology	Description
Ischaemia, often with infection, 64% (very rare in upper limb)	• Inability to reconstruct distal disease or failure of reconstruction • Delay in relieving acute or critical ischaemia • Extensive necrosis or an otherwise useless limb, e.g. joint deformities • Poor general health and no prospect of walking • In advanced gangrene, concomitant arterial reconstruction may allow a lesser amputation, e.g. below knee versus above knee
Uncomplicated diabetic neuropathy, 20%	Local amputations should be all that is needed but it is likely that too many major amputations are performed for neuropathic diabetic foot. Education and surveillance of diabetics could largely eliminate major diabetic foot disorders
Trauma and its consequences, 9% (main cause of upper-limb amputations)	Severed or trapped limbs, extensive nerve and vessel damage, and crush injuries, together with secondary infection (primarily gas gangrene) are the main reasons for amputation after trauma
Malignancies, 4% (also affect upper limb)	Primarily sarcomas. This figure is being reduced by the current trend to excise osteosarcomas and replace with a prosthesis for bone, preserving the limb
Paralysis and deformities, 3% (occasionally in upper limb)	Gross deformities and 'floppy' paralysed limbs, or limbs with intolerable pain are often better amputated

estimate as statistics are based on referral numbers to limb-fitting centres. About 25 per cent of new amputees have diabetes (neuropathy and arterial insufficiency) and 75 per cent are non-diabetic. However, it is likely that too many major amputations are still being done in diabetics who have lesions that could heal with local amputation only. It is also certain that too many above-knee amputations are still being performed for ischaemia, although the ratio is gradually improving (see Table 23.14). Whereas the average ratio of above-knee to below-knee amputations is currently about 1 : 1, several British units have published a below-knee amputation rate for all comers of better than 70 per cent. It should be noted that this includes a minor surgical revision rate of about 10 per cent before final healing is achieved. Table 23.14 demonstrates that arterial insufficiency (which is largely atherosclerotic) is the predominant cause of lower-limb amputation, with diabetic foot complications following. Other causes are rare.

Amputation in arterial insufficiency

Economics of amputation compared with reconstructive surgery

A major lower-limb amputation causes considerable handicap to a patient, particularly an elderly one. No amputation prosthesis can function like a normal limb and, in particular, an above-knee prosthesis makes enormous demands on a patient in terms of putting it on, energy expenditure in use, slowness of walking, and discomfort. Indeed, full rehabilitation of the elderly, including normal walking, is almost never achieved.

The cost of an amputation in the first year, including hospital and rehabilitation charges is difficult to quantify precisely, but amounts to between £15 000 and £45 000, compared with the cost of an average arterial reconstruction of around £2500–£5000, including graft surveillance and secondary procedures. If more limbs could be saved by earlier diagnosis and more

Table 23.15 Assessing level of amputation in ischaemia

Factor	Assessment
In diabetics, what is the relative contribution of neuropathy and arterial insufficiency?	In diabetics with gangrene or ulceration, the extent of ischaemia is the major determinant of the level of amputation. 'Pure' neuropathy can be treated by local excision of dead tissue, whereas ischaemia requires arterial reconstruction and/or major amputation
What is the extent of necrosis?	The extent of gangrene helps determine the level of amputation. If skin is poorly perfused or necrotic at the proposed level of amputation, it will undoubtedly fail
Is there infection present?	Amputation must remove all infected and necrotic tissue and the wound be left open
What is the severity and extent of ischaemia?	• Extent of necrosis and trophic skin changes • Palpability of peripheral pulses: if foot pulses are confirmed as palpable, critical ischaemia is very unlikely • Doppler pressures: low ankle and toe arterial systolic pressure confirm clinical findings • Limb blood flow measurements: these are largely research tools and have little application in daily clinical practice. Examples include clearance of injected radioisotopes and plethysmography • Arteriography: this does not show the extent of ischaemia but can help determine whether reconstruction is possible • Tissue oxygen saturation using needle oxygen saturation probes: this is another research tool with little clinical application • Findings at operation: 　(a) if necrotic tissue or pus is found at the proposed level of amputation, healing at this level is unlikely. However, if the changes are not extensive, a provisional guillotine amputation at this level may be appropriate, with revision to the most suitable level after a few days 　(b) Provided the muscle looks healthy, neither the amount of bleeding from the cut muscle nor the patency of major blood vessels are useful indicators of healing potential
Mobility of the knee joint	Fixed flexion deformity of more than 15º makes a functional below-knee amputation stump unlikely. This is usually caused by fibrosis of flexor muscles, resulting from disuse and posture occasioned by chronic pain
What level of amputation to perform at the same time as reconstructive surgery	• If amputation is to be performed immediately after reconstructive surgery, the level of amputation will be determined by how much useful tissue would remain after removing all dead tissue. This may be best determined at operation although a provisional amputation should be performed if there is doubt • Whether a partially necrotic foot should be retained depends on whether it is likely to become a functional entity; necrosis proximal to the metatarsal heads suggests that a below-knee amputation is likely to be the best choice

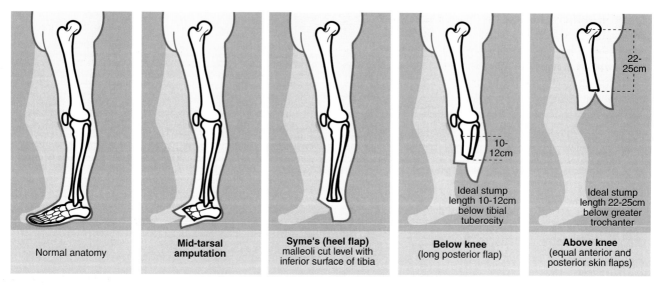

Figure 23.14 Sites of election for lower-limb amputations.

effective treatment, this would represent efficient use of scarce resources.

Indications for amputation in arterial insufficiency

When reconstructive surgery is inappropriate

Reconstructive arterial surgery may not be feasible or even technically possible in some patients with critical ischaemia, especially those with diffuse distal arterial disease. In some, reconstructive surgery may have failed either immediately or months or years later. For all of these, there may be no alternative to amputation. If there is substantial tissue necrosis and a functionally useless foot, or if there is deep spreading infection, reconstructive surgery is futile if employed to save the whole limb, and early amputation is the best choice.

Toxic effects of a dead limb

It is important to remember that a dead limb, particularly if infected, can cause an apparently non-specific decline in a patient. The patient becomes less alert, blood pressure may fall, and renal function declines. This process is mediated by the release of free radicals and cytokines from the necrotic limb and will result in death of the patient within a few days. However, timely amputation can immediately reverse the process. Thus, amputation should not be unreasonably deferred once the decision to amputate has been taken.

Talking to the patient

The need for amputation should be discussed gently with the patient, if possible giving him or her a day or two to discuss and come to terms with this disfiguring operation before it is performed. Like mastectomy, the obvious and visible disfigurement of an amputation has profound psychological effects and needs to be handled gently and sympathetically.

Assessing level of amputation in ischaemia

No test can reliably determine at what level an amputation will heal, although when a series of amputations is looked at in retrospect, a number of tests could have predicted about 70 per

Table 23.16 Lower-limb amputations in England and Wales: evolving proportion of below-knee to above-knee amputations

	1973	1982	1986	1994	1998
Above knee	70%	60%	50%	40%	43%
Below knee	30%	40%	50%	60%	60%

Table 23.17 Lower-limb amputations in England and Wales: changing proportions of above-knee to below-knee amputations in diabetic and non-diabetic patients

Level of amputation		1973	1982	1998
Above knee	Diabetic	484	415	155
	Non-diabetic	2470	2484	1601
Below knee	Diabetic	408	768	430
	Non-diabetic	755	1157	1889
Total (all causes)		4117	4824	4075

Note that the total numbers of above-knee amputations has fallen but the number of below-knee amputations have risen, so that the overall number of amputations has not changed substantially.

cent of the BK amputations which actually healed. However, they would have wrongly predicted that 30 per cent of those that did heal would not have healed. Thus, the level of amputation is determined essentially by clinical evaluation (Table 23.15), bearing in mind the 'sites of election' preferred by prosthetists, shown in Fig. 23.14.

Preservation of the knee

Tables 23.16 and 23.17 show the changing proportion of above- and below-knee amputations in diabetic and non-diabetic patients.

Amputation technique

Level of amputation

The main principles that guide the level of amputation are:

- Painfully ischaemic and necrotic tissue must all be removed.

- Infection must be eliminated.

- Primary skin healing must be facilitated. The amputation must be made through healthy tissue. If not, there is a high risk of wound breakdown and chronic ulceration, requiring further amputation at a higher level. When amputation is for peripheral ischaemia, it is almost always necessary to amputate at mid-tibial level or above to ensure healing.

- In most cases, aim to fit a functional and easy-to-use prosthesis. The choice of amputation level must take into account the fitting of a prosthetic limb. For this purpose, the mid–tibia (below knee) and lower femoral levels (above knee) are preferred. These sites of election provide adequate clearance for the prosthetist to include an artificial joint which is essential for satisfactory walking. If the patient's knee joint can be saved, the functional success of a prosthesis is much better. With recent improvements in prostheses, there has been a renewal of interest in through-knee amputation, but most limb fitters regard it as a poor amputation and published results report a high failure rate of healing.

Developments in amputation technique

The traditional 'guillotine' amputation of the battlefield simply sliced off the limb, leaving the wound to heal by secondary intention. This reduced the risk of fatal gas gangrene or tetanus but left a poor result for fitting an artificial limb prosthesis.

Box 23.6 Properties of the ideal amputation stump

- Healed with minimal scar tissue. The skin wound should not be bound down to the deep tissues which would cause tearing with shear forces within a limb prosthesis.
- Pain free.
- The skin and hypodermis should be supple and mobile but not floppy. The deep fascia of both flaps should be healed together.
- The stump should be conical to allow a prosthetic bucket to slide on without trauma and be retained without excessive movement.
- The joint above should not be in flexion deformity and should be reasonably mobile.
- The stump should be capable of being fitted with a satisfactory prosthesis which the patient is able to use to achieve the aims of everyday life.

Amputation techniques in recent years have changed considerably, with the intention of producing a healed, well-shaped, and 'padded' stump after the primary operation. For below-knee amputations, a long posterior flap of muscle and skin is now wrapped forward over the amputated bone and the fascia sutured in place. The muscle brings an improved blood supply and the technique results in more reliable healing and a suitably shaped and cushioned stump.

For above-knee amputations, a myoplastic flap technique is used in which the bony amputation level is proximal to the muscular and cutaneous amputation level. This allows the muscles to be sutured over the exposed bone end, adductors to abductors and flexors to extensors, after which the short anterior and posterior fascial and skin flaps are closed over the muscle.

Forefoot amputations are mainly used in neuropathic diabetic foot problems, but may be appropriate after arterial reconstruction. Symes or trans-malleolar amputation is regarded by many as inferior in functional capacity to a good below-knee amputation, but does have the advantage that it can be used without footwear at night to respond to urgent calls of nature.

Results of amputation

The success rate of rehabilitation of amputees is disappointingly small. The worst results are achieved in older, infirm patients, particularly if undergoing above-knee amputation. It is safe to

---

Table 23.18 Problems with lower-limb amputations

Problem	Notes
Ischaemic pain in stump	Arterial reconstruction or amputation at a higher level
Non-healing stump or later ulceration of stump	Arterial reconstruction to improve perfusion, local refashioning or amputation at a higher level, depending on severity of problem
Phantom limb sensations and phantom limb pain	All amputees experience odd or distorted sensations but true phantom limb pain is rare. The latter is more likely to develop if the patient has suffered prolonged ischaemic pain before amputation and is extremely difficult to treat
Patient unable to cope with prosthesis	Modify prosthesis or aim to make patient 'wheelchair independent' and perhaps provide a lightweight cosmetic prosthesis

assume that such patients are unlikely ever to walk satisfactorily again. These results should be considered if there is an option to revascularize an ischaemic limb which would otherwise be amputated, and add weight to the economic argument that successful arterial surgery is overall cheaper than amputation.

In one series of unselected amputation patients, 12 per cent died in hospital and only half were accepted for walking training. Using standardized indices of 'activities of daily living' and observing the time taken to walk 10 metres, it was found that only one-third were successful walkers (of whom 90 per cent took more than 30 seconds to walk 10 m), one-third were partial or 'party trick' walkers, and one-third were not walking at all. When tested for pulse rate recovery, peak flow, and grip strength, partial walkers were found to be weaker and slower as well as older than successful walkers.

In another series, 2 years after below-knee amputation, one-third had died, only one-third were walking (although 90 per cent had walked at some time), and one-third were wheelchair dependent. Similarly, 2 years after above-knee amputation, one-third had died, one-quarter were walking (one-third having walked at some time), and nearly half were wheelchair bound.

Potential problems with lower-limb amputations are listed in Table 23.18.

Prostheses and limb fitting

Aims of limb fitting

Ideally, a patient for amputation is professionally counselled before operation by an experienced physiotherapist, for example, and has a chance to meet other amputees. When the patient attends a limb-fitting centre, the most important decision concerns the level of function that is to be aimed for. The general fitness of the patient, the patient's ability to cope with a prosthesis, and the suitability of the stump, together with progress under rehabilitation will determine the scheme of rehabilitation, as follows:

◆ High performance approaching normal function required in a young patient after amputation for trauma.

◆ Good walking ability within and outside the house such as for a patient of average fitness and competence.

◆ Occasional walking within the home but fundamentally wheelchair dependent, for an elderly, unfit patient.

◆ No attempt at limb fitting for an unfit patient who is handicapped in other ways, such as blindness. The patient will be wholly wheelchair dependent. In this case, rehabilitation aims to help the patient transfer between wheelchair and chair or bed. A light, foam, non-functional cosmetic limb is often provided.

The initial prosthesis

Where a functional prosthesis is planned, some form of artificial limb should be provided as soon as practicable after amputation, to allow early mobilization. This prevents loss of the proprioception and balance involved in walking and reduces the likelihood of flexion deformities of knee and hip.

A temporary limb with a pneumatic socket for stump fitting can often be used for early walking training, even before the wound is fully healed. If the healing of a below-knee amputation is likely to be prolonged, a 'bypass' prosthesis, such as an above-knee/below-knee pylon, can be provided while awaiting healing. The formerly common temporary pylons are rarely needed nowadays with the widespread use of modular prostheses, which can be provided earlier than before.

Elements of a limb prostheses

An artificial limb consists of a socket into which the stump fits, a foot and ankle combination distally, a connecting structure (strut), and for above-knee prostheses, a joint and its control mechanism to replace the knee. Most modern prostheses are of modular construction and can be assembled rapidly, using off-the-shelf components which are coupled to an individually moulded socket.

The components of a prosthesis include:

◆ **The 'structure'**—this may be exoskeletal or endoskeletal. Exoskeletal prostheses are made of light sheet metal or wood and provide both support and cosmetic shape. The more modern endoskeletal type consists of a metal or composite (e.g. carbon fibre) strut with attached end fittings. The strut is padded with foam to give it shape and covered with skin-like synthetic material. The strut must maintain precise alignment of socket and foot and may incorporate a means of fine adjustment for this purpose.

◆ **The socket**—this transmits forces between the stump and the prosthesis in vertical and transverse planes as well as in rotation. The shape of the socket deviates from the shape of the stump, after taking into account the contained bone, the different compressibility of tissues and areas tolerant of or sensitive to pressure. Sockets are designed to be either predominantly proximal bearing, predominantly distal bearing, or total bearing, according to where the body weight is intended to be mainly borne on the prosthesis. Some sockets provide the only attachment ('suspension') to the patient. In others, additional support is needed using suspensory elements around shoulders, waist, pelvis, or thigh.

◆ **The ankle and foot unit**—this unit needs to transfer forces between patient and ground in a stable manner and modify these forces during the gait cycle. Thus, the anterior part of the foot needs to be flexible to allow it to bend appropriately during 'push off', and the ideal ankle joint needs to allow flexion and extension with an appropriate degree of resistance, together with a small amount of rotation.

◆ **The knee joint.** The working of the normal knee is complex and, to replace it, a functional prosthesis requires complex mechanical equivalents. When standing, the knee joint needs to lock automatically. This can be achieved by designing the long axis to pass in front of the knee centre when the hip is extended. The knee should also be stable but with 8–12° flexion to allow walking over uneven surfaces. This is controlled by a mechanical or hydraulic stabilizer. In walking, the swing phase of knee flexion comes into operation. This is controlled and buffered by a separate pneumatic or hydraulic device which relies on restricted transfer of air or oil through small orifices in a closed system.

Above-knee prostheses

The endoskeletal type is preferred in developed countries but exoskeletal types are used for established amputees unwilling to change, those who work in wet or dirty environments or who kneel a lot, dwellers or travellers in developing countries (for reasons of maintenance), and those with extremely thin legs.

The socket for either type is usually constructed of soft, flexible plastic, lining a rigid plastic support frame. This type is easy to construct by modern methods but needs relining when the stump volume changes. Metal sockets are expensive to manufacture but are cool to wear and can be expanded or contracted to match changes in stump dimensions. Wood is a good material but prostheses are labour intensive to produce. Leather sockets become hardened with prolonged use.

Modern above-knee sockets are designed to bear the body weight largely on the ischial tuberosity. This is a considerable functional improvement on the 'conventional' or plug-fit socket. There are several variations on this theme: the 'H' socket is triangular in section with an ischial seat to carry the weight. Counterpressure is provided from the antero-lateral side to maintain the tuberosity on the seat. The 'Q' (quadrilateral) and the 'E-Q' (Euro-quadrilateral) sockets are variations which include greater clearance for anatomical structures, particularly the adductor longus tendon.

Sockets are made to provide total contact with the skin of the stump. This prevents stump congestion and assists suspension. Many above-knee prostheses do not need external suspension and are kept in place by muscle contraction and suction. To do this the stump volume must be stable and the contour smooth; muscle control must be good and the patient must be reasonably agile. Finally, the stump must be of adequate length. When external suspension is required, there is a wide range of options which can be matched to the individual patient's needs.

Several different types of knee joint and ankle/foot combination are available. The choices depend on the sophistication of the limb-fitting services available, the demands the patient is likely to make on the prosthesis, and economic factors.

Below-knee prostheses

The most advanced knee prostheses are patellar tendon bearing (PTB) but cannot be used in all circumstances. PTB prosthesis are not appropriate if there is a bulbous stump, a short stump (bone section less than 5 cm below medial hamstring insertion), a scarred stump, flexion deformity of the knee, ligamentous or muscular instability of the knee, stump pain on weight bearing, or an absent patella.

PTB limbs are usually endoskeletal modular prostheses with a soft foam finish. The socket is usually plastic (e.g. glass-reinforced plastic (GRP) or polypropylene). The socket is a snug fit with a patellar tendon bar which transmits the main weight.

This fills the entire space between the patella and tibial tubercle. It is flared posteriorly to accommodate the hamstring tendons. A removable liner is often included to provide cushioning and potential for adjustment.

Below-knee prostheses generally require suspension. The most common is a supracondylar belt which straps around the lower thigh. A promising recent development is the silicone-lined suction socket. This incorporates a valve built into the socket which allows air to evacuate when weight is borne to generate suction. This type does not require additional suspension.

Rehabilitation and walking training for the new amputee

If practicable, the patient should undergo a week of preparation before amputation. This includes learning the exercises that will be required after amputation and undergoing physiotherapy to mobilize stiff or contracted joints.

Walking training using a pneumatic walking aid should start within 2 weeks of amputation. After the definitive prosthesis is fitted, patients benefit from a period of instruction in a rehabilitation department, preferably as an inpatient. This includes how to put the limb on and take it off, how to balance when standing between parallel bars, and how to transfer weight from one leg to the other. The patient practices lifting the prosthesis off the floor and making strides from 'toe off' to heel contact.

Later, the patient begins walking between parallel bars, aiming for a stable stance and gait pattern. Progress is gradually made to walking without bars using other aids such as a walking frame, crutches, and eventually walking sticks.

The estimated costs of rehabilitation are given in Table 23.19.

Table 23.19 The cost of rehabilitation after amputation

At a conservative estimate, the cost of getting an amputee walking might be:	
Two weeks' inpatient rehabilitation	£3000
12 physiotherapy visits	£200
Limb prosthesis	£1000
Basic wheelchair	£200
Home modifications	£250
Total	**£4650**
The cost of achieving wheelchair mobility is little different:	
Electric wheelchair	£1500
Home modifications	£3000
Total	**£4500**

Bibliography

Amputation

Kaufman, J.L. (1955). Alternative methods for below-knee amputation: reappraisal of the Kendrick procedure. *J. Am. Coll. Surg.*, **181**, 511–6.

Burgess, E.M., Romano, R.L. (1968). The management of lower extremity amputees using immediate postsurgical prostheses. *Clin. Orthop.*, **57**, 137–56.

Robinson, K.P., Hoile, R., Coddington, T. (1982). Skew flap myoplastic below-knee amputation: a preliminary report. *Br. Surg.*, **69**, 554–7.

Aneurysms

Cappeller, W.A. Holzel, D., Hinz, M.H., and Lauterjung, L. (1998). Germany. Ten-year results following elective surgery for abdominal aortic aneurysm. *Angiology*, **17**, (4), 234–40. [Retrospective study with 5–12-year follow-up on 521 (95.6%) of 545 consecutive operations. Hospital mortality was 6.4% and cumulative survival 65% at 5 years and 41% at 10 years. The mean survival was 95.1 months. Patients who had undergone aorto-coronary bypass had a better long-term outcome.]

The UK Small Aneurysm Trial Participants (1998). Mortality results for randomised controlled trial of early elective surgery or ultrasonographic surveillance for small abdominal aortic aneurysms. *Lancet*, **352**, 1649–55. [1090 patients with symptomless AAA of 4.0–5.5 cm aged 60–76 were randomized to elective surgery or ultrasonographic surveillance and followed up for 4.6 years. 309 patients died but mortality did not differ between the groups at 2, 4, or 6 years. Age, sex, or size did not modify the hazard ratio. Early surgery does not provide a long-term survival advantage for small AAAs.]

Choksy, S.W., William, A.B.M., Quick, C.R.G. (1999). Ruptured abdominal aortic aneurysm in the Huntingdon District: a 10 year experience. *Ann. R. Coll. Surg. Engl.*, **81**, 27–31.

Carotid artery disease

European Carotid Surgery Trial Collaborative Group (1991). MRC European carotid surgery trial: interim results for symptomatic patients with severe (70–99%) or with mild (0–29%) carotid stenosis. *Lancet*, **337**, 1235–41.

North American Symptomatic Carotid Endarterectomy Trial Collaborative Group (1991). Beneficial effects for endarterectomy in symptomatic patients with high grade stenoses. *N. Eng. J. Med.*, **325**, 445–53.

Executive committee for the asymptomatic carotid atherosclerosis study (1995). Endarterectomy for asymptomatic carotid artery stenosis. *JAMA*, **273**, 1421–61.

Ellis, M., Greenhalgh, R. (1987). Management of the asymptomatic carotid bruit. *J. Vasc. Surg.*, **5**, 869–73.

Thrombolysis

Chesterman, C.N., Sharp, A.A. (1971). Arterial thrombolysis. *Lancet*, **2**, 264–5.

Dotter, C.T., Rosch, J., Seaman, A.J., Dennis, D., Massey, W.H. (1972). Streptokinase treatment of thromboembolic disease. *Radiol.*, **102**, 283–90.

Hughes, C. (1958). Aeterial repair during the Korean War. *Ann. Surg.*, **147**, 555–61.

Perry, M.O. (1993). Vascular trauma, pp. 630–47 In *Vascular Surgery*, (ed. Moore, W.S.), W.B. Saunders, Philadelphia.

Bongard, F., Wilson, S., Perry, M. (1991).Vascular injuries in surgical practice. Appleton and Lange, Norwalk, CT.

General

Gruntzig, A., Hopff, H. (1974). [Percutaneous recanalization after chronic arterial occlusion with a new dilator-catheter. *Dtsch Med Wochenschr*, **99**, 2502–11.

Swebel, W. (1992). *Introduction to vascular sonography*, (3rd edn). WB. Saunders, Philadelphia.

Campbell, W.B. (1996). *Complications in arterial surgery.* Butterworth Heinemann, Oxford.

Fowkes, F.G.R. (1990). *Epidemiology of peripheral vascular disease.* Springer Verlag, Berlin.

Greenhalgh, R.M. and Fowkes, F.G.R. (1996). *Trials and tribulations of vascular surgery.* WB. Saunders, London.

Hosley, E. (1988). Treating claudication in five words. *BMJ*, **2962**, 1483–4.

MacKinnan, S.E. (1996). Thoracic outlet syndrome. *Seminars in thoracic and cardiovascular surgery*, **8**, 175–228.

Morris, G., Friend, P., Vassallo, D., Farrington, M., Leapman, S., and Quick, C.R.G. (1994). Antibiotic irrigation and conservative surgery for major aortic graft infection. *J. Vasc. Surg.*, **20**, 88–95.

Beattie, D.K., Golledge, J., Greenhalgh, R.M., and Davies, A.H. (1997). Quality of life assessment in vascular disease: towards a consensus. *Europ. J. Vasc. Endovasc. Surg.*, **13**, 9–13.

Davies, A.H., Beard, J., and Wyatt, M.G. (1999). *Essential vascular surgery*. W.B. Saunders, London.

CHAPTER 24

Thyroid, parathyroid, and salivary glands

Anjan K. Banerjee and Clive R. Quick

1 Introduction

1.1 Specialties involved in head and neck surgery

Head and neck surgery cannot be regarded as a coherent specialty because surgeons from several disciplines treat disorders in this region without many strict guidelines (Table 24.1). Even for a single condition such as a parotid swelling, a patient may come under the care of a general surgeon, an ENT surgeon, or a plastic surgeon, according to local practice and the preference of the referring doctor.

However, certain areas are treated virtually exclusively by certain specialists. For example, surgical intracranial disease is managed entirely by neurosurgeons (except for occasional life-saving emergency burr holes for extradural haemorrhage). Certain ENT surgeons specialize in the surgery of acoustic neuromas but usually operate alongside a neurosurgeon for these procedures. Eye and orbital surgery is the exclusive province of the ophthalmic surgeon, and facial fractures come under the care of the oral surgeon, as does most surgery to do with the teeth, alveolar margin, or jaws.

This chapter aims to cover those aspects of head and neck surgery that traditionally come under the care of general surgeons. No attempt has been made to cover specialist ENT surgery, ophthalmology, neurosurgery, oral surgery, or plastic surgery, except where the fields are likely to overlap, or a knowledge of the specialty is required in order to make an informed referral.

The head and neck present particular hazards when operating because of the concentration of vital structures in the area with the potential risk of inadvertent damage. However, if the surgeon has a detailed knowledge of the local anatomy, this is rewarded by the satisfaction of finding there is little anatomical variation and that all the structures are where they should be!

The head and neck have an excellent blood supply which confers the advantages of rapid healing with minimal scarring and a low risk of infection. However, this profuse blood supply means that operations can be haemorrhagic and the view is easily obscured, leading to potential iatrogenic damage of vital structures unless particular care is taken to arrest haemorrhage from even the smallest vessels. Special perioperative measures are sometimes taken to reduce vascularity, for example employing **hypotensive anaesthesia** for parotidectomy or the use of subcutaneous injections of weak adrenaline (epinephrine) solution prior to thyroidectomy.

Endocrine disorders of the thyroid and parathyroid tend to be managed jointly by physician and surgeon, to decide whether surgery is appropriate and the optimum time for intervention for thyrotoxicosis, for example. Most patients with hyperparathyroidism require surgical exploration of the neck, a procedure best performed by a surgeon with special experience.

Head and neck cancer (pharynx, sinuses, oral cavity, and jaws) is usually managed jointly by ENT surgeons, oral surgeons, and radiotherapists, although cancers of salivary glands and thyroid usually come under the care of general surgeons with an interest in the area, or endocrine surgeons.

1.2 Clinical diagnosis of a lump in the neck

The clinical diagnosis of lumps in the neck will not be covered in detail here but the following is an *aide-mémoire* of history taking, clinical examination, and investigation:

History

- Country of origin of the patient—is this likely to be a tropical disease, TB, or endemic goitre?

- Type of patient—age, sex, smoking habit, occupation, previous malignant disease, including lymphoma.

- Rate of growth of the lump.

- Neurological deficit—facial weakness, dribbling, hoarseness.

- Family history—particularly for thyroid disease.

Examination

For detailed examination of the thyroid see next Section 2. In general, try to work out the organ of origin of the lump. During

Table 24.1 Specialists treating head and neck disorders

General surgeons	Abscesses, lymph nodes, thyroid
Endocrine surgeons	Thyroid and parathyroid
Otorhinolaryngologists (ENT surgeons)	Ear, nose, pharynx, larynx, facial sinuses. Sub-specialists treat head and neck cancer, acoustic neuromas, parotid, thyroid, etc.
Plastic and reconstructive surgeons	Skin, sometimes thyroid, salivary glands
Ophthalmic surgeons	Eye and orbit, eyelids, lachrymal apparatus
Neurosurgeons	Cranium, cranial nerves
Vascular surgeons	Carotid atherosclerosis, aneurysms, and tumours
Orthopaedic surgeons and rheumatologists	Arthritis, spinal fractures
Maxillofacial and dental surgeons	Teeth and mouth, facial fractures, salivary glands

examination, consciously consider the following characteristics of the lump:

- situation of lump and tissue layer of origin—relate to nearby anatomy (e.g. skin, muscles, arteries, salivary glands)

- size;

- shape;

- surface—including temperature;

- fixation both to skin and deeply;

- consistency—use only soft, firm, or hard;

- fluctuation;

- pulsation;

- bruit—thyroid, carotid area;

- neurological dysfunction—facial nerve, recurrent laryngeal;

- lymph nodes in field of drainage.

2 Differential diagnosis of common lumps in the neck

2.1 Lymph-node enlargement

Lymph-node enlargement is the most common cause of a lump in the neck. It is most often caused by acute infections of the upper respiratory tract, which are characterized clinically by a transient tender enlargement of lymph nodes, usually in the upper anterior triangle of the neck (jugulo-digastric node). Note that in children and young people, lymph nodes may remain moderately enlarged long after the initiating cause has resolved.

A non-tender lymph node may be a more significant clinical finding and is more likely to be associated with either primary or secondary lymphatic malignancy.

Acute or chronic local infection

- Bacterial and viral pharyngitis and tonsillitis (particularly if chronic or recurrent).

- Suppuration and wounds.

- Dental infection (apical/gingival/periodontal).

- Tuberculosis and other mycobacterial infection.

- Other granulomatous diseases (e.g. cat-scratch disease).

- Actinomycosis.

Acute or chronic systemic infection (generalized lymphadenopathy)

- Rubella.

- Infectious mononucleosis (glandular fever).

- AIDS-related lymphadenopathy.

- Secondary syphilis.

Malignant disease

- Primary: lymphomas—cervical adenopathy is a common first presentation.

- Metastatic: metastasis down from primary cancer of mouth, pharynx, oesophagus or air passages; metastasis up from breast, lung, abdominal viscera (Troisier's sign/Virchow's node).

2.2 Examination of the patient with thyroid enlargement

The patient should be examined sitting up, both from in front and from behind. The main points to consider are:

1. Is the thyroid enlarged?

2. Is the enlargement generalized or solitary?

3. Is the patient hyper- or hypothyroid?

4. Is there a retrosternal extension?

5. Is there a vocal cord palsy?

6. Are there any eye signs?

2.3 Salivary swellings

Differential diagnosis includes:

- Stone in duct or gland.

- Retention cyst.

- Neoplasm—adenolymphoma, pleomorphic adenoma, adenocystic carcinoma, acinic cell carcinoma.

- Chronic sialadenitis.

- Autoimmune disorders (e.g. Sjögren's syndrome—expect lachrymal gland enlargement and dry mouth and eyes).

- Acute parotitis or abscess.

- 'Mikulicz disease' (now thought to be a low-grade lymphoma).

2.4 Skin and subcutaneous lumps

- Epidermal (sebaceous) cyst.

- Malignancy: BCC, SCC, malignant melanoma, skin metastasis.

- Pyogenic granuloma.

- Kerato-acanthoma.

- Congenital swellings:

   (a) cystic hygroma in a child or young person;

   (b) branchial cyst;

(c) thyroglossal cyst;

(d) dermoid cyst.

◆ Cervical rib (expect to feel prominent subclavian arterial pulsation overlying it).

◆ Benign neoplasms (e.g. lipoma).

2.5 Some rarities

◆ Arterial

(a) carotid body tumour/chemodectoma (may be able to palpate this bimanually in tonsillar fossa);

(b) carotid artery aneurysm (very rare).

◆ Pharyngeal pouch.

◆ Laryngocoele.

◆ Bony tumours and abnormalities of the jaws and teeth.

◆ Other malignancies (e.g. carcinoma of maxillary antrum).

3 Principles of investigative techniques

3.1 Introduction

As in other fields, the choice of special investigations employed in this area depends on how robust is the diagnosis reached by clinical examination and what is available locally. For example, a sebaceous cyst of the scalp is readily recognized by its clinical features, the diagnosis is confirmed on excision, and no special investigations are required. In contrast, 'alerting' symptoms such as facial pain associated with a nerve palsy but in the absence of a obvious lump may require a battery of investigations before the diagnosis becomes clear. The extent and type of investigation varies according to the presentation. For example, each of the following presentations requires a markedly different route of investigation: skin lumps, recurrent salivary gland swelling, facial pain, fixed lymph-node swelling in the neck, oral ulcers, hoarseness with thyroid swelling, and facial palsy with parotid swelling.

3.2 Blood tests

Thyroid

Blood tests are useful for determining:

◆ the state of endogenous drive of the thyroid gland, by measuring the thyroid stimulating hormone (TSH) level;

◆ whether the patient is euthyroid, hypothyroid, or hyperthyroid by measuring the free (i.e. non-protein-bound) plasma thyroxine (fT_4) and sometimes the plasma tri-iodothyronine (T_3).

When patients are taking thyroxine replacement or antithyroid drugs for hyperthyroidism, these blood tests need to be interpreted with care, particularly after surgery for thyroid cancer when replacement T_4 is administered to suppress endogenous output.

Low normal levels of T_4 with high TSH may be found in cases of early hypothyroidism. Patients systemically unwell from other disorders may have a low T_4 as well a low TSH (**sick euthyroid syndrome**).

Parathyroid

Standard blood tests include plasma calcium studies and parathormone (PTH) assay. Selective venous sampling is reserved for revision parathyroid surgery. In this technique, selective venous sampling and assay of venous samples for parathormone aids localization of ectopic parathyroid tissue. The diagnosis of primary, secondary, and tertiary hyperparathyroidism may be suspected from renal function tests, and plasma phosphate and calcium levels.

3.3 Plain X-rays

In head and neck disease generally, the types of plain X-rays used include: lateral or lateral oblique of the jaws, oral pantomography, 30° occipito-mental, intraoral films for jaw lesions, and occlusal film for suspected submandibular duct stone. Plain X-rays may be indicated as follows:

◆ for suspected fractures of the skull or jaws;

◆ for swellings of the jaws to show whether there is bony involvement;

◆ to determine whether there is opacification of the paranasal sinuses consistent with fluid or soft-tissue masses;

◆ for teeth and possible tooth-related problems, such as apical abscesses;

◆ for suspected salivary stones—radiology of the floor of the mouth and parotid duct area (salivary stones are usually calcified);

◆ to demonstrate tracheal compression or deviation in the presence of a possible retrosternal goitre—thoracic outlet (inlet) X-rays;

◆ as part of the work-up for a patient with abnormal lymph nodes in the neck or with arm symptoms suspicious of cervical rib—chest X-ray;

◆ chest—particularly if TB is suspected or the patient is hoarse (possible malignant carinal nodes from carcinoma of lung);

◆ CT scanning—for suspected malignancy anywhere in head and neck. Particularly useful for retrosternal thyroid, sinuses.

3.4 Contrast X-rays

◆ Sialography, for salivary duct and gland lesions.

◆ Arteriography, for aneurysm and chemodectoma (possibly therapeutic embolization).

- For localizing abnormal parathyroid glands, highly selective angiography may be performed with direct injection into the superior or inferior thyroid arteries and internal mammary arteries. Digital subtraction of the angiograms may also be performed. These radiological methods may give a distinctive contrast 'blush' in adenomas or hyperplastic glands.

3.5 Ultrasonography

B-mode ultrasound scanning is valuable for thyroid swellings. It can show whether a lesion is cystic, mixed solid and cystic, or solid, and can readily distinguish solitary from multiple nodules. Ultrasound-guided fine-needle aspiration (FNA) or biopsy of thyroid nodules is often employed. Duplex Doppler (combined B-mode and Doppler) is useful for delineating arterial anatomy, for example, in suspected aneurysms in the neck.

3.6 Endoscopy

Endoscopy in the head and neck is usually performed with flexible fibre-optic instruments, but occasionally rigid instruments, such as a sinoscope, are employed. This technique is invaluable for direct visualization and biopsy of pharynx, larynx, nasal cavity, oesophagus, and air passages. A rigid mediastinoscope is sometimes used to biopsy nodes in the mediastinum via a small incision.

Pharynx

Fibre-optic flexible endoscopy of the entire pharynx is now part of daily practice in otolaryngology (ENT). For general surgeons, the main application is in a patient with an obviously malignant node in the neck to seek a primary cancer in the pharynx. The 'silent' area of the nasopharynx often gives rise to tiny primaries which metastasize before the primary cancer causes symptoms. Sometimes these are so tiny that they are not even visible on fibre endoscopy and can only be shown on blind, deep biopsies of the fossa of Rosenmüller, performed via a rigid endoscope under general anaesthesia.

Larynx

Where there is any doubt about vocal-cord function prior to surgery and, ideally, prior to any form of thyroid or parathyroid surgery, both vocal cords should be examined for normal function and documented to be so. This is to ensure that any loss of function after operation will not be attributed to the operation if it was known to be present beforehand.

Gastrointestinal

High dysphagia may require endoscopic examination of the pharynx and the upper oesophagus. This is usually performed using flexible instruments as the need for rigid instruments has largely been superseded.

3.7 Histology and cytology

Histological examination should be performed on all surgical specimens, and other tissues or cells removed to ensure that

unexpected malignancies do not pass unnoticed until too late. Occasionally unusual types of tumour are discovered which may radically alter the treatment proposed.

Specimens are obtained in the form of fine-needle aspirates, core biopsies, incision biopsies (e.g. large skin lesion or ulcer), excision biopsies (e.g. lymph node), or surgical specimens.

3.8 Fine-needle aspiration cytology

Tissue diagnosis using fine-needle aspiration cytology (FNAC) is increasingly popular for the diagnosis of thyroid nodules, following successful studies in Scandinavia and elsewhere. FNA is also employed for recently changed nodules in multinodular goitres. Given appropriate technique and a well-trained cytologist, up to 90 per cent of thyroid nodules can be successfully categorized by this method. The rate of false negatives and false positives is acceptable and the number of unnecessary operations performed on benign lesions is reduced as a result of this diagnostic information. If a colloid nodule is diagnosed, operative excision is not necessary unless the nodule causes compressive symptoms or cosmetic deformity.

Fine-needle aspiration cytology enables recognition of:

- **Colloid goitre** (the most common cause of a thyroid nodule). The slides show an abundance of colloid material and some atrophic follicular cells.

- **Thyroid cysts.** If fluid alone is aspirated and the lump disappears, a cyst is the likely diagnosis. The fluid should be examined cytologically and, if benign, the patient examined in a few weeks to ensure that the lump has not reappeared.

- **Neoplasms.** Thyroid neoplasms are often soft, but may be firm or hard. Thus the palpation characteristics are generally unhelpful in making the diagnosis and a tissue diagnosis must be obtained. FNAC is the method of first choice in most cases, although some centres favour core biopsy, using for example, the slender variety of Trucut biopsy needle.

The use of FNAC for suspected thyroid malignancy

Follicular carcinomas cannot be distinguished cytologically from benign follicular adenomas because both display sheets of follicular cells with infrequent metastases. Lesions with this cytological appearance must be removed surgically, although most will be benign. Lesions which are obviously malignant on cytology include papillary, medullary, and anaplastic carcinomas. Note, however, that most lymphomas are inadequately sampled by FNA.

Incision biopsy is occasionally used for diagnosing generalized thyroid enlargement where the chances of malignancy are low or lymphoma is suspected.

Papillary carcinoma

This is the most common thyroid malignancy. It is usually confined to one lobe but may be multicentric. Papillary carcinoma frequently metastasizes to local lymph nodes but this does not necessarily make the prognosis worse. The diagnosis can usually be made confidently on a satisfactory FNA specimen

Follicular neoplasms

Follicular neoplasms include follicular adenoma and follicular carcinoma. **Follicular carcinoma** is the second most common thyroid malignancy. FNA alone cannot distinguish between adenoma and carcinoma as the cells look intrinsically benign and similar in both lesions. The diagnosis of malignancy is based on whether there is capsular invasion and invasion of blood vessels, and can only be determined from histological specimens taken from many parts of the tumour which include the capsule.

If a follicular neoplasm is found on FNA, radioiodine scanning can be used to distinguish between 'cold' nodules (absent uptake), which have a 20 per cent chance of being follicular carcinoma, and those with normal or increased iodine uptake, which are almost invariably benign. However, most surgeons prefer excision as the safest option.

Medullary carcinoma

Medullary carcinomas make up about 10 per cent of thyroid carcinomas and arise from thyroid C (calcitonin-secreting) cells. Medullary carcinomas have a characteristic appearance on FNAC. If the plasma calcitonin is also elevated, the diagnosis is confirmed. Some of these patients have multiple endocrine neoplasia type II (MEN II) and in these, phaeochromocytoma should be excluded before operation for thyroid carcinoma. There is often a strong family history in MEN II syndrome.

Anaplastic carcinoma

Anaplastic carcinomas constitute about 5 per cent of thyroid carcinomas and is found chiefly in elderly people. This tumour behaves extremely aggressively, infiltrating neck structures widely. FNAC demonstrates widespread areas of necrosis or fibrosis with few viable cells, making it difficult to obtain representative samples. Thus, many specimens may need to be obtained. It may be difficult to distinguish anaplastic small-cell carcinoma from poorly differentiated lymphoma and an open biopsy may be required to make this important distinction between a potentially curable condition on the one hand, and a hopeless condition on the other.

Thyroid lymphoma

This is relatively uncommon and may occur as part of a more generalized lymphoma or remain localized in the thyroid. The normal thyroid contains aggregations of lymphoid tissue which may become malignant. They are prominent in Hashimoto's disease but the incidence of lymphoma in these patients is probably no higher than normal. FNA is unreliable for diagnosing lymphoma, which usually requires open incision biopsy.

Metastatic carcinoma

Occasionally tumours remote from the thyroid metastasize into the gland and this may explain certain unusual cytological findings. FNAC is also sometimes used as a preliminary inves-tigation of lymph-node enlargement in the neck, particularly if a patient develops a doubtful lymph node swelling during follow-up after treatment for a local carcinoma.

Limitations of fine-needle aspiration

◆ The absence of malignant cells in the aspirate does not exclude a malignancy, because of the possibility of inaccurate targeting of the needle.

◆ The presence of malignant cells within the aspirate indicates the nature of the underlying disease but does not indicate the degree of malignancy. For example, it will not differentiate between carcinoma in situ and invasive carcinoma. This type of information would be obtained if a core of tissue was removed by a Trucut needle biopsy.

Technique of fine-needle aspiration

◆ The area to be needled is fixed between the index finger and thumb. The skin is cleaned with a spirit swab and the needle with a syringe already attached is introduced directly into the lump.

◆ Cells are aspirated from the lesion by continued suction on the syringe while the needle is passed through the mass.

◆ On withdrawing the needle the aspirate is expressed onto two clean glass slides and smeared. One slide is dried in air and the other is fixed with an alcohol-based fixative. Each slide is labelled with the patient's name, age, and identification number. They are then delivered to the cytologist as soon as possible.

3.9 Radioisotope scans

Principles of the use of radioisotopes for diagnostic scanning

◆ Organ- or tissue-specific 'tracers' are combined with a radioactive label.

◆ The tracer is distributed systemically, usually by an intravenous injection, and selectively picked up by the tissue of interest. The distribution of the tracer is measured by a gamma camera.

◆ Scans can be static or dynamic. Static scans measure the quantity of radioactive label in an area at a predetermined time after injection. Dynamic scans continually measure the level of isotope and provide the rate at which the organ or tissue takes up and subsequently discharges the tracer.

The precise dose of radioiodine used is calculated for each patient, based on weight and clinical indication. Diagnostic scanning requires the lowest dose, treatment for thyrotoxicosis needs intermediate doses, while ablative treatment for cancer needs the highest doses. Caution needs to be exercised since MBq and mCi are commonly confused; note that 1 Curie = 3.71×10^{10} Becquerel.

Examples of common doses of radioiodine used for various situations:

- diagnostic thyroid scan: 1–2 mCi;

- therapy for thyrotoxicosis: 5–10 mCi;

- ablative treatment for cancer: 50–150 mCi (depending on weight of thyroid gland remnant). Up to 200 mCi may be used for metastatic disease.

Thyroid

Technetium and iodine scans are sometimes employed for imaging the thyroid. Technetium scanning can be carried out easily in any unit with nuclear medicine facilities, but radio-iodine scanning requires more elaborate preparation of the isotopes. It is often more useful diagnostically, giving some information about thyroid function. Active thyroid tissue avidly takes up iodine and this property is the basis for using intravenous iodine radioisotopes to image the thyroid gland. Nowadays, these scans are largely qualitative as the need for measuring quantitative uptake to diagnose hyperthyroidism has been superseded by simpler tests, for example, by accurate measurements of plasma free thyroxine.

Ultrasonography and fine-needle aspiration cytology have replaced other former applications of isotope scanning, but the technique may still be useful in certain cases to determine whether a solid nodule (or multiple nodules) is cold (i.e. adenoma or carcinoma), warm (normal thyroid tissue), or hot (toxic nodule). As described earlier, where fine-needle aspiration is the local investigation of first choice, isotope scanning may be indicated after a follicular neoplasm has been diagnosed to exclude cases where carcinoma is extremely unlikely. When radioiodine therapy is planned after surgery for treating thyroid carcinoma, a pre-liminary scan is employed to identify tissue that takes up iodine and is therefore likely to respond to radioiodine ablative therapy.

Parathyroid

Thallium-201 is taken up by thyroid and parathyroid tissue whereas technetium-99m is taken up only by the thyroid. If both isotopes are used separately on the same patient, a subtraction scan can be performed to remove the thyroid image, leaving the parathyroid image. This is sometimes used in an attempt to locate the parathyroid glands. However, the technique is not highly reliable, with the most common cause of a false positive being co-existing thyroid disease: thyroid adenomas show reduced trapping of ^{99m}Tc with avid uptake of ^{201}Tl and may therefore be indistinguishable from parathyroid adenomas. A tracer specific for parathyroid tissue would be a great advantage and one possibility under investigation is the use of phenothia-zinium dyes such as methylene blue, labelled with radioiodine. ^{99m}Tc-labelled sestamibi (**Cardiolite**) is a non-specific tracer similar in behaviour to ^{201}Tl. Used with iodine-123, it has the advantage of producing better images.

Parathyroid ultrasonography is heavily dependent on the ex-perience of the operator. Parathyroid tumours are typically hypo-echoic or virtually anechoic when small. Sensitivity in identifying pathological parathyroid glands is a function of tumour size, operator experience, and discrimination of equipment.

Dynamic CT scanning (rapid scanning performed during the infusion of contrast media) is valuable in enhancing visual-ization of both thyroid and parathyroid tissue and for defining surrounding vascular structures. A particular indication is for guiding needles for fine-needle aspiration of cells for both parathyroid hormone assay and cytology.

Magnetic resonance imaging may have a future in this area. Already, T_1- and T_2-weighted and gadolinium–DTPA studies have proved useful in selected cases.

3.10 CT and MRI scanning

These forms of imaging have greatly improved the diagnostic accuracy of lesions deep within the head and neck region. For example, previously 'hidden' areas, such as the retropharynx and the nasopharynx, can be examined usefully by these tomo-graphic techniques. CT scanning is useful to investigate the extent of a retrosternal goitre, and, if malignant, to assess whether it is invading the trachea or great vessels.

MRI is becoming the standard for investigating the central nervous system but is not yet universally available. With increasingly sophisticated image capture and processing, mag-netic resonance imaging and magnetic resonance angiography (which does not require contrast) are likely to have increasing application in head and neck disorders.

CT scanning can be used to guide biopsies of solid lesions which would otherwise be inaccessible from the surface. The histological nature of head and neck tumours determines to a great extent the way they are optimally managed, and is there-fore an important diagnostic entity. For example, a lymphoma may best be treated with chemotherapy, a metastatic squamous carcinoma by radiotherapy, and a sarcoma may require com-bination treatment or may not be amenable to any treatment. The histology of a lymph node which proves to be metastatic often give helpful clues as to the identity of the primary tumour.

3.11 Arteriography

Carotid atherosclerosis

This method is still used selectively for symptomatic carotid atherosclerosis. Nowadays, however, the prime method of inves-tigation is duplex Doppler ultrasonography. At present, only when a stenosis has been judged to be greater than 70 per cent by duplex scanning is there proven benefit for carotid surgery and thus only this group is likely to be considered for arte-riography. Many surgeons are now prepared to operate on the results of the duplex scan alone, given its great sensitivity and specificity in specialist hands, and given the risks of stroke inherent in carotid arteriography.

Suspected carotid body tumours

Any firm mass in close proximity to the carotid bifurcation should suggest this diagnosis. Carotid body tumours are of two main types: **chemodectomas** and **ganglioneuromas**. The first is highly vascular, with a characteristic pattern of vascularity seen on arteriography. Ganglioneuromas are not highly vascular and cannot be diagnosed confidently by this means. Magnetic resonance angiography may prove to be the best investigation for either condition.

Major arteriovenous malformations

Arteriography can be used to demonstrate the main feeding vessels, which may be amenable to embolization by super-selective cannulation. Embolization can be employed to prepare the patient for excisional surgery by devascularizing the lesion, or as treatment in itself.

4 Avoiding inadvertent damage when operating on the neck

4.1 Introduction

The neck is a complex concentration of anatomical structures. There are several important nerves that can be inadvertently damaged unless the surgeon is closely aware of where these nerves lie in relation to the field of operation (Fig. 24.1). Many of these nerves lie deeply and are only at risk during particular operations. Nevertheless, superficial nerves can be damaged during operations on subcutaneous tissues, which are often carried out by relatively inexperienced surgical staff. These include the mandibular branch of the facial nerve and the spinal accessory nerve in the posterior triangle. The latter is commonly related intimately to an enlarged lymph node.

4.2 Mandibular branch of the facial nerve

This is the lowest but one of the branches of the facial nerve. After it emerges from the lower extremity of the parotid, it loops downwards, about 2 cm below the lower border of the mandible, lying superficial to the deep cervical fascia. In order to avoid nerve damage, any incision close to the lower border of the mandible should be placed at least two finger breadths below the mandible; the incision should pass perpendicularly down to the deep cervical fascia through the platysma muscle. Placing the incision in this way should avoid dividing of the nerve, but care still needs to be taken to avoid neuropraxia caused by undue retraction on the upper skin flap. Damage to the mandibular branch of the facial nerve results in paralysis of the depressor anguli oris muscle, which causes drooping of the corner of the mouth and an asymmetrical smile.

4.3 The spinal accessory nerve

This nerve runs diagonally across the posterior triangle of the neck, emerging one-third of the way down the posterior border of the sternomastoid muscle. Lymph node biopsy is the most common operation performed in the posterior triangle of the neck and the surgeon must be aware of the position of this nerve if

damage is to be avoided. Wherever possible, node biopsy should be performed under general anaesthesia by an experienced surgeon. This allows better control and visibility, enabling safer dissection. The incision should be large enough to allow the nerve to be identified and any dissection of lymph nodes should keep close to the node. Section of the spinal accessory nerve causes shoulder drop and weakness of the deltopectoral girdle.

4.4 The recurrent laryngeal nerve and thyroid surgery

The recurrent laryngeal nerve needs to be identified and preserved in virtually all thyroid operations (see Fig. 24.1). The nerve emerges from the mediastinum and passes upwards in the tracheo-oesophageal groove to pass close to the terminal branches of the inferior thyroid artery. The nerve may pass superficial to the artery, deep to it, or pass between the branches. The nerve is best found just below the inferior thyroid artery because here it is lies apart from the thyroid. Once found, the thyroidectomy can continue in a plane anterior to the nerve. In difficult cases, it is possible to operate within the thyroid capsule (unless a lobe is being removed for malignant disease), thereby ensuring an extra layer of tissue between the surgeon and the nerve.

4.5 The facial nerve and parotid surgery

In superficial or total parotidectomy, it is essential to locate the facial nerve. The nerve should be located proximal to where it divides into its trunks, and the safest technique is to locate it at the stylomastoid foramen and then trace it forwards. Dissection in this area is never easy and although apparently well represented in operative diagrams, the only reliable way to learn the technique is to be taught by a surgeon skilled in parotid surgery.

During superficial parotidectomy, the greater auricular nerve is located in the subcutaneous tissue as it runs forwards across the anterior border of the sternomastoid muscle. This nerve usually has to be sacrificed during the operation and results in anaesthesia of the earlobe and the outer surface of the pinna. This fact must be mentioned preoperatively when obtaining consent, and the discussion recorded in the patient's notes.

4.6 Lingual and hypoglossal nerves during removal of the submandibular gland

The operative details of this procedure are described later in this chapter. The **hypoglossal nerve** lies in the deep part of the dissection for removal of a submandibular gland and, although not embedded in the gland, it is at risk if there are any adhesions caused by inflammatory changes in the gland. The nerve lies just superior to the hyoid and inferior to the stylohyoid muscle and is not usually seen during the course of submandibular gland excision. The **lingual nerve** is closely related to the deep portion of the submandibular gland and duct and must be identified and freed from these structures as the deep part of the gland is dissected towards the origin of its duct. If a stone is present in the deep part of the gland, this can prove to be a difficult dissection.

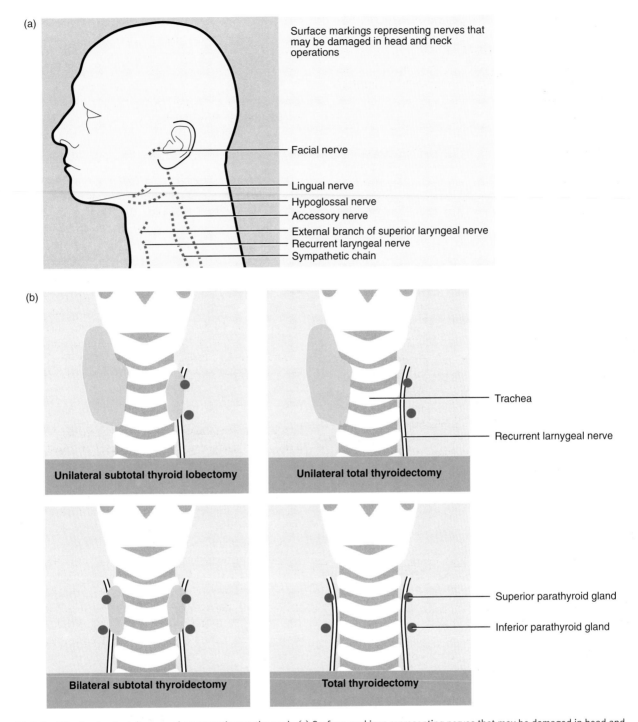

Figure 24.1 Avoiding inadvertent damage when operating on the neck. (a) Surface markings representing nerves that may be damaged in head and neck operations. (b) Structures at particular risk with different types of thyroidectomy.

4.7 Horner's syndrome

Horner's syndrome (Table 24.2) can be caused by iatrogenic damage to the cervical sympathetic plexus. It can occur as a complication of a cervical (thoraco-dorsal) sympathectomy in which the upper part of the stellate ganglion is damaged. It also occasionally occurs after thyroidectomy in which lateral retraction of the carotid sheath has produced a neuropraxia of the cervical sympathetic fibres as they run up towards the eye.

Primary causes of Horner's syndrome

◆ Lesions in the cavernous sinus or orbit.

◆ Lesions adjacent to the carotid artery (e.g. thrombosis, aneurysm).

Table 24.2 Clinical features of Horner's syndrome

Loss of sweating on the skin of the head and neck (anhidrosis)
Sunken eyeball (enophthalmos)
Small pupil (meiosis)
Drooping of the upper eyelid (ptosis)

- Lesions of the cervical sympathetic chain.
- Invasion of the T1 root (Pancoast tumour of the lung).
- Lesions within the cervical spinal cord (e.g. syringobulbia, intraspinal tumour).
- Brainstem lesions (e.g. infarction, demyelination).

5 Thyroid surgery

5.1 Clinical approach to a patient presenting with a goitre

Thyroid swellings can be classified clinically into diffuse, multinodular, or solitary. The surgeon should determine whether the patient is clinically euthyroid or hyperthyroid by examining the pulse rate and rhythm, the eyes for exophthalmos and lid lag, and the hands for tremor and excessive sweating.

Based on these clinical findings most patients can be placed into one of six categories:

- Diffuse goitre/euthyroid = physiological goitre or autoimmune thyroiditis.
- Diffuse goitre/hyperthyroid = primary hyperthyroidism. This is the only thyroid pathology which will be associated with exophthalmos and lid lag.
- Multinodular goitre/euthyroid = multinodular goitre caused by long-standing relative lack of iodine.
- Multinodular goitre/hyperthyroid = this is rare and is occasionally seen when a multinodular goitre is treated with iodine.
- Solitary nodule/euthyroid = this might include a series of pathological conditions such as multinodular disease, cysts which may be degenerate adenomas, thyroid adenoma, and thyroid carcinoma.
- Solitary thyroid nodule/hyperthyroid = a functioning adenoma which is virtually always benign.

5.2 Thyroid disorders

The solitary thyroid nodule

A solitary thyroid nodule is a single, discrete mass of abnormal tissue in an otherwise normal thyroid. If the diagnosis is based on clinical examination alone, it is not possible to be certain that the apparently normal part of the thyroid is pathologically

Table 24.3 The causes of a clinically solitary thyroid nodule in a euthyroid patient

Dominant nodule in a multinodular gland
Thyroid cyst
Papillary or follicular adenoma
Papillary or follicular carcinoma
Medullary carcinoma

normal. The most common cause of a solitary thyroid nodule is probably a **dominant nodule** in a multinodular goitre (Table 24.3). The importance of a dominant nodule is that it may harbour a carcinoma and it not easy to determine which nodule may contain a carcinoma short of removing the thyroid lobe. Most solitary nodules occur in a euthyroid patient. Less commonly, an autonomous 'hot' nodule may be found in a euthyroid patient, with suppression of TSH production, or a hot nodule may cause hyperthyroidism.

Clinical presentation

Patients usually present after they or a friend has noticed a lump in their neck. Most solitary nodules do not become large and they rarely cause compressive symptoms. However, patients may have a feeling of constriction in the neck or difficulty in swallowing. A solitary nodule is usually easily palpable and a note should be made of its size, position, and texture, in particular whether it is hard or associated with local enlargement of lymph nodes. However, it should be noted that patients are often referred with a suspected thyroid nodule, which turns out to be a normal anatomical feature such as the end of the hyoid bone or the thyroid cartilage.

Investigation of a solitary nodule

Summarized in Table 24.4.

Ultrasonography

This is the most useful initial test because a skilled ultrasonographer can distinguish a solitary solid nodule (one which may turn out to be a malignancy) from a thyroid cyst and from a dominant nodule in a multinodular gland. Ultrasonography

Table 24.4 Investigation of a thyroid nodule — summary

Circulating thyroid stimulating hormone (TSH) and thyroid hormone levels (T_4 and sometimes T_3). Hyperthyroidism must be reversed before surgery
Ultrasonography — is a nodule solid or cystic? Is the remaining thyroid normal or multinodular?
Thyroid autoantibodies (thyroglobulin and thyroid follicular microsomes) — for autoimmune thyroiditis
Radioisotope scans, e.g. technetium, ^{131}I. 'Cold' nodules have a greater chance of malignancy
Fine-needle aspiration for cytology — colloid nodule, cyst, papillary carcinoma, follicular lesion (distinguishing adenoma and carcinoma not possible), non-diagnostic

enables the remaining thyroid to be studied and a decision made as to whether it is normal thyroid or multinodular.

Radioisotope scans

This used to be the prime investigation for solitary thyroid nodules because 'cold' nodules (i.e. those which did not take up radioactive iodine) are more likely to be malignant. Radioisotope scans are used more selectively now because of the improved accuracy of ultrasound scanning and particularly because of the proven benefit of fine-needle aspiration cytology. Toxic adenomas represent one condition where isotope scans may be useful.

Fine-needle aspiration cytology

Fine-needle aspiration cytology can help to determine the cause of a solitary thyroid nodule. Local expertise needs to be accumulated for reliable interpretation of thyroid cytology. Early on, the rate of false positives and false negatives is likely to be high. As experience develops, FNAC becomes the most useful first investigation for suspected thyroid malignancy.

FNAC in thyroid disease may give the following results:

- non-diagnostic (blood, no epithelial cells);

- normal thyroid cells;

- probably colloid nodule;

- papillary carcinoma—papillary cell clusters with abnormal nuclei; psammoma bodies are strong indicators that the lesion is a papillary carcinoma;

- follicular cells—adenoma or carcinoma.

It is not possible to distinguish between benign and malignant follicular lesions on aspiration cytology because the distinction is based on finding invasion of vessels or thyroid capsule by the tumour. This can only be determined on precise, multisection histology.

Preoperative nuclear DNA analysis

It is possible to analyse the DNA content of the cells removed by fine-needle aspiration. On the basis of nuclear DNA content analysis measured by flow cytometry, malignant tumours can be classified into two major types, namely euploid and aneuploid tumours. It has been found that euploid tumours generally have a low malignant potential, as indicated by slow growth rate and long patient survival time. However, this test remains experimental in thyroid disease.

Management of the solitary thyroid nodule

Patients often present with what appears to be a solitary thyroid nodule, and management of the 'solitary nodule' is a popular examination question.

Typically, the patient presents with an asymptomatic lump in the anterior triangle of the neck, which has often been present for years and has recently been noticed by a friend or relative. Occasionally, the patient has mild symptoms of dyspnoea or stridor, often when lying on one side in bed. There may be a family history of thyroid disease. Unless the lesion can be definitely categorized as a thyroid cyst, a colloid nodule, or part of a multinodular gland, the patient should be advised to have the thyroid nodule removed surgically to obtain a specific diagnosis. The usual operative procedure is either a partial or complete lobectomy. This removes the offending lump and delivers the whole specimen for histology. If it proves to be a benign tumour then no further treatment is required. If it is malignant then further decisions need to be taken.

Diagnostic questions to be answered about a clinically solitary thyroid nodule

- Is it a true solitary nodule? Many apparently solitary nodules are part of a multinodular goitre. This can be determined accurately by ultrasound scanning.

- Could this be part of an autoimmune process (i.e. Hashimoto's disease)? Plasma autoantibodies are tested and high levels of antithyroglobulin activity or antimitochondrial activity are diagnostic. Under these circumstances, the gland should be scanned after administering a diagnostic dose of radioiodine. If there is a **cold nodule**, this should be managed as for any cold nodule: the next stage would usually be fine-needle aspiration for cytology. If the nodule is **warm** (i.e. like normal thyroid tissue), no surgery is indicated as there is no risk of malignancy and the gland is very likely to fail spontaneously later; this would be hastened by surgery.

- Thyroid hormone status. Is the patient hyper- or hypothyroid? TSH level and free plasma T_4 is likely to give the answer. Most patients with solitary nodules are euthyroid.

- What is the likely pathology? Fluid-filled lesions (cysts) on ultrasound have a very low risk of malignancy. These can usually be aspirated and will disappear, although they may refill.

Two common groups have a particular risk of malignancy:

- An elderly patient presenting with a firm mass in the thyroid is likely to have an anaplastic carcinoma.

- A new nodule developing in a long-standing multinodular goitre must be treated with suspicion as malignant transformation may occur.

In most patients, the risk of a solitary nodule being malignant is 1 : 10. If the nodule is also 'cold' on isotope scanning the risk increases to 1 : 6. If a non-cystic swelling needs to be removed because it is cosmetically unacceptable or because it is retrosternal (there is a risk of sudden enlargement due to haemorrhage which can cause respiratory embarrassment), then no further diagnostic procedures are necessary. Most other lesions should be considered for fine-needle aspiration cytology. There is a case for all nodules to be sampled in this way so that surgeon and laboratory gain experience in the technique.

When cytology is suspicious of malignancy, the nodule (or lobe if large) should be removed and the specimen examined histologically. If cytology of a good specimen is negative, surgery may be avoided, although periodic follow-up is prudent.

Occasionally, in a euthyroid patient, a solitary nodule will prove to be 'hot'. In this case, autogenous TSH is low as secretion from the nodule causes feedback suppression of the rest of the gland. Even less commonly, a hot nodule produces sufficient thyroid hormone for the patient to become hyperthyroid (i.e. a toxic nodule). Excision will effect a cure. Rarely, a thyroid carcinoma can present as a hot nodule.

Surgery for a solitary nodule

The standard preoperative preparation for excision of a thyroid lesion is required (i.e. exclude Hashimoto's disease, check that both vocal cords are functioning properly, and discuss the possibility of permanent recurrent laryngeal nerve damage before operation (risk 1 : 100 to 1 : 1000)). If the patient is euthyroid, no other special preparation is necessary. There are no special requirements for anaesthesia other than the advisability of an endotracheal tube or laryngeal mask according to anaesthetic choice.

Retrosternal goitre

Seventy-five to 90 per cent of goitres extending into the thorax lie anterior to the major vessels and the recurrent laryngeal nerves. Their blood supply usually arises from the normal place in the neck, rather than in the chest. Anteriorly placed goitres can normally be delivered out of the thorax without thoracotomy once the lobe has been fully mobilized in the neck. In particularly large goitres, the capsule may be breached and the goitre removed piecemeal, reducing the bulk and allowing delivery. In cases of proven or suspected malignancy, or adherent benign lesions, a median sternotomy may be required. Posteriorly placed goitres have sometimes been approached primarily through the neck and chest.

Particular areas of difficulty to be considered are control of the blood supply (usually from the neck but sometimes capsular vascularization in the chest) and identification of the recurrent laryngeal nerves.

Primary thyroid cancers

Presentation of carcinoma of the thyroid

- Discrete solitary thyroid nodule.

- Incidental cytological or histological finding.

- Suspicious nodule found during surgery for benign condition and subjected to frozen section.

- Generalized goitre with recent change.

- Discrete cervical lymph node mass without apparent thyroid mass.

- Diffuse central neck mass causing pressure symptoms.

- Distant metastases.

Papillary carcinoma

Papillary carcinoma may occur at any age but is most common during the first three decades and is sometimes seen in childhood. It may present as a mass in the thyroid or, less commonly, as a solid swelling in a lymph node draining the thyroid, with the primary being impalpable. Occult and intrathyroid varieties, in particular, have an excellent prognosis, with 5-year survival above 95 per cent. Note that papillary carcinomas classically spread via lymph nodes but are unusual in that this does not usually worsen the prognosis.

Types of papillary carcinoma

- Occult: the tumour is not palpable and is less than 1.5 cm in diameter.

- Intrathyroid: the tumour is larger but lies within the substance of the gland. Tumours that are reported as 'papillary with a follicular component' tend to behave as papillary.

- Extrathyroid: the tumour is locally invasive and has breached the capsule of the gland and invaded local structures such as the larynx, trachea, and oesophagus. Spread to lymph nodes does not, on its own, categorize a papillary tumour as extrathyroid; the definition depends on the degree of local invasion.

Management of papillary carcinoma

There are two main schools of thought governing management strategy: the first approach favours total thyroidectomy with identification and preservation of parathyroids. The rationale behind this is that the disease may be multifocal through any part of the thyroid. The alternative, and less favoured, approach is to perform a total lobectomy and removal of the isthmus (see below). If other foci are present and are not removed, the 5-year mortality rises to above 10 per cent.

If neck nodes are involved, the favoured approach is to remove any that are involved individually, a technique known as 'cherry picking'. Some authorities advocate formal block dissection of the ipsilateral nodes, but the most recent data suggest that this gives no advantage and represents a more major procedure.

After total thyroidectomy, a radioiodine whole-body scan is performed to seek residual thyroid tissue in the neck and any functioning metastases. If there is any uptake, therapeutic doses of radioiodine are administered. If total thyroidectomy has not been performed, this approach is not possible as the residual gland takes up the diagnostic iodine.

In appropriate cases, scanning is repeated 6 monthly for 2 years and then annually for 5 years. All patients are given T_4 sufficient to suppress TSH as there is evidence that TSH stimulates the tumour. A dose of 100–150 μg daily is sufficient for most adults. TSH levels should be checked from time to time to ensure that TSH is suppressed and to confirm that the patient is complying with the treatment. T_3 needs to be substituted for T_4 a week before scanning.

A sensitive radioimmunoassay for plasma thyroglobulin has been developed; levels above 50 ng/ml suggest the presence of functioning thyroid tissue and hence recurrent disease. It is a cheaper and more efficient means of follow-up than scanning with radioiodine and does not require stopping suppression therapy beforehand.

The alternative approach to the treatment of papillary cancer advises total lobectomy on the affected side with excision of the isthmus. Radioiodine is not used for scanning or therapy and reliance is placed on thyroid hormone replacement to suppress TSH and to allow regression, even of established metastases. This method has advantages in avoiding the morbidity of total thyroidectomy, particularly for the non-specialist surgeon, and it also avoids the risk of hypocalcaemia. It is difficult to judge the merits of the two approaches: confusion arises because of differing pathological interpretations between centres. The more radical approach is undoubtedly preferable in extrathyroidal disease or with papillary thyroid carcinoma arising as a result of previous cervical radiotherapy.

Follicular carcinoma

Follicular carcinoma has a predilection for the 30–50 year old group. The average 5-year survival is 60 per cent, and the 10-year survival, 50 per cent. Follicular carcinoma classically spreads via the bloodstream and is associated with secondaries in bone and lung. The poorer prognosis may justify a more radical approach than for papillary carcinoma. Total thyroidectomy with preservation of the parathyroids and removal of any affected nodes is desirable. If total thyroidectomy is not performed, it is impossible to do total body scanning as the radioiodine will be taken up preferentially in remaining thyroid rather than by metastases. A similar follow-up scheme of serial scanning or plasma thyroglobulin assay is used in the same way as for papillary cancers (see above).

Types of follicular thyroid carcinoma:

(1) minimally angio-invasive;

(2) angio-invasive tumours. These microscopically show tumour within the thyroid blood vessels.

Total lobectomy versus completion thyroidectomy for well-differentiated thyroid cancer

How does the surgeon decide whether further surgery is required when treating a patient with a carcinoma of the thyroid?

◆ There is no evidence to prove that total thyroidectomy produces a improved survival when compared with lobectomy. The case is often made that the disease is multifocal and hence total thyroid removal is indicated, but survival figures do not support this concept.

◆ The advantage of removing the whole thyroid is that radioactive iodine can then be used to scan for and treat recurrences. The ability for metastases to take up radioactive iodine is a variable one and is more often a feature of follicular carcinoma.

A case can be made for performing a completion thyroidectomy in patients where the histology indicates a likelihood of progressive disease (i.e. an extrathyroid papillary carcinoma). However, in follicular carcinoma the contralateral lobe

Table 24.5 Lahey Clinic differentiated thyroid cancer risk group

Low-risk group	All younger patients without distant metastases (men < 41; women < 51)
	All older patients with:
	(1) intrathyroidal papillary cancer or follicular cancer with minor capsular involvement;
	(2) primary cancers < 5 cm in diameter;
	(3) no distant metastases
High-risk group	All patients with distant metastases
	All older patients with:
	(1) extrathyroidal papillary cancer or follicular cancer with major tumour capsular involvement
	(2) primary cancers > 5 cm

usually has to be removed at a second operation as frozen section cannot distinguish between follicular adenoma and follicular carcinoma. The second procedure is usually performed about 6 weeks after the first and the procedure is much easier if the opposite lobe was left undisturbed. It will be clear from this account that if a conservative approach is followed for papillary carcinoma, routine frozen section for thyroid surgery is unnecessary. It should be mentioned that some authorities have calculated tumour prognostic indices from age, stage, tumour grade, and vascular invasion to classify a group of patients with follicular carcinoma under 45 years of age who only require ipsilateral total thyroid lobectomy, so-called 'minimal follicular cancer' (Table 24.5). However, this policy is followed only in a minority of centres.

Suppression of TSH in therapy of well-differentiated thyroid cancer

It is standard practice to treat patients after surgery for well-differentiated thyroid cancers with T_4 with the intention of maintaining plasma thyroxine just above the upper limit of normal. This minimizes endogenous TSH drive by negative feedback and reduces stimulation of the thyroid, minimizing recurrences.

Anaplastic carcinoma

Anaplastic carcinoma occurs in elderly people and grows rapidly into neighbouring structures, including the strap muscles and trachea. Very few patients survive a year. There is rapidly progressive swelling of the neck on one or both sides, voice changes due to involvement of the recurrent laryngeal nerves, and stridor from tracheal compression. Wherever possible, some attempt should be made to relieve respiratory obstruction. This is best achieved by internal stenting rather than surgery. Unfortunately, anaplastic thyroid cancer is insensitive to radiotherapy and chemotherapy so palliative care is all that can usefully be offered.

Medullary carcinoma

Medullary thyroid carcinoma arises from the thyroid C cells. It was first recognized as a separate entity in 1959 and was previously described in the same group as anaplastic tumours, which may have accounted for the occasional long survivor of the latter group in earlier series.

It is a rare tumour and is associated with high blood levels of calcitonin. It may arise spontaneously or be part of multiple endocrine neoplasia (MEN) type II, when it may be associated with phaeochromocytoma and parathyroid adenoma (type IIa) or mucosal neuromas and Marfanoid habitus (type IIb). Five-year survival is 50 per cent. Treatment is by total thyroidectomy with parathyroid identification and preservation. Some authorities recommend prophylactic dissection of the lymph nodes of the central compartment of the neck, including those of the superior mediastinum. Thyroxine is given for replacement therapy only, since the tumour is not stimulated by TSH. The tumour is not responsive to radiotherapy or chemotherapy. Follow-up of the patient and screening of first-degree relatives (if part of MEN) is by serial measurement of plasma calcitonin and urinary vanillylmandelic acid. Recently, the gene for MEN type IIa has been identified on chromosome 12 and this will allow more precise opportunistic screening of first-degree relatives.

Thyroid lymphoma

The prognosis depends on the degree of extrathyroid spread. Lymphoma is the only thyroid tumour which is radiosensitive. It is relatively rare and is most often seen in association with severe long-standing autoimmune thyroiditis (Hashimoto's disease). Five-year survival is not meaningful, because of the advanced age of many patients. The histological diagnosis can be difficult between lymphoma, severe autoimmune thyroiditis, and anaplastic carcinoma. If a thyroid lymphoma is suspected early during operation for thyroid malignancy, thyroidectomy need not be undertaken unless it is essential for decompression. Radiotherapy to the neck, together with adjuvant chemotherapy if there is evidence of spread, effects a high cure rate.

Radiotherapy for thyroid carcinoma

Indications for radiotherapy in thyroid cancer are:

- **Radioactive ablation of thyroid remnants**. Residual thyroid tissue can normally be detected by iodine scintigraphy even after a radical thyroid resection. Ablation of this thyroid remnant is feasible if more than 0.5 per cent of the iodine is concentrated in the remaining thyroid. Some centres will ablate patients only in high-risk categories (see Table 24.5). Monitoring may be performed with whole-body iodine scans or plasma thyroglobulin assay.

- **Radioactive iodine therapy for metastatic disease**. Only about 60–70 per cent of metastases from follicular or papillary tumours concentrate iodine, and it is more likely in younger patients. Pulmonary and lymph-node metastases have a higher response rate than skeletal metastases. An iodine-uptake scan is undertaken when patients have stopped thyroxine and have a plasma TSH greater than 50 IU/l. Standard doses of 150–200 mCi are usually prescribed.

External-beam radiotherapy

External-beam radiotherapy is well established in thyroid lymphoma and is useful for the treatment of the compression symptoms. Careful iso-dose plans are made for the patient using a single anterior field of 20–30 MeV. Its use in inoperable macroscopic follicular and papillary tumours is more contentious, but local control can be maintained for a number of years. In younger patients with papillary tumours radiotherapy should perhaps be avoided because of its role in the aetiology of such tumours.

Thyroglossal cyst

Embryologically, a thyroglossal cyst involves cystic change in a persistent remnant of the embryonic thyroglossal tract. The thyroid develops at the junction of the anterior two-thirds and posterior one-third of the tongue (**tuberculum impar**) and descends through the tongue, forming a tract in close relation to the hyoid bone before reaching its final position in the neck. Thyroglossal cysts can be located at any point along this line of descent but most commonly are below the level of the thyroid cartilage in the midline.

Clinical features

A rounded cystic swelling is found in the midline which moves upward on swallowing and also on protrusion of the tongue. The cyst may contain functioning thyroid tissue, but more commonly is lined by flattened cuboidal epithelium. Occasionally, thyroid cancers develop within the cyst, almost invariably of papillary type. Although congenital in origin, thyroglossal cysts usually manifest later in life as they fill with secretions.

The differential diagnosis of anterior midline cervical swellings is as follows:

- laryngocoele: often found in wind-instrument players, essentially a 'blow out' of the laryngeal membrane;

- plunging ranula: normally a sublingual mucous retention cyst; rarely this can occur in the lower midline of the neck;

- midline dermoid cyst;

- chondroma of the laryngeal or thyroid cartilage;

- inclusion dermoid;

- superficial midline epidermoid cyst;

- subhyoid bursa;

- dental abscess from lower incisor tooth;

- submental lymph-node enlargement.

Pharyngeal pouch is sometimes described as a midline lesion but in reality lies to one side of the midline.

Investigations

Ultrasonography of the neck confirms a midline swelling deep to the platysma. If functioning thyroid tissue is suspected, a hot spot may be seen on a ^{99m}Tc scan or a ^{131}I radioisotope scan. The rare thyroid carcinoma in a thyroglossal cyst will result in a cold nodule.

Excision of thyroglossal cyst

- The patient is placed 20° head up with the neck extended.

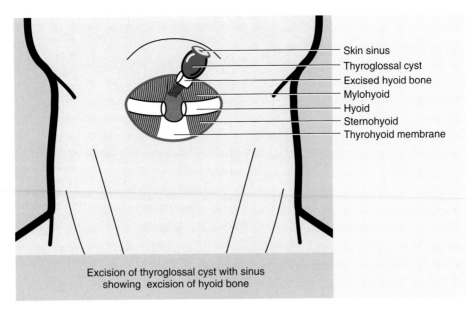

Skin sinus
Thyroglossal cyst
Excised hyoid bone
Mylohyoid
Hyoid
Sternohyoid
Thyrohyoid membrane

Excision of thyroglossal cyst with sinus
showing excision of hyoid bone

Figure 24.2 Operation for thyroglossal cyst.

◆ The skin and platysma may be infiltrated with dilute adrenaline (epinephrine) solution 1 : 250 000 and a transverse skin incision made and platysma flaps elevated. The cyst is carefully dissected out and the fistula track is traced upwards in the midline to the body of the hyoid.

◆ The central muscle attachments to the hyoid are raised with a periosteal elevator and the body of the hyoid carefully excised with a pair of bone shears (Fig. 24.2). The track deep to the hyoid is usually a fibrous band that gradually peters out. This is excised as far as possible. The wound is closed with a suction drain in layers. The drain can usually be removed and the patient discharged the following day.

Thyroiditis

Autoimmune (Hashimoto's) thyroiditis

This condition is almost certainly of autoimmune aetiology. Histologically, it is characterized by destruction of thyroid follicles by lymphocytic infiltration, frequently organized into lymphoid follicles and with a variable degree of fibrous replacement of destroyed acini. The thyroid follicular cells undergo change to eosinophilic Askanazy cells.

Thyroid microsomal and antithyroglobulin antibody titres are markedly raised, usually above 1 : 6400. Mild elevation can occur in Graves' disease but this condition is characterized by thyroid stimulating antibodies (TSI) and antiophthalmic antibodies. This overlap is of interest, since some patients with Graves' disease have foci of lymphocytic thyroiditis present.

In Hashimoto's disease the typical patient is female (M : F, 1 : 4), often postmenopausal, with a thyroid swelling which is firm to palpation and either diffuse or predominantly affecting one side. The patient may be hyper- or euthyroid in the early stages of the illness but will almost inevitably become hypothyroid later. The diagnosis depends on the positive antibody titres but

10 per cent may be negative or equivocal. Radionuclide scanning and ultrasonography may be suggestive but not diagnostic. The hypothyroid phase responds well to replacement therapy. Surgery is usually reserved for compressive symptoms or, if malignant change is suspected, total lobectomy is usually performed. In the toxic phase, surgery or radioiodine is to be avoided since all patients will eventually become hypothyroid.

Reidel's thyroiditis

This very rare condition is not autoimmune in origin but is associated with a group of miscellaneous fibrosing diseases around the body, including retroperitoneal fibrosis, sclerosing cholangitis, fibrosing mediastinitis, Peyronie's disease, and hepatic fibrosis. There is usually painless enlargement of the thyroid gland which is woody hard to palpation. Pressure symptoms may be present and tracheal compression. Males and females are equally affected and thyroid antibodies are negative. Surgical treatment may be required to decompress the trachea; a conservative approach limited to excision of the isthmus is adequate.

Subacute (de Quervain's) thyroiditis

This rare condition presents with or following a flu-like illness with pain and swelling of the thyroid gland. The pain radiates into the neck towards the ears. The gland is tender to palpation. There is an elevated ESR, transiently elevated thyroid antibodies, and raised T_4 in the acute phase, with a reduced uptake of radioiodine in the isotope scan.

The condition may be viral in aetiology (usually paramyxovirus). If the condition persists, mild hypothyroidism is the rule, but the disease usually runs a self-limiting course with a return to normal thyroid function and autoantibodies. Rarely, the condition runs a remitting and relapsing course which responds with a short course of steroids. Surgery is not indicated.

Table 24.6 Causes of hyperthyroidism

Graves' disease (diffuse toxic goitre)	
Toxic nodular goitre	Multinodular (Plummer's disease)
	Single toxic adenoma
Nodular goitre with Graves' disease	
Well-differentiated thyroid carcinoma	
Early stages of Hashimoto's disease	
Excess thyroid stimulating hormone	Inappropriate TSH secretion by pituitary tumour
	Non-tumorous
	Choriocarcinoma, hydatidiform mole
	Embryonal testicular carcinoma
Extraneous thyroid hormone	Intentional (factitious)
	Overenthusiastic therapy
	During T_3 suppression test
	Metastatic thyroid cancer
	Struma ovarii
Transient thyroiditis following irradiation	

Acute bacterial thyroiditis

Specific infective pyogenic and tuberculous thyroiditis have been reported but are rare. Treatment is with antibiotics and surgical drainage.

Hyperthyroidism

The causes of hyperthyroidism are summarized in Table 24.6. Primary thyrotoxicosis (Graves' disease) is an autoimmune condition which has a genetic predisposition. The hyperthyroidism is due to the presence of a circulating immunoglobulin (TSI) that binds to the TSH receptors of thyroid follicular cells.

Clinical features

A goitre may be felt. The skin is hot and damp. The nails may have onycholysis and alopecia. The eyes show signs of lid retraction, lid lag, ophthalmoplegia and exophthalmos. These have been devised into a mnemonic classification—'NO SPECS':

- No physical signs/symptoms;

- Only signs/no symptoms: lid retraction/lid lag/proptosis less than 22 mm;

- Soft tissue involvement: symptoms and signs;

- Proptosis greater than 2.2 mm;

- Extraocular muscle involvement(ophthalmoplegia);

- Corneal injury;

- Sight loss (optic nerve involvement).

Cardiovascular features include palpitations, tachycardia, atrial fibrillation, and, rarely, high output cardiac failure. Neuromuscular irritability and proximal myopathy with wasting can occur. Anorexia, nausea, vomiting, weight loss, and diarrhoea are other features. Oligomenorrhoea or amenorrhoea is also seen. The diagnosis is made on clinical examination and special investigations described above.

Treatment of hyperthyroidism

Three methods of treatment of thyrotoxicosis are antithyroid drugs, radioiodine, and surgery.

Antithyroid drugs

Carbimazole impairs secretion and synthesis of T_4 by the thyroid. In general, a high initial dose is used (20 mg twice daily) to bring the patient under control, after which the dose can be reduced to 10 mg once or twice daily for maintenance. Medical therapy may be continued for 18 months, although some surgeons discontinue medication after 6–12 months. After this, over half of the patients relapse. The patient must be warned of two important side-effects of therapy, namely skin rash and sore throat. The latter may be a harbinger of leucopenia and agranulocytosis, which in 0.01 per cent may lead to marrow failure. If the patient fails to tolerate these drugs, **propylthiouracil** may be used, up to 1.2 g/day in divided doses. This has the additional effect of blocking peripheral de-iodination of T_4 to T_3. In a small number of patients, perchlorate may be used, which blocks the uptake of iodine into the thyroid.

In the early phase of thyrotoxicosis, a beta-blocker such as propranolol may be added to block the peripheral action of catecholamines, which would otherwise be enhanced by the raised level of thyroxine. Antithyroid drugs and beta-blockers are also used to control thyrotoxic patients prior to surgery. Lugol's iodine may be used to reduce gland vascularity prior to surgery. In general, antithyroid drugs are useful in patients unfit or unwilling to undergo surgery, for the control of toxic patients, and in transient hyperthyroidism (e.g. hashitoxicosis). These drugs can be used safely in pregnancy at a low dose to avoid neonatal or fetal thyroid suppression. Some physicians treat primary thyrotoxicosis with high doses of carbimazole (30 mg twice daily) plus a replacement dose of T_4 ('**block and replace**').

Radioiodine

Radioiodine is the most widely employed treatment for thyrotoxicosis and can be used safely in young adults. An intermediate dose (400 MBq) may be used to suppress thyroid function. At least 25 per cent of patients require treatment for resulting hypothyroidism and this proportion will increase with time. Its use should be avoided in women who might be pregnant. Radioiodine is particularly useful for recurrent thyrotoxicosis after subtotal thyroidectomy.

Surgery

In experienced hands the morbidity of subtotal thyroidectomy is small. The indications for surgery include:

- recurrence after treatment with antithyroid drugs;

- patient preference;

- occupational pressures—some patients require to be made euthyroid rapidly;

- large goitres with pressure symptoms;

- thyrotoxicosis due to functioning multinodular goitre or toxic adenoma (although the latter group also respond to lower doses of radioiodine);

- possibility of malignancy.

The preparation for surgery, operative details and complications of surgery are described elsewhere in the chapter.

5.3 Thyroidectomy

Aims of thyroidectomy

The amount of thyroid tissue to be removed depends on the morphology of the gland and on the histopathology:

- Unilateral total lobectomy is indicated for many solitary thyroid nodules, especially if large.

- Unilateral subtotal lobectomy indicated for small, anteriorly placed nodules.

- Bilateral subtotal thyroidectomy indicated for Graves' disease. Some surgeons prefer to perform a total lobectomy on one side and a subtotal lobectomy on the other.

- Bilateral total lobectomy (total thyroidectomy) in cases of aggressive follicular, papillary, and medullary thyroid carcinoma. The current trend is towards total thyroidectomy for large multinodular glands to prevent the otherwise inevitable regrowth.

The surgical approach used is similar for all of these operations; for the purpose of simplicity, a right thyroid lobectomy will be described later.

Preparation of the patient

Informed consent must be obtained by explaining the nature of the operation and the important potential complications. Particular attention needs to given to explaining possible voice changes due to recurrent or external laryngeal nerve injury. With this in mind, it is customary to examine the vocal cords before surgery.

The patient should be clinically and biochemically euthyroid. This can virtually always be achieved with a combination of antithyroid drugs and beta-blockers. Some surgeons use Lugol's iodine, 0.2–0.5 ml three times a day for 10 days, before operation on thyrotoxic patients as a means of reducing the blood flow to the thyroid and hence limiting blood loss. However, there is no general agreement that this is beneficial or necessary.

Surgical exposure

Position on the operating table

The operation is nearly always performed under general anaesthesia with endotracheal intubation and muscle relaxation. The patient lies supine, with the upper part of the body elevated about 20° upward and the lower part parallel to the ground ('armchair position') in order to reduce engorgement in the large veins of the neck. A sandbag is placed in the interscapular region and the neck is extended to make the thyroid gland more prominent. The head is supported on a head ring (Fig. 24.3).

Following skin preparation, the subcutaneous tissues of the anterior part of the neck can be infiltrated with adrenaline (epinephrine) in normal saline 1 : 250 000. This can be useful to simplify dissection of the subplatysmal tissues and reduce blood loss at this stage of the operation. However, many anaesthetists are wary of the technique because of the risk of inducing cardiac arrhythmias.

Some surgeons like to use loupe magnifiers for thyroid surgery, in order to see clearly the danger points around the parathyroid glands and the recurrent laryngeal nerves (Fig. 24.4).

Skin incision

A standard 'collar' incision is used, even for small nodules. The skin incision is placed in a suitable skin crease if possible, 3 cm (two fingers' breadths) above the sternum and the medial aspects of the clavicles, and extending from one sternomastoid muscle to the other. The incision is deepened through the platysma.

Access to the thyroid gland

The cervical fascia containing the anterior jugular veins and the strap muscles of the neck shield the surgeon from the anterior surface of the thyroid gland. The surgeon has the choice of gaining access to the thyroid either via a midline vertical incision through the fascia between the strap muscles (the conventional approach) or of dividing the strap muscles in a transverse direction and ligating the anterior jugular veins then developing the flaps beneath the strap muscles. This alternative approach is employed routinely in parts of continental Europe and

(a)

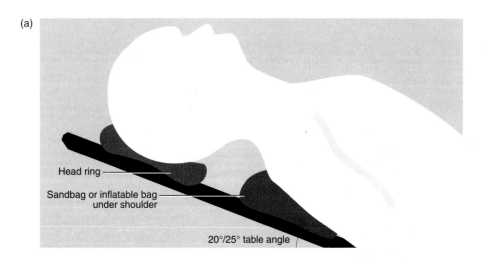

Head ring

Sandbag or inflatable bag
under shoulder

20°/25° table angle

(b)

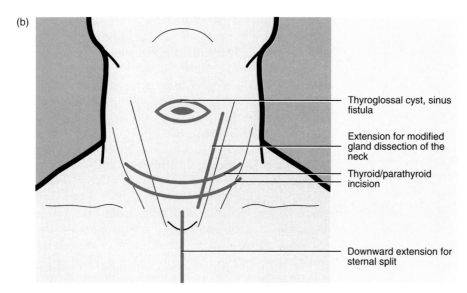

Thyroglossal cyst, sinus
fistula

Extension for modified
gland dissection of the
neck

Thyroid/parathyroid
incision

Downward extension for
sternal split

(c)

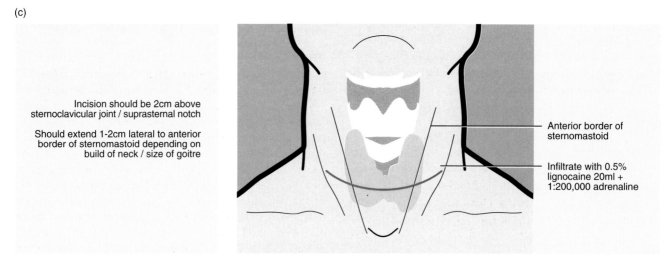

Incision should be 2cm above
sternoclavicular joint / suprasternal notch

Should extend 1-2cm lateral to anterior
border of sternomastoid depending on
build of neck / size of goitre

Anterior border of
sternomastoid

Infiltrate with 0.5%
lignocaine 20ml +
1:200,000 adrenaline

Figure 24.3 Surgical exposure for thyroidectomy and related operations: (a) positioning the patient on the table; (b) choice of incision; (c) standard collar incision.

(a)

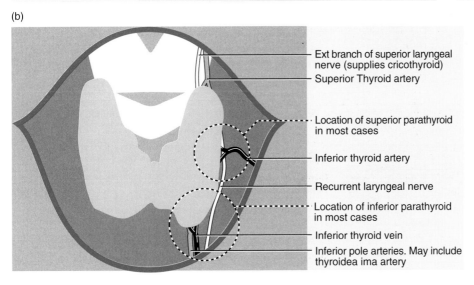

Thyroid cartilage

Anterior jugular vein

Sternohyoid

Sternocleidomastoid

Suprasternal notch

Skin flaps are elevated by blunt dissection.

The straps are separated.

Helpful for the first assistant to put traction away from the midline with a gauze swab.

The sternohyoid and sternothyroids are elevated off the thyroid lobe.

N.B. The sternothyroid is often stuck closely to the thyroid capsule and needs separating to enter the correct plane.

For large goitres the strap muscles may be divided.

(b)

Ext branch of superior laryngeal nerve (supplies cricothyroid)

Superior Thyroid artery

Location of superior parathyroid in most cases

Inferior thyroid artery

Recurrent laryngeal nerve

Location of inferior parathyroid in most cases

Inferior thyroid vein

Inferior pole arteries. May include thyroidea ima artery

Figure 24.4 (a) Exposure of the thyroid at operation. (b) Dissection of the lateral thyroid lobe.

elsewhere, and is favoured by some surgeons whenever access is likely to prove difficult.

In the conventional approach, the platysma is grasped in two Allis forceps and a subplatysmal dissection performed, avoiding the large anterior jugular veins, to elevate the upper flap to the prominence of the thyroid cartilage. An inferior flap is developed in the same way down to the suprasternal notch. The skin flaps are then kept apart in a self-retaining Joll's retractor (Fig. 24.4).

If division of the strap muscles is required, stay sutures are placed on either side of the proposed line of division to assist later closure. The transsection is made towards the cranial end of the muscle to limit denervation palsy of the sternohyoid and sternothyroids. Division may be preferable if the gland is very large.

Redo thyroidectomy presents particular problems of access; on occasions, a deliberate lateral approach to the thyroid lobe is preferred, entering just medial to the anterior border of the sternomastoid and dividing the strap muscles may provide better access.

Lateral mobilization of the thyroid lobe

The secret of success at all stages of thyroid surgery is to ensure that the correct plane is entered. At this point, the plane lies over the surface of the thyroid; if the sternothyroid is not recognized, too superficial a plane can be entered. To mobilize the lateral part of the lobe, the dissection is largely performed bluntly with gentle teasing apart of the filmy connective tissue to minimize risk of damage to the recurrent laryngeal nerve. Some surgeons completely ban the use of diathermy once inside the strap muscles. However, others favour the judicious use of bipolar diathermy.

The middle thyroid vein enters the antero-lateral border of the lobe and needs to be secured with an absorbable ligature and divided. The position of the vein is a useful marker for the inferior thyroid artery which lies immediately posterior to the vein as it emerges from behind the common carotid artery. The thyroid lobe is retracted medially by hand, maintaining grip with a swab, and dissection continues posteriorly to identify the common carotid artery and then the inferior thyroid artery as it passes at an angle from the superio-lateral aspect of the operating field into the posterior part of the thyroid lobe (Fig. 24.4b). The inferior thyroid artery is cleared of all remaining surrounding tissue laterally to avoid damage to the recurrent laryngeal nerve. An absorbable suture is placed around the cleaned inferior thyroid artery and tied in continuity. Ligation and division of the inferior thyroid arteries is usually unnecessary. Gentle lateral retraction of the common carotid artery allows the inferior thyroid artery to be identified and ligated as far laterally as possible. Care should be taken to avoid damage to the cervical sympathetic chain at this stage as a Horner's syndrome may be provoked. The recurrent laryngeal nerve can be identified at this stage or else following mobilization of the superior pole of the thyroid.

Partial lobectomy

Some nodules (for example, those in the isthmus) are sited so that the recurrent laryngeal is in no danger even if it is not identified, but most partial lobectomies are performed more safely if the nerve is identified as it meanders near the division of the inferior thyroid artery. After this, the area to be excised can be mobilized from the trachea, marked out with artery forceps, and excised with a scalpel. The cut ends of thyroid are oversewn with absorbable sutures to prevent haemorrhage. The wound are usually closed with suction drainage for 24 hours.

Total lobectomy

If the preoperative diagnosis is suspicious of carcinoma, or if the diagnosis is multinodular goitre, many surgeons recommend removing the entire thyroid, together with the isthmus.

Mobilization of the superior pole of the thyroid gland

Full mobilization of the thyroid can only be obtained after division of the upper pole vessels. The sternomastoid muscle is retracted in an upward direction and the superior pole of the thyroid is pulled gently downwards to reveal the superior thyroid

artery and vein. These vessels always enter the superior pole of the thyroid on its anterior surface. Even in large glands which extend high into the neck, these vessels can be found low down on the anterior surface (see Fig. 24.5). They are identified and doubly ligated low down with absorbable sutures, incorporating some of the upper pole of the thyroid in the ligature to minimize risk to the external laryngeal branch of the superior laryngeal nerve. Following division of the pedicle, it is then possible to mobilize the upward extending thyroid gland without danger of major haemorrhage. If the arterial ligature should slip, then it is possible to contain the haemorrhage by packing the wound and by intermittent pressure on the common carotid artery in the depths of the wound.

Identifying the recurrent laryngeal nerve

This is an essential manoeuvre in thyroidectomy. The preferred place to look for the nerve is at the inferior aspect of the thyroid gland, where it is most likely to be lying in the tracheo-oesophageal groove. It can be identified as a white cord, often with a small blood vessel running on its surface, and it can sometimes be palpated in the tracheo-oesophageal groove. However, it needs to be seen rather than felt in order to be confident of its identity. Many surgeons prefer to identify the recurrent laryngeal nerve prior to ligation of the inferior thyroid artery. The importance of identifying the nerve is that it allows the surgeon to protect the nerve at all times, particularly when removing the thyroid lobe, and it gives the surgeon the confidence of working in a plane which is always anterior to the position of the recurrent laryngeal nerve (Fig. 24.4b).

Removal of the thyroid lobe

The vessels supplying and draining the lower pole are ligated and the upper and lower parathyroids are sought and preserved. For benign disease, it is usually possible to remove the lobe by intracapsular dissection. The advantage of dissecting inside the

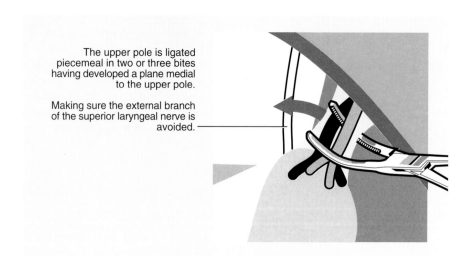

The upper pole is ligated piecemeal in two or three bites having developed a plane medial to the upper pole.

Making sure the external branch of the superior laryngeal nerve is avoided.

Figure 24.5 Superior pole vessels of the thyroid.

capsule is that it offers an additional protective mechanism against damage to the recurrent laryngeal nerve because the nerve lies outside the capsule. Haemostats are applied to the capsule of the gland two-thirds of the way back to the posterior surface of the thyroid. Incising the capsule anteriorly to the clips allows an intracapsular dissection. The dissection continues medially towards the trachea where the isthmus is marked. The whole lobe is dissected free from the trachea, the isthmus divided on the opposite side, and the lobe removed. The lobe it is examined for possible adherent parathyroid tissue and, if any is found, it is removed and implanted in one of the sterno-mastoid muscles as an autotransplant.

Haemostasis

It is essential that the operative field is dry before wound closure. Closure should not be performed until normal blood pressure has been regained to ensure that there are no bleeding points. It is important to avoid any manoeuvre that may damage the recurrent laryngeal nerve when achieving haemostasis. This includes excessive diathermy and the suturing of the thyroid capsule under tension to the tracheal tissues. The latter is a manoeuvre which is often used to obtain haemostasis and can prove very useful in vascular glands, particularly if surgery is being carried out for thyrotoxicosis. However, it should not be used routinely because it does have the possible complication of stretching the recurrent laryngeal nerve and causing neuro-praxia, as well as causing potential damage to the trachea.

Wound closure

The wound is closed in layers and usually a suction drain placed in the operative bed. Skin closure is achieved either using a sub-cuticular stitch or Michel clips, depending on the surgeon's preference. Postoperatively the patient is nursed at an angle of 45° to avoid venous engorgement in the neck.

Postoperative recovery

As the patient wakes up and the endotracheal tube is removed, the anaesthetist should visually check that both cords are moving normally. Some anaesthetists use a laryngeal mask and check the cords with a flexible bronchoscope before extubation. At this point, inadvertent damage to the recurrent laryngeal nerve or nerves may become apparent.

Patients rarely need intravenous fluids after surgery and the suction drain can usually be removed after 24 hours. No more than a day or two needs to be spent in hospital after operation.

Problems during thyroidectomy

Failure to identify recurrent laryngeal nerves

These authors advocate identification of the recurrent nerve as best practice in virtually all thyroid surgery. If the right-side nerve cannot be identified, the rare non-recurrent form must be considered. This occurs in about 1 per cent of patients, but only on the right side. Note that a non-recurrent nerve may be mistaken for a right inferior thyroid artery and ligated.

A different approach when a recurrent laryngeal nerve cannot be located is to restrict the plane of dissection closely to the thyroid capsule, thus avoiding contact with the nerve.

Inadvertent division of the recurrent laryngeal nerve

If the nerve is divided, re-anastomosis should be attempted using fine monofilament sutures but, unfortunately, this rarely succeeds. Various palliative surgical approaches are available to treat symptomatic vocal cord palsy:

1. Unilateral vocal fold palsy:

    (a) Teflon injection into the vocal folds;

    (b) subchondral thyroplasty;

    (c) nerve anastomoses and neuromuscular transplants.

2. Bilateral vocal cord palsy (abductors paralysed, causing respiratory obstruction):

    (a) permanent tracheostomy;

    (b) nerve or nerve/muscle transplantation;

    (c) vocal fold lateralization procedures.

Postoperative complications of thyroidectomy

Bleeding and airway obstruction

The main surgical hazard after operation is a slipped ligature causing postoperative haemorrhage in the neck deep to the strap muscles. This can cause pressure effects on the trachea or larynx and also laryngeal oedema, giving rise to airway obstruction. If there is clinical evidence of airway obstruction as indicated by inspiratory stridor, the patient should be re-intubated and the haematoma evacuated in the operating theatre if time allows. If not, emergency opening of the wound must take place on the ward. Thus, junior doctors looking after the patient need to be briefed about the mechanics of the wound closure in order to achieve this. Instruments for this purpose should be placed beside the patient's bed. Although this is a very rare compli-cation, steps to overcome it must not be neglected.

Airway obstruction due to tracheal collapse

This is a rare cause of postoperative airway obstruction and is usually associated with very large and long-standing multi-nodular goitres weakening the tracheal cartilages by prolonged pressure atrophy ('tracheomalacia'). On removing such a gland, the trachea collapses, causing respiratory obstruction. This is an emergency requiring immediate re-intubation for 3 or 4 days. After this, the condition usually resolves. In not, tracheostomy or tracheal stenting is required, at least temporarily.

Recurrent laryngeal nerve damage

This is an extremely serious but usually avoidable complication. When unilateral damage has occurred, there is postoperative hoarseness, but if bilateral damage has occurred, there is likely to be laryngeal obstruction requiring tracheostomy. Damage is best avoided by clearly visualizing the nerves at surgery. When nerves which are damaged (neuropraxia) rather than divided, return of function can be expected after a few months. The chance of this occurring are much higher if the nerves have been seen clearly at operation.

Hypocalcaemia

The calcium level should be measured within 48 hours of thyroid surgery to check for parathyroid damage. Parathyroid dysfunction is probably most often due to interference with their blood supply, rendering them ischaemic, although sometimes parathyroids are inadvertently removed. This is a rare complication of thyroid surgery and for there to be permanent hypocalcaemia, all four glands need to have been removed or damaged. Monitoring the plasma calcium postoperatively in all patients after thyroid surgery is a wise precaution. Hypocalcaemia which is transient and not associated with any unpleasant symptoms does not need treatment. However, if there is numbness, paraesthesiae, neuromuscular excitability, or tetany associated with hypocalcaemia, immediate relief can be obtained by intravenous injection of 10 ml of 10 per cent calcium gluconate plus oral calcium. If the hypocalcaemia continues, it is necessary to add vitamin D to the oral calcium in the form of 1α-hydroxycholecalciferol on a daily basis.

Hypothyroidism

This can complicate of any thyroid surgery but is seen particularly where the remaining thyroid tissue is slowly destroyed by the process of autoimmune thyroiditis. This occurs in Hashimoto's disease, which itself rarely requires surgery, or in the thyroid remnant following a thyroidectomy for Graves' disease. The risk of developing hypothyroidism is much higher if the preoperative thyroid antibodies are positive and the histological picture of the thyroid specimen shows lymphoid infiltration. Treatment with oral thyroxine replacement is essential and can be started as soon as plasma TSH levels become elevated.

'Thyroid storm' or thyroid crisis

This is a rare complication and occurs most often in hyperthyroid patients who are poorly prepared for surgery. It is caused by the release of excess thyroid hormones as a result of gland manipulation. The clinical picture can be life threatening and reflects an acute and severe exacerbation of hyperthyroidism. Clinically, patients may be dyspnoeic, tachycardic, hyperpyrexial, restless, and confused, and there may be vomiting and diarrhoea. Treatment is with large doses of antithyroid drugs and potassium iodide, together with beta-blockade and digoxin for the toxic cardiac effects. The hyperpyrexia is treated by cooling and phenothiazines such as Largactil®. In extreme cases, the patient may require plasmapheresis to reduce the level of circulating T_4 and T_3.

Thyroid crisis (storm) is a very rare emergency. The specific treatment includes intravenous fluids, external cooling, and a variety of drug treatments:

- beta-adrenoceptor blockade with propranolol 1–5 mg as a slow intravenous injection four times a day then 40–80 mg four times a day orally;

- inhibition of thyroid hormone synthesis with either propylthiouracil 150–300 mg three times a day orally or via a nasogastric tube, or carbimazole 15–30 mg three times a day;

- inhibition of thyroid hormone release by potassium iodide 100 mg four times a day orally or Lugol's iodine 20 drops three times a day orally;

- hydrocortisone 100 mg intravenously four times a day.

Other complications of thyroidectomy

Haemorrhage, major or minor, causes an uncomfortable haematoma, and wound infection is rare. Subtle changes in voice quality are common after thyroidectomy. For most patients this is not of serious consequence but a singer may be profoundly affected. Careful preoperative discussions are vital.

6 Parathyroid surgery

6.1 Anatomy of the parathyroid glands

Normal parathyroid glands vary in number, location, and macroscopic appearance. From a surgical point of view the surgeon is concerned with the following aspects of parathyroid anatomy:

- whether the parathyroid glands seen at surgery are normal;

- where in the neck the surgeon should look for the glands;

- the relationship of the parathyroid glands to the recurrent laryngeal nerve;

- where the surgeon should look if one or more of the normal glands are missing.

Normal parathyroid glands are about 2 mm across and yellowish brown in colour. Their variable position is a direct result of the embryological derivation of the four parathyroid glands. The upper pair (together with the corresponding thyroid lobe) originate from the fourth branchial pouches, whereas the third branchial pouch differentiates into the lower pair of parathyroid glands and the two lobes of the thymus. Eighty per cent of patients have four parathyroid glands: the upper pair are usually located near the point where the recurrent laryngeal nerve enters the larynx. The lower pair are more variable in location and may be found anywhere between the inferior thyroid artery and the thymus. This pair can be the most elusive because of ectopic positions. All four glands may be in close relationship to the recurrent laryngeal nerve and the nerve must be identified and protected from damage in all parathyroid operations.

If it is not possible to find four parathyroid glands at neck exploration, then the most frequent area of ectopic location for the superior parathyroid glands are retropharyngeal or retro-oesophageal. If an inferior parathyroid gland is missing, a wide area may need to be explored, extending from the carotid artery bifurcation down into the mediastinum, including locations within the thymus gland.

6.2 Physiology of the parathyroids

Calcium haemostasis depends mainly on parathormone, the hormone produced by the parathyroid cells, on vitamin D synthesized by the kidney, and on calcitonin secreted by the C cells of the thyroid gland.

More than 90 per cent of the total body calcium is in bone and undergoes constant dynamic metabolism. In the extracellular fluid, less than 50 per cent calcium is in a free or ionized form, with most of the rest bound to plasma proteins (mainly albumin), and a small portion in soluble form. The concentration of calcium in the extracellular fluid needs to be maintained within very narrow limits. Any reduction in plasma calcium level is detected by the parathyroid glands which respond by secreting parathormone. This stimulates bone resorption and thereby moves calcium from bone into plasma. The effects of parathormone are as shown in Table 24.7.

In hyperparathyroidism, it used to be thought that pathological parathyroid tissue secreted excess parathormone in an autonomous fashion, independent of the extracellular calcium concentration. This is no longer thought to be true. It appears that in patients with primary hyperparathyroidism, the suppression of parathormone output normally associated with an increase in the level of circulating calcium occurs at a higher level. The defect therefore is the sensitivity of the parathyroids to a high calcium level, which should provide negative feedback to decrease their output of parathormone. The threshold level of plasma calcium is thus raised.

6.3 Primary hyperparathyroidism

Introduction

Primary hyperparathyroidism results in an increase in plasma calcium arising from a parathyroid adenoma or hyperplasia of all four glands. The diagnosis has been made more frequently because of automated plasma biochemical screening. Hypercalcaemia has been detected in many apparently asymptomatic individuals. Although described as asymptomatic, on close questioning many of these patients admit to symptoms of fatigue, weakness, depression, nocturia, polyuria, polydipsia,

Table 24.7 The effects of parathormone

Increases plasma calcium levels
Lowers plasma phosphate by increasing the renal clearance of phosphate
Increases bone remodelling by stimulating osteoblast and osteoclast activity
Increases urinary bicarbonate excretion, stimulates 1-hydroxylase activity in the kidney and converts 25-hydroxyvitamin D into the most active form of vitamin D (1,25-dihydroxyvitamin D_3)

Table 24.8 Other syndromes associated with primary hyperparathyroidism

Nephrolithiasis
Hypertension
Gout and pseudogout
Peptic ulcer disease
Bouts of acute pancreatitis

arthralgia, and constipation, and these symptoms can often be improved by surgery. The more extreme cases are associated with severe absorptive bone disease, renal stones, and peptic ulceration (Table 24.8), and now form the minority of cases of primary hyperparathyroidism.

Management of a patient with an elevated plasma calcium

It is important to confirm the presence of hypercalcaemia in a sequence of blood tests with correction for the level of plasma albumin. The diagnosis of primary hyperparathyroidism is made by exclusion of the causes listed in Table 24.9 and demonstrating elevated levels of parathormone in the peripheral blood. Additional helpful biochemical tests may include a decreased plasma phosphate and a mild hyperchloraemic acidosis.

In essence, a diagnosis of primary hyperparathyroidism should be considered in a patient with a raised plasma calcium with the following characteristics:

- a raised parathormone level;
- no metastatic bone disease;
- a normal chest X-ray, excluding sarcoidosis and carcinoma of the bronchus;
- normal plasma proteins to exclude multiple myeloma;
- a normal ESR to exclude the likelihood of multiple myeloma.

Causes of primary hyperparathyroidism

Most cases occur spontaneously and are not accompanied by other endocrine disorders. Nevertheless, primary hyperpara-

Table 24.9 Differential diagnosis of a raised plasma calcium

Metastatic bone disease
Multiple myeloma
Carcinoma of the bronchus with ectopic production of parathormone by the tumour
Sarcoidosis
Abnormally increased intake of vitamin D, milk, or calcium
Thiazide diuretics
Addison's disease
Thyrotoxicosis
Familial hypocalciuric hypercalcaemia

thyroidism is the most common manifestation of the hereditary **MEN I** or **Wermer's syndrome**, which includes parathyroid hyperplasia or adenoma, pituitary and pancreatic tumours, carcinoid tumours, and multiple lipomata. Primary hyperparathyroidism is also part of the **MEN IIa** or **Sipple syndrome**, which includes parathyroid hyperplasia or adenomas, C-cell hyperplasia or medullary carcinoma of the thyroid, and phaeochromocytoma. In these cases the phaeochromocytomas are usually bilateral. Primary hyperparathyroidism occurs rarely in **MEN IIb syndrome**.

Treatment of primary hyperparathyroidism

It is well established that bone disease occurring as a result of primary hyperparathyroidism can be corrected by surgical removal of the offending parathyroid gland or glands. However, it is not proven that hyperparathyroid hypertension or renal disease can be reversed by returning the patient's plasma calcium to normal. Nevertheless, most physicians would advise surgery if a patient presented with hyperparathyroid renal disease.

There has been considerable discussion about the advice to be given to patients who are incidentally found to have a raised plasma calcium and who fall into the asymptomatic group. The advice to operate is based on an understanding that early correction of hypercalcaemia will clear any non-specific symptoms and protect against the future development of hypertension and renal disease.

In general, the accepted indications for operative intervention are symptoms related to the skeleton, kidneys, or gastrointestinal tract, and for patients who have vague symptoms of ill-health likely to be associated with hypercalcaemia or an excessively raised corrected calcium (>3).

Preoperative localization of parathyroid tumours

Eighty per cent of hyperparathyroidism is caused by a solitary adenoma. However, it is difficult to predict the likelihood of there being four hyperplastic glands. A family history of endocrine disorders and, in particular, parathyroid disease may indicate the likelihood of hyperplasia. The incidence of carcinoma is 1 per cent and can be suspected if the plasma calcium is extremely high and associated with severe bone disease.

The occasional difficulty in finding the offending gland or glands at surgery has led to a series of investigations being employed in an attempt to locate the tumour preoperatively. None of these tests is ideal. Many specialist surgeons believe that the only localization needed is surgical exploration in the hands of an experienced parathyroid surgeon.

Table 24.10 Techniques for imaging the parathyroid glands

Ultrasonography

CT scanning

Thallium-technetium isotope subtraction scanning

Sestamabi technetium scanning

The simplest of these tests is ultrasound (Table 24.10) and in the hands of a good ultrasonographer it is possible to pick up most parathyroid tumours. The more sophisticated tests including venous sampling and parathormone estimations need not be used prior to a first exploration of the neck but held in reserve for difficult cases where a parathyroid tumour has not been found at the first operation, or when hypercalcaemia recurs.

The surgical strategy

The aim of parathyroid surgery is to find and remove the offending parathyroid tissue. In most cases, this will be a solitary adenoma. It can confidently be expected that the plasma calcium will return to normal if the tumour is removed. In most cases, it is a straightforward matter to locate a solitary tumour.

Decision making during the course of parathyroid surgery

1. If a solitary adenoma has been located by preoperative ultrasound scanning of the neck and surgical exploration confirms this, the surgeon has to decide whether there is any need to explore the neck further. If the other ipsilateral parathyroid is not enlarged, is it safe to assume that the surgeon is dealing with single-gland disease and can avoid exploring the opposite side of the neck? The statistical prevalence of single-gland disease and the very rare occurrence of a double adenoma (which may be confused with hyperplasia) makes the conservative approach to exploration of the neck attractive. Exploring both sides of the neck increase the likelihood of damage to the recurrent laryngeal nerves and routine exploration of all four parathyroids may lead to an increase incidence of postoperative hypocalcaemia. Nevertheless, current teaching advocates identification of all four parathyroids, even in single-gland disease.

2. If two enlarged glands are found on exploration of one side of the neck, the underlying pathology is likely to be hyperplasia. It is then necessary to explore the contralateral side. If hyperplasia is confirmed, then treatment remains controversial. Some surgeons advocate removing three and a half glands; others advocate removing all four glands and implanting a small part of chopped up gland in a forearm pouch which can be removed easily if hypercalcaemia recurs. Yet others advocate removing all parathyroid tissue and cryopreserving some tissue for reimplantation if hypoparathyroidism occurs. Hyperplasia of the four glands is most likely to be seen in the multiple endocrine neoplasia syndromes, chronic renal insufficiency, and familial hyperparathyroidism.

3. If an abnormal gland cannot be located readily, then a search of the usual ectopic sites needs to be made (Table 24.11, Fig. 24.6). If an adenoma cannot be found in any of these sites, then the operation is terminated. Unless the surgeon has definite evidence of a mediastinal tumour then there is no indication for performing a mediastinotomy during the first exploration of the neck.

Table 24.11 Ectopic sites for parathyroid adenomas

In the thymus or thyro-thymic ligament

High in the neck

Posterior to the oesophagus

In the carotid sheath

Beneath the thyroid capsule or within the thyroid itself

In the mediastinum

In the tracheo-oesophageal groove

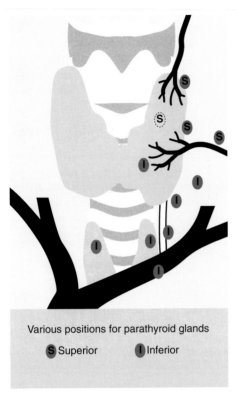

Various positions for parathyroid glands

S Superior   **I** Inferior

Figure 24.6 Ectopic sites for parathyroid adenomas.

Strategy for neck exploration for hyperparathyroidism

1. Look for the recurrent laryngeal nerve.

2. Look for the upper parathyroid (in a 2 cm radius, 1 cm above the junction of the recurrent laryngeal nerve and the inferior thyroid artery).

3. Look in the tracheo-oesophageal groove, retro-oesophageal and retropharyngeal spaces.

4. Look for lower parathyroids, from inferior thyroid pole to thymus (thyro-thymic ligament).

5. Perform transcervical thymectomy.

6. Look in the carotid sheath.

7. Perform thyroid lobectomy.

8. Usually stop; rarely, split sternum and explore mediastinum and pericardium. Usually the wound is closed and the patient

sent later for selective venous sampling or elaborate radioisotopic studies (e.g. sestamibi technetium scans).

Exploration of the neck rarely demonstrates two grossly enlarged glands and two normal glands weighing less than 50 mg. This may be a true 'double adenoma', and removal of both enlarged glands and biopsy of the normal glands will cure the condition. However, this presentation can be mistaken for asymmetrical hyperplasia, particularly in MEN I patients.

Parathyroid carcinoma is very rare and is manifest as a solid mass on neck exploration in the area of the parathyroid. The ipsilateral lobe of the thyroid may be involved and there may be lymph-node involvement. It is important not to break into the mass; thus a radical excision of the ipsilateral lobe of the thyroid and parathyroid glands should be performed. Most of these patients have severe hypercalcaemia preoperatively. Chemotherapy is not effective, and bisphosphonates may give temporary relief.

Microadenomas of the parathyroid have been reported. These are functioning adenomas within a normal parathyroid gland. Such patients are often diagnosed on re-exploration. If an adenomatous parathyroid is disrupted at operation, seedlings of recurrent adenoma may occur in the neck.

Re-exploration of the neck for hyperparathyroidism

If hypercalcaemia recurs or persists after parathyroid surgery, no further surgery should be carried out until the cause has been definitively established. When hypercalcaemia persists or recurs within 6 months of surgery it is usually caused by a missed abnormal gland. Before further surgery it is best to attempt pre-operative localization, because if the main techniques do not reveal an adenoma, the surgeon will be very fortunate to find one at a re-exploration. Techniques to be considered for mapping the likely sites of abnormal parathyroid tissue include ultrasonography, radioisotope scanning using either ^{201}Tl–^{99m}Tc subtraction scanning or ^{99m}Tc-labelled sestamibi. Other techniques include digital subtraction, highly selective angiography and selective venous catheterization with PTH sampling.

The results of these tests will help decide whether the patient needs exploration of the neck via the old operative scar, or of the mediastinum through a median sternotomy. A major risk factor in re-do operations is damage to the recurrent laryngeal nerve or to the normal parathyroid glands. In general, every effort should be made to locate the parathyroid abnormality at the first operation in order to avoid the real problems of re-do surgery.

6.4 Secondary and tertiary hyperparathyroidism

Secondary hyperparathyroidism develops in response to chronic hypocalcaemia in patients with chronic renal failure or intestinal malabsorption. It is characterized by normocalcaemia, hyperplasia of all four parathyroids, and an elevated level of circulating parathormone. The continuing stimulus to the four parathyroids eventually results in a state of autonomy, with either an exacerbation of the hyperplastic state or the development of adenomas. The patient develops an autonomous hypercalcaemia, usually associated with the onset of severe bone disease. Patients should normally undergo a total or subtotal parathyroidectomy, as described earlier.

In patients with secondary hyperparathyroidism due to chronic renal failure, the hyperparathyroidism usually begins to disappear 6–12 months after successful renal transplantation. If the patient remains hypercalcaemic after this period, parathyroid function is likely to have become irreversibly autonomous (tertiary hyperparathyroidism) and parathyroidectomy is needed.

7 Salivary glands

7.1 Submandibular gland

Submandibular calculus

Submandibular duct stone typically presents with a history of intermittent unilateral swelling beneath the angle of the jaw. The swelling is often uncomfortable but rarely painful unless the gland becomes infected. Symptoms come and go and last for a variable period. Typically the submandibular gland remains moderately enlarged but every few days, swells further during and after a meal. Swelling persists as long as the duct remains obstructed, from a few hours to several weeks.

Diagnosis is made if the submandibular gland is enlarged on palpation and a stone can be felt in the line of the duct in the floor of the mouth on bimanual palpation. It is confirmed by plain X-ray, of which the most useful is an occlusal film. Here, the plate is placed horizontally in the mouth and the beam directed vertically from below the jaw. Stones in the anterior part of the duct are usually palpable, but posterior stones within the gland are not. The latter may also be missed on X-ray unless good-quality films are taken and examined skilfully.

Treatment

Duct stones should be removed because symptoms are likely to recur and there is the ever-present risk of infection in the obstructed gland. Anterior stones can be removed from within the mouth but posterior stones and gland stones usually require excision of the submandibular gland via an external submandibular incision. Thus, the indication for the latter operation would need to be more pressing than for the former as both anaesthesia and surgery are much more invasive.

Removal of submandibular duct stones may be carried out under local anaesthesia using a lingual nerve block, or more commonly, under general anaesthesia on a day-case basis.

Under general anaesthesia, the patient will have an endotracheal tube passed via a nasal approach and the pharynx is packed with gauze to prevent inhalation of blood and debris. The jaws are held gently apart with a rubber prop or 'bite block' unless the patient is edentulous, and a sucker must be to hand.

If possible, confirm the diagnosis at operation by bimanual palpation, starting at the back and milking the stone forwards.

If the stone can be palpated or moved to the anterior part of the duct, it has been taught that the proximal part of the duct should be encircled with a suture to prevent the stone shifting posteriorly, but in practice this is rarely possible because the duct falls away so rapidly from the floor of the mouth. The incision is along the course of the duct and should allow the stone to be lifted out. Sometimes, the stone has a spiky surface and is embedded in the duct wall. The incision is left open and will close remarkably quickly, leaving a small fistula if the duct orifice is stenosed.

If the stone cannot be found or disappears backwards out of reach when the duct is opened, the approach needs to be changed. Now, the duct orifice should be cannulated with a lachrymal probe and the orifice opened out with pointed scissors. Usually, the orifice is narrow and the duct behind it markedly dilated. The stone may sometimes be retrieved with grasping forceps but if not, the stone will usually be passed spontaneously later if salivary flow is encouraged with citrus fruit or juice. If the stone is not retrieved at operation, the patient must be informed and warned to try and retrieve the stone later. A further X-ray should be performed for medico-legal safety about 2 weeks later to confirm whether the stone remains or has gone. There is no special postoperative care other than gentle mouthwashes for blood.

There are no common complications and results are good if the above precautions are adhered to.

Excision of a submandibular gland

This operation is indicated in patients who have stones impacted in the deep part of the submandibular gland, or in the rare case of tumours affecting the submandibular gland. The main risks of this procedure are damage to the mandibular branch of the facial nerve, damage to the lingual nerve, and haemorrhage from the facial artery.

The patient lies supine on the operating table with the head, supported on a rubber ring, turned away from the side of the lesion. The incision is made over the submandibular gland at least 2 cm below and parallel to the lower border of the mandible (Fig. 24.7b). The platysma muscle is divided in the line of the incision to expose the fascia enclosing the submandibular gland. In this way damage to the mandibular branch of the facial nerve can be avoided. An operative plane is then developed between the gland and the fascia and the superficial part of the gland is fully mobilized from the underlying mylohyoid muscle (Fig. 24.7a).

The posterior aspect of the gland is carefully separated from the surrounding tissues and it is here that the facial artery and vein may be found closely applied to the posterior part of the gland. The vessels are either separated from the gland or divided after ligation (Fig. 24.7c). After freeing the posterior border, the gland can be turned back on itself to reveal the deeper structures which include the hyoid bone, hyoglossus muscle, and the

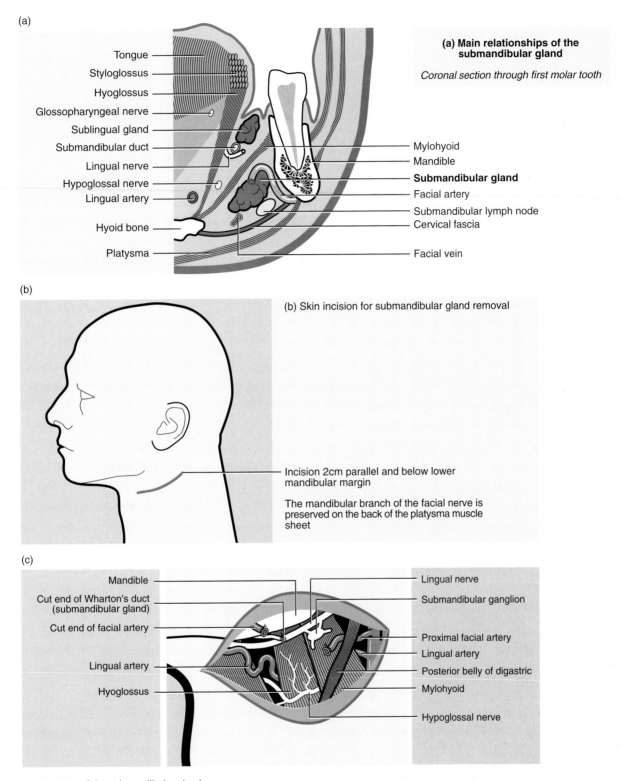

(a)

Tongue —
Styloglossus —
Hyoglossus —
Glossopharyngeal nerve —
Sublingual gland —
Submandibular duct —
Lingual nerve —
Hypoglossal nerve —
Lingual artery —
Hyoid bone —
Platysma —

(a) Main relationships of the submandibular gland

Coronal section through first molar tooth

— Mylohyoid
— Mandible
— **Submandibular gland**
— Facial artery
— Submandibular lymph node
— Cervical fascia
— Facial vein

(b)

(b) Skin incision for submandibular gland removal

— Incision 2cm parallel and below lower mandibular margin

The mandibular branch of the facial nerve is preserved on the back of the platysma muscle sheet

(c)

Mandible —
Cut end of Wharton's duct (submandibular gland) —
Cut end of facial artery —
Lingual artery —
Hyoglossus —

— Lingual nerve
— Submandibular ganglion
— Proximal facial artery
— Lingual artery
— Posterior belly of digastric
— Mylohyoid
— Hypoglossal nerve

Figure 24.7 Excision of the submandibular gland.

lingual nerve (Fig. 24.7a). On a deeper plane lies the hypoglossal nerve. The deep part of the gland is then separated from the deep portion of the mylohyoid muscle and it is here that the lingual nerve is found lying superior to the deep part of the gland as the submandibular duct emerges from it. The mylohyoid is retracted anteriorly, the duct identified and ligated. This part of the operation maybe difficult owing to local inflammation caused by stone disease.

7.2 Parotid gland

Swellings of the parotid gland

Parotid gland swellings may be neoplastic or non-neoplastic. The former group may be further divided into benign, intermediate, and malignant tumours.

Non-neoplastic swellings

- The most common swelling is caused by sialadenitis and perhaps sialectasis, sometimes associated with parotid duct calculi.

- Infective causes—the most common is mumps parotitis. The history is often diagnostic. It may be associated with orchitis and pancreatitis. Bacteria can produce an acute suppurative parotitis, often associated with poor dental hygiene.

- In association with alcoholic hepatitis.

- Connective tissue diseases, most commonly Sjögren's disease and systemic sclerosis, but occasionally associated with other vasculitides and systemic lupus erythematosus (SLE).

- Cystic parotid swellings have been reported in HIV.

- TB and syphilis.

- Epidermal cysts.

Benign tumours

Monomorphic adenomas

- The most common monomorphic adenoma is the **adeno-lymphoma**, which is encapsulated and occurs in older men. It is bilateral in approximately 10 per cent. It does not recur if enucleated but will do so if incompletely excised. It is said to occur exclusively in smokers.

- **Oncocytoma** is a slowly growing tumour characterized by large, pale-staining oncocytes. It does not recur after removal.

Miscellaneous

Haemangiomas, lipomas, fibromas, and lymph-node tumours can all arise within the substance of the gland.

Intermediate-grade tumours

- Pleomorphic adenoma ('mixed parotid tumour'). Many authorities regard this as benign but it behaves with some degree of local invasion, particularly if incompletely excised. Thirty to 40 per cent of parotid tumours are pleomorphic adenomas.

- Well-differentiated mucoepidermoid tumour.

- Acinic-cell tumour.

Malignant tumours

- Poorly differentiated mucoepidermoid tumour.

- Adenocarcinoma.

- Squamous carcinoma arising in pleomorphic adenoma.

- Adenoid cystic tumour. This is malignant, particularly with a propensity to spread along the perineural sheaths.

- Sarcomas: these are rare but can arise in connective tissue.

- Malignant melanoma: the most common malignant parotid tumour in pale-skinned people in sunny climates.

- Metastatic tumours.

More than 90 per cent of salivary gland tumours arise in the parotid. The submandibular, sublingual, and other minor salivary glands account for the remainder. The proportion of malignant tumours, particularly the acinic cell tumour, increases in non-parotid gland tumours.

Clinical assessment

Traditionally, history and clinical examination have proved the mainstay of diagnosis. Certainly, the site, size and progression of the swelling, together with systemic symptoms and signs, often give a clue. Adenolymphoma is most common in elderly men, bilateral in 10 per cent of patients, and slow growing; facial nerve involvement ipsilaterally suggests infiltration with a malignant parotid tumour. Benign and intermediate tumours are all slow growing and the size of the tumour mass is related to the length of the history, which may be several years. Tumours arising in the deep lobe are often diagnosed much later, unless they bulge into the palate or tonsillar region.

Malignant tumours may be characterized by rapid growth, hardness, skin attachment and ulceration, deep fixity, and lymph-node enlargement. Facial nerve involvement leads to rapid diagnosis. However, in the early stages of development these tumours infiltrate sensory nerves and produce vague pain in the distribution of the great auricular and auriculo-temporal nerves. The combination of pain and enlargement of the parotid must be treated with suspicion of malignancy. However, in many patients diagnosis is not achieved until surgery. Incorrect pre-operative diagnosis may result in either overtreatment for benign disease or insufficiently radical treatment for malignant disease.

Specific investigations for parotid swellings

Fine-needle aspiration cytology

FNAC is simple, cheap, and effective, and has high accuracy and low false-positive and false-negative rates. The technique may be performed easily without local anaesthesia in the outpatient department. However, many surgeons find it unhelpful as the diagnosis is rarely robust.

Sialography

Sialography may be used to diagnose non-calculous salivary gland disease if the space-occupying lesion distorts the pattern of salivary ducts. The main use of sialography is to demonstrate diffuse parotid salivary disease, such as Sjögren's syndrome or calculous disease of the parotid. Briefly, sialography is performed by careful introduction of either a plastic or metal cannula into the opening of the parotid duct of Stensen opposite the upper second molar tooth. An appropriate water-soluble contrast medium is injected and radiographs are taken in lateral and oblique views to demonstrate the whole length of the duct.

Isotope scintigraphy

Isotope scintigraphy is a potentially useful technique in that adenolymphomas and oxyphil-cell adenomas will selectively take up technetium-99m and iodine-123. Cystic hygroma, parotid haemangioma, and mucoepidermoid tumour have also been reported to have characteristic appearances. Thermography and ultrasound have also been used, but they are too non-specific, except in detecting rare parotid cysts.

Computed tomography

Computed tomography (CT) is useful in showing the exact site and size of lesions suspected to be malignant lying within the parotid, as well as indicating extraparotid mass lesions. CT, in combination with FNAC, allows more accurate preoperative assessment which, in turn, permits a more conservative or a non-operative approach to management, thereby minimizing treatment-induced morbidity.

Magnetic resonance imaging

MRI studies have shown that both spin-echo T_1-weighted images and T_2-weighted images, and short tau inversion recovery (STIR) sequence are useful in differentiating benign tumours from malignant tumours with a resolution of 6 mm, but the histological grade may not be predicted accurately.

Clinical management of a parotid swelling

Benign tumours of the parotid are most often treated by superficial parotidectomy. However, some surgeons favour precision enucleation if malignancy is unlikely. This gives reduced morbidity and probably as good a cure rate as the more radical operation. Deep parotid swellings (diagnosed by CT or MRI) require a more extensive procedure, although the facial nerve can usually be spared.

If malignant neoplasms are diagnosed, surgery or radiotherapy may be appropriate. If surgery is the choice, total parotidectomy (with or without sparing of the facial nerve) or radical parotidectomy (together with cervical lymph-node block dissection) may be appropriate.

Patients with recurrent parotid swelling without a mass, and with salivary secretion rates of less than 0.5 ml/min, or with the main duct grossly dilated, may be treated by parotid duct ligation or parotidectomy. Milder cases may be treated by stimulation of parotid secretion, often simply achieved by sucking acidic sweets.

Operative technique: superficial parotidectomy

Proper informed consent must be obtained. The patient is anaesthetized and intubated with the head on a ring and turned away from the side of operation, with the head end of the table tilted up 20°. A cotton-wool pledget may be placed in the external auditory meatus. An S-shaped incision is made immediately anterior to the ipsilateral pinna, curving backwards under the earlobe and straight forwards and downwards at the anterior border of the sternomastoid for 2–3 cm (Fig. 24.8a). The incision is deepened in the upper and lower third of the incision, leaving a bridge of undisturbed tissue over the stylomastoid foramen and facial nerve trunk in the middle third. In the lower third the greater auricular nerve is met quite superficially. Although this can be preserved, it is often useful to excise 2 cm and preserve it in saline in case a cable graft is required to repair a damaged facial nerve. A clear plane can be found anterior to the sternomastoid; this is deepened until the posterior belly of the digastric is visible. The bridge of tissue is now dealt with by inserting a pair of curved artery forceps, opening them, and carefully dividing tissues superficial to the blades.

Locating the facial nerve trunk

The triangular cartilaginous part of the external auditory meatus acts as a pointer; the stylomastoid foramen lies 3–6 mm deep to its apex (Fig. 24.8b). The stylomastoid vein sits immediately superficial to the nerve. Venous bleeding suggests that the nerve is close and diathermy must be avoided. Once the main trunk is identified, the upper and lower trunks and branches are dissected using artery forceps to open a plane along and superficial to each of the facial nerve branches from behind forwards and above downwards. Although the retromandibular vein lies deep to the nerve, particularly in the lower part of the gland, superficial communicating branches may need to be ligated to prevent troublesome bleeding. Only when the nerve is exposed should the skin flap be raised from the superficial surface of the parotid. The reason for this approach is that deep tumours may stretch the nerve superficially and if the skin flap is raised before tracing the facial nerve, inadvertent damage may ensue. The parotid duct can be ligated with an absorbable ligature and the superficial part of the gland excised. A suction drain is advisable, and the wound is closed with a continuous suture to platysma and a subcuticular absorbable suture. A pressure dressing may be useful. The drain is removed at 48 hours and the patient discharged.

Complications of parotidectomy

- Haematoma.

- Facial nerve palsy: may be temporary or permanent. If damage is recognized at surgery, it should be repaired. Grade III (complete) palsy is unusual in non-malignant parotid disease.

- Frey's syndrome: 'gustatory sweating' is probably caused by reconnection of the secretomotor facial nerve salivary parasympathetic fibres into the cut ends of the greater auricular nerve. This can be troublesome and is avoided by enucleation rather than superficial parotidectomy, or possibly by removing a good segment of the latter nerve if it is sacrificed.

- Parotid duct fistula: avoided by ligating the duct.

(a)

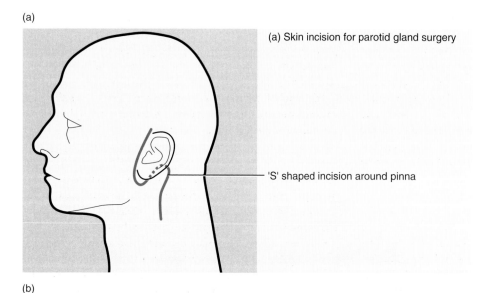

(a) Skin incision for parotid gland surgery

'S' shaped incision around pinna

(b)

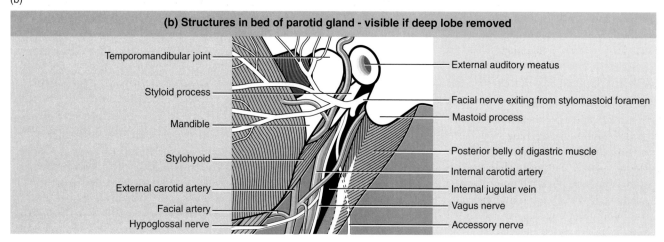

(b) Structures in bed of parotid gland - visible if deep lobe removed

Temporomandibular joint

Styloid process

Mandible

Stylohyoid

External carotid artery

Facial artery

Hypoglossal nerve

External auditory meatus

Facial nerve exiting from stylomastoid foramen

Mastoid process

Posterior belly of digastric muscle

Internal carotid artery

Internal jugular vein

Vagus nerve

Accessory nerve

Figure 24.8 Superficial parotidectomy.

8 Other lumps and sinuses in the neck

8.1 Branchial cyst

This lateral neck swelling is commonly found at the anterior border of the sternomastoid. It undoubtedly arises as a remnant of the branchial arch/cleft system but its precise aetiology remains in doubt. It may represent a persistent, unobliterated third branchial arch remnant, or a persistent cervical sinus may be responsible.

Clinical features

Sixty per cent occur in men and the peak age of incidence is during the third decade. Two-thirds are anterior to the sterno-mastoid in the upper third of the neck and the remainder are in other areas, either opposite the middle or lower thirds of the sternomastoids, the parotid area, adjacent to the pharynx, or in the posterior triangle.

The common presentation is a sudden onset of pain and swelling (continuous or intermittent). Less commonly, there are symptoms of infection or a sensation of pressure.

Branchial cysts are usually lined by stratified squamous epithelium. More than 80 per cent have lymphoid tissue in the wall, which may be due to chronic infection or may indicate a common origin with lymph nodes. Branchial cysts contain serous fluid which glistens with cholesterol crystals when absorbed on a swab.

Investigations

The diagnosis of branchial cyst is easily confirmed on ultra-sonography. Aspiration of fluid is sometimes successful in treating branchial cysts, but may be painful. If a chemodectoma is suspected because of direct or transmitted pulsation or solid con-sistency on clinical examination, a carotid duplex scan is helpful.

Excision of branchial cyst

With the patient positioned with a head-up tilt and the head turned to the opposite side, a horizontal skin incision is made at the level of the lesion through the platysma and flaps are raised to the upper and lower margins of the lump. The deep investing cervical fascia is incised over the lump parallel to the anterior border of the sternomastoid. The cyst is dissected out; immediately deep to the cyst lie the origin of the external and internal carotid arteries and the vagus nerve. The cyst is related superiorly to the middle constrictor muscle and hypoglossal and glossopharyngeal nerves. The entire lining of the cyst should be removed intact because if fragments of the wall are left, the cyst may recur. The incision is closed in layers, usually with a suction drain.

8.2 Branchial sinus and fistula

Sinuses or fistulas originating from the third branchial arch are the most common. The lesions usually present in childhood or adolescence with recurrent discharge of clear fluid from tiny openings anterior to the inferior end of the sternomastoid. A branchial sinus is a blind-ending tract of variable length; a branchial fistula communicates with the pharynx. Differentiation is by contrast sinography.

Excision of branchial sinus or fistula

With the patient positioned with a head-up tilt and with the head turned to the opposite side, an elliptical skin crease incision is made around the opening of the sinus. The incision is deepened through the subcutaneous tissue and platysma. Traction is placed on the skin ellipse with tissue forceps and the track may then be felt as a fibrous cord running upwards along the anterior border of the sternomastoid deep to the investing cervical fascia. If the track extends higher in the neck than can comfortably be reached through the initial incision, a second incision is made parallel to and above the first at the level of the hyoid, and the mobilized track drawn upwards through the second incision. The usual course of the track is to pass between the external and internal carotid arteries and then deep to the posterior belly of the digastric muscle. Part of the digastric may be excised to allow the track to be followed upwards to its termination. Deep to the posterior belly of the digastric, the track lies superficial to the middle constrictor muscle of the pharynx and care must be taken to avoid damage to either the hypoglossal or glossopharyngeal nerves at this point. The entire track can then be excised. The wound is closed in layers and a small suction drain is sometimes used.

8.3 Chemodectoma

Nests of non-chromaffin paraganglionic cells derived from the neural crest normally occur in the carotid bulb, the jugular bulb, in the cavity of the middle ear, in the ganglion nodosum of the vagus nerve, adjacent to the major thoracic arteries, and in the ciliary ganglion of the orbit. Chemodectoma of the carotid body is more common in populations living at high altitude, probably because chronic hypoxia leads to carotid body hyperplasia. The usual age of presentation is between 35 and 50 years.

In 10 per cent of cases, there is a strong family history. In these, there is a tendency to bilateral tumours and concurrent phaeochromocytoma. Clinically, the globular or ovoid tumour is firmly adherent to the bifurcation of the carotid artery, but is seldom more than 4 or 5 cm in diameter.

Histological examination shows large, uniform epithelioid cells surrounded by a vascular stroma. There are capillaries in the fibrous septa between the cell nests.

Clinical features

Presentation is with a painless lump in the neck. There is often a history of several years and this helps to differentiate a carotid body tumour from a lymphoma or a metastatic lymph node enlargement, but is compatible with a branchial cyst. The tumour is usually at the bifurcation of the carotid artery and can cause displacement and separation of the internal and external carotids (grade II tumour) or complete encasement (grade III tumour). The mass is firm and rubbery and usually demonstrates transmitted rather than expansile pulsation. A bruit may be present and the mass may decrease in size as a result of carotid compression before refilling in stages with each pulsation. Rarely, patients complain of mild dysphagia or discomfort. Large tumours may involve the ninth to twelfth cranial nerves or the sympathetic chain, causing a Horner's syndrome.

Investigations

The diagnosis is often made at the time of inadvertent open biopsy of a suspected lymph node enlargement but should be suspected beforehand from its clinical features and ultra-sonographic findings. More information may be obtained from carotid duplex scanning or CT scanning, but an angiogram with fast injection and rapid serial films is perhaps the most useful next investigation. In the capillary phase of arteriography, there is an internal blush and the draining veins are usually dilated. Differentiation between a chemodectoma and a glomus vagale tumour is made by the more superior position of the latter and its relative lack of vascularity. Angiography is also useful to determine the extent of the tumour, to see if there is separation of the internal and external carotid arteries, and also to see if there is cross-circulation from the other side.

Treatment

Resection of carotid body tumours has always carried risks, but operative mortality has fallen with a better understanding of the physiology of cerebral blood flow, advances in arterial surgical techniques, and carotid bypass and hypothermia where necessary. Removal is indicated for tumours which are clinically or histologically malignant and are resectable, for patients under 50 years of age with a small or medium-sized tumour, or for a tumour which has extended into the pharynx or palate and is interfering with swallowing, speaking, or breathing. Surgery is performed using a similar approach and incision to that used for carotid endarterectomy and a shunt may be employed. For inoperable tumours, radiotherapy may be used for palliation.

Other tumours which may present in a similar way to carotid body tumours are **ganglioneuromas** (closely related to chemodectomas) and **Schwann cell tumours** (neurofibromas and schwannomas). Removal of these is generally less hazardous as regards damage to the carotid artery and inadvertent embolization. If one of these tumours is malignant, *en bloc* dissection of neck nodes may be indicated.

8.4 Cystic hygroma

This is a congenital lymphatic swelling which presents as a fluctuant, transilluminable swelling in infants. The lesion sometimes regresses spontaneously but often requires surgical excision. It is situated laterally over the sternomastoid muscle.

8.5 Cervical rib

This may present as a swelling in the supraclavicular fossa but more commonly produces a thoracic outlet syndrome, affecting either the subclavian artery or the brachial plexus.

9 Conclusion

This chapter has dealt with an overview suitable for the non-specialist in endocrine and head and neck surgery. Of necessity, some of the controversial areas (e.g. pathophysiology and adjuvant therapy) have been greatly simplified. The interested reader is invited to consult one or more of the specialist texts listed below. Future developments will involve more accurate non-invasive diagnosis, based on molecular techniques. The operative techniques are likely to be unaffected by the revolution in minimal access surgery, although, particularly in parathyroidectomy, such approaches have been described as being feasible.

This field offers opportunities for worthwhile surgical research and will continue to provide clinical challenges for the general surgeon.

Bibliography

Banerjee, A.K. and Cooper J.C. (1995). Non-surgical treatment of multinodular non-toxic goitre. *Postgrad. Med. J.*, **71**, 643. [A brief review of the role of thyroxine suppression in controlling the size of multinodular goitre, thus avoiding surgery.]

Banerjee, A.K., Ubhi, C.S., and Pegg, C.A.S. (1994). Diagnostic approaches to parotid swellings. *Br. J. Hosp. Med.*, **51**, 516–21. [A review of modern methods of achieving accurate preoperative diagnosis.]

Char, D.H. (1990). *Thyroid eye disease*, (2nd edn). Churchill Livingstone, London. [A detailed book on this important area.]

Cusick, E.L., MacIntosh, C.A., Krukowski, Z.H., *et al.* (1990). Management of isolated thyroid swellings : a prospective six year study of fine needle aspiration cytology in diagnosis. *BMJ*, **301**, 318–21.

Kark, A.E., Kissin, M.W., Auerbach, R., and Meikle, M. (1984). Voice changes after thyroidectomy: role of the external laryngeal nerve. *BMJ*, **289**, 1412–15.

Lynn, J. and Bloom, S.R. (1993). *Surgical endocrinology*, (2nd edn). Butterworth–Heinemann, Oxford. [An authoritative text in surgical endocrinology: an important reference for the specialist endocrine surgeon and for candidates offering endocrine surgery as a special interest for the Intercollegiate examination.]

Lynn, J., Gamvros, O.I., and Taylor, S. (1981). Medullary carcinoma of the thyroid. *World J. Surg.*, **5**, 27–32. [A key review of this rare but important condition.]

Owen, E.R.T.C., Banerjee, A.K., Kissin, M., and Kark, A.E. (1989). Complications of parotid surgery: the need for selectivity. *Br. J. Surg.*, **76**, 1034–5.

Owen, E.R.T.C., Banerjee, A.K., Pritchard, A.J.N., Hudson, E.A., and Kark, A.E. (189). Role of fine needle aspiration cytology and computed tomography in the diagnosis of parotid swellings. *Br. J. Surg.*, **76**, 1273–4.

Russell, R.C.G. (1986). Thyroidectomy. *Br. J. Hosp. Med.*, **35**, 327–30. [A clear review of the operative details.]

Senapati, A. and Young, A.E. (1990). Parathyroid transplantation. *Br. J. Surg.*, **77**, 1171–4.

Shaha, A. and Jaffe, B.M. (1988). Complications of thyroid surgery performed by residents. *Surgery*, **104**, 1109–14. [Useful reading for registrars performing thyroid surgery.]

Shaw, J.H.F., Holden, A., and Sage, M. (1989). Thyroid lymphoma. *Br. J. Surg.*, **76**, 895–7.

Wade, J.S.H. (1985). Vulnerability of the recurrent laryngeal nerves at thyroidectomy. *Br. J. Surg.*, **43**, 164–80. [A classic review of this complication.]

Weetman, A.P. and McGregor, A.M. (1984). Autoimmune thyroid disease: developments in our understanding. *Endocrine Rev.*, **5**, 309–55. [Important review article to be read by surgeons managing such patients.]

Wheeler, M.H. (1996). Investigation of the solitary thyroid nodule. *Clin. Endocrinol.*, **44**, 245–7.

CHAPTER 25

Breast surgery

Christobel Saunders with John McGregor

1 Introduction

When a woman presents with a breast problem, concern about malignancy is often uppermost in her mind. Virtually every woman who discovers a breast problem assumes the worst, despite the fact that less than 10 per cent of breast pathology is malignant.

The surgeon's initial role is to rapidly and accurately establish the diagnosis and to advise the patient about the options for treatment. The most important diagnostic error to avoid is wrongly labelling a lesion benign when it later turns out to be malignant. This means that when dealing with persistent, non-cyclical, breast symptoms, undefined breast lumps, or questionable lesions on imaging, a high degree of suspicion should be employed. Where clinical appearance and other investigations are equivocal, biopsy must be the final arbiter.

Diagnostic techniques less invasive than open biopsy have progressively improved in recent years in their sensitivity and specificity, so that a definitive diagnosis can now be reached in most cases without the need for open biopsy. Techniques include high resolution ultrasound scanning, mammography, fine-needle aspiration cytology, and core-cut or Trucut biopsy. Fine-needle aspiration cytology (FNAC) can be obtained with precision from small lesions discovered on ultrasound scanning or mammography, using **stereotactic localization** of the aspiration needle under ultrasound or mammographic control.

The classification of benign lesions has been the considerably clarified by the ANDI concept (abnormalities of normal development and involution), which places benign changes in the breast on a spectrum from normal to individual pathological entities. In benign disease, most patients only need reassurance that their symptoms are not due to cancer, and symptomatic treatment.

The profile of breast cancer and its treatment is very high, with continual media coverage and public interest. The National Breast Cancer Screening programme and the establishment of multidisciplinary specialist Breast Units has also raised public awareness, and perhaps anxiety levels about breast cancer, and has certainly improved the quality of care of breast cancer patients throughout the country.

2 Symptoms of breast disease

2.1 Breast pain

Cyclical breast pain is a symptom experienced to a greater or lesser extent by most women, at least during occasional menstrual cycles. Cyclical pain is more common between the mid-20s and the menopause, and usually takes the form of a sensation of fullness and heaviness in the week or so before menstruation. The pain is often unilateral and is associated with breast tenderness, which may be either generalized, or localized to the upper outer quadrant. The cause of cyclical breast pain is unknown, but is assumed to be related to the balance of various hormones—prolactin, oestrogen, progesterone, and perhaps gonadotrophins. Patients often tolerate cyclical breast pain but present for help when the pain or tenderness becomes persistent and starts to interfere with life. Non-cyclical mastalgia is likely to be of similar aetiology and most commonly occurs perimeno-pausally (and, of course, in some women on hormone replacement therapy (HRT)). Pain is rarely a symptom of cancer, but pain does not exclude a diagnosis of cancer.

2.2 A breast 'lump' or lumpiness

A lump may have been detected by the patient herself (usually by chance, e.g. in the shower, although occasionally during self-examination) or may have been found during a well-woman check or in a Family Planning Clinic. An episode of breast pain or localized tenderness may have drawn the patient's attention to an area which appears lumpy. Sometimes, a patient reports an episode of trauma to the breast which has drawn her attention to a lump which usually proves to have been a pre-existing lump.

On clinical examination, a discrete lump may be found. Often, however, a patch of breast tissue which is clearly different from normal is found, or else there may be an indistinct area of thickening or nodularity or 'lumpiness'. Nodularity is most often found in the upper outer quadrant of the breast where more glandular tissue is concentrated. Sometimes no abnormality is palpable, yet the patient is certain an abnormality is present. Under these circumstances, the clinician should take the history seriously and search hard to exclude an underlying cancer, using the range of diagnostic methods.

The probability of particular pathological diagnoses being present depends on a variety of factors, of which the most important are the patient's age (Fig. 25.1) and the clinical findings (Fig. 25.2). The common diagnoses are as follows.

Fibroadenoma

This is a discrete, smooth, rounded, freely mobile swelling most commonly found in the age group 20–30 years. It does not contain fluid on aspiration. It is commonly known as a 'breast mouse' because of its extreme mobility.

Benign nodularity and mastalgia

The patient is usually between 30 and 45 years. The condition is often unilateral and the patient's attention is often brought to the area by pain, which is usually cyclical but sometimes continuous. On examination, the affected area, usually in the outer upper quadrant of the breast, is often tender and thickened, or nodular with an indistinct edge.

Breast cyst

Cysts form part of the spectrum of benign breast disorders classified under the ANDI concept, described later. Breast cysts occur in perimenopausal women and often appear with alarming rapidity. They are smooth, rounded swellings which are often multiple and may appear very hard or tense. Aspiration causes miraculous disappearance of the lump. Cyst contents range from clear yellowish to dark-green, murky fluid. Malignancy is occasionally associated with breast cysts and so a diagnostic system must be employed which avoids missing malignancy (described later).

Carcinoma

Carcinomas are usually but not always painless. Characteristic features of carcinoma are hardness of the lump on palpation, skin changes suggesting invasion, tethering of the lump to skin

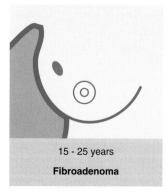
15 - 25 years
Fibroadenoma

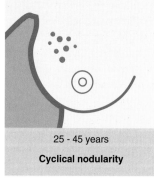
25 - 45 years
Cyclical nodularity

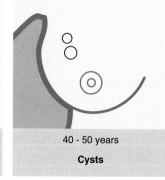
40 - 50 years
Cysts

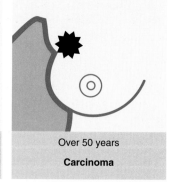
Over 50 years
Carcinoma

Figure 25.1 The likely causes of a breast lump at a given age.

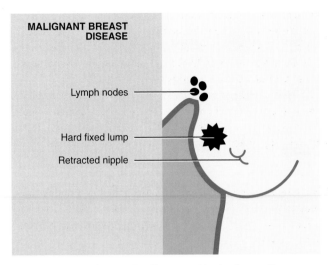

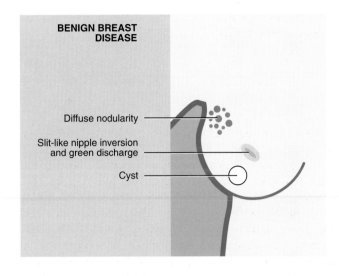

Figure 25.2 Clinical signs of malignant and benign breast disease.

or underlying structures, and enlargement of regional lymph nodes. Early carcinomas may be clinically indistinguishable from benign lumps and thus all breast lumps need to have malignancy excluded. It is best to assume any woman over the age of 40 presenting with a breast lump has a carcinoma until proved otherwise.

2.3 Nipple disorders

Recent nipple inversion is the most common complaint, but occasionally the texture of the nipple skin has changed, as may occur for example in Paget's disease.

Nipple inversion

Nipple inversion is not abnormal when dating from puberty. When it occurs for the first time in middle age, nipple inversion nearly always results from either an underlying carcinoma or else fibrosis associated with **mammary duct ectasia**.

Alteration in the texture of the nipple

'Eczema' of the nipple, with the skin becoming thick, red, and scaly may represent simple eczema, but the possibility of Paget's disease must be considered. Paget's disease is malignant infiltration of the nipple in continuity with an underlying intraduct carcinoma and is more likely in older women. Simple eczema is most likely in a lactating woman.

Nipple discharge

Nipple discharge is nearly always associated with benign breast disease but occasionally it heralds an intraduct papilloma or carcinoma, particularly if the discharge contains blood. An underlying lump is suspicious of carcinoma and in most cases, mammography is desirable.

Most discharges are clear or greenish. Clear discharge is of no significance, whereas greenish discharge probably indicates mammary duct ectasia. Blood may be obvious but, if not, the discharge should be tested for blood using a urine-testing 'dip stick'. If there is sufficient, the discharge can be sent for cytological assessment.

3 Investigation of breast disease

The history of a patient with a breast problem directs the clinician towards a specific diagnosis but it is rarely diagnostic in itself. The findings on clinical examination (Table 25.1) and the age of the patient are likely to be of greater importance. Subsequent investigations are directed towards establishing an accurate tissue diagnosis and excluding disease elsewhere in the breasts (Fig. 25.3).

3.1 Fine-needle aspiration for cytology

Breast cysts

Aspiration of cysts produces an immediate cure (not always long-term), relieves anxiety, and indicates almost certainly the

Table 25.1 Important questions in taking a breast history

Primary complaint
Duration
Cyclical changes in symptoms
Age
Pain
Menstrual history
Parity and age of patient when children were born
Current and past hormonal therapy
Family history of carcinoma of the breast, particularly first- and second-degree relatives
Previous breast disease
Previous frequent diagnostic chest X-rays or radiotherapy to chest

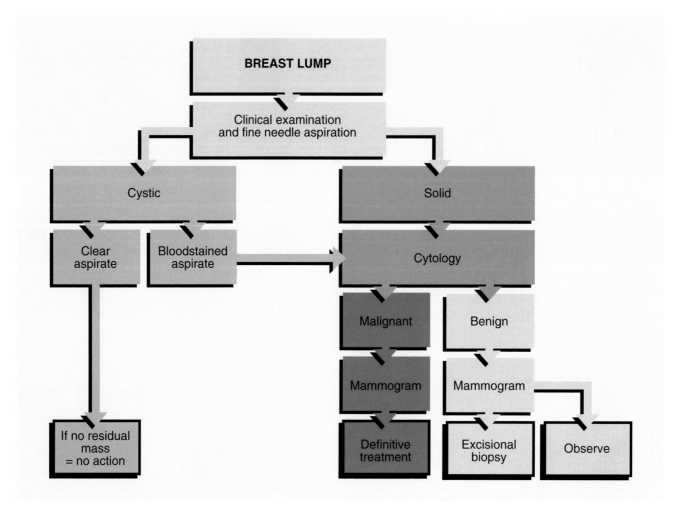

Figure 25.3 Investigation of a breast lump.

benign nature of the disease. Cyst fluid does not usually need to be sent for cytological examination. The presence of a residual lump after cyst aspiration, bloody aspirate, or recurrence of the cyst could mean that there is an associated malignancy, and excision biopsy is recommended. Some radiologists prefer that cysts are not aspirated before breast imaging as the images may be distorted, making exclusion of carcinoma more difficult.

Solid lesions

The solid nature of a breast lump may only become apparent when attempting aspiration. If no fluid is obtained, then FNA specimens should be obtained for cytology. Local routines vary, but standard techniques should be used to obtain the specimens and prepare and fix the slides. Cells viewed in this way allow the pathologist to comment on their cytological morphology (Fig. 25.4) and to give an opinion as to their nature.

Several grades are recognized, as follows:

◆ C0: an acellular sample of no diagnostic value;

◆ C1: inadequate material for diagnosis, usually because only blood or stromal cells are seen;

◆ C2: normal;

◆ C3: atypical, probably benign;

◆ C4: atypical, possibly malignant;

◆ C5: definitely malignant.

It is worth repeating the aspiration if any result except benign (C2) or malignant (C5) is obtained, or if the cytology does not correspond with the clinical impression. A pathologist may even be able to specify the type of lesion from the cytological appearance of the aspirate, for example a fibroadenoma.

The need to biopsy the affected area is determined by the cytological assessment. If cells are reported as definitely malignant then no inference can be made as to whether this represents a carcinoma in situ or an invasive tumour. This can only be differentiated by obtaining a tissue specimen by core biopsy or by excision.

3.2 Core-cut or Trucut® biopsy

This is usually done under local anaesthesia. Core biopsy specimens provide more diagnostic material than FNA specimens and retain the tissue architecture. This allows the pathologist to differentiate between in situ and invasive cancer.

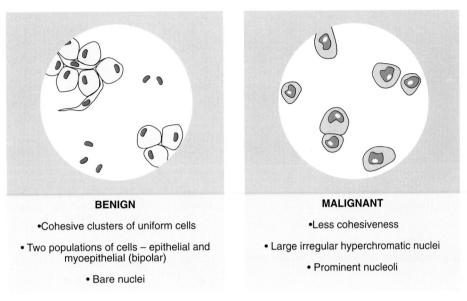

BENIGN

•Cohesive clusters of uniform cells

• Two populations of cells – epithelial and myoepithelial (bipolar)

• Bare nuclei

MALIGNANT

•Less cohesiveness

• Large irregular hyperchromatic nuclei

• Prominent nucleoli

Figure 25.4 Cytological findings in benign and malignant breast disease.

3.3 Mammography

Soft-tissue X-ray films of the breasts allow assessment of the structure and orientation of the fibroglandular element of the breasts. The young breast is dense and the contrast between fat and glandular tissue is less obvious because most of the breast tissue is glandular. This increased density makes it more difficult for abnormalities to be seen. Mammography is regarded as most suitable for imaging the breast undergoing involutionary change where the relative fat content is increased. Mammography should normally be restricted to patients older than 40 except where a palpable lesion is present.

3.4 Ultrasonography

This is not reliable enough to use as a screening test but is useful to determine whether a palpable lump is solid or cystic, and to look for other lumps in young breasts. Many breast clinics now have an ultrasound machine in the clinic with which the surgeon can accurately locate a lump and aspirate it under ultrasound guidance.

4 Treatment aims in breast disease

4.1 Benign breast disease

Anomalies of normal development and involution (ANDI)

This classification is a framework upon which to build a picture of benign breast disease which encompasses most benign conditions (Fig. 25.5). It allows a clearer understanding of

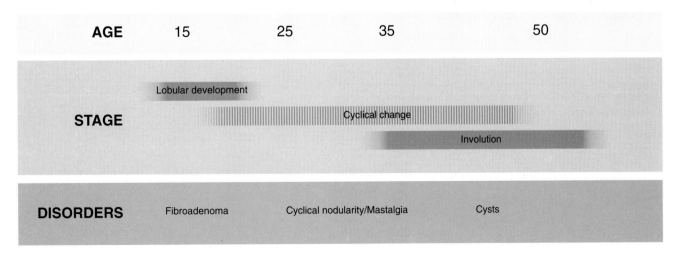

Figure 25.5 Abnormalities of normal involution and development (the ANDI concept).

benign disorders by placing them on a spectrum from 'normal' to pathological. Treatment is directed only towards those that are pathological.

Fibroadenoma

This benign lump, usually found in young women, requires no treatment if the patient is aged under 30 and the lesion is small, asymptomatic, and not enlarging rapidly. Many fibroadenomas disappear without treatment over a few years. If, however, the patient is over 30, the lump causes symptoms, or the patient requests removal, excision biopsy should be performed.

Breast lumpiness and tenderness

This is a common complaint and in patients younger than 40 is virtually always due to benign breast disease. The pain and discomfort is more often positioned in the upper outer quadrant of the breast and can be associated with thickening of the breast tissue in this area. The cause of the problem is not well understood but is regarded as 'hormonal' in aetiology. The symptoms are often cyclical and are worse just prior to menstruation. Non-cyclical breast pain also occurs, most commonly around the menopause, presumably because cycles are less regular. The most important aspect of treatment is to ensure that the problem is benign. 'Triple assessment', which involves clinical examination, imaging with ultrasound or mammography or both, and fine-needle aspiration cytology of any lesions detected, serves to reassure patient and surgeon. If all three show that the condition is benign, there is no need for open biopsy. Treatment of unequivocal benign breast disease is largely symptomatic (Table 25.2).

Breast cysts

Cysts are virtually all associated with other benign disease within the same spectrum elsewhere in the breast. For example, multiple cysts of varying sizes are invariably detectable on ultrasonography. Symptomatic cysts are treated by needle aspiration and patients should be reviewed at about 6 weeks to ensure that the cyst has not recurred.

Scheme for management of a breast cyst

1. Aspirate the cyst. Some units prefer this to be performed during ultrasound imaging. Excision biopsy is not needed if the lump disappears completely and there is no blood in the aspirate.

Table 25.2 Treatments for breast tenderness

Reassurance
Advice regarding a well-fitting bra
Oil of evening primrose
Change of oral contraceptive or HRT
Danazol (androgenic side-effects are frequent)
Tamoxifen
Experimental treatment such as Zoladex®, Restandol®, hypnotherapy

2. If aspirated before imaging in a women over 50, arrange for mammography and breast ultrasound to check the remaining breast architecture.

3. Reassess after 6 weeks. If there are no worrying features, a second aspiration may be performed using the same criteria. Excision is advised if the cyst has recurred once or twice.

Nipple discharge

This may be the only symptom but it is important to assess the breasts for any underlying lesion such as a palpable breast lump or a mammographic abnormality. If an underlying lesion is found, it is sensible to concentrate on the breast lesion and the nipple discharge becomes of secondary importance. If the nipple discharge is the only symptom and the breast is judged to be otherwise normal, then a nipple discharge can be dealt with as shown in Fig. 25.6.

The inverted nipple of late onset

This has been included as a benign problem but the most serious cause is an underlying carcinoma which draws the nipple inwards. If this proves to be the case, then it is managed in the same way as other malignant breast lesions.

The alternative diagnosis is **mammary duct ectasia**—a condition characterized by chronic duct dilatation and fibrosis. It is most commonly seen in women in their 40s and 50s and causes a slit-like inversion of the nipple (as opposed to the indrawing of carcinoma). A related condition is **periductal mastitis**—subareolar chronic inflammation and infection. This is seen in a somewhat younger age group. The consequences of these conditions include:

- subareolar abscess or mammillary fistula, most common in periductal mastitis;

- inverted nipple and nipple discharge, most common in duct ectasia.

Clinical assessment of the breast and mammography should allow an accurate clinical diagnosis to be made. Smoking is common in women with these conditions and may be contributory. No active treatment is usually required for duct ectasia apart from advice about giving up smoking. The chronic inflammation associated with periductal mastitis sometimes needs surgery. If so, it is important that this is satisfactorily performed in the first instance or the problem will recur.

Surgical management of ductal complications

Subareolar abscess

This presents urgently and usually requires prompt surgical drainage. If seen in the phase of periareolar inflammation without pus formation, antibiotics can be used. Organisms are frequently sensitive to metronidazole.

Mammillary fistula

Subareolar excision of the breast duct system is needed.

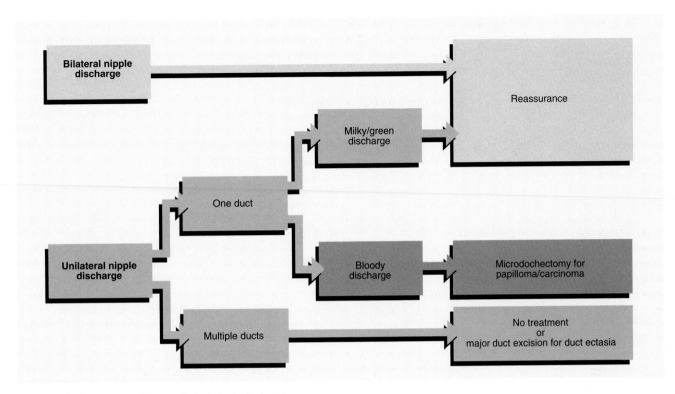

Figure 25.6 Management of uncomplicated nipple discharge.

Inverted nipple

This is a difficult condition to treat and there is a likelihood of recurrence. Congenitally inverted nipples may be everted by division of the underlying ducts, but breast feeding becomes impossible.

Skin changes in the nipple and areola

The usual cause of this is Paget's disease and it is important to search for an underlying neoplasm which should either be palpable or visible on mammography. Scrapings from the eczematous area can be examined cytologically or incision biopsy performed. In either case, characteristic giant Paget's cells should be detectable. If malignancy is excluded, a diagnosis of nipple eczema can be made and treated with local corticosteroids.

Congenital breast diseases

Accessory nipples with or without breast tissue are common and are usually found along the 'milk-line'. Accessory breast tissue may undergo hypertrophy during pregnancy and may even lactate. Extreme differences in the size of the breasts may also occur. Breasts are rarely completely symmetrical so perceived problems may range from a small difference within the normal range to Poland's syndrome, where one breast is absent entirely.

Pregnancy-related breast disorders

Lactational mastitis with formation of breast abscesses is usually due to infection by skin flora via cracked nipples. Abscesses require early surgical incision and drainage to avoid destruction of breast tissue. An important role of the midwife and health visitor is preventing these and other breast problems during lactation. Milk-filled cysts or **galactocoeles**, may form in the lactating breast and require only aspiration. Incision is unwise and may lead to a milk fistula.

Patients at high risk of breast cancer

Certain types of benign breast disease have an increased likelihood of developing malignant breast lesions. An increasing number of patients with benign breast disease are managed without resort to open biopsy. As a result, some predisposed to malignancy inevitably fail to be identified by the usual combination of mammography and FNAC. However, in cases where formal histology is obtained and reported as benign, surgeons need to be aware of the relative risk of future malignancy in various diagnoses. These are listed in Table 25.3.

A family history of breast cancer may be an important risk factor, particularly if one or more first-degree relatives has had the disease under the age of 40 or has had bilateral breast cancer. About 5 per cent of women with breast cancer have a genetic predisposition to the disease, and we are now able to identify 'breast cancer genes'. The BRCA1 gene on the 17q chromosome has been clearly identified and about 80 per cent of women with this gene will develop breast cancer by the age of 70. There is also a familial association with ovarian cancer. Other genetic abnormalities are also recognized as being associated with breast cancer, for example the TP53 gene.

Table 25.3 Relative risk of malignancy associated with benign and borderline pathological entities

Non-proliferative lesions, no increased risk	Cysts Apocrine metaplasia Duct ectasia Mild ductal epithelial hyperplasia Benign calcifications Fibroadenoma Harmartoma
Proliferative lesions without atypia with no increased risk	Sclerosing adenosis Single intraduct papilloma
Proliferative lesions without atypia, with increased risk of carcinoma in up to 1:3	Multiple intraduct papillomas
Atypical proliferative lesions (with some but not all the features of carcinoma in situ), at least fourfold increase in the risk of invasive breast cancer in the future	Atypical lobular hyperplasia Atypical ductal hyperplasia: 10–15% develop invasive cancer within 10–15 years

High-risk benign disease and a family history of breast cancer have an additive effect on increasing risk.

4.2 Prevention of breast cancer

A number of trials are under way looking at chemoprevention of breast cancer using tamoxifen or retinoids. In the UK, women who have a strong family history of breast cancer or who have a high-risk benign or borderline lesion (including atypical hyperplasia and lobular carcinoma in situ) are eligible. Some women with a very strong family history of breast cancer seek secure preventative treatment and may be considered for prophylactic mastectomies. No other 'lifestyle' preventative measures have been shown to be beneficial.

4.3 Non-invasive breast malignancy: carcinoma in situ

Distinguishing between small areas of pre-invasive cancer and hyperplastic but benign breast tissue is often difficult on histological analysis. However, the entity of pre-invasive carcinoma is clearly recognized and is found with increasing frequency as a result of the National Breast Screening Programme. In this, up to 20 per cent of newly detected cancers are pre-invasive. Most of these are ductal carcinoma in situ (DCIS). Lobular carcinoma in situ (LCIS) is usually a chance finding at biopsy, representing less than 1 per cent of cancers. DCIS occasionally presents symptomatically with a lump, nipple discharge, or in association with Paget's disease, but most are found on mammographic screening or in tissue adjoining an excised invasive breast cancer. Up to half of DCIS lesions can be expected to progress to invasive cancer without treatment; however, adequate treatment can provide cure in 98 per cent of cases. For those with extensive disease, this is likely to mean mastectomy, and the role of adjuvant tamoxifen and radiotherapy is still under debate. Axillary surgery is not indicated when invasive cancer is not detected. Lobular carcinoma in situ is almost always asymptomatic and is often bilateral. It has a lower risk of future invasive cancer than DCIS and treatment tends to be less radical. Fifteen to 20 per cent of affected women go on to develop carcinoma in one or the other breast. Currently, treatment is most often watchful waiting but some patients may wish to be considered for prophylactic bilateral mastectomies. LCIS patients are also eligible for chemoprevention studies in breast cancer.

5 Screening for breast cancer: the practical approach

See Chapter 1 for further details.

5.1 Introduction

The aim of screening for breast cancer is to reduce cause-specific mortality and morbidity from the disease. An incidental benefit is that detecting breast cancers when they are smaller allows more women the opportunity of conservative surgery. Whatever the benefits of the screening programme in 'curing' or preventing breast cancer and in prolonging the lives of sufferers, immense fringe benefits have accrued from the widespread introduction of integrated breast cancer units. The overall quality of management of the 'worried well' as well as the diagnosis and treatment of early and symptomatic breast cancers has improved out of all recognition in recent years in UK as a result.

5.2 The screening method

Screening has been targeted at women between the ages of 50 and 64. Women younger than 50 are not screened because there is as yet little statistical proof that improvement in mortality can be achieved. The cost-benefits of screening women over the age of 64 are not optimal and thus this is not routinely undertaken.

The recommended method of screening is to ask women to attend at 3-yearly intervals for a 'single' view mammogram. Recent studies have shown an advantage of screening with both an oblique and cranio-caudal view and this is likely to become the norm. There is uncertainty whether a 3-year interval between screens is sufficiently frequent as there is an increase in **interval cancers** appearing between 2 and 3 years after screening. This suggests that screening should be increased to every 2 years. In the second screening round, it has been found that the type of cancer detected is likely to be the more aggressive in its behaviour.

5.3 Maintaining a high standard of care in the screening unit

The chief problem associated with screening for breast cancer is the anxiety which is induced whenever an abnormality is detected. This can be limited in two ways: first the accuracy of mammographic interpretation should be high, ensuring that all cancers are spotted (high specificity) but the number of doubtful lesions requiring further investigation is minimized (high sensitivity). An acceptable benign to malignant biopsy rate is less than 1.5 : 1 and the minimum accepted detection rate of cancers should be 5 per 1000 people screened (Table 25.4). Secondly, when an abnormality is seen, advice and treatment must follow quickly (Table 25.5). This requires a well-organized unit with staff dedicated to providing expertise in patient support, radiology, cytological interpretation, and surgical treatment. The team approach is an important ingredient in the success and popularity of a unit.

The risk of inducing carcinogenesis by mammography has been calculated as one chance per million mammograms performed.

Types of lesion detected

Mammography

- **Microcalcifications**: not all are malignant, but the following features are suggestive of cancer:

  (a) clusters of more than five microcalcifications;

  (b) morphology suggestive of a ductal distribution, i.e. longitudinal and branched;

  (c) fine rather than course;

Table 25.5 Management of mammographic screening-detected abnormalities

Stage 1	Mammographic screening of women between the ages of 50 and 64
Stage 2	Recall of patients with mammographic abnormalities. 7% of women have some abnormality on a one-view mammographic screen
Stage 3	Further radiological views of abnormal areas; may include magnified views
Stage 4	FNAC of impalpable lesions and rapid cytological opinion. About 1% need FNAC and half of these need localization and surgery, approximately 6:1000 screened
Stage 5	Immediate referral for surgery if appropriate. If cytology is benign, but clinical or radiological suspicion remains, excision biopsy is advised
Stage 6	Stereotactic localization of the abnormality and surgical removal of the marked lesion, with 1–2 cm of surrounding breast tissue. Specimen X-rayed to ensure that the radiological abnormality has been removed

  (d) wide variation in shape (polymorphism);

  (e) increased calcification when compared with a previous mammogram.

- **Parenchymal disturbances**: these can be round, smooth lesions if benign, or stellate lesions, usually with an irregular border, suggesting carcinoma.

- **A mixture of the two.**

Histopathology

Lesions removed may be of four types:

(1) benign;

(2) atypical cells but benign—atypical hyperplasia;

(3) carcinoma in situ (CIS);

(4) invasive carcinoma.

5.4 Management of the screen-detected lesion

Cytological (FNAC) or histological diagnosis of the lesion (using a core-cut needle) is desirable before surgery is planned. This

Table 25.4 Standards set and achievements of the UK National Breast Screening Programme

Criterion	Required standard	Result achieved by 1995
Attendance rate	>70% of those invited	71.5%
Recall rate for further investigation	<10%	7.1%
Biopsy rate	<1.5%	1%
Cancer detection rate	>5/1000 screened	6.3/1000 screened
Benign/malignant ratio	<1.5 : 1	0.61 : 1
Cancers >1 cm	>20%	20.9%

allows the patient to be prepared for the appropriate treatment and helps the surgeon to plan the best operation. In many cases a screen-detected lesion is palpable. However, if it is not, the lesion must be localized prior to excision. The preferred method is under mammographic control, passing a hooked wire into the area of the abnormality via a needle held perpendicular to the skin surface. The patient is taken to the operating theatre soon afterwards for excision of the area around the end of the wire. Finally, the specimen is X-rayed before the patient is woken up to ensure that the lesion has been properly removed.

Carcinoma in situ

About 17 per cent of screen-detected lesions are found to be ductal carcinoma in situ. In contrast, only about 4 per cent of symptomatic breast lumps are in situ cancer. The clinical significance of DCIS is that it indicates breast tissue at risk of becoming invasive carcinoma. Without treatment, the incidence of progression to invasive carcinoma within 20 years is 30–50 per cent. With carcinoma in situ, the clinical questions that need to be answered are:

- What treatment offers the best chance of preventing future development of invasive carcinoma?

- If local treatment is used, should this be bilateral? (Particularly important in the case of LCIS.)

- What is the best method of surveillance in patients known to be at risk?

The answers to these questions are not entirely known and clinical trials are currently addressing them. Mastectomy is accepted as appropriate for most cases with widespread DCIS and offers an almost 100 per cent cure. If it appears radiologically that DCIS is confined to a small area of the breast, conservative surgery may be curative, although it must be ensured that the margins are histologically clear after excision. Provided there is no invasive component to the disease, there is no indication for treatment of the axilla.

Radiotherapy may reduce the 5 per cent recurrence rate after local excision of DCIS but its role in pre-invasive carcinoma in general is still uncertain. Tamoxifen is also of unproven benefit in DCIS, but it is thought to be protective against recurrences and reduces the incidence of new lesions in the contralateral breast. It is somewhat paradoxical that patients with small invasive carcinomas are usually considered for breast-conserving surgery whereas those with pre-malignant lesions, many of which are unlikely to become symptomatic in the patient's lifetime, are asked to consider total mastectomy. However, until better treatments are developed, this remains the recommended course of action.

Invasive carcinoma

Some screen-detected cancers are likely to be the earliest invasive cancers one sees in clinical practice. If prognosis is directly related to the size of the lesion (and this is generally true, but by no means absolute), lesions less than 1 cm in diameter detected on screening should have a particularly good prognosis. The principles of management are similar to those used for symptomatic 'early' breast cancer except when the surrounding breast tissue is replaced by areas of carcinoma in situ. In these circumstances, mastectomy may be the best treatment to enhance local control and minimize recurrence.

6 Primary symptomatic malignant breast disease

6.1 Introduction

Breast cancer is a common malignancy. One woman in 12 will develop the disease and about half of these will die from it. Despite its high incidence, there is still controversy over the optimum method of treating the disease in an individual. However, an increasing fund of experimental and laboratory data is being put into practice in large clinical trials. Meta-analysis of these trials allows reasonably accurate predictions of outcome of the treatments available for breast cancer in patients with different prognostic indicators. It is important to understand the basis on which treatment decisions are made; these are discussed below.

Treatment can be considered under the heading of local therapies, which include surgery and radiotherapy, and systemic treatment aimed at eliminating micrometastases or controlling overt metastases. Wherever possible, treatment aims to eradicate the disease and effect a 'cure'. In order to achieve this, it is usually necessary to treat the breast and also to give systemic therapy. There are two prerequisites in predicting whether cure is likely:

1. Staging: the degree of tumour spread needs to be known (i.e. whether the disease is localized to the breast, involves lymph nodes, or has spread systemically).

2. Therapy: there has to be treatment available which is effective against disease in these sites.

The relative lack of improvement in the results of treatment for breast cancer despite enormous research and clinical efforts is because current treatments probably have little influence on the biological behaviour of breast cancer once it has become invasive. We cannot reliably determine the degree of spread, particularly of micrometastases, and treatment against systemic disease may slow the process but probably never cures it.

However, treatment is worthwhile provided the aims are realistic and if it is tailored to the individual. To understand the principles of treatment and to facilitate a logical approach, it is necessary to understand the broad concepts of the biological behaviour of cancers and to be aware of the indices of tumour activity employed to predict the likelihood of tumour spread and the rate of progression—the **prognostic indicators**.

6.2 Biological activity of breast cancer

Introduction

All malignancies are characterized by the potential to invade local tissues, spread to regional lymph nodes, and to spread sys-

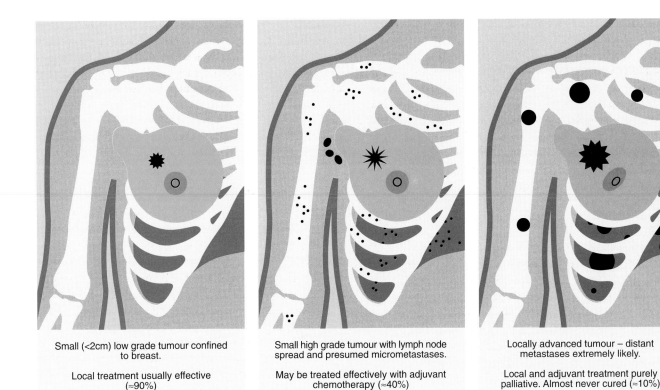

| Small (<2cm) low grade tumour confined to breast. | Small high grade tumour with lymph node spread and presumed micrometastases. | Locally advanced tumour – distant metastases extremely likely. |

Small (<2cm) low grade tumour confined to breast.

Local treatment usually effective (≈90%)

Small high grade tumour with lymph node spread and presumed micrometastases.

May be treated effectively with adjuvant chemotherapy (≈40%)

Locally advanced tumour – distant metastases extremely likely.

Local and adjuvant treatment purely palliative. Almost never cured (≈10%)

Figure 25.7 The biological behaviour of breast cancers.

temically, for example, by vascular invasion. In clinical practice, it is difficult to assess the degree of spread reliably, in the knowledge that some cancers remain localized while others spread systemically early in their growth cycle. The clinical implication is that patients with disease that remains localized will not die from it and can be treated adequately by local treatment alone. Unfortunately, the proportion of cases with disease limited to the breast is very small and problems arising from systemic spread can be anticipated in a large proportion of women with the disease. The tumour biology may be illustrated by a number of possible scenarios (Fig. 25.7).

Clinical types of breast cancer

1. Potentially curable 'early' breast cancer. Patients with small tumours (less than 2 cm diameter) confined to the breast with no regional or distant metastases, particularly tumours of 'special histological type', for example **tubular carcinomas**. This group of patients is expected to have a survival similar to women without breast cancer and may be cured by local treatment alone. Unfortunately, about one-third of patients who appear to fall into this group at presentation subsequently develop metastases.

2. Patients with 'early' breast cancer who initially appeared to have localized disease but who subsequently develop distant metastases. It can be inferred that patients in this group already have micrometastases at their original presentation which are clinically and radiologically undetectable. The most

reliable prognostic indicator of this scenario is involvement of axillary lymph nodes at diagnosis.

3. Patients with a primary breast lesion and clinical evidence of metastatic disease (e.g. in the liver, lung, or bone). These patients are incurable by local treatment and systemic treatment and generally have a very poor prognosis with 5-year survival between 15 and 25 per cent.

Early and late breast cancer

The term 'early breast cancer' describes disease which is apparently confined to the breast (without involvement of local lymph nodes) and which is technically resectable. The disease is described as advanced or late if there are signs of local invasion of the skin or chest wall, involvement of local lymph nodes, or evidence of distant spread. However, the term 'early' is not a useful one because of the strong and unpredictable possibility of micrometastases. The presence of involved regional lymph nodes is the most important prognostic indicator that the disease has strong metastatic potential.

6.3 Aims of treatment

Disease in the breast and regional lymph nodes must be eradicated to avoid the unpleasant sequelae of uncontrolled local disease such as ulceration and infection. The treatment methods employed are determined by assessment of the local disease, but decisions on effective local treatment should not be compromised because of detectable systemic disease unless life expectancy is very short.

Management of established systemic disease

Once systemic disease is apparent, all treatment has to be regarded as palliative. Systemic drug therapy is used to treat asymptomatic disease in the usual secondary sites of bone, liver, and lung, with supplementary treatments aimed at specific problems, such as bone pain, pathological fractures, and pleural or peritoneal effusions or cerebral metastases.

The palliative nature of this treatment means that its effectiveness is measured in terms of improving symptoms and quality of life rather than long-term cure.

Decisions regarding the use of adjuvant therapy

The aim of adjuvant therapy in early breast cancer is to eradicate systemic micrometastases or to substantially slow their progress. The effectiveness of such therapy cannot be determined by the response of individual patients because of the inaccuracy of determining which patients have micrometastases. Thus adjuvant regimens have to be assessed in clinical trials. The measurable end points used to assess effectiveness are improvements in mortality rates (overall survival), the lengthening of the 'disease-free' intervals (recurrence-free survival), and maintenance of a good quality of life.

In breast cancer both hormonal and chemotherapy are used as adjuvant therapy. The potential benefits of the treatment have to be measured against possible side-effects and this equation is pivotal when chemotherapy is being considered. As adjuvant therapy has serious side-effects, it is sensible to use it selectively. Attempts have to be made to identify patients most likely to have micrometastases and thus likely to benefit most from chemotherapy. The proportional improvement in survival with adjuvant treatment is similar regardless of the stage of breast cancer, thus, if the patient has an excellent chance of survival without therapy, the added benefit of a toxic adjuvant treatment (chemotherapy) becomes very small and is probably not worthwhile. However, if the adjuvant therapy has a low toxicity (as is the case for tamoxifen) then all patients can be treated irrespective of the likelihood of micrometastases. Figure 25.8 illustrates the relative improvements in outcome of various form of adjuvant therapy.

Evaluating the likelihood of a patient having distant micrometastases

If distant metastases are present at diagnosis, this overrides all other prognostic indices in predicting an adverse outcome. In patients with no evidence of distant metastases, there is no single factor which can reliably predict the likelihood of present or future micrometastases; however, the state of involvement of the axillary lymph nodes and the number of nodes involved is the single most useful predictive factor for long-term survival (Table 25.6). Other putative prognostic indicators are of practical value only in node-negative patients because positivity is such a powerful predictor. Node-negative patients at high risk of recurrence would thus be the preferred group for aggressive chemotherapy. Prognostic indicators are useful if they coherently present either a good prognosis or a bad prognosis, but indicators are often mixed, some adverse and some favourable. In these patients, clinical judgement is required when considering adjuvant therapy. Commonly used prognostic indicators are listed in Table 25.7.

The management of disease in the breast and axilla

If left untreated, a cancer of the breast will enlarge and infiltrate the pectoralis muscle and the overlying skin. At some point it spreads to the regional axillary lymph nodes, which progressively become fixed and later ulcerate the axillary skin. The first duty is to ensure that the patient has the best chance of local control of the disease. There is no single treatment which is suitable for all primary breast cancers, and the multiplicity of treatment regimens can be confusing for the trainee. Information that needs to be collected prior to deciding about definitive local treatment:

1. Obtain a definite tissue diagnosis by cytology or needle biopsy.

2. Decide whether the cancer is 'operable' (i.e. no involvement of significant areas of skin or fixity to chest wall or fixed axillary nodes).

Table 25.7 Indicators of a good prognosis in breast cancer

No involved lymph nodes
Tumour less than 1 cm in diameter
Well-differentiated histology
No vascular or lymphatic invasion

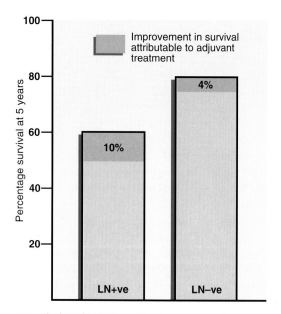

Figure 25.8 The benefit of adjuvant treatment in breast cancer.

Table 25.6 Prognostic indicators in breast cancer

	5-year survival % (disease-free survival %)	10-year survival
Presence of distant metastases[a]	10	0
Involvement of axillary lymph nodes		
Negative	78 (60)	65
1–3 positive	60 (50)	50
4 or more positive	30 (21)	30
5-year probability of tumour recurrence		
Diameter of primary tumour		
Less than 1 cm	6%	
Less than 2 cm	11%	
Histological nuclear grading		
Grade I (well differentiated)	Best	
Grade II (intermediate)	Intermediate	
Grade III (anaplastic)	Worst	
Histology		
• Infiltrating ductal and infiltrating lobular carcinoma have a similar prognosis	5-year recurrence rate 0–20% 10-year recurrence rate 5–25%	
• Special histological types': tubular, colloid, medullary	Prognosis usually much better than ductal or lobular	
• Vascular invasion (usually venous) or lymphatic invasion, often associated with nodal metastases, anaplasia, and other poor prognostic factors	Survival 59% if node negative, 12% if node positive	
Proliferation indices		
Flow cytometry measures how rapidly a tumour is dividing, by measuring: (1) the percentage of cells in the S phase of the DNA replication cycle; and (2) the total amount of extra DNA in the cancer cells (aneuploidy)	High S phase (particularly) and aneuploidy predict short disease-free interval and poor survival	
Hormone receptor status		
Oestrogen receptor (ER) indicates potential response to endocrine therapy; Progesterone receptor (PgR status may predict response better in premenopausal women	if negative, <10% respond; if positive, >60% respond.	
Assessment of oncogenes and tumour suppressor genes, cathepsin-D, growth factors, etc. These are currently experimental	unknown as yet	

[a] If distant metastases are present at diagnosis, this overrides all other prognostic indices. Other prognostic indicators are useful only in node-negative patients.

3. Decide whether conservative surgery is practicable or if mastectomy is needed (Table 25.8). If the tumour is large and widely infiltrating, is primary chemotherapy or radiotherapy desirable to shrink the tumour? Options after this include no surgery, conservative surgery, or mastectomy.

Table 25.8 Indications for mastectomy in operable breast cancer

Diffuse disease of intraductal or invasive type

Multiple primary lesions

Large primary >5 cm in diameter

Cosmetically unacceptable result of local excision

Patient preference

Technical problems with radiotherapy

Recurrence after radiotherapy

Possibly tumours with bad prognostic indicators

4. Discuss treatment options with the patient and obtain her views. Even if conservative surgery is possible, the patient may opt for mastectomy with or without reconstruction.

Obtaining local control of the disease

Local control is achieved if the disease can be eradicated from the breast and local draining lymphatics and lymph nodes. Local control is a goal in all patients with breast cancer, whatever the stage, because without it, uncontrolled local disease will occur and seriously impair the patient's quality of life. Most discussions about treating breast cancer revolve around how local control can best be achieved. For most patients, surgery, with or without local irradiation, is the preferred treatment.

Surgery (Table 25.9) and radiotherapy (Table 25.10) are used individually or in combination in the local control of breast cancer. There are various combinations of treatment, but as a

Table 25.9 Surgical options to obtain local control of breast cancer

Wide local excision (2 cm clearance of the tumour) ± axillary lymph-node dissection

Formal quadrantectomy ± axillary lymph-node dissection

Mastectomy ± axillary lymph-node dissection

There is no longer a case for radical mastectomy with resection of chest wall muscles unless these are involved and cannot be treated adequately with radiotherapy.

Table 25.10 Radiotherapy to obtain local control of breast cancer

Irradiation to the chest wall and remaining breast tissue, PLUS

Irradiation to axillary lymph nodes if not removed surgically[a]

'Top-up' dose of irradiation to the site of the primary tumour (external beam or radioactive needles, e.g. iridium)

[a] There is rarely a case for surgical excision of lymph nodes plus radiotherapy to the axilla because of the high incidence of side-effects, including lymphoedema and brachial plexus neuralgia.

general principle, the more extensive the local surgery the less the need for additional radiotherapy. However, in most cases, wide local excision or quadrantectomy alone is insufficient treatment for this disease because of an unacceptable rate of local recurrence.

It is important to choose treatment combinations that allow the chest wall and axilla to receive sufficient treatment to minimize recurrence but not so much as to cause the fibrotic and necrotic sequelae of overtreatment, such as rib necrosis, lung fibrosis and, possibly, coronary heart disease.

6.4 Practical aspects of surgery for breast cancer

Position on the table

The patient should lie supine on the operating table with the arm on the affected side abducted to 90°. The arm can be secured in position if the breast alone is to be operated upon. For axillary dissection, the breast and lateral chest wall should be prepared as far as the posterior axillary line and the arm draped so it can be moved during the course of the procedure to facilitate the dissection.

Treatment of the breast tumour

Wide local excision or quadrantectomy

The aim is to remove the entire tumour with a margin of normal breast tissue. Contraindications to this choice of treatment are large tumours involving more than one quadrant of the breast and smaller tumours which are situated centrally and where adequate surgery would leave a cosmetically unacceptable result.

Conservative surgery followed by radiotherapy has a slightly greater risk of local recurrence than mastectomy but broadly similar results in terms of overall survival.

Table 25.11 Levels of axillary dissection

Level I: low axilla, up to the lateral border of pectoralis minor

Level II: mid axilla, deep to pectoralis minor up to the interpectoral (Ritter's) node

Level III: apical axilla, medial to pectoralis minor, including infraclavicular area

Mastectomy

The chief advantage of mastectomy is that it usually avoids the need for radiotherapy.

Management of the axilla

Information about whether the axillary lymph nodes are involved with tumour is valuable in determining the prognosis and to help decide whether adjuvant therapy should be employed. This can be obtained only by surgical dissection. The surgeon needs to decide whether to sample the nodes or to perform a diagnostic and therapeutic clearance. Three levels of clearance are recognized: for this purpose the axilla is divided into three levels in relation to the lower and upper borders of pectoralis minor muscle (Table 25.11).

Surgery to the axilla

Node sampling

Removal of nodes from the axillary tail and lower part of the axilla (level I) provides histological information on the state of these nodes, but the amount of axilla cleared is too small to be regarded as therapeutic. Its only use is for staging the disease. However, up to 25 per cent of cases will have false-negative results because nodes in the upper part of the axilla occasionally contain tumour without involving the lower nodes. Many now regard node sampling as inadequate.

Axillary clearance

Axillary clearance is an integral part of the radical and Patey-type mastectomies and is usually combined with wide local excision of breast carcinoma. Surgical dissection of the axilla should never be combined with radical axillary radiotherapy because this combination results in the highest incidence of brachial plexus complications and lymphoedema.

Should every patient with breast cancer have an axillary dissection?

The aims of axillary dissection are for diagnosis (to determine axillary lymph-node involvement to prognosticate and to aid decisions about adjuvant therapy) and therapy (an alternative therapy to axillary radiotherapy).

Ideally, all patients with local breast cancer should have an axillary dissection, at least for statistical purposes of response to treatment. In practice, sensible compromises can often be made without it. If chemotherapy is not to be given because of age or other infirmity whatever the result of node dissection, most surgeons would not dissect the axilla. If the axilla is clinically clear, no treatment is given, and if there is clinical evidence of involvement, axillary radiotherapy is given.

Adjuvant treatment with tamoxifen has minimal side-effects and is now accepted as beneficial in virtually all patients with breast cancer, and its use does not depend on axillary node status. The little that is lost in diagnostic accuracy is gained in reduced morbidity of surgery.

However, in premenopausal women, chemotherapy may be indicated only for node-positive disease and so nodal status needs to be obtained. Axillary clearance is desirable to improve the accuracy of staging and to avoid the need for future irradiation of the axilla.

6.5 Radiotherapy and adjuvant therapy

Radiotherapy in breast cancer

Axillary radiotherapy is technically difficult and carries an increased risk of shoulder stiffness compared with surgical clearance and a similar risk of lymphoedema (less than 2 per cent of cases).

Radiotherapy is used in the primary treatment of breast cancer as follows:

1. For the breast when there is a large tumour infiltrating skin or chest wall (neoadjuvant therapy). Surgery may be performed later.

2. For the breast and chest wall after wide local excision of a primary breast tumour.

3. Some surgeons advocate axillary irradiation following mastectomy if the axillary nodes have been sampled and found to be positive for secondary deposits. In most of these cases, some form of systemic adjuvant therapy is desirable because involved nodes are a marker of systemic micrometastases.

Adjuvant therapy in early breast cancer

As a result of the analysis of huge volumes of data generated from clinical trials in early breast cancer, the benefits of adjuvant systemic therapy are now quantifiable. Most patients are likely to

be offered some form of adjuvant treatment. Tamoxifen is given to most postmenopausal women for 5 years and, more recently, has been offered increasingly to premenopausal women since benefit has been shown to accrue. Combination chemotherapy gives a similar survival advantage but toxic side-effects potentially limit its use to younger women with a poor prognosis, as predicted by their lymph-node status and tumour histology. Improved drugs and systems of delivery have widened the range of patients suitable for chemotherapy but, while modest improvements have been shown for disease-free survival, the ultimate aim of curing metastatic cancer remains elusive. Figure 25.9 illustrates the survival benefits of adjuvant therapy.

7 The management of locally advanced breast cancer

Locally advanced breast cancer has one or more of the following characteristics:

- invasion of overlying skin and/or dermal lymphatics (peau d'orange);

- fixation to the chest wall;

- an inflammatory type of breast cancer;

- involved and fixed axillary lymph nodes.

Any of these findings indicates that the tumour has spread systemically and the eventual prognosis is poor. Local treatments are needed for local control and radiotherapy may be more appropriate than surgery. Local treatments alone are unlikely to be adequate and systemic treatment is required from the start.

7.1 Treatment of symptomatic systemic spread of breast cancer

Patients present with secondary disease at the initial presentation or later following initial treatment. Treatment is essentially similar in either case. The most common sites for

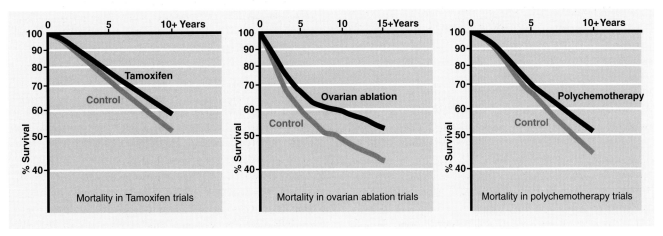

Figure 25.9 Survival graphs with various forms of adjuvant therapy.

metastases are lung, liver, brain (visceral), and bone (osseous). Once the disease has reached this stage all treatment is palliative. Although cure cannot be achieved, it may be possible to give symptomatic relief or even induce remissions of months or years, so all hope should not be abandoned.

Hormonal therapy

The cytokinetics of breast cancer are complex; however, it is known that a proportion of breast cancer cells are dependent on the hormonal environment for their continued growth. Changes in the hormonal environment can cause tumours to regress for a period. Control, however, is only temporary and is eventually followed by relapse in weeks, months, or years. This is probably because breast cancers contain a mixed population of cells, some of which are hormone sensitive. Simplistically, relapse occurs when cells insensitive to the hormone treatment proliferate and cause clinical symptoms. At this point the treatment needs to be stopped and alternatives considered.

In clinical practice, it would be useful to be able to predict the likelihood of a cancer being hormone sensitive. Oestrogen (estrogen) receptors (ERs) and progesterone receptors (PgRs) can both be measured to give some insight into the potential responsiveness of the tumour. However, these tests are not 'all or nothing' and there is a range of receptor concentrations which arise from the differing cell populations within the tumour. Cancers which are strongly ER positive are likely to respond to hormonal therapy, both in the adjuvant setting and in the treatment of metastatic disease. However, even ER-negative tumours have about a 15 per cent response rate. In addition, it should be noted that the ER status of the primary tumour is not always the same as that of the secondary tumour. Thus hormonal receptor studies remain a useful but not essential guide to responsiveness to hormonal therapy.

In practice, osseous metastases are most likely to respond to hormonal manipulation, and visceral deposits sometimes respond to hormonal therapy.

Hormonal manipulation

Drug therapy

As described above, ER status gives some indication of the potential response to hormone therapy. Tamoxifen is effective and has a low morbidity, so this is the usual starting drug. Even if it has already been used as adjuvant treatment, it is worth starting treatment with this provided the cancer did not progress while the patient was on tamoxifen. Tumour response can be inferred from symptomatic improvement, reduction in the size of metastases on X-ray or ultrasound scans, or improved patient well being. Any decision to change hormonal therapy is based on clinical judgement. It is customary to graduate through different preparations, as shown in Table 25.12.

Table 25.12 Hormonal drug therapy for breast cancer treatment

Oestrogen receptor antagonist: tamoxifen
Progestogens: Megace®/Provera®
Aromatase inhibitor, e.g. 4-hydroxyandrostenedione

Endocrine surgery

A surgical approach to modifying the hormonal milieu is rarely employed these days as the available drugs are, for the most part, as effective as any surgical procedure. Before tamoxifen, patients often underwent bilateral oophorectomy and occasionally bilateral adrenalectomy, or even hypophysectomy for systemic spread of breast cancer. Even in their heyday, adrenalectomy and, particularly, hypophysectomy caused severe side-effects for marginal benefit. Nowadays, the gonadotrophin-releasing hormone analogue, goserelin (Zoladex®), is sometimes used to cause reversible ovarian ablation.

Chemotherapy

Palliative chemotherapy is most effective if the treatment modality has not been used before; however, the introduction of new second-line chemotherapeutic agents such as Taxol® may improve results.

Local radiotherapy

This provides excellent palliation for localized painful bony deposits or pathological fractures and is often used.

Treatment of pleural effusions and ascites

These may need intermittent drainage and sometimes chemical or surgical pleurodesis.

Palliative care

The palliative care team provides much needed symptom control in patients with multiple problems associated with advanced disease.

8 Psychological support of patients undergoing breast surgery

Psychological morbidity following breast cancer surgery is common. Many studies have demonstrated that substantial anxiety and depression occur in 20–50 per cent of patients within 1 year of operation. Concerns about prognosis, potentially mutilating surgery, loss of body image, and sexual problems all contribute to this morbidity. The emotional aspects of care are particularly sensitive and it is obligatory to explain exactly what is happening to the patient from the first encounter. There is now more openness about discussing the diagnosis, treatment options, and the prognosis, partly because patients are far more knowledgeable as a result of media publicity. Research has shown that up to one-third of patients want to participate actively in decisions about treatment, and that most benefit from a fully informed discussion. Patients often express preferences for particular forms of treatment, and provided the likely outcome of the patient's preferred treatment as compared with others is made known, it is often possible to accommodate these wishes.

8.1 Breast counselling

Breast-care and counselling nurses are now an integral part of most specialist units and can do much to lessen the impact of the diagnosis and treatment on the patient's psychological well being. There are accumulating data to suggest that an experienced breast-care nurse can significantly reduce psychological morbidity among breast cancer patients. The nurse has many roles to play. By liaising with the clinician at both the initial consultation and preoperative ward round, she is able discuss treatment with the patient and her partner and resolve misunderstandings. The breast nurse can help with physical rehabilitation postoperatively, for example, explaining and fitting prostheses after mastectomy. Most importantly, however, she is a trained ear to whom patients can express their hidden fears and anxieties. She can support the patient and the family through the acute psychological distress associated with diagnosis, surgery, and many forms of adjuvant therapy, particularly chemotherapy. Thereafter she is available to support patients long after they have left hospital. A contact telephone number is usually provided for patients to call at almost any time. In addition, the breast-care nurse is able to provide continuity when the patient returns for outpatient review, often to be seen by different clinicians.

However, the clinician's role is also important. Team work, involving the surgeon, oncologist, breast-care nurse, and ward nurses, is crucial to avoid giving confusing or potentially misleading information to patients.

Most women are distraught and fear the worst when they discover a breast lump. The anxiety is compounded by any delay, and efforts should be made to see patients with breast lumps at the earliest available outpatient clinic.

Uncertainty increases psychological morbidity and the first consultation with the clinician must be informative. This means it should be conducted in a manner which the patient (and her partner) can understand. If the clinician thinks the lump is likely to be malignant, then the patient should be informed. Many patients are less anxious after being told they have cancer, as some of the uncertainty is over, despite their worst fear being realized. Positive factors such as the smallness of the tumour should be emphasized, but false reassurances should be avoided.

Increasingly, specialist breast clinics have immediate access to mammography and fine-needle aspiration cytology, and rapid diagnosis increases the accuracy of information given to the patient at the first consultation. However, breast cancer is only one of the serious diagnoses doctors are required to treat, and equitable provision of care should not be forgotten in achieving excellence in this one field.

Once the diagnosis has been made, the clinician should give the patient and partner an outline of the intended surgical procedure and be available to answer questions about subsequent treatment. The period between outpatient consultation and admission for surgery should be minimized if practicable, as delay increases anxiety levels, even though it has little impact on outcome.

In the clinic and at the preoperative ward round, adequate time should be set aside to explain the surgical procedure, and the patient should be allowed to express her own wishes and concerns. In many instances, the discussion focuses on the choice between mastectomy or lumpectomy. The patient should never go to the operating theatre without a clear impression of what is going to happen.

Most patients will be discharged from hospital before histology results are available, and should therefore be reviewed as soon as possible to avoid further uncertainty. Many patients already know that axillary lymph node involvement has implications for prognosis and further treatment. The postoperative consultation should be honest and informative, outlining the nature and reasoning behind any additional treatment suggested. If the patient is to be recruited into a clinical trial of adjuvant therapy, this has to be adequately explained. The opportunity should be taken to emphasize positive factors, such as completeness of surgical excision or favourable nodal status.

8.2 Maintaining the body image after breast surgery

The absence of a breast carries a double burden: it is a constant reminder of the disease as well as a major disfigurement. Attempts to compensate for mastectomy have always formed part of the treatment scheme in malignant breast disease. The move towards more limited surgery was partly stimulated by realization of the adverse psychological effects mastectomy can produce. Despite this, one-third of patients suffer from serious depression and/or anxiety for months or years following the treatment of breast carcinoma, irrespective of the extent of the surgery.

If a patient is planned to undergo mastectomy, she should at least be offered the option of an external prosthesis and may be considered for breast reconstruction.

Mastectomy prostheses

Immediately after surgery, a temporary prosthesis consisting of a lightweight foam- or fibre-filled pad covered with cotton to fit within the bra can be employed before discharge from hospital. This is unsuitable for the rigours of everyday life and needs to be replaced later by a permanent prosthesis. The lightweight prosthesis can be retained for nightwear.

Silicone prostheses are covered with a waterproof polyurethane skin and can even be used with swimwear. The permanent prosthesis is usually fitted 6 weeks or so after surgery, allowing time for the wound to settle. The fitter should be experienced in selecting the correct shape and size, because a badly fitted prosthesis is worse than none.

Breast reconstruction

Most woman who have undergone mastectomy can potentially be offered breast reconstruction. Even if the prognosis is relatively poor, reconstruction may be a valuable part of improving the patient's quality of life. This type of surgery is increasingly being offered by the trained breast surgeon or is performed in partnership with a plastic surgeon. Breast reconstruction may be done immediately or delayed until treatment is complete and the patient has had a chance to come to terms with her altered body image.

Silicone implants

Placing a subpectoral silicone prosthesis is the easiest form of breast reconstruction. Following a total mastectomy, the prosthesis needs to be placed deep to the pectoral muscles. The prosthesis can be made of silicone gel, an inflatable silicone envelope filled with saline, or a combination prosthesis with a centre of gel surrounded by a saline-filled envelope. The pectoral muscles and chest wall skin may need to be expanded to allow a prosthesis to be fitted to match the opposite breast. Pre-implant tissue expanders consist of a saline-filled bag which is gradually increased in volume by incremental saline injections. This is later replaced by a permanent silicone prosthesis. Alternatively, a combined tissue expander and prosthesis of the Becker type can be employed.

The expander is placed beneath the pectoralis major muscle. The muscle is first split along its length to create a cavity in which to implant the device. Contraindications to reconstruction by tissue expansion include chest wall irradiation, where there will be considerable fibrosis of the tissues. In addition, it is difficult to produce a large 'breast' mass by tissue expansion.

Complications of implant insertion include:

◆ Capsular contraction is the most common complication. Contraction of a fibrous sheath which forms around the implant leads to distortion of the reconstructed breast and often causes discomfort. In general, it appears to be less of a problem with the newer, textured prosthesis than with the original smooth implants.

◆ Implant rupture may lead to leakage of silicone gel, and this can cause diagnostic difficulties as to the nature of breast lumps around a prosthesis. More recently there has been concern regarding the carcinogenic potential of silicone in the breast, but there is no strong evidence to support this. Overall, rupture affects approximately 1 per cent of all prostheses.

◆ Infection is a disaster which almost always necessitates removing the prosthesis. For this reason, prophylactic antibiotics are indicated at the time of reconstruction.

Myocutaneous flaps

The principle of a myocutaneous flap (e.g. latissimus dorsi or transverse rectus abdominis muscle (TRAM); Fig. 25.10) is to transfer a segment of muscle with its overlying skin to the mastectomy site. It allows compensation for removal of a large breast or even part of the chest wall. A myocutaneous flap is also required in circumstances where reconstruction by tissue expansion is not feasible; for example, where the chest wall skin is tight, scarred, or damaged by radiation therapy, or in instances where the pectoral muscles have been removed. The latissimus dorsi flap requires a prosthesis to be placed under the muscle to equalize the breast sizes (Fig. 25.10). The muscle is detached from its origin and rotated on its insertion along with the overlying skin. Blood supply comes from the thoracodorsal pedicle, which must be carefully preserved. Alternatively, a transverse rectus abdominis myocutaneous (TRAM) flap can provide sufficient tissue such that an implant is not required. The flap can either be rotated on the superior epigastric vessels or anastomosed as a free flap using microvascular techniques. A TRAM flap has the advantage that it produces the most normal-looking and -feeling breast.

The most commonly encountered problem with this form of reconstruction is flap necrosis and the highest incidence of failure occurs with rotated TRAM flaps. Other complications include abdominal wall hernias owing to removal of the rectus abdominis muscle.

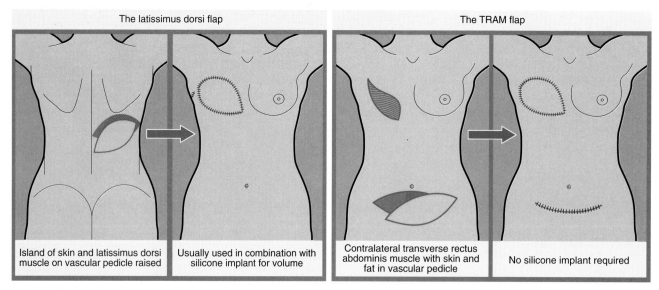

The latissimus dorsi flap		The TRAM flap	
Island of skin and latissimus dorsi muscle on vascular pedicle raised	Usually used in combination with silicone implant for volume	Contralateral transverse rectus abdominis muscle with skin and fat in vascular pedicle	No silicone implant required

Figure 25.10 Latissimus dorsi and TRAM flap reconstruction after mastectomy.

Nipple and areola reconstruction

The nipple and areola can be reconstructed from skin taken from the opposite nipple, the labia, or the inner aspect of the thigh. Most plastic surgeons prefer to leave this until after the breast reconstruction and any contralateral surgery has healed, to enable symmetrical positioning of the 'new' nipple and areola. Tattooing the areola afterwards may improve its cosmetic appearance. Commercially produced 'false' nipples are also available.

The opposite breast

In some patients there is a need to alter the contralateral breast to obtain a better match with the reconstructed side. Procedures such as reduction mammoplasty or breast elevation may be necessary. Conversely, it may be necessary to consider augmentation mammoplasty in a patient with small breasts to match the reconstructed side.

9 Follow-up for treated breast cancer

Excess mortality from breast cancer occurs up to 35 years after diagnosis and some surgeons follow up patients for life. However, most recurrences occur within the first 2 years, with a progressive fall off afterwards thereafter. Thus a reasonable policy might be 3-monthly review up until 2 years and 6-monthly or yearly follow-up to 5 or 10 years.

Recurrence is often difficult to detect, both clinically and radiologically, particularly in an irradiated breast. Thus, detection of recurrence needs to rely on a combination of clinical experience, mammography, and FNAC. Incision biopsy may be needed if the diagnostic problem cannot be resolved in other ways.

9.1 Detecting a second primary in the contralateral breast

The risk of developing a second primary breast cancer is six times greater than for unaffected women and is greatest for women who develop their first cancer under the age of 40. The risk appears to be diminished by about 40 per cent by the use of tamoxifen. The contralateral breast should be subject to regular clinical examination, with mammography annually or 2 yearly.

Bibliography

Barr, L.C. and Baum, M. (1992). Time to abandon TNM staging of breast cancer? *Lancet*, **339**, (9798), 915–17.

Bartelink, H. (1988). Radiotherapy in the management of early breast cancer, a review. *Eur. J. Cancer Clin. Oncol.*, **24**, (1), 77–82.

Dixon, M. and Sainsbury, R. (1993). *Handbook of diseases of the breast*. Churchill Livingstone, London.

Duffy, S.W., Tabor, L., Fagerberg, G. Gad, A., Grontoft, O., Sorth, M.C., Day, N.E. (1991). Breast screening, prognostic factors and survival: results from the Swedish two county study. *B.J. Cancer*, **64**, 1133–8.

Early Breast Cancer Triallists Collaborative Group (1992). Systemic treatment of early breast cancer by hormonal, cytotoxic or immunological therapy. *Lancet*, **339**, 1–15; 71–85.

Fentiman, I.S. (1988). Surgery in the management of early breast cancer, a review. *Eur. J. Cancer Clin. Oncol.*, **24**, (1), 73–6.

Haagenson, C.D. (1986). *Diseases of the breast*, 3rd Ed W.B. Saunders, Philadelphia.

Hortobagyi, G.N. (1992). Overview of new treatments for breast cancer. *Breast Cancer Res. Treat.*, **21**, 3–13.

Muss, H.B. (1992). Endocrine therapy for advanced breast cancer, a review. *Breast Cancer Res. Treat.*, **21**, 15–26.

Rubens, R.D. (1988). Adjuvant systemic treatment for early breast cancer, a review. *Eur. J. Cancer Clin. Oncol.*, **24**, (1), 83–7.

CHAPTER 26

External hernias

M.L. Da Costa and H.P. Redmond

1 Introduction

A hernia is defined as the protrusion of an organ or viscus, or part of one, through a defect in its containing cavity. This definition covers not only the common varieties of hernias (inguinal, femoral, incisional, umbilical), but also herniation of other organs, such as the brain through fascial defects or foramina in the cranium with raised intracranial pressure.

Seventy-five per cent of all hernias are inguinal (50 per cent indirect and 25 per cent direct). Incisional and ventral hernias account for 10 per cent; femoral, 8 per cent; umbilical, 4 per cent; and, finally, the rarer forms, 3 per cent (Table 26.1). Eighty-six per cent of all groin hernias occur in males, but 84 per cent of all femoral hernias occur in females. Despite this, inguinal hernias are still more common than the femoral variety in women.

Table 26.1 Incidence of different types of hernia

Type of hernia	Percentage
Inguinal	75
indirect	50
direct	25
Incisional and ventral	10
Femoral	8
Umbilical	4
Rare (e.g. Spigelian, obturator)	3

2 Anatomy

2.1 Anterior abdominal wall and related structures

The anterior abdominal wall is a muscular, multilaminar, layered structure, comprising skin, fat, fascia, several muscles with their aponeuroses, and peritoneum.

The sheets of muscles sweep round from both sides of the abdomen to meet in the midline at the linea alba. In doing so, the aponeuroses of these muscles form a tough **rectus sheath** which encloses the rectus abdominis muscle.

The external oblique muscle originates from the outer surfaces of the lower eight ribs and the anterior half of the iliac crest. The muscle transforms into an aponeurotic sheet as it approaches the midline and forms the anterior wall of the rectus sheath. Medially, it is attached above to the xiphisternum, along the length of the linea alba in the midline and below to the pubis. There is deficiency in the aponeurosis over the pubic crest, which forms the triangular **superficial inguinal ring**. Through this, the spermatic cord in the male and the round ligament in the female pass out of the inguinal canal. The lower rolled edge of the aponeurosis is free and is attached laterally to the anterior superior iliac spine and medially to the pubic tubercle, to form the inguinal ligament.

The internal oblique muscle originates from the thoraco-lumbar fascia, the anterior two-thirds of the iliac crest, and the lateral two-thirds of the inguinal ligament. It becomes aponeurotic medially and splits to form two leaves of the rectus sheath from the xiphoid process to 2.5 cm below the umbilicus. The two leaves of the aponeurosis from each side meet in the midline to form the **linea alba**. Below the umbilicus, the entire aponeurosis passes anteriorly and, above this point, the transverse free posterior edge is known as the **semicircular fold of Douglas** or the **arcuate ligament**.

The transversus abdominis originates from the lower six costal cartilages, the thoraco-lumbar fascia, the iliac crest, and the lateral one-third of the inguinal ligament. The medial attachments are similar to those of the internal oblique; its aponeurosis passes posteriorly only down to the level of the arcuate ligament, after which it passes entirely anteriorly.

The lowermost fibres of the internal oblique and transversus abdominis fuse together to form the strong, so-called **conjoint tendon** in only 5 per cent of cases. This arches over the inguinal canal, anterior to the lower part of the rectus sheath, to attach to the pubic crest and pecten pubis. Much more commonly, the transversus abdominis fuses with the internal oblique and the anterior wall of the rectus sheath deep to the superficial ring. In this situation, it is the free lower edge of transversus abdominis which forms an arch, or **falx inguinalis**, above the floor of the inguinal canal. In the rest, there is simply the fused inferior edges of the two muscles, sometimes known as the **conjoint musculature**. This constitutes the upper margin of the area through which all forms of inguinal hernias protrude. It also forms an important structure in all anatomical repairs of inguinal hernias.

Anatomists describe the **transversalis fascia** as a sheet of loose areolar tissue lying between transversus abdominis and extraperitoneal fat, which is continuous with pelvic and iliac fascias inferiorly, blends with the inferior diaphragmatic fascia superiorly, and fuses with the anterior laminar of the thoraco-lumbar fascia posteriorly. However, in surgical terms, the transversalis fascia is only of importance where it is thickened and fibrous, in the inguinal region. Here it forms a distinct fibrous sheet which fills in the D-shaped defect beneath the falx inguinalis, medial to the deep inguinal ring. It also thickens and strengthens the inferomedial margin of the **deep inguinal ring**.

The deep inguinal ring is a defect in the transversalis fascia, lying at a point 1.25 cm above the inguinal ligament and midway between the anterior superior iliac spine and the pubic symphysis (not the pubic tubercle as students commonly relate). It is found directly above the femoral pulse. Its relations are the lower margin of transversus abdominis superiorly, the inferior epigastric vessels, and interfoveolar ligament (when present) medially. The latter structure is a thickening of the transversalis fascia, reinforcing the medial portion of the deep ring. Lytle (1970) proposed that medial traction on the ring by the internal oblique when intra-abdominal pressure rises acts as a valve, shutting off the deep ring.

The **iliopubic tract** is another fascial condensation of the transversalis fascia. This arises from the iliopubic arch and is inserted into the anterior superior iliac spine and internal lip of the wing of the ilium. It extends inferomedially above and slightly behind the inguinal ligament and arches over the femoral vessels, forming the anterior portion of the **femoral sheath**. It then fans out to insert into the superior border of the pubic ramus, the pubic tubercle, and body of the pubis. A lateral portion of this sheet curves down to the pubic ramus immediately after the ligament passes over the femoral vessels, and recurves to form the medial boundary of the femoral canal, thus completing the femoral canal.

Hasselbach's triangle is classically described as being bounded superiorly by the rectus sheath, inferiorly by the inguinal ligament and laterally by the inferior epigastric vessels. This area is inherently weak as the posterior wall is formed solely by the transversalis fascia. However, none of these boundaries lies in the same plane and thus provide no useful understanding of the anatomy or basis of surgical repairs of inguinal hernias.

The periosteum of the pelvis along the iliopectineal line is fused with another fascial condensation of the transversalis fascia and iliopubic tract which forms the lacunar (Cooper's) ligament. It is constantly present and strong. It was originally described by Sir Astley Cooper, but he failed to anticipate how significant this structure would become in the repair of hernias of the groin.

Thus the four anatomical structures that form the basis of sound repair of inguinal hernias have been described: the deep crural arch, the transversalis aponeurotic arch (or the conjoint tendon when present), the lacunar (Cooper's) ligament, and the iliopubic tract.

2.2 The inguinal canal

The inguinal canal is usually about 4 cm long and extends from the deep to the superficial ring and, in the adult, runs an oblique course. It slants inferomedially and lies above and parallel to the inguinal ligament. In this canal lies the spermatic cord in the male and the round ligament of the uterus in the female.

The layers from superficial to deep are: the skin, the superficial (Scarpa's) fascia, and the external oblique fascia. The lateral one-third is formed by the muscular fibres of the internal oblique. The posterior wall is formed by the reflected border of the inguinal ligament inferiorly, the falx inguinalis superiorly, and the floor is made up of the transversalis fascia, the preperitoneal fat, and finally the peritoneum. Superiorly arching over the canal is the transversus aponeurotic arch, and the inguinal ligament lies inferiorly, the lower portion of the transversalis fascia fusing with it. The inferomedial border is formed by the strong lacunar (Cooper's) ligament.

2.3 Spermatic cord

This lies in the inguinal canal, entering from the peritoneal cavity via the deep inguinal ring. The ilio-inguinal nerve lies superficial and inferior to it. As the cord traverses the inguinal canal it successively acquires its coverings from the layers of the anterior abdominal wall. The internal spermatic fascia is derived from the transversalis fascia and is a thin, loose covering. The internal oblique gives it the cremasteric muscle and fascia, composed of skeletal muscle fibres and loose connective tissue. A thin, fibrous layer continuous with the aponeurosis of the external oblique forms its outer layer as it passes through the superficial ring: the external spermatic fascia. Again, in surgical terms, these structures are not recognizable individually—essentially, the cord is covered in the cremaster muscle and some loose connective tissue.

The spermatic cord is composed of the following structures embedded in loose **connective tissue**:

◆ **arteries:** testicular, cremasteric, and artery to vas deferens;

◆ **veins:** testicular, which is formed by the confluence of the pampiniform plexus of veins at the level of the superficial ring;

◆ **lymphatic vessels;**

◆ **nerves:** the genital branch of the genitofemoral, the cremasteric, and testicular sympathetic plexus and filaments from the pelvic plexus accompanying the deferential artery; and

◆ **vas (ductus) deferens.**

2.4 The round ligament in the female

This narrow, flat band arises from the lateral uterine angle, enters the inguinal canal through the deep inguinal ring, traverses the canal, and splits into strands which merge with connective tissue in the labium majus. It is accompanied by blood vessels, lymphatics, and nerves and, like the spermatic cord, this structure derives its coverings from the layers of the anterior abdominal wall as it passes through the inguinal canal.

2.5 Femoral canal

This passage occupies the most medial compartment in the femoral sheath; the other structures, from lateral to medial, are the femoral artery and vein. This canal is approximately 1.25 cm long and is conical in shape, directed caudally. The upper end is the femoral ring. The canal contains lymph vessels connecting the deep inguinal group to the external iliac chain of nodes and a lymph node (of Cloquet), all of which are embedded in areolar tissue, probably to allow the femoral vein to distend.

The boundaries of the femoral canal are the inguinal ligament anteriorly, pectineus muscle and 'fascia' posteriorly, the femoral vein laterally, and the strong, unyielding lacunar ligament medially. This last structure plays an important role in the complications arising from femoral hernias. The spermatic cord (male) or round ligament (female) lies just above the anterior margin of the canal, and the inferior epigastric vessels lie near the anterolateral rim. The femoral canal is larger in the female owing to the wider pelvis and the smaller femoral vessels.

3   Physiology of the inguinal canal

The integrity of the inguinal canal is maintained by its obliquity and the structural arrangements of the wall.

First, the deep and superficial rings do not coincide. Secondly, the internal oblique and transversus abdominis act at the deep ring to close it like a sphincter when the abdominal wall contracts. Transversus abdominis pulls the deep crural arch superiorly and laterally. This serves to close the internal ring and also to pull the deep ring up and outwards under cover of the internal oblique. Thus surgical repair of the inguinal canal must not fix the transversalis fascia to any overlying layer which would interfere with this action. Thirdly, increases in intra-abdominal pressure push the posterior wall against the anterior wall, thus closing off the canal and strengthening deficiencies in its structure. Finally, the transversus aponeurotic arch or conjoint tendon acts in a shutter fashion on contraction. The normally arching structure flattens out and approximates the roof to the floor.

4   Aetiology of inguinal hernias

Most classifications place inguinal hernias as either congenital or acquired. Indirect inguinal hernias in the young are due to a fully or partially patent processus vaginalis which is normally obliterated soon after birth. In contrast, indirect hernias in the elderly are acquired, although, as already described, there are potential weaknesses in the inguinal area, particularly in males. With advancing years, the abdominal wall muscles become attenuated and defects develop. In a small proportion of patients, there is some condition causing persistent or intermittently increased intra-abdominal pressure, for example, chronic cough from obstructive airways disease; straining on micturition due to prostatic enlargement; straining at defecation, perhaps heralding a colonic neoplasm or ascites. However, the importance of raised intra-abdominal pressure has been overstated in student teaching.

Direct inguinal hernias may also be considered as a congenital failure of the shutter mechanism of the transversus aponeurotic arch. It may be that this structure lies in a higher position than normal and contraction fails to approximate the arch to the floor of the canal. Recent advances in our understanding of collagen synthesis have revealed defective hydroxyproline in the anterior rectus sheath near inguinal hernias in adults. This inherent collagen defect may explain recurrent hernias in some patients despite careful repairs by experienced surgeons (or it may not!).

More pragmatic classifications for inguinal hernias have been devised which incorporate the anatomical defects with the type of repair suitable for their management (Table 26.2).

5   Composition of a hernia

A typical hernia is described as having a sac with its contents and coverings. The sac is then described as consisting of a mouth, neck, body, and fundus. The nature of the neck varies between

Table 26.2 Anatomical classification of inguinal hernias (Gilbert)

Indirect	Type I	Snug internal ring and intact canal floor
	Type II	One finger-breadth internal ring, intact canal floor
	Type III	Two finger-breadth internal ring, defective canal floor
Direct	Type IV	Floor completely defective, no sac anterior to canal floor, internal ring intact
	Type V	Defect one finger-breadth or less, intact internal ring

different types of hernia as well as within the same types of hernia. There may be a narrow or a wide neck, or no neck at all. This has obvious importance with regard to the potential for complications with hernias. A narrow neck predisposes to incarceration and strangulation, as is common in umbilical and femoral hernias. The body of a hernia sac also varies in size and content, and may even be empty.

An abdominal hernia may contain fluid consisting of clear peritoneal exudate, or bloodstained fluid when the hernia is strangulated. The sac may also contain any mobile viscus or part of a viscus. The most common are:

◆ Omentum: this is found in most abdominal hernias, either alone or in combination with other abdominal contents.

◆ Bowel: usually small bowel but can include large bowel. Usually, the entire diameter of bowel protrudes through the abdominal wall defect, potentially compromising the entire lumen; sometimes only a portion of the diameter is involved, usually the antimesenteric border. This is known as a Richter's hernia and is common in femoral hernias.

◆ Bladder: rare but occurs in direct inguinal hernias.

◆ Ovary with or without its corresponding Fallopian tube.

◆ Meckel's diverticulum: this forms a **Littre's hernia**.

Hernias may be **diffuse**, as in some direct inguinal and lumbar hernias, or more commonly **funicular**. This form of hernia occurs when the organ or viscus passes through a relatively tight or constricting defect. Examples of funicular hernias are most indirect inguinal and femoral hernias.

Reducible hernias can reduce spontaneously (for example when lying down) or else by applying manual pressure. Bowel is characteristically difficult to reduce initially but then becomes easier and reduces completely, often with a gurgle. Omentum, however, is initially easy to reduce but becomes more difficult as reduction continues and final reduction is often impossible. This occurs because omentum is often adherent to the inside of the sac. **Irreducible hernias** cannot be returned through the fascial defect by manipulation. These are then known as **incarcerated** if there is no compromise to blood supply of the organ or viscus, **obstructed** if the lumen of the viscus is occluded, or **strangulated** when occlusion of the blood supply occurs. The two latter forms may progress to infarction and perforation of the viscus if prolonged and unrelieved. Clinically, a hernia should only be described as incarcerated if it is chronically irreducible with no acute change in size or symptoms. An acute hernia should be considered to be strangulated until proved otherwise, so that remedial action is not postponed by giving it an anodyne label.

6 Inguinal hernias

6.1 History

Inguinal hernias commonly manifest as an asymptomatic lump in the groin. The patient may notice that it becomes bigger or more prominent with coughing, straining, or lifting heavy objects. This bulging may be accompanied by pain. The hernia may reduce spontaneously, especially on lying down, or the patient may, over time, develop ways to reduce the hernia manually. Another common symptom is a complaint of a dragging sensation or dull ache that occurs in the groin which may radiate down into the testis. This may be due to traction of the hernia on sensitive peritoneum or on the spermatic cord. Indirect hernias tend to cause more symptoms than direct hernias.

6.2 Physical signs and examination technique

Inguinal hernias are sometimes described as lying above and medial to the pubic tubercle. This is both inaccurate and unhelpful as it defines only the position of the body or fundus of the hernia and not the neck of the sac. The key to clinical examination of groin hernias is the inguinal ligament: inguinal hernias arise above the inguinal ligament whereas femoral hernias arise below it. The pubic tubercle is a useful bony landmark for the medial end of the ligament, but the anterior superior spine needs to be defined as well, to define its lateral end. The pubic tubercle can best be found by following the pubic crest laterally from the symphysis pubis, or by following the inguinal ligament from the anterior superior iliac spine infero-medially to it. The technique of invaginating the scrotal skin to palpate the pubic tubercle or to place the pulp of the examining little finger into the superficial ring should be avoided as it causes pain and yields little extra information.

The patient should always be examined both standing and supine. On standing, look for a lump and, if not visible, ask the patient to strain or cough. A lump that is already present will bulge more prominently and a small hernia may become evident with this manoeuvre. If the lump extends into the scrotum, it is almost certainly an indirect hernia. It is also said that if the swelling is elliptical and follows an oblique course on coughing it tends to favour the diagnosis of an indirect hernia. Direct hernias tend not tend to descend into the scrotum, appear symmetrical and hemispherical in outline, and reduce spontaneously on lying down.

Despite all these traditionally described signs, inguinal hernias can be difficult to recognize if small, and differentiating between direct and indirect hernias is highly unreliable. Both types can occur together and cause further clinical diagnostic difficulty. It is probably of little importance to distinguish clinically between direct and indirect hernias as most hernias should be repaired if possible, and diagnosis at operation is straightforward.

Place a hand over the swelling and ask the patient to cough, seeking a cough impulse. In the case of a swelling appearing to extend into the scrotum, differentiation from a scrotal swelling must be made. If the examining hand can 'get above' the swelling, it is scrotal and not a hernia.

Reducibility should be sought next. The patient should first be asked if the hernia is reducible and, if it is, to demonstrate how it is done. Taxis by the clinician should be slow and gentle to avoid discomfort. Once reduced, if the hernia can be controlled by finger pressure over the deep ring, it is likely to be indirect. Taxis should not be attempted if there are signs of obstruction, inflammation and oedema of the overlying skin, or peritonitis.

A hernia do not, as a rule, transilluminate, and percussion over it should be hyperresonant. Auscultation of the lump should yield bowel sounds if the hernia contains bowel and there is no obstruction.

6.3 Differential diagnosis of an inguinal swelling

◆ Scrotal swellings: including testicular swellings, hydrocoele of the testis or cord, varicocoele or haematoma following trauma, or spontaneous haemorrhage in patients on anticoagulants.

◆ 'Lipoma of the cord': this results from herniation of preperitoneal fat through the deep ring into the spermatic cord, and distinction may only be possible at operation.

◆ Groin lymphadenopathy or abscess.

◆ Undescended testis. Undescended testes lying in the inguinal canal may be mistaken for a hernia, even in adults. This emphasizes the importance for examining the scrotum in all cases of groin hernias.

◆ Femoral hernia turning up along the inguinal ligament: as the termination of Scarpa's fascia in the upper thigh will not allow an enlarging femoral hernia to extend inferiorly, the hernia progresses instead along the inguinal ligament laterally and can be mistaken for an inguinal hernia. This underlines the importance of determining the relation of the neck of the sac to the pubic tubercle. In practice, femoral hernias rarely attain a size large enough for this to occur.

◆ Groin pain of obscure aetiology: this can pose a difficult clinical problem. Herniography may help to rule out a hernia as the cause of pain.

6.4 Management of inguinal hernias

All inguinal hernias should be repaired unless there are specific contraindications against doing so. This is based on the fact that complications of obstruction and strangulation outweigh the risks of surgery in most patients. Although direct inguinal hernias do not carry a high risk of incarceration and its sequelae, it is difficult to distinguish accurately between indirect and direct hernias. The morbidity and mortality from emergency operations for such complications are high. Repair in elderly patients can be safely carried out after good optimization of general health and the use of local or regional anaesthesia.

Painful, tender, irreducible hernias should be treated immediately. Fit patients should have their hernias repaired operatively. If unfit, resuscitation should be attempted, followed by reassessment. If the patient is still a substantial operative risk, manual reduction can be attempted. Sedation, muscle relaxants, and adequate analgesia should be given prior to attempting taxis. Leaving the patient reclined, tilted head downwards, for a period may cause spontaneous reduction or may aid taxis. If reduction is successful, the hernia should be repaired during the same hospital admission. Careful observation should follow and if there are any signs of peritonitis or suspicion of infarcted bowel, leucocytosis or pyrexia, laparotomy should be performed. If repair is carried out after reduction and bloodstained fluid is found in the sac, the abdomen should be explored, as this may be a sign of strangulated, and possibly non-viable, bowel.

6.5 Principles of operative treatment

Any significant medical conditions that pose anaesthetic problems or may contribute to failure of the repair should be identified and corrected as far as possible. These include cardiorespiratory disease, unstable diabetes mellitus, chronic cough, prostatic disease, and suspected colonic neoplasm. Prostatic construction poses a threat of urinary retention postoperatively as well as a predisposition to urinary tract infections.

At operation, an indirect hernia lies anterior to the cord structures but within the cremasteric sheath. This sheath should be 'circumcised' at the neck after mobilizing the cord to the deep ring, and then 'sleeved' distally. This gives a clear view of the cord contents and allows the sac to be recognized and separated from the cord down to the deep ring. This is essential to allow for proper excision of the sac and adequate access for repair of the wall. The sac should be opened, the contents inspected and reduced, and the sac ligated and excised. If the hernia is a **sliding** type, there is no true sac and the hernia consists of retroperitoneal structures such as bladder or colon 'sliding' through the defect. In this case, the hernia is simply reduced before repair. Children and adolescents generally have no substantial weakness in the posterior wall and a herniotomy and tightening of the deep ring (Lytle's procedure) will usually suffice. Adults, on the other hand, usually require some form of herniorrhaphy or hernioplasty to reconstitute the anatomy of the canal (see below). In women, the round ligament can be ligated and divided to allow for complete closure of the deep ring. Recurrent hernias in males occasionally require orchidectomy because of previous cord damage and very occasionally to close the deep ring for a sound repair.

For direct inguinal hernias, it is vital to confirm that no indirect hernia exists, as failure to recognize an indirect hernia will invariably lead to recurrence and possibly litigation. Even if the hernia is obviously direct, the cord must be inspected as described earlier. In every case, a peritoneal remnant can be seen anterior to the cord at the neck. Provided this does not constitute a sac, the operator can be sure there is no indirect hernia and this finding should be recorded in the operation notes. In direct hernias, good repair of the posterior wall is imperative, but most surgeons would regard it as equally important with indirect hernias. Indeed, apart from the treatment of the indirect sac, the same repair technique can be used. The aim should be to reconstitute the normal anatomy as far as possible with minimal tension. Only aponeurotic or fascial structures should be used in the repair, for lasting strength. If the neck of the direct hernia is so wide as to preclude a tension-free repair, a relaxing incision in the anterior rectus sheath (Tanner slide) or a mesh repair can be performed.

Suture materials should be chosen to achieve a balance between avoiding complications from the use of foreign materials and providing the lasting tensile strength required to allow sound consolidation of scar tissue. Non-absorbable materials should be used, usually nylon or polypropylene. The potential drawback is the risk of infection, sinus formation, and tissue reaction. Prosthetic mesh repairs (hernioplasties) were initially thought to increase the incidence of these complications, but the problem of local reaction to prosthetic materials has been all but eliminated by modern synthetics such as polypropylene and expanded polytetrafluoroethylene (PTFE). Lichtenstein (1993) published the results of over 3000 primary mesh repairs without increased infective complications over established methods of repair and with an impressively low recurrence rate of 1.3 per cent. Other authors have been able to reproduce the low recurrence rates, and the ease of teaching and learning this mesh technique is one of its chief merits.

In general, bilateral inguinal hernias should not be dealt with by open operation at the same time in adults, because the tension exerted on the repairs is believed to predispose to recurrences. Children and young adults can have bilateral operations, however, as repair of the wall is not usually required and it avoids a second admission and anaesthetic.

Early recurrences are usually due to failure of the operative procedure: either a concurrent hernia was missed or there was a failure to repair the defect adequately. Late recurrences are usually due to progressive weakening of the muscles and fascia with age. Repeated recurrences, especially if repair has been carried out meticulously by an experienced surgeon, suggest there may be a collagen defect. Recurrent hernias, particularly if symptomatic, should be treated early, as the defects are usually tight and unyielding due to dense scar tissue and there is a high risk of complications.

6.6 Inguinal hernias in children

Herniotomy in children is a safe and effective procedure and can be performed as a day case in most patients. If the child is less than 7 years old, the deep and superficial rings will still overlap, the obliquity of the inguinal canal not yet having developed. Thus approaching the inguinal canal does not require an extensive incision and the external oblique aponeurosis need not be breached.

A skin-crease incision is made just above the pubic tubercle. The subcutaneous tissue and fascia is divided down to the external oblique aponeurosis and the superficial ring is identified. The external spermatic fascia is divided and the spermatic cord and testis delivered by gentle blunt dissection.

The coverings of the cord are now split and dissected off the cord using dissecting forceps or gauze dissection. The hernial sac lies anterior to the vas and its vessels and will appear white and opalescent. If the sac is complete (extending into the scrotum), it is dissected off the cord structures and its proximal part clamped and divided distal to the clamp. The fundus can be left open *in situ* and causes no adverse effects. Traction is applied to the clamp and the proximal part of the sac is traced to the inguinal ring. The sac is twisted round several times to reduce any abdominal contents, its neck suture ligated, and the redundant sac excised. If the sac is incomplete and the fundus easily found, the dissection is started from the fundus and traced proximally to the ring.

It is imperative to replace the testis properly in the scrotum after the operation and to check the alignment of the testicular vessels to avoid torsion. Some surgeons advocate placing the testis in a dartos pouch. Closure is effected using absorbable deep sutures in Scarpa's fascia and an absorbable subcuticular suture to close the skin.

6.7 Operative repair of inguinal hernias in adults

The aim of operative hernia repairs should be to achieve a life-time recurrence rate of less than 1 per cent (Devlin 1979). The operation consists of two components: the identification, ligation, and excision of the sac (herniotomy); and the repair of the inguinal canal (herniorrhaphy) if indicated.

Herniotomy prior to reconstruction of the inguinal canal

The skin incision is made l cm above and parallel to the inguinal ligament. It begins over the deep ring and extends down to just above the pubic tubercle. Hooking the incision down over the pubic tubercle can provide good access to the spermatic cord emerging through the external ring (Devlin 1979). The skin and subcutaneous tissues are divided down to the external oblique aponeurosis, ligating all large vessels and coagulating smaller ones. Haemostasis has to be meticulous to prevent haematoma formation and the risk of infection.

Some authors recommend opening the deep fascia of the thigh to gain access to the femoral canal at this point, to exclude a concomitant femoral hernia; however, this can be achieved later if desired, via the posterior wall of the inguinal canal after opening the transversalis fascia. The external oblique aponeurosis is opened along the line of its fibres through the superficial ring and laterally past the deep ring, taking great care not to divide the ilio-inguinal nerve. The two flaps are raised by gauze and finger dissection to visualize the conjoint musculature superiorly and the deep, upturned edge of the inguinal ligament inferiorly.

Having identified the ilio-inguinal nerve, it must be preserved; one way of doing so is by retraction over a haemostat clipped to the upper or lower edge of the external oblique and everted away from the wound. The cord structures are now exposed as described earlier. Another technique is to split the coverings longitudinally and progressively dissect them off the cord by a combination of sharp and blunt dissection. Excessive stripping of fat from the cord should be avoided as this can predispose to testicular oedema and hydrocoele. However, if a so-called lipoma of the cord is found, it should be excised after mobilizing it from the cord down to the deep ring. This allows the cord to be slender at its neck.. An indirect sac should come into view and can be grasped by haemostats to facilitate further dissection off the cord. The sac should be freed from the cord structures right up to the deep ring where the transversalis fascia is seen to condense. Identifying this is of paramount importance for the next stage of repairing the posterior wall of the canal.

Indirect sac

The sac is opened and any contents reduced. Small bowel or omentum tethered by adhesions are taken down and reduced into the peritoneal cavity. The sac is then transfixed (i.e. sutured and ligated) close to the deep ring and the redundant sac excised.

Sliding hernia

Also known as a **hernia en glissade**, this form of hernia can cause problems if not recognized and managed correctly. In this condition, part of the sac, most commonly the posterior wall, is formed by the wall of a viscus which is usually retroperitoneal. It usually contains the caecum and appendix on the right side or the sigmoid colon on the left. Bladder can herniate on either side.

No attempt should be made to dissect the viscus from the sac as this might result in compromise of its blood supply or breaching of its wall. Any redundant peritoneum is cleared from around the viscus and the sac closed with a pursestring suture. The hernia is then reduced behind the transversalis fascia. Another method of dealing with this form of hernia is to resect a U-shaped cuff of peritoneum around the viscus, leaving a fringe of peritoneum on either side. These fringes are then sutured together over the organ and the resultant defect in the sac closed. However, given the anatomy, there appears little advantage in doing more than simply reducing the entire sac.

Direct sac

This form of hernia is commonly of the diffuse variety, bulging through Hasselbach's triangle. Uncommonly, it can present as a distinct sac with a narrow neck, probably arising as a result of heavy lifting forcing abdominal contents to rupture through transversalis fascia. In the former type, the sac does not need to be excised, but in the latter it needs to be dissected out and the neck ligated after formal reduction of its contents.

Pantaloon hernia

This is a combination of both a direct and an indirect hernia. The sac is delivered lateral to the inferior epigastric vessels (Hoguet manoeuvre) and the hernia dealt with as for an indirect hernia. One of the standard repair techniques deals with both hernias.

Herniorrhaphy

There are many different types of repairs. However, most are variations or corruptions of the repairs described by Marcy (1871) and Bassini (1884). Both these herniologists appreciated the anatomy and physiology of the inguinal canal and stressed the need for tension-free reconstruction of the anatomy of the inguinal canal with preservation of its function. Marcy described closure of the patulous deep ring using transversalis fascia to stabilize the posterior wall and the defective deep ring. Bassini not only improved on Marcy's idea but also subjected his operations to prospective follow-up. He dissected the indirect sac and closed it. The transversalis fascia was then divided from the deep ring down to the pubic tubercle and the 'triple layer' consisting of this layer, the transversus aponeurosis, and the internal oblique was sutured to the upturned edge of the external oblique aponeurosis. This manoeuvre not only reinforced the posterior wall but also maintained the obliquity of the canal.

The general principles of haemostasis and infection as expounded by Halsted are integral to successful hernia repair. He initially skeletonized the spermatic cord and transplanted the cord subcutaneously, but later abandoned this after an unacceptably high rate of testicular atrophy and hydrocoele. Halsted has also been credited with recognizing the value of the anterior relaxing incision first described by Woffler (1892) and popularized by Tanner (1942) in the UK.

The principles that have been extracted from the experience and experimentation of the early and contemporary herniologists can be summed up as follows:

♦ Good visualization of the deep ring and either division of the transversalis fascia for reconstruction of the posterior wall as suggested by Marcy and Bassini or incorporating this fascia using a darn. The repair of the transversalis fascia and tightening the deep ring are important as the area of weakness, namely the deep ring, is patulous in indirect hernias.

♦ Marcy and Bassini, and later Halsted, stressed preservation of the obliquity of the canal as integral to its function. Double breasting (imbrication) of the posterior wall is reported to give improved results (Wyllys Andrews 1895). The general principles of meticulous haemostasis and avoidance of infection and tissue trauma are essential to successful hernia repair.

7 Techniques of individual types of hernia repair

7.1 Anaesthesia

Local, spinal, epidural, or general anaesthesia can be used. Description of the latter three forms of anaesthesia are beyond the realms of this text but the technique of local anaesthesia will be described.

The anaesthetic solution of choice is 0.5 per cent lignocaine (lidocaine) with 1 : 200 000 adrenaline (epinephrine). This dilute solution allows a large volume of up to 100 ml to be used, facilitating adequate spread of solution. Care should be exercised when using adrenaline (epinephrine) based solutions in the elderly, and they may be best avoided in those with known cardiac problems. The contrary view is that they may be safer in these patients provided great care is taken to ensure that the drug is not injected intravenously. Bupivacaine (0.25 per cent) to a maximum dose of 2 mg/kg body weight can also be used as this gives more prolonged anaesthesia over the area but takes a longer time to exert its full effect.

The ilio-inguinal nerve can be blocked by infiltrating the area approximately 2.5 cm medial to the anterior superior iliac spine on the side of the proposed repair. Local anaesthetic is then infiltrated into the skin and subcutaneous tissues along the line of the incision. This is continued through the external oblique aponeurosis as it floods the inguinal canal and promotes anaesthesia of the cord. During the operation, layers of the cord and the peritoneum forming the sac should be infiltrated with local anaesthetic. This is particularly important as traction on the sensitive peritoneum causes pain. The periosteum overlying

Table 26.3 Results of the Shouldice repair (adapted from Kingsnorth)

Author	Indirect recurrences (%)	Direct recurrences (%)	Total recurrences (%)	Total number of cases
Glasgow 1954–1986	0.9	1.1	3.5	20485
Devlin 1970–1982	0.8			718
Barwell 1974–1991	0.8	2.6	3.0	2512
Berliner 1972–1983	1.6		5.9	2513
1980–1983	1.1			1017
Shouldice trainees 1945–1990	0.5		1.5	20271

the pubic tubercle should be injected with a generous amount of anaesthetic before the repair proceeds.

7.2 Shouldice repair

Advocates of this well-established method of repair consider this to be the most successful procedure in terms of low recurrence rates (Table 26.3). It originated at the Shouldice Clinic in Canada, a clinic dedicated solely to hernia repair. At the clinic, a thorough training in the technique is mandatory, together with many cases performed under supervision. Such a careful training and such great experience for each operator could be expected to produce excellent results. The question is whether operators with less rigorous training can produce equivalent results; this should be a cornerstone in evaluating any method of hernia repair.

The Shouldice technique is perhaps underpractised in the UK and Ireland, and this may be because of the relative complexity of the technique. Advocates of the Lichtenstein technique (see below) claim that this technique is easier to teach and learn and gives excellent results with little experience.

The crucial features of the Shouldice procedure are proper visualization of the transversalis fascia, followed by its repair, as was first stressed by Bassini but, interestingly, lost in later modifications of his technique.

As the coverings of the cord are dissected, the condensation of the transversalis fascia at the deep ring should be identified. It is then possible to lift it off the pre-peritoneal fat and divide it from the deep ring as far as the pubic tubercle. Care must be taken not to damage the inferior epigastric vessels while doing so. The cremasteric vessels are related to the lower flap of the transversalis fascia, as they originate from the inferior epigastric vessels, and they should be ligated and divided. This is because excessive manipulation of flap can tear these vessels and cause troublesome bleeding. The lower flap should be mobilized inferiorly to clearly visualize the iliopubic tract and allow examination of the femoral canal to exclude a concomitant femoral hernia.

The repair is then carried out using a double-breasting technique using a non-absorbable suture—nowadays polypropylene or nylon are preferred, although Shouldice originally used stainless-steel wire. The upper flap has strength at the 'white line' where the transversalis fascia lies deep to the edge of the transversus abdominis or conjoint tendon. Suturing is started at the pubic tubercle by anchoring the lower lateral flap to the upper medial flap at the level of the 'white line'. The suturing continues to the deep ring, thus tightening it to comfortably admit the tip of the little finger. The direction of the suturing is then changed to continue back towards the pubic tubercle. The edge of the upper lateral flap is now sutured to the iliopubic tract of the lower medial flap. This suture is then tied to itself at the pubic tubercle. In suturing fascia, the sutures should be placed at slightly different levels in the fascia so as to prevent splitting.

The wall is now reinforced by suturing the conjoint musculature to the inguinal ligament. Starting laterally at the margin of the deep ring, bites are taken of the deep upturned edge of the inguinal ligament and the deep tendinous surface of the conjoint musculature. This is carried out to the pubic tubercle and then proceeds laterally again by picking up conjoint musculature and external oblique aponeurosis just above the inguinal ligament. Suturing must always be snug but never tight.

The cord and nerve are replaced in the canal and the external oblique aponeurosis closed over it by double-breasting, starting medially and suturing the lower lateral flap to the upper medial flap. On return, the upper lateral flap is sutured to the lower medial flap. The subcutaneous layer is closed by absorbable interrupted sutures to Scarpa's fascia, followed by an absorbable subcuticular suture to skin or skin clips.

7.3 Nylon darn (Moloney 1958)

This consists of a criss-crossing lattice of nylon to strengthen the posterior wall of the canal. Suturing starts at the pubic tubercle, where a knot is tied after picking up the periosteum over the tubercle, and the suture end is kept long in a haemostat. The suturing is then carried out laterally, picking up conjoint musculature at two or three levels in an in-and-out fashion up and down and then the upturned edge of the inguinal ligament. This continues to the deep ring to tighten it enough to admit the tip of the little finger. The suture is then locked and the direction changed, to head back towards the pubic tubercle, criss-crossing the previous layer of sutures. The suture is then tied to the long end of the knot at the tubercle. The lattice forms an architectural support for connective tissue on healing, thus lending strength to the posterior wall.

7.4 Lichtenstein procedure

Usher (1958) was the first to propose the use of synthetic mesh to reinforce the posterior wall of the inguinal canal. At this time polyethylene was used and there were considerable problems with prosthetic reaction and mesh infection that hindered its acceptance and widespread use. Lichtenstein (1974) revived the concept and has popularized a repair using a polypropylene mesh. Other synthetics available include Dacron and expanded polytetrafluoroethylene (PTFE). Lichtenstein (1989) reported on a series of 1000 consecutive cases with no recurrences or infective complications. The main criticism of this paper was the short follow-up period. Almost all the cases were performed under local anaesthesia as day cases. Over the next 4 years further results of this procedure were published; Lichtenstein (1992) reported the results from five centres using his 'tension-free repair', quoting an overall recurrence rate of 0.2 per cent and an infection rate of 0.03 per cent. A personal series of 3125 repairs was published by Lichtenstein in 1993, with only four recurrences identified. These results were compared with cases from 70 other centres, totalling over 23 000 repairs, and similar recurrence and infection rates were found.

A single dose of intravenous amoxicillin with clavulanate (Augmentin®) is recommended to be administered at induction, to minimize the risk of infection of the prosthetic material. After excising the sac, attention is turned to the posterior wall. The conjoint musculature superiorly, and the inguinal ligament inferiorly, are cleared of all excess tissue to display the wall clearly. The repair consists of a synthetic mesh placed and stitched (or tacked using titanium staples) to cover the posterior wall of the canal. Laterally, it wraps around the cord at the deep ring, thus supporting this defect. A 15 × 7.5 cm patch of polypropylene mesh is fashioned to fit snugly over the posterior wall, stretching from the pubic tubercle and the conjoint musculature above it, across to beyond the deep ring. A slit is made in the mesh from its lateral margin to just beyond the deep ring to enable the mesh to wrap round the cord but maintaining a buttress around the deep ring.

The lower medial end is sutured or stapled to the pubic tubercle, followed by the upper medial end to the conjoint musculature above. The mesh is then attached progressively along its upper edge to the conjoint musculature and the lower edge to the inguinal ligament. The two flaps created around the deep ring are stapled or stitched together around the cord and to the posterior wall. Many surgeons use a continuous 2/0 polypropylene suture along the inguinal ligament and interrupted sutures of the same material to the upper border and to the posterior wall.

This repair is ideal for day cases as dissection and disturbance of the tissues is minimal and there is no increase in muscle tension inherent in Bassini-type repairs. Infection rates are low despite the apparent risk, and recurrences are low if the procedure is performed correctly. Postoperative pain is much less than for the Shouldice or Bassini techniques and return to full activity consequently more rapid.

7.5 Laparoscopic hernia repair

The advent of minimal access surgery in the late 1980s has changed the many people's perception of the management of several procedures traditionally treated by open surgical techniques. Laparoscopic cholecystectomy is now a firmly established and generally accepted technique, but laparoscopic hernia repair has a less clearly defined role. Surgeons are cautious about embracing this technique as follow-up periods are not yet long enough to compare its longevity with established open repairs. The early laparoscopic repairs were performed transperitoneally, in contrast to all current open techniques. This led to many complications with adhesions and herniation through port sites. This has led to the evolution of the extraperitoneal (properitoneal) approach to laparoscopic inguinal hernia repair.

A further disadvantage for all laparoscopic techniques is that they cannot yet be performed under local anaesthesia. The obvious advantage to laparoscopic techniques is that the approach to the posterior wall of the inguinal canal is direct and both inguinal and femoral hernial orifices can be examined at the same time. In addition, bilateral repairs can be performed if necessary without any additional discomfort to the patient and with very little increase in operating time. This repair is also tension-free, which potentially reduces the chances of recurrence, and also permits a faster return to normal activity.

Ger (1982) first proposed laparoscopic hernial repair, based on observations made during open inguinal hernia repairs. One patient in the series had the hernial opening closed with staples laparoscopically, marking the first laparoscopic hernia repair. Ger *et al.* (1990) also developed a stapling device for laparoscopic closure of the hernial sac. Laparoscopic mesh repair was first proposed by Bogjavalenski (1989), using polypropylene mesh placed in the indirect inguinal hernial sac. Since then many different repairs have been proposed, for example Shultz (1990), Corbitt (1991, 1993), Toy and Smoot (1991), Arregui (1992), and McKernan and Laws (1993).

As detailed descriptions of the various techniques are best left to specialized works, a brief description of two contrasting methods, and the more recently described extraperitoneal mesh technique (EPMR), will be included.

Transabdominal preperitoneal repair (TAPP)

This technique was first described by Arregui (1992). The procedure is performed under general anaesthesia, and a suitable antibiotic should be administered prophylactically at the time of induction of anaesthesia as foreign material is going to be placed in the groin. Urinary catheterization is not mandatory if the patient empties the bladder prior to going to theatre. A carbon dioxide pneumoperitoneum is established and maintained at a pressure of between 12 and 15 mmHg and the patient placed in the Trendelenburg (head down) position at 15–30°. A three-port technique with ports placed is used: a 10 mm port is placed infra-umbilically for the viewing endoscope; a 5 mm port is placed at the level of the umbilicus and in the mid-clavicular line on the side of the hernia for operating instruments; and a 12.5 mm port established in the corresponding position on the opposite side for operating instruments (by means of a 5 mm reducer) and for passing the stapler. Other authors (Darzi and Monson 1994) have proposed a modification of this widely used pattern of port placement as they argue that this method causes undue problems with manipulation of the instruments and that the assistant and operating surgeon are not ideally placed for comfortable and easy operating. Their modification involves the placement of a 12 mm port infra-umbilically for instrumentation by means of a 5 mm reducer, and for the stapler; a 10 mm port in the right iliac fossa at the level of the umbilicus at the mid-clavicular line for the camera; and the 5 mm port for the endoscopic graspers only, placed in the same position on the opposite side for a left inguinal hernia, more medial and lower for bilateral hernias, and even lower and medial for a right inguinal hernia, so that the left iliac fossa and the umbilical port are always running parallel to each other, thus preventing criss-crossing of instruments. In this situation, the surgeon stands on the patient's left for all hernias, and the placement of the camera, and the two instrument ports ensure that at no time do the three ports cross one another.

Indirect inguinal hernia

The indirect sac is first reduced by means of a grasping forceps placed through the right-hand port. A second grasping forceps placed through the left-hand port is used to aid full reduction of the sac. The right grasping forceps is then replaced by diathermy scissors to allow the peritoneum over the superolateral aspect of the sac to be incised, thus avoiding the inferior epigastric vessels, the testicular vessels, and the vas. The incision in the peritoneum is then carried over the anterior surface of the sac and then laterally towards the anterior superior iliac spine. All the time, the potential properitoneal space is developed by blunt and sharp dissection. Attention is now turned to the medial aspect of the sac by manipulating the sac to the patient's lateral side. By this time the anterior, lateral, and medial margins of the sac should be clearly displayed. Finally, the posterior aspect of the sac is dealt with by gently stripping the tissue containing the vas and testicular vessels away from the sac. The sac, once free, can either be entirely removed or the sac divided across, pulling the proximal part into the peritoneal cavity. To set the stage for successful and secure placement of the mesh, the vas and testicular vessels must be dissected off the peritoneum. At the end of this dissection, the peritoneum should be freed from the overlying transversalis fascia antero-laterally, the deep ring, and inferior epigastric vessels, to create a 'space' for the mesh to lie in. Next, the pubic tubercle and ramus have to clearly demonstrated. This is achieved by blunt dissection of the tissues away from the pubic ramus as the grasping forceps in the opposite hand sweeps the tissues medially. The tubercle is easily sought by tracing the exposed pubic ramus down to it.

Most laparoscopists would advocate rolling up of the mesh to push it through the 12.5 mm port, but grasping the corner and pushing it through the port unrolled seems to work just as well or even better, as there is often a struggle to unroll the mesh, making correct placement difficult. The mesh is orientated with its long axis running across the inguinal region, ensuring that the deep ring, as well as the area of Hasselbach's triangle, are adequately covered. Stapling proceeds first to the pubic tubercle, along the inferior pubic ramus, then just medial, followed by just lateral to the inferior epigastric vessels. The mesh is then fixed superolaterally. Stapling should not extend into the psoas muscle laterally for fear of trapping the lateral cutaneous nerve of the thigh. To seat the mesh in place, the peritoneum is stapled closed over it.

The 12.5 mm port is removed, followed by the 5 mm port under direct vision to ensure that no bleeding is occurring. The authors close the fascial defects at the two larger port sites with 0-gauge polyglactin on a J-needle, and skin with an absorbable subcuticular suture.

Direct inguinal hernias

Again, dissection is started superiorly after the sac has been reduced. The peritoneal 'window' is created laterally as before across the obliterated umbilical artery and the deep ring towards the anterior superior iliac spine. Then the vas and testicular vessels are carefully dissected off the peritoneum. It is crucial to enter the plane anterior to the peritoneum of the direct sac, and posterior to the transversalis fascia, so that the mesh will cover the weak defect in the posterior wall of the inguinal canal. The mesh is then introduced through the port as before, and

stapling is carried out as previously described, after which the peritoneum is closed over the mesh.

Extraperitoneal mesh repair (EPMR)

A detailed description of this repair is beyond the scope of this book and the reader is referred to more specialized texts for a complete discussion.

Basically, transgression of the peritoneal cavity is avoided by developing the properitoneal space by means of insufflation or by employing a balloon dissector. Thus potential complications of entering the peritoneal cavity and creating a pneumoperitoneum are avoided. This technique is more technically demanding for several reasons: first, the anatomy of the inguinal canal from this approach is unfamiliar to most surgeons; secondly, operating space, and so manoeuvrability is quite limited; thirdly, securing the mesh in place is difficult from this approach.

A three-port technique is used with a 12 mm port infra-umbilically, a 5 mm port suprapubically in the midline, and a 10 mm port in the midline between the two others. An infra-umbilical incision is made and the dissection carried down to the fascia and between the rectus muscles. A tunnel is created in the properitoneal space, aiming towards the pubic bone to allow the placement of a 12 mm trocar. The extraperitoneal space can then be developed, either by insufflation of carbon dioxide at a pressure of up to 12 mmHg or by means of a specially designed balloon dissector incorporated into a trocar (e.g. Auto Suture, UK). The properitoneal space is developed bluntly to allow further placement of the 10 mm and 5 mm trocars under direct vision.

Dissection of the hernia commences at the symphysis pubis and moves along the line of Cooper's ligament. The dissection proceeds to the external iliac vessels, exposing any direct inguinal hernia defect, then continues superiorly to reach the deep ring and any indirect hernia orifice. Either the entire sac is dissected off the cord structures and dealt with, or the neck is dissected off the cord and divided, leaving the distal part *in situ*.

The mesh is delivered through the 12 mm port and positioned over the defect. Stapling starts at Cooper's ligament and the iliopubic tract and continues onto the transversus abdominis and finally the lateral border of the rectus muscle. The instruments are withdrawn and the skin incisions closed.

7.6 Recurrent hernias

These are usually due to faulty technique (missed sac or poor repair) or to obesity or other causes of persistently raised intra-abdominal pressure (coughing, straining at stool or micturition) in early cases, and probably collagen abnormalities or natural thinning and weakening of the muscles and fascia in late cases.

Removal of the spermatic cord and complete obliteration of the deep ring would appear to offer the best chance of complete cure of a recurrent hernia. However, this is not acceptable to most men and a **properitoneal (posterior) approach** is probably the best choice of repair, especially in situations where there have been multiple previous attempts at repair. Other situations where a posterior approach is recommended are a previously infected repair or persistent neuralgia in a previous repair with prosthetic material, simultaneous repair of bilateral recurrences, and testicular atrophy on the contralateral side. The incidence of the latter complication is markedly reduced by the posterior approach.

In the open properitoneal approach, a lower midline or transverse abdominal incision is performed. For the transverse approach, an incision is made 3 cm above the inguinal ligament on the side of the hernia. All three muscle layers are incised in the same direction, taking care not to open the peritoneum. The posterior wall of the canal can now be inspected and any indirect sac can be dealt with. The posterior wall is then repaired from its deep surface, and the deep ring can also be tightened using one or two interrupted sutures.

7.7 The relaxing incision

This manoeuvre is recommended during any Bassini type of repair (including Shouldice) in which a tension-free approximation of the conjoint musculature to the inguinal ligament cannot be achieved. The relaxing incision was popularized by Reinhoff (1940) in the US and Tanner (1942) in the UK, and is popularly known as the 'Tanner slide'. There have been no reports of pararectal herniation or herniation through the midline, provided the technique carried out correctly.

In cases where the transversalis fascia is weak, a variant can be used, employing the mobilized rectus sheath as a flap to buttress the repair (**Halsted technique**).

The relaxing incision is performed as follows. The external oblique is cleared as far as the midline. An incision is made in the rectus sheath approximately 1.5 cm from the midline, starting 0.5 cm above the pubic crest, and curves laterally and upward for 7–8 cm. Several important points should be noted:

- the iliohypogastric nerve must be avoided;

- good haemostasis is imperative to avoid haematoma formation;

- the midline and lateral edge of the rectus sheath should not be crossed by the incision, in order to prevent herniation.

7.8 Strangulation and obstruction of a hernia

This represents an emergency, and operative intervention should be carried out early. However, the patient is often elderly and is likely to be dehydrated by the time attention is sought, and thus adequate resuscitation must be carried out prior to surgery. This entails intravenous fluid replacement, urinary catheterization to monitor urinary output, nasogastric intubation, and correction of any remediable medical problems.

A groin approach can be employed, as for elective repair. However, if there is difficulty, the abdomen should be opened by a midline incision and the bowel dealt with through the peritoneal cavity. Alternatively, the approach can be through a midline incision in the first instance to reduce the hernia and

inspect the bowel or other abdominal contents involved. Infarcted bowel or bowel of doubtful viability or necrotic omentum can then be resected. Approach through the usual groin incision does not allow adequate access, and dubious bowel or omentum may be missed.

8 Femoral hernia

8.1 Introduction

Protrusion of a peritoneal sac through the femoral canal medial to the femoral vessels forms a femoral hernia. This variety of hernia is far less common than the inguinal variety in both sexes, but is proportionately more common in females.

The aetiology of femoral hernia is still obscure. The femoral canal is wider in females because of the wider pelvis and the smaller femoral vessels. Other associations are:

- parity: these hernias are more common in parous than nulliparous females;

- age: femoral hernias occur with greater frequency in middle-aged and elderly women;

- weight loss: in elderly women is weight loss is associated with femoral hernia, perhaps as a result of loss of fat in the femoral canal;

- increased intra-abdominal pressure: a result of coughing or straining.

Richter's hernia

This refers to a knuckle of bowel, usually small bowel, with only a portion of its circumference pinched at the neck, usually at its antimesenteric border. Richter's hernias are common in strangulated femoral hernias and symptoms are usually of incomplete obstruction. It may be difficult to diagnose preoperatively, but is potentially dangerous as the strangulated portion quickly infarcts, making it liable to perforate.

Management depends on the condition of the bowel after release. Wrapping the segment in warm packs for several minutes will help decide whether the compromised bowel is viable. The non-viable portion of bowel may need to be resected and anastomosed end to end, but a limited wedge resection of the non-viable portion may be possible.

8.2 Management of femoral hernia

Operation is virtually always indicated. If reducible or asymptomatic, this should be performed on the next available elective list. If symptomatic, even if the hernia is not strangulated, operation is imperative as soon as possible. This is because there is a high incidence of strangulation in femoral hernias, and these complications carry a high morbidity in the elderly.

There are two traditional approaches: the low approach and two varieties of high approach. The former is ideal for elective repairs, and the latter approaches, for complicated femoral hernias. If local anaesthesia is used, a solution of 0.5 per cent lignocaine (lidocaine) with 1 : 200 000 adrenaline (epinephrine) can be used, to a total volume of 100 ml in a healthy adult.

Low approach or crural operation (Lockwood)

A 5–6 cm incision is made directly over the hernia below and parallel to the inguinal ligament. This is carried through skin and subcutaneous tissue down to the coverings of the sac. These comprise the cribriform fascia over the femoral vessels, extra-peritoneal fat, and finally peritoneum. It is important to clear the extraperitoneal fat down to the neck of the sac first. Then gentle gauze dissection of the sac is performed until the peritoneum is visible and can be traced down to its neck. The boundaries of the ring are then identified clearly: the lacunar ligament medially, the femoral vein laterally, the inguinal ligament anteriorly, and the pectineus muscle posteriorly. The upper border of the pubis should be palpated to delineate the upper limit of pectineus. The lateral boundary should always be kept in mind as the femoral vein is easily damaged, with profuse haemorrhage.

The sac is then opened and the contents reduced. Adhesions, if present, are also taken down to facilitate the reduction. The neck is then transfixed under tension and excess sac excised. The stump is allowed to retract, provided there is no bleeding.

Repair of the canal

Some surgeons prefer to use a J-shaped needle to repair the canal as the narrow space imposes constraints on manoeuvrability. Others find this no particular advantage. In any case, an 0 or 2/0 non-absorbable suture is employed. A technique favoured by the authors for repair is as follows: the femoral vein is gently retracted laterally and the first suture taken through the pectineus from its deep surface to superficial surface laterally, just next to the retracted vein. This stitch is carried through the inguinal ligament from superficial to deep at the same level as the pectineal suture. The suture then returns to take a bite in the pectineal ligament, as the first stitch, at a point halfway between it and the lacunar ligament, continuing to take the inguinal ligament as before at the same level. The stitch is then tied, approximating the pectineal to the inguinal ligament, thus closing off the femoral canal. This repair is obviously under a certain amount of tension and healing will be slow and relatively ineffective. Devlin recommends supporting this repair with a flap of pectineal fascia mobilized from the surface of pectineus inferior to the canal. This flap is sutured using 2/0 polypropylene up onto the external oblique aponeurosis and down both sides to cover the repair and relieving tension on the primary closure. Some surgeons find that this pectineal fascia is inadequate to use in this way.

The operation is completed by closing the subcutaneous tissue and skin.

High approaches

Inguinal approach (Lothiessen repair)

An inguinal incision is made to gain access to the inguinal canal. The transversalis fascia is divided as in the Shouldice procedure and the inferior flap mobilized to gain access to the femoral canal. The sac is then delivered up into the canal and dealt with as usual.

Repair of the femoral canal is achieved by using 2/0 polypropylene suture to approximate the pectineal ligament to the inguinal ligament, as before, but this time approaching it superiorly. This is then followed by a formal repair of the posterior wall of the inguinal canal.

The advantage of this approach is that there is good access to the canal and sac, especially in strangulated hernias. However, it is a technically difficult operation and has the disadvantage of opening, and thus breaching, an otherwise intact inguinal canal.

McEvedy procedure

This procedure does not traverse the inguinal canal but allows for repair of the canal and gives sufficient access to enable a strangulated hernia to be dealt with adequately.

A curved vertical incision is made along the lateral edge of the rectus muscle down to the pubic tubercle and through the aponeurotic layers, to allow the rectus muscle to be retracted medially. Dissection continues to clear the properitoneal fat from the peritoneum (extraperitoneally), thus exposing the femoral sac, which can be delivered up into the operating field. If this proves difficult, the skin incision can be carried inferiorly to allow manipulation of the hernia from both above and below. The sac is dealt with as usual.

The repair again picks up pectineal ligament to inguinal ligament or conjoint musculature to close the canal, and the incision is closed in layers. It should be noted that this approach is equivalent to a laparotomy in its recovery time, whereas the low approach is a much lesser procedure.

Midline approach (Henry)

This gives excellent access to both femoral canals through one incision and allows simultaneous repair of bilateral femoral hernias. It is a difficult approach and should be attempted only by an experienced surgeon.

A vertical suprapubic midline incision is made through all layers to the peritoneum, retracting the recti laterally. The properitoneal plane is developed bilaterally by blunt dissection to expose the femoral canals and the sacs dealt with as usual. If strangulation is present, the peritoneum can easily be opened and the hernial contents dealt with as necessary.

Closure of the canal is achieved by approximation of the pectineal ligament to the inguinal ligament or conjoint musculature.

8.3 Strangulated femoral hernias

General principles of adequate fluid resuscitation, monitoring, and medical optimization should be adhered to first. Operative repair is best carried out under general anaesthesia. The most reliable approaches are the high approaches previously described, as they offer good access for delivering the strangulated contents and subsequently dealing with them. The other alternative, preferred by many experienced surgeons, is via the low approach which, if difficulty is encountered, can be alleviated by a midline abdominal incision to allow access to the peritoneal cavity.

9 Umbilical hernia

True umbilical hernias result from protrusion of a peritoneal sac through a defect in the umbilical cicatrix. This is thought to be commonly caused by infection of the area postpartum (**omphalitis**), resulting in a weak umbilical scar. Infantile umbilical hernias commonly regress spontaneously by the age of 2 or 3 years, but if persistent should be repaired surgically as the neck is usually tight and the hernia prone to strangulation.

The origin of hernias in the umbilical area in adults is a subject of dichotomous views. Many are due to a defect in the linea alba near the umbilical cicatrix, and are thus correctly termed **paraumbilical hernias**. These are more commonly found in obese patients, those with pelvic floor prolapses and hiatus hernias, and in black races. However, a substantial proportion (probably more than 50 per cent) of adult umbilical hernias prove to be true umbilical hernias at operation.

The surgical technique for repairing paraumbilical and large umbilical hernias that has stood the test of time is the **Mayo repair** (Mayo 1898) in which the defect in the fascial layer is closed in a vertical, double-breasting fashion.

9.1 Umbilical hernias in infants and children

This usually manifests as a lump that is more prominent when the child cries or strains. Its is otherwise asymptomatic and causes more concern to the parents than to the child.

The majority of infantile hernias close spontaneously by the second or third year of life but rarely close after this age. If the neck is greater than 1.5 cm wide at any age, this will fail to close spontaneously. Both of these are indications for recommending repair.

Principles of surgical management

The hernial sac is excised in the same way as with other types of hernias. The defect in the linea alba can be closed in most cases by a simple direct repair using a non-absorbable suture (e.g. 2/0 polypropylene). Some surgeons prefer to employ the Mayo double-breasting technique. The umbilicus should be reconstituted as an inverted structure by suturing its centre to the abdominal wall. This is for psychosocial reasons in most, but for religious reasons in others.

Operative technique for the Mayo repair

A curved transverse incision is performed subumbilically. A skin flap containing the umbilicus is raised and the hernial sac carefully dissected off the flap. Dissection of the sac is continued down to the neck and the defect in the linea alba clearly defined. If the defect is small and the hernial contents cannot be reduced, the defect should be enlarged transversely from each side of the defect.

The sac is then opened, its contents reduced and the neck transfixed with 2/0 polyglactin. Redundant sac is excised and the stump inspected for bleeding before being allowed to retract.

Non-absorbable 2/0 polypropylene sutures are used to close the fascial defect. An interrupted horizontal mattress suture employed, bites in the upper flap being placed farther from the edge than in the lower flap to establish double-breasting when they are tied. Three to four sutures are usually required, depending on the size of the defect and whether it had to be extended. These are not tied until all the sutures have been put in place.

After tying this layer of sutures, the upper flap is then stitched to the anterior surface of the lower flap with interrupted or continuous polypropylene sutures.

Interrupted 2/0 polyglactin sutures are used to close the subcutaneous tissue. A tacking stitch is used to approximate the underside of the umbilicus to the linea alba to preserve its shape. The skin is then closed with an absorbable suture (e.g. 4/0 polyglycolate).

9.2 Umbilical hernia in the adult

True umbilical hernias in adults should be repaired as the incidence of obstruction and strangulation is high.

Paraumbilical hernias may be asymptomatic or present with a symptomatic swelling around the umbilicus. Long-standing hernias become irreducible as a result of adhesions forming in the sac. They enlarge, stretching the overlying skin, causing atrophy and, later, ulceration. Bowel may become obstructed or strangulated within part of the sac rather than at the neck, which itself is often wide. When this occurs, there may be very little in the way of systemic symptoms or abdominal tenderness, but the key is that the patient is obstructed and the hernia has become reddened. This requires early operation after a suitable period of resuscitation. Very large hernias may be difficult to manage as the abdomen may not have the capacity to allow reduction of the contents at operation.

Principles of management

Paraumbilical hernias should generally be repaired unless the patient is very obese, or medically unfit to withstand general anaesthesia. Any skin infection should be dealt with before operation, and it is recommended that closure be effected by subcuticular sutures, adhesive strips, or skin clips, as suture tracts may become infected. Very large hernias may be judged irreducible without causing cardiopulmonary compromise. If operation is essential, a pneumoperitoneum can be induced, increasing the volume daily until operation.

Operative procedures

If the hernia is small, a subumbilical approach may be used to preserve the umbilicus. However, large paraumbilical hernias may require excision of the umbilicus and thus the patient should be warned that this may occur.

If the subumbilical approach is not used, a fusiform incision is made around the umbilicus. It is advisable not to excise too generously at the start, as excess skin can be trimmed before closure. The ellipse of skin and subcutaneous tissue is excised carefully to avoid damage to the underlying sac. Haemostasis has to be meticulous throughout the procedure.

The sac is identified and the skin and subcutaneous tissue overlying it excised. The neck is found and the entire margin of the defect clearly displayed. The defect is now enlarged transversely in both directions through the anterior and posterior layers of the rectus sheath, retracting the recti carefully so as not to tear the inferior epigastric vessels. The sac is then opened and the contents inspected and reduced. Omentum and colon are the most common contents, and more often than not, dense adhesions fix these contents within the sac. Careful adhesiolysis should be performed to free all the contents in order to reduced them. Haemostasis is vital and omentum that cannot be freed should be excised. Finger-guided dissection may be helpful in freeing the neck of abdominal contents, after which the sac can be opened generously to allow the remaining adhesiolysis. The sac is then transfixed and excess sac excised.

The repair is performed using 0 or 2/0 polypropylene in an interrupted horizontal mattress technique, as previously described. However, more sutures are required because of the larger defect, and the bites in the upper flap should be taken 2–4 cm from the edge, and 1–2 cm from the edge of the lower flap. These should not be tied until all the sutures have been placed, and as the tying proceeds, the assistant should hold the adjacent suture under tension to facilitate tying and to ensure even tension along the suture line. This is further ensured by placing the sutures at different levels along the suture line. The edge of the upper flap is then sutured to the anterior surface of the lower flap, either with interrupted or a continuous stitch.

Closed suction drainage is employed in the space beneath the subcutaneous tissue, and this layer is closed with interrupted 2/0 polyglactin sutures.

10 Incisional hernia

This form of hernia is the next most common after inguinal hernias and is the result of herniation through a previous surgical incision. The overall incidence is difficult to determine, partly as a result of underreporting of minor degrees of hernia and partly because of a relatively high incidence among lower abdominal incisions performed for gynaecological procedures which are not counted in surgical audits. The incidence for all abdominal wounds is probably around 6–7 per cent at 5 years.

Gerdy is credited with describing the first repair in 1836, followed by Maydl in 1886. Biological prosthetic materials were used at first to strengthen repairs, not only in incisional hernias but also in inguinal hernia repairs. Materials included fascia lata (Kirschner 1910) and fascial strips (Gallie and LeMesurier 1923), as well as tendons, skin grafts, and strips of skin. More recently, non-biological prosthetic materials have been used. Early types included stainless steel and tantalum gauze. These have been superseded by polyester (Marlex®) and polypropylene mesh.

10.1 Aetiological factors in the development of incisional hernias

Local factors

◆ Poor wound closure technique: probably the most important factor and includes use of an inadequate total length of continuous suture material caused by placing sutures too far apart and/or too near the edge; knots untying; sutures breaking; sutures too tight causing necrosis of wound edges.

◆ Wound infection: in most series this is held responsible for up to 60 per cent of incisional hernias.

◆ Wound haematoma.

◆ Multiple incisions through the same scar or close to it—particularly if performed less than 6 months after the previous incision.

◆ Placement of drainage tubes through the incision.

◆ Incorrect choice of suture material for closure (e.g. catgut).

◆ Type of incision: lower abdominal incisions appear to have a higher incidence than upper abdominal incisions; midline incisions heal better than paramedian incisions in most series. Vertical incisions may have a higher incidence of incisional hernia than transverse incisions.

◆ Early partial wound dehiscence.

◆ Persistently raised intra-abdominal pressure after operation: this include coughing as a result of chest infection, urinary retention secondary to prostatic obstruction, constipation, and prolonged ileus.

General factors

◆ Anaemia

◆ Uraemia

◆ Hypoprotinaemia and malnutrition

◆ Jaundice

◆ Malignancy

◆ Obesity

◆ Immunosuppressive therapy (e.g. corticosteroids, cyclophosphamide, and azathioprine).

10.2 Symptoms of incisional hernias

Incisional hernias are usually asymptomatic but become more visible with coughing or straining. Mild symptoms of aching, especially on straining, may be evident and cause a patient to seek advice. The incidence of obstruction and strangulation is relatively rare because the necks of these hernias are usually wide. However, with time large, pendulous hernias develop multiple adhesions and loculations within the sac, which may make the sac irreducible or cause symptoms of obstruction, requiring surgery. The contents are most commonly omentum and small bowel or colon.

10.3 Management of incisional hernias

Surgical repair of incisional hernias has a high failure rate, particularly for recurrent incisional hernia. Therefore, definite indications for surgery are required before embarking on these procedures. Many incisional hernias cause minimal symptoms and surgery is clearly not essential and may be best avoided. Some patients benefit from surgical intervention. Clearly, obstruction and strangulation are absolute indications for intervention. Contraindications to surgical repair are:

◆ **Gross obesity**: this makes the operation technically difficult and predisposes the patient to a high incidence of post-operative complications and recurrence.

◆ **Wound infection**: this may be in the form of deep, persistent stitch sinus or, indeed, multiple stitch sinuses after the use of non-absorbable suture material or skin infection, especially in long-standing large, pendulous hernias in which the overlying skin is stretched and atrophic or even ulcerated.

◆ All infection should be treated aggressively with regular cleansing and dressings and no repair attempted until the infection has been eradicated and allowed to settle for 2–3 months. Deep suture sinuses should be laid open and the offending stitches removed. The wound is then left to heal by secondary intention. If repair is needed, this should follow several months later.

◆ **Chronically raised intra-abdominal pressure**: any cause of increased intra-abdominal pressure should be treated first. These includes prostatic obstruction, constipation, and chronic cough.

10.4 Operative principles of incisional hernia repair

Restoration of the normal anatomy should be attempted as much as possible and the repair should be tension-free. Only aponeurotic and fascial structures should be included in the repair as only these layers possess the requisite strength. If there is a gross deficiency of these layers, an alternative should be sought in the form of a prosthetic mesh. Non-absorbable sutures should be used to hold the repair together as the fascia heals and develops its own inherent strength slowly. Jenkins (1976) determined that the optimal length of suture material to effect closure of a fascial defect is determined by the distance of the sutures from the edge (1 cm), the distance apart (1 cm), and to the length of the wound. On this basis, the length of suture used should be at least four times the length of the wound.

Persistently raised intra-abdominal pressure postoperatively should be avoided. As mentioned before, such preoperative conditions should be corrected before repair is undertaken. Chest infections should be prevented by stopping smoking 2–3 weeks prior to surgery, aggressive chest physiotherapy, and early mobilization. Constipation should be avoided, and prolonged ileus can be prevented or limited by avoiding opening the peritoneum if possible, or by minimal handling of bowel. Finally, very large incisional hernias may not be amenable to repair immediately as the abdomen may not be able to accommodate the returned contents without significant cardio-respiratory compromise. This should be anticipated and weekly carbon dioxide insufflation through a trocar may be required prior to surgical repair.

10.5 Operative repair

The choice of technique depends on the surgeon's preference and nature of the hernia. The range includes simple closure, the Mayo-type repair, the keel technique, and prosthetic mesh repair.

Simple closure

This repair is suitable only for hernias in which the fascial defect is small and which can be closed without undue tension. A skin incision is made to excise the scar and any surrounding redundant skin.

The scar and subcutaneous tissue is gently undermined and excised carefully, avoiding the sac which often lies close to the surface. The sac is identified and dissected down to the neck to fully define the fascial defect.

The sac is opened and any adhesions taken down. If strangulation or obstruction is present, small bowel may require resection and non-viable omentum excised. Colon that is compromised should be resected, but it is safest to exteriorize the ends as a colostomy and a mucous fistula. The sac is then excised and the peritoneal defect closed with 2/0 polyglactin.

Attention is now turned to repair of the fascial defect. Dissection should proceed outwards from the margins of the defect until normal fascia can be visualized to a width of at least 3 cm around the entire circumference. A direct repair or a Mayo repair is then performed, in the latter by double-breasting the fascial flaps with 0 nylon or polypropylene. Sutures should not be greater than 0.5 cm apart and the suture line should be staggered to stabilized the repair.

A suction drain is usually placed down to this suture line and the subcutaneous tissue and skin closed in the usual way. It is wise to cover the operation with a single dose of prophylactic antibiotics.

Keel technique

This refers to the inversion of the peritoneal sac without opening it by layer upon layer of continuous absorbable suture. It is the procedure of choice in large, diffuse sacs in which the contents are not obstructed or strangulated, and the fascia can be approximated without undue tension.

Once the fascial margins are defined, the sac is left unopened. An absorbable suture is run in a continuous horizontal mattress fashion, starting from one end of the defect. On reaching the other end the sutures are then placed at a different level and so on until the fascial layer is reached. Tightening the suture as it progresses causes inversion of the sac in a fashion that resembles the keel of a ship. The fascial layers are then repaired as previously described.

Mesh repair

This is employed for large, diffuse hernias where fascial loss prevents tension-free approximation. The initial dissection is as already described and the sac opened or a keel procedure performed. If the peritoneal defect is too large to close, omentum should be used to overlie the bowel as synthetic material must not be placed in direct contact with abdominal viscera.

A mesh polyester (Marlex®) or polypropylene mesh is fashioned in the shape of a rectangle 4 cm longer at each end and 2 cm beyond the lateral margins of the defect (Devlin).

Each side of mesh is sutured using three rows of sutures, the first at the edge of the defect, the next l cm from the edge, and the final row to secure the edge of the mesh 3 cm from the edge. This may be performed on a single sheet of mesh or, alternatively, the mesh is divided into two longitudinally, each half sutures separately to the abdominal wall and, finally, an assistant brings the edges of the two halves of mesh together to allow the surgeon to suture them together in the middle.

Suction drainage is employed over this mesh and the subcutaneous tissues, and skin closed as usual.

11 Epigastric hernia

This presents as a small swelling in the midline at one or more site between the xiphoid process and umbilicus. It is due to protrusion of preperitoneal fat through small defects in the linea alba. Many remain at this stage, but if the defect enlarges, it tends to drag peritoneum with it, producing a true hernia. The neck is usually too small to allow herniation of intra-abdominal viscera but the sac may contain omentum.

Epigastric hernias may be asymptomatic or there may be attacks of pain and tenderness. This is caused by the narrowness of the neck, which pinches peritoneum, especially during exertion. These symptoms may be mistaken for peptic ulcer disease.

On examination, the lump may be obvious in the midline between the xiphoid and umbilicus, especially in oblique view. Palpation with the pulp of the finger drawn along the midline usually reveals the lump, which is sometimes reducible or tender.

11.1 Operative repair of epigastric hernias

Even in the face of a clinically evident epigastric hernia, symptoms may demand a preliminary gastroscopy to rule out a peptic ulcer.

A vertical or transverse incision is made over the lump. The nub of preperitoneal fat or the true sac is isolated by gauze dissection down to the defect in the linea alba. This is usually very small and should be widened transversely. The fat is then incised to exclude a true sac; if none is present, the pedicle is ligated and the fat excised. If a sac is present, it should be opened and the contents inspected. Any dubious omentum is excised. The sac is then ligated and excised.

The repair is either by direct suture or one based on the Mayo procedure to double-breast the defect. The subcutaneous tissue and skin are then closed in the usual manner.

12 Uncommon hernias

12.1 Obturator hernia

An obturator hernia is formed by protrusion of a sac through the obturator foramen. It is more common in thin females over 60 years of age. This form of hernia is difficult to diagnose and is usually discovered during a laparotomy for intestinal obstruction. The swelling is usually not clinically obviously because it is hidden under pectineus, but if suspected, a fullness may be detected in the femoral triangle at a lower level than the site at which a femoral hernia would be expected. Compression of the obturator nerve by the hernia occurs in about 50 per cent of cases and this causes pain or paraesthesia at the knee or along the inside of the thigh. The limb is usually held in semi-flexion, and passive and active movements of the hip joint elicit pain. Symptomatic obturator hernias are often strangulated and of the Richter variety.

Operative management

Bladder catheterization is advisable in this situation. When obstructed or strangulated, a lower midline laparotomy incision is performed. When the hernia is found, reduction is carried out by gently stretching the obturator fascia with the operator's fingers or forceps. If this does not work, the fascia can be incised carefully parallel to the obturator vessels and nerves. The bowel is dealt with as necessary. Recurrence is prevented in the female by suturing the broad ligament over the obturator foramen. Alternatively, a polyester patch can be used to close the foramen.

12.2 Interstitial hernia (interparietal hernia)

The sac associated with an inguinal hernia may come to lie between layers of the abdominal wall, either external and internal obliques or internal oblique and transversus abdominis. Bowel obstruction may be the first sign of this form of hernia and there may be no clinically detectable swelling. Sufferers are usually male. Laparotomy may be performed to make the diagnosis and the sac can be reduced and dealt with.

12.3 Spigelian hernia

This hernia occurs through a pararectus defect, usually at the level of the arcuate line. Men and women are equally affected and the patient is usually obese and over 50 years of age. The hernia may be difficult to palpate if it lies deep to the internal oblique muscle, but if it passes between this and the external oblique muscles it is easier to detect clinically. The lump should be carefully marked preoperatively otherwise it may be impossible to detect during the procedure. The hernia should be dissected out to delineate the defect clearly, the sac dealt with in the usual way, and the defect closed with a non-absorbable 2/0 polypropylene suture.

12.4 Lumbar hernia

The most common lumbar hernia occurs through the **inferior lumbar triangle of Petit**, which is bounded by the iliac crest inferiorly, the edge of the external oblique laterall, and the latissimus dorsi medially. A more unusual form occurs through the **superior lumbar triangle**, defined by the twelfth rib superiorly, the sacrospinalis medially, and the internal oblique laterally. Symptoms are usually non-existent to mild, comprising mostly vague backache or a dragging sensation. This can be treated conservatively as the neck is wide and problems unusual. If a large incisional lumbar hernia occurs as a result of an operation for access to the kidney, an operative repair employing fascial flaps needs to be performed or a synthetic mesh sutured in place.

12.5 Littre's hernia

This is an interesting variant of a femoral hernia in which an inflamed Meckel's diverticulum is found within the sac. This can occur in any age group and is impossible to diagnose preoperatively. A tender groin swelling prompts an exploration and the Meckel's diverticulum is either excised or the segment of bowel containing the diverticulum is resected with a primary anastomosis, followed by closure of the defect.

12.6 Maydl's hernia

This hernia was first described in 1895, and comprises a W-shaped segment of bowel contained in a hernia. The segment that becomes compromised is the intra-abdominal apex of the 'W' and may be easily missed if the small bowel is not thoroughly checked.

12.7 Perineal hernia

This is an internal incisional hernia through the pelvic floor and may follow gynaecological or obstetric procedures, or extensive rectal surgery. Unless the hernia is strangulated, symptoms are minimal and a perineal bulge may be the only complaint. If operation is advised, a bidirectional approach is employed: first, the sac is dissected out by an incision directly over it. Then a laparotomy incision allows the neck of the sac to be approached and the sac dealt with. The pelvic floor is then repaired.

12.8 Sciatic hernia

This is formed by the protrusion of a sac through the **lesser sciatic foramen**. Differential diagnoses of a swelling in this area include lipoma, liposarcoma, neuroma tuberculous abscess, or a gluteal aneurysm. Most of these swellings beneath the gluteus maximus should be explored after ultrasonography and CT or MRI scanning have been performed to determine the cause of swelling.

12.9 Gluteal hernia

Herniation through the greater sciatic foramen causes a gluteal hernia and the management is similar to that for a sciatic hernia.

Bibliography

A series of articles in: *Surgical Clinics of North America* (1998), vol. 78

Abrahamson, J. Etiology and pathophysiology of primary and recurrent groin hernia formation, pp. 953–72, vi.

Bendavid, R. Complications of groin hernia surgery, pp. 1089–103.

Crawford, D.L. and Phillips, E.H. Laparoscopic repair and groin hernia surgery, pp. 1047–62.

Kurzer, M., Belsham, P.A., and Kark, A.E. The Lichtenstein repair, pp. 1025–46.

O'Riordan, D.C. and Kingsnorth, A.N. (1998). Audit of patient outcomes after herniorrhaphy. *Surg. Clin. North. Am.*, **78**, 1129–39.

Patino, J.F., Garcia-Herreros, L.G., and Zundel, N. Inguinal hernia repair. The Nyhus posterior preperitoneal operation, pp. 1063–74.

Robbins, A.W. and Rutkow, I.M. Mesh plug repair and groin hernia surgery, pp. 1007–23, vi–vii.

Rutkow, I.M. and Robbins, A.W. Classification systems and groin hernias, pp. 1117–27, viii.

Others

Amid, P.K., Shulman, A.G., Lichtenstein, I.L. (1996). Open tension-free repair of inguinal hernias: the Lichtenstein technique. *Eur. J. Surg.*, **162**, 447–53.

Amid, P.K., Shulman, A.G., Lichtenstein, I.L. (1994). Local anesthesia for inguinal hernia repair step-by-step procedure. *Ann. Surg.*, **220**, 735–7.

Amid, P.K., Shulman, A.G., Lichtenstein, I.L. (1994). A critical comparison of laparoscopic hernia repair with Lichtenstein tension-free hernioplasty. *Med. J. Aust.*, **161**, 239–41.

Cueto, J., Vazquez, J.A., Solis, M.A., Valdez, G., Valencia, S., and Weber, A. (1998). Bowel obstruction in the postoperative period of laparoscopic inguinal hernia repair (TAPP): review of the literature. *J. Soc. Laparoendosc. Surg.*, **2**, (3), 277–80.

Halsted (1893). *Bull. Johns Hopkins Hosp.*, **4**, 17.

Jones, R.L. and Wingate, J.P. (1998). Herniography in the investigation of groin pain in adults. *Clin. Radiol.*, **53**, (11), 805–8.

Kapur, P., Caty, M.G., and Glick, P.L. (1998). Pediatric hernias and hydroceles. *Pediatr. Clin. North America*, **45**, (4), 773–89.

Kingsnorth, A.N. (1994). Hernia repair. *Lancet*, **343**, 1500–1.

Kingsnorth, A.N. (1996). Laparoscopic versus open repair of inguinal hernia. Hernia repair should be individualised to the patient. *BMJ.*, **3**, 310.

Kingsnorth, A.N., Porter, C.S., Bennett, D.H., Walker, A.J., Hyland, M.E., Sodergren, S. (2000). Lichtenstein patch or Perfix plug-and-patch in inguinal hernia: a prospective double-blind randomized controlled trial of short-term outcome. *Surgery*, **127**, 276–83.

Krahenbuhl, L., Schafer, M., Feodorovici, M.A., and Buchler, M.W. (1998). Laparoscopic hernia surgery: an overview. *Dig. Surg.*, **15**, (2), 158–66.

Lichtenstein, I.L., Shulman, A.G., Amid, P.K. (1993). The cause, prevention, and treatment of recurrent groin hernia. *Surg. Clin. North. Am.*, **73**, 529–44.

Lichtenstein, I.L., Shulman, A.G., Amid, P.K., Montllor, M.M. (1989). The tension-free hernioplasty. *Am. J. Surg.*, **157**, 188–93.

Lichtenstein, I.L. (1987). Herniorrhaphy. A personal experience with 6,321 cases. *Am. J. Surg.*, **153**, 53–9.

Lucas, S.W. and Arregui, M.E. (1999). Minimally invasive surgery for inguinal hernia. *World J. Surg.*, **23**, (4), 350–5.

McGreevy, J.M. (1998). Groin hernia and surgical truth [editorial]. *Am. J. Surg.*, **176**, (4), 301–4.Shulman, A.G., Amid, P.K., Lichtenstein, I.L. (1994). Returning to work after herniorrhaphy. *BMJ*, **309**, 216–7.

Index